Scrotal US & contents - 76870

90378 - Synagis injection

1st d, 99233 mod. 21 } jaundice
2nd d, 99233 mod. 25

99211 nurse visit
99024 post-op No charge
99000 handling specimens.
96372 injection only
99058 - Emergency basic

OTHER PMIC TITLES OF INTEREST

CODING AND REIMBURSEMENT TITLES

Collections Made Easy!
CPT Coders Choice®, Thumb Indexed
CPT & HCPCS Coding Made Easy!
CPT Easy Links
CPT Plus!
DRG Plus!
E/M Coding Made Easy!
Getting Paid for What You Do
HCPCS Coders Choice®, Color Coded, Thumb Indexed
Health Insurance Carrier Directory
HIPAA Compliance Manual
ICD-9-CM, Coders Choice®, Thumb Indexed
ICD-9-CM Coding for Physicians' Offices
ICD-9-CM Coding Made Easy!
ICD-9-CM, Home Health Edition
Medical Fees in the United States
Medicare Compliance Manual
Medicare Rules & Regulations
Physicians Fee Guide
Reimbursement Manual for the Medical Office

PRACTICE MANAGEMENT TITLES

Accounts Receivable Management for the Medical Practice
Achieving Profitability With a Medical Office System
Encyclopedia of Practice and Financial Management
Managed Care Organizations
Managing Medical Office Personnel
Marketing Strategies for Physicians
Medical Marketing Handbook
Medical Office Policy Manual
Medical Practice Forms
Medical Practice Handbook
Medical Staff Privileges
Negotiating Managed Care Contracts
Patient Satisfaction
Performance Standards for the Laboratory
Professional and Practice Development
Promoting Your Medical Practice
Starting in Medical Practice
Working With Insurance and Managed Care Plans

AVAILABLE FROM YOUR LOCAL MEDICAL BOOK STORE OR CALL 1-800-MED-SHOP

OTHER PMIC TITLES OF INTEREST

CPT®•PLUS!

A Comprehensive Guide To Current Procedural Terminology

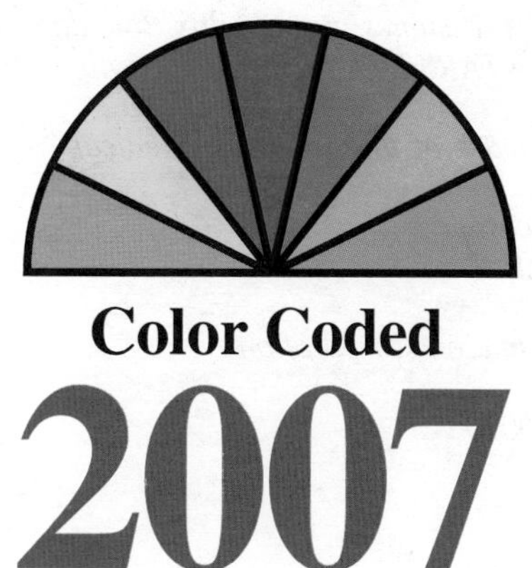

Color Coded

2007

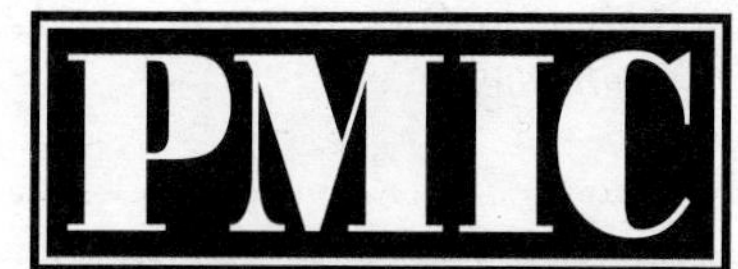

ISBN 1-57066-406-4 (Soft cover)
ISBN 1-57066-407-2 (Spiral)

Practice Management Information Corporation
4727 Wilshire Boulevard
Los Angeles, California 90010
1-800-MED-SHOP
http://pmiconline.com/

Printed in China

INTRODUCTION

CPT® PLUS! 2007 is an enhanced CPT® coding resource which includes all official CPT 2007 codes and complete descriptions plus comprehensive CPT coding instructions, full-color anatomical illustrations, a unique color-coding system to help identify CPT codes subject to special coding rules, and a new and improved alphabetic index.

The CPT coding system includes over 7,900 codes and descriptions for reporting medical services, procedures, supplies and materials. Accurate CPT coding provides an efficient method of communicating medical services and procedures among health care providers, health care facilities, and third party payers and enhances the health care provider's control of the reimbursement process.

The CPT coding system is revised annually by the American Medical Association (AMA). Each year hundreds of additions, changes and deletions are made the CPT coding system. These changes become effective on January 1st. CPT is required by federal law for all health insurance claim forms filed with Medicare, Medicaid, CHAMPUS and Federal Employee Health Plans and is accepted or required by all other third party payers.

CPT® PLUS! 2007 provides valuable instructions, coding tips, and other information to help providers maximize reimbursement while minimizing audit liability. Our objective is to make CPT coding faster, easier and more accurate for medical office, healthcare facility and third party payer coding and billing staff, while setting a new standard for CPT coding references.

James B. Davis, Publisher

DISCLAIMER

This publication is designed to offer basic information regarding coding and reporting of medical services, supplies and procedures using the CPT coding system. The information presented is based on a thorough analysis of the CPT coding system and the experience and interpretations of the editors. Though all of the information has been carefully researched and checked for accuracy and completeness, neither the editors nor the publisher accept any responsibility or liability with regard to errors, omissions, misuse or misinterpretation.

CONTENTS

CPT CODING FUNDAMENTALS

CPT® is an acronym for Current Procedural Terminology. Physicians' Current Procedural Terminology, Fourth Edition, known as CPT-4 or more commonly CPT, is a systematic listing of codes and descriptions which classify medical services and procedures. CPT codes are used by physicians, hospitals, and other health care professionals, to report specific medical, surgical and diagnostic services and procedures for statistical and third party payment purposes.

The CPT coding system is maintained by the American Medical Association (AMA) and a revised edition of the CPT book is published each fall. The new CPT codes become effective on January 1st of the following year. The revisions in each new edition are prepared by the CPT Editorial Panel with the assistance of physicians representing all specialties of medicine.

A thorough understanding of the CPT coding system is essential in order to provide accurate reporting of medical services and procedures, maximize payments from third parties, minimize denials, rejections and reductions from third parties, and to protect the medical practice from audit liability.

KEY POINTS REGARDING THE CPT CODING SYSTEM

- *CPT codes describe medical procedures, services and supplies.*
- *All CPT codes are five digit codes.*
- *CPT codes are mandated by federal law for Medicare, Medicaid, CHAMPUS and Federal Employee Health Plan (FEHP) reporting and are accepted or required by all other third party payers.*
- *CPT codes are self-definitive, eg. with the exception of CPT codes for unlisted procedures and/or the few CPT codes which include the term specify in the description, each CPT code number represents the universal definition of the service or procedure.*
- *CPT codes are revised and updated annually by the AMA and the revisions become effective each January 1st. Hundreds of CPT codes are added, changed or deleted each year. All health care professionals, third party payers, and health care facilities must maintain copies of the current code books.*
- *Accurate CPT coding provides an efficient method of communicating medical, surgical and diagnostic services and procedures among health care professionals, health care facilities, and third party payers.*

- *Accurate CPT coding enhances the health care provider's control of the reimbursement process.*

STRUCTURE OF THE CPT CODING SYSTEM

The CPT coding system includes over 7,900 codes and definitions for medical services, procedures and diagnostic tests. Each procedure or service is identified by a five digit code, followed by the definition.

The CPT coding system is divided into eight ***SECTIONS****. The eight sections of are:*

Evaluation and Management	*99201-99499*
Anesthesiology	*00100-01999, 99100-99140*
Surgery	*10021-69990*
Radiology	*70010-79999*
Pathology and Laboratory	*80048-89356*
Medicine	*90281-99199, 99500-99602*
Category II Performance Measurement	*0001F-4018F*
Category III Emerging Technology	*0003T-0140T*

Each section of the CPT book includes subsections with anatomic, procedural, condition, or descriptor subheadings. The Evaluation and Management (E/M) section is presented first because 1) these codes are used by virtually all health care providers and 2) are the most frequently used CPT codes.

HOW TO USE THE CPT CODING SYSTEM

A provider or coder using the CPT coding system first chooses the name and associated code of the procedure or service which most accurately identifies and describes the service(s) performed. The provider or coder then chooses names and codes for additional services or procedures. If necessary, modifiers are chosen and added to the selected service and procedure codes. All services or procedures coded must also be documented in the patient's medical record.

According to CPT, "The listing of a service or procedure and its code number in a specific section of the CPT book does not restrict its use to a specific specialty group. Any procedure or service in any section of the CPT coding system may be used to designate the services rendered by any qualified physician or other qualified health care professional."

The codes and descriptions listed in the CPT coding system are those that are generally consistent with contemporary medical practice and being performed by health care professionals in clinical practice. Inclusion in the CPT coding system does not represent endorsement by the American Medical Association of any particular diagnostic or therapeutic procedure. In addition, inclusion or exclusion of a procedure does not imply any health insurance coverage or reimbursement policy.

CPT FORMAT AND CONVENTIONS

DESCRIPTIONS

The descriptions associated with CPT codes have been developed by the AMA to provide complete descriptions of medical services and procedures.

Many CPT descriptions include the definition of basic procedures followed by supplemental descriptions for variations or modifications of the basic procedure. In the CPT coding book, the basic procedure description ends with a semicolon (;), followed by the additional description.

If a CPT description includes the same basic procedure as the preceding listing, the basic procedure is not listed. Only the supplemental description is listed, preceded by an indentation. For example:

25100 Arthrotomy, wrist joint; with biopsy

25105   with synovectomy

SYMBOLS

● *A filled BLACK CIRCLE preceding a CPT code indicates that the code is new to this revision of the CPT coding system. A symbol key appears on all left-hand pages.*

▲ *A filled BLACK TRIANGLE preceding a CPT code indicates that there is a revision to the description. Wherever possible, the revised text is identified with underlining.*

( ) *CPT codes enclosed within parenthesis have been deleted from the CPT coding system and should no longer be used.*

\+ *A bold plus sign preceding a CPT code indicates that the code is an "add-on" code and must be listed in addition to the main CPT code.*

⃠ *This symbol preceding a CPT code indicates that the code is exempt from the use of modifier -51.*

⊙ *This symbol preceding a CPT code indicates that the procedure includes conscious sedation as a part of providing the procedure and that the conscious sedation codes, 99141 or 99142, should not be reported separately.*

Note that a CPT code may be preceded by the add-on, star symbol or modifier-51 exempt symbol, in addition to new or changed code symbols.

COLOR CODING

Separate procedure. A procedure or service that is normally performed as an integral component of a total service or procedure. CPT codes identified as separate procedure codes should not be coded in addition to the basic procedure code of which it is considered an integral component.

However, if the procedure or service that is usually designated as a separate procedure is performed independently or is considered to be unrelated or distinct from other procedures or services provided at that time, the separate procedure may be coded by itself. The modifier -59 should be added to the separate procedure code to indicate that the procedure is not considered to be a component of another procedure, but is a distinct, independent procedure.

Unlisted code. Descriptions include the term "unlisted." Use only when a CPT code which specifically describes the service or procedure is unavailable. A report is usually required by third party payers.

Nonspecific code. Descriptions include the term "specify" instructing the coder to include additional information such as the quadrant, the nerve, the muscle, the level of spine, the number of joints, the type of study, the method of dosimetry, the hormone, the receptor, the assay method, the type of kit, the material injected, the type of tests, the number of tests, the doses provided.

CCI comprehensive code. Indicates codes identified as comprehensive codes in the Comprehensive Coding Initiative, revised annually. Per CMS rules, all identifiable component procedures are included in the comprehensive code and should not be billed separately to Medicare.

ITALICIZED AND NON-ITALICIZED TEXT

Italicized text is used throughout this publication to distinguish information authored, contributed or otherwise provided by PMIC.

Non-italicized text is used to distinguish information reproduced verbatim from CPT 2007, published by the American Medical Association.

SECTION OVERVIEWS

Specific guidelines are presented at the beginning of each of the six sections of the CPT coding system. The guidelines define items that are necessary to interpret and report the procedures and services contained in that section. CPT guidelines also provide explanations regarding terms that apply only to a particular section.

This page intentionally left blank.

CODING & BILLING ISSUES

Most billing, coding and reporting issues involving the CPT® coding system apply generally to all medical specialties and professions. However, there are some specialty specific issues defined in each section of the CPT coding system that apply only to the specific medical specialty represented.

SUPPORTING DOCUMENTATION

Documentation in the patient's medical report must clearly support the procedures, services and supplies coded on the health insurance claim form. Most medical chart reviewers take the position that if something is not documented in the medical record, then the service or procedure was not performed and therefore is not subject to reimbursement.

If a medical practice is selected for an audit by Medicare or other third party payer, the accuracy and completeness of the documentation of the medical records, or lack thereof, will have a significant impact on the outcome of the audit. The current emphasis on "fraud" and "abuse" by Medicare, Medicaid and private third party payer necessitates a review of documentation by all health care professionals.

SPECIAL MEDICARE CONSIDERATIONS

To satisfy Medicare requirements, there must be sufficient documentation in the medical record to verify the services coded and the level of care required. Section 1833(e) of Title XVIII, Social Security Act requires "available information that documents a claim." If there is no documentation to justify the services or level of care, the claim cannot be considered for Medicare benefits.

If there is insufficient documentation to support claims that have already been paid by Medicare, the reimbursement will be considered an overpayment and a refund will be requested by Medicare. Medicare has the authority to review any information, including medical records, when such information pertains to a Medicare claim.

UNLISTED PROCEDURES OR SERVICES

There are services or procedures performed by health care professionals that are not found in the CPT coding system. These services or procedures may be either new procedures which have not yet been assigned a CPT code or simply a variation of a procedure which precludes using the existing CPT code. Each section of the CPT coding system includes codes for reporting these unlisted procedures.

Unlisted procedure codes should not be coded unless the coder has reviewed the CPT coding system carefully to ensure that a more specific code is not available. If a specific CPT code is not located, check for HCPCS codes that may be reportable.

As a rule, a report needs to be enclosed with the health insurance claim form when reporting unlisted procedure codes. Because unlisted procedure codes are subject to manual medical review, payment is usually slower than for normal processing time.

CPT ADDITIONS, CHANGES, AND DELETIONS

Each year hundreds of codes are added, changed or deleted from the CPT coding system. A summary of these changes is found in Appendix B of the CPT code book, which provides a quick reference for coding review. In addition to the summary, these modifications are identified throughout the CPT code book.

ADDITIONS TO THE CPT CODING SYSTEM

New codes are added to the CPT coding system each year. New CPT codes are identified with a small black circle placed to the left of the code number. Examples of new codes found in CPT 2007 include:

● **33203** Insertion of epicardial electrode(s); endoscopic approach (eg, thoracoscopy, pericardioscopy)

● **86788** Antibody; West Nile virus, IgM

CHANGES TO CPT CODE DEFINITIONS

Each year the definitions of many CPT codes are revised. CPT codes with changed definitions are identified with a small black triangle placed to the left of the code number. Examples of CPT codes with changed definitions in CPT 2007 include:

▲ **17000** Destruction (eg, laser surgery, electrosurgery, cryosurgery, chemosurgery, surgical curettement), premalignant lesions (eg, actinic keratoses); first lesion

▲ **19361** Breast reconstruction with latissimus dorsi flap, without prosthetic implant

The only way to determine exactly what part of the definition has been changed is to compare the current changed definition with the definition from the previous edition of the CPT code book.

DELETIONS FROM THE CPT CODING SYSTEM

Each year some CPT codes are deleted. Deleted CPT codes, and references to replacement codes, are enclosed within parentheses. Examples of CPT codes deleted from CPT 2007 include:

(15000 deleted 2007 edition, see 15002, 15004.)

(76003 deleted 2007 edition, see 77002)

NEW SECTIONS AND SUBSECTIONS

New sections and subsections are frequently added to the CPT coding system to reflect changes in technology or medical practice and to provide additional code sequences for special purposes.

Anticoagulant Management	99363-99364
Mastectomy Procedures	19300-19307
Radiologic Guidance	77001-77032
Breast Mammography	77051-77059
Stereotactic Radiation Treatment Delivery	77371-77373
Ventilator Management	94002-94005
Functional Brain Mapping	96020
Medical Genetics and Genetic Counseling	96040

CATEGORY II PERFORMANCE MEASUREMENT CODES

Category II, Performance Measurement CPT codes, are designed to facilitate outcomes research. This new section was introduced in the 2005 CPT updates. Category II codes include the letter "F" as the fifth digit of the five digit CPT code. These codes are optional, and are not a substitute for Category I codes.

CATEGORY III EMERGING TECHNOLOGY CODES

Emerging technology codes are temporary codes for emerging technology, services and procedures. These codes are designed to permit data collection and assessment of new technologies. All Category III codes include the letter "T" as the fifth digit of the five digit CPT code. The inclusion of a specific service or procedure in this section does not imply or endorse clinical efficacy, safety, or applicability to clinical practice.

CPT 2007 ADDITIONS, CHANGES, AND DELETIONS

Following is a summary listing all additions, deletions, and revisions applicable to CPT 2007 codes. The descriptors of the codes listed as "grammatical change" have not been substantially changed, but involve placement of the semicolon, or other punctuation, or a similar minor change.

Evaluation and Management

99251 Code revised

99252 Code revised

99253 Code revised

99254 Code revised

99255 Code revised

99363 Code added

99364 Code added

Anesthesia

00625 Code added

00626 Code added

01995 Code deleted

Surgery

15000 Code deleted

15001 Code deleted

15002 Code added

15003 Code added

15004 Code added

15005 Code added

15731 Code added

15830 Code added

15831 Code deleted

15847 Code added

17000 Code revised

17004 Code revised

17110 Code revised

17304 Code deleted

17305 Code deleted

17306 Code deleted

17307 Code deleted

17310 Code deleted

17311 Code added

17312 Code added

17313 Code added

17314 Code added

17315 Code added

19105 Code added

19120 Code revised

19140 Code deleted

19160 Code deleted

19162 Code deleted

19180 Code deleted

19182 Code deleted

19200 Code deleted

19220 Code deleted

19240 Code deleted

19300 Code added

19301 Code added

19302 Code added

19303 Code added

19304 Code added

19305 Code added

19306 Code added

19307 Code added

19361 Code revised

21300 Code deleted

22526 Code added

22527 Code added

22857	Code added
22862	Code added
22865	Code added
25109	Code added
25600	Code revised
25606	Code added
25607	Code added
25608	Code added
25609	Code added
25611	Code deleted
25620	Code deleted
26170	Code revised
26180	Code revised
26504	Code deleted
27315	Code deleted
27320	Code deleted
27325	Code added
27326	Code added
28030	Code deleted
28055	Code added
31700	Code deleted
31708	Code deleted
31710	Code deleted
32998	Code added
33200	Code deleted
33201	Code deleted
33202	Code added
33203	Code added
33245	Code deleted
33246	Code deleted
33253	Code deleted
33254	Code added
33255	Code added
33256	Code added
33265	Code added
33266	Code added
33675	Code added
33676	Code added
33677	Code added
33681	Code revised
33724	Code added
33726	Code added
35301	Code revised
35302	Code added
35303	Code added
35304	Code added
35305	Code added
35306	Code added
35381	Code revised
35501	Code revised
35506	Code revised
35507	Code deleted
35509	Code revised
35537	Code added
35538	Code added
35539	Code added
35540	Code added
35541	Code deleted

35546	Code deleted
35601	Code revised
35637	Code added
35638	Code added
35641	Code deleted
35883	Code added
35884	Code added
37210	Code added
43647	Code added
43648	Code added
43881	Code added
43882	Code added
44152	Code deleted
44153	Code deleted
44157	Code added
44158	Code added
44211	Code revised
47716	Code deleted
47719	Code added
48005	Code deleted
48105	Code added
48180	Code deleted
48548	Code added
49085	Code deleted
49324	Code added
49325	Code added
49326	Code added
49402	Code added
49435	Code added
49436	Code added
51720	Code revised
52204	Code revised
54150	Code revised
54152	Code deleted
54160	Code revised
54161	Code revised
54820	Code deleted
54865	Code added
55859	Code deleted
55875	Code added
55876	Code added
56442	Code added
56720	Code deleted
57296	Code added
57558	Code added
57820	Code deleted
58541	Code added
58542	Code added
58543	Code added
58544	Code added
58548	Code added
58950	Code revised
58957	Code added
58958	Code added
61107	Code revised
61210	Code revised
64590	Code revised
64595	Code revised

64910 Code added

64911 Code added

67346 Code added

67350 Code deleted

Radiology

70540 Code revised

70554 Code added

70555 Code added

71275 Code revised

72291 Code added

72292 Code added

75998 Code deleted

76003 Code deleted

76005 Code deleted

76006 Code deleted

76012 Code deleted

76013 Code deleted

76020 Code deleted

76040 Code deleted

76061 Code deleted

76062 Code deleted

76065 Code deleted

76066 Code deleted

76070 Code deleted

76071 Code deleted

76075 Code deleted

76076 Code deleted

76077 Code deleted

76078 Code deleted

76082 Code deleted

76083 Code deleted

76086 Code deleted

76088 Code deleted

76090 Code deleted

76091 Code deleted

76092 Code deleted

76093 Code deleted

76094 Code deleted

76095 Code deleted

76096 Code deleted

76355 Code deleted

76360 Code deleted

76362 Code deleted

76370 Code deleted

76393 Code deleted

76394 Code deleted

76400 Code deleted

76536 Code revised

76604 Code revised

76645 Code revised

76700 Code revised

76770 Code revised

76776 Code added

76778 Code deleted

76813 Code added

76814 Code added

76856 Code revised

76880 Code revised

76940 Code revised

76986 Code deleted

76998 Code added

77001 Code added

77002 Code added

77003 Code added

77011 Code added

77012 Code added

77013 Code added

77014 Code added

77021 Code added

77022 Code added

77031 Code added

77032 Code added

77051 Code added

77052 Code added

77053 Code added

77054 Code added

77055 Code added

77056 Code added

77057 Code added

77058 Code added

77059 Code added

77071 Code added

77072 Code added

77073 Code added

77074 Code added

77075 Code added

77076 Code added

77077 Code added

77078 Code added

77079 Code added

77080 Code added

77081 Code added

77082 Code added

77083 Code added

77084 Code added

77371 Code added

77372 Code added

77373 Code added

77435 Code added

78700 Code revised

78704 Code deleted

78707 Code revised

78708 Code revised

78709 Code revised

78710 Code revised

78715 Code deleted

78730 Code revised

78760 Code deleted

78761 Code revised

Pathology and Laboratory

82107 Code added

83698 Code added

83913 Code added

86788 Code added

86789 Code added

87088 Code revised

87305 Code added

87498 Code added

87640 Code added

87641 Code added

87653 Code added

87808 Code added

88106 Code revised

88107 Code revised

89060 Code revised

Medicine

90655 Code revised

90656 Code revised

90657 Code revised

90658 Code revised

90669 Code revised

90700 Code revised

90702 Code revised

90714 Code revised

90715 Code revised

90718 Code revised

90732 Code revised

90761 Code revised

90766 Code revised

91060 Code deleted

91111 Code added

92025 Code added

92573 Code deleted

92640 Code added

94002 Code added

94003 Code added

94004 Code added

94005 Code added

94610 Code added

94620 Code revised

94644 Code added

94645 Code added

94656 Code deleted

94657 Code deleted

94774 Code added

94775 Code added

94776 Code added

94777 Code added

95012 Code added

95078 Code deleted

96020 Code added

96040 Code added

96415 Code revised

96423 Code revised

96904 Code added

Category II Codes

0001F Code revised

0012F Code added

1000F Code revised

1001F Code deleted

1015F Code added

1018F Code added

1019F Code added

1022F Code added

1026F	Code added
1030F	Code added
1034F	Code added
1035F	Code added
1036F	Code added
1038F	Code added
1039F	Code added
2003F	Code deleted
2010F	Code added
2014F	Code added
2018F	Code added
2022F	Code added
2024F	Code added
2026F	Code added
2028F	Code added
3000F	Code deleted
3002F	Code deleted
3006F	Code added
3011F	Code added
3014F	Code added
3017F	Code added
3020F	Code added
3021F	Code added
3022F	Code added
3023F	Code added
3025F	Code added
3027F	Code added
3028F	Code added
3035F	Code added
3037F	Code added
3040F	Code added
3042F	Code added
3046F	Code added
3047F	Code added
3048F	Code added
3049F	Code added
3050F	Code added
3060F	Code added
3061F	Code added
3062F	Code added
3066F	Code added
3072F	Code added
3076F	Code added
3077F	Code added
3078F	Code added
3079F	Code added
3080F	Code added
4009F	Code revised
4015F	Code revised
4025F	Code added
4030F	Code added
4033F	Code added
4035F	Code added
4037F	Code added
4040F	Code added
4045F	Code added
4050F	Code added
6005F	Code added

Category III Codes

0003T Code deleted

0008T Code deleted

0018T Code deleted

0021T Code deleted

0044T Code deleted

0045T Code deleted

0062T Code revised

0082T Code deleted

0083T Code deleted

0090T Code revised

0091T Code deleted

0093T Code revised

0094T Code deleted

0096T Code revised

0097T Code deleted

0120T Code deleted

0141T Code added

0142T Code added

0143T Code added

0144T Code added

0145T Code added

0146T Code added

0147T Code added

0148T Code added

0149T Code added

0150T Code added

0151T Code added

0153T Code added

0154T Code added

0155T Code added

0156T Code added

0157T Code added

0158T Code added

0159T Code added

0160T Code added

0161T Code added

0162T Code added

0163T Code added

0164T Code added

0165T Code added

0166T Code added

0167T Code added

0168T Code added

0169T Code added

0170T Code added

STARRED PROCEDURES

Starred procedure designation was removed from CPT 2004.

INSTRUCTIONAL NOTES

Notes found in the CPT coding system give instructions for using codes. When selecting a code, look for instructions in the section guidelines for any additional information necessary to code accurately. Also, instructional notes take the form of parenthetical statements and paragraphs, which may appear at the beginning of subsections, headings and subheadings, or above and below the code itself.

DEFINITION OF NEW AND ESTABLISHED PATIENT

Solely for the purposes of distinguishing between new and established patients, professional services are those face-to-face services rendered by a physician and coded by a specific cpt code(s). A new patient is one who has not received any professional services from the physician or another physician of the same specialty who belongs to the same group practice, within the past three years.

An established patient is one who has received professional services from the physician or another physician of the same specialty who belongs to the same group practice, within the past three years.

In the instance where a physician is on call for or covering for another physician, the patient's encounter will be classified as it would have been by the physician who is not available.

No distinction is made between new and established patients in the emergency department. Evaluation and Management services in the emergency department category may be coded for any new or established patient who presents for treatment in the emergency department.

PLACE (LOCATION) OF SERVICE

The CPT coding system makes specific distinctions for place (location) of service for CPT codes defined in the evaluation and management section. The place of service may have considerable impact on reimbursement. The following list gives CPT code ranges for some specific places of service:

Office or Other Outpatient Services	*99201-99215*
Hospital Inpatient Services	*99221-99239*
Emergency Department	*99281-99288*
Nursing Facility Services	*99304-99318*
Domiciliary, Rest Home, or Custodial Care Services	*99324-99337*
Domiciliary, Rest Home, or Home Care Plan Oversight Services	*99339-99340*
Home Services	*99341-99350*

HOSPITAL CARE

Hospital services frequently cause reimbursement problems for health care professionals. The three most common coding errors are:

- *More than one physician submits an initial hospital care code for the same patient.*
- *Follow-up hospital visits are coded incorrectly.*
- *Concurrent care visits by multiple specialists are coded improperly.*

If more than one physician is involved in the process of hospitalizing a patient, for example, surgeon and internist, the physicians must decide which is going to actually admit the patient and report the admission services on the health insurance claim form. If both do, the first health insurance claim form to arrive will be processed and paid, and the second will be rejected.

There are valid reasons for visiting a patient more than once daily while hospitalized, however, many physicians and even some insurance billers do not know that subsequent hospital visit codes are for "daily" services. When a physician visits the patient twice in one day, providing a brief level of service each time, the physician or insurance biller may incorrectly report two hospital visit services for the same day, instead of a higher level code incorporating both visits.

Reporting multiple hospital visits provided on the same day separately on the health insurance claim form usually results in either the entire claim being returned for clarification, or the second visit being denied as an apparent duplication. Unfortunately, insurance billers who are unclear on the proper coding of same day hospital visits may simply accept the rejection without question and write-off the unpaid visit as uncollectible.

The CPT coding system clearly defines subsequent hospital care as "per day", meaning daily services. If the physician visits the patient twice in one day, providing the equivalent of "brief" services each time, report the service using the appropriate evaluation and management code that defines the cumulative level of service provided.

HOSPITAL DISCHARGE

The CPT codes for hospital discharge services are evaluation and management code 99238 and 99239, defined as Hospital Discharge Day Management. Hospital discharge services include final examination of the patient, discussion of the hospital stay, instructions for continuing care, and preparation of discharge records. Many health insurance companies do not recognize and/or do not reimburse this CPT code.

Options for the use of these codes include the use of one of the other hospital daily services codes from the evaluation and management series 99231-99233 and perhaps using a code that has a higher value than the routine hospital visit.

REFERRAL

A referral is the transfer of the total care or specific portion of care of a patient from one physician to another. A referral is not a request for consultation. If a patient is referred to the physician for total care or a portion of their care, use evaluation and management visit codes, and other CPT codes if appropriate, to report the services provided. If a patient is sent to the physician for a consultation, use evaluation and management consultation codes to report the services provided.

SEPARATE OR MULTIPLE PROCEDURES

It is appropriate to designate multiple procedures that are rendered on the same date by separate entries. For example: if a proctosigmoidoscopy was performed in addition to a hospital visit, the proctosigmoidoscopy would be considered a SEPARATE procedure and listed in addition to the hospital visit on the health insurance claim form. Another example would be individual medical psychotherapy rendered in addition to a brief subsequent hospital service. In this instance, both services would be coded.

SUPPLIES AND MATERIALS SUPPLIED BY THE PHYSICIAN

The CPT coding system includes specific codes for identifying certain supplies and materials provided by the physician. These supply codes are used to report supplies and materials that are not included in the definition of the basic service.

CPT CODES FOR SUPPLIES AND MATERIALS

92310-92371 Supply of spectacles, contact lenses, low vision aids and ocular prosthesis.

95144-95170 Provision of antigens for allergen immunotherapy.

99070 Supplies and materials (except spectacles) provided by the physician.

99071 Educational supplies, such as books, tapes, and pamphlets, provided by the physician for the patient's education at cost to physician.

PURCHASED DIAGNOSTIC SERVICES

It is common for physicians to bill patients and health insurance companies for diagnostic services that were procured or ordered on behalf of the patient but not actually provided by the ordering physician. It is also common for the ordering physician to "mark-up" the fee for the purchased service prior to billing. This is referred to as global billing.

Medical equipment companies, particularly those offering electrocardiography, pulmonary diagnostic equipment, and other diagnostic equipment, have used this global billing concept in the past as a method of selling physicians a new "profit center" for their practice. Some even provided technicians, who were not employees of the practice, to perform the diagnostic tests in the physicians office. OBRA 1987 placed severe restrictions on global billing of certain diagnostic tests as of March 1, 1988.

The Medicare regulations apply to diagnostic tests other than clinical laboratory tests including, but not limited to: EKGs, EEGs, cardiac monitoring, X-rays and ultrasound. Global billing is allowed only when the billing physician personally performs or supervises the diagnostic procedure. To qualify under the supervision definition, the person performing the test must be an employee or the physician or group. Ownership interest in an outside supplier does not meet the supervision requirement.

Billing for purchased services under the new requirement is complicated. The provider must provide the supplier's name, address, provider number and net charge on the health insurance claim form. In addition, a HCPCS Level III modifier must be coded to indicate that the service was purchased. Billing for global services usually will also require a HCPCS Level III modifier to indicate that the service was not purchased. This requirement does not apply to the professional component of these services if provided separately.

Providers should discontinue billing for the technical component of diagnostic services that were not provided or supervised by the provider as defined in this regulation for the following reasons:

1. *The provider is no longer making any profit on these procedures;*
2. *Operating costs are higher due to the increased reporting requirements; and*
3. *Risk of audit liability is increased if these services are not coded properly.*

UNBUNDLING

Unbundling is defined as reporting multiple CPT codes when one CPT code is sufficient. For example, it is considered unbundling if incidental surgical procedures are coded separately, or office visits for uncomplicated follow-up care are separately coded. This practice often happens unintentionally. However, most third-party payers currently have software in place to catch unbundling when it occurs. When physicians continually break out or itemize services in this manner, they often find themselves under close scrutiny and even the focus of an audit by the insurance company. It is most important to know the guidelines to prevent unbundling when coding and billing for services and/or procedures.

CONSCIOUS SEDATION

Conscious sedation induces an altered state of consciousness that minimizes pain and discomfort through the use of pain relievers and sedatives. Patients who receive conscious sedation usually are able to speak and respond to verbal cues throughout the procedure, communicating any discomfort they experience to the provider. A brief period of amnesia may erase any memory of the procedure. Conscious sedation is administered in hospitals, outpatient facilities, for example ambulatory surgery centers, and doctors offices to facilitate procedures such as the following:

- *Breast biopsy*
- *Vasectomy*
- *Minor foot surgery*
- *Minor bone fracture repair*
- *Plastic/reconstructive surgery*
- *Dental prosthetic/reconstructive surgery*
- *Endoscopy*

Procedures That Include Conscious Sedation

Beginning with CPT 2006, surgical and medical procedures that include conscious sedation as part of the procedure were identified with a ⊙ symbol to the left of the CPT code. Because these surgical and medical procedures include conscious sedation, the CPT codes for conscious sedation, 99143-99145, should not be reported separately. Following is a list of surgical and medical CPT codes that include conscious sedation:

19298	33249	43216	43272
20982	35470	43217	43453
22526	35471	43219	43456
22527	35472	43220	43458
31615	35473	43226	43750
31620	35474	43227	44360
31622	35475	43228	44361
31623	35476	43231	44363
31624	36555	43232	44364
31625	36557	43234	44365
31628	36558	43235	44366
31629	36560	43236	44369
31635	36561	43237	44370
31645	36563	43238	44372
31646	36565	43239	44373
31656	36566	43240	44376
31725	36568	43241	44377
32019	36570	43242	44378
32020	36571	43243	44379
32201	36576	43244	44380
33010	36578	43245	44382
33011	36581	43246	44383
33206	36582	43247	44385
33207	36583	43248	44386
33208	36585	43249	44388
33210	36590	43250	44389
33211	36870	43251	44390
33212	37184	43255	44391
33213	37185	43256	44392
33214	37186	43257	44393
33216	37187	43258	44394
33217	37188	43259	44397
33218	37203	43260	44500
33220	37210	43261	44901
33222	37215	43262	45303
33223	37216	43263	45305
33233	43200	43264	45307
33234	43201	43265	45308
33235	43202	43267	45309
33240	43204	43268	45315
33241	43205	43269	45317
33244	43215	43271	*continued*

45320	47011	92982	93541
45321	48511	92984	93542
45327	49021	92986	93543
45332	49041	92987	93544
45333	49061	92995	93545
45334	50021	92996	93555
45335	50382	93312	93556
45337	50384	93313	93561
45338	50387	93314	93562
45339	50592	93315	93571
45340	58823	93316	93572
45341	66720	93317	93609
45342	69300	93318	93613
45345	77600	93501	93615
45355	77605	93505	93616
45378	77610	93508	93618
45379	77615	93510	93619
45380	92953	93511	93620
45381	92960	93514	93621
45382	92961	93524	93622
45383	92973	93526	93624
45384	92974	93527	93640
45385	92975	93528	93641
45386	92978	93529	93642
45387	92979	93530	93650
45391	92980	93539	93651
45392	92981	93540	93652

This page intentionally left blank.

CPT MODIFIERS

The CPT® coding system includes two-digit modifier codes which are used to report that a service or procedure has been "altered or modified by some specific circumstance" without altering or modifying the basic definition or CPT code.

The proper use of CPT modifiers can speed up claim processing and increase reimbursement, while the improper use of CPT modifiers may result in claim delays or claim denials. In addition, using certain CPT modifiers, for example -22, too frequently may trigger a claims audit.

CPT MODIFIERS

-21 Prolonged evaluation and management services

When the face-to-face or floor/unit service(s) provided is prolonged or otherwise greater than that usually required for the highest level of evaluation and management service within a given category, it may be identified by adding modifier '-21' to the evaluation and management code number. A report may also be appropriate.

-22 Unusual procedural services

When the service(s) provided is greater than that usually required for the listed procedure, it may be identified by adding modifier '-22' to the procedure number. A report may also be appropriate.

Modifier -22 is frequently abused and misused. Some physicians routinely add modifier -22 to CPT procedure codes with the expectation that higher reimbursement will be forthcoming. Many third party payers routinely ignore an undocumented modifier -22 on health insurance claim forms for the same reason.

In most cases, it is more appropriate to choose a CPT code of a higher value than to use modifier -22. If the provider reports modifier -22, documentation in the form of a cover letter or report must be provided with the health insurance claim form to explain the situation or circumstances that make the procedure(s) unusual.

-23 Unusual anesthesia

Occasionally, a procedure, which usually requires either no anesthesia or local anesthesia, because of unusual circumstances must be done under general anesthesia. This circumstance may be reported by adding the modifier '-23' to the procedure code of the basic service.

-24 Unrelated evaluation and management service by the same physician during a postoperative period

The physician may need to indicate that an evaluation and management service was performed during a postoperative period for a reason(s) unrelated to the original procedure. This circumstance may be reported by adding the modifier '-24' to the appropriate level of E/M service.

-25 Significant, separately identifiable evaluation and management service by the same physician on the same day of a procedure or other service

The physician may need to indicate that on the day a procedure or service identified by a CPT code was performed, the patient's condition required a significant, separately identifiable E/M service above and beyond the other service provided or beyond the usual preoperative and postoperative care associated with the procedure that was performed. The E/M service may be prompted by the symptom or condition for which the procedure and/or service was provided. As such, different diagnoses are not required for reporting of the E/M services on the same date. This circumstance may be reported by adding the modifier '-25' to the appropriate level of E/M service.

Note: This modifier is not used to report an E/M service that resulted in a decision to perform surgery. See modifier '-57.'

-26 Professional component

Certain procedures are a combination of a physician component and a technical component. When the physician component is reported separately, the service may be identified by adding the modifier '-26' to the usual procedure number.

-27 Multiple outpatient hospital evaluation and management encounters on the same date

For hospital outpatient reporting purposes, utilization of hospital resources related to separate and distinct E/M encounters performed in multiple outpatient hospital settings on the same date may be reported by adding the modifier '-27' to each appropriate level outpatient and/or emergency department E/M code(s).

This modifier provides a means of reporting circumstances involving evaluation and management services provided by physician(s) in more than one (multiple) outpatient hospital setting(s) (eg, hospital emergency department, clinic).

Note: This modifier is not to be used for physician reporting of multiple E/M services performed by the same physician on the same date. For physician reporting of all outpatient evaluation and management services provided by the same physician on the same date and performed in multiple outpatient setting(s) (eg, hospital emergency department, clinic), see Evaluation and Management, Emergency Department, or Preventive Medicine Services codes.

-32 Mandated services

Services related to mandated consultation and/or related services (eg, PRO, third party payer, governmental, legislative or regulatory requirement) may be identified by adding the modifier '-32' to the basic procedure.

Occasionally a consultation and/or related service may be mandated by a third party (eg, peer review organization, third party payer, governmental, legislative or regulatory requirement).

HCPCS modifier -SF is reported instead of CPT modifier -32 if the patient is a Medicare patient.

-47 Anesthesia by surgeon

Regional or general anesthesia provided by the surgeon may be reported by adding the modifier '-47' to the basic service. (This does not include local anesthesia.)

Note: Modifier '-47' would not be used as a modifier for the Anesthesia procedures.

-50 Bilateral procedure

Unless otherwise identified in the listings, bilateral procedures that are performed at the same operative session, should be identified by adding the modifier '-50' to the appropriate five digit code.

This modifier is reported when bilateral procedures requiring a separate incision are performed during the SAME operative session. Proper reporting of this modifier on the CMS1500 health insurance claim form requires the CPT procedure code to be listed two times: first with no modifier, and the second time with modifier -50.

This modifier may not be used if the definition of the basic procedure code includes the term "bilateral."

-51 Multiple procedures

When multiple procedures, other than E/M services, are performed at the same session by the same provider, the primary procedure or service may be reported as listed. The additional procedure(s) or service(s) may be identified by appending the modifier '-51' to the additional procedure or service code(s).

Note: This modifier should not be appended to designated "add-on" codes.

-52 Reduced services

Under certain circumstances a service or procedure is partially reduced or eliminated at the physician's discretion. Under these circumstances the service provided can be identified by its usual procedure number and the addition of the modifier '-52' signifying that the service is reduced. This provides a means of reporting reduced services without disturbing the identification of the basic service.

Note: For hospital outpatient reporting of a previously scheduled procedure/service that is partially reduced or canceled as a result of extenuating circumstances or those that threaten the well-being of the patient prior to or after administration of anesthesia, see modifiers '-73' and '-74' (see modifiers approved for ASC hospital outpatient use).

The intended use of this modifier is to report the reduction of a service without affecting provider profiles maintained by health insurance companies.

Modifier -52 is another frequently misused modifier. Some medical practices mistakenly use modifier -52 to mean "reduced fee" and use it as a discounting method. Not only is this incorrect, the provider may seriously damage their provider profile with health insurance companies. The proper use for modifier -52 is to report that a service was not completed, or some part of a multiple-part service was not performed. A fee reduction may be in order as well; however that is not the primary purpose of the modifier.

-53 Discontinued procedure

Under certain circumstances, the physician may elect to terminate a surgical or diagnostic procedure. Due to extenuating circumstances or those that threaten the well being of the patient, it may be necessary to indicate that a surgical or diagnostic procedure was started but discontinued. This circumstance may be reported by adding the modifier '-53' to the code reported by the physician for the discontinued procedure.

Note: This modifier is not used to report the elective cancellation of a procedure prior to the patient's anesthesia induction and/or surgical preparation in the operating suite. For hospital outpatient/ambulatory surgery center (ASC) reporting of a previously scheduled procedure/service that is partially reduced or cancelled as a result of extenuating circumstances or those that threaten the well-being of the patient prior to or after administration of anesthesia, see modifiers '-73' and '-74' (see modifiers approved for ASC hospital outpatient use).

-54 Surgical care only

When one physician performs a surgical procedure and another provides preoperative and/or postoperative management, surgical services may be identified by adding the modifier '-54' to the usual procedure number.

-55 Postoperative management only

When one physician performed the postoperative management and another physician performed the surgical procedure, the postoperative component may be identified by adding the modifier '-55' to the usual procedure number.

-56 Preoperative management only

When one physician performed the preoperative care and evaluation and another physician performed the surgical procedure, the preoperative component may be identified by adding the modifier '-56' to the usual procedure number.

-57 Decision for surgery

An evaluation and management service that resulted in the initial decision to perform the surgery may be identified by adding the modifier '-57' to the appropriate level of E/M service.

-58 Staged or related procedure or service by the same physician during the postoperative period

The physician may need to indicate that the performance of a procedure or service during the postoperative period was: a) planned prospectively at the time of the original procedure (staged); b) more extensive than the original procedure; or c) for therapy following a diagnostic surgical procedure. This circumstance may be reported by adding the modifier '-58' to the staged or related procedure.

Note: This modifier is not used to report the treatment of a problem that requires a return to the operating room.

-59 Distinct Procedural Service

Under certain circumstances the physician may need to indicate that a procedure or service was distinct or independent from other services performed on the same day. Modifier '-59' is used to identify procedures/ services that are not normally reported together, but are appropriate under the circumstances. This may represent a different session or patient encounter, different procedure or surgery, different site or organ system, separate incision/excision, separate lesion, or separate injury (or area of injury in extensive injuries) not ordinarily encountered or performed on the same day by the same physician.

However, when another already established modifier is appropriate it should be used rather than modifier '-59.' Only if no more descriptive modifier is available, and the use of modifier '-59' best explains the circumstances, should modifier '-59' be used.

-62 Two surgeons

When two surgeons work together as primary surgeons performing distinct part(s) of a procedure, each surgeon should report his/her distinct operative work by adding the modifier '-62' to the procedure code and any associated add-on code(s) for that procedure as long as both surgeons continue to work together as primary surgeons.

Each surgeon should report the co-surgery once using the same procedure code. If additional procedure(s) (including add-on procedure(s) are performed during the same surgical session, separate code(s) may also be reported with the modifier '-62' added.

Note: If a co-surgeon acts as an assistant in the performance of additional procedure(s) during the same surgical session, those services may be reported using separate procedure code(s) with the modifier '-80' or modifier '-82' added, as appropriate.

-63 Procedure performed on infants less than 4 kg

Procedures performed on neonates and infants up to a present body weight of 4 kg may involve significantly increased complexity and physician work commonly associated with these patients. This circumstance may be reported by adding the modifier '-63' to the procedure number.

Note: Unless otherwise designated, this modifier may only be appended to procedures/services listed in the 20000-69999 code series. Modifier '-63' should not be appended to any CPT codes listed in the Evaluation and Management Services, Anesthesia, Radiology, Pathology/Laboratory, or Medicine sections.

-66 Surgical team

Under some circumstances, highly complex procedures (requiring the concomitant services of several physicians, often of different specialties, plus other highly skilled specialy trained personnel, various types of complex equipment) are carried out under the "surgical team" concept. Such circumstances may be identified by each participating physician with the addition of the modifier '-66' to the basic procedure number used for reporting services.

-73 Discontinued out-patient hospital/ambulatory surgery center (ASC) procedure prior to the administration of anesthesia

Due to extenuating circumstances or those that threaten the well being of the patient, the physician may cancel a surgical or diagnostic procedure subsequent to the patient's surgical preparation (including sedation when provided, and being taken to the room where the procedure is to be performed), but prior to the administration of anesthesia (local, regional block(s) or general). Under these circumstances, the intended service that is prepared for but cancelled can be reported by its usual procedure number and the addition of the modifier '-73.'

Note: The elective cancellation of a service prior to the administration of anesthesia and/or surgical preparation of the patient should not be reported. For physician reporting of a discontinued procedure, see modifier '-53.'

-74 Discontinued out-patient hospital/ambulatory surgery center (ASC) procedure after administration of anesthesia

Due to extenuating circumstances or those that threaten the well being of the patient, the physician may terminate a surgical or diagnostic procedure after the administration of anesthesia (local, regional block(s), general) or after the procedure was started (incision made, intubation started, scope inserted, etc.). Under these circumstances, the procedure started but terminated can be reported by its usual procedure number and the addition of the modifier '-74.'

Note: The elective cancellation of a service prior to the administration of anesthesia and/or surgical preparation of the patient should not be reported. For physician reporting of a discontinued procedure, see modifier '-53.'

-76 Repeat procedure by same physician

The physician may need to indicate that a procedure or service was repeated subsequent to the original procedure or service. This circumstance may be reported by adding the modifier '-76' to the repeated procedure/service.

-77 Repeat procedure by another physician

The physician may need to indicate that a basic procedure or service performed by another physician had to be repeated. This situation may be reported by adding modifier '-77' to the repeated procedure/service.

-78 Return to the operating room for a related procedure during the postoperative period

The physician may need to indicate that another procedure was performed during the postoperative period of the initial procedure. When this subsequent procedure is related to the first, and requires the use of the operating room, it may be reported by adding the modifier '-78' to the related procedure. (For repeat procedures on the same day, see '-76.')

-79 Unrelated procedure or service by the same physician during the postoperative period

The physician may need to indicate that the performance of a procedure or service during the postoperative period was unrelated to the original procedure. This circumstance may be reported by using the modifier '-79.' (For repeat procedures on the same day, see '-76.')

-80 Assistant surgeon

Surgical assistant services may be identified by adding the modifier '-80' to the usual procedure number(s).

-81 Minimum assistant surgeon

Minimum surgical assistant services are identified by adding the modifier '-81' to the usual procedure number.

-82 Assistant surgeon (when qualified resident surgeon not available)

The unavailability of a qualified resident surgeon is a prerequisite for use of modifier '-82' appended to the usual procedure code number(s).

-90 Reference (outside) laboratory

When laboratory procedures are performed by a party other than the treating or reporting physician, the procedure may be identified by adding the modifier '-90' to the usual procedure number.

-91 Repeat clinical diagnostic laboratory test

In the course of treatment of the patient, it may be necessary to repeat the same laboratory test on the same day to obtain subsequent (multiple) test results. Under these circumstances, the laboratory test performed can be identified by its usual procedure number and the addition of modifier '-91.'

Note: This modifier may not be used when tests are rerun to confirm initial results; due to testing problems with specimens or equipment; or for any other reason when a normal, one-time, reportable result is all that is required.

This modifier may not be used when other code(s) describe a series of tests results (eg, glucose tolerance tests, evocative/suppression testing). This modifier may only be used for laboratory test(s) performed more than once on the same day on the same patient.

-99 Multiple modifiers

Under certain circumstances two or more modifiers may be necessary to completely delineate a service. In such situations modifier '-99' should be added to the basic procedure, and other applicable modifiers may be listed as part of the description of the service.

ANESTHESIA PHYSICAL STATUS MODIFIERS

P1 A normal healthy patient

P2 A patient with mild systemic disease

P3 A patient with severe systemic disease

P4 A patient with severe systemic disaease that is a constant threat to life

P5 A moribund patient who is not expected to survive without the operation

P6 A declared brain-dead patient whose organs are being removed for donor purposes

GENETIC TESTING CODE MODIFIERS

The following modifiers are used with molecular laboratory procedures related to genetic testing. These modifiers should be used with CPT and HCPCS codes to provide diagnostic granularity of service. This allows providers to submit complete and precise genetic testing information without altering test descriptors.

The genetic testing code modifiers are categorized by mutation. The first digit identifies the disease category and the second digit identifies gene type.

Neoplasia (solid tumor)

0A BRCA1 (Hereditary breast/ovarian cancer)

0B BRCA2 (Hereditary breast cancer)

0C Neurofibromin (Neurofibromatosis, type 1)

0D Merlin (Neurofibromatosis, type 2)

0E c-RET (Multiple endocrine neoplasia, types 2A/B, familial medullary thyroid carcinoma)

0F VHL (Von Hippel Lindau disease)

0G SDHD (Hereditary paraganglioma)

0H SDHB (Hereditary paraganglioma)

0I Her-2/neu

0J MLH1 (HNPCC)

0K MSH2 (HNPCC)

0L APC (Hereditary polyposis coli)

0M Rb (Retinoblastoma)

1Z Solid tumor, not otherwise specified

Neoplasia (lymphoid/hemotopoetic)

2A AML1 - also ETO (Acute myeloid leukemia)

2B BCR - also ABL (Chronic myeloid, acute lymphoid leukemia)

2C CGF1

2D CBF beta (Leukemia)

2E MML (Leukemia)

2F PML/RAR alpha (Promyelocytic leukemia)

2G TEL (Leukemia)

2H bcl-2 (Lymphoma)

2I bcl-1 (Lymphoma)

2J c-myc (Lymphoma)

2K IgH (Lymphoma/leukemia)

2Z Lymphoid/hematopoetic neoplasia, not otherwise specified

Non-neoplastic hematology/coagulation

3A Factor V (Leiden, others) (Hypercoagulable state)

3B FACC (Fanconi anemia)

3C FACD (Fanconi Anemia)

3D Beta globin (Thalassemia)

3E Alpha globin (Thalassemia)

3F MTHFR (Elevated homocysteine)

3G Prothrombin (Factor II, 20210A) (Hypercoagulable state)

3H Factor VIII (Hemophilia A/VWF)

3I Factor IX (Hemophilia B)

3J Beta globin

3Z Non-neoplastic hematology/coagulation, not otherwise specified

Histocompatibility/blood typing

4A HLA-A

4B HLA-B

4C HLA-C

4D HLA-D

4E HLA-DR

4F HLA-DQ

4G HLA-DP

4H Kell

4Z Histocompatibility/blood typing, not otherwise specified

Neurologic, non-neoplastic

5A Aspartoacylase A (Canavan disease)

5B FMR-1 (Fragile X, FRAXA, syndrome)

5C Frataxin (Freidreich's ataxia)

5D Huntington (Huntington's disease)

5E GABRA (Prader Willi-Angelman syndrome)

5F Connexin-26 (GJB2) (Hereditary deafness)

5G Connexin-32 (X-linked Charcot-Marie-Tooth disease)

5H SNRPN (Prader Willi-Angelman syndrome)

5I Ataxin-1 (Spinocerebellar ataxia, type 1)

5J Ataxin-2 (Spinocerebellar ataxia, type 2)

5K Ataxin-3 (Spinocerebellar ataxia, type 3, Machado-Joseph disease)

5L CACNA1A ((Spinocerebellar ataxia, type 6)

5M Ataxin-7 (Spinocerebellar ataxia, type 7)

5N PMP-22 (Charcot-Marie-Tooth disease, type 1A)

5O MECP2 (Rett syndrome)

5Z Neurologic, non-neoplastic, not otherwise specified

Muscular, on-neoplastic

6A Dystrophin (Duchenne/Becker muscular dystrophy)

6B CMPK (Myotonic dystrophy, type 1)

6C ZNF-9 (Myotonic dystrophy, type 2)

6D SMN (Autosomal recessive spinal muscular atrophy)

6Z Muscular, not otherwise specified

Metabolic, other

7A Apolipoprotein E (Cardiovascular disease, Alzheimer's disease)

7B Sphingomyelin phosphodiesterase (Nieman-Pick disease)

7C Acid Beta Glucosidase (Gaucher disease)

7D HFE (Hemochromatosis)

7E Hexosaminidase A (Tay-Sachs disease)

7Z Metabolic, other, not otherwise specified

Metabolic, transport

8A CFTR (Cystic fibrosis)

8Z Metabolic, transport, not otherwise specified

Metabolic-parmacogenetics

9A TPMT (thiopurine methyltransferase) (patients on antimetabolite therapy)

9L Metabolic-pharmacogenetics, not otherwise specified

Dysmorphology

9M FGFR1 (Pfeiffer and Kallmann syndromes)

9N FGFR2 (Crouzon, Jackson-Weiss, Apert, Saethre-Chotzen syndromes)

9O FGFR3 (Achondroplasia, Hypochondroplasia, Thanatophoric dysplasia, types I and II, Crouzon syndrome with acanthosis nigricans, Muencke syndromes)

9P TWIST (Saethre-Chotzen syndrome)

9Q CATCH-22 (22q11 deletion syndromes)

9Z Dysmorphology, not otherwise specified

HCPCS MODIFIERS

HCPCS modifiers, defined and managed by The Centers for Medicare and Medicaid Services (CMS), are two digit modifier codes which may be either alpha (all letters) or alphanumeric (letters plus numbers). Some HCPCS modifiers may be used with CPT codes to modify procedures and services on health insurance claim forms filed for Medicare patients. See the most current edition of HCPCS for a complete list.

ANATOMICAL ILLUSTRATIONS

A fundamental knowledge and understanding of basic human anatomy and physiology is a prerequisite for accurate CPT© procedure coding. While a comprehensive treatment of anatomy and physiology is beyond the scope of this text, the large scale, full color anatomical illustrations on the following pages are designed to facilitate the procedure coding process for both beginning and experienced coders.

The illustrations provide an anatomical perspective of procedure coding by providing a side-by-side view of the major systems of the human body and a corresponding list of the most common CPT procedural categories used to report medical, surgical and diagnostic services performed on the illustrated system.

The CPT procedural categories listed on the left facing page of each anatomical illustration are code ranges only and should not be used for coding. These categories are provided as "pointers" to the appropriate section of CPT, where the definitive code may be found.

PLATE 1. SKIN AND SUBCUTANEOUS TISSUE - MALE

SKIN, SUBCUTANEOUS AND ACCESSORY STRUCTURES	
Incision and Drainage	10040-10180
Excision—Debridement	11000-11044
Paring or Cutting	11055-11057
Biopsy	11100-11101
Removal of Skin Tags	11200-11201
Shaving of Lesions	11300-11313
Excision-Benign Lesions	11400-11471
Excision-Malignant Lesions	11600-11646
Nails	11719-11765
Repair (Closure)	
Repair-Simple	12001-12021
Repair-Intermediate	12031-12057
Repair-Complex	13100-13160
Adjacent Tissue Transfer	14000-14350
Free Skin Grafts	15000-15400
Flaps (Skin and/or Deep Tissues)	15570-15999
Burns	16000-16036
Destruction	
Destruction, Benign or Premalignant Lesions	17000-17250
Destruction, Malignant Lesions	17260-17286
Mohs' Micrographic Surgery	17304-17310
Other Destruction Procedures	17340-17999
Laboratory Services	
Skin Tests, Immunology	86485-86586
Skin Tests, Allergy	95010-95199
Visit and Medicine Services	
E/M Services	99201-99499
Special Dermatological Procedures	96900-96999

Male Figure
(Anterior View)

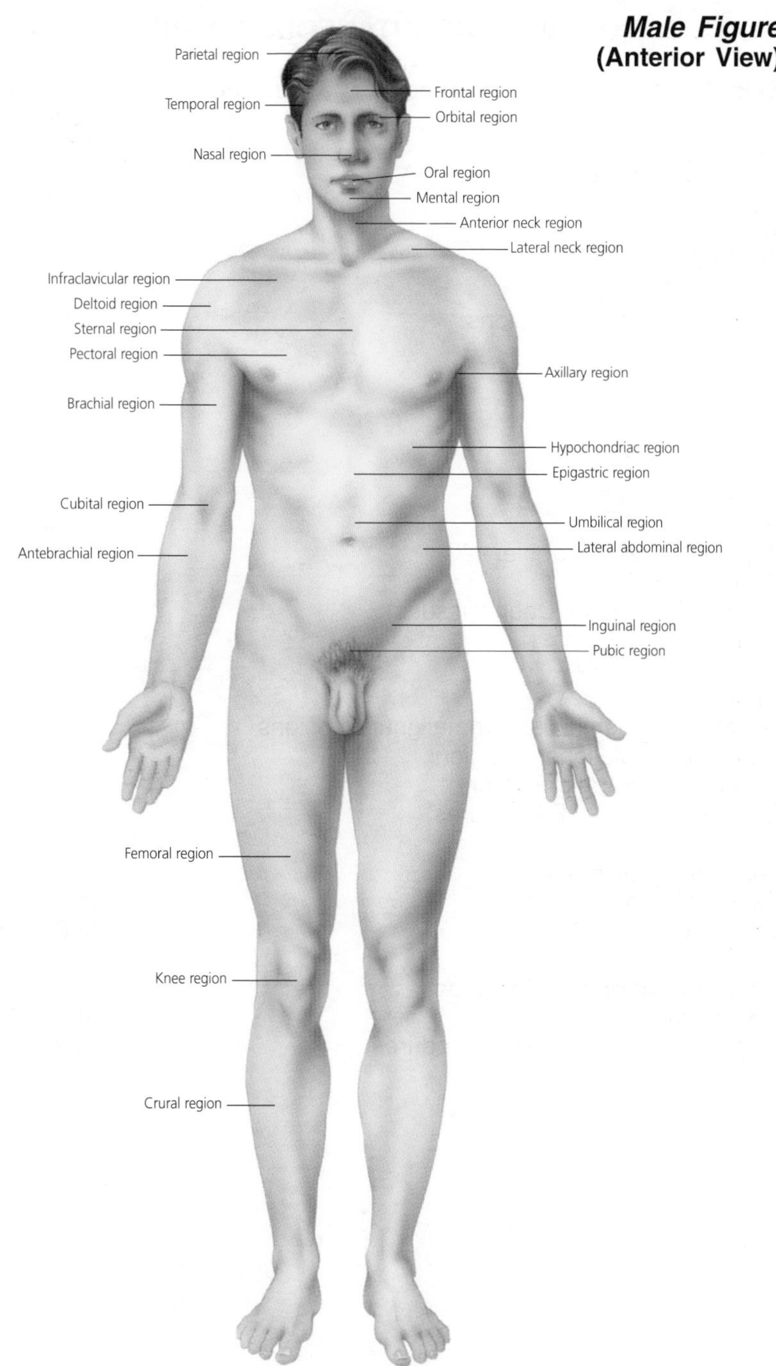

PLATE 2. SKIN AND SUBCUTANEOUS TISSUE - FEMALE

Skin, Subcutaneous and Accessory Structures	
Incision and Drainage	10040-10180
Excision-Debridement	11000-11044
Paring or Cutting	11055-11057
Biopsy	11100-11101
Removal of Skin Tags	11200-11201
Shaving of Lesions	11300-11313
Excision-Benign Lesions	11400-11471
Excision-Malignant Lesions	11600-11646
Nails	11719-11765
Repair (Closure)	
Repair-Simple	12001-12021
Repair-Intermediate	12031-12057
Repair-Complex	13100-13160
Adjacent Tissue Transfer	14000-14350
Free Skin Grafts	15000-15400
Flaps (Skin and/or Deep Tissues)	15570-15999
Burns	16000-16036
Destruction	
Destruction, Benign or Premalignant Lesions	17000-17250
Destruction, Malignant Lesions	17260-17286
Mohs' Micrographic Surgery	17304-17310
Other Destruction Procedures	17340-17999
Laboratory Services	
Skin Tests, Immunology	86485-86586
Skin Tests, Allergy	95010-95199
Visit and Medicine Services	
E/M Services	99201-99499
Special Dermatological Procedures	96900-96999

Female Figure
(Anterior View)

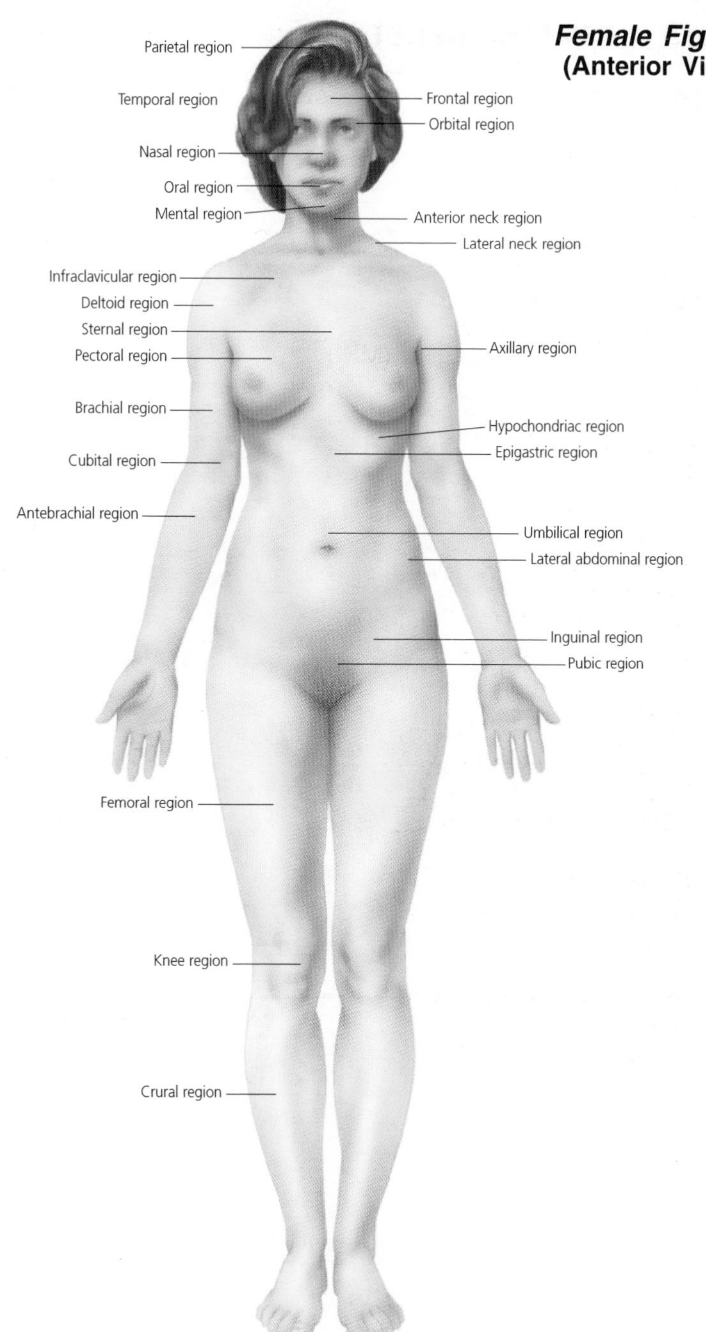

PLATE 3. FEMALE BREAST

Breast	
Incision	19000-19030
Excision	19100-19272
Introduction	19290-19295
Repair and/or Reconstruction	19316-19396
Other Procedures	19499
Radiology Services	
Mammography	76082-76092
Magnetic Resonance Imaging (MRI)	76093-76094
Stereotactic Localization	76095
Ultrasound	76645
E/M Services	99201-99499

Female Breast

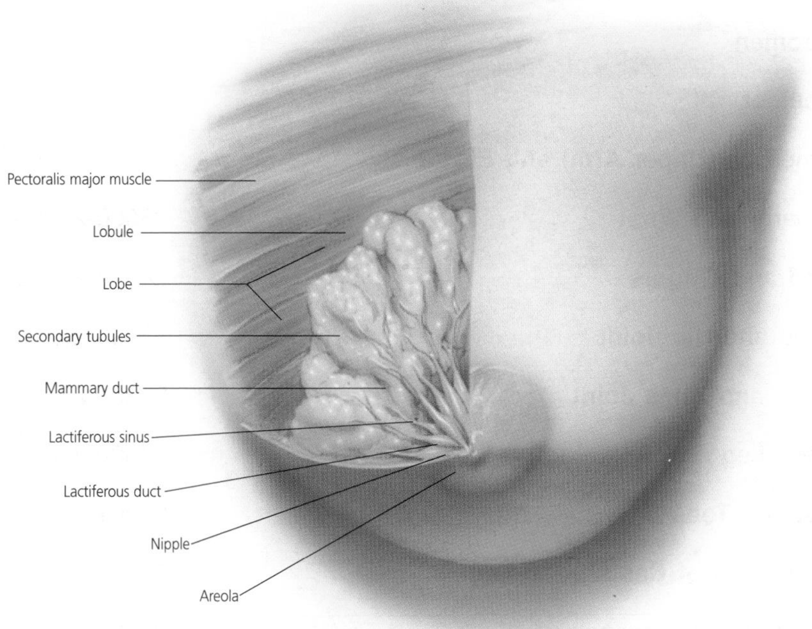

PLATE 4. MUSCULAR SYSTEM AND CONNECTIVE TISSUE - ANTERIOR VIEW

General	20000-20999
Head	21010-21499
Neck (Soft Tissues) and Thorax	21501-21899
Back and Flank	21920-21935
Spine (Vertebral Column)	22100-22899
Abdomen	22900-22999
Shoulder	23000-23929
Humerous (Upper Arm) and Elbow	23930-24999
Forearm and Wrist	25000-25999
Hand and Fingers	26010-26989
Pelvis and Hip Joint	26990-27299
Femur and Knee Joint	27301-27599
Lower Leg and Ankle Joint	27600-27899
Foot and Toes	28001-28899
Application of Casts/Strapping	29000-29799
Endoscopy/Arthroscopy	29800-29999
E/M Services	99201-99499

Muscular System (Anterior View)

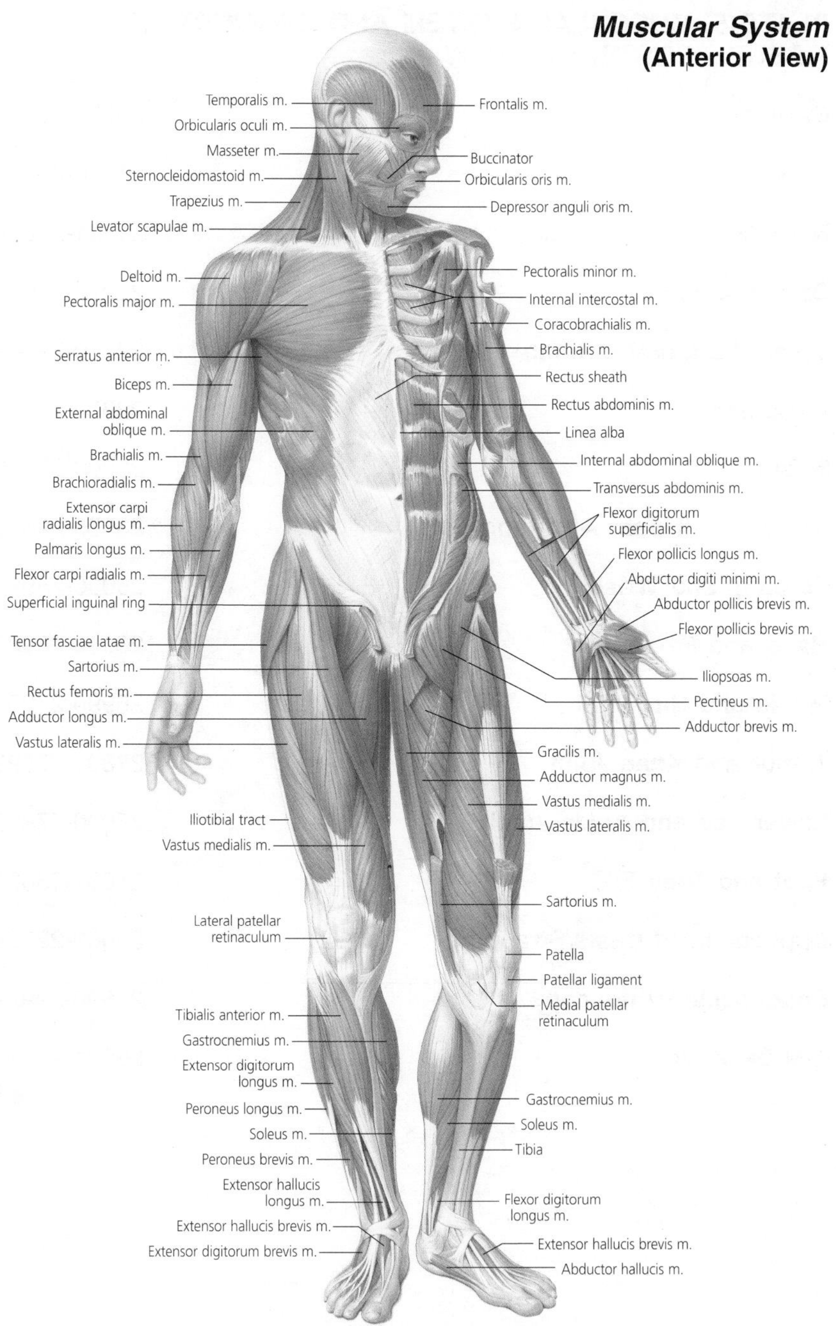

PLATE 5. MUSCULAR SYSTEM AND CONNECTIVE TISSUE - POSTERIOR VIEW

General	20000-20999
Head	21010-21499
Neck (Soft Tissues) and Thorax	21501-21899
Back and Flank	21920-21935
Spine (Vertebral Column)	22100-22899
Abdomen	22900-22999
Shoulder	23000-23929
Humerous (Upper Arm) and Elbow	23930-24999
Forearm and Wrist	25000-25999
Hand and Fingers	26010-26989
Pelvis and Hip Joint	26990-27299
Femur and Knee Joint	27301-27599
Lower Leg and Ankle Joint	27600-27899
Foot and Toes	28001-28899
Application of Casts/Strapping	29000-29799
Endoscopy/Arthroscopy	29800-29999
E/M Services	99201-99499

Muscular System
(Posterior View)

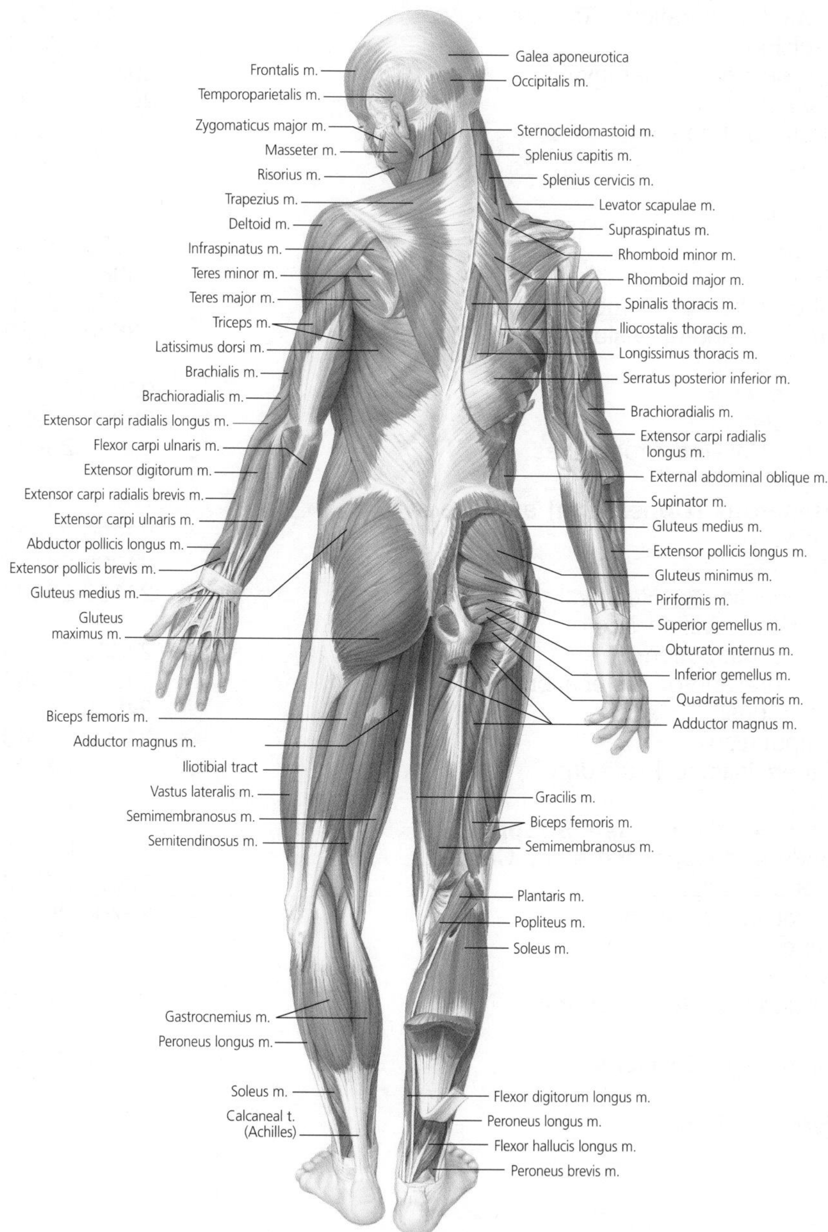

PLATE 6. MUSCULAR SYSTEM - SHOULDER AND ELBOW

General	
Wound exploration - Trauma	20100-20103
Excision	20150-20251
Introduction or Removal	20500-20694
Replantation	20802-20838
Grafts of Implants	20900-20938
Other	20950-20999
Shoulder	
Incision	23000-23044
Excision	23065-23222
Introduction or Removal	23330-23350
Fracture and/or Dislocation	23500-23680
Manipulation	23700
Arthrodesis	23800-23802
Amputation	23900-23921
Other/Unlisted Procedures	23929
Humerous (Upper Arm) and Elbow	
Incision	23930-24006
Excision	24065-24155
Introduction or Removal	24160-24220
Repair, Revision and/or Reconstruction	24300-24498
Fracture and/or Dislocation	24500-24685
Arthrodesis	24800-24802
Amputation	24900-24940
Other/Unlisted Procedure	24999
Application of Casts/Strapping	
Body and Upper Extremity Casts and Strapping	29000-29280
Removal or Repair	29700-29750
Other	29799
Endoscopy/Arthroscopy	29805-29838
Radiology Services	73000-73225
E/M Services	99201-99499

Shoulder and Elbow
(Anterior View)

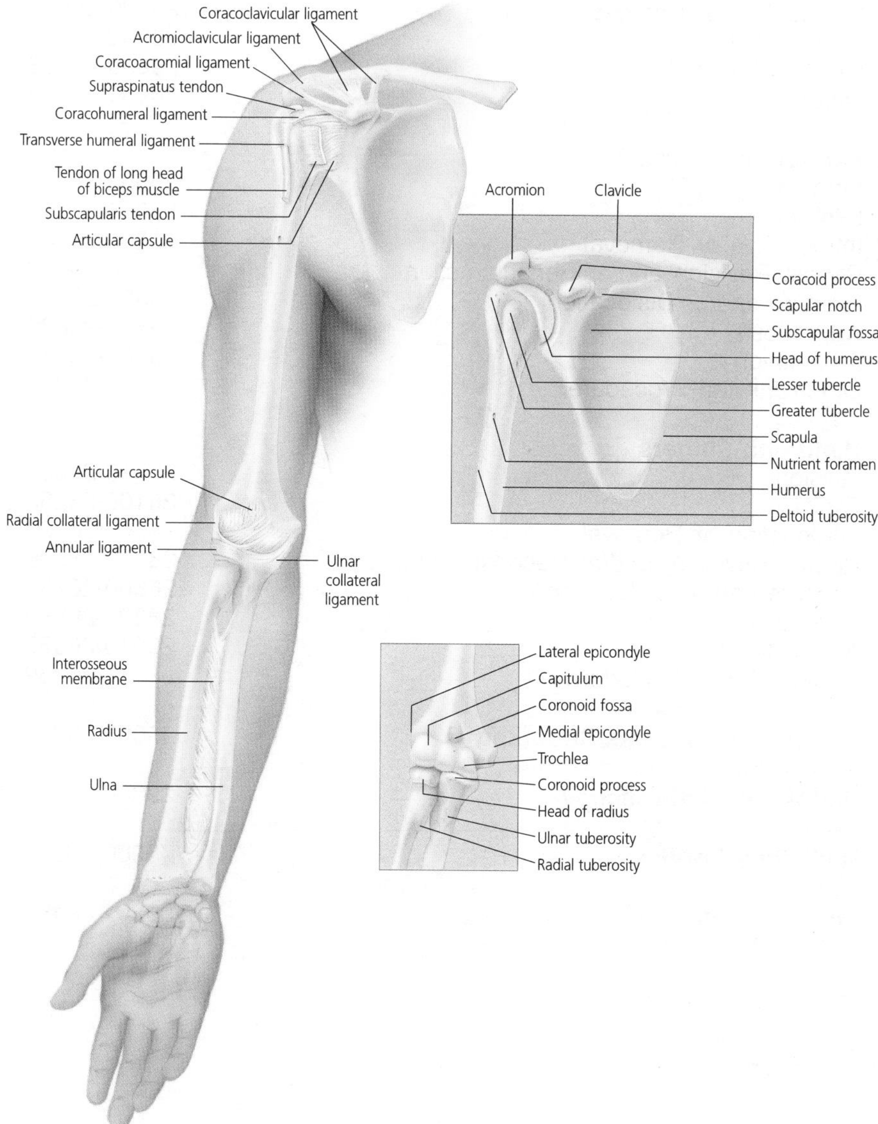

PLATE 7. MUSCULAR SYSTEM - HAND AND WRIST

General	
Wound exploration - Trauma	20100-20103
Excision	20105-20251
Introduction or Removal	20500-20694
Replantation	20802-20838
Grafts of Implants	20900-20938
Other	20950-20999
Forearm and Wrist	
Incision	25000-25040
Excision	25065-25240
Introduction or Removal	25246-25259
Repair, Revision and/or Reconstruction	25260-25492
Fracture and/or Dislocation	25500-25695
Arthrodesis	25800-25830
Amputation	25900-25931
Other/Unlisted Procedure	25999
Hand and Fingers	
Incision	26010-26080
Excision	26100-26262
Introduction or Removal	26320
Repair, Revision, and/or Reconstruction	26340-26596
Fracture and/or Dislocation	26600-26785
Arthrodesis	26820-26863
Amputation	26910-26952
Other/Unlisted Procedure	26989
Application of Casts/Strapping	29000-29280
Endoscopy/Arthroscopy	29840-29848
Radiology Services	73000-73225
E/M Services	99201-99499

Hand and Wrist

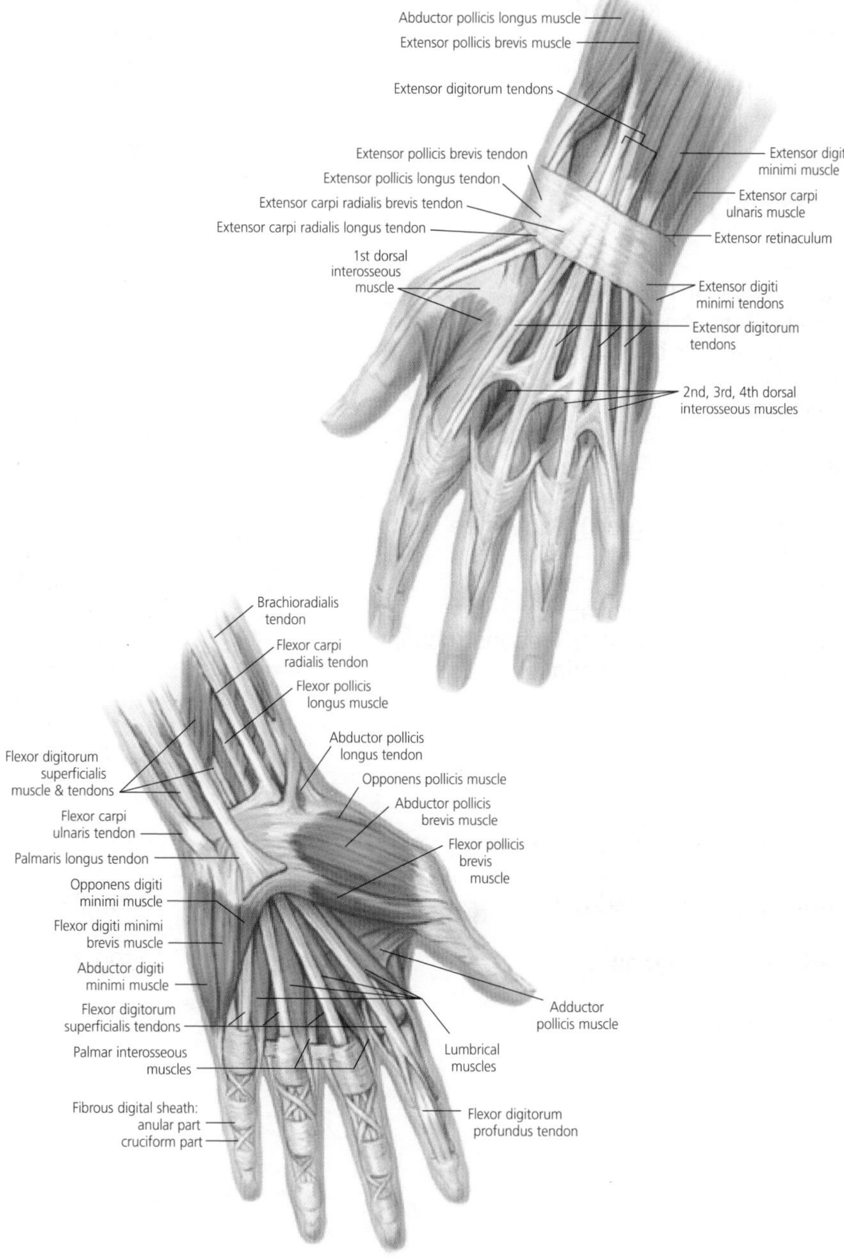

PLATE 8. MUSCULOSKELETAL SYSTEM - HIP AND KNEE

General	
Wound exploration - Trauma	20100-20103
Excision	20150-20251
Introduction or Removal	20500-20694
Replantation	20802-20838
Grafts of Implants	20900-20938
Other	20950-20999
Pelvis and Hip Joint	
Incision	26990-27036
Excision	27040-27080
Introduction or Removal	27086-27096
Repair, Revision, and/or Reconstruction	27097-27187
Fracture and/or dislocation	27193-27266
Manipulation	27275
Arthrodesis	27280-27286
Amputation	27290-27295
Other/Unlisted Procedure	27299
Femur (Thigh Region) and Knee Joint	
Incision	27301-27320
Excision	27323-27365
Introduction or Removal	27370-37372
Repair, Revision, and/or Reconstruction	27380-27499
Fracture and/or Dislocation	27500-27566
Manipulation	27570
Arthrodesis	27580
Amputation	27590-27598
Other/Unlisted Procedure	27599
Application of Casts/Strapping	29305-29590
Endoscopy/Arthroscopy	29850-29889
Radiology Services	73500-73725
E/M Services	99201-99499

Hip and Knee
(Anterior View)

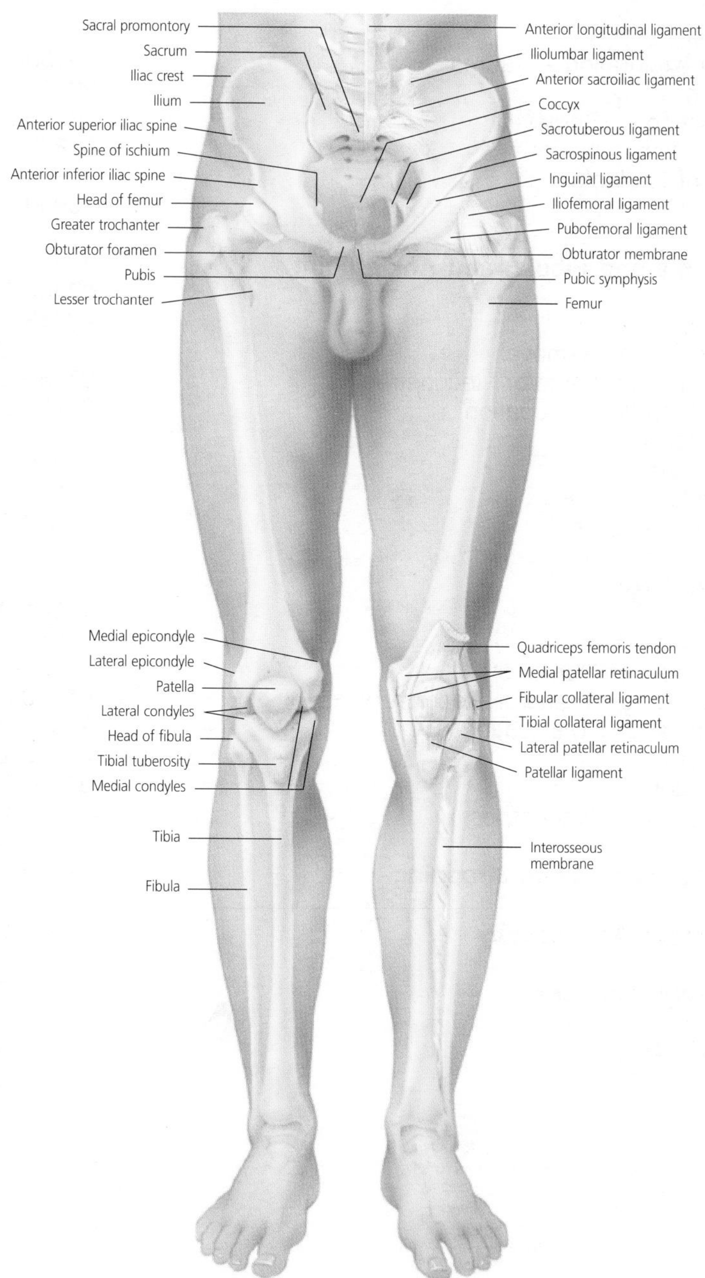

PLATE 9. MUSCULOSKELETAL SYSTEM - FOOT AND ANKLE

General	
Wound exploration - Trauma	20100-20103
Excision	20150-20251
Introduction or Removal	20500-20694
Replantation	20802-20838
Grafts of Implants	20900-20938
Other	20950-20999

Leg (Tibia and Fibula) and Ankle Joint	
Incision	27600-27612
Excision	27613-27647
Introduction or Removal	27648
Repair, Revision and/or Reconstruction	27650-27745
Fracture and/or Dislocation	27750-27848
Manipulation	27860
Arthrodesis	27870-27871
Amputation	27880-27889
Other Procedures	27892-27899

Foot and Toes	
Incision	28001-28035
Excision	28043-28175
Introduction or Removal	28190-28193
Repair, Revision, and/or Reconstruction	28200-28360
Fracture and/or Dislocation	28400-28675
Arthrodesis	28705-28760
Amputation	28800-28825
Other/Unlisted Procedures	28899

Application of Casts/Strapping	29305-29590
Endoscopy/Arthroscopy	29891-29999
Radiology Services	73500-73725
E/M Services	99201-99499

Foot and Ankle

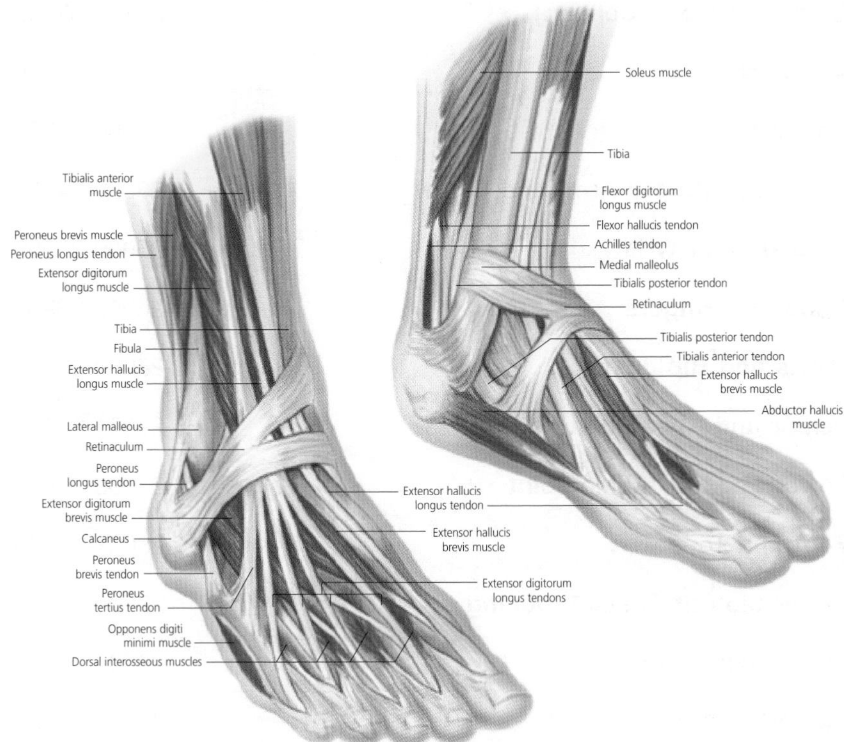

PLATE 10. SKELETAL SYSTEM - ANTERIOR VIEW

General	20100-20999
Head	21010-21499
Neck (Soft Tissues) and Thorax	21501-21899
Back and Flank	21920-21935
Spine (Vertebral Column)	22100-22899
Abdomen	22900-22999
Shoulder	23000-23929
Humerous (Upper Arm) and Elbow	23930-24999
Forearm and Wrist	25000-25999
Hand and Fingers	26010-26989
Pelvis and Hip Joint	26990-27299
Femur and Knee Joint	27301-27599
Lower Leg and Ankle Joint	27600-27899
Foot and Toes	28001-28899
Application of Casts/Strapping	29000-29799
Endoscopy/Arthroscopy	29800-29999
Radiology Services	70010-73725
E/M Services	99201-99499

Skeletal System
(Anterior View)

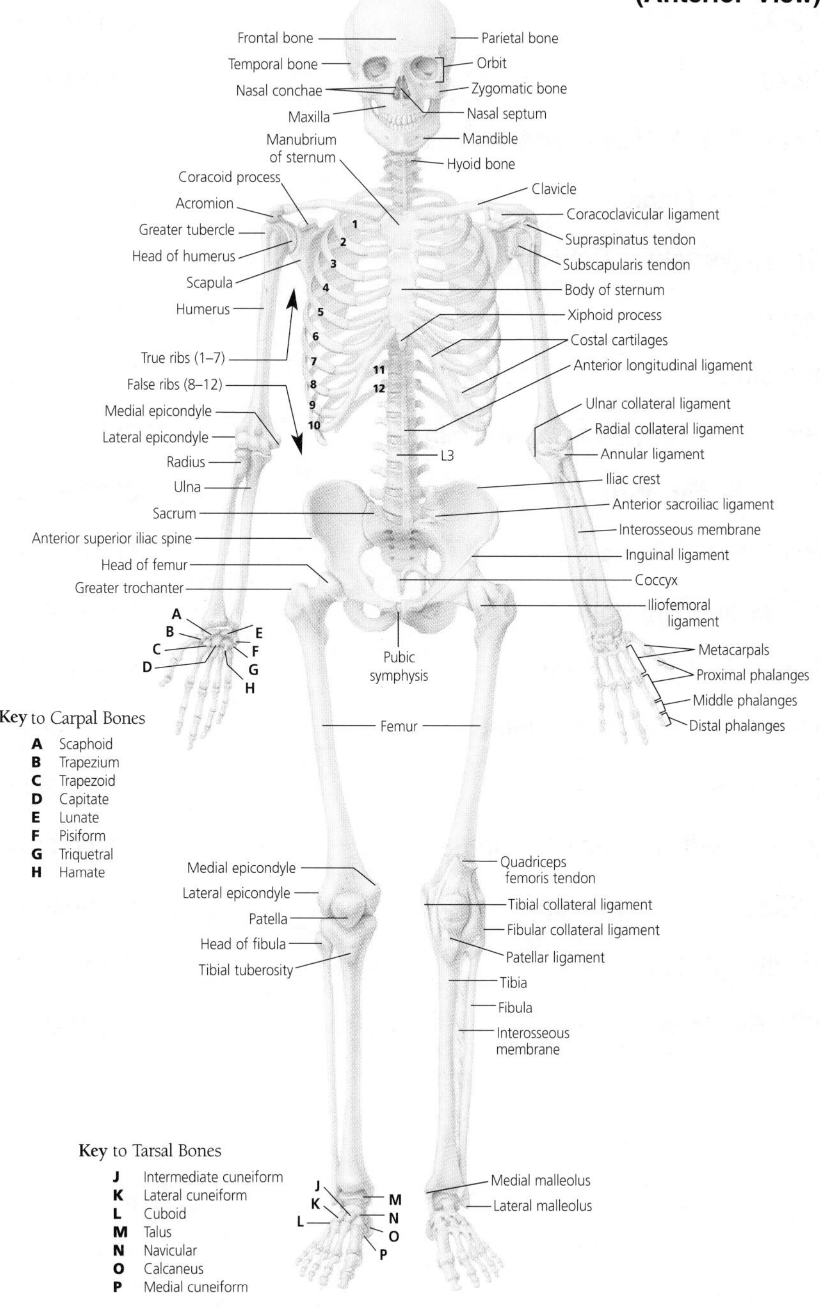

Key to Carpal Bones

- **A** Scaphoid
- **B** Trapezium
- **C** Trapezoid
- **D** Capitate
- **E** Lunate
- **F** Pisiform
- **G** Triquetral
- **H** Hamate

Key to Tarsal Bones

- **J** Intermediate cuneiform
- **K** Lateral cuneiform
- **L** Cuboid
- **M** Talus
- **N** Navicular
- **O** Calcaneus
- **P** Medial cuneiform

PLATE 11. SKELETAL SYSTEM - POSTERIOR VIEW

General	20100-20999
Head	21010-21499
Neck (Soft Tissues) and Thorax	21501-21899
Back and Flank	21920-21935
Spine (Vertebral Column)	22100-22899
Abdomen	22900-22999
Shoulder	23000-23929
Humerous (Upper Arm) and Elbow	23930-24999
Forearm and Wrist	25000-25999
Hand and Fingers	26010-26989
Pelvis and Hip Joint	26990-27299
Femur and Knee Joint	27301-27599
Lower Leg and Ankle Joint	27600-27899
Foot and Toes	28001-28899
Application of Casts/Strapping	29000-29799
Endoscopy/Arthroscopy	29800-29999
Radiology Services	70010-73725
E/M Services	99201-99499

Skeletal System
(Posterior View)

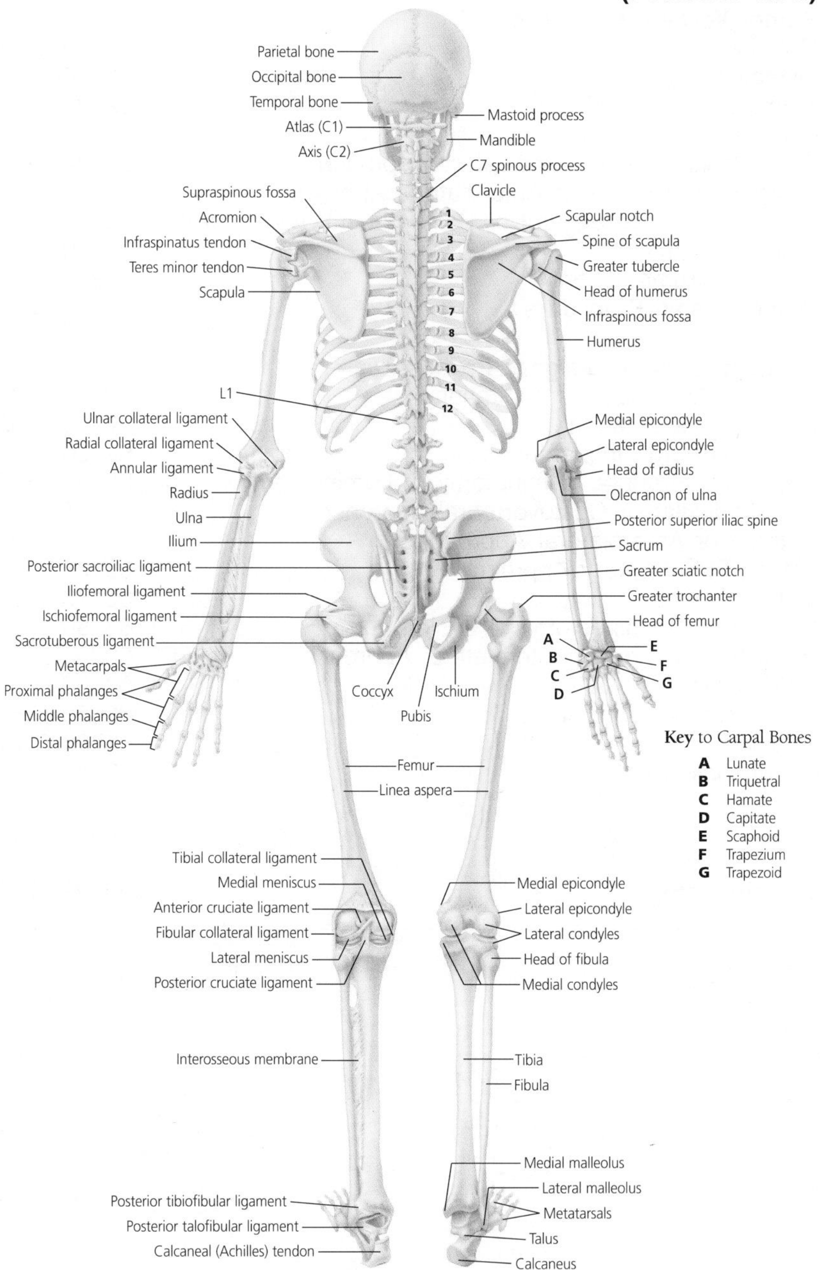

Key to Carpal Bones

A Lunate
B Triquetral
C Hamate
D Capitate
E Scaphoid
F Trapezium
G Trapezoid

PLATE 12. SKELETAL SYSTEM - VERTEBRAL COLUMN

Spine (Vertebral Column)	
Excision	22100-22116
Osteotomy	22210-22226
Fracture and/or Dislocation	22305-22328
Manipulation	22505
Arthrodesis-Lateral Extracavitary Approach	22532-22534
Arthrodesis-Anterior or Anterolateral Approach	22548-22585
Arthrodesis-Posterolateral or Posterolateral Approach	22590-22632
Spine Deformity	22800-22819
Spinal Instrumentation	22840-22855
Other/Unlisted Procedures	22899

Nervous System Surgery Procedures	
Injection, Drainage, or Aspiration	62263-62319
Catheter Implantation	62350-62355
Reservoir/Pump Implantation	62360-62368
Posterior Extradural Laminotomy or Laminectomy	63001-63048
Transpedicular or Costovertebral Approach	63055-63066
Anterior or Anterolateral Approach	63075-63091
Lateral Extracavitary Approach	63101-63103
Incision	63170-63200
Excision by Laminectomy of Lesion	63250-63290
Excision, Anterior or Anterolateral Approach	63300-63308
Stereotaxis	63600-63615
Neurostimulators (Spinal)	63650-63688
Repair	63700-63710
Shunt, Spinal CSF	63740-63746

Radiology Services	72010-72295
E/M Services	99201-99499

Vertebral Column
(Lateral View)

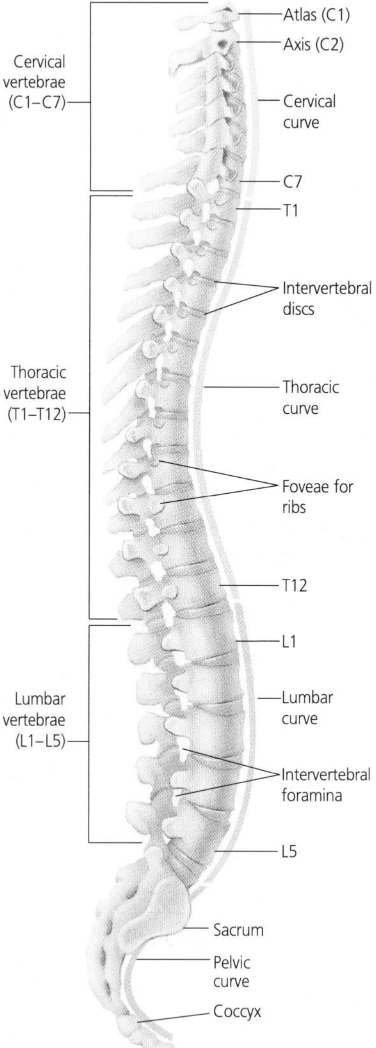

PLATE 13. RESPIRATORY SYSTEM

Nose	
Incision	30000-30020
Excision	30100-30160
Introduction	30200-30220
Removal of Foreign Body	30300-30320
Repair	30400-30630
Destruction	30801-30802
Other	30901-30999
Accessory Sinuses	
Incision	31000-31090
Excision	31200-31230
Endoscopy	31231-31294
Other	31299
Larynx	
Excision	31300-31420
Introduction	31500-31502
Endoscopy	31505-31579
Repair	31580-31590
Destruction	31595
Other	31599
Trachea and Bronchi	
Incision	31600-31614
Endoscopy	31615-31656
Introduction	31700-31730
Repair	31750-31830
Lungs and Pleura	
Incision	32000-32225
Excision	32310-32540
Endoscopy	32601-32665
Repair	32800-32820
Lung Transplantation	32850-32854
Surgical Collapse Therapy; Thoracoplasty	32900-32960
Radiology Services/Chest	71010-71555
E/M Services	99201-99499

Respiratory System

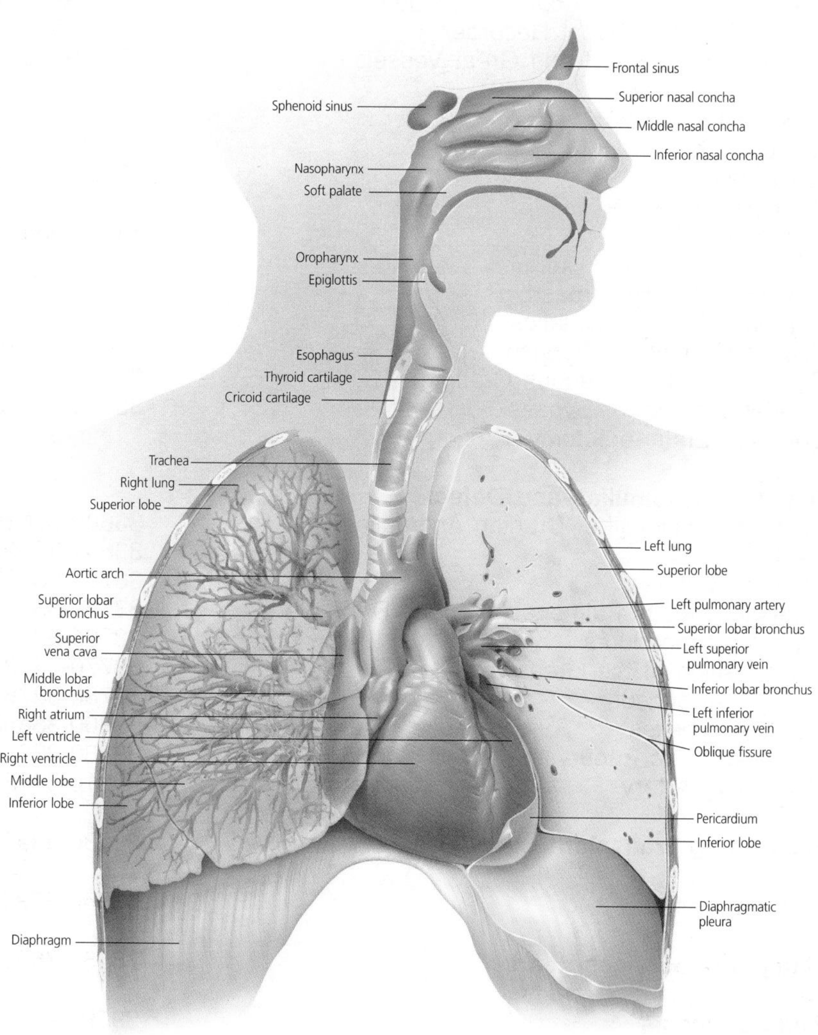

©Scientific Publishing Ltd., Rolling Meadows, IL

PLATE 14. HEART AND PERICARDIUM

General	
Pericardium	33010-33050
Cardiac Tumor	33120-33130
Pacemaker or Defibrillator	33200-33249
Electrophysiologic Operative Procedures	33250-33261
Patient Activated Event Recorder	33282-33284
Wounds of the Heart and Great Vessels	33300-33335
Cardiac Valves	
Aortic Valve	33400-33417
Mitral Valve	33420-33430
Tricuspid Valve	33460-33468
Pulmonary Valve	33470-33478
Coronary Artery Bypass	
Coronary Artery Anomalies	33500-33506
Venous Grafting for Bypass	33510-33516
Combined Arterial-Venous Grafting	33517-33530
Arterial Grafting for Bypass	33533-33545
Coronary Endarterectomy	33572
Repair of Anomalies and Defects	
Single Ventricle/Other Cardiac Anomalies	33600-33619
Septal Defect	33641-33697
Sinus of Valsalva	33702-33722
Total Anomalous Pulmonary Venous Drainage	33730-33732
Shunting Procedures	33735-33767
Transposition of the Great Vessels	33770-33781
Truncus Arteriosus	33786-33788
Aortic Anomalies	33800-33853
Thoracic Aortic Aneurysm	33860-33877
Pulmonary Artery	33910-33924
Heart/Lung Transplant	33930-33945
Cardiac Assist	33960-33980
Radiology Services/Heart	75552-75556
E/M Services	99201-99499

Heart
ernal View)

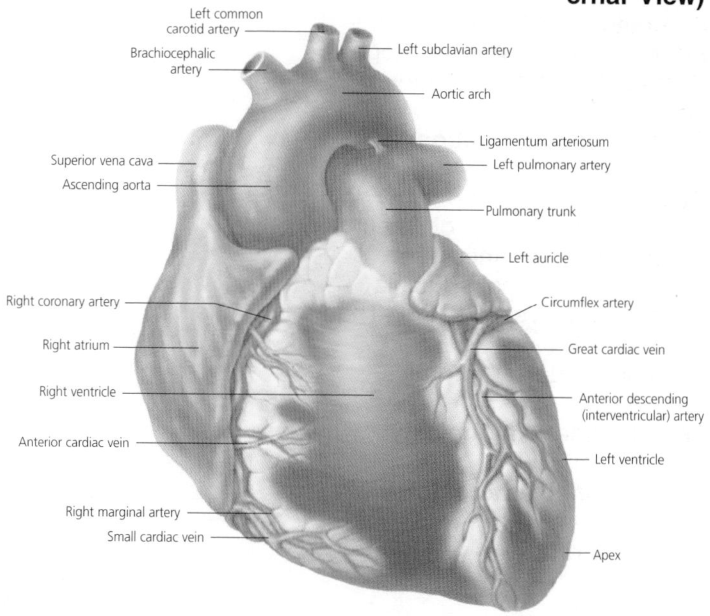

Heart
(Internal View)

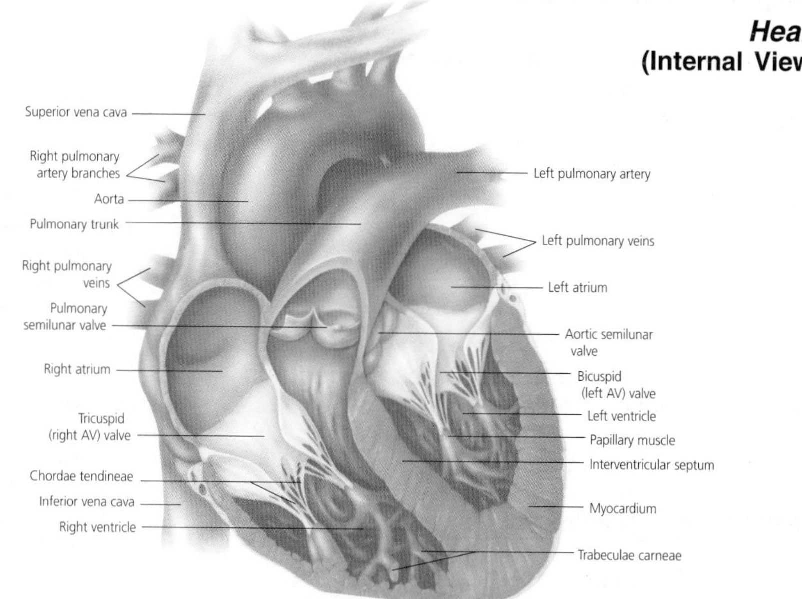

PLATE 15. CIRCULATORY SYSTEM

Embolectomy/Thrombectomy	
Arterial, With or Without Repair	34001-34203
Venous, Direct or w/Catheter	34401-34490
Venous Reconstruction	34501-34530
Repair	
Endovascular Repair of Aneurysm	34800-34900
Direct Repair of Aneurysm	35001-35162
Repair Arteriovenous Fistula	35180-35190
Repair Blood Vessel Other Than for Fistula	35201-35286
Thromboendarterectomy	35301-35390
Transluminal Angioplasty	35450-35476
Transluminal Atherectomy	35480-35495
Bypass Graft	
Vein	35500-35572
In-situ Vein	35582-35587
Composite Grafts	35681-35683
Transposition and Exploration/Revision	
Arterial Transposition	35691-35697
Exploration/Revision	35700-35907
Vascular Injection Procedures	
Intravenous	36000-36015
Intra-Arterial/Intra-Aortic	36100-36299
Venous	36400-36597
Arterial	36600-36660
Intraosseous	36680
Cannulization or Shunt and Other Procedures	
Intervascular Cannulization or Shunt	36800-36870
Portal Decompression Procedures	37140-37183
Transcatheter Procedures	37195-37209
Intravascular Ultrasound Services	37250-37251
Ligation and Other Procedures	37565-37799
Radiology Services	75600-75996
E/M Services	99201-99499

Vascular System

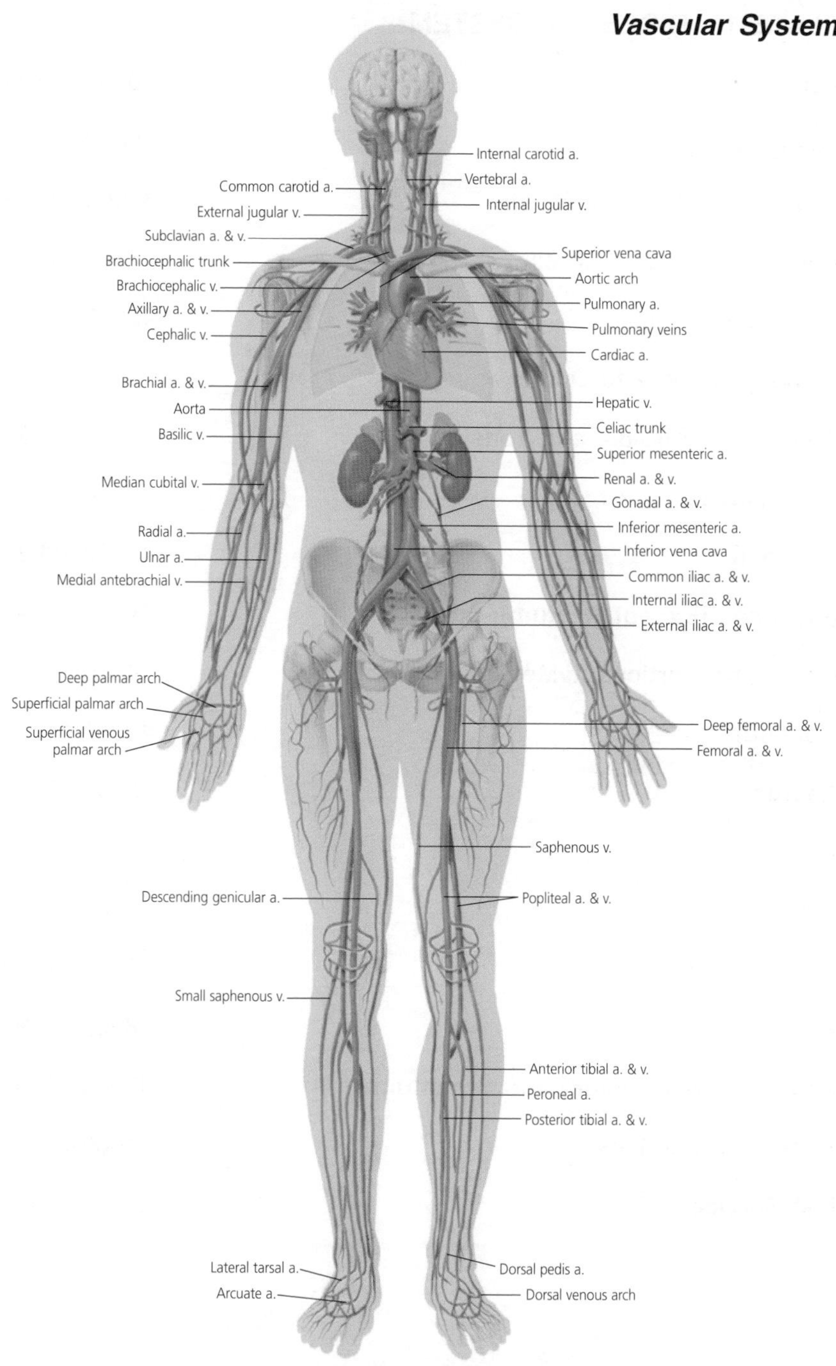

PLATE 16. DIGESTIVE SYSTEM

Lips	40490-40799
Vestibule of Mouth	40800-40899
Tongue and Floor of Mouth	41000-41599
Dentoalveolar Structures	41800-41899
Palate and Uvula	42000-42299
Salivary Gland and Ducts	42300-42699
Pharynx, Adenoids, and Tonsils	42700-42999
Esophagus	43020-43499
Stomach	43500-43999
Intestines (Except Rectum)	44005-44799
Meckel's Diverticulum/Mesentery	44800-44899
Appendix	44900-44979
Rectum	45000-45999
Anus	46020-46999
Liver	47000-47399
Biliary Tract	47400-47999
Pancreas	48000-48999
Abdomen, Peritoneum and Omentum	49000-49999
Radiology Services	74000-74363
E/M Services	99201-99499

Digestive System

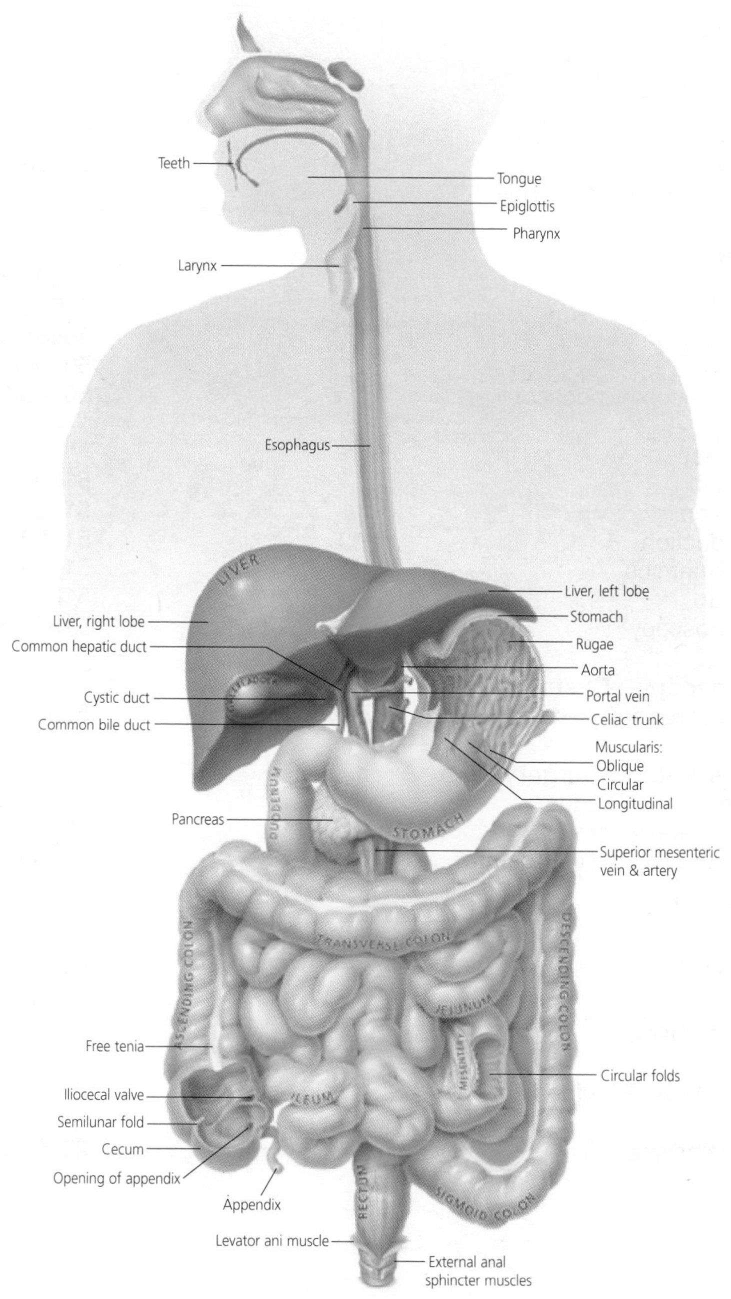

©Practice Management Information Corp., Los Angeles, CA

PLATE 17. GENITOURINARY SYSTEM

Kidney	
Incision	50010-50135
Excision	50200-50290
Renal Transplantation	50300-50380
Introduction	50390-50398
Repair	50400-50540
Laparoscopy/Endoscopy	50541-50580
Ureter	
Incision	50600-50630
Excision	50650-50660
Introduction	50684-50690
Repair	50700-50940
Laparoscopy/Endoscopy	50945-50980
Bladder	
Incision	51000-51080
Excision	51500-51597
Introduction	51600-51720
Urodynamics	51725-51798
Repair	51800-51980
Laparoscopy	51990-51992
Endoscopy—Cystoscopy—Urethroscopy—Cystourethroscopy	52000-52010
Transurethral Surgery	
Urethra and Bladder	52204-52318
Ureter and Pelvis	52320-52355
Vesical Neck and Prostate	52400-52700
Urethra	
Incision	53000-53085
Excision	53200-53275
Repair	53400-53520
Manipulation	53600-53665
Radiology Services	74400-74485
E/M Services	99201-99499

Urinary System

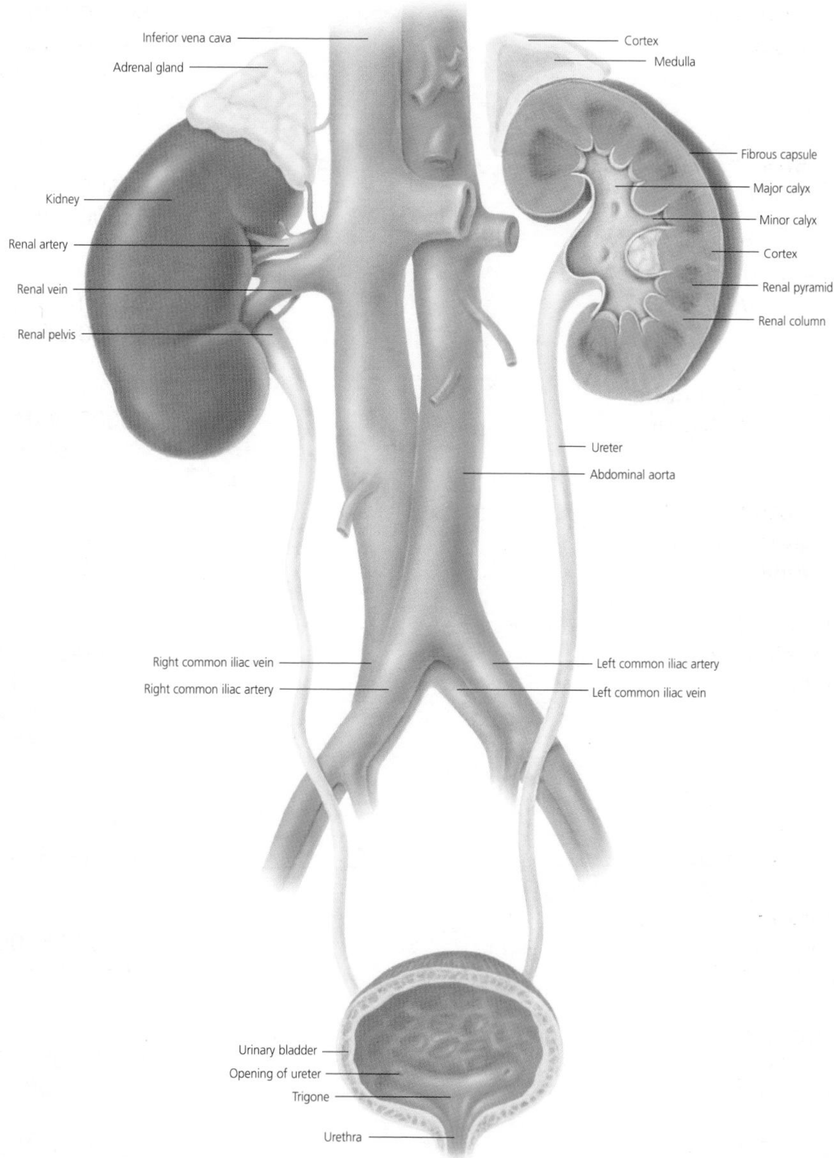

PLATE 18. MALE REPRODUCTIVE SYSTEM

Penis	
Incision	54000-54015
Destruction	54050-54065
Excision	54100-54164
Introduction	54200-54250
Repair	54300-54440
Testis	
Excision	54500-54560
Repair	54600-54680
Epididymis	
Incision/Excision	54700-54861
Repair	54900-54901
Tunica Vaginalis	
Incision/Excision	55000-55041
Repair	55060
Scrotum	
Incision/Excision	55100-55150
Repair	55175-55180
Vas Deferens	
Incision/Excision	55200-55250
Introduction	55300
Repair	55400
Suture	55450
Spermatic Cord	
Excision	55500-55540
Laparoscopy	55550-55559
Seminal Vesicles	
Incision	55600-55605
Excision	55650-55680
Prostate	
Incision	55700-55725
Excision	55801-55865
E/M Services	99201-99499

Male Reproductive System

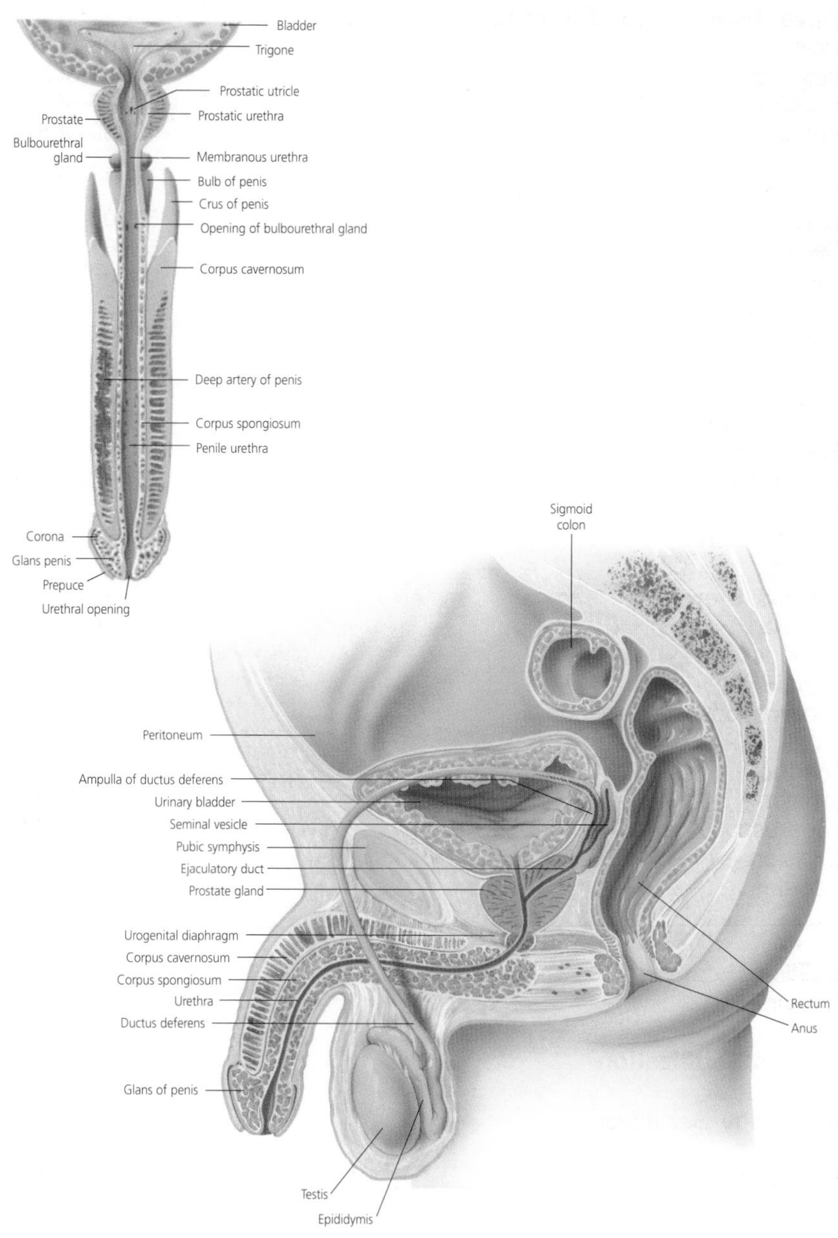

PLATE 19. FEMALE REPRODUCTIVE SYSTEM

Vulva, Perineum and Introitus	
Incision	56405-56441
Destruction	56501-56515
Excision	56605-56740
Repair	56800-56810
Vagina	
Incision	57000-57023
Destruction	57061-57065
Excision	57100-57135
Introduction	57150-57180
Repair	57200-57335
Manipulation	57400-57415
Cervix Uteri	
Endoscopy	57452-57461
Excision	57500-57556
Repair	57700-57720
Manipulation	57800-57820
Corpus Uteri	
Excision	58100-58294
Introduction	58300-58353
Repair	58400-58540
Laparoscopy/Hysteroscopy	58545-58579
Oviduct	
Incision	58600-58615
Laparoscopy	58660-58679
Excision	58700-58720
Repair	58740-58770
Ovary	
Incision	58800-58825
Excision	58900-58960
In Vitro Fertilization	58970-58976
Radiology Services	74710-74775
E/M Services	99201-99499

Female Reproductive System

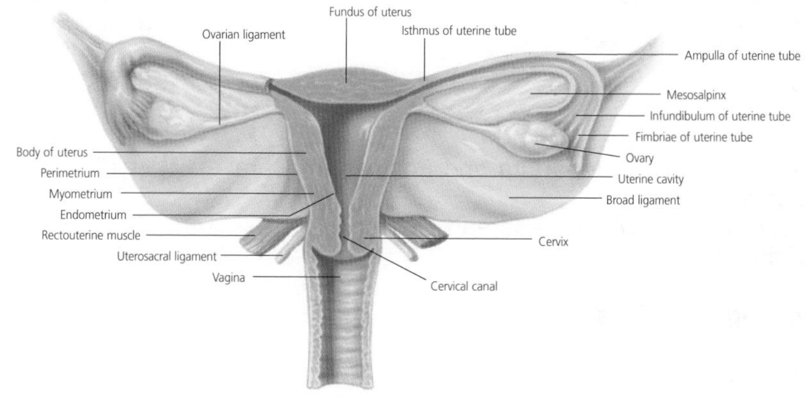

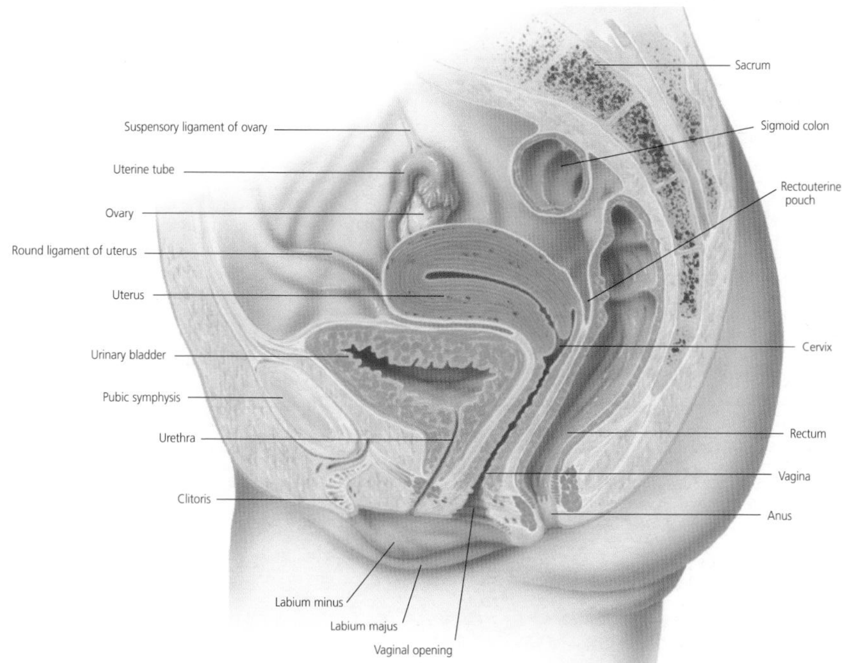

PLATE 20. PREGNANCY, CHILDBIRTH AND THE PUERPERIUM

Antepartum Services	
Antepartum Services	59000-59076
Excision	59100-59160
Introduction	59200
Repair	59300-59350
Delivery	
Vaginal Delivery, Antepartum and Postpartum Care	59400-59430
Cesarean Delivery	59510-59525
Delivery after Previous Cesarean Delivery	59610-59622
Abortion	59812-59857
Radiology Services	74710-74775
E/M Services	
E/M Services	99201-99499
Newborn Care	99431-99440

Female Reproductive System: Pregnancy
(Lateral View)

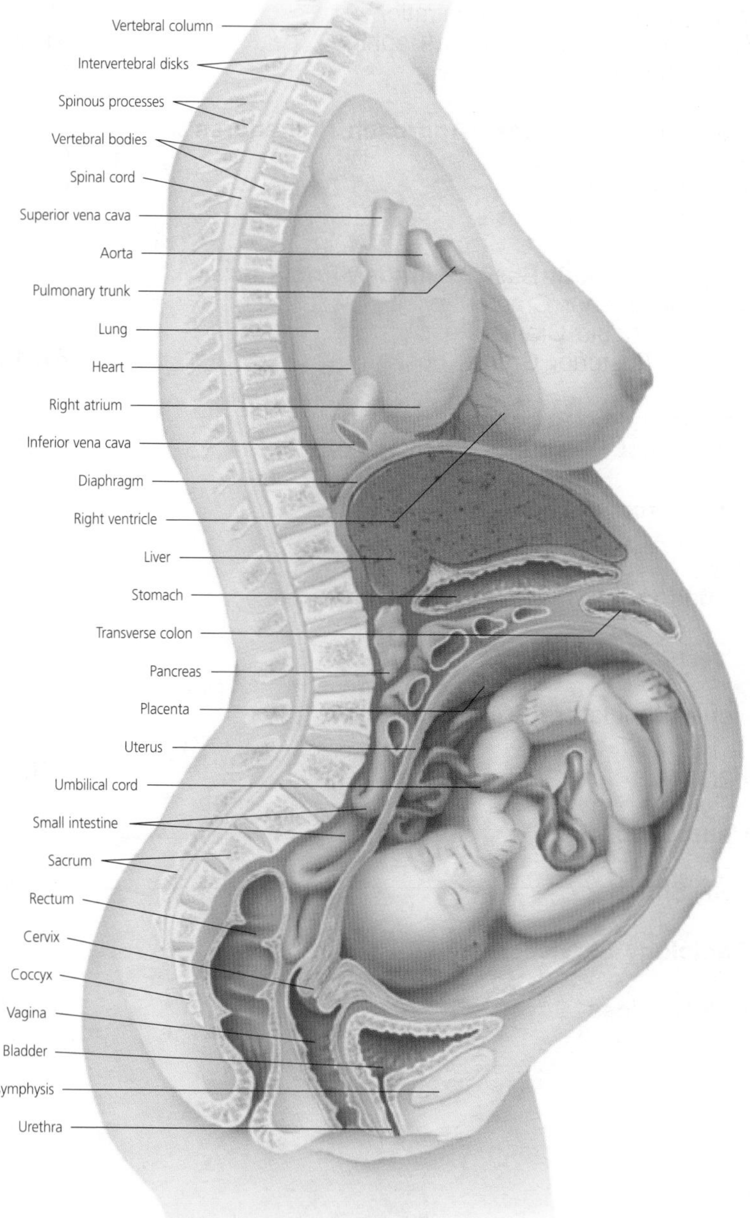

PLATE 21. NERVOUS SYSTEM - BRAIN

Skull, Meninges, and Brain	
Injection, Drainage, or Aspiration	61000-61070
Twist Drill, Burr Hole(s), or Trephine	61105-61253
Craniectomy or Craniotomy	61304-61576
Surgery of Skull Base Approach Procedures	
Anterior Cranial Fossa	61580-61586
Middle Cranial Fossa	61590-61592
Posterior Cranial Fossa	61595-61598
Surgery of Skull Base Definitive Procedures	
Base of Anterior Cranial Fossa	61600-61601
Base of Middle Cranial Fossa	61605-61613
Base of Posterior Cranial Fossa	61615-61616
Repair and/or Reconstruction of Surgical Defects of Skull Base	61618-61619
Endovascular Therapy	61623-61626
Surgery for Aneurysm, Arterio-Venous Malformation or Vascular Disease	61680-61711
Stereotaxis	61720-61795
Neurostimulators (Intra-Cranial)	61850-61888
Repair	62000-62148
Neuroendoscopy	62160-62165
CSF Shunt	62180-62258
Radiology Services	70010-70559
E/M Services	99201-99499

Brain
(Base View)

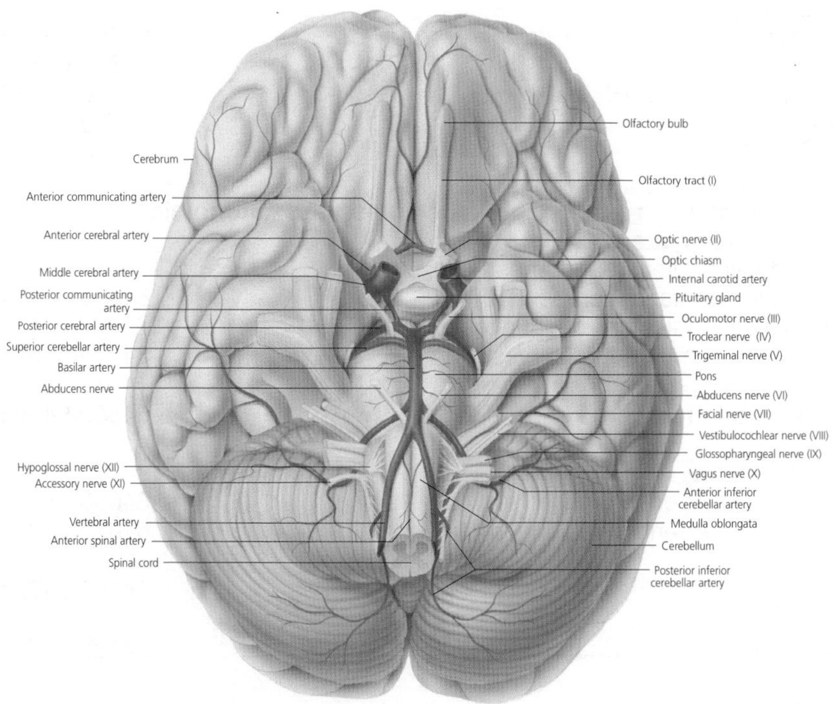

PLATE 22. NERVOUS SYSTEM

Spine and Spinal Cord

Injection, Drainage or Aspiration	62263-62319
Catheter Implantation	62350-62368
Posterior Extradural Laminotomy or Laminectomy	63001-63048
Transpedicular or Costovertebral Approach	63055-63066
Anterior or Anterolateral Approach	63075-63091
Incision	63170-63200
Excision by Laminectomy of Lesion	63250-63290
Excision, Anterior or Anterolateral Approach Intraspinal Lesion	63300-63308
Stereotaxis	63600-63615
Neurostimulators (Spinal)	63650-63688
Repair	63700-63710
Shunt, Spinal CSF	63740-63746

Extracranial Nerves, Peripheral Nerves and Autonomic Nervous System

Introduction/Injection of Anesthetic Agent Somatic Nerves	64400-64484
Introduction/Injection of Anesthetic Agent Sympathetic Nerves	64505-64530

Neurostimulators	64550-64595

Destruction

Neurolytic Agent Somatic Nerves	64600-64640
Neurolytic Agent Sympathetic Nerves	64680-64681

Neuroplasty	64702-64727
Transection or Avulsion	64732-64772

Excision

Somatic Nerves	64774-64795
Sympathetic Nerves	64802-64823

Neurorrhaphy

Without Nerve Graft	64831-64876
With Nerve Graft	64885-64907

E/M Services	99201-99499

Nervous System

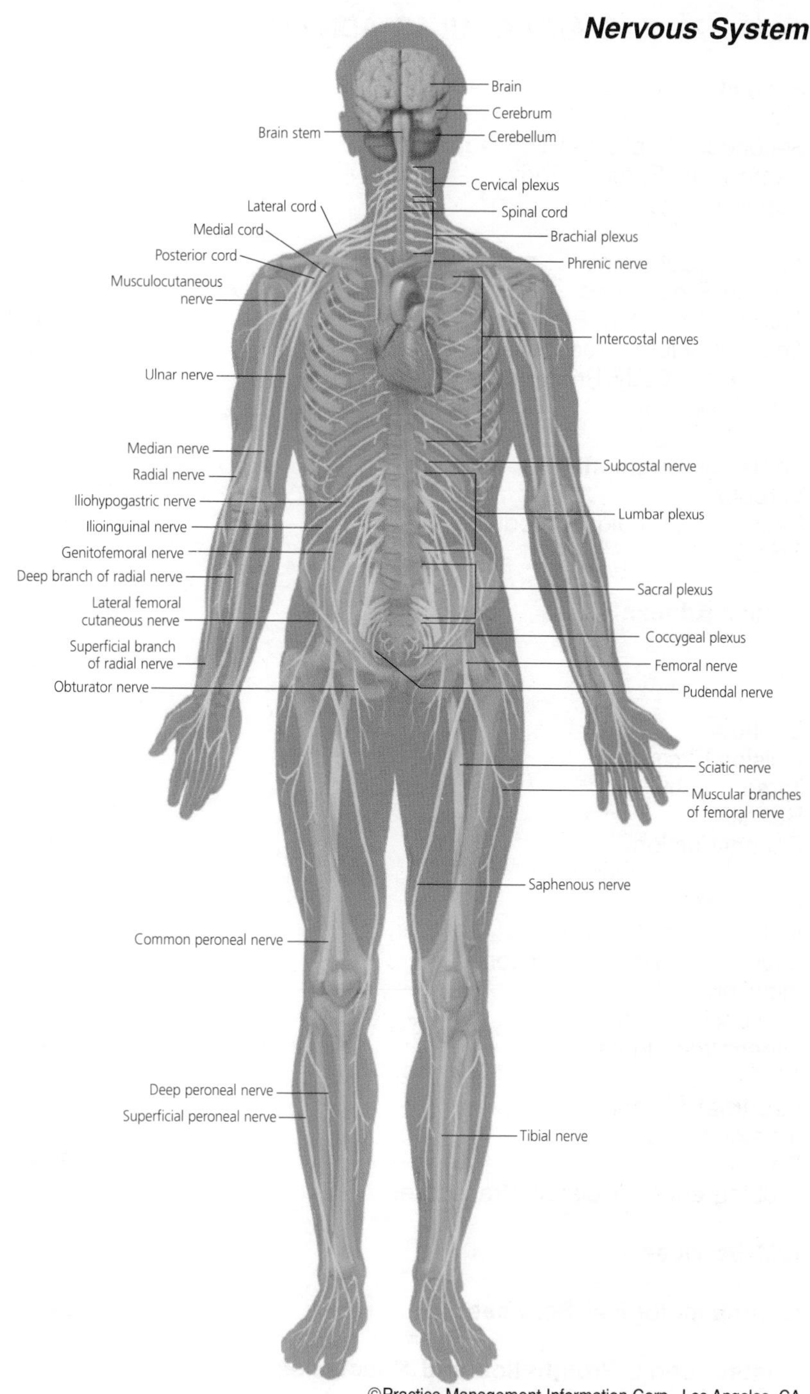

PLATE 23. EYE AND OCULAR ADNEXA

Eyeball	
Removal of Eye	65091-65114
Secondary Implant(s) Procedures	65125-65175
Removal of Foreign Body	65205-65265
Repair of Laceration	65270-65290
Anterior Segment	
Cornea Procedures	65400-65782
Anterior Chamber Procedures	65800-66030
Anterior Sclera Procedures	66130-66250
Iris, Ciliary Body Procedures	66500-66770
Lens Procedures	66820-66990
Posterior Segment	
Vitreous	67005-67040
Retina or Choroid Procedures	67101-67228
Sclera	67250-67255
Ocular Adnexa	67311-67399
Orbit	67400-67599
Eyelids	
Incision/Excision	67700-67850
Tarsorrhaphy	67875-67882
Repair	67900-67924
Reconstruction	67930-67975
Conjunctiva	
Incision and Drainage	68020-68040
Excision and/or Destruction	68100-68135
Injection	68200
Conjunctivoplasty	68320-68340
Other Procedures	68360-68399
Lacrimal System	
Incision/Excision	68400-68550
Repair	68700-68770
Probing and/or Related Procedures	68801-68850
E/M Services	99201-99499
Ophthalmological Services	92002-92287
Contact Lens, Prosthetics and Spectacles	92310-92396

Right Eye
(Horizontal Section)

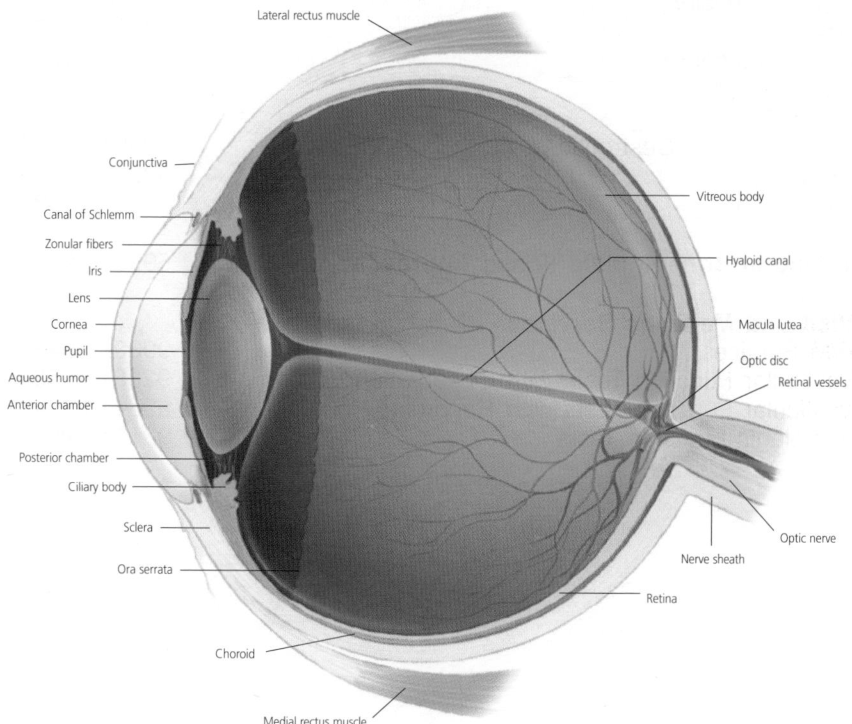

PLATE 24. AUDITORY SYSTEM

External Ear	
Incision	69000-69090
Excision	69100-69155
Removal of Foreign Body	69200-69222
Repair	69300-69320
Middle Ear	
Introduction	69400-69410
Incision/Excision	69420-69554
Repair	69601-69676
Other Procedures	69700-69799
Inner Ear	
Incision and/or Destruction	69801-69840
Excision	69905-69915
Introduction	69930
Temporal Bone, Middle Fossa Approach	69950-69970
Visit and Medicine Services	
E/M Services	99201-99499
Vestibular Function Tests with Observation	92531-92534
Vestibular Function Tests with Recording	92541-92548
Audiologic Function Tests	92551-92597

The Ear

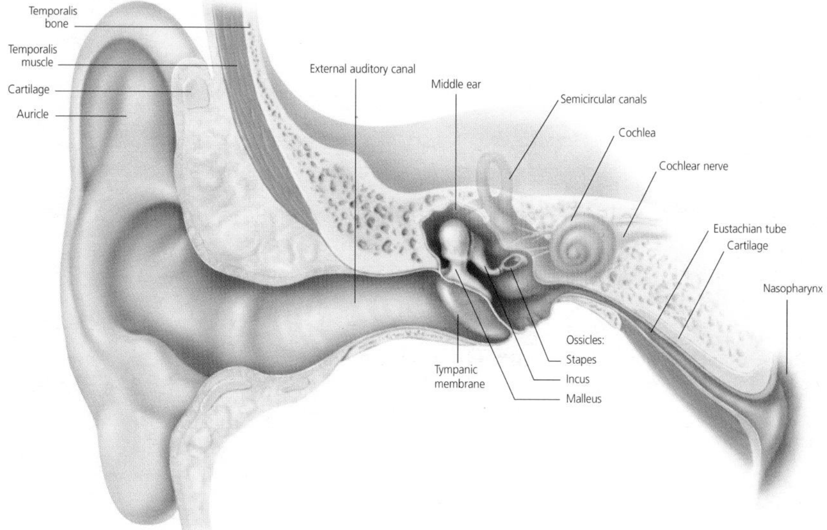

©Scientific Publishing Ltd., Rolling Meadows, IL

This page intentionally left blank.

EVALUATION & MANAGEMENT GUIDELINES

EVALUATION AND MANAGEMENT (E/M) SERVICES OVERVIEW

The first section of the CPT coding system is the evaluation and management (E/M) section, which includes procedure codes for visits and special care services. Within each subsection, the CPT codes are arranged first by patient category, then by the level of service.

The evaluation and management section of the CPT coding system includes codes for reporting visits, consultations, prolonged service, case management services, preventive medicine services, newborn care, and special services. The section is divided into categories such as office visits, hospital visits and consultations. Most of the categories are further divided into two or more subcategories.

The subcategories for evaluation and management services are further classified into levels of service that are identified by specific codes. The level of service classification is important because the physician work required to provide the service varies by the type of service, the place of service, and the patient's clinical status.

The basic format of the evaluation and management service codes and definitions is the same for most categories.

- *A unique five-digit CPT code number is listed*
- *The place and/or type of service is specified, for example "office consultation"*
- *The content of the service is defined, eg. "comprehensive history and comprehensive examination"*
- *The nature of the presenting problem(s) usually associated with a given level is described.*
- *The time typically required to provide the service is specified.*

EVALUATION AND MANAGEMENT SERVICES SUBSECTIONS

The Evaluation and Management section of the CPT book is divided into the following subsections:

Office or Other Outpatient Services	99201-99215
Hospital Observation Services	99217-99220
Hospital Inpatient Services	99221-99239
Consultations	99241-99255
Emergency Department Services	99281-99288
Pediatric Critical Care Patient Transport	99289-99290
Critical Care Services	99291-99292
Inpatient and Pediatric Critical Care Services	99293-99294
Inpatient Neonatal Critical Care	99295-99296
Continuing Intensive Care Services	99298-99300
Nursing Facility Services	99304-99318
Domiciliary, Rest Home, or Custodial Care Services	99324-99328
Domiciliary, Rest Home, or Home Care Plan Oversight	99339-99340
Home Services	99341-99350
Prolonged Services	99354-99360
Case Management Services	99361-99373
Care Plan Oversight Services	99374-99380
Preventive Medicine Services	99381-99429
Newborn Care Services	99431-99440
Special Evaluation and Management Services	99450-99456
Other Evaluation and Management Services	99499

All of these subsections have extensive notes that should be reviewed carefully prior to selecting codes for services located within the section.

EVALUATION AND MANAGEMENT SERVICES GUIDELINES

In addition to the information presented in the introduction, several other items unique to the Evaluation and Management codes are defined or identified in the guidelines.

CLASSIFICATION OF EVALUATION AND MANAGEMENT SERVICES

The Evaluation and Management section is divided into broad categories such as office visits, hospital visits, and consultations. Most of the categories are further divided into two or more subcategories (subsections) of evaluation and management services. For example, there are two subcategories of office visits (new patient and established patient) and there are two subcategories of hospital visits (initial and subsequent).

The subcategories of evaluation and management services are further classified into levels of evaluation and management services that are identified by specific codes. This classification is important because the nature of physician work varies by type of service, place of service, and the patient's status.

The basic format of the levels of evaluation and management services is the same for most categories. First, a unique code number is listed. Second, the place and/or type of service is specified, eg, office consultation. Third, the content of the service is defined, eg, comprehensive history and comprehensive examination. Fourth, the nature of the presenting problem(s) usually associated with a given level is described. Fifth, the time typically required to provide the service is specified.

DEFINITIONS OF COMMONLY USED TERMS

Certain key words and phrases are used throughout the Evaluation and Management section. The following definitions are intended to reduce the potential for differing interpretations and to increase the consistency of reporting by physicians in differing specialties.

NEW AND ESTABLISHED PATIENTS

Solely for the purposes of distinguishing between new and established patients, professional services are those face-to-face services rendered by a physician and coded by a specific CPT code(s). A new patient is one who has not received any professional services from the physician or another physician of the same specialty who belongs to the same group practice, within the past three years.

An established patient is one who has received professional services from the physician or another physician of the same specialty who belongs to the same group practice, within the past three years.

In the instance where a physician is on call for or covering for another physician, the patient's encounter will be classified as it would have been by the physician who is not available.

No distinction is made between new and established patients in the emergency department. Evaluation and Management services in the emergency department category may be coded for any new or established patient who presents for treatment in the emergency department.

CHIEF COMPLAINT

A concise statement describing the symptom, problem, condition, diagnosis or other factor that is the reason for the encounter, usually stated in the patient's words.

CONCURRENT CARE

Concurrent care is the provision of similar services, eg, hospital visits, to the same patient by more than one physician on the same day. When concurrent care is provided, no special reporting is required. Modifier '-75' has been deleted.

COUNSELING

Counseling is a discussion with a patient and/or family concerning one or more of the following areas:

- diagnostic results, impressions, and/or recommended diagnostic studies;
- prognosis;
- risks and benefits of management (treatment) options;
- instructions for management (treatment) and/or follow-up;
- importance of compliance with chosen management (treatment) options;
- risk factor reduction; and
- patient and family education. (For psychotherapy, see 90804-90857)

FAMILY HISTORY

A review of medical events in the patient's family that includes significant information about:

- the health status or cause of death of parents, siblings, and children;
- specific diseases related to problems identified in the chief complaint or history of the present illness, and/or system review;
- diseases of family members which may be hereditary or place the patient at risk.

HISTORY OF PRESENT ILLNESS

A chronological description of the development of the patient's present illness from the first sign and/or symptom to the present. This includes a description of location, quality, severity, timing, context, modifying factors and associated signs and symptoms significantly related to the presenting problem(s).

LEVELS OF EVALUATION AND MANAGEMENT SERVICES

Within each category or subcategory of evaluation and management service, there are three to five levels of evaluation and management services available for reporting purposes. Levels of evaluation and management services are not interchangeable among the different categories or subcategories of service. For example, the first level of evaluation and management services in the subcategory of office visit, new patient, does not have the same definition as the first level of evaluation and management services in the subcategory of office visit, established patient.

The levels of evaluation and management services include examinations, evaluations, treatments, conferences with or concerning patients, preventive pediatric and adult health supervision, and similar medical services, such as the determination of the need and/or location for appropriate care. Medical screening includes the history, examination, and medical decision making required to determine the need and/or location for appropriate care and treatment of the patient (eg, office and other outpatient setting, emergency department, nursing facility, etc.). The levels of evaluation and management services encompass the wide variations in skill, effort, time, responsibility and medical knowledge required for the prevention or diagnosis and treatment of illness or injury and the promotion of optimal health. Each level of evaluation and management services may be used by all physicians.

The descriptors for the levels of evaluation and management services recognize seven components, six of which are used in defining the levels of evaluation and management services. These components are:

- history;
- examination;
- medical decision making;
- counseling;
- coordination of care;
- nature of presenting problem; and
- time.

The first three of these components (history, examination, and medical decision making) are considered the key components in selecting a level of evaluation and management services. (See "determine the extent of history obtained")

The next three components (counseling, coordination of care, and the nature of the presenting problem) are considered contributory factors in the majority of encounters. Although the first two of these contributory factors are important evaluation and management services, it is not required that these services be provided at every patient encounter.

Coordination of care with other providers or agencies without a patient encounter on that day is coded using the case management codes.

The final component, time, is discussed in detail.

Any specifically identifiable procedure (ie, identified with a specific cpt code) performed on or subsequent to the date of initial or subsequent "Evaluation and management services" should be coded separately. The actual performance and/or interpretation of diagnostic tests/studies ordered during a patient encounter are not included in the levels of evaluation and management services. Physician performance of diagnostic tests/studies for which specific CPT codes are available may be coded separately, in addition to the appropriate evaluation and management code. The physician's interpretation of the results of diagnostic tests/studies (ie, professional component) with preparation of a separate distinctly identifiable signed written report may also be coded separately, using the appropriate CPT code with the modifier '-26' appended.

The physician may need to indicate that on the day a procedure or service identified by a CPT code was performed, the patient's condition required a significant separately identifiable evaluation and management service above and beyond other services provided or beyond the usual preservice and postservice care associated with the procedure that was performed. The evaluation and management service may be caused or prompted by the symptoms or condition for which the procedure and/or service was provided. This circumstance may be coded by adding the modifier '-25' to the appropriate level of evaluation and management service. As such, different diagnoses are not required for reporting of the procedure and the evaluation and management services on the same date.

NATURE OF PRESENTING PROBLEM

A presenting problem is a disease, condition, illness, injury, symptom, sign, finding, complaint, or other reason for encounter, with or without a diagnosis being established at the time of the encounter. The evaluation and management codes recognize five types of presenting problems that are defined as follows:

Minimal: a problem that may not require the presence of the physician, but service is provided under the physician's supervision.

Self-limited or minor: a problem that runs a definite and prescribed course, is transient in nature, and is not likely to permanently alter health status or has a good prognosis with management/compliance.

Low severity: a problem where the risk of morbidity without treatment is low; there is little to no risk of mortality without treatment; full recovery without functional impairment is expected.

Moderate severity: a problem where the risk of morbidity without treatment is moderate; there is moderate risk of mortality without treatment; uncertain prognosis or increased probability of prolonged functional impairment.

High severity: a problem where the risk of morbidity without treatment is high to extreme; there is a moderate to high risk of mortality without treatment or high probability of severe, prolonged functional impairment.

PAST HISTORY

A review of the patient's past experiences with illnesses, injuries, and treatments that includes significant information about:

- prior major illnesses and injuries;
- prior operations;
- prior hospitalizations;
- current medications;
- allergies (eg, drug, food);
- age appropriate immunization status;
- age appropriate feeding/dietary status.

SOCIAL HISTORY

An age appropriate review of past and current activities that includes significant information about:

- marital status and/or living arrangements;
- current employment;
- occupational history;
- use of drugs, alcohol, and tobacco;
- level of education;
- sexual history;
- other relevant social factors

SYSTEM REVIEW (REVIEW OF SYSTEMS)

An inventory of body systems obtained through a series of questions seeking to identify signs and/or symptoms which the patient may be experiencing or has experienced. For the purposes of CPT the following elements of a system review have been identified:

- Constitutional symptoms (fever, weight loss, etc.)
- Eyes
- Ears, nose, mouth, throat
- Cardiovascular
- Respiratory
- Gastrointestinal

- Genitourinary
- Musculoskeletal
- Integumentary (skin and/or breast)
- Neurological
- Psychiatric
- Endocrine
- Hematologic/lymphatic
- Allergic/immunologic

The review of systems helps define the problem, clarify the differential diagnosis, identify needed testing, or serves as baseline data on other systems that might be affected by any possible management options.

TIME

The inclusion of time in the definitions of levels of evaluation and management services has been implicit in prior editions of CPT. The inclusion of time as an explicit factor beginning in CPT 1992 is done to assist physicians in selecting the most appropriate level of evaluation and management services. It should be recognized that the specific times expressed in the visit code descriptors are averages, and therefore represent a range of times which may be higher or lower depending on actual clinical circumstances.

Time is not a descriptive component for the emergency department levels of evaluation and management services because emergency department services are typically provided on a variable intensity basis, often involving multiple encounters with several patients over an extended period of time. Therefore, it is often difficult for physicians to provide accurate estimates of the time spent face-to-face with the patient.

Studies to establish levels of evaluation and management services employed surveys of practicing physicians to obtain data on the amount of time and work associated with typical evaluation and management services. Since "work" is not easily quantifiable, the codes must rely on other objective, verifiable measures that correlate with physicians' estimates of their "work". It has been demonstrated that physicians' estimations of intraservice time (as explained on the next page), both within and across specialties, is a variable that is predictive of the "work" of evaluation and management services. This same research has shown there is a strong relationship between intra-service time and total time for evaluation and management services. Intra-service time, rather than total time, was chosen for inclusion with the codes because of its relative ease of measurement and because of its direct correlation with measurements of the total amount of time and work associated with typical evaluation and management services.

Intra-service times are defined as face-to-face time for office and other outpatient visits and as unit/floor time for hospital and other inpatient visits. This distinction is necessary because most of the work of typical office visits takes place during the face-to-face time with the patient, while most of the work of typical hospital visits takes place during the time spent on the patient's floor or unit.

Face-to-face time (office and other outpatient visits and office consultations): for coding purposes, face-to-face time for these services is defined as only that time that the physician spends face-to-face with the patient and/or family. This includes the time in which the physician performs such tasks as obtaining a history, performing an examination, and counseling the patient.

Physicians also spend time doing work before or after the face-to-face time with the patient, performing such tasks as reviewing records and tests, arranging for further services, and communicating further with other professionals and the patient through written reports and telephone contact.

This non-face-to-face time for office services—also called pre- and post-encounter time—is not included in the time component described in the evaluation and management codes. However, the pre- and post-face-to-face work associated with an encounter was included in calculating the total work of typical services in physician surveys.

Thus, the face-to-face time associated with the services described by any evaluation and management code is a valid proxy for the total work done before, during, and after the visit.

Unit/floor time (hospital observation services, inpatient hospital care, initial and follow-up hospital consultations, nursing facility): for reporting purposes, intra-service time for these services is defined as unit/floor time, which includes the time that the physician is present on the patient's hospital unit and at the bedside rendering services for that patient. This includes the time in which the physician establishes and/or reviews the patient's chart, examines the patient, writes notes and communicates with other professionals and the patient's family.

In the hospital, pre- and post-time includes time spent off the patient's floor performing such tasks as reviewing pathology and radiology findings in another part of the hospital. This pre- and post-visit time is not included in the time component described in these codes. However, the pre- and post-work performed during the time spent off the floor or unit was included in calculating the total work of typical services in physician surveys. Thus, the unit/floor time associated with the services described by any code is a valid proxy for the total work done before, during, and after the visit.

UNLISTED SERVICE

An evaluation and management service may be provided that is not listed in this section of CPT. When reporting such a service, the appropriate "Unlisted" code may be used to indicate the service, identifying it by "Special Report", as discussed in the following paragraph. The "Unlisted Services" and accompanying codes for the evaluation and management section are as follows:

99429 Unlisted preventive medicine service
99499 Unlisted evaluation and management service

RESULTS/TESTING/REPORTS

Results are the technical component of a service. Testing leads to results; results lead to interpretation. Reports are the work product of the interpretation of numerous test results.

SPECIAL REPORT

An unlisted service or one that is unusual, variable, or new may require a special report demonstrating the medical appropriateness of the service. Pertinent information should include an adequate definition or description of the nature, extent, and need for the procedure; and the time, effort, and equipment necessary to provide the service. Additional items which may be included are complexity of symptoms, final diagnosis, pertinent physical findings, diagnostic and therapeutic procedures, concurrent problems, and follow-up care.

CLINICAL EXAMPLES

Clinical examples of the codes for evaluation and management services are included in the CPT code book to assist physicians in understanding the meaning of the descriptors and selecting the correct code. The clinical examples are listed in Appendix C of the CPT code book. Each example was developed by physicians in the specialties shown.

The same problem, when seen by physicians in different specialties, may involve different amounts of work. Therefore, the appropriate level of encounter should be coded using the descriptors rather than the examples.

INSTRUCTIONS FOR SELECTING A LEVEL OF EVALUATION AND MANAGEMENT SERVICE

IDENTIFY THE CATEGORY AND SUBCATEGORY OF SERVICE

The categories and subcategories of codes available for reporting evaluation and management services are shown in Table 1 on the following page.

Table 1: Categories and subcategories of service

Category/subcategory	Code Numbers
Office or other outpatient services	
New patient	99201-99205
Established patient	99211-99215
Hospital observation discharge services	99217
Hospital observation services	99218-99220
Hospital observation or inpatient care services (including admission and discharge services)	99234-99236
Hospital inpatient services	
Initial hospital care	99221-99223
Subsequent hospital care	99231-99233
Hospital discharge services	99238-99239
Consultations	
Office consultations	99241-99245
Initial inpatient consultations	99251-99255
Emergency department services	99281-99288
Pediatric patient transport	99289-99290
Critical care services	
Adult (over 24 months of age)	99291-99292
Pediatric	99293-99294
Neonatal	99295-99296
Continuing Intensive Care Services	99298-99300
Nursing facility services	
Initial nursing facility care	99304-99306
Subsequent nursing facility care	99307-99310
Nursing facility discharge services	99315-99316
Other nursing facility services	99318
Domiciliary, rest home or custodial care services	
New patient	99324-99328
Established patient	99334-99337
Domiciliary, rest home or home care plan oversight services	99339-99340
Home services	
New patient	99341-99345
Established patient	99347-99350
Prolonged services	
With direct patient contact	99354-99357
Without direct patient contact	99358-99359
Standby services	99360
Case management services	
Team conferences	99361-99362
Telephone calls	99371-99373
Care plan oversight services	99374-99380
Preventive medicine services	
New patient	99381-99387
Established patient	99391-99397
Individual counseling	99401-99404
Group counseling	99411-99412
Other	99420-99429
Newborn care	99431-99440
Special E/M services	99450-99456
Other E/M services	99499

REVIEW THE REPORTING INSTRUCTIONS FOR THE SELECTED CATEGORY OR SUBCATEGORY

Most of the categories and many of the subcategories of service have special guidelines or instructions unique to that category or subcategory. Where these are indicated, eg, "Inpatient Hospital Care," special instructions will be presented preceding the levels of evaluation and management services.

REVIEW THE LEVEL OF EVALUATION AND MANAGEMENT SERVICE DESCRIPTORS AND EXAMPLES IN THE SELECTED CATEGORY OR SUBCATEGORY

The descriptors for the levels of evaluation and management services recognize seven components, six of which are used in defining the levels of evaluation and management services. These components are:

- history;
- examination;
- medical decision making;
- counseling;
- coordination of care;
- nature of presenting problem; and
- time.

The first three of these components (ie, history, examination, and medical decision making) should be considered the key components in selecting the level of evaluation and management services. An exception to this rule is in the case of visits which consist predominantly of counseling or coordination of care.

The nature of the presenting problem and time are provided in some levels to assist the physician in determining the appropriate level of E/M service.

DETERMINE THE EXTENT OF HISTORY OBTAINED

The extent of the history is dependent upon clinical judgment and on the nature of presenting problems(s). The levels of evaluation and management services recognize four types of history that are defined as follows:

Problem focused: chief complaint; brief history of present illness or problem.

Expanded problem focused: chief complaint; brief history of present illness; problem pertinent system review.

Detailed: chief complaint; extended history of present illness; problem pertinent system review extended to include a review of a limited number of additional systems; pertinent past, family, and/or social history directly related to the patient's problems.

Comprehensive: chief complaint; extended history of present illness; review of systems which is directly related to the problem(s) identified in the history of the present illness plus a review of all additional body systems; complete past, family, and social history.

The comprehensive history obtained as part of the preventive medicine evaluation and management service is not problem-oriented and does not involve a chief complaint or present illness. It does, however, include a comprehensive system review and comprehensive or interval past, family, and social history as well as a comprehensive assessment/history of pertinent risk factors.

DETERMINE THE EXTENT OF EXAMINATION PERFORMED

The extent of the examination performed is dependent on clinical judgment and on the nature of the presenting problem(s). The levels of evaluation and management services recognize four types of examination that are defined as follows:

Problem focused: a limited examination of the affected body area or organ system.

Expanded problem focused: a limited examination of the affected body area or organ system and other symptomatic or related organ system(s).

Detailed: an extended examination of the affected body area(s) and other symptomatic or related organ system(s).

Comprehensive: a general multi-system examination or a complete examination of a single organ system. Note: the comprehensive examination performed as part of the preventive medicine evaluation and management service is multisystem, but its extent is based on age and risk factors identified.

For the purposes of these CPT definitions, the following body areas are recognized:

- Head, including the face
- Neck
- Chest, including breasts and axilla
- Abdomen
- Genitalia, groin, buttocks
- Back
- Each extremity

For the purposes of these CPT definitions, the following organ systems are recognized:

- Eyes

- Ears, nose, mouth, and throat
- Cardiovascular
- Respiratory
- Gastrointestinal
- Genitourinary
- Musculoskeletal
- Skin
- Neurologic
- Psychiatric
- Hematologic/lymphatic/immunologic

DETERMINE COMPLEXITY OF MEDICAL DECISION MAKING

Medical decision making refers to the complexity of establishing a diagnosis and/or selecting a management option as measured by:

- the number of possible diagnoses and/or the number of management options that must be considered;
- the amount and/or complexity of medical records, diagnostic tests, and/or other information that must be obtained, reviewed, and analyzed; and
- the risk of significant complications, morbidity, and/or mortality, as well as comorbidities, associated with the patient's presenting problems(s), the diagnostic procedure(s) and/or the possible management options.

Four types of medical decision making are recognized: straightforward; low complexity; moderate complexity; and high complexity. To qualify for a given type of decision making, two of the three elements in Table 2 below must be met or exceeded.

Table 2: Complexity of Medical Decision Making

Number of diagnoses or management options	Amount and/or complexity of data to be reviewed	Risk of complications and/or morbidity or mortality	Type of decision making
Minimal	Minimal or none	Minimal	**Straightforward**
Limited	Limited	Low	**Low complexity**
Multiple	Moderate	Moderate	**Moderate complexity**
Extensive	Extensive	High	**High complexity**

Comorbidities/underlying diseases, in and of themselves, are not considered in selecting a level of evaluation and management services unless their presence significantly increases the complexity of the medical decision making.

SELECT THE APPROPRIATE LEVEL OF EVALUATION AND MANAGEMENT SERVICES BASED ON THE FOLLOWING

1. For the following categories/subcategories, all of the key components, (ie, history, examination, and medical decision making), must meet or exceed the stated requirements to qualify for a particular level of evaluation and management service: office, new patient; hospital observation services; initial hospital care; office consultations; initial inpatient consultations; confirmatory consultations; emergency department services; comprehensive nursing facility assessments; domiciliary care, new patient; and home, new patient.

2. For the following categories/subcategories, two of the three key components (ie, history, examination, and medical decision making) must meet or exceed the stated requirements to qualify for a particular level of evaluation and management services: office, established patient; subsequent hospital care; follow-up inpatient consultations; subsequent nursing facility care; domiciliary care, established patient; and home, established patient.

3. When counseling and/or coordination of care dominates (more than 50%) the physician/patient and/or family encounter (face-to-face time in the office or other outpatient setting or floor/unit time in the hospital or nursing facility), then time may be considered the key or controlling factor to qualify for a particular level of evaluation and management services. This includes time spent with parties who have assumed responsibility for the care of the patient or decision making whether or not they are family members (eg, foster parents, person acting in locum parentis, legal guardian). The extent of counseling and/or coordination of care must be documented in the medical record.

OTHER DEFINITIONS OF NATURE OF THE PRESENTING PROBLEM

In addition to the above five specific definitions found in the CPT coding system, there are other definitions found in the E.M Service codes used to report Subsequent Hospital Care and Follow-Up Inpatient Consultations. See Table 3 for these additional definitions.

DIAGNOSTIC TESTS OR STUDIES

The performance of diagnostic tests or studies for which specific CPT codes are available is not included in the levels of evaluation and management services. Any diagnostic tests or studies performed by the physician for which specific CPT codes are available should be coded separately, in addition to the appropriate evaluation and management service code.

Table 3: Other Definitions of Nature of Presenting Problems

Evaluation and Management Codes	*Nature of Presenting Problem(s) Defined*	*Equivalent To*
99231 or 99261	*Stable, recovering or improving*	*Self-limited or minor*
99232 or 99262	*Inadequate response or minor complication*	*Low to moderate severity*
99233 or 99263	*Significant complication or new problem*	*Moderate to high severity*

EVALUATION AND MANAGEMENT SERVICES MODIFIERS

Evaluation and management services may be modified under certain circumstances. When applicable, the modifying circumstance should be identified by reporting the appropriate modifier code in addition to the basic service. Modifiers which may be used with evaluation and management service codes are:

-21 Prolonged evaluation and management services

-24 Unrelated evaluation and management service by the same physician during a postoperative period

-25 Significant, separately identifiable evaluation and management service by the same physician on the same day of the procedure or other service

-32 Mandated services

-52 Reduced services

-57 Decision for surgery

HOW TO CHOOSE EVALUATION AND MANAGEMENT CODE(S)

Choosing the correct evaluation and management service code to report is a nine step process. The most important steps, in terms of both reimbursement and audit liability, are verifying compliance and documentation.

1. ***Identify the Category of Service***

   Where was the patient seen and what category of services were provided?

   ☐ *Office or Other Outpatient Services*

- ☐ *Hospital Observation Services*
- ☐ *Hospital Inpatient Services*
- ☐ *Consultations*
- ☐ *Emergency Department Services*
- ☐ *Pediatric Patient Transport*
- ☐ *Critical Care Services*
- ☐ *Neonatal Intensive Care*
- ☐ *Nursing Facility Services*
- ☐ *Domiciliary, Rest Home or Custodial Care Services*
- ☐ *Home Services*
- ☐ *Prolonged Services*
- ☐ *Standby Services*
- ☐ *Case Management Services*
- ☐ *Care Plan Oversight Services*
- ☐ *Preventive Medicine Services*
- ☐ *Special or Other E/M Services*

2. *Identify the Subcategory of Service*

Is the patient a new patient or established patient?
Is the service initial care, subsequent care or follow-up?

- ☐ *New Patient*
- ☐ *Established Patient*
- ☐ *Initial Care*
- ☐ *Subsequent Care*
- ☐ *Follow-up*

3. *Determine the Extent of History Obtained*

What level of history was taken on this patient?

- ☐ *Problem Focused*
- ☐ *Expanded Problem Focused*
- ☐ *Detailed*
- ☐ *Comprehensive*

4. *Determine the Extent of Examination Performed*

What level of physician examination was performed?

- ☐ *Problem Focused*
- ☐ *Expanded Problem Focused*
- ☐ *Detailed*
- ☐ *Comprehensive*

5. *Determine the Complexity of Medical Decision Making*

What level of medical decision making was required?

- ☐ *Straightforward*
- ☐ *Low Complexity*
- ☐ *Moderate Complexity*
- ☐ *High Complexity*

6. *Record the Approximate Amount of Time*

How much time was spent either face-to-face with the patient for office visits and consults, or unit or floor time for hospital care, hospital consults, and nursing facilities?

If counseling and/or coordination of care exceeds 50 percent of the total face-to-face physician/patient encounter, then TIME is considered to be the key or controlling factor which qualifies the choice of a particular level of evaluation and management service. The extent of counseling and/or coordination of care must be documented in the medical record.

7. *Verify Compliance with Reporting Requirements*

All Three Key Components Required

To report services for new patients, initial care, office or confirmatory consultations, emergency department services, and comprehensive nursing facility assessments, all three key components must meet or exceed the stated requirements.

- ☐ *History component met or exceeded*
- ☐ *Examination component met or exceeded*
- ☐ *Medical decision making component met or exceeded*

Two of Three Key Components Required

To report services to established patients, subsequent or follow-up care, two of the three key components must meet or exceed the stated requirements.

- ☐ *History component met or exceeded; and/or*
- ☐ *Examination component met or exceeded; and/or*
- ☐ *Medical decision making component met or exceeded*

8. *Verify Documentation*

Make sure that the medical record includes proper documentation of the history, examination, medical decision making, the nature of the problem(s), the approximate amount of time, and when appropriate, the extent of counseling and/or coordination of care.

9. *Assign the Code*

The following is an example of the code selection process.

EXAMPLE OF THE CODE SELECTION PROCESS

1. Category of Service	*Office*
2. Subcategory	*New patient*
3. History	*Problem focused*
4. Examination	*Problem focused*
5. Medical Decision Making	*Straightforward*
6. Intra-service Time	*10 minutes*
7. Key Components	*Met or exceeded*
8. Documentation	*Met or exceeded*
9. Assign the Code	***99201***

EVALUATION AND MANAGEMENT SERVICES DOCUMENTATION GUIDELINES

Documentation in the medical record of all services provided is critical for reimbursement and audit liability. If the provider reported a service or procedure on the health insurance claim form but did not document it, or document it completely, in the patient's medical records, from the point of view of Medicare or private health insurance company auditors, the service was not performed, can't be reported, and therefore will not be paid for.

Millions of dollars are reclaimed from physicians and other medical professionals annually by Medicare and other third party payers because the medical record documentation does not support the services and procedures reported. Providers can protect their medical practices from audit liability by following the most current documentation guidelines published by CMS.

The following documentation guidelines for evaluation and management services were developed jointly by the American Medical Association (AMA) and CMS. The stated goal of CMS in publishing these guidelines is to provide physicians and health insurance claims reviewers with advice about preparing or reviewing documentation for evaluation and management services.

In developing and testing the validity of these guidelines, special emphasis was placed on assuring that they:

- *are consistent with the clinical descriptors and definitions contained in CPT,*

- *would be widely accepted by clinicians and minimize any changes in record-keeping practices; and*
- *would be interpreted and applied uniformly by users across the country.*

WHAT IS DOCUMENTATION AND WHY IS IT IMPORTANT?

Medical record documentation is required to record pertinent facts, findings, and observations about an individual's health history including past and present illnesses, examinations, tests, treatments, and outcomes. The medical record chronologically documents the care of the patient and is an important element contributing to high quality care. The medical record facilitates:

- *the ability of the physician and other medical professionals to evaluate and plan the patient's immediate treatment, and to monitor his/her health care over time;*
- *communication and continuity of care among physicians and other medical professionals involved in the patient's care;*
- *accurate and timely claims review and payment;*
- *appropriate utilization review and quality of care evaluations; and*
- *collection of data that may be useful for research and education.*

An appropriately documented medical record can reduce many of the hassles associated with claims processing and may serve as a legal document to verify the care provided, if necessary.

WHAT DO THIRD PARTY PAYERS WANT AND WHY?

Because payers have a contractual obligation to enrollees, they may require reasonable documentation that services are consistent with the insurance coverage provided. They may request information to validate:

- *the site of service;*
- *the medical necessity and appropriateness of the diagnostic and/or therapeutic services provided; and/or*
- *that services provided have been accurately reported.*

GENERAL PRINCIPLES OF MEDICAL RECORD DOCUMENTATION

The principles of documentation listed below are applicable to all types of medical and surgical services in all settings. For evaluation and management (E/M) services, the nature and amount of physician work and documentation varies by type of service, place of service and the patient's status. The general principles listed below may be modified to account for these variable circumstances in providing evaluation and management services.

1. *The medical record should be complete and legible.*

2. *The documentation of each patient encounter should include:*

   - *the reason for the encounter as well as relevant history, physical examination findings and prior diagnostic test results;*
   - *an assessment, clinical impression or diagnosis;*
   - *a plan for care; and*
   - *the date and legible identity of the observer.*

3. *If not documented, the rationale for ordering diagnostic and other ancillary services should be easily inferred.*

4. *Past and present diagnoses should be accessible to the treating and/or consulting physician.*

5. *Appropriate health risk factors should be identified.*

6. *The patient's progress, response to and changes in treatment, and revision of diagnosis should be documented.*

7. *CPT and ICD-9-CM codes reported on the health insurance claim form or patient billing statement should be supported by the documentation in the medical record.*

DOCUMENTATION OF EVALUATION AND MANAGEMENT SERVICES

This section provides definitions and documentation guidelines for the three key components of evaluation and management services and for visits which consist predominately of counseling or coordination of care. The three key components—history, examination, and medical decision making—appear in the descriptors for office and other outpatient services, hospital observation services, hospital inpatient services, consultations, emergency department services, nursing facility services, domiciliary care services, and home services. Note that Documentation Guidelines are identified by the symbol •DG.

The E/M descriptors recognize seven components which are used in defining the levels of service. These components are:

- *History*
- *Examination*
- *Medical decision making*
- *Counseling*
- *Coordination of care*

- *Nature of presenting problem*
- *Time*

The first three (i.e., history, examination and medical decision making) are the key components in selecting the level of evaluation and management services. However, with visits that consist predominantly of counseling or coordination of care, time is the key or controlling factor to qualify for a particular level of evaluation and management service.

Because the level of evaluation and management service is dependent on two or three key components, performance and documentation of one component (e.g., examination) at the highest level does not necessarily mean that the encounter in its entirety qualifies for the highest level of evaluation and management service.

These documentation guidelines for evaluation and management services reflect the needs of the typical adult population. For certain groups of patients, the recorded information may vary slightly from that described here.

Specifically, the medical records of infants, children, adolescents and pregnant women may have additional or modified information recorded in each history and examination area.

As an example, newborn records may include under history of the present illness, the details of the mother's pregnancy and the infant's status at birth; social history focused on family structure; family history focused on congenital anomalies and hereditary disorders in the family. In addition, the content of a pediatric examination will vary with the age and development of the child. Although not specifically defined in these documentation guidelines, these patient group variations on history and examination are appropriate.

DOCUMENTATION OF HISTORY

The levels of evaluation and management services are based on four types of history (Problem Focused, Expanded Problem Focused, Detailed, and Comprehensive). Each type of history includes some or all of the following elements:

- *Chief complaint*
- *History of present illness*
- *Review of systems*
- *Past, family and/or social history*

The extent of history of present illness, review of systems and past, family and/or social history that is obtained and documented is dependent upon clinical judgement and the nature of the presenting problem(s).

Present History	*Review of Systems*	*Past, Family or Social History*	*Type of History*
Brief	*N/A*	*N/A*	*Problem Focused*
Brief	*Problem Pertinent*	*N/A*	*Expanded Problem Focused*
Extended	*Extended*	*Pertinent*	*Detailed*
Extended	*Complete*	*Complete*	*Comprehensive*

The above chart shows the progression of the elements required for each type of history. To qualify for a given type of history all three elements in the table must be met. (A chief complaint is indicated at all levels.)

•DG: *The chief complaint, review of systems and past, family and/or social history may be listed as separate elements of history, or they may be included in the description of the history of the present illness.*

•DG: *A review of systems and/or a past, family and/or social history obtained during an earlier encounter does not need to be re-recorded if there is evidence that the physician reviewed and updated the previous information. This may occur when a physician updates his or her own record or in an institutional setting or group practice where many physicians use a common record. The review and update may be documented by:*

- *describing any new review of systems and/or past, family and/or social history information or noting there has been no change in the information; and*
- *noting the date and location of the earlier review of systems and/or past, family and/or social history.*

•DG: *The review of systems and/or past, family and/or social history may be recorded by ancillary staff or on a form completed by the patient. To document that the physician reviewed the information, there must be a notation supplementing or confirming the information recorded by others.*

•DG: *If the physician is unable to obtain a history from the patient or other source, the record should describe the patient's condition or other circumstance which precludes obtaining a history.*

Definitions and specific documentation guidelines for each of the elements of history are listed below.

CHIEF COMPLAINT

The chief complaint is "a concise statement describing the symptom, problem, condition, diagnosis, or other factor that is the reason for the encounter, usually stated in the patient's words."

•*DG: The medical record should clearly reflect the chief complaint.*

HISTORY OF PRESENT ILLNESS

The history of present illness is "a chronological description of the development of the patient's present illness from the first sign and/or symptom to the present." *It includes the following elements:*

- *Location*
- *Quality*
- *Severity*
- *Duration*
- *Timing*
- *Context*
- *Modifying factors*
- *Associated signs and symptoms*

***Brief** and **extended** history of present illnesses are distinguished by the amount of detail needed to accurately characterize the clinical problem(s). A **brief** history of present illness consists of one to three elements of the history of present illness.*

•*DG: The medical record should describe at least one to three elements of the present illness (history of present illness).*

*An **extended** history of present illness consists of at least four elements of the history of present illness or the status of at least three chronic or inactive conditions.*

•*DG: Medical record should describe at least four elements of the present illness (history of present illness), or the status of at least three chronic or inactive conditions.*

REVIEW OF SYSTEMS

A review of systems is "an inventory of body systems obtained through a series of questions seeking to identify signs and/or symptoms which the patient may be experiencing or has experienced." *For purposes of review of systems, the following systems are recognized:*

- *Constitutional symptoms (e.g., fever, weight loss)*
- *Eyes*
- *Ears, Nose, Mouth, Throat*
- *Neck*
- *Cardiovascular*
- *Respiratory*
- *Gastrointestinal*
- *Genitourinary*
- *Musculoskeletal*
- *Integumentary (skin and/or breast)*
- *Neurological*
- *Psychiatric*
- *Endocrine*
- *Hematologic/Lymphatic*
- *Allergic/Immunologic*

*A **problem pertinent** review of systems inquires about the system directly related to the problem(s) identified in the history of present illness.*

•DG: *The patient's positive responses and pertinent negatives for the system related to the problem should be documented.*

*An **extended** review of systems inquires about the system directly related to the problem(s) identified in the history of present illness and a limited number of additional systems.*

•DG: *The patient's positive responses and pertinent negatives for two to nine systems should be documented.*

*A **complete** review of systems inquires about the system(s) directly related to the problem(s) identified in the history of present illness plus all additional body systems.*

•DG: *At least ten organ systems must be reviewed. Those systems with positive or pertinent negative responses must be individually documented. For the remaining systems, a notation indicating all other systems are negative is permissible. In the absence of such a notation, at least ten systems must be individually documented.*

PAST, FAMILY AND/OR SOCIAL HISTORY

The past, family and/or social history consists of a review of the following areas:

- *Past history: the patient's past experiences with illnesses, operations, injuries and treatments.*
- *Family history: a review of medical events in the patient's family, including diseases which may be hereditary or place the patient at risk.*
- *Social history: an age appropriate review of past and current activities.*

For certain categories of evaluation and management services that include only an interval history, it is not necessary to record information about the past, family and/or social history. Those categories are subsequent hospital care, follow-up inpatient consultations and subsequent nursing facility care.

A ***pertinent*** *past, family and/or social history is a review of the history area(s) directly related to the problem(s) identified in the history of present illness.*

•***DG:*** *At least one specific item from any of the three history areas must be documented for a pertinent past, family and/or social history*

A ***complete*** *past, family and/or social history is of a review of two or all three of the past, family and/or social history areas, depending on the category of the evaluation and management service. A review of all three history areas is required for services that by their nature include a comprehensive assessment or reassessment of the patient. A review of two of the three history areas is sufficient for other services.*

•***DG:*** *At least one specific item from two of the three history areas must be documented for a complete past, family and/or social history for the following categories of evaluation and management services: office or other outpatient services, established patient; emergency department; domiciliary care, established patient; and home care, established patient.*

•***DG:*** *At least one specific item from each of the three history areas must be documented for a complete past, family and/or social history for the following categories of evaluation and management services: office or other outpatient services, new patient; hospital observation services; hospital inpatient services, initial care; consultations; comprehensive nursing facility assessments; domiciliary care, new patient; and home care, new patient.*

DOCUMENTATION OF EXAMINATION

The levels of E/M services are based on four types of examination:

- *Problem Focused* — "a limited examination of the affected body area or organ system."
- *Expanded Problem Focused* — "a limited examination of the affected body area or organ system and any other symptomatic or related body organ system(s)."
- *Detailed* — "an extended examination of the affected body area(s) and other symptomatic or related organ system(s)."
- *Comprehensive* — "a general multi-system examination, or complete examination of a single organ system."

These types of examinations have been defined for general multi-system and the following single organ systems:

- *Cardiovascular*
- *Ears, Nose, Mouth and Throat*
- *Eyes*
- *Genitourinary (Female)*
- *Genitourinary (Male)*
- *Hematologic/Lymphatic/Immunologic*
- *Musculoskeletal*
- *Neurological*
- *Psychiatric*
- *Respiratory*
- *Skin*

A general multi-system examination or a single organ system examination may be performed by any physician regardless of specialty. The type (general multi-system or single organ system) and content of examination are selected by the examining physician and are based upon clinical judgement, the patient's history, and the nature of the presenting problem(s).

The content and documentation requirements for each type and level of examination are summarized below and described in detail in tables beginning on page 116. In the tables, organ systems and body areas recognized by CPT for purposes of describing examinations are shown in the left column. The content, or individual elements, of the examination pertaining to that body area or organ system are identified by bullets (●) in the right column.

Parenthetical examples, (e.g., ...), have been used for clarification and to provide guidance regarding documentation. Documentation for each element must satisfy any numeric requirements (such as "Measurement of any three of the following seven...") included in the description of the element. Elements with multiple components but with no specific numeric requirement (such as "Examination of liver and spleen") require documentation of at least one component. It is possible for a given examination to be expanded beyond what is defined here. When that occurs, findings related to the additional systems and/or areas should be documented.

•***DG:*** *Specific abnormal and relevant negative findings of the examination of the affected or symptomatic body area(s) or organ system(s) should be documented. A notation of "abnormal" without elaboration is insufficient.*

•***DG:*** *Abnormal or unexpected findings of the examination of any asymptomatic body area(s) or organ system(s) should be described.*

•***DG:*** *A brief statement or notation indicating "negative" or "normal" is sufficient to document normal findings related to unaffected area(s) or asymptomatic organ system(s).*

GENERAL MULTI-SYSTEM EXAMINATIONS

To qualify for a given level of multi-system examination, the following content and documentation requirements should be met:

- *Problem Focused Examination — should include performance and documentation of one to five elements identified by a bullet (•) in one or more organ system(s) or body area(s).*
- *Expanded Problem Focused Examination — should include performance and documentation of at least six elements identified by a bullet (•) in one or more organ system(s) or body area(s).*
- *Detailed Examination — should include at least six organ systems or body areas. For each system/area selected, performance and documentation of at least two elements identified by a bullet (•) is expected. Alternatively, a detailed examination may include performance and documentation of at least twelve elements identified by a bullet (•) in two or more organ systems or body areas.*
- *Comprehensive Examination — should include at least nine organ systems or body areas. For each system/area selected, all elements of the examination identified by a bullet (•) should be performed, unless specific directions limit the content of the examination. For each area/system, documentation of at least two elements identified by a bullet is expected.*

SINGLE ORGAN SYSTEM EXAMINATIONS

Variations among single organ system examinations in the organ systems and body areas identified in the left columns and in the elements of the examinations described in the right columns reflect differing emphases among specialties. To qualify for a given level of single organ system examination, the following content and documentation requirements should be met:

- *Problem Focused Examination — should include performance and documentation of one to five elements identified by a bullet (•), whether in a box with a shaded or unshaded border.*
- *Expanded Problem Focused Examination — should include performance and documentation of at least six elements identified by a bullet (•), whether in a box with a shaded or unshaded border.*
- *Detailed Examination — examinations other than the eye and psychiatric examinations should include performance and documentation of at least twelve elements identified by a bullet (•), whether in box with a shaded or unshaded border.*

  Eye and psychiatric examinations should include the performance and documentation of at least nine elements identified by a bullet (•), whether in a box with a shaded or unshaded border.
- *Comprehensive Examination — should include performance of all elements identified by a bullet (•), whether in a shaded or unshaded box. Documentation of every element in each box with a shaded border and at least one element in each box with an unshaded border is expected.*

Documentation of every element in each box with a shaded border and at least one element in each box with an unshaded border is expected.

GENERAL MULTI-SYSTEM EXAMINATION

SYSTEM/BODY AREA	*ELEMENTS OF EXAMINATION*
Constitutional	• *Measurement of any three of the following seven vital signs: 1) sitting or standing blood pressure, 2) supine blood pressure, 3) pulse rate and regularity, 4) respiration, 5) temperature, 6) height, 7) weight (May be measured and recorded by ancillary staff)* • *General appearance of patient (e.g., development, nutrition, body habitus, deformities, attention to grooming)*
Eyes	• *Inspection of conjunctivae and lids* • *Examination of pupils and irises (e.g., reaction to light and accommodation, size and symmetry)* • *Ophthalmoscopic examination of optic discs (e.g., size, C/D ratio, appearance) and posterior segments (e.g., vessel changes, exudates, hemorrhages)*
Ears, Nose, Mouth, Throat	• *External inspection of ears and nose (e.g., overall and appearance, scars, lesions, masses)* • *Otoscopic examination of external auditory canals and tympanic membranes* • *Assessment of hearing (e.g., whispered voice, finger rub, tuning fork)* • *Inspection of nasal mucosa, septum and turbinates* • *Inspection of lips, teeth and gums* • *Examination of oropharynx: oral mucosa, salivary glands, hard and soft palates, tongue, tonsils and posterior pharynx*
Neck	• *Examination of neck (e.g., masses, overall appearance, symmetry, tracheal position, crepitus)* • *Examination of thyroid (e.g., enlargement, tenderness, mass)*

Respiratory	• *Assessment of respiratory effort (e.g., intercostal retractions, use of accessory muscles, diaphragmatic movement)* • *Percussion of chest (e.g., dullness, flatness, hyperresonance)* • *Palpation of chest (e.g., tactile fremitus)* • *Auscultation of lungs (e.g., breath sounds, adventitious sounds, rubs)*
Cardiovascular	• *Palpation of heart (e.g., location, size, thrills)* • *Auscultation of heart with notation of abnormal sounds and murmurs* *Examination of:* • *Carotid arteries (e.g., pulse amplitude, bruits)* • *Abdominal aorta (e.g., size, dbruits)* • *Femoral arteries (e.g., pulse amplitude, bruits)* • *Pedal pulses (e.g., pulse amplitude)* • *Extremities for edema and/or varicosities*
Chest (Breasts)	• *Inspection of breasts (e.g., symmetry, nipple discharge)* • *Palpation of breasts and axillae (e.g., masses or lumps, tenderness)*
Gastrointestinal (Abdomen)	• *Examination of abdomen with notation of presence of masses or tenderness* • *Examination of liver and spleen* • *Examination for presence or absence of hernia* • *Examination (when indicated) of anus, perineum and rectum, including sphincter tone, presence of hemorrhoids, rectal masses* • *Obtain stool sample for occult blood test when indicated*
Genitourinary Male	• *Examination of the scrotal contents (e.g., hydrocele, spermatocele, tenderness of cord, testicular mass)* *continued*

	• *Examination of the penis* • *Digital rectal examination of prostate gland (e.g., size, symmetry, nodularity, tenderness)*
Genitourinary Female	• *Pelvic examination (with or without specimen collection for smears and cultures), including:* • *Examination of external genitalia (e.g., general appearance, hair distribution, lesions) and vagina (e.g., general appearance, estrogen effect, discharge, lesions, pelvic support, cystocele, rectocele)* • *Examination of urethra (e.g., masses, tenderness, scarring)* • *Examination of bladder (e.g., fullness, masses, tenderness)* • *Cervix (e.g., general appearance, lesions, discharge)* • *Uterus (e.g., size, contour, position, mobility, tenderness, consistency, descent or support)* • *Adnexa/parametria (e.g., masses, tenderness, organomegaly, nodularity)*
Lymphatic	*Palpation of lymph nodes in two or more areas:* • *Neck* • *Axillae* • *Groin* • *Other*
Musculoskeletal	• *Examination of gait and station* • *Inspection and/or palpation of digits and nails (eg clubbing, cyanosis, inflammatory conditions, petechiae, ischemia, infections, nodes)* • *Examination of joints, bones and muscles of one or more of the following six areas: 1) head and neck; 2) spine, ribs and pelvis; 3) right upper extremity; 4) left upper extremity; 5) right lower extremity; and 6) left lower*

	extremity. The examination of a given area includes: • *Inspection and/or palpation with notation of presence of any misalignment, asymmetry, crepitation, defects, tenderness, masses, effusions* • *Assessment of range of motion with notation of any pain, crepitation or contracture* • *Assessment of stability with notation of any dislocation (luxation), subluxation or laxity* • *Assessment of muscle strength and tone (e.g., flaccid, cog wheel, spastic) with notation of any atrophy or abnormal movements*
Skin	• *Inspection of skin and subcutaneous tissue (e.g., rashes, lesions, ulcers)* • *Palpation of skin and subcutaneous tissue (e.g., induration, subcutaneous nodules, tightening)*
Neurologic	• *Test cranial nerves with notation of any deficits* • *Examination of deep tendon reflexes with notation of pathological reflexes (e.g., Babinski)* • *Examination of sensation (e.g., by touch, pin, vibration, proprioception)*
Psychiatric	• *Description of patient's judgment and insight* *Brief assessment of mental status including:* • *Orientation to time, place and person* • *Recent and remote memory* • *Mood and affect (e.g., depression, anxiety, agitation)*

CONTENT AND DOCUMENTATION REQUIREMENTS

Level of Exam	*Perform and Document:*
Problem Focused	*One to five elements identified by a bullet.*
Expanded Problem Focused	*At least six elements identified by a bullet.*
Detailed	*At least two elements identified by a bullet from each of six areas/systems OR at least twelve elements identified by a bullet in two or more areas/systems.*
Comprehensive	*Perform all elements identified by a bullet in at least nine organ systems or body areas and document at least two elements identified by a bullet from each of nine areas/systems.*

CARDIOVASCULAR EXAMINATION

SYSTEM/BODY AREA	*ELEMENTS OF EXAMINATION*
Constitutional	• *Measurement of any three of the following seven vital signs: 1) sitting or standing blood pressure, 2) supine blood pressure, 3) pulse rate and regularity, 4) respiration, 5) temperature, 6) height, 7) weight (May be measured and recorded by ancillary staff)* • *General appearance of patient (e.g., development, nutrition, body habitus, deformities, attention to grooming)*
Head and Face	
Eyes	• *Inspection of conjunctivae and lids (e.g., xanthelasma)*
Ears, Nose, Mouth and Throat	• *Inspection of teeth, gums and palate* • *Inspection of oral mucosa with notation of presence of pallor or cyanosis*
Neck	• *Examination of jugular veins (e.g., distension; a, v or cannon a waves)* • *Examination of thyroid (e.g., enlargement, tenderness, mass)*
Respiratory	• *Assessment of respiratory effort (e.g., intercostal retractions, use of accessory muscles, diaphragmatic movement)* • *Auscultation of lungs (e.g., breath sounds, adventitious sounds, rubs)*
Cardiovascular	• *Palpation of heart (e.g., location, size and forcefulness of the point of maximal impact; thrills; lifts; palpable S3 or S4)* • *Auscultation of heart including sounds, abnormal sounds and murmurs*

continued

	• *Measurement of blood pressure in two or more extremities when indicated (e.g., aortic dissection, coarctation)* *Examination of:* • *Carotid arteries (e.g., waveform, pulse amplitude, bruits, apical-carotid delay)* • *Abdominal aorta (e.g., size, bruits)* • *Femoral arteries (e.g., pulse amplitude, bruits)* • *Pedal pulses (e.g., pulse amplitude)* • *Extremities for peripheral edema and/or varicosities*
Chest (Breasts)	
Gastrointestinal (Abdomen)	• *Examination of abdomen with notation of presence (Abdomen) of masses or tenderness* • *Examination of liver and spleen* • *Obtain stool sample for occult blood from patients who are being considered for thrombolytic or anticoagulant therapy*
Genitourinary	
Lymphatic	
Musculoskeletal	• *Examination of the back with notation of kyphosis or scoliosis* • *Examination of gait with notation of ability to undergo exercise testing and/or participation in exercise programs* • *Assessment of muscle strength and tone (e.g., flaccid, cog wheel, spastic) with notation of any atrophy and abnormal movements*

Extremities	• *Inspection and palpation of digits and nails (e.g., clubbing, cyanosis, inflammation, petechiae, ischemia, infections, Osler's nodes)*
Skin	• *Inspection and/or palpation of skin and subcutaneous tissue (e.g., stasis dermatitis, ulcers, scars, xanthomas)*
Neurological/Psychiatric	*Brief assessment of mental status including:* • *Orientation to time, place and person* • *Mood and affect (e.g., depression, anxiety, agitation)*

CONTENT AND DOCUMENTATION REQUIREMENTS

Level of Exam	***Perform and Document:***
Problem Focused	*One to five elements identified by a bullet.*
Expanded Problem Focused	*At least six elements identified by a bullet.*
Detailed	*At least twelve elements identified by a bullet.*
Comprehensive	*Perform all elements identified by a bullet; document every element in each box with a shaded border and at least one element in each box with an unshaded border.*

EAR, NOSE AND THROAT EXAMINATION

SYSTEM/BODY AREA	*ELEMENTS OF EXAMINATION*
Constitutional	• *Measurement of any three of the following seven vital signs: 1) sitting or standing blood pressure, 2) supine blood pressure, 3) pulse rate and regularity, 4) respiration, 5) temperature, 6) height, 7) weight (May be measured and recorded by ancillary staff)* • *General appearance of patient (e.g., development, nutrition, body habitus, deformities, attention to grooming)* • *Assessment of ability to communicate (e.g., use of sign language or other communication aids) and quality of voice*
Head and Face	• *Inspection of head and face (e.g., overall appearance, scars, lesions and masses)* • *Palpation and/or percussion of face with notation of presence or absence of sinus tenderness* • *Examination of salivary glands* • *Assessment of facial strength*
Eyes	• *Test ocular motility including primary gaze alignment*
Ears, Nose, Mouth and Throat	• *Otoscopic examination of external auditory canals and tympanic membranes including pneumo-otoscopy with notation of mobility of membranes* • *Assessment of hearing with tuning forks and clinical speech reception thresholds (e.g., whispered voice, finger rub)* • *External inspection of ears and nose (e.g., overall appearance, scars, lesions and masses)* • *Inspection of nasal mucosa, septum and turbinates* *continued*

	• *Inspection of lips, teeth and gums* • *Examination of oropharynx: oral mucosa, hard and soft palates, tongue, tonsils and posterior pharynx (e.g., asymmetry, lesions, hydration of mucosal surfaces)* • *Inspection of pharyngeal walls and pyriform sinuses (e.g., pooling of saliva, asymmetry, lesions)* • *Examination by mirror of larynx including the condition of the epiglottis, false vocal cords, true vocal cords and mobility of larynx (Use of mirror not required in children)* • *Examination by mirror of nasopharynx including appearance of the mucosa, adenoids, posterior choanae and eustachian tubes (Use of mirror not required in children)*
Neck	• *Examination of neck (e.g., masses, overall appearance, symmetry, tracheal position, crepitus)* • *Examination of thyroid (e.g., enlargement, tenderness, mass)*
Respiratory	• *Inspection of chest including symmetry, expansion and/or assessment of respiratory effort (e.g., intercostal retractions, use of accessory muscles, diaphragmatic movement)* • *Auscultation of lungs (e.g., breath sounds, adventitious sounds, rubs)*
Cardiovascular	• *Auscultation of heart with notation of abnormal sounds and murmurs* • *Examination of peripheral vascular system by observation (e.g., swelling, varicosities) and palpation (e.g., pulses, temperature, edema, tenderness)*
Chest (Breasts)	
Gastrointestinal (Abdomen)	

Genitourinary	
Lymphatic	• *Palpation of lymph nodes in neck, axillae, groin and/or other location*
Musculoskeletal	
Extremities	
Skin	
Neurological/Psychiatric	• *Test cranial nerves with notation of any deficits* *Brief assessment of mental status including:* • *Orientation to time, place and person* • *Mood and affect (e.g., depression, anxiety, agitation)*

CONTENT AND DOCUMENTATION REQUIREMENTS

Level of Exam	*Perform and Document:*
Problem Focused	*One to five elements identified by a bullet.*
Expanded Problem Focused	*At least six elements identified by a bullet.*
Detailed	*At least twelve elements identified by a bullet.*
Comprehensive	*Perform all elements identified by a bullet; document every element in each box with a shaded border and at least one element in each box with an unshaded border.*

EYE EXAMINATION

SYSTEM/BODY AREA	*ELEMENTS OF EXAMINATION*
Constitutional	
Head and Face	
Eyes	• *Test visual acuity (Does not include determination of refractive error)* • *Gross visual field testing by confrontation* • *Test ocular motility including primary gaze alignment* • *Inspection of bulbar and palpebral conjunctivae* • *Examination of ocular adnexae including lids (e.g., ptosis or lagophthalmos), lacrimal glands, lacrimal drainage, orbits and preauricular lymph nodes* • *Examination of pupils and irises including shape, direct and consensual reaction (afferent pupil), size (e.g., anisocoria) and morphology* • *Slit lamp examination of the corneas including epithelium, stroma, endothelium, and tear film* • *Slit lamp examination of the anterior chambers including depth, cells, and flare* • *Slit lamp examination of the lenses including clarity, anterior and posterior capsule, cortex, and nucleus* • *Measurement of intraocular pressures (except in children and patients with trauma or infectious disease)* • *Ophthalmoscopic examination through dilated pupils (unless contraindicated) of* • *Optic discs including size, C/D ratio, appearance (e.g., atrophy, cupping, tumor elevation) and nerve fiber layer* • *Posterior segments including retina and vessels (e.g., exudates and hemorrhages)*

Ears, Nose, Mouth and Throat	
Neck	
Respiratory	
Cardiovascular	
Chest (Breasts)	
Gastrointestinal (Abdomen)	
Genitourinary	
Lymphatic	
Musculoskeletal	
Extremities	
Skin	
Neurological/Psychiatric	*Brief assessment of mental status including:* • *Orientation to time, place and person* • *Mood and affect (e.g., depression, anxiety, agitation)*

CONTENT AND DOCUMENTATION REQUIREMENTS

Level of Exam	***Perform and Document:***
Problem Focused	*One to five elements identified by a bullet.*
Expanded Problem Focused	*At least six elements identified by a bullet.*
Detailed	*At least nine elements identified by a bullet.*
Comprehensive	*Perform all elements identified by a bullet; document every element in each box with a shaded border and at least one element in each box with an unshaded border.*

GENITOURINARY EXAMINATION

SYSTEM/BODY AREA	*ELEMENTS OF EXAMINATION*
Constitutional	• *Measurement of any three of the following seven vital signs: 1) sitting or standing blood pressure, 2) supine blood pressure, 3) pulse rate and regularity, 4) respiration, 5) temperature, 6) height, 7) weight (May be measured and recorded by ancillary staff)* • *General appearance of patient (e.g., development, nutrition, body habitus, deformities, attention to grooming)*
Head and Face	
Eyes	
Ears, Nose, Mouth and Throat	
Neck	• *Examination of neck (e.g., masses, overall appearance, symmetry, tracheal position, crepitus)* • *Examination of thyroid (e.g., enlargement, tenderness, mass)*
Respiratory	• *Assessment of respiratory effort (e.g., intercostal retractions, use of accessory muscles, diaphragmatic movement)* • *Auscultation of lungs (e.g., breath sounds, adventitious sounds, rubs)*
Cardiovascular	• *Auscultation of heart with notation of abnormal sounds and murmurs* • *Examination of peripheral vascular system by observation (e.g., swelling, varicosities) and palpation (e.g., pulses, temperature, edema, tenderness)*
Chest (Breasts)	*[See genitourinary (female)]*

Gastrointestinal (Abdomen)	• *Examination of abdomen with notation of presence of masses or tenderness* • *Examination for presence or absence of hernia* • *Examination of liver and spleen* • *Obtain stool sample for occult blood test when indicated*
Genitourinary (male)	• *Inspection of anus and perineum* *Examination (with or without specimen collection for smears and cultures) of genitalia including:* • *Scrotum (e.g., lesions, cysts, rashes)* • *Epididymides (e.g., size, symmetry, masses)* • *Testes (e.g., size, symmetry, masses)* • *Urethral meatus (e.g., size, location, lesions, discharge)* • *Penis (e.g., lesions, presence or absence of foreskin, foreskin retractability, plaque, masses, scarring, deformities)* *Digital rectal examination including:* • *Prostate gland (e.g., size, symmetry, nodularity, tenderness)* • *Seminal vesicles (e.g., symmetry, tenderness, masses, enlargement)*
Genitourinary (female)	*Includes at least seven of the following eleven elements identified by bullets:* • *Inspection and palpation of breasts (e.g., masses or lumps, tenderness, symmetry, nipple discharge)* • *Digital rectal examination including sphincter tone, presence of hemorrhoids, rectal masses* *Pelvic examination (with or without specimen collection for smears and cultures) including:*

	• *External genitalia (e.g., general appearance, hair distribution, lesions)* • *Urethral meatus (e.g., size, location, lesions, prolapse)* • *Urethra (e.g., masses, tenderness, scarring)* • *Bladder (e.g., fullness, masses, tenderness)* • *Vagina (e.g., general appearance, estrogen effect, discharge, lesions, pelvic support, cystocele, rectocele)* • *Cervix (e.g., general appearance, lesions, discharge)* • *Uterus (e.g., size, contour, position, mobility, tenderness, consistency, descent or support)* • *Adnexa/parametria (e.g., masses, tenderness, organomegaly, nodularity)* • *Anus and perineum*
Lymphatic	• *Palpation of lymph nodes in neck, axillae, groin and/or other location*
Musculoskeletal	
Extremities	
Skin	• *Inspection and/or palpation of skin and subcutaneous tissue (e.g., rashes, lesions, ulcers)*
Neurological/Psychiatric	*Brief assessment of mental status including:* • *Orientation (e.g., time, place and person) and* • *Mood and affect (e.g., depression, anxiety, agitation)*

CONTENT AND DOCUMENTATION REQUIREMENTS

Level of Exam	***Perform and Document:***
Problem Focused	*One to five elements identified by a bullet.*
Expanded Problem Focused	*At least six elements identified by a bullet.*
Detailed	*At least twelve elements identified by a bullet.*
Comprehensive	*Perform all elements identified by a bullet; document every element in each box with a shaded border and at least one element in each box with an unshaded border.*

HEMATOLOGIC, LYMPHATIC, AND/OR IMMUNOLOGIC EXAMINATION

SYSTEM/BODY AREA	*ELEMENTS OF EXAMINATION*
Constitutional	• *Measurement of any three of the following seven vital signs: 1) sitting or standing blood pressure, 2) supine blood pressure, 3) pulse rate and regularity, 4) respiration, 5) temperature, 6) height, 7) weight (May be measured and recorded by ancillary staff)* • *General appearance of patient (e.g., development, nutrition, body habitus, deformities, attention to grooming)*
Head and Face	• *Palpation and/or percussion of face with notation of presence or absence of sinus tenderness*
Eyes	• *Inspection of conjunctivae and lids*
Ears, Nose, Mouth and Throat	• *Otoscopic examination of external auditory canals and tympanic membranes* • *Inspection of nasal mucosa, septum and turbinates* • *Inspection of teeth and gums* • *Examination of oropharynx (e.g., oral muc hard and soft palates, tongue, tonsils, posterior pharynx)*
Neck	• *Examination of neck (e.g., masses, overall appearance, symmetry, tracheal position, crepitus)* • *Examination of thyroid (e.g., enlargement, tenderness, mass)*
Respiratory	• *Assessment of respiratory effort (e.g., intercostal retractions, use of accessory muscles, diaphragmatic movement)* • *Auscultation of lungs (e.g., breath sounds, adventitious sounds, rubs)*

Cardiovascular	• *Auscultation of heart with notation of abnormal sounds and murmurs* • *Examination of peripheral vascular system by observation (e.g., swelling, varicosities) and palpation (e.g., pulses, temperature, edema, tenderness)*
Chest (Breasts)	
Gastrointestinal (Abdomen)	• *Examination of abdomen with notation of presence of masses or tenderness*
Genitourinary	
Lymphatic	• *Palpation of lymph nodes in neck, axillae, groin, and/or other location*
Musculoskeletal	
Extremities	• *Inspection and palpation of digits and nails (e.g., clubbing, cyanosis, inflammation, petechiae, ischemia, infections, nodes)*
Skin	• *Inspection and/or palpation of skin and subcutaneous tissue (e.g., rashes, lesions, ulcers, ecchymoses, bruises)*
Neurological/Psychiatric	*Brief assessment of mental status including:* • *Orientation to time, place and person* • *Mood and affect (e.g., depression, anxiety, agitation)*

CONTENT AND DOCUMENTATION REQUIREMENTS

Level of Exam	*Perform and Document:*
Problem Focused	*One to five elements identified by a bullet.*
Expanded Problem Focused	*At least six elements identified by a bullet.*
Detailed	*At least twelve elements identified by a bullet.*
Comprehensive	*Perform all elements identified by a bullet; document every element in each box with a shaded border and at least one element in each box with an unshaded border.*

MUSCULOSKELETAL EXAMINATION

SYSTEM/BODY AREA	*ELEMENTS OF EXAMINATION*
Constitutional	• *Measurement of any three of the following seven vital signs: 1) sitting or standing blood pressure, 2) supine blood pressure, 3) pulse rate and regularity, 4) respiration, 5) temperature, 6) height, 7) weight (May be measured and recorded by ancillary staff)* • *General appearance of patient (e.g., development, nutrition, body habitus, deformities, attention to grooming)*
Head and Face	
Eyes	
Ears, Nose, Mouth and Throat	
Neck	
Respiratory	
Cardiovascular	• *Examination of peripheral vascular system by observation (e.g., swelling, varicosities) and palpation (e.g., pulses, temperature, edema, tenderness)*
Chest (Breasts)	
Gastrointestinal (Abdomen)	
Genitourinary	
Lymphatic	• *Palpation of lymph nodes in neck, axillae, groin and/or other location*

Musculoskeletal	• *Examination of gait and station* • *Examination of joint(s), bone(s) and muscle(s)/ tendon(s) of four of the following six areas: 1) head and neck; 2) spine, ribs and pelvis; 3) right upper extremity; 4) left upper extremity; 5) right lower extremity; and 6) left lower extremity. The examination of a given area includes:* • *Inspection, percussion and/or palpation with notation of any misalignment, asymmetry, crepitation, defects, tenderness, masses or effusions* • *Assessment of range of motion with notation of any pain (e.g., straight leg raising), crepitation or contracture* • *Assessment of stability with notation of any dislocation (luxation), subluxation or laxity* • *Assessment of muscle strength and tone (e.g., flaccid, cog wheel, spastic) with notation of any atrophy or abnormal movements*

NOTE: For the comprehensive level of examination, all four of the elements identified by a bullet must be performed and documented for each of four anatomic areas. For the three lower levels of examination, each element is counted separately for each body area. For example, assessing range of motion in two extremities constitutes two elements.

Extremities	*[See musculoskeletal and skin]*
Skin	• *Inspection and/or palpation of skin and subcutaneous tissue (e.g., scars, rashes, lesions, cafe-au-lait spots, ulcers) in four of the following six areas: 1) head and neck; 2) trunk; 3) right upper extremity; 4) left upper extremity; 5) right lower extremity; and 6) left lower extremity.*

NOTE: For the comprehensive level, all four areas must be examined and documented. For the three lower levels, each body area is counted separately. For example, inspection and/or palpation of the skin and subcutaneous tissue of two extremities constitutes two elements.

Neurological/Psychiatric	• *Test coordination (e.g., finger/nose, heel/knee/shin, rapid alternating movements in the upper and lower extremities, evaluation of fine motor coordination in young children)* • *Examination of deep tendon reflexes and/or nerve stretch test with notation of pathological reflexes (e.g., Babinski)* • *Examination of sensation (e.g., by touch, pin, vibration, proprioception)* *Brief assessment of mental status including* • *Orientation to time, place and person* • *Mood and affect (e.g., depression, anxiety, agitation)*

CONTENT AND DOCUMENTATION REQUIREMENTS

Level of Exam	***Perform and Document:***
Problem Focused	*One to five elements identified by a bullet.*
Expanded Problem Focused	*At least six elements identified by a bullet.*
Detailed	*At least twelve elements identified by a bullet.*
Comprehensive	*Perform all elements identified by a bullet; document every element in each box with a shaded border and at least one element in each box with an unshaded border.*

NEUROLOGICAL EXAMINATION

SYSTEM/BODY AREA	*ELEMENTS OF EXAMINATION*
Constitutional	• *Measurement of any three of the following seven vital signs: 1) sitting or standing blood pressure, 2) supine blood pressure, 3) pulse rate and regularity, 4) respiration, 5) temperature, 6) height, 7) weight (May be measured and recorded by ancillary staff)* • *General appearance of patient (e.g., development, nutrition, body habitus, deformities, attention to grooming)*
Head and Face	
Eyes	• *Ophthalmoscopic examination of optic discs (e.g., size, C/D ratio, appearance) and posterior segments (e.g., vessel changes, exudates, hemorrhages)*
Ears, Nose, Mouth and Throat	
Neck	
Respiratory	
Cardiovascular	• *Examination of carotid arteries (e.g., pulse amplitude, bruits)* • *Auscultation of heart with notation of abnormal sounds and murmurs* • *Examination of peripheral vascular system by observation (e.g., swelling, varicosities) and palpation (e.g., pulses, temperature, edema, tenderness)*
Chest (Breasts)	
Gastrointestinal (Abdomen)	
Genitourinary	
Lymphatic	

Musculoskeletal	• *Examination of gait and station* *Assessment of motor function including:* • *Muscle strength in upper and lower extremities* • *Muscle tone in upper and lower extremities (e.g., flaccid, cog wheel, spastic) with notation of any atrophy or abnormal movements (e.g., fasciculation, tardive dyskinesia)*
Extremities	*[See musculoskeletal]*
Skin	
Neurological/Psychiatric	*Evaluation of higher integrative functions including:* • *Orientation to time, place and person* • *Recent and remote memory* • *Attention span and concentration* • *Language (e.g., naming objects, repeating phrases, spontaneous speech)* • *Fund of knowledge (e.g., awareness of current events, past history, vocabulary)* *Test the following cranial nerves:* • *2nd cranial nerve (e.g., visual acuity, visual fields, fundi)* • *3rd, 4th and 6th cranial nerves (e.g., pupils, eye movements)* • *5th cranial nerve (e.g., facial sensation, corneal reflexes)* • *7th cranial nerve (e.g., facial symmetry, strength)* • *8th cranial nerve (e.g., hearing with tuning fork, whispered voice and/or finger rub)* • *9th cranial nerve (e.g., spontaneous or reflex palate movement)* *continued*

- *11th cranial nerve (e.g., shoulder shrug strength)*
- *12th cranial nerve (e.g., tongue protrusion)*
- *Examination of sensation (e.g., by touch, pin, vibration, proprioception)*
- *Examination of deep tendon reflexes in upper and lower extremities with notation of pathological reflexes (e.g., Babinski)*
- *Test coordination (e.g., finger/nose, heel/knee/shin, rapid alternating movements in the upper and lower extremities, evaluation of fine motor coordination in young children)*

CONTENT AND DOCUMENTATION REQUIREMENTS

Level of Exam	***Perform and Document:***
Problem Focused	*One to five elements identified by a bullet.*
Expanded Problem Focused	*At least six elements identified by a bullet.*
Detailed	*At least twelve elements identified by a bullet.*
Comprehensive	*Perform all elements identified by a bullet; document every element in each box with a shaded border and at least one element in each box with an unshaded border.*

PSYCHIATRIC EXAMINATION

SYSTEM/BODY AREA	*ELEMENTS OF EXAMINATION*
Constitutional	• *Measurement of any three of the following seven vital signs: 1) sitting or standing blood pressure, 2) supine blood pressure, 3) pulse rate and regularity, 4) respiration, 5) temperature, 6) height, 7) weight (May be measured and recorded by ancillary staff)* • *General appearance of patient (e.g., development, nutrition, body habitus, deformities, attention to grooming)*
Head and Face	
Eyes	
Ears, Nose, Mouth and Throat	
Neck	
Respiratory	
Cardiovascular	
Chest (Breasts)	
Gastrointestinal (Abdomen)	
Genitourinary	
Lymphatic	
Musculoskeletal	• *Assessment of muscle strength and tone (e.g., flaccid, cog wheel, spastic) with notation of any atrophy and abnormal movements* • *Examination of gait and station*
Extremities	
Skin	

Neurological

Psychiatric	• *Description of speech including: rate; volume; articulation; coherence; and spontaneity with notation of abnormalities (e.g., perseveration, paucity of language)* • *Description of thought processes including: rate of thoughts; content of thoughts (e.g., logical vs. illogical, tangential); abstract reasoning; and computation* • *Description of associations (e.g., loose, tangential, circumstantial, intact)* • *Description of abnormal or psychotic thoughts including: hallucinations; delusions; preoccupation with violence; homicidal or suicidal ideation; and obsessions* • *Description of the patient's judgment (e.g., concerning everyday activities and social situations) and insight (e.g., concerning psychiatric condition)* *Complete mental status examination including:* • *Orientation to time, place and person* • *Recent and remote memory* • *Attention span and concentration* • *Language (e.g., naming objects, repeating phrases)* • *Fund of knowledge (e.g., awareness of current events, past history, vocabulary)* • *Mood and affect (e.g., depression, anxiety, agitation, hypomania, lability)*

CONTENT AND DOCUMENTATION REQUIREMENTS

Level of Exam	***Perform and Document:***
Problem Focused	*One to five elements identified by a bullet.*
Expanded Problem Focused	*At least six elements identified by a bullet.*
Detailed	*At least nine elements identified by a bullet.*
Comprehensive	*Perform all elements identified by a bullet; document every element in each box with a shaded border and at least one element in each box with an unshaded border.*

RESPIRATORY EXAMINATION

SYSTEM/BODY AREA	*ELEMENTS OF EXAMINATION*
Constitutional	• *Measurement of any three of the following seven vital signs: 1) sitting or standing blood pressure, 2) supine blood pressure, 3) pulse rate and regularity, 4) respiration, 5) temperature, 6) height, 7) weight (May be measured and recorded by ancillary staff)* • *General appearance of patient (e.g., development, nutrition, body habitus, deformities, attention to grooming)*
Head and Face	
Eyes	
Ears, Nose, Mouth and Throat	• *Inspection of nasal mucosa, septum and turbinates* • *Inspection of teeth and gums* • *Examination of oropharynx (e.g., oral mucosa, hard and soft palates, tongue, tonsils and posterior pharynx)*
Neck	• *Examination of neck (e.g., masses, overall appearance, symmetry, tracheal position, crepitus)* • *Examination of thyroid (e.g., enlargement, tenderness, mass)* • *Examination of jugular veins (e.g., distension; a, v or cannon a waves)*
Respiratory	• *Inspection of chest with notation of symmetry and expansion* • *Assessment of respiratory effort (e.g., intercostal retractions, use of accessory muscles, diaphragmatic movement)* • *Percussion of chest (e.g., dullness, flatness, hyperresonance)* *continued*

	• *Palpation of chest (e.g., tactile fremitus)* • *Auscultation of lungs (e.g., breath sounds, adventitious sounds, rubs)*
Cardiovascular	• *Auscultation of heart including sounds, abnormal sounds and murmurs* • *Examination of peripheral vascular system by observation (e.g., swelling, varicosities) and palpation (e.g., pulses, temperature, edema, tenderness)*
Chest (Breasts)	
Gastrointestinal (Abdomen)	• *Examination of abdomen with notation of presence of masses or tenderness* • *Examination of liver and spleen*
Genitourinary	
Lymphatic	• *Palpation of lymph nodes in neck, axillae, groin and/or other location*
Musculoskeletal	• *Assessment of muscle strength and tone (e.g., flaccid, cog wheel, spastic) with notation of any atrophy and abnormal movements* • *Examination of gait and station*
Extremities	• *Inspection and palpation of digits and nails (e.g., clubbing, cyanosis, inflammation, petechiae, ischemia, infections, nodes)*
Skin	• *Inspection and/or palpation of skin and subcutaneous tissue (e.g., rashes, lesions, ulcers)*
Neurological/Psychiatric	*Brief assessment of mental status including:* • *Orientation to time, place and person* • *Mood and affect (e.g., depression, anxiety, agitation)*

CONTENT AND DOCUMENTATION REQUIREMENTS

Level of Exam	***Perform and Document:***
Problem Focused	*One to five elements identified by a bullet.*
Expanded Problem Focused	*At least six elements identified by a bullet.*
Detailed	*At least twelve elements identified by a bullet.*
Comprehensive	*Perform all elements identified by a bullet; document every element in each box with a shaded border and at least one element in each box with an unshaded border.*

SKIN EXAMINATION

SYSTEM/BODY AREA	*ELEMENTS OF EXAMINATION*
Constitutional	• *Measurement of any three of the following seven vital signs: 1) sitting or standing blood pressure, 2) supine blood pressure, 3) pulse rate and regularity, 4) respiration, 5) temperature, 6) height, 7) weight (May be measured and recorded by ancillary staff)* • *General appearance of patient (e.g., development, nutrition, body habitus, deformities, attention to grooming)*
Head and Face	
Eyes	• *Inspection of conjunctivae and lids*
Ears, Nose, Mouth and Throat	• *Inspection of lips, teeth and gums* • *Examination of oropharynx (e.g., oral mucosa, hard and soft palates, tongue, tonsils, posterior pharynx)*
Neck	• *Examination of thyroid (e.g., enlargement, tenderness, mass)*
Respiratory	
Cardiovascular	• *Examination of peripheral vascular system by observation (e.g., swelling, varicosities) and palpation (e.g., pulses, temperature, edema, tenderness)*
Chest (Breasts)	
Gastrointestinal (Abdomen)	• *Examination of liver and spleen* • *Examination of anus for condyloma and other lesions*
Genitourinary	

Lymphatic	• *Palpation of lymph nodes in neck, axillae, groin and/or other location*
Musculoskeletal	
Extremities	• *Inspection and palpation of digits and nails (e.g., clubbing, cyanosis, inflammation, petechiae, ischemia, infections, nodes)*
Skin	• *Palpation of scalp and inspection of hair of scalp, eyebrows, face, chest, pubic area (when indicated) and extremities* *Inspection and/or palpation of skin and subcutaneous tissue (e.g., rashes, lesions, ulcers, susceptibility to and presence of photo damage) in eight of the following ten areas:* • *Head, including the face and* • *Neck* • *Chest, including breasts and axillae* • *Abdomen* • *Genitalia, groin, buttocks* • *Back* • *Right upper extremity* • *Left upper extremity* • *Right lower extremity* • *Left lower extremity*

NOTE: For the comprehensive level, the examination of at least eight anatomic areas must be performed and documented. For the three lower levels of examination, each body area is counted separately. For example, inspection and/or palpation of the skin and subcutaneous tissue of the right upper extremity and the left upper extremity constitutes two elements.

• *Inspection of eccrine and apocrine glands of skin and subcutaneous tissue with identification and location of any hyperhidrosis, chromhidroses or bromhidrosis*

Neurological/Psychiatric	*Brief assessment of mental status including:* • *Orientation to time, place and person* • *Mood and affect (e.g., depression, anxiety, agitation)*

CONTENT AND DOCUMENTATION REQUIREMENTS

Level of Exam	***Perform and Document:***
Problem Focused	*One to five elements identified by a bullet.*
Expanded Problem Focused	*At least six elements identified by a bullet.*
Detailed	*At least twelve elements identified by a bullet.*
Comprehensive	*Perform all elements identified by a bullet; document every element in each box with a shaded border and at least one element in each box with an unshaded border.*

DOCUMENTATION OF THE COMPLEXITY OF MEDICAL DECISION MAKING

The levels of evaluation and management services recognize four types of medical decision making (straight-forward, low complexity, moderate complexity and high complexity). Medical decision making refers to the complexity of establishing a diagnosis and/or selecting a management option as measured by:

- the number of possible diagnoses and/or the number of management options that must be considered;
- the amount and/or complexity of medical records, diagnostic tests, and/or other information that must be obtained, reviewed and analyzed; and
- the risk of significant complications, morbidity and/or mortality, as well as comorbidities, associated with the patient's presenting problem(s), the diagnostic procedure(s) and/or the possible management options.

The following chart illustrates the progression of the elements required for each level of medical decision making. To qualify for a given type of decision making, two of the three elements in the table must be either met or exceeded.

NUMBER OF DIAGNOSES OR MANAGEMENT OPTIONS

The number of possible diagnoses and/or the number of management options that must be considered is based on the number and types of problems addressed during the encounter, the complexity of establishing a diagnosis and the management decisions that are made by the physician.

Generally, decision making with respect to a diagnosed problem is easier than that for an identified but undiagnosed problem. The number and type of diagnostic tests employed may be an indicator of the number of possible diagnoses. Problems which are improving or resolving are less complex than those which are worsening or failing to change as expected. The need to seek advice from others is another indicator of complexity of diagnostic or management problems.

•***DG:*** *For each encounter, an assessment, clinical impression, or diagnosis should be documented. It may be explicitly stated or implied in documented decisions regarding management plans and/or further evaluation.*

- *For a presenting problem with an established diagnosis, the record should reflect whether the problem is: a) improved, well controlled, resolving or resolved; or, b) inadequately controlled, worsening, or failing to change as expected.*
- *For a presenting problem without an established diagnosis, the assessment or clinical impression may be stated in the form of differential diagnoses or as a "possible", "probable", or "rule out" (R/O) diagnosis.*

Number of Diagnoses	Amount of Data to Review	Risk of Complication	Type of Decision Making
Minimal	*Minimal or None*	*Minimal*	***Straightforward***
Limited	*Limited*	*Low*	***Low Complexity***
Multiple	*Moderate*	*Moderate*	***Moderate Complexity***
Extensive	*Extensive*	*High*	***High Complexity***

Each of the elements of medical decision making is described below

•**DG:** *The initiation of, or changes in, treatment should be documented. Treatment includes a wide range of management options including patient instructions, nursing instructions, therapies, and medications.*

•**DG:** *If referrals are made, consultations requested or advice sought, the record should indicate to whom or where the referral or consultation is made or from whom the advice is requested.*

AMOUNT AND/OR COMPLEXITY OF DATA TO BE REVIEWED

The amount and complexity of data to be reviewed is based on the types of diagnostic testing ordered or reviewed. A decision to obtain and review old medical records and/or obtain history from sources other than the patient increases the amount and complexity of data to be reviewed.

Discussion of contradictory or unexpected test results with the physician who performed or interpreted the test is an indication of the complexity of data being reviewed. On occasion the physician who ordered a test may personally review the image, tracing or specimen to supplement information from the physician who prepared the test report or interpretation; this is another indication of the complexity of data being reviewed.

•**DG:** *If a diagnostic service (test or procedure) is ordered, planned, scheduled, or performed at the time of the evaluation and management encounter, the type of service, e.g., lab or x-ray, should be documented.*

•**DG:** *The review of lab, radiology and/or other diagnostic tests should be documented. A simple notation such as "WBC elevated" or "chest x-ray unremarkable" is acceptable. Alternatively, the review may be documented by initialing and dating the report containing the test results.*

•**DG:** *A decision to obtain old records or decision to obtain additional history from the family, caretaker or other source to supplement that obtained from the patient should be documented.*

•DG: *Relevant findings from the review of old records, and/or the receipt of additional history from the family, caretaker or other source to supplement that obtained from the patient should be documented. If there is no relevant information beyond that already obtained, that fact should be documented. A notation of "Old records reviewed" or "additional history obtained from family" without elaboration is insufficient.*

•DG: *The results of discussion of laboratory, radiology or other diagnostic tests with the physician who performed or interpreted the study should be documented.*

•DG: *The direct visualization and independent interpretation of an image, tracing or specimen previously or subsequently interpreted by another physician should be documented.*

RISK OF SIGNIFICANT COMPLICATIONS, MORBIDITY AND/OR MORTALITY

The risk of significant complications, morbidity, and/or mortality is based on the risks associated with the presenting problem(s), the diagnostic procedure(s), and the possible management options.

•DG: *Comorbidities/underlying diseases or other factors that increase the complexity of medical decision making by increasing the risk of complications, morbidity, and/or mortality should be documented.*

•DG: *If a surgical or invasive diagnostic procedure is ordered, planned or scheduled at the time of the evaluation and management encounter, the type of procedure, e.g., laparoscopy, should be documented.*

•DG: *If a surgical or invasive diagnostic procedure is performed at the time of the evaluation and management encounter, the specific procedure should be documented.*

•DG: *The referral for or decision to perform a surgical or invasive diagnostic procedure on an urgent basis should be documented or implied.*

The Table of Risk on the following page may be used to help determine whether the risk of significant complications, morbidity, and/or mortality is minimal, low, moderate, or high. Because the determination of risk is complex and not readily quantifiable, the table includes common clinical examples rather than absolute measures of risk. The assessment of risk of the presenting problem(s) is based on the risk related to the disease process anticipated between the present encounter and the next one. The assessment of risk of selecting diagnostic procedures and management options is based on the risk during and immediately following any procedures or treatment. The highest level of risk in any one category (presenting problem(s), diagnostic procedure(s), or management options) determines the overall risk.

DOCUMENTATION OF AN ENCOUNTER DOMINATED BY COUNSELING OR COORDINATION OF CARE

In the case where counseling and/or coordination of care dominates (more than 50%) of the physician/patient and/or family encounter (face-to-face time in the office or other or outpatient setting, floor/unit time in the hospital or nursing facility), time is considered the key or controlling factor to qualify for a particular level of evaluation and management services.

•DG: *If the physician elects to report the level of service based on counseling and/or coordination of care, the total length of time of the encounter (face-to-face or floor time, as appropriate) should be documented and the record should describe the counseling and/or activities to coordinate care.*

TABLE OF RISK

LEVEL OF RISK	*PRESENTING PROBLEM(S)*	*DIAGNOSTIC PROCEDURES*	*MANAGEMENT OPTIONS*
Minimal	• *One self-limited or minor problem, (eg, cold, insect bite, tinea corporis)*	• *Laboratory tests requiring venipuncture* • *Chest x-rays* • *EKG/EEG* • *Urinalysis* • *Ultrasound, (eg, echocardiography)* • *KOH prep*	• *Rest* • *Gargles* • *Elastic bandages* • *Superficial dressings*
Low	• *Two or more self-limited or minor problems* • *One stable chronic illness, (eg, well controlled hypertension, non-insulin dependent diabetes, cataract, BPH)* • *Acute uncomplicated illness or injury, (eg, cystitis, allergic rhinitis, simple sprain)*	• *Physiologic tests not under stress, (eg, pulmonary function tests)* • *Non-cardiovascular imaging studies with contrast,(eg, barium enema)* • *Superficial needle biopsies* • *Clinical laboratory tests requiring arterial puncture* • *Skin biopsies*	• *Over-the-counter drugs* • *Minor surgery with no identified risk factors* • *Physical therapy* • *Occupational therapy* • *IV fluids without additives*

continued

TABLE OF RISK (continued)

LEVEL OF RISK	PRESENTING PROBLEM(S)	DIAGNOSTIC PROCEDURES	MANAGEMENT OPTIONS
Moderate	• *One or more chronic illnesses with mild exacerbation, progression, or side effects of treatment* • *Two or more stable chronic illnesses* • *Undiagnosed new problem with uncertain prognosis, (eg, lump in breast)* • *Acute illness with systemic symptoms, (eg, pyelonephritis, pneumonitis, colitis)* • *Acute complicated injury, (eg, head injury with brief loss of consciousness)*	• *Physiologic tests under stress, (eg, cardiac stress test, fetal contraction stress test)* • *Diagnostic endoscopies with no identified risk factors* • *Deep needle or incisional biopsy* • *Cardiovascular imaging studies with contrast and no identified risk factors, (eg, arteriogram, cardiac catheterization)* • *Obtain fluid from body cavity, (eg, lumbar puncture, thoracentesis, culdocentesis)*	• *Minor surgery with identified risk factors* • *Elective major surgery (open, percutaneous or endoscopic) with no identified risk factors* • *Prescription drug management* • *Therapeutic nuclear medicine* • *IV fluids with additives* • *Closed treatment of fracture or dislocation without manipulation*
High	• *One or more chronic illnesses with severe exacerbation, progression, or side effects of treatment* • *Acute or chronic illnesses or injuries that pose a threat to life or bodily function, (eg, multiple trauma, acute MI, pulmonary embolus, severe respiratory distress, progressive severe rheumatoid arthritis, psychiatric illness with potential threat to self or others, peritonitis, acute renal failure)* • *An abrupt change in neurologic status, (eg, seizure, TIA, weakness, sensory loss)*	• *Cardiovascular imaging studies with contrast with identified risk factors* • *Cardiac electrophysiological tests* • *Diagnostic endoscopies with identified risk factors* • *Discography*	• *Elective major surgery (open, percutaneous or endoscopic) with identified risk factors* • *Emergency major surgery (open, percutaneous or endoscopic)* • *Parenteral controlled substances* • *Drug therapy requiring intensive monitoring for toxicity* • *Decision not to resuscitate or to de-escalate care because of poor prognosis*

This page intentionally left blank.

EVALUATION AND MANAGEMENT

E/M 99200

OFFICE OR OTHER OUTPATIENT SERVICES

The following codes are used to report E./M services provided to new and established patients in the office or other outpatient facility, including the emergency department when the physician is not assigned to the emergency department. The key coding issues are the extent of history obtained, the extent of examination performed, and the complexity of medical decision making. Additional reporting issues include counseling and/or coordination of care, the nature of presenting problem(s), and the duration of face-to-face time spent with the patient and/or family.

To report services provided to a patient who is admitted to a hospital or nursing facility in the course of an encounter in the office or other ambulatory facility, see the notes for initial hospital inpatient care in the Hospital Inpatient Services section below or initial nursing facility care in the Nursing Facility Services section.

CODING RULES

1. *A patient is considered an outpatient until admitted as an inpatient to a health care facility.*

2. *If outpatient evaluation and management services are provided in conjunction with, or result in, an inpatient admission, the service is reported using CPT codes for initial hospital care.*

3. *CPT codes in this section may also be used to report the services provided by a physician to a patient in an observation area of a hospital.*

4. *Laboratory tests, radiology services, and diagnostic or therapeutic procedures performed in conjunction with evaluation and management services are reported in addition to the basic evaluation and management service.*

5. *Supplies and materials provided by the physician over and above those usually included with the evaluation and management or other services rendered may be listed separately. List all drugs, trays, supplies and materials provided.*

Separate Procedure | Unlisted Procedure | 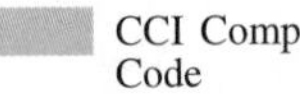 CCI Comp. Code | 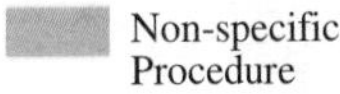 Non-specific Procedure

NEW PATIENT

99201 Office or other outpatient visit for the evaluation and management of a new patient, which requires these three key components:

- a problem focused history;
- a problem focused examination; and
- straightforward medical decision making.

Counseling and/or coordination of care with other providers or agencies are provided consistent with the nature of the problem(s) and the patient's and/or family's needs.

Usually, the presenting problems are self limited or minor. Physicians typically spend 10 minutes face-to-face with the patient and/or family.

99202 Office or other outpatient visit for the evaluation and management of a new patient, which requires these three key components:

- an expanded problem focused history;
- an expanded problem focused examination; and
- straightforward medical decision making.

Counseling and/or coordination of care with other providers or agencies are provided consistent with the nature of the problem(s) and the patient's and/or family's needs.

Usually, the presenting problem(s) are of low to moderate severity. Physicians typically spend 20 minutes face-to-face with the patient and/or family.

99203 Office or other outpatient visit for the evaluation and management of a new patient, which requires these three key components:

- a detailed history;
- a detailed examination; and
- medical decision making of low complexity.

Counseling and/or coordination of care with other providers or agencies are provided consistent with the nature of the problem(s) and the patient's and/or family's needs.

Usually, the presenting problem(s) are of moderate severity. Physicians typically spend 30 minutes face-to-face with the patient and/or family.

99204 Office or other outpatient visit for the evaluation and management of a new patient, which requires these three key components:

- a comprehensive history;
- a comprehensive examination; and
- medical decision making of moderate complexity.

Counseling and/or coordination of care with other providers or agencies are provided consistent with the nature of the problem(s) and the patient's and/or family's needs.

Usually, the presenting problem(s) are of moderate to high severity. Physicians typically spend 45 minutes face-to-face with the patient and/or family.

99205 Office or other outpatient visit for the evaluation and management of a new patient, which requires these three key components:

- a comprehensive history;
- a comprehensive examination; and
- medical decision making of high complexity.

Counseling and/or coordination of care with other providers or agencies are provided consistent with the nature of the problem(s) and the patient's and/or family's needs.

Usually, the presenting problem(s) are of moderate to high severity. Physicians typically spend 60 minutes face-to-face with the patient and/or family.

ESTABLISHED PATIENT

99211 Office or other outpatient visit for the evaluation and management of an established patient, that may not require the presence of a physician. Usually, the presenting problem(s) are minimal. Typically, 5 minutes are spent performing or supervising these services.

99212 Office or other outpatient visit for the evaluation and management of an established patient, which requires at least two of these three key components:

- a problem focused history;
- a problem focused examination;
- straightforward medical decision making.

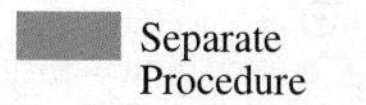
Separate Procedure

Unlisted Procedure

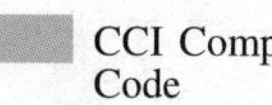
CCI Comp. Code

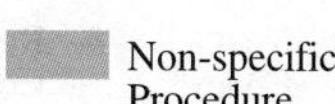
Non-specific Procedure

Counseling and/or coordination of care with other providers or agencies are provided consistent with the nature of the problem(s) and the patient's and/or family's needs.

Usually, the presenting problem(s) are self limited or minor. Physicians typically 10 minutes face-to-face with the patient and/or family.

99213 Office or other outpatient visit for the evaluation and management of an established patient, which requires at least two of these three key components:

- an expanded problem focused history;
- an expanded problem focused examination;
- medical decision making of low complexity.

Counseling and coordination of care with other providers or agencies are provided consistent with the nature of the problem(s) and the patient's and/or family's needs.

Usually, the presenting problem(s) are of low to moderate severity. Physicians typically spend 15 minutes face-to-face with the patient and/or family.

99214 Office or other outpatient visit for the evaluation and management of an established patient, which requires at least two of these three key components:

- a detailed history;
- a detailed examination;
- medical decision making of moderate complexity.

Counseling and/or coordination of care with other providers or agencies are provided consistent with the nature of the problem(s) and the patient's and/or family's needs.

Usually, the presenting problem(s) are of moderate to high severity. Physicians typically spend 25 minutes face-to-face with the patient and/or family.

99215 Office or other outpatient visit for the evaluation and management of an established patient, which requires at least two of these three key components:

- a comprehensive history;
- a comprehensive examination;
- medical decision making of high complexity.

Counseling and/or coordination of care with other providers or agencies are provided consistent with the nature of the problem(s) and the patient's and/or family's needs.

Usually, the presenting problem(s) are of moderate to high severity. Physicians typically spend 40 minutes face-to-face with the patient and/or family.

HOSPITAL OBSERVATION SERVICES

Occasionally a physician will watch or "observe" a patient in an area of an inpatient hospital designated as an "observation" area. This area is frequently located in or near the emergency room, and the observation typically after any acute care is rendered.

The purpose of the observation is to determine if the patient's condition requires inpatient hospitalization. Patients considered under observation status may be discharged from the observation area or admitted to the hospital as an inpatient.

All observation care services are "per day" and should be coded only once per date of service. CPT code 99217 is used to report all services provided on discharge from "observation status" if the discharge is on other than the initial date of "observation status."

OBSERVATION CARE DISCHARGE SERVICES

Observation care discharge of a patient from "observation status" includes final examination of the patient, discussion of the hospital stay, instructions for continuing care, and preparation of dishcarge records. For observation or inpatient hospital care including the admission and discharge of the patient on the same date, see codes 99234-99236 as appropriate.

99217 Observation care discharge day management (This code is to be utilized by the physician to report all services provided to a patient on discharge from "observation status" if the discharge is on other than the initial date of "observation status." To report services to a patient designated as "observation status" or "inpatient status" and discharged on the same date, use codes for Observation or Inpatient Care Services [including Admission and Discharge Services, 99234-99236 as appropriate]).

discharge

INITIAL OBSERVATION CARE

NEW OR ESTABLISHED PATIENT

The following codes are used to report the encounter(s) by the supervising physician with the patient when designated as "observation status." This refers to the initiation of observation status, supervision of the care plan for observation, and

Separate Procedure | Unlisted Procedure | CCI Comp. Code | Non-specific Procedure

performance of periodic reassessments. For observation encounters by other physicians, see Office or Other Outpatient Consultation codes (99241-99245).

99218 Initial observation care, per day, for the evaluation and management of a patient which requires these three key components:

- a detailed or comprehensive history;
- a detailed or comprehensive examination; and
- medical decision making that is straightforward or of low complexity.

Counseling and/or coordination of care with other providers or agencies are provided consistent with the nature of the problem(s) and the patient's and/or family's needs.

Usually, the problem(s) requiring admission to "observation status" are of low severity.

99219 Initial observation care, per day, for the evaluation and management of a patient, which requires these three key components:

- a comprehensive history;
- a comprehensive examination; and
- medical decision making of moderate complexity.

Counseling and/or coordination of care with other providers or agencies are provided consistent with the nature of the problem(s) and the patient's and/or family's needs.

Usually, the problem(s) requiring admission to "observation status" are of moderate severity.

99220 Initial observation care, per day, for the evaluation and management of a patient, which requires these three key components:

- a comprehensive history;
- a comprehensive examination; and
- medical decision making of high complexity.

Counseling and/or coordination of care with other providers or agencies are provided consistent with the nature of the problem(s) and the patient's and/or family's needs.

Usually, the problem(s) requiring admission to "observation status" are of high severity.

HOSPITAL INPATIENT SERVICES

Hospital inpatient services refer to hospital visits during the course of an inpatient hospital stay. The services may be provided by the patient's primary physician and/or other physicians in the event of multiple illnesses or injuries. Evaluation and management codes 99221-99239 are used to report services provided in the hospital. The key coding issues are the extent of history obtained, the extent of examination performed, and the complexity of medical decision making. Additional reporting issues include counseling and/or coordination of care, the nature of presenting problem(s), and the time spent at the bedside and on the patient's facility floor or unit.

CODING RULES

1. *CPT codes defined as Initial Hospital Care are used to report the first hospital inpatient encounter with the patient by the admitting physician.*

2. *The admitting physician should report all service related to the admission provided in all other locations.*

3. *For observation care or inpatient hospital care services provided to patients who are admitted and discharged on the same date, report with CPT codes 99234-99236 from the Observation or Inpatient Care services subsections.*

INITIAL HOSPITAL CARE

NEW OR ESTABLISHED PATIENT

The following codes are used to report the first hospital inpatient encounter with the patient by the admitting physician. For initial inpatient encounters by physicians other than the admitting physician, see initial inpatient consultation codes (99251-99255) or subsequent hospital care codes (99231-99233) as appropriate.

99221 Initial hospital care, per day, for the evaluation and management of a patient which requires these three key components:

- a detailed or comprehensive history;
- a detailed or comprehensive examination; and
- medical decision making that is straightforward or of low complexity.

Counseling and/or coordination of care with other providers or agencies are provided consistent with the nature of the problem(s) and the patient's and/or family's needs.

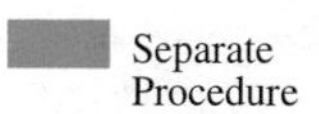 Separate Procedure 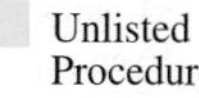 Unlisted Procedure 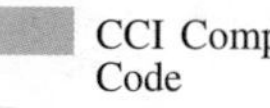 CCI Comp. Code 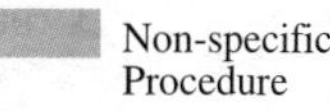 Non-specific Procedure

Usually, the problem(s) requiring admission are of low severity. Physicians typically spend 30 minutes at the bedside and on the patient's hospital floor or unit.

99222 Initial hospital care, per day, for the evaluation and management of a patient, which requires these three key components:

- a comprehensive history;
- a comprehensive examination; and
- medical decision making of moderate complexity.

Counseling and/or coordination of care with other providers or agencies are provided consistent with the nature of the problem(s) and the patient's and/or family's needs.

Usually, the problem(s) requiring admission are of moderate severity. Physicians typically spend 50 minutes at the bedside and on the patient's hospital floor or unit.

99223 Initial hospital care, per day, for the evaluation and management of a patient, which requires these three key components:

- a comprehensive history;
- a comprehensive examination; and
- medical decision making of high complexity.

Counseling and/or coordination of care with other providers or agencies are provided consistent with the nature of the problem(s) and the patient's and/or family's needs.

Usually, the problem(s) requiring admission are of high severity. Physicians typically spend 70 minutes at the bedside and on the patient's hospital floor or unit.

SUBSEQUENT HOSPITAL CARE – follow up subsequent inpatient

All levels of subsequent hospital care include reviewing the medical record and reviewing the results of diagnostic studies and changes in the patient's status (i.e., changes in history, physical condition and response to management) since the last assessment by the physician.

99231 Subsequent hospital care, per day, for the evaluation and management of a patient, which requires at least two of these three key components:

- a problem focused interval history;
- a problem focused examination;

- medical decision making that is straightforward or of low complexity.

Counseling and/or coordination of care with other providers or agencies are provided consistent with the nature of the problem(s) and the patient's and/or family's needs.

Usually, the patient is stable, recovering or improving. Physicians typically spend 15 minutes at the bedside and on the patient's hospital floor or unit.

99232 Subsequent hospital care, per day, for the evaluation and management of a patient, which requires at least two of these three key components:

- an expanded problem focused interval history;
- an expanded problem focused examination;
- medical decision making of moderate complexity.

Counseling and/or coordination of care with other providers or agencies are provided consistent with the nature of the problem(s) and the patient's and/or family's needs.

Usually, the patient is responding inadequately to therapy or has developed a minor complication. Physicians typically spend 25 minutes at the bedside and on the patient's hospital floor or unit.

99233 Subsequent hospital care, per day, for the evaluation and management of a patient, which requires at least two of these three key components:

- a detailed interval history;
- a detailed examination;
- medical decision making of high complexity.

Counseling and/or coordination of care with other providers or agencies are provided consistent with the nature of the problem(s) and the patient's and/or family's needs.

Usually, the patient is unstable or has developed a significant complication or a significant new problem. Physicians typically spend 35 minutes at the bedside and on the patient's hospital floor or unit.

OBSERVATION OR INPATIENT CARE SERVICES (INCLUDING ADMISSION AND DISCHARGE SERVICES)

The following codes are used to report observation or inpatient hospital care services provided to patients admitted and discharged on the same date of sevice. Then a patient is admitted to the hospital from observation status on the same date, the physician should report only the initial hospital care code. The initial hospital care code reported by the admitting physician should include the services related to the observation status services he/she provided on the same date of inpatient admission.

For patients admitted to observation or inpatient care and discharged on a different date, see codes 99218-99220 and 99217, or 99221-99223 and 99238, 99239.

99234 Observation or inpatient hospital care, for the evaluation and management of a patient including admission and discharge on the same date which requires these three key components:

- a detailed or comprehensive history;
- a detailed or comprehensive examination; and
- medical decision making that is straightforward or of low complexity.

Counseling and/or coordination of care with other providers or agencies are provided consistent with the nature of the problem(s) and the patient's and/or family's needs.

Usually the presenting problem(s) requiring admission are of low severity.

99235 Observation or inpatient hospital care, for the evaluation and management of a patient including admission and discharge on the same date which requires these three key components:

- a comprehensive history;
- a comprehensive examination; and
- medical decision making of moderate complexity.

Counseling and/or coordination of care with other providers or agencies are provided consistent with the nature of the problem(s) and the patient's and/or family's needs.

Usually the presenting problem(s) requiring admission are of moderate severity.

99236 Observation or inpatient hospital care, for the evaluation and management of a patient including admission and discharge on the same date which requires these three key components:

- a comprehensive history;

- a comprehensive examination; and
- medical decision making of high complexity.

Counseling and/or coordination of care with other providers or agencies are provided consistent with the nature of the problem(s) and the patient's and/or family's needs.

Usually the presenting problem(s) requiring admission are of high severity.

HOSPITAL DISCHARGE SERVICES

99238 Hospital discharge day management; 30 minutes or less

99239 Hospital discharge day management; more than 30 minutes

(These codes are to be utilized by the physician to report all services provided to a patient on the date of discharge, if other than the initial date of inpatient status. To report services to a patient who is admitted as an inpatient, and discharged on the same date, see codes 99234-99236 for observation or inpatient hospital care including the admission and discharge of the patient on the same date. To report concurrent care services provided by a physician(s) other than the attending physician, use subsequent hospital care codes (99231-99233) on the day of discharge.)

(For Observation Care Discharge, use 99217)

(For observation or inpatient hospital care including the admission and discharge of the patient on the same date, see 99234-99236)

(For Nursing Facility Care Discharge, 99315, 99316)

(For discharge services provided to newborns admitted and discharged on the same date, use 99435)

CONSULTATIONS

- medicare don't use.

A consultation is the process of taking a history, performing a physical examination, and ordering and interpreting appropriate diagnostic tests, for the purpose of rendering an expert opinion about a patient's illness and/or injury.

A consultation may be requested by a patient's primary physician, by the patient or by a third party, such as a review organization.

The key coding issues are the location of the service, the extent of history obtained, the extent of examination performed, and the complexity of medical decision making. Additional reporting issues include counseling and/or coordination of care, the nature of presenting problem(s), and the time, depending on location, spent either face-to-face with the patient and/or family or at the bedside and on the patient's facility floor or unit.

A "consultation" initiated by a patient and/or family, and not requested by a physician or other appropriate source, is not reported using the consultation codes by may be reported using the office visit, home service, or domiciliary/rest home care codes, as appropriate.

If a consultation is mandated, eg, by a third-party payer, modifier 32 should also be reported.

CODING RULES

1. *The request for a consultation from the attending physician or other appropriate source, and the need for a consultation must be documented in the patient's medical record.*

2. *The consulting physician must document all services provided and the resulting opinion in the patient's medical record.*

3. *Modifier -32 must be added to the consulting service CPT code if a confirmatory consultation is required by a third party, such as a PRO.*

4. *If the consulting physician assumes responsibility for the continuing care of the patient, the service is no longer considered a consultation, and any subsequent visit services rendered are coded using evaluation and management codes.*

OFFICE OR OTHER OUTPATIENT CONSULTATIONS

NEW OR ESTABLISHED PATIENT

99241 Office consultation for a new or established patient, which requires these three key components:

- a problem focused history;
- a problem focused examination; and
- straightforward medical decision making.

Counseling and/or coordination of care with other providers or agencies are provided consistent with the nature of the problem(s) and the patient's and/or family's needs.

Usually, the presenting problem(s) are self limited or minor. Physicians typically spend 15 minutes face-to-face with the patient and/or family.

99242 Office consultation for a new or established patient, which requires these three key components:

- an expanded problem focused history;
- an expanded problem focused examination; and
- straightforward medical decision making.

Counseling and/or coordination of care with other providers or agencies are provided consistent with the nature of the problem(s) and the patient's and/or family's needs.

Usually, the presenting problem(s) are of low severity. Physicians typically spend 30 minutes face-to-face with the patient and/or family.

99243 Office consultation for a new or established patient, which requires these three key components:

- a detailed history;
- a detailed examination; and
- medical decision making of low complexity.

Counseling and/or coordination of care with other providers or agencies are provided consistent with the nature of the problem(s) and the patient's and/or family's needs.

Usually, the presenting problem(s) are of moderate severity. Physicians typically spend 40 minutes face-to-face with the patient and/or family.

99244 Office consultation for a new or established patient, which requires these three key components:

- a comprehensive history;
- a comprehensive examination; and
- medical decision making of moderate complexity.

Counseling and/or coordination of care with other providers or agencies are provided consistent with the nature of the problem(s) and the patient's and/or family's needs.

Usually, the presenting problem(s) are of moderate to high severity. Physicians typically spend 60 minutes face-to-face with the patient and/or family.

99245 Office consultation for a new or established patient, which requires these three key components:

- a comprehensive history;
- a comprehensive examination; and
- medical decision making of high complexity.

Counseling and/or coordination of care with other providers or agencies are provided consistent with the nature of the problem(s) and the patient's and/or family's needs.

Usually, the presenting problem(s) are of moderate to high severity. Physicians typically spend 80 minutes face-to-face with the patient and/or family.

INPATIENT CONSULTATIONS hospital

NEW OR ESTABLISHED PATIENT

The following CPT codes are used to report physician consultations provided to hospital inpatients, residents of nursing facilities, or patients in a partial hospital setting. Only one consultation should be reported by a consultant per admission. Subsequent services during the same admission are reported using Subsequent Hospital Care codes (99231-99233) or Subsequent Nursing Facility Care codes (99307-99310), including services to complete the initial consultation, monitor progress, revise recommendations, or address new problems.

▲ **99251** Inpatient consultation for a new or established patient, which requires these three key components:

- a problem focused history;
- a problem focused examination; and
- straightforward medical decision making.

Counseling and/or coordination of care with other providers or agencies are provided consistent with the nature of the problem(s) and the patient's and/or family's needs.

Usually, the presenting problem(s) are self limited or minor. Physicians typically spend 20 minutes at the bedside and on the patient's hospital floor or unit.

▲ **99252** Inpatient consultation for a new or established patient, which requires these three key components:

- an expanded problem focused history;
- an expanded problem focused examination; and
- straightforward medical decision making.

● New Code ▲ Revised Code + Add-On Code ⃠ Modifier -51 Exempt ⊙ Conscious Sedation

Counseling and/or coordination of care with other providers or agencies are provided consistent with the nature of the problem(s) and the patient's and/or family's needs.

Usually, the presenting problem(s) are of low severity. Physicians typically spend 40 minutes at the bedside and on the patient's hospital floor or unit.

▲ **99253** Inpatient consultation for a new or established patient, which requires these three key components:

- a detailed history;
- a detailed examination; and
- medical decision making of low complexity.

Counseling and/or coordination of care with other providers or agencies are provided consistent with the nature of the problem(s) and the patient's and/or family's needs.

Usually, the presenting problem(s) are of moderate severity. Physicians typically spend 55 minutes at the bedside and on the patient's hospital floor or unit.

▲ **99254** Inpatient consultation for a new or established patient, which requires three key components:

- a comprehensive history;
- a comprehensive examination; and
- medical decision making of moderate complexity.

Counseling and/or coordination of care with other providers or agencies are provided consistent with the nature of the problem(s) and the patient's and/or family's needs.

Usually, the presenting problem(s) are of moderate to high severity. Physicians typically spend 80 minutes at the bedside and on the patient's hospital floor or unit.

▲ **99255** Inpatient consultation for a new or established patient, which requires these three key components:

- a comprehensive history;
- a comprehensive examination; and
- medical decision making of high complexity.

Counseling and/or coordination of care with other providers or agencies are provided consistent with the nature of the problem(s) and the patient's and/or family's needs.

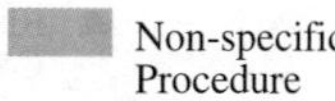

Usually, the presenting problem(s) are of moderate to high severity. Physicians typically spend 110 minutes at the bedside and on the patient's hospital floor or unit.

EMERGENCY DEPARTMENT SERVICES

Does not inpatient

Evaluation and management codes 99281-99288 are used to report services provided to new or established patients in the emergency department. The emergency department is defined as a facility for the treatment of patients with emergent conditions. The emergency department must be attached to a hospital and operate on a 24/7 basis.

The key coding issues for evaluation and management emergency services are the extent of history obtained, the extent of examination performed, and the complexity of medical decision making. Additional reporting issues include counseling and/or coordination of care, and the nature of presenting problem(s).

Time is not a descriptive component for evaluation and management services provided in the emergency department. These services are typically provided on a variable intensity basis, often involving multiple encounters with several patients over an extended period of time. Therefore, it is difficult for physicians to provide accurate estimates of the time spent face-to-face with the patient in the emergency department.

CODING RULES

1. *No distinction is made between new and established patients in the emergency department.*

2. *If the emergency department is used for observation or inpatient care services, report using codes from the Observation Care services subsection of the CPT coding system.*

3. *For critical care services provided in the emergency department, use the appropriate codes from the Critical Care subsection of the CPT coding system.*

EMERGENCY DEPARTMENT SERVICES

NEW OR ESTABLISHED PATIENT

(99261 deleted 2006 edition. To report, see 99231-99233, 99307-99310)

(99262 deleted 2006 edition. To report, see 99231-99233, 99307-99310)

(99263 deleted 2006 edition. To report, see 99231-99233, 99307-99310)

● New Code ▲ Revised Code + Add-On Code ⊘ Modifier -51 Exempt ⊙ Conscious Sedation

(99271 deleted 2006 edition. To report, see the appropriate E/M service code for the setting and type of service (eg, consultation))

(99272 deleted 2006 edition. To report, see the appropriate E/M service code for the setting and type of service (eg, consultation))

(99273 deleted 2006 edition. To report, see the appropriate E/M service code for the setting and type of service (eg, consultation))

(99274 deleted 2006 edition. To report, see the appropriate E/M service code for the setting and type of service (eg, consultation))

(99275 deleted 2006 edition. To report, see the appropriate E/M service code for the setting and type of service (eg, consultation))

99281 Emergency department visit for the evaluation and management of a patient, which requires these three key components:

- a problem focused history;
- a problem focused examination; and
- straightforward medical decision making.

Counseling and/or coordination of care with other providers or agencies are provided consistent with the nature of the problem(s) and the patient's and/or family's needs.

Usually, the presenting problem(s) are self limited or minor.

99282 Emergency department visit for the evaluation and management of a patient, which requires these three key components:

- an expanded problem focused history;
- an expanded problem focused examination; and
- medical decision making of low complexity.

Counseling and/or coordination of care with other providers or agencies are provided consistent with the nature of the problem(s) and the patient's and/or family's needs.

Usually, the presenting problem(s) are of low to moderate severity.

99283 Emergency department visit for the evaluation and management of a patient, which requires these three key components:

- an expanded problem focused history;
- an expanded problem focused examination; and
- medical decision making of moderate complexity.

Separate Procedure | Unlisted Procedure | CCI Comp. Code | Non-specific Procedure

Counseling and/or coordination of care with other providers or agencies are provided consistent with the nature of the problem(s) and the patient's and/or family's needs.

Usually, the presenting problem(s) are of moderate severity.

99284 Emergency department visit for the evaluation and management of a patient, which requires these three key components:

- a detailed history;
- a detailed examination; and
- medical decision making of moderate complexity.

Counseling and/or coordination of care with other providers or agencies are provided consistent with the nature of the problem(s) and the patient's and/or family's needs.

Usually, the presenting problem(s) are of high severity, and require urgent evaluation by the physician but do not pose an immediate significant threat to life or physiologic function.

99285 Emergency department visit for the evaluation and management of a patient, which requires these three key components within the constraints imposed by the urgency of the patient's clinical condition and/or mental status:

- a comprehensive history;
- a comprehensive examination; and
- medical decision making of high complexity.

Counseling and/or coordination of care with other providers or agencies are provided consistent with the nature of the problem(s) and the patient's and/or family's needs.

Usually, the presenting problem(s) are of high severity and pose an immediate significant threat to life or physiologic function.

OTHER EMERGENCY SERVICES

99288 Physician direction of emergency medical systems (EMS) emergency care, advanced life support

PEDIATRIC CRITICAL CARE PATIENT TRANSPORT

The following codes 99289 and 99290 are used to report the physical attendance and direct fact-to-face care by a physician during the interfacility transport of a critically ill or critically injured pediatric patient. For the purpose of reporting codes 99298 and 99290, face-to-face care begins when the physician assumes primary responsibility of the pediatric patient at the referring hospital/facility, and ends when the receiving hospital/facility accepts responsibility for the pediatric patient's care.

99289 Critical care services delivered by a physician, face-to-face, during an interfacility transport of critically ill or critically injured pediatric patient, 24 months of age or less; first 30-74 minutes of hands on care during transport

\+ **99290** each additional 30 minutes (List separately in addition to code for primary service)

(Use 99290 in conjunction with 99289)

(Critical care of less than 30 minutes total duration should be reported with the appropriate E/M code)

CRITICAL CARE SERVICES

Critical care includes the care of critically ill patients in a variety of medical emergencies that requires the constant attention of the physician. Cardiac arrest, shock, bleeding, respiratory failure, postoperative complications, or a critically ill neonate are examples of medical emergencies defined in CPT. Critical care is usually, but not always, given in a critical area, such as the coronary care unit, intensive care unit, respiratory care unit, or the emergency care facility.

CPT codes listed in this section are intended to include cardiopulmonary resuscitation (CPR) and the variety of services commonly employed with this procedure as well as other acute emergency situations. Other services, such as catheter placement, cardiac output measurement, dialysis management, control of gastrointestinal hemorrhage, cardioversion, etc. are considered to be included when reporting critical care services under these time-based CPT codes.

Evaluation and management codes 99291-99292 are used to report services for specific conditions (usually) provided in a critical care area. Key coding issues include the condition of the patient (supported by diagnostic coding), the service(s) provided, and the amount of time spent. Follow-up critical care services may be reported using either evaluation and management codes from this section or hospital evaluation and management codes from the series 99231-99233.

CODING RULES

1. *The critical care CPT codes are used to report the total duration of time spent by a physician providing constant attention to a critically ill patient.*

2. *Critical care code 99291 is used to report the first hour of critical care on a given day. It may be reported only once per day even if the time spent is not continuous on that day.*

3. *Critical care 99292 is used to report each additional 30 minutes beyond the first hour.*

4. *Other procedures which are not considered included in the critical care services, for example, suturing of lacerations, setting of fractures, reduction of joint dislocations, lumbar puncture, peritoneal lavage and bladder tap, are reported separately.*

CORRECT CODING CHART FOR CRITICAL CARE SERVICES base on time

DURATION OF CRITICAL CARE	CODE(S) TO REPORT
less than 30 minutes	appropriate E/M codes
30- 74 minutes	99291 once
75-104 minutes	99291 once and 99292 once
105-134 minutes	99291 once and 99292 twice
135-164 minutes	99291 once and 99292 three times
165-194 minutes	99291 once and 99292 four times
194 minutes or longer	99291 and 99292 as appropriate (see illustrated reporting examples above)

CRITICAL CARE SERVICES

99291 Critical care, evaluation and management of the critically ill or critically injured patient; first 30-74 minutes

+ **99292** each additional 30 minutes (List separately in addition to code for primary service)

(Use 99292 in conjunction with 99291)

INPATIENT NEONATAL AND PEDIATRIC CRITICAL CARE SERVICES

Neonatal intensive care refers to services, including management, monitoring and treatment, provided to a critically ill newborn or infant, usually in the neonatal intensive care unit (NICU). Counseling of parents, case management services and personal direct supervision of the NICU team are bundled into these codes.

CODING RULES

1. *Neonatal intensive care services start with the date of admission and are coded only once per day, per patient.*

2. *Once the neonate is no longer considered to be critically ill, report with CPT codes for subsequent hospital care instead of neonatal intensive care.*

3. *Neonatal intensive care CPT codes are coded in addition to physician stand-by code 99360 or newborn resuscitation code 99440 when the physician is present for the delivery and newborn resuscitation is required.*

4. *Procedures which are routinely performed as part of NICU care are included in the bundled NICU codes. These routine procedures include: venous/arterial catheterization, bladder catheterization, intubation, lumbar puncture, mechanical ventilation/CPAP, IV and/or blood transfusions, and monitoring.*

5. *Codes 99295 and 99256 are used to report services provided to a critically ill neonate through the first 28 days of life.*

6. *Codes 99293 ad 99294 are used to report services provided to a critically ill neonate from 29 days old through 24 months old.*

INPATIENT PEDIATRIC CRITICAL CARE

99293 Initial inpatient pediatric critical care, per day, for the evaluation and management of a critically ill infant or young child, 29 days through 24 months of age

99294 Subsequent inpatient pediatric critical care, per day, for the evaluation and management of a critically ill infant or young child, 29 days through 24 months of age

INPATIENT NEONATAL CRITICAL CARE

99295 Initial inpatient neonatal critical care, per day, for the evaluation and management of a critically ill neonate, 28 days of age or less

This code is reserved for the date of admission for neonates who are critically ill. Critically ill neonates require cardiac and/or respiratory support (including ventilator or nasal CPAP when indicated), continuous or frequent vital sign monitoring, laboratory and blood gas interpretations, follow-up physician reevaluations, and constant observation by the health care team under direct physician supervision. Immediate preoperative evaluation and stabilization of neonates with life threatening surgical or cardiac conditions are included under this code. Neonates with life threatening surgical or cardiac conditions are included under this code.

Care for neonates who require an intensive care setting but who are not critically ill is reported using the initial hospital care codes (99221-99223).

99296 Subsequent inpatient neonatal critical care, per day, for the evaluation and management of a critically ill neonate, 28 days of age or less.

A critically ill and unstable neonate will require cardiac and/or respiratory support (including ventilator or nasal CPAP when indicated), continuous or frequent vital sign monitoring, laboratory and blood gas interpretations, follow-up physician re-evaluations throughout a 24-hour period, and constant observation by the health care team under direct physician supervision. In addition, most will require frequent ventilator changes, intravenous fluid alterations, and/or early initiation of parenteral nutrition. Neonates in the immediate post-operative period or those who become critically ill and unstable during the hospital stay will commonly qualify for this level of care.

CONTINUING INTENSIVE CARE SERVICES

99298 Subsequent intensive care, per day, for the evaluation and management of the recovering very low birth weight infant (present body weight less than 1500 grams).

Infants with present body weight less than 1500 grams who are no longer critically ill continue to require intensive cardiac and respiratory monitoring, continuous and/or frequent vital sign monitoring, heat maintenance, enteral and/or parenteral nutritional adjustments, laboratory and oxygen monitoring and constant observation by the health care team under direct physician supervision.

99299 Subsequent intensive care, per day, for the evaluation and management of the recovering low birth weight infant (present body weight of 1500-2500 grams).

Infants with present body weight of 1500-2500 grams who are no longer critically ill continue to require intensive cardiac and respiratory monitoring, continuous and/or frequent vital sign monitoring, heat maintenance, enteral and/or parenteral nutritional adjustments, laboratory and oxygen monitoring, and constant observation by the health care team under direct physician supervision.

99300 Subsequent intensive care, per day, for the evaluation and management of the recovering infant (present body weight of 2501-5000 grams)

NURSING FACILITY SERVICES

A patient may be transferred from an inpatient hospital to a nursing facility for supervised care when the patient no longer requires the skill levels of the inpatient hospital. Evaluation and management service codes 99304-99310 are used to report services provided in nursing facilities. The key coding issues are the extent of history obtained, the extent of examination performed, and the complexity of medical decision making. Additional reporting issues include counseling and/or coordination of care, the nature of presenting problem(s), and the time spent at the bedside and on the patient's facility floor or unit.

These CPT codes are also used to report evaluation and management services provided to a patient in a psychiatric residential treatment center. If procedures such as medical psychotherapy are provided in addition to evaluation and management services, these are coded in addition to the evaluation and management services.

CPT codes in this section apply to Comprehensive Nursing Facility Assessments and Subsequent Nursing Facility care. Both subcategories apply to new and established patients. Comprehensive Assessments may be performed at one or more sites during the assessment process; including the hospital, the office, a nursing facility, a domiciliary facility and/or the patient's home.

(For care plan oversight services provided to nursing facility residents, see 99379-99380)

CODING RULES

1. *If a patient is admitted to the nursing facility after receiving services in the physician's office or hospital emergency department, all evaluation and management services are considered inclusive in the initial nursing facility care.*

2. *With the exception of hospital discharge services, evaluation and management service on the same date provided in locations other than the nursing facility that are related to the admission should not be coded separately.*

3. *When reporting these CPT codes to Medicare include the HCPCS Level II modifier -SP or -MP, or HCPCS Level III modifier if specified by the local Medicare carrier.*

INITIAL NURSING FACILITY CARE

NEW OR ESTABLISHED PATIENT

(For nursing facility care discharge, see 99315, 99316)

Typical unit times have not been established for 99304-99306

(99301 deleted 2006 edition.)

(99302 deleted 2006 edition.)

(99303 deleted 2006 edition.)

99304 Initial nursing facility care, per day, for the evaluation and management of a patient which requires these three key components:

- a detailed or comprehensive history;
- a detailed or comprehensive examination;
- and medical decision making that is straightforward or of low complexity.

Counseling and/or coordination of care with other providers or agencies are provided consistent with the nature of the problem(s) and the patient's and/or family's needs.

Usually, the problem(s) requiring admission are of low severity.

99305 Initial nursing facility care, per day, for the evaluation and management of a patient which requires these three key components:

● New Code ▲ Revised Code + Add-On Code ⊘ Modifier -51 Exempt ⊙ Conscious Sedation

- a comprehensive history;
- a comprehensive examination;
- and medical decision making of moderate complexity.

Counseling and/or coordination of care with other providers or agencies are provided consistent with the nature of the problem(s) and the patient's and/or family's needs.

Usually, the problem(s) requiring admission are of moderate severity.

99306 Initial nursing facility care, per day, for the evaluation and management of a patient, which requires these three key components:

- a comprehensive history;
- a comprehensive examination;
- and medical decision making of high complexity.

Counseling and/or coordination of care with other providers or agencies are provided consistent with the nature of the problem(s) and the patient's and/or family's needs.

Usually, the problem(s) requiring admission are of high severity.

SUBSEQUENT NURSING FACILITY CARE

follow up

NEW OR ESTABLISHED PATIENT

99307 Subsequent nursing facility care, per day, for the evaluation and management of a patient, which requires at least two of these three key components:

- a problem focused interval history;
- a problem focused examination;
- straightforward medical decision making.

Counseling and/or coordination of care with other providers or agencies are provided consistent with the nature of the problem(s) and the patient's and/or family's needs.

Usually, the patient is stable, recovering, or improving.

99308 Subsequent nursing facility care, per day, for the evaluation and management of a patient, which requires at least two of these three key components:

- an expanded problem focused interval history;
- an expanded problem focused examination;

- medical decision making of low complexity.

Counseling and/or coordination of care with other providers or agencies are provided consistent with the nature of the problem(s) and the patient's and/or family's needs.

Usually, the patient is responding inadequately to therapy or has developed a minor complication.

99309 Subsequent nursing facility care, per day, for the evaluation and management of a patient, which requires at least two of these three key components:

- a detailed interval history;
- a detailed examination;
- medical decision making of moderate complexity.

Counseling and/or coordination of care with other providers or agencies are provided consistent with the nature of the problem(s) and the patient's and/or family's needs.

Usually, the patient has developed a significant complication or a significant new problem.

99310 Subsequent nursing facility care, per day, for the evaluation and management of a patient, which requires at least two of these three key components:

- a comprehensive interval history;
- a comprehensive examination;
- medical decision making of high complexity.

Counseling and/or coordination of care with other providers or agencies are provided consistent with the nature of the problem(s) and the patient's and/or family's needs.

The patient may be unstable or may have developed a significant new problem requiring immediate physician attention.

(99311 deleted 2006 edition.)

(99312 deleted 2006 edition.)

(99313 deleted 2006 edition.)

NURSING FACILITY DISCHARGE SERVICES

99315 Nursing facility discharge day management; 30 minutes or less

99316 more than 30 minutes

OTHER NURSING FACILITY SERVICES

99318 Evaluation and management of a patient involving an annual nursing facility assessment, which requires these three key components:

- a detailed interval history;
- a comprehensive examination;
- and medical decision making that is of low to moderate complexity.

Counseling and/or coordination of care with other providers or agencies are provided consistent with the nature of the problem(s) and the patient's and/or family's needs.

Usually, the patient is stable, recovering, or improving.

(Do not report 99318 on the same date of service as nursing facility services codes 99304-99316)

DOMICILIARY, REST HOME (eg, BOARDING HOME), OR CUSTODIAL CARE SERVICES

E/M service codes 99324-99340 are used to report services provided to a new or established patient in domiciliary, rest home or custodial care facility. The key coding issues are the extent of history obtained, the extent of examination performed, and the complexity of medical decision making. Additional reporting issues include counseling and/or coordination of care, and the nature of presenting problems.

When reporting these CPT codes to Medicare include HCPCS modifier -SP or -MP to indicate single or multiple patients seen during the visit. Consult the local Medicare intermediary before using these modifiers.

(For care plan oversight services provided to a patient in a domiciliary facility under the care of a home health agency, see 99374-99375)

(For care plan oversight services provided to a patient in a domiciliary facility under the individual supervision of a physician, see 99339, 99340)

NEW PATIENT

(99321 deleted 2006 edition.)

(99322 deleted 2006 edition.)

(99323 deleted 2006 edition.)

99324 Domiciliary or rest home visit for the evaluation and management of a new patient, which requires these three key components:

- a problem focused history;
- a problem focused examination; and
- straightforward medical decision making.

Counseling and/or coordination of care with other providers or agencies are provided consistent with the nature of the problem(s) and the patient's and/or family's needs.

Usually, the presenting problem(s) are of low severity. Physicians typically spend 20 minutes with the patient and/or family or caregiver.

99325 Domiciliary or rest home visit for the evaluation and management of a new patient, which requires these three key components:

- an expanded problem focused history;
- an expanded problem focused examination; and
- medical decision making of low complexity.

Counseling and/or coordination of care with other providers or agencies are provided consistent with the nature of the problem(s) and the patient's and/or family's needs.

Usually, the presenting problem(s) are of moderate severity. Physicians typically spend 30 minutes with the patient and/or family or caregiver.

99326 Domiciliary or rest home visit for the evaluation and management of a new patient, which requires these three key components:

- a detailed history;
- a detailed examination; and
- medical decision making of moderate complexity.

Counseling and/or coordination of care with other providers or agencies are provided consistent with the nature of the problem(s) and the patient's and/or family's needs.

Usually, the presenting problem(s) are of moderate to high severity. Physicians typically spend 45 minutes with the patient and/or family or caregiver.

99327 Domiciliary or rest home visit for the evaluation and management of a new patient, which requires these three key components:

- a comprehensive history;
- a comprehensive examination; and
- medical decision making of moderate complexity.

Counseling and/or coordination of care with other providers or agencies are provided consistent with the nature of the problem(s) and the patient's and/or family's needs.

Usually, the presenting problem(s) are of high severity. Physicians typically spend 60 minutes with the patient and/or family or caregiver.

99328 Domiciliary or rest home visit for the evaluation and management of a new patient, which requires these three key components:

- a comprehensive history;
- a comprehensive examination; and
- medical decision making of high complexity.

Counseling and/or coordination of care with other providers or agencies are provided consistent with the nature of the problem(s) and the patient's and/or family's needs.

Usually, the patient is unstable or has developed a significant new problem requiring immediate physician attention. Physicians typically spend 75 minutes with the patient and/or family or caregiver.

ESTABLISHED PATIENT

(99331 deleted 2006 edition.)

(99332 deleted 2006 edition.)

(99333 deleted 2006 edition.)

99334 Domiciliary or rest home visit for the evaluation and management of an established patient, which requires at least two of these three key components:

- a problem focused interval history;
- a problem focused examination;
- straightforward medical decision making.

Counseling and/or coordination of care with other providers or agencies are provided consistent with the nature of the problem(s) and the patient's and/or family's needs.

Usually, the presenting problem(s) are self-limited or minor. Physicians typically spend 15 minutes with the patient and/or family or caregiver.

99335 Domiciliary or rest home visit for the evaluation and management of an established patient, which requires at least two of these three key components:

- an expanded problem focused interval history;
- an expanded problem focused examination;
- medical decision making of low complexity.

Counseling and/or coordination of care with other providers or agencies are provided consistent with the nature of the problem(s) and the patient's and/or family's needs.

Usually, the presenting problem(s) are of low to moderate severity. Physicians typically spend 25 minutes with the patient and/or family or caregiver.

99336 Domiciliary or rest home visit for the evaluation and management of an established patient, which requires at least two of these three key components:

- a detailed interval history;
- a detailed examination;
- medical decision making of moderate complexity.

Counseling and/or coordination of care with other providers or agencies are provided consistent with the nature of the problem(s) and the patient's and/or family's needs.

Usually, the presenting problem(s) are of moderate to high severity. Physicians typically spend 40 minutes with the patient and/or family or caregiver.

99337 Domiciliary or rest home visit for the evaluation and management of an established patient, which requires at least two of these three key components:

- a comprehensive interval history;
- a comprehensive examination;
- and medical decision making of moderate to high complexity.

Counseling and/or coordination of care with other providers or agencies are provided consistent with the nature of the problem(s) and the patient's and/or family's needs.

Usually, the presenting problem(s) are of moderate to high severity. The patient may be unstable or may have developed a significant new problem requiring immediate physician attention. Physicians typically spend 60 minutes with the patient and/or family or caregiver.

DOMICILIARY, REST HOME (eg, ASSISTED LIVING FACILITY), OR HOME CARE PLAN OVERSIGHT SERVICES

(For instructions on the use of 99339, 99340, see introductory notes for 99374-99380)

(For care plan oversight services for patients under the care of a home health agency, hospice, or nursing facility, see 99374-99380)

99339 Individual physician supervision of a patient (patient not present) in home, domiciliary or rest home (eg, assisted living facility) requiring complex and multidisciplinary care modalities involving regular physician development and/or revision of care plans, review of subsequent reports of patient status, review of related laboratory and other studies, communication (including telephone calls) for purposes of assessment or care decisions with health care professional(s), family member(s), surrogate decision maker(s) (eg, legal guardian) and/or key caregiver(s) involved in patient's care, integration of new information into the medical treatment plan and/or adjustment of medical therapy, within a calendar month; 15-29 minutes

99340 30 minutes or more

(Do not report 99339, 99340 for patients under the care of a home health agency, enrolled in a hospice program, or for nursing facility residents)

HOME SERVICES - house call

Evaluation and management codes 99341-99350 are used to report services provided to new and established patients in the patient's home. The key coding issues are the extent of history obtained, the extent of examination performed, and the complexity of medical decision making. Additional reporting issues include counseling and/or coordination of care, and the nature of presenting problem(s).

(For care plan oversight services provided to a patient in the home under the care of a home health agency, see 99374-99375)

(For care plan oversight services provided to a patient in the home under the individual supervision of a physician, see 99339, 99340)

NEW PATIENT

99341 Home visit for the evaluation and management of a new patient, which requires these three key components:

- a problem focused history;
- a problem focused examination; and
- straightforward medical decision making.

Counseling and/or coordination of care with other providers or agencies are provided consistent with the nature of the problem(s) and the patient's and/or family's needs.

Usually, the presenting problem(s) are of low severity. Physicians typically spend 20 minutes face-to-face with the patient and/or family.

99342 Home visit for the evaluation and management of a new patient, which requires these three key components:

- an expanded problem focused history;
- an expanded problem focused examination; and
- medical decision making of low complexity.

Counseling and/or coordination of care with other providers or agencies are provided consistent with the nature of the problem(s) and the patient's and/or family's needs.

Usually, the presenting problem(s) are of moderate severity. Physicians typically spend 30 minutes face-to-face with the patient and/or family.

99343 Home visit for the evaluation and management of a new patient, which requires these three key components:

- a detailed history;
- a detailed examination; and
- medical decision making of moderate complexity.

Counseling and/or coordination of care with other providers or agencies are provided consistent with the nature of the problem(s) and the patient's and/or family's needs.

Usually, the presenting problem(s) are of moderate to high severity. Physicians typically spend 45 minutes face-to-face with the patient and/or family.

99344 Home visit for the evaluation and management of a new patient, which requires these three components:

- a comprehensive history;
- a comprehensive examination; and
- medical decision making of moderate complexity.

Counseling and/or coordination of care with other providers or agencies are provided consistent with the nature of the problem(s) and the patient's and/or family's needs.

Usually, the presenting problem(s) are of high severity. Physicians typically spend 60 minutes face-to-face with the patient and/or family.

99345 Home visit for the evaluation and management of a new patient, which requires these three key components:

- a comprehensive history;
- a comprehensive examination; and
- medical decision making of high complexity.

Counseling and/or coordination of care with other providers or agencies are provided consistent with the nature of the problem(s) and the patient's and/or family's needs.

Usually, the patient is unstable or has developed a significant new problem requiring immediate physician attention. Physicians typically spend 75 minutes face-to-face with the patient and/or family.

ESTABLISHED PATIENT

99347 Home visit for the evaluation and management of an established patient, which requires at least two of these three key components:

- a problem focused interval history;
- a problem focused examination;
- straightforward medical decision making.

Counseling and/or coordination of care with other providers or agencies are provided consistent with the nature of the problem(s) and the patient's and/or family's needs.

Usually, the presenting problem(s) are self-limited or minor. Physicians typically spend 15 minutes face-to-face with the patient and/or family.

99348 Home visit for the evaluation and management of an established patient, which requires at least two of these three key components:

- an expanded problem focused interval history;
- an expanded problem focused examination;
- medical decision making of low complexity.

Counseling and/or coordination of care with other providers or agencies are provided consistent with the nature of the problem(s) and the patient's and/or family's needs.

Usually, the presenting problem(s) are of low to moderate severity. Physicians typically spend 25 minutes face-to-face with the patient and/or family.

99349 Home visit for the evaluation and management of an established patient, which requires at least two of these three key components:

- a detailed interval history;
- a detailed examination;
- medical decision making of moderate complexity.

Counseling and/or coordination of care with other providers or agencies are provided consistent with the nature of the problem(s) and the patient's and/or family's needs.

Usually, the presenting problem(s) are moderate to high severity. Physicians typically spend 40 minutes face-to-face with the patient and/or family.

● New Code ▲ Revised Code + Add-On Code ⊘ Modifier -51 Exempt ⊙ Conscious Sedation

99350 Home visit for the evaluation and management of an established patient, which requires at least two of these three key components:

- a comprehensive interval history;
- a comprehensive examination;
- medical decision making of moderate to high complexity.

Counseling and/or coordination of care with other providers or agencies are provided consistent with the nature of the problem(s) and the patient's and/or family's needs.

Usually, the presenting problem(s) are of moderate to high severity. The patient may be unstable or may have developed a significant new problem requiring immediate physician attention. Physicians typically spend 60 minutes face-to-face with the patient and/or family.

PROLONGED SERVICES

Evaluation and management service CPT codes 99354-99360 are used to report inpatient or outpatient services which include prolonged service or physician standby service that is beyond the usual service. The key coding issues are the location of the service, whether the service is direct (face-to-face) or not direct, and the total duration of the prolonged service.

CODING RULES

1. *Prolonged services are reported in addition to other physician services.*
2. *Prolonged services involving direct (face-to-face) time are reported as cumulative time on a given date, even if the time is not continuous.*
3. *If the total duration of prolonged services is less than 30 minutes, the prolonged service is not reported.*

CORRECT CODING FOR PROLONGED SERVICES

DURATION OF PROLONGED SERVICE	CODE(S) TO REPORT
less than 30 minutes	not reported separately
30- 74 minutes	99354 once
75-104 minutes	99354 once and 99355 once
105-134 minutes	99354 once and 99355 twice
135-164 minutes	99354 once and 99355 three times
165-194 minutes	99354 once and 99355 four times

PROLONGED PHYSICIAN SERVICE WITH DIRECT (FACE-TO-FACE) PATIENT CONTACT

+ **99354** Prolonged physician service in the office or other outpatient setting requiring direct (face-to-face) patient contact beyond the usual service (eg, prolonged care and treatment of an acute asthmatic patient in an outpatient setting); first hour (List separately in addition to code for office or other outpatient Evaluation and Management service)

(Use in conjunction with codes 99201-99215, 99241-99245, 99304-99350)

+ **99355** each additional 30 minutes (List separately in addition to code for prolonged physician service)

(Use 99355 in conjunction with 99354)

+ **99356** Prolonged physician service in the inpatient setting, requiring direct (face-to-face) patient contact beyond the usual service (eg, maternal fetal monitoring for high risk delivery or other physiological monitoring, prolonged care of an acutely ill inpatient); first hour (List separately in addition to code for inpatient Evaluation and Management service)

(Use 99356 in conjunction with codes 99221-99233, 99251-99255)

+ **99357** each additional 30 minutes (List separately in addition to code for prolonged physician service)

(Use 99357 in conjunction with 99356)

PROLONGED PHYSICIAN SERVICE WITHOUT DIRECT (FACE-TO-FACE) PATIENT CONTACT

+ **99358** Prolonged evaluation and management service before and/or after direct (face-to-face) patient care (eg, review of extensive records and tests, communication with other professionals and/or the patient/family); first hour (List separately in addition to code(s) for other physician service(s) and/or inpatient or outpatient Evaluation and Management service)

+ **99359** each additional 30 minutes (List separately in addition to code for prolonged physician service)

(Use 99359 in conjunction with 99358)

(To report telephone calls, see 99371-99373)

PHYSICIAN STANDBY SERVICES

99360 Physician standby service, requiring prolonged physician attendance, each 30 minutes (eg, operative standby, standby for frozen section, for cesarean/high risk delivery, for monitoring EEG)

(For hospital mandated on call services, see 99026, 99027)

(99360 may be reported in addition to 99431, 99440 as appropriate)

(Do not report 99360 in conjunction with 99436)

CASE MANAGEMENT SERVICES

Case management is a process wherein a physician is responsible for direct care of the patient and has the additional responsibility of coordinating all other services provided to the patient. Case management services may be provided during medical conferences, or by telephone. The key coding issues are the type of service, the amount of time spent, and the level of service provided.

TEAM CONFERENCES

99361 Medical conference by a physician with interdisciplinary team of health professionals or representatives of community agencies to coordinate activities of patient care (patient not present); approximately 30 minutes

99362 approximately 60 minutes

ANTICOAGULANT MANAGEMENT

Anticoagulant services are intented to describe the outpatient management of warfarin therapy, including ordering, review and interpretation of International Normalized Ratio (INR) testing, communication with patient, and dosage adjustments as appropriate.

These services are outpatient services only. When anticoagulation therapy is initiated or continued in the inpatient or observation setting, a new period begins after discharge and is reported with 99364. Do not report 99363-99364 with 99217-99239, 99291-99300, 99304-99318 or other codes for physician review, interpretation, and patient management of home INR testing for a patient with mechanical heart valves.

Any period less than 60 continuous outpatient days is not reported. If less than the specified minimum number of services per period are performed, do not report the anticoagulation management services (99363-99364).

● **99363** Anticoagulant management for an outpatient taking warfarin, physician review and interpretation of International Normalized Ratio (INR) testing, patient instructions, dosage adjustment (as needed), and ordering of additional tests; initial 90 days of therapy (must include a minimum of 8 INR measurements)

● **99364** Anticoagulant management for an outpatient taking warfarin, physician review and interpretation of International Normalized Ratio (INR) testing, patient instructions, dosage adjustment (as needed), and ordering of additional tests; each subsequent 90 days of therapy (must include a minimum of 3 INR measurements)

TELEPHONE CALLS

99371 Telephone call by a physician to patient or for consultation or medical management or for coordinating medical management with other health care professionals (eg, nurses, therapists, social workers, nutritionists, physicians, pharmacists); simple or brief (eg, to report on tests and/or laboratory results, to clarify or alter previous instructions, to integrate new information from other health professionals into the medical treatment plan, or to adjust therapy)

99372 intermediate (eg, to provide advice to an established patient on a new problem, to initiate therapy that can be handled by telephone, to discuss test results in detail, to coordinate medical management of a new problem in an established patient, to discuss and evaluate new information and details, or to initiate new plan of care)

99373 complex or lengthy (eg, lengthy counseling session with anxious or distraught patient, detailed or prolonged discussion with family members regarding seriously ill patient, lengthy communication necessary to coordinate complex services of several different health professionals working on different aspects of the total patient care plan)

CARE PLAN OVERSIGHT SERVICES

Care plans prepared and/or reviewed by a physician are frequently required for patients under the care of home health agencies, hospices, or residing in nursing facilities. Evaluation and management service codes 99374-99380 are used to report care plan oversight services. The key coding issues are the location of service, the complexity of the plan, and the amount of physician time provided within a 30-day period.

● New Code ▲ Revised Code + Add-On Code ⃠ Modifier -51 Exempt ⊙ Conscious Sedation

CODING RULES

1. *Evaluation and management services are not inclusive of care plan oversight services. Care plan oversight is coded separately.*

2. *Care plan oversight services may be coded only by a single physician for each patient during a specific period of time.*

(For care plan oversight services of patients in the home, domiciliary, or rest home (eg, assisted living facility) under the individual supervision of a physician, see 99339, 99340)

99374 Physician supervision of a patient under care of home health agency (patient not present) in home, domiciliary or equivalent environment (eg, Alzheimer's facility) requiring complex and multidisciplinary care modalities involving regular physician development and/or revision of care plans, review of subsequent reports of patient status, review of related laboratory and other studies, communication (including telephone calls) for purposes of assessment or care decisions with health care professional(s), family member(s), surrogate decision maker(s) (eg., legal guardian) and/or key caregiver(s) involved in patient's care, integration of new information into the medical treatment plan and/or adjustment of medical therapy, within a calendar month; 15-29 minutes

99375 30 minutes or more

99377 Physician supervision of a hospice patient (patient not present) requiring complex and multidisciplinary care modalities involving regular physician development and/or revision of care plans, review of subsequent reports of patient status, review of related laboratory and other studies, communication (including telephone calls) for purposes of assessment or care decisions with health care professional(s), family member(s), surrogate decision maker(s) (eg, legal guardian) and/or key caregiver(s) involved in patient's care, integration of new information into the medical treatment plan and/or adjustment of medical therapy, within a calendar month; 15-29 minutes

99378 30 minutes or more

99379 Physician supervision of a nursing facility patient (patient not present) requiring complex and multidisciplinary care modalities involving regular physician development and/or revision of care plans, review of subsequent reports of patient status, review of related laboratory and other studies, communication (including telephone calls) for purposes of assessment or care decisions with health care professional(s), family member(s), surrogate

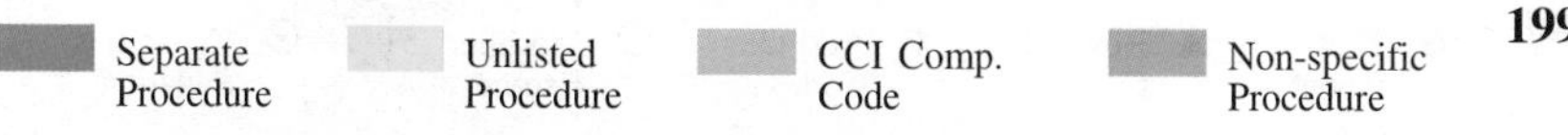

decision maker(s) (eg, legal guardian) and/or key caregiver(s) involved in patient's care, integration of new information into the medical treatment plan and/or adjustment of medical therapy, within a calendar month; 15-29 minutes

99380 30 minutes or more

PREVENTIVE MEDICINE SERVICES

Preventive medicine services codes are used to report routine evaluation and management of adults and children in the absence of patient complaints or counseling and/or risk factor reduction intervention services to healthy individuals. The key coding issues are whether the patient is a new patient or established patient, the age of the patient, the circumstances of the examination, and the nature of any abnormalities encountered, and for counseling services, whether the service was provided to an individual or to a group and the amount of time spent counseling.

CODING RULES

1. *The selection of Preventive Medicine codes is mostly dependent upon the age of the patient.*

2. *Preventive medicine codes are coded only in the absence of illness. If illness, injury is discovered during provision of a preventive medicine service, office/outpatient evaluation and management codes are coded.*

3. *Immunizations and diagnostic studies involving laboratory or radiology, or other procedures are not included in the preventive medicine service and should be coded separately.*

NEW PATIENT

99381 Initial comprehensive preventive medicine evaluation and management of an individual including an age and gender appropriate history, examination, counseling/anticipatory guidance/risk factor reduction interventions, and the ordering of appropriate immunization(s), laboratory/diagnostic procedures, new patient; infant (age under 1 year)

99382 early childhood (age 1 through 4 years)

99383 late childhood (age 5 through 11 years)

99384 adolescent (age 12 through 17 years)

99385 18-39 years

● New Code ▲ Revised Code + Add-On Code ⊘ Modifier -51 Exempt ⊙ Conscious Sedation

99386 40-64 years

99387 65 years and over

ESTABLISHED PATIENT

99391 Periodic comprehensive preventive medicine reevaluation and management of an individual including an age and gender appropriate history, examination, counseling/anticipatory guidance/risk factor reduction interventions, and the ordering of appropriate immunization(s), laboratory/diagnostic procedures, established patient; infant (age under 1 year)

99392 early childhood (age 1 through 4 years)

99393 late childhood (age 5 through 11 years)

99394 adolescent (age 12 through 17 years)

99395 18-39 years

99396 40-64 years

99397 65 years and over

COUNSELING AND/OR RISK FACTOR REDUCTION INTERVENTION

NEW OR ESTABLISHED PATIENT

Preventive Medicine, Individual Counseling

99401 Preventive medicine counseling and/or risk factor reduction intervention(s) provided to an individual (separate procedure); approximately 15 minutes

99402 approximately 30 minutes

99403 approximately 45 minutes

99404 approximately 60 minutes

Preventive Medicine, Group Counseling

99411 Preventive medicine counseling and/or risk factor reduction intervention(s) provided to individuals in a group setting (separate procedure); approximately 30 minutes

99412 approximately 60 minutes

Other Preventive Medicine Services

99420 Administration and interpretation of health risk assessment instrument (eg, health hazard appraisal)

99429 Unlisted preventive medicine service

NEWBORN CARE SERVICES

99431 History and examination of the normal newborn infant, initiation of diagnostic and treatment programs and preparation of hospital records. (This code should also be used for birthing room deliveries.)

99432 Normal newborn care in other than hospital or birthing room setting, including physical examination of baby and conference(s) with parent(s)

99433 Subsequent hospital care, for the evaluation and management of a normal newborn, per day

99435 History and examination of the normal newborn infant, including the preparation of medical records. (This code should only be used for newborns assessed and discharged from the hospital or birthing room on the same date.)

99436 Attendance at delivery (when requested by delivering physician) and initial stabilization of newborn

(99436 may be reported in addition to 99431)

(Do not report 99436 in conjunction with 99440)

99440 Newborn resuscitation: provision of positive pressure ventilation and/or chest compressions in the presence of acute inadequate ventilation and/or cardiac output

SPECIAL EVALUATION AND MANAGEMENT SERVICES

The following codes are used to report evaluations performed to establish baseline information prior to life or disability insurance certificates being issued. This service is performed in the office or other setting, and applies to both new and established patients.

BASIC LIFE AND/OR DISABILITY EVALUATION SERVICES

99450 Basic life and/or disability examination that includes:

- measurement of height, weight and blood pressure;
- completion of a medical history following a life insurance pro forma;
- collection of blood sample and/or urinalysis complying with "chain of custody" protocols; and
- completion of necessary documentation/certificates.

WORK RELATED OR MEDICAL DISABILITY EVALUATION SERVICES

99455 Work related or medical disability examination by the treating physician that includes:

- completion of a medical history commensurate with the patient's condition;
- performance of an examination commensurate with the patient's condition;
- formulation of a diagnosis, assessment of capabilities and stability, and calculation of impairment;
- development of future medical treatment plan; and
- completion of necessary documentation/certificates and report.

99456 Work related or medical disability examination by other than the treating physician that includes:

- completion of a medical history commensurate with the patient's condition;
- performance of an examination commensurate with the patient's condition;
- formulation of a diagnosis, assessment of capabilities and stability, and calculation of impairment;

- development of future medical treatment plan; and
- completion of necessary documentation/certificates and report.

(Do not report 99455, 99456 with 99080 for the completion of Workman's Compensation forms)

OTHER EVALUATION AND MANAGEMENT SERVICES

99499 Unlisted evaluation and management service

● New Code ▲ Revised Code + Add-On Code ⊘ Modifier -51 Exempt ⊙ Conscious Sedation

ANESTHESIA

ANESTHESIA OVERVIEW

The second section of the CPT coding system is the anesthesia section, which includes service codes for the delivery of anesthesia. Within each subsection, the CPT codes are arranged by anatomical site.

The Anesthesiologist provides pain relief and maintenance, or restoration, of a stable condition during and immediately following an operation, an obstetric or diagnostic procedure. The Anesthesiologist assesses the risk of the patient undergoing surgery and optimizes the patient's condition prior to, during, and after surgery.

ANES 00100

Reporting of anesthesia services is dependent on the third party payer involved. Anesthesia services covered by Medicare are coded using codes from the ANESTHESIA section of the CPT coding system. For most other third party payers, anesthesia services are coded using codes from the SURGERY section of the CPT coding system to describe the major surgical procedure.

Anesthesia services may be coded by anesthesiologists or anesthetists working under the supervision of the anesthesiologist. Anesthesia services include pre- and post-op visits, anesthesia delivery, giving fluids and/or blood needed during a procedure, and monitoring. Anesthesia delivery includes general, regional, supplementing local anesthesia, and other supportive services.

To report moderate (conscious) sedation provided by a physician also performing the service for which conscious sedation is being provided, see codes 99143-99145.

For the procedures listed in Appendix G, when a second physician other than the health care professional performing the diagnostic or therapeutic services provides moderate (conscious) sedation in the facility setting (eg, hospital, outpatient hospital/ambulatory surgery center, skilled nursing facility), the second physician reports the associated moderate sedation procedure/service 99148-99150; when these services are performed by the second physician in the nonfacility setting (eg, physician office, freestanding imaging center), codes 99148-99150 would not be reported. Moderate sedation does not include minimal sedation (anxiolysis), deep sedation, or monitored anesthesia care (00100-01999).

KEY POINTS ABOUT ANESTHESIA CODING

1. *Time recording for anesthesia services starts with patient preparation for anesthesia induction and ends when the anesthesiologist or anesthetist has*

completed his/her services and transfers responsibility for postoperative supervision.

2. *Consultations and/or other evaluation and management services which are not included in the administration or supervising the administration of anesthesia, regardless of location provided, are reporting using CPT codes from the evaluation and management section of the CPT book.*

3. *Any supplies and/or materials provided by the anesthesiologist or anesthetist which are not considered to be included in the standard service may be coded separately.*

4. *Multiple procedures provided on the same date of service should be coded separately.*

5. *Any service which may be considered rare, unusual, variable or not defined should be supported with a special report which clearly defines the need for the unusual service. These services are generally coded with an unlisted CPT code or by adding modifier -22 to the CPT code which defines the procedure.*

ANESTHESIA SERVICE MODIFIERS

A physical status modifier must be added to all CPT codes when reporting anesthesia services. The physical status modifier defines the physical condition of the patient and ranges from a normal health patient to a declared brain-dead patient whose organs are being harvested for a transplant.

PHYSICAL STATUS MODIFIERS

-P1 A normal healthy patient.

-P2 A patient with a mild systemic disease.

-P3 A patient with severe systemic disease.

-P4 A patient with severe systemic disease that is a constant threat to life.

-P5 A moribund patient who is not expected to survive without the operation.

-P6 A declared brain-dead patient whose organs are being removed for donor purposes.

OTHER ANESTHESIA SERVICE MODIFIERS

Under certain circumstances, medical services and procedures may need to be further modified. Other CPT coding system modifiers commonly used with ANESTHESIA services include:

-22 Unusual services

-23 Anesthesia

-32 Mandated services

-51 Multiple procedures

QUALIFYING CIRCUMSTANCES FOR ANESTHESIA

In the case of difficult and/or extraordinary circumstances such as extreme youth or age, extraordinary condition of the patient, and/or unusual risk factors it may be appropriate to report one or more of the following qualifying circumstances in addition to the anesthesia services.

+ **99100** Anesthesia for patient of extreme age, under one year and over seventy

  (For procedure performed on infants less than 1 year of age at time of surgery, see 00833, 00834)

+ **99116** Anesthesia complicated by utilization of total body hypothermia

+ **99135** Anesthesia complicated by utilization of controlled hypotension

+ **99140** Anesthesia complicated by emergency conditions (specify) (List separately in addition to code for primary anesthesia procedure)

  (An emergency is defined as existing when delay in treatment of the patient would lead to a significant increase in the threat to life or body part.)

This page intentionally left blank.

ANESTHESIA CODES

HEAD

00100 Anesthesia for procedures on salivary glands, including biopsy

00102 Anesthesia for procedures on plastic repair of cleft lip

00103 Anesthesia for reconstructive procedures of eyelid (eg, blepharoplasty, ptosis surgery)

00104 Anesthesia for electroconvulsive therapy

00120 Anesthesia for procedures on external, middle, and inner ear including biopsy; not otherwise specified

00124 otoscopy

00126 tympanotomy

00140 Anesthesia for procedures on eye; not otherwise specified

00142 lens surgery

00144 corneal transplant

00145 vitreoretinal surgery

00147 iridectomy

00148 ophthalmoscopy

00160 Anesthesia for procedures on nose and accessory sinuses; not otherwise specified

00162 radical surgery

00164 biopsy, soft tissue

00170 Anesthesia for intraoral procedures, including biopsy; not otherwise specified

00172 repair of cleft palate

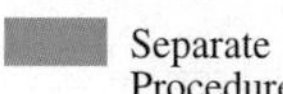 Separate Procedure 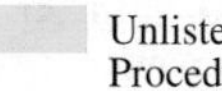 Unlisted Procedure 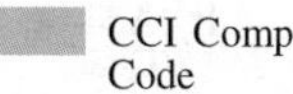 CCI Comp. Code Non-specific Procedure

00174 excision of retropharyngeal tumor

00176 radical surgery

00190 Anesthesia for procedures on facial bones or skull; not otherwise specified

00192 radical surgery (including prognathism)

00210 Anesthesia for intracranial procedures; not otherwise specified

00212 subdural taps

00214 burr holes, including ventriculography

00215 cranioplasty or elevation of depressed skull fracture, extradural (simple or compound)

00216 vascular procedures

00218 procedures in sitting position

00220 cerebrospinal fluid shunting procedures

00222 electrocoagulation of intracranial nerve

NECK

00300 Anesthesia for all procedures on the integumentary system, muscles and nerves of head, neck, and posterior trunk, not otherwise specified

00320 Anesthesia for all procedures on esophagus, thyroid, larynx, trachea and lymphatic system of neck; not otherwise specified, age 1 year or older

00322 needle biopsy of thyroid

(For procedures on cervical spine and cord, see 00600, 00604, 00670)

00326 Anesthesia for all procedures on the larynx and trachea in children less than 1 year of age

(Do not report 00326 in conjunction with code 99100)

00350 Anesthesia for procedures on major vessels of neck; not otherwise specified

00352 simple ligation

(For arteriography, use 01916)

THORAX (CHEST WALL AND SHOULDER GIRDLE)

00400 Anesthesia for procedures on the integumentary system on the extremities, anterior trunk and perineum; not otherwise specified

00402 reconstructive procedures on breast (eg, reduction or augmentation mammoplasty, muscle flaps)

00404 radical or modified radical procedures on breast

00406 radical or modified radical procedures on breast with internal mammary node dissection

00410 electrical conversion of arrhythmias

00450 Anesthesia for procedures on clavicle and scapula; not otherwise specified

00452 radical surgery

00454 biopsy of clavicle

00470 Anesthesia for partial rib resection; not otherwise specified

00472 thoracoplasty (any type)

00474 radical procedures (eg, pectus excavatum)

INTRATHORACIC

00500 Anesthesia for all procedures on esophagus

00520 Anesthesia for closed chest procedures; (including bronchoscopy) not otherwise specified

00522 needle biopsy of pleura

00524 pneumocentesis

00528 mediastinoscopy and diagnostic thoracoscopy not utilizing one lung ventilation

(For tracheobronchial reconstruction, use 00539)

00529 mediastinoscopy and diagnostic thoracoscopy utilizing one lung ventilation

00530 Anesthesia for permanent transvenous pacemaker insertion

00532 Anesthesia for access to central venous circulation

00534 Anesthesia for transvenous insertion or replacement of pacing cardioverter/defibrillator

(For transthoracic approach, use 00560)

00537 Anesthesia for cardiac electrophysiologic procedures including radiofrequency ablation

00539 Anesthesia for tracheobronchial reconstruction

00540 Anesthesia for thoracotomy procedures involving lungs, pleura, diaphragm, and mediastinum (including surgical thoracoscopy); not otherwise specified

00541 utilizing one lung ventilation

(For thoracic spine and cord anesthesia procedures via an anterior transthoracic approach, see 00625-00626)

00542 decortication

(00544 deleted 2004 edition. To report, use 00542)

00546 pulmonary resection with thoracoplasty

00548 intrathoracic procedures on the trachea and bronchi

00550 Anesthesia for sternal debridement

00560 Anesthesia for procedures on heart, pericardial sac, and great vessels of chest; without pump oxygenator

00561 with pump oxygenator, under one year of age

● New Code ▲ Revised Code + Add-On Code ⃠ Modifier -51 Exempt ⊙ Conscious Sedation

(Do not report 00561 in conjunction with 99100, 99116, and 99135)

00562 with pump oxygenator

00563 with pump oxygenator with hypothermic circulatory arrest

00566 Anesthesia for direct coronary artery bypass grafting without pump oxygenator

00580 Anesthesia for heart transplant or heart/lung transplant

SPINE AND SPINAL CORD

00600 Anesthesia for procedures on cervical spine and cord; not otherwise specified

(For myelography and diskography, see radiological procedures 01905)

00604 procedures with patient in the sitting position

00620 Anesthesia for procedures on thoracic spine and cord; not otherwise specified

00622 thoracolumbar sympathectomy

● **00625** Anesthesia for procedures on the thoracic spine and cord, via an anterior transthoracic approach; not utilizing one lung ventilation

● **00626** utilizing one lung ventilation

(For anesthesia for thoractomy procedures other than spinal, see 00540-00541)

00630 Anesthesia for procedures in lumbar region; not otherwise specified

00632 lumbar sympathectomy

00634 chemonucleolysis

00635 diagnostic or therapeutic lumbar puncture

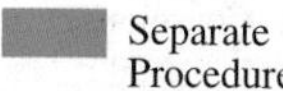
Separate Procedure
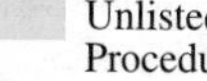
Unlisted Procedure
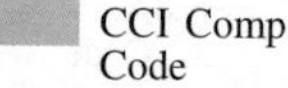
CCI Comp. Code
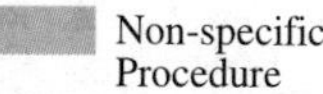
Non-specific Procedure

00640 Anesthesia for manipulation of the spine or for closed procedures on the cervical, thoracic or lumbar spine

00670 Anesthesia for extensive spine and spinal cord procedures (eg, spinal instrumentation or vascular procedures)

UPPER ABDOMEN

00700 Anesthesia for procedures on upper anterior abdominal wall; not otherwise specified

00702 percutaneous liver biopsy

00730 Anesthesia for procedures on upper posterior abdominal wall

00740 Anesthesia for upper gastrointestinal endoscopic procedures, endoscope introduced proximal to duodenum

00750 Anesthesia for hernia repairs in upper abdomen; not otherwise specified

00752 lumbar and ventral (incisional) hernias and/or wound dehiscence

00754 omphalocele

00756 transabdominal repair of diaphragmatic hernia

00770 Anesthesia for all procedures on major abdominal blood vessels

00790 Anesthesia for intraperitoneal procedures in upper abdomen including laparoscopy; not otherwise specified

00792 partial hepatectomy or management of liver hemorrhage (excluding liver biopsy)

00794 pancreatectomy, partial or total (eg, Whipple procedure)

00796 liver transplant (recipient)

(For harvesting of liver, use 01990)

00797 gastric restrictive procedure for morbid obesity

LOWER ABDOMEN

00800 Anesthesia for procedures on lower anterior abdominal wall; not otherwise specified

00802 panniculectomy

00810 Anesthesia for lower intestinal endoscopic procedures, endoscope introduced distal to duodenum

00820 Anesthesia for procedures on lower posterior abdominal wall

00830 Anesthesia for hernia repairs in lower abdomen; not otherwise specified

00832 ventral and incisional hernias

(For hernia repairs in the infant 1 year of age or younger, see 00834, 00836)

00834 Anesthesia for hernia repairs in the lower abdomen not otherwise specified, under 1 year of age

(Do not report 00834 in conjunction with code 99100)

00836 Anesthesia for hernia repairs in the lower abdomen not otherwise specified, infants less than 37 weeks gestational age at birth and less than 50 weeks gestational age at time of surgery

(Do not report 00836 in conjunction with code 99100)

00840 Anesthesia for intraperitoneal procedures in lower abdomen including laparoscopy; not otherwise specified

00842 amniocentesis

00844 abdominoperineal resection

00846 radical hysterectomy

00848 pelvic exenteration

00851 tubal ligation/transection

00860 Anesthesia for extraperitoneal procedures in lower abdomen, including urinary tract; not otherwise specified

00862 renal procedures, including upper 1/3 of ureter, or donor nephrectomy

00864 total cystectomy

00865 radical prostatectomy (suprapubic, retropubic)

00866 adrenalectomy

00868 renal transplant (recipient)

(For donor nephrectomy, use 00862)

(For harvesting kidney from brain-dead patient, use 01990)

00870 cystolithotomy

00872 Anesthesia for lithotripsy, extracorporeal shock wave; with water bath

00873 without water bath

00880 Anesthesia for procedures on major lower abdominal vessels; not otherwise specified

00882 inferior vena cava ligation

PERINEUM

(For perineal procedures on the integumentary system, muscles and nerves, see 00300, 00400)

00902 Anesthesia for; anorectal procedure

00904 radical perineal procedure

00906 vulvectomy

00908 perineal prostatectomy

00910 Anesthesia for transurethral procedures (including urethrocystoscopy); not otherwise specified

00912 transurethral resection of bladder tumor(s)

00914 transurethral resection of prostate

00916 post-transurethral resection bleeding

00918 with fragmentation, manipulation and/or removal of ureteral calculus

00920 Anesthesia for procedures on male genitalia (including open urethral procedures); not otherwise specified

00921 vasectomy, unilateral or bilateral

00922 seminal vesicles

00924 undescended testis, unilateral or bilateral

00926 radical orchiectomy, inguinal

00928 radical orchiectomy, abdominal

00930 orchiopexy, unilateral or bilateral

00932 complete amputation of penis

00934 radical amputation of penis with bilateral inguinal lymphadenectomy

00936 radical amputation of penis with bilateral inguinal and iliac lymphadenectomy

00938 insertion of penile prosthesis (perineal approach)

00940 Anesthesia for vaginal procedures (including biopsy of labia, vagina, cervix or endometrium); not otherwise specified

00942 colpotomy, vaginectomy, colporrhaphy and open urethral procedures

00944 vaginal hysterectomy

00948 cervical cerclage

00950 culdoscopy

00952 hysteroscopy and/or hysterosalpingography

PELVIS (EXCEPT HIP)

01112 Anesthesia for bone marrow aspiration and/or biopsy, anterior or posterior iliac crest

01120 Anesthesia for procedures on bony pelvis

01130 Anesthesia for body cast application or revision

01140 Anesthesia for interpelviabdominal (hindquarter) amputation

01150 Anesthesia for radical procedures for tumor of pelvis, except hindquarter amputation

01160 Anesthesia for closed procedures involving symphysis pubis or sacroiliac joint

01170 Anesthesia for open procedures involving symphysis pubis or sacroiliac joint

01173 Anesthesia for open repair of fracture disruption of pelvis or column fracture involving acetabulum

01180 Anesthesia for obturator neurectomy; extrapelvic

01190 intrapelvic

UPPER LEG (EXCEPT KNEE)

01200 Anesthesia for all closed procedures involving hip joint

01202 Anesthesia for arthroscopic procedures of hip joint

01210 Anesthesia for open procedures involving hip joint; not otherwise specified

01212 hip disarticulation

01214 total hip arthroplasty

01215 revision of total hip arthroplasty

01220 Anesthesia for all closed procedures involving upper 2/3 of femur

● New Code ▲ Revised Code + Add-On Code ⃠ Modifier -51 Exempt ⊙ Conscious Sedation

01230 Anesthesia for open procedures involving upper 2/3 of femur; not otherwise specified

01232 amputation

01234 radical resection

01250 Anesthesia for all procedures on nerves, muscles, tendons, fascia, and bursae of upper leg

01260 Anesthesia for all procedures involving veins of upper leg, including exploration

01270 Anesthesia for procedures involving arteries of upper leg, including bypass graft; not otherwise specified

01272 femoral artery ligation

01274 femoral artery embolectomy

KNEE AND POPLITEAL AREA

01320 Anesthesia for all procedures on nerves, muscles, tendons, fascia, and bursae of knee and/or popliteal area

01340 Anesthesia for all closed procedures on lower 1/3 of femur

01360 Anesthesia for all open procedures on lower 1/3 of femur

01380 Anesthesia for all closed procedures on knee joint

01382 Anesthesia for diagnostic arthroscopic procedures of knee joint

01390 Anesthesia for all closed procedures on upper ends of tibia, fibula, and/or patella

01392 Anesthesia for all open procedures on upper ends of tibia, fibula, and/or patella

01400 Anesthesia for open or surgical arthroscopic procedures on knee joint; not otherwise specified

01402 total knee arthroplasty

01404 disarticulation at knee

01420 Anesthesia for all cast applications, removal, or repair involving knee joint

01430 Anesthesia for procedures on veins of knee and popliteal area; not otherwise specified

01432 arteriovenous fistula

01440 Anesthesia for procedures on arteries of knee and popliteal area; not otherwise specified

01442 popliteal thromboendarterectomy, with or without patch graft

01444 popliteal excision and graft or repair for occlusion or aneurysm

LOWER LEG (BELOW KNEE, INCLUDES ANKLE AND FOOT)

01462 Anesthesia for all closed procedures on lower leg, ankle, and foot

01464 Anesthesia for arthroscopic procedures of ankle and/or foot

01470 Anesthesia for procedures on nerves, muscles, tendons, and fascia of lower leg, ankle, and foot; not otherwise specified

01472 repair of ruptured Achilles tendon, with or without graft

01474 gastrocnemius recession (eg, Strayer procedure)

01480 Anesthesia for open procedures on bones of lower leg, ankle, and foot; not otherwise specified

01482 radical resection (including below knee amputation)

01484 osteotomy or osteoplasty of tibia and/or fibula

01486 total ankle replacement

01490 Anesthesia for lower leg cast application, removal, or repair

01500 Anesthesia for procedures on arteries of lower leg, including bypass graft; not otherwise specified

01502 embolectomy, direct or with catheter

01520 Anesthesia for procedures on veins of lower leg; not otherwise specified

01522 venous thrombectomy, direct or with catheter

SHOULDER AND AXILLA

Includes humeral head and neck, sternoclavicular joint, acromioclavicular joint, and shoulder joint

01610 Anesthesia for all procedures on nerves, muscles, tendons, fascia, and bursae of shoulder and axilla

01620 Anesthesia for all closed procedures on humeral head and neck, sternoclavicular joint, acromioclavicular joint, and shoulder joint

01622 Anesthesia for diagnostic arthroscopic procedures of shoulder joint

01630 Anesthesia for open or surgical arthroscopic procedures on humeral head and neck, sternoclavicular joint, acromioclavicular joint, and shoulder joint; not otherwise specified

01632 radical resection

01634 shoulder disarticulation

01636 interthoracoscapular (forequarter) amputation

01638 total shoulder replacement

01650 Anesthesia for procedures on arteries of shoulder and axilla; not otherwise specified

01652 axillary-brachial aneurysm

01654 bypass graft

01656 axillary-femoral bypass graft

01670 Anesthesia for all procedures on veins of shoulder and axilla

01680 Anesthesia for shoulder cast application, removal or repair; not otherwise specified

01682 shoulder spica

UPPER ARM AND ELBOW

01710 Anesthesia for procedures on nerves, muscles, tendons, fascia, and bursae of upper arm and elbow; not otherwise specified

01712 tenotomy, elbow to shoulder, open

01714 tenoplasty, elbow to shoulder

01716 tenodesis, rupture of long tendon of biceps

01730 Anesthesia for all closed procedures on humerus and elbow

01732 Anesthesia for diagnostic arthroscopic procedures of elbow joint

01740 Anesthesia for open or surgical arthroscopic procedures of the elbow; not otherwise specified

01742 osteotomy of humerus

01744 repair of nonunion or malunion of humerus

01756 radical procedures

01758 excision of cyst or tumor of humerus

01760 total elbow replacement

01770 Anesthesia for procedures on arteries of upper arm and elbow; not otherwise specified

01772 embolectomy

01780 Anesthesia for procedures on veins of upper arm and elbow; not otherwise specified

01782 phleborrhaphy

FOREARM, WRIST, AND HAND

01810 Anesthesia for all procedures on nerves, muscles, tendons, fascia, and bursae of forearm, wrist, and hand

01820 Anesthesia for all closed procedures on radius, ulna, wrist, or hand bones

01829 Anesthesia for diagnostic arthroscopic procedures on the wrist

01830 Anesthesia for open or surgical arthroscopic/endoscopic procedures on distal radius, distal ulna, wrist, or hand joints; not otherwise specified

01832 total wrist replacement

01840 Anesthesia for procedures on arteries of forearm, wrist, and hand; not otherwise specified

01842 embolectomy

01844 Anesthesia for vascular shunt, or shunt revision, any type (eg, dialysis)

01850 Anesthesia for procedures on veins of forearm, wrist, and hand; not otherwise specified

01852 phleborrhaphy

01860 Anesthesia for forearm, wrist, or hand cast application, removal, or repair

RADIOLOGICAL PROCEDURES

01905 Anesthesia for myelography, diskography, vertebroplasty

01916 Anesthesia for diagnostic arteriography/venography

(Do not report 01916 in conjunction with therapeutic codes 01924-01926, 01930-01933)

01920 Anesthesia for cardiac catheterization including coronary angiography and ventriculography (not to include Swan-Ganz catheter)

01922 Anesthesia for non-invasive imaging or radiation therapy

01924 Anesthesia for therapeutic interventional radiologic procedures involving the arterial system; not otherwise specified

01925 carotid or coronary

01926 intracranial, intracardiac, or aortic

01930 Anesthesia for therapeutic interventional radiologic procedures involving the venous/lymphatic system (not to include access to the central circulation); not otherwise specified

01931 intrahepatic or portal circulation (eg, transcutaneous porto-caval shunt (TIPS))

01932 intrathoracic or jugular

01933 intracranial

BURN EXCISIONS OR DEBRIDEMENT

01951 Anesthesia for second and third degree burn excision or debridement with or without skin grafting, any site, for total body surface area (TBSA) treated during anesthesia and surgery; less than four percent total body surface area

01952 between four and nine percent of total body surface area

+ **01953** each additional nine percent total body surface area or part thereof (List separately in addition to code for primary procedure)

(Use 01953 in conjunction with code 01952)

OBSTETRIC

01958 Anesthesia for external cephalic version procedure

01960 Anesthesia for vaginal delivery only

01961 Anesthesia for cesarean delivery only

01962 Anesthesia for urgent hysterectomy following delivery

01963 Anesthesia for cesarean hysterectomy without any labor analgesia/anesthesia care

(01964 deleted 2006 edition. To report, see 01965, 01966)

01965 Anesthesia for incomplete or missed abortion procedures

01966 Anesthesia for induced abortion procedures

01967 Neuraxial labor analgesia/anesthesia for planned vaginal delivery (this includes any repeat subarachnoid needle placement and drug injection and/or any necessary replacement of an epidural catheter during labor)

+ **01968** Anesthesia for cesarean delivery following neuraxial labor analgesia/anesthesia (List separately in addition to code for primary procedure performed)

(Use 01968 in conjunction with code 01967)

+ **01969** Anesthesia for cesarean hysterectomy following neuraxial labor analgesia/anesthesia (List separately in addition to code for primary procedure performed)

(Use 01969 in conjunction with code 01967)

OTHER PROCEDURES

01990 Physiological support for harvesting of organ(s) from brain-dead patient

01991 Anesthesia for diagnostic or therapeutic nerve blocks and injections (when block or injection is performed by a different provider); other than the prone position

01992 prone position

(Do not report code 01991 or 01992 in conjunction with 99141)

(When regional intravenous administration of local anesthetic agent or other medication in the upper or lower extremity is used as the anesthetic for a surgical procedure, report the appropriate anesthesia code. To report a Bier block for pain management, use 64999. For intra-arterial or intravenous injections, see 90773, 90774.)

(For intra-arterial or intravenous therapy for pain management, see 90773, 90774)

(01995 deleted 2007 edition.)

01996 Daily hospital management of epidural or subarachnoid continuous drug administration

(Report code 01996 for daily hospital management of continuous epidural or subarachnoid drug administration performed after insertion of an epidural or subarachnoid catheter placed primarily for anesthesia administration during an operative session, but retained for post-operative pain management)

01999 Unlisted anesthesia procedure(s)

● New Code ▲ Revised Code + Add-On Code ⃠ Modifier -51 Exempt ⊙ Conscious Sedation

SURGERY

SURGERY SECTION OVERVIEW

The third section of the CPT coding system is the surgery section, and it includes surgical procedure codes for all body areas. Within each subsection, the CPT codes are arranged by anatomical site.

It is essential to understand the organization of the CPT surgery section in order to locate the correct procedure code. Understanding other or alternative terms which may apply to a procedure, injury, illness or condition may also make the location of the appropriate procedure easier and faster.

All procedures listed in the surgery section of the CPT book include local, metacarpal/digital block or topical anesthesia if used, the surgical procedure, and normal uncomplicated follow-up care. For diagnostic surgical procedures, follow-up care includes only the care related to recovery from the diagnostic procedure. For therapeutic surgical procedures, follow-up care includes only the care which would usually be included in the surgical service. Any complications resulting in additional services are not considered to be included and should be coded separately.

KEY POINTS ABOUT SURGERY SERVICES

- *Evaluation and management services provided by surgeons in the office, home or hospital, plus consultations and other medical services are coded using evaluation and management service codes.*
- *Any supplies and/or materials provided by the surgeon which are not considered to be included in the standard service may be coded separately.*

GLOBAL SURGICAL PACKAGE

Third-party payers differ in their definition of a surgical or global surgical package concept. Medicare defines the global surgical package as follows:

- *The surgeon's initial evaluation or consultation will be paid separately.*
- *There is a one day preoperative period covered under the global surgical package.*
- *Included in the package are all intraoperative services that are considered to be usual and necessary. Separate billing of these services would be considered unbundling.*
- *Any treatment of complications by the surgeon not requiring a return to the operating room is included in the package.*

- *The surgical package contains a standard 90-day postoperative period which includes all visits to the physician during that time unless the visit is for a totally different reason than that for the surgery.*
- *In cases of organ transplant, immunosuppressive therapy is not included in the global package.*
- *Minor surgical procedures are those with a 0 or 10-day postoperative period, and are excluded from the surgical package definition.*

SPECIAL REPORT

Surgical procedures which are new, unusual or vary significantly from the standard definition may require a special report. When preparing reports to accompany health insurance claim forms the provider should include a description of the nature, extent, and need for the procedure, and the time, effort, and equipment necessary to provides the service. Try to keep these reports as brief and simple as possible. Additional items which may be needed are:

- *complexity of symptoms*
- *final diagnosis*
- *pertinent physical findings*
- *diagnostic and therapeutic procedures*
- *concurrent problems*
- *follow-up care*

MULTIPLE SURGICAL PROCEDURES

It is common for several surgical procedures to be performed at the same operative session. When multiple procedures are performed on the same day or at the same session, the "major" procedure or service is listed first followed by secondary, additional, or "lessor" procedures or services. CPT modifier -51 is added to all procedures following the first one.

Reporting multiple procedures incorrectly may have a serious impact on reimbursement from health insurance payers. An inexperienced health insurance biller may simply list the procedures on the health insurance claim form in the order dictated or described in the operative report.

There are two critical decisions related to reporting multiple surgical procedures correctly; namely: 1) The order in which the procedures are listed on the health insurance claim form, and 2) whether or not to list the additional procedures with full or reduced fees.

ORDER OF LISTING MULTIPLE PROCEDURES

The first procedure to be listed when reporting services under the multiple procedure rule is the procedure with the highest fee. Additional procedures should be listed in descending order by fee. Modifier -51 should be added to each additional procedure.

All third party payers will reduce the allowance for the additional procedures, typically by 50 percent for the second procedure, and 50 to 75 percent for the third and subsequent procedures. Listing the procedures in descending order by fee minimizes the possibility of an incorrect reduction.

21. DIAGNOSIS OR NATURE OF ILLNESS OR INJURY. (RELATE ITEMS 1,2,3 OR 4 TO ITEM 24E BY LINE)

1. 952.10   3. ___.__

2. ___.__   4. ___.__

24	A DATE(S) OF SERVICE FROM MM	DD	YY	FROM MM	DD	YY	B Place of Service	C Type of Service	D PROCEDURES, SERVICES, OR SUPPLIES (Explain Unusual Circumstances) CPT/HCPCS	MODIFIER	E DIAGNOSIS CODE
1	06	15	07				21		63046		
2	06	15	07				21		62223	51	
3											
4											

BILLING FULL VERSUS REDUCED FEES

The full fee should be listed for each procedure coded on the health insurance claim form as part of multiple surgical procedures. Third party payers will automatically reduce the allowances for the additional procedures by a specific formula. Listing all multiple procedures with full fees in descending fee order (the procedure with the highest fee first, the procedure with the next highest fee second, et cetera) will result in the maximum total allowable reimbursement for the provider or the insured.

After the maximum benefit has been paid by the health insurance company, the balance remaining, less any patient co-insurance or deductible requirements, should be written off. Note that billing practices vary in different areas of the country. Providers should continue to use the method that is customary or required by third party payers in the provider's practice location.

SEPARATE PROCEDURE

Some surgical procedures are considered to be an integral part of a more extensive surgical procedure. In this circumstance, the integral procedure is not coded. When the integral procedure is performed independently and is unrelated to other services, it should be listed as a "separate procedure."

SURGERY SUBSECTIONS

The SURGERY section of the CPT coding system is divided into 17 subsections:

Integumentary System	10040-19499
Musculoskeletal System	20000-29999
Respiratory System	30000-32999
Cardiovascular System	33010-37799
Hemic and Lymphatic Systems	38100-38999
Mediastinum and Diaphragm	39000-39599
Digestive System	40490-49999
Urinary System	50010-53899
Male Genital System	54000-55899
Intersex Surgery	55970-55980
Female Genital Surgery	56405-58999
Maternity Care and Delivery	59000-59899
Endocrine System	60000-60699
Nervous System	61000-64999
Eye and Ocular Adnexa	65091-68899
Auditory System	69000-69979
Operating Microscope	69990

Each sub-section of the SURGERY section of the CPT coding system is divided into organs then into procedures involving anatomic sites. Each anatomic site is further separated into surgical processes such as incision, excision, repair, removal, amputation, etc.

SURGERY SECTION MODIFIERS

Due to various circumstances, surgical procedures may be considered to be modified in comparison to the full or complete procedure. Modified procedures are identified by reporting a two-digit modifier to the CPT procedure code(s). The following CPT modifiers may be coded with surgical procedures:

-22 Unusual Procedural Services

-26 Professional Component

-32 Mandated Services

-47 Anesthesia by Surgeon

-50 Bilateral Procedure

-51 Multiple Procedures

-52 Reduced Services

-54 Surgical Care Only

-55 Postoperative Management Only

-56 Preoperative Management Only

-57 Decision for Surgery

-58 Staged or Related Procedure or Service by the Same Physician During the Postoperative Period

-62 Two Surgeons

-66 Surgical Team

-76 Repeat Procedure by Same Physician

-77 Repeat Procedure by Another Physician

-78 Return to the Operating Room for a Related Procedure During the Postoperative Period

-79 Unrelated Procedure or Service by the Same Physician During the Postoperative Period

-80 Assistant Surgeon

-81 Minimum Assistant Surgeon

-82 Assistant Surgeon (when qualified resident surgeon not available)

-90 Reference (Outside) Laboratory

-99 Multiple modifiers

ADD-ON CODES

Many surgical procedures are performed secondary to primary surgical procedures. These procedures are classified as "additional" or "supplemental" procedures and are designated as "add-on" codes in the CPT coding system. "Add-on" CPT codes are identified in the CPT code book by a black plus sign "+" placed to the left of the code number.

Many of the CPT "Add-on" codes are further identified by phrases included within the descriptions of the definition of the CPT code or include the phrase "(List separately in addition to primary procedure)" following the definition. Examples of CPT codes identified as "add-on" codes in CPT 2007 include:

+ 11008 Removal of prosthetic material or mesh, abdominal wall for necrotizing soft tissue infection (list separately in addition to code for primary procedure)

+ 15116 Epidermal autograft, face, scalp, eyelids, mouth, neck, ears, orbits, genitalia, hands, feet, and/or multiple digits; each additional 100 sq cm, or each additional one percent of body area of infants and children, or part thereof (List separately in addition to code for primary procedure)

STARRED PROCEDURES

CPT used to define minor surgical procedures by placing a star (*) after the procedure code number. This designation was removed in CPT 2004.

MEDICAL AND SURGICAL SUPPLIES

HCPCS Level II codes for medical and surgical supplies, A4000-A4999, may be used to report supplies and materials provided to Medicare patients if the supplies and materials are not considered to be included with or part of the basic service(s) or procedure(s).

SURGERY CODES

GENERAL

10021 Fine needle aspiration; without imaging guidance

10022 with imaging guidance

(For radiological supervision and interpretation, see 76942, 77002, 77012, 77021)

(For percutaneous needle biopsy other than fine needle aspiration, see 20206 for muscle, 32400 for pleura, 32405 for lung or mediastinum, 42400 for salivary gland, 47000, 47001 for liver, 48102 for pancreas, 49180 for abdominal or retroperitoneal mass, 60100 for thyroid, 62269 for spinal cord)

(For evaluation of fine needle aspirate, see 88172, 88173)

This page intentionally left blank.

● New Code ▲ Revised Code + Add-On Code ⊘ Modifier -51 Exempt ⊙ Conscious Sedation

INTEGUMENTARY SYSTEM

SKIN, SUBCUTANEOUS AND ACCESSORY STRUCTURES

INCISION AND DRAINAGE

(For excision, see 11400, et seq)

10040 Acne surgery (eg, marsupialization, opening or removal of multiple milia, comedones, cysts, pustules)

10060 Incision and drainage of abscess (eg, carbuncle, suppurative hidradenitis, cutaneous or subcutaneous abscess, cyst, furuncle, or paronychia); simple or single

10061 complicated or multiple

10080 Incision and drainage of pilonidal cyst; simple

10081 complicated

(For excision of pilonidal cyst, see 11770-11772)

10120 Incision and removal of foreign body, subcutaneous tissues; simple

10121 complicated

(To report wound exploration due to penetrating trauma without laparotomy or thoracotomy, see 20100-20103, as appropriate)

(To report debridement associated with open fracture(s) and/or dislocation(s), use 11010-11012, as appropriate)

10140 Incision and drainage of hematoma, seroma or fluid collection

(If imaging guidance is performed, see 76942, 77012, 77021)

10160 Puncture aspiration of abscess, hematoma, bulla, or cyst

(If imaging guidance is performed, see 76942, 77012, 77021)

10180 Incision and drainage, complex, postoperative wound infection

(For secondary closure of surgical wound, see 12020, 12021, 13160)

INTEG 10000

EXCISION-DEBRIDEMENT

(For dermabrasions, see 15780-15783)

(For nail debridement, see 11720-11721)

(For burn(s), see 16000-16035)

11000 Debridement of extensive eczematous or infected skin; up to 10% of body surface

(For abdominal wall or genitalia debridement for necrotizing soft tissue infection, see 11004-11006)

+ **11001** each additional 10% of the body surface (List separately in addition to code for primary procedure)

(Use 11001 in conjunction with code 11000)

11004 Debridement of skin, subcutaneous tissue, muscle and fascia for necrotizing soft tissue infection; external genitalia and perineum

11005 abdominal wall, with or without fascial closure

11006 external genitalia, perineum and abdominal wall, with or without fascial closure

+ **11008** Removal of prosthetic material or mesh, abdominal wall for necrotizing soft tissue infection (list separately in addition to code for primary procedure)

(Use 11008 in conjunction with 11004-11006)

(Do not report 11008 in conjunction with 11000-11001, 11010-11044)

(Report skin grafts or flaps separately when performed for closure at the same session as 11004-11008)

(When insertion of mesh is used for closure, use 49568)

(If orchiectomy is performed, use 54520)

(If testicular transplantation is performed, use 54680)

11010 Debridement including removal of foreign material associated with open fracture(s) and/or dislocation(s); skin and subcutaneous tissues

11011 skin, subcutaneous tissue, muscle fascia, and muscle

11012 skin, subcutaneous tissue, muscle fascia, muscle, and bone

11040 Debridement; skin, partial thickness

11041 skin, full thickness

11042 skin, and subcutaneous tissue

11043 skin, subcutaneous tissue, and muscle

11044 skin, subcutaneous tissue, muscle, and bone

(Do not report 11040-11044 in conjunction with 97597-97602)

PARING OR CUTTING

(To report destruction, see 17000-17004)

11055 Paring or cutting of benign hyperkeratotic lesion (eg, corn or callus); single lesion

11056 two to four lesions

11057 more than four lesions

BIOPSY

(For biopsy of conjunctiva, use 68100; eyelid, use 67810)

11100 Biopsy of skin, subcutaneous tissue and/or mucous membrane (including simple closure), unless otherwise listed; single lesion

+ 11101 each separate/additional lesion (List separately in addition to code for primary procedure)

(Use 11101 in conjunction with code 11100)

REMOVAL OF SKIN TAGS

11200 Removal of skin tags, multiple fibrocutaneous tags, any area; up to and including 15 lesions

+ 11201 each additional ten lesions (List separately in addition to code for primary procedure)

(Use 11201 in conjunction with code 11200)

SHAVING OF EPIDERMAL OR DERMAL LESIONS

Many of the procedure codes listed in the integumentary system subsection of the CPT manual are designated in centimeters or square centimeters. Many physicians document sizes using inches or millimeters. Make sure to verify, and convert if necessary, measurements before assigning a code.

To be able to code lesion removal appropriately, the site, size in centimeters, method of removal and morphology must be documented in the medical record. Always code morphology from the pathology report.

Excision of lesion codes are determined by the diameter of the actual lesion, not the specimen sent to pathology. However, the size of the specimen can be used when the size of the lesion cannot be located in the operative report or elsewhere in the medical record.

When more than one dimension of a lesion is provided in the documentation, select the code based on the largest size. For example, if the dimensions indicated are 3 cm x 2 cm x 1.5 cm, the lesion should be coded as 3 cm. Excision of benign and malignant lesions includes anesthesia and simple repair of the defect site.

11300 Shaving of epidermal or dermal lesion, single lesion, trunk, arms or legs; lesion diameter 0.5 cm or less

11301 lesion diameter 0.6 to 1.0 cm

11302 lesion diameter 1.1 to 2.0 cm

11303 lesion diameter over 2.0 cm

11305 Shaving of epidermal or dermal lesion, single lesion, scalp, neck, hands, feet, genitalia; lesion diameter 0.5 cm or less

11306 lesion diameter 0.6 to 1.0 cm

11307 lesion diameter 1.1 to 2.0 cm

11308 lesion diameter over 2.0 cm

11310 Shaving of epidermal or dermal lesion, single lesion, face, ears, eyelids, nose, lips, mucous membrane; lesion diameter 0.5 cm or less

11311 lesion diameter 0.6 to 1.0 cm

11312 lesion diameter 1.1 to 2.0 cm

11313 lesion diameter over 2.0 cm

EXCISION OF BENIGN LESIONS

Excision (including simple closure) of benign lesions of skin (eg., neoplasm, cicatricial, fibrous, inflammatory, congenital, cystic lesions) includes local anesthesia. See appropriate size and area below. For shave removal, see 11300 et seq., and for electrosurgical and other methods, see 17000 et seq..

For excision of benign lesions requiring more than simple closure, ie, requiring intermediate or complex closure, report 11400-11466 in addition to appropriate intermediate (12031-12057) or complex closure (13100-13153) codes. For reconstructive closure, see 11400-14300, 15000-15261, 15570-15770.

11400 Excision, benign lesion including margins, except skin tag (unless listed elsewhere), trunk, arms or legs; excised diameter 0.5 cm or less

11401 excised diameter 0.6 to 1.0 cm

11402 excised diameter 1.1 to 2.0 cm

11403 excised diameter 2.1 to 3.0 cm

11404 excised diameter 3.1 to 4.0 cm

11406 excised diameter over 4.0 cm

(For unusual or complicated excision, add modifier -22)

11420 Excision, benign lesion including margins, except skin tag (unless listed elsewhere), scalp, neck, hands, feet, genitalia; excised diameter 0.5 cm or less

11421 excised diameter 0.6 to 1.0 cm

11422 excised diameter 1.1 to 2.0 cm

11423 excised diameter 2.1 to 3.0 cm

11424 excised diameter 3.1 to 4.0 cm

11426 excised diameter over 4.0 cm

(For unusual or complicated excision, add modifier -22)

11440 Excision, other benign lesion including margins (unless listed elsewhere), face, ears, eyelids, nose, lips, mucous membrane; excised diameter 0.5 cm or less

11441 excised diameter 0.6 to 1.0 cm

11442 excised diameter 1.1 to 2.0 cm

11443 excised diameter 2.1 to 3.0 cm

11444 excised diameter 3.1 to 4.0 cm

11446 excised diameter over 4.0 cm

(For unusual or complicated excision, add modifier -22)

(For eyelids involving more than skin, see also 67800 et seq.)

11450 Excision of skin and subcutaneous tissue for hidradenitis, axillary; with simple or intermediate repair

11451 with complex repair

11462 Excision of skin and subcutaneous tissue for hidradenitis, inguinal; with simple or intermediate repair

11463 with complex repair

11470 Excision of skin and subcutaneous tissue for hidradenitis, perianal, perineal, or umbilical; with simple or intermediate repair

11471 with complex repair

(When skin graft or flap is used for closure, use appropriate procedure code in addition)

(For bilateral procedure, add modifier -50)

EXCISION OF MALIGNANT LESIONS

For excision of malignant lesions requiring more than simple closure, i.e., requiring intermediate or complex closure, report 11600-11646 in addition to appropriate intermediate (12031-12057) or complex closure (13100-13153) codes. For reconstructive closure, see 14000-14300, 15000-15261, 15570-15770.

11600 Excision, malignant lesion including margins, trunk, arms, or legs; excised diameter 0.5 cm or less

11601 excised diameter 0.6 to 1.0 cm

11602 excised diameter 1.1 to 2.0 cm

11603 excised diameter 2.1 to 3.0 cm

11604 excised diameter 3.1 to 4.0 cm

11606 excised diameter over 4.0 cm

11620 Excision, malignant lesion including margins, scalp, neck, hands, feet, genitalia; excised diameter 0.5 cm or less

11621 excised diameter 0.6 to 1.0 cm

11622 excised diameter 1.1 to 2.0 cm

11623 excised diameter 2.1 to 3.0 cm

11624 excised diameter 3.1 to 4.0 cm

11626 excised diameter over 4.0 cm

11640 Excision, malignant lesion including margins, face, ears, eyelids, nose, lips; excised diameter 0.5 cm or less

11641 excised diameter 0.6 to 1.0 cm

11642 excised diameter 1.1 to 2.0 cm

11643 excised diameter 2.1 to 3.0 cm

11644 excised diameter 3.1 to 4.0 cm

11646 excised diameter over 4.0 cm

(For eyelids involving more than skin, see also 67800 et seq)

NAILS

(For drainage of paronychia or onychia, see 10060, 10061)

11719 Trimming of nondystrophic nails, any number

11720 Debridement of nail(s) by any method(s); one to five

11721 six or more

11730 Avulsion of nail plate, partial or complete, simple; single

+ **11732** each additional nail plate (List separately in addition to code for primary procedure)

(Use 11732 in conjunction with code 11730)

11740 Evacuation of subungual hematoma

11750 Excision of nail and nail matrix, partial or complete, (eg, ingrown or deformed nail) for permanent removal;

11752 with amputation of tuft of distal phalanx

(For skin graft, if used, use 15050)

11755 Biopsy of nail unit (eg, plate, bed, matrix, hyponychium, proximal and lateral nail folds) (separate procedure)

11760 Repair of nail bed

11762 Reconstruction of nail bed with graft

11765 Wedge excision of skin of nail fold (eg, for ingrown toenail)

PILONIDAL CYST

11770 Excision of pilonidal cyst or sinus; simple

11771 extensive

11772 complicated

(For incision of pilonidal cyst, see 10080, 10081)

INTRODUCTION

11900 Injection, intralesional; up to and including seven lesions

11901 more than seven lesions

(11900, 11901 are not to be used for preoperative local anesthetic injection)

(For veins, see 36470, 36471)

(For intralesional chemotherapy administration, see 96405, 96406)

11920 Tattooing, intradermal introduction of insoluble opaque pigments to correct color defects of skin, including micropigmentation; 6.0 sq cm or less

11921 6.1 to 20.0 sq cm

+ 11922 each additional 20.0 sq cm (List separately in addition to code for primary procedure)

(Use 11922 in conjunction with code 11921)

11950 Subcutaneous injection of filling material (eg, collagen); 1 cc or less

11951 1.1 to 5.0 cc

11952 5.1 to 10.0 cc

11954 over 10.0 cc

11960 Insertion of tissue expander(s) for other than breast, including subsequent expansion

(For breast reconstruction with tissue expander(s), use 19357)

11970 Replacement of tissue expander with permanent prosthesis

11971 Removal of tissue expander(s) without insertion of prosthesis

11975 Insertion, implantable contraceptive capsules

11976 Removal, implantable contraceptive capsules

11977 Removal with reinsertion, implantable contraceptive capsules

11980 Subcutaneous hormone pellet implantation (implantation of estradiol and/or testosterone pellets beneath the skin)

11981 Insertion, non-biodegradable drug delivery implant

11982 Removal, non-biodegradable drug delivery implant

11983 Removal with reinsertion, non-biodegradable drug delivery implant

REPAIR (CLOSURE)

To be able to code wound repair appropriately, the site, length of wound in centimeters and type of repair must be documented in the medical record. Review the definitions of simple, intermediate and complex repair in the current CPT coding system.

Simple repair is used when the wound is superficial, eg., involving primarily epidermis or dermis, or subcutaneous tissues without significant involvement of deeper structures, and requires simple one layer closure. This includes local anesthesia and chemical or electrocauterization of wounds not closed.

Intermediate repair includes the repair of wounds that, in addition to the above, require layered closure of one or more of the deeper layers of subcutaneous tissue and superficial (non-muscle) fascia, in addition to the skin (epidermal and dermal) closure. Single-layer closure of heavily contaminated wounds that have required extensive cleaning or removal of particulate matter also constitutes intermediate repair.

Complex repair includes the repair of wounds requiring more than layered closure, viz., scar revision, debridement (eg., traumatic lacerations or avulsions), extensive undermining, stents or retention sutures. Necessary preparation includes creation of a defect for repairs (eg., excision of a scar requiring complex repair) or the debridement of complicated lacerations or avulsions. Complex repair does not include excision of benign (11400-11446) or malignant (11600-11646) lesions.

Multiple wound repairs from the same body site (category of codes) that were repaired using the same type of closure (simple, intermediate, or complex) should be coded as one wound. Add the measurements of each wound and assign a single code for the repair.

Simple exploration of nerves, blood vessels or tendons exposed in an open wound are integral part of the wound repair treatment and should not be coded separately. If the wound requires enlargement, extension of dissection, debridement, removal of foreign body, ligation or coagulation of minor subcutaneous and/or muscular blood vessel(s), of the subcutaneous tissue, muscle fascia, and/or muscle, not requiring thoracotomy or laparotomy, use wound exploration codes (20100-20103), as appropriate.

REPAIR — SIMPLE

Sum of lengths of repairs for each group of anatomic sites.

12001 Simple repair of superficial wounds of scalp, neck, axillae, external genitalia, trunk and/or extremities (including hands and feet); 2.5 cm or less

12002 2.6 cm to 7.5 cm

12004 7.6 cm to 12.5 cm

12005 12.6 cm to 20.0 cm

12006 20.1 cm to 30.0 cm

12007 over 30.0 cm

12011 Simple repair of superficial wounds of face, ears, eyelids, nose, lips and/or mucous membranes; 2.5 cm or less

12013 2.6 cm to 5.0 cm

12014 5.1 cm to 7.5 cm

12015 7.6 cm to 12.5 cm

12016 12.6 cm to 20.0 cm

12017 20.1 cm to 30.0 cm

12018 over 30.0 cm

12020 Treatment of superficial wound dehiscence; simple closure

12021 with packing

(For extensive or complicated secondary wound closure, use 13160)

REPAIR — INTERMEDIATE

Sum of lengths of repairs for each group of anatomic sites.

12031 Layer closure of wounds of scalp, axillae, trunk and/or extremities (excluding hands and feet); 2.5 cm or less

12032 2.6 cm to 7.5 cm

12034 7.6 cm to 12.5 cm

12035 12.6 cm to 20.0 cm

12036 20.1 cm to 30.0 cm

12037 over 30.0 cm

12041 Layer closure of wounds of neck, hands, feet and/or external genitalia; 2.5 cm or less

12042 2.6 cm to 7.5 cm

12044 7.6 cm to 12.5 cm

12045 12.6 cm to 20.0 cm

12046 20.1 cm to 30.0 cm

12047 over 30.0 cm

12051 Layer closure of wounds of face, ears, eyelids, nose, lips and/or mucous membranes; 2.5 cm or less

12052 2.6 cm to 5.0 cm

12053 5.1 cm to 7.5 cm

12054 7.6 cm to 12.5 cm

12055 12.6 cm to 20.0 cm

12056 20.1 cm to 30.0 cm

12057 over 30.0 cm

REPAIR — COMPLEX

Reconstructive procedures, complicated wound closure.

Sum of lengths of repairs for each group of anatomic sites.

(For full thickness repair of lip or eyelid, see respective anatomical subsections)

13100 Repair, complex, trunk; 1.1 cm to 2.5 cm

(For 1.0 cm or less, see simple or intermediate repairs)

13101 2.6 cm to 7.5 cm

+ **13102** each additional 5 cm or less (List separately in addition to code for primary procedure)

(Use 13102 in conjunction with code 13101)

13120 Repair, complex, scalp, arms, and/or legs; 1.1 cm to 2.5 cm

(For 1.0 cm or less, see simple or intermediate repairs)

13121 2.6 cm to 7.5 cm

+ **13122** each additional 5 cm or less (List separately in addition to code for primary procedure)

(Use 13122 in conjunction with 13121)

13131 Repair, complex, forehead, cheeks, chin, mouth, neck, axillae, genitalia, hands and/or feet; 1.1 cm to 2.5 cm

(For 1.0 cm or less, see simple or intermediate repairs)

13132 2.6 cm to 7.5 cm

+ **13133** each additional 5 cm or less (List separately in addition to code for primary procedure)

(Use 13133 in conjunction with 13132)

13150 Repair, complex, eyelids, nose, ears and/or lips; 1.0 cm or less

(See also 40650-40654, 67961-67975)

13151 1.1 cm to 2.5 cm

13152 2.6 cm to 7.5 cm

+ **13153** each additional 5 cm or less (List separately in addition to code for primary procedure)

(Use 13153 in conjunction with code 13152)

13160 Secondary closure of surgical wound or dehiscence, extensive or complicated

(For packing or simple secondary wound closure, see 12020, 12021)

ADJACENT TISSUE TRANSFER OR REARRANGEMENT

Codes for adjacent tissue transfer or rearrangement (14000-14350) are determined by the size and location of the defect site. Excision of lesions performed prior to an adjacent tissue transfer or rearrangement are included in codes 14000 to 14350.

14000 Adjacent tissue transfer or rearrangement, trunk; defect 10 sq cm or less

14001 defect 10.1 sq cm to 30.0 sq cm

14020 Adjacent tissue transfer or rearrangement, scalp, arms and/or legs; defect 10 sq cm or less

14021 defect 10.1 sq cm to 30.0 sq cm

14040 Adjacent tissue transfer or rearrangement, forehead, cheeks, chin, mouth, neck, axillae, genitalia, hands and/or feet; defect 10 sq cm or less

14041 defect 10.1 sq cm to 30.0 sq cm

14060 Adjacent tissue transfer or rearrangement, eyelids, nose, ears and/or lips; defect 10 sq cm or less

14061 defect 10.1 sq cm to 30.0 sq cm

(For eyelid, full thickness, see 67961 et seq)

14300 Adjacent tissue transfer or rearrangement, more than 30 sq cm, unusual or complicated, any area

14350 Filleted finger or toe flap, including preparation of recipient site

SKIN REPLACEMENT SURGERY AND SKIN SUBSTITUTES

Free skin grafts are coded by type (split or full), location, and size. For a specific location, a primary code is defined and followed by a supplemental code for additional coverage area. As a result of this coding scheme, for a given area of involvement, the initial code is limited to one unit of service; the supplemental code may have multiple units of service depending on the area to be covered. Because, for a specific area, only one type of skin graft is typically applied, the primary free skin graft CPT codes (15100, 15120, 15200, 15220, 15240, 15260) are mutually exclusive to one another. If multiple areas require different grafts, a modifier indicating different sites should be used (anatomic or modifier -59).

Generally, debridement of non-intact skin (CPT codes 11000-11042) in anticipation of a skin graft is necessary prior to application of the skin graft and is included in the skin graft (CPT codes 15050-15400). When skin is intact, however, and the graft is being performed after excisional preparation of intact skin, the CPT code 15000 (Excisional preparation) is separately reported. CPT code 15000 is not to be used to describe debridement of non-intact, necrotic or infected skin, nor is its use indicated with other lesion removal codes.

1. *CPT codes 15350 (application of allograft) and 15400 (application of xenograft) are part of all other graft codes and are not to be separately reported with other grafts (CPT codes 15050 - 15261) for graft placement at the same site.*

2. *The CPT code 67911 describes the "Correction of lid retraction;" a parenthetical notation is added advising that, if autogenous graft materials are used, tissue graft codes 20920, 20922 or 20926 can be reported. Accordingly, all other procedures necessary to accomplish the service are included.*

Use 15002-15005 for initial wound recipient site preparation.

Codes 15002-15005 describe burn and wound preparation or incisional or excisional release of scar contracture resulting in an open wound requiring a skin graft. Codes 15100-15431 describe the application of skin replacements and skin substitutes. The following definition should be applied to those codes that reference "100 sq cm or 1% of body area of infants and children" when determining the involvement of body size: The measurement of 100 sq cm is applicable to adults and children age 10 and older; percentages of body surface area apply to infants and children younger than the age of 10.

These codes are not intended to be reported for simple graft application alone or application stabilized with dressings (eg., by simple gauze wrap). The skin substitute/graft is anchored using the surgeon's choice of fixation. When services are performed in the office, the supply of the skin substitute/graft should be reported separately. Routine dressing supplies are not reported separately.

(For microvascular flaps, see 15756-15758)

Surgical Preparation

(15000 deleted 2007 edition, see 15002, 15004.)

(15001 deleted 2007 edition, see 15003, 15005.)

● **15002** Surgical preparation or creation of recipient site by excision of open wounds, burn eschar, or scar (including subcutaneous tissues), or incisional release of scar contracture, trunk, arms,

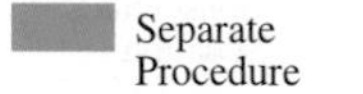

legs; first 100 sq cm or 1% of body area of infants and children

●+15003 Surgical preparation or creation of recipient site by excision of open wounds, burn eschar, or scar (including subcutaneous tissues), or incisional release of scar contracture, trunk, arms, legs; each additional 100 sq cm or each additional 1% of body area of infants and children (List separately in addition to code for primary procedure)

(Use 15003 in conjunction with 15002)

● 15004 Surgical preparation or creation of recipient site by excision of open wounds, burn eschar, or scar (including subcutaneous tissues), or incisional release of scar contracture, face, scalp, eyelids, mouth, neck, ears, orbits, genitalia, hands, feet and/or multiple digits; 1500405 first 100 sq cm or 1% of body area of infants and children

●+15005 Surgical preparation or creation of recipient site by excision of open wounds, burn eschar, or scar (including subcutaneous tissues), or incisional release of scar contracture, face, scalp, eyelids, mouth, neck, ears, orbits, genitalia, hands, feet and/or multiple digits; each additional 100 sq cm or each additional 1% of body area of infants and children (List separately in addition to code for primary procedure)

(Use 15005 in conjunction with 15004)

(Report 15002-15005 in conjunction with code for appropriate skin grafts or replacements [15050-15261, 15330-15336]. List the graft or replacement separately by its procedure number when the graft, immediate or delayed, is applied)

(For excision of benign lesions, see 11400-11471)

(For excision of malignant lesions, see 11600-11646)

(For excision to prepare or create recipient site with dressings or materials not listed in 15040-15431, use 15002-15005 only)

(For excision with immediate skin grafting, use 15002-15005 in conjunction with 15050-15261)

(For excision with immediate allograft skin placement, use 15002-15005 in conjunction with 15300-15336 and 15360-15366)

(For excision with immediate xenogenic dermis placement, use 15002-15005 in conjunction with 15400-15421)

● New Code ▲ Revised Code + Add-On Code ⊘ Modifier -51 Exempt ⊙ Conscious Sedation

Grafts

Autograft/Tissue Cultured Autograft

15040 Harvest of skin for tissue cultured skin autograft, 100 sq cm or less

15050 Pinch graft, single or multiple, to cover small ulcer, tip of digit, or other minimal open area (except on face), up to defect size 2 cm diameter

15100 Split-thickness autograft, trunk, arms, legs; first 100 sq cm or less, or one percent of body area of infants and children (except 15050)

+ 15101 each additional 100 sq cm, or each additional one percent of body area of infants and children, or part thereof (List separately in addition to code for primary procedure)

(Use 15101 in conjunction with code 15100)

15110 Epidermal autograft, trunk, arms, legs; first 100 sq cm or less, or one percent of body area of infants and children

+ 15111 each additional 100 sq cm, or each additional one percent of body area of infants and children, or part thereof (List separately in addition to code for primary procedure)

(Use 15111 in conjunction with 15110)

15115 Epidermal autograft, face, scalp, eyelids, mouth, neck, ears, orbits, genitalia, hands, feet, and/or multiple digits; first 100 sq cm or less, or one percent of body area of infants and children

+ 15116 each additional 100 sq cm, or each additional one percent of body area of infants and children, or part thereof (List separately in addition to code for primary procedure)

(Use 15116 in conjunction with 15115)

15120 Split-thickness autograft, face, scalp, eyelids, mouth, neck, ears, orbits, genitalia, hands, feet, and/or multiple digits; first 100 sq cm or less, or one percent of body area of infants and children (except 15050)

+ 15121 each additional 100 sq cm, or each additional one percent of body area of infants and children, or part thereof (List separately in addition to code for primary procedure)

(Use 15121 in conjunction with code 15120)

(For eyelids, see also 67961 et seq)

15130 Dermal autograft, trunk, arms, legs; first 100 sq cm or less, or one percent of body area of infants and children

+ 15131 each additional 100 sq cm, or each additional one percent of body area of infants and children, or part thereof (List separately in addition to code for primary procedure)

(Use 15131 in conjunction with 15130)

15135 Dermal autograft, face, scalp, eyelids, mouth, neck, ears, orbits, genitalia, hands, feet, and/or multiple digits; first 100 sq cm or less, or one percent of body area of infants and children

+ 15136 each additional 100 sq cm, or each additional one percent of body area of infants and children, or part thereof (List separately in addition to code for primary procedure)

(Use 15136 in conjunction with 15135)

15150 Tissue cultured epidermal autograft, trunk, arms, legs; first 25 sq cm or less

+ 15151 additional 1 sq cm to 75 sq cm (List separately in addition to code for primary procedure)

(Do not report 15151 more than once per session)

(Use 15151 in conjunction with 15150)

+ 15152 each additional 100 sq cm, or each additional one percent of body area of infants and children, or part thereof (List separately in addition to code for primary procedure)

(Use 15152 in conjunction with 15151)

15155 Tissue cultured epidermal autograft, face, scalp, eyelids, mouth, neck, ears, orbits, genitalia, hands, feet, and/or multiple digits; first 25 sq cm or less

+ 15156 additional 1 sq cm to 75 sq cm (List separately in addition to code for primary procedure)

(Do not report 15156 more than once per session)

(Use 15156 in conjunction with 15155)

+ 15157 each additional 100 sq cm, or each additional one percent of body area of infants and children, or part thereof (List separately in addition to code for primary procedure)

(Use 15157 in conjunction with 15156)

Acellular Dermal Replacement

15170 Acellular dermal replacement, trunk, arms, legs; first 100 sq cm or less, or one percent of body area of infants and children

+ 15171 each additional 100 sq cm, or each additional one percent of body area of infants and children, or part thereof (List separately in addition to code for primary procedure)

(Use 15171 in conjunction with 15170)

15175 Acellular dermal replacement, face, scalp, eyelids, mouth, neck, ears, orbits, genitalia, hands, feet, and/or multiple digits; first 100 sq cm or less, or one percent of body area of infants and children

+ 15176 each additional 100 sq cm, or each additional one percent of body area of infants and children, or part thereof (List separately in addition to code for primary procedure)

(Use 15176 in conjunction with 15175)

15200 Full thickness graft, free, including direct closure of donor site, trunk; 20 sq cm or less

+ 15201 each additional 20 sq cm (List separately in addition to code for primary procedure)

(Use 15201 in conjunction with 15200)

15220 Full thickness graft, free, including direct closure of donor site, scalp, arms, and/or legs; 20 sq cm or less

+ 15221 each additional 20 sq cm (List separately in addition to code for primary procedure)

(Use 15221 in conjunction with 15220)

15240 Full thickness graft, free, including direct closure of donor site, forehead, cheeks, chin, mouth, neck, axillae, genitalia, hands, and/or feet; 20 sq cm or less

(For finger tip graft, use 15050)

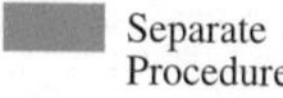
Separate Procedure
Unlisted Procedure
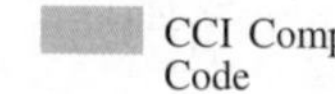
CCI Comp. Code
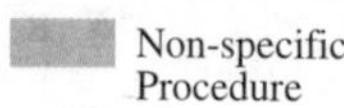
Non-specific Procedure

(For repair of syndactyly, fingers, see 26560-26562)

+ 15241 each additional 20 sq cm (List separately in addition to code for primary procedure)

(Use 15241 in conjunction with code 15240)

15260 Full thickness graft, free, including direct closure of donor site, nose, ears, eyelids, and/or lips; 20 sq cm or less

+ 15261 each additional 20 sq cm (List separately in addition to code for primary procedure)

(Use 15261 in conjunction with code 15260)

(For eyelids, see also 67961 et seq)

(Repair of donor site requiring skin graft or local flaps, to be added as additional separate procedure)

Allograft/Tissue Cultured Allogeneic Skin Substitute

Application of a non-autologous human skin graft (ie, homograft) from a donor to a part of the recipient's body to resurface an area damaged by burns, traumatic injury, soft tissue infection and/or tissue necrosis or surgery.

15300 Allograft skin for temporary wound closure, trunk, arms, legs; first 100 sq cm or less, or one percent of body area of infants and children

+ 15301 each additional 100 sq cm, or each additional one percent of body area of infants and children, or part thereof (List separately in addition to code for primary procedure)

(Use 15301 in conjunction with 15300)

15320 Allograft skin for temporary wound closure, face, scalp, eyelids, mouth, neck, ears, orbits, genitalia, hands, feet, and/or multiple digits; first 100 sq cm or less, or one percent of body area of infants and children

+ 15321 each additional 100 sq cm, or each additional one percent of body area of infants and children, or part thereof (List separately in addition to code for primary procedure)

(Use 15321 in conjunction with 15320)

15330 Acellular dermal allograft, trunk, arms, legs; first 100 sq cm or less, or one percent of body area of infants and children

+ **15331** each additional 100 sq cm, or each additional one percent of body area of infants and children, or part thereof (List separately in addition to code for primary procedure)

(Use 15331 in conjunction with 15330)

15335 Acellular dermal allograft, face, scalp, eyelids, mouth, neck, ears, orbits, genitalia, hands, feet, and/or multiple digits; first 100 sq cm or less, or one percent of body area of infants and children

+ **15336** each additional 100 sq cm, or each additional one percent of body area of infants and children, or part thereof (List separately in addition to code for primary procedure)

(Use 15336 in conjunction with 15335)

15340 Tissue cultured allogeneic skin substitute; first 25 sq cm or less

+ **15341** each additional 25 sq cm

(Use 15341 in conjunction with 15340)

(Do not report 15340, 15341 in conjunction with 11040-11042, 15002-15005)

(15342 deleted 2006 edition. To report, see 15170, 15175, 15340, 15360, 15365)

(15343 deleted 2006 edition. To report, see 15171, 15176, 15341, 15361, 15366)

(15350 deleted 2006 edition. To report, see 15300, 15320, 15330, 15335)

(15351 deleted 2006 edition. To report, see 15301, 15321, 15331, 15336)

15360 Tissue cultured allogeneic dermal substitute; trunk, arms, legs; first 100 sq cm or less, or one percent of body area of infants and children

+ **15361** each additional 100 sq cm, or each additional one percent of body area of infants and children, or part thereof (List separately in addition to code for primary procedure)

(Use 15361 in conjunction with 15360)

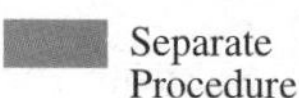 Separate Procedure 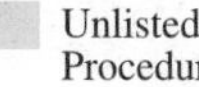 Unlisted Procedure 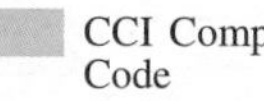 CCI Comp. Code 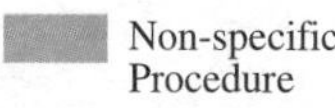 Non-specific Procedure

15365 Tissue cultured allogeneic dermal substitute, face, scalp, eyelids, mouth, neck, ears, orbits, genitalia, hands, feet, and/or multiple digits; first 100 sq cm or less, or one percent of body area of infants and children

+ 15366 each additional 100 sq cm, or each additional one percent of body area of infants and children, or part thereof (List separately in addition to code for primary procedure)

(Use 15366 in conjunction with 15365)

Xenograft

Application of a non-human skin graft or biologic wound dressing (eg, porcine tissue or pigskin) to a part of the recipient's body following debridement of the burn wound or area of traumatic injury, soft tissue infection and/or tissue necrosis, or surgery.

15400 Xenograft, skin (dermal), for temporary wound closure; trunk, arms, legs; first 100 sq cm or less, or one percent of body area of infants and children

+ 15401 each additional 100 sq cm, or each additional one percent of body area of infants and children, or part thereof (List separately in addition to code for primary procedure)

(Use 15401 in conjunction with code 15400)

15420 Xenograft skin (dermal), for temporary wound closure, face, scalp, eyelids, mouth, neck, ears, orbits, genitalia, hands, feet, and/or multiple digits; first 100 sq cm or less, or one percent of body area of infants and children

+ 15421 each additional 100 sq cm, or each additional one percent of body area of infants and children, or part thereof (List separately in addition to code for primary procedure)

(Use 15421 in conjunction with 15420)

15430 Acellular xenograft implant; first 100 sq cm or less, or one percent of body area of infants and children

+ 15431 each additional 100 sq cm, or each additional one percent of body area of infants and children, or part thereof (List separately in addition to code for primary procedure)

(Use 15431 in conjunction with 15430)

(Do not report 15430, 15431 in conjunction with 11040-11042, 15002-15005, 0170T)

● New Code ▲ Revised Code + Add-On Code ⃠ Modifier -51 Exempt ⊙ Conscious Sedation

FLAPS (SKIN AND/OR DEEP TISSUES)

Flap grafts (CPT codes 15570-15576) include excision of lesions at the same site (CPT codes 11400-11646).

(For microvascular flaps, see 15756-15758)

(For flaps without inclusion of a vascular pedicle, see 15570-15576)

(For adjacent tissue transfer flaps, see 14000-14300)

15570 Formation of direct or tubed pedicle, with or without transfer; trunk

15572 scalp, arms, or legs

15574 forehead, cheeks, chin, mouth, neck, axillae, genitalia, hands or feet

15576 eyelids, nose, ears, lips, or intraoral

15600 Delay of flap or sectioning of flap (division and inset); at trunk

15610 at scalp, arms, or legs

15620 at forehead, cheeks, chin, neck, axillae, genitalia, hands, or feet

15630 at eyelids, nose, ears, or lips

15650 Transfer, intermediate, of any pedicle flap (eg, abdomen to wrist, Walking tube), any location

(For eyelids, nose, ears, or lips, see also anatomical area)

(For revision, defatting or rearranging of transferred pedicle flap or skin graft, see 13100-14300)

(Procedures 15732-15738 are described by donor site of the muscle, myocutaneous, or fasciocutaneous flap)

● **15731** Forehead flap with preservation of vascular pedicle (eg, axial pattern flap, paramedian forehead flap)

(For muscle, myocutaneous, or fasciocutaneous flap of the head or neck, see 15732)

15732 Muscle, myocutaneous, or fasciocutaneous flap; head and neck (eg, temporalis, masseter muscle, sternocleidomastoid, levator scapulae)

(For forehead flap with preservation of vascular pedicle, use 15731)

15734 trunk

15736 upper extremity

15738 lower extremity

OTHER FLAPS AND GRAFTS

15740 Flap; island pedicle

15750 neurovascular pedicle

15756 Free muscle or myocutaneous flap with microvascular anastomosis

(Do not report code 69990 in addition to code 15756)

15757 Free skin flap with microvascular anastomosis

(Do not report code 69990 in addition to code 15757)

15758 Free fascial flap with microvascular anastomosis

(Do not report code 69990 in addition to code 15758)

15760 Graft; composite (eg, full thickness of external ear or nasal ala), including primary closure, donor area

15770 derma-fat-fascia

15775 Punch graft for hair transplant; 1 to 15 punch grafts

15776 more than 15 punch grafts

(For strip transplant, use 15220)

OTHER PROCEDURES

15780 Dermabrasion; total face (eg, for acne scarring, fine wrinkling, rhytids, general keratosis)

15781 segmental, face

15782 regional, other than face

15783 superficial, any site, (eg, tattoo removal)

15786 Abrasion; single lesion (eg, keratosis, scar)

+ **15787** each additional four lesions or less (List separately in addition to code for primary procedure)

(Use 15787 in conjunction with code 15786)

15788 Chemical peel, facial; epidermal

15789 dermal

15792 Chemical peel, nonfacial; epidermal

15793 dermal

(15810 deleted 2006 edition.)

(15811 deleted 2006 edition.)

15819 Cervicoplasty

15820 Blepharoplasty, lower eyelid;

15821 with extensive herniated fat pad

15822 Blepharoplasty, upper eyelid;

15823 with excessive skin weighting down lid

(For bilateral blepharoplasty, add modifier -50)

15824 Rhytidectomy; forehead

(For repair of brow ptosis, use 67900)

15825 neck with platysmal tightening (platysmal flap, P-flap)

15826 glabellar frown lines

15828 cheek, chin, and neck

Separate Procedure | Unlisted Procedure | CCI Comp. Code | Non-specific Procedure

15829 superficial musculoaponeurotic system (SMAS) flap

(For bilateral rhytidectomy, add modifier -50)

● **15830** Excision, excessive skin and subcutaneous tissue (includes lipectomy); abdomen, infraumbilical panniculectomy

(Do not report 15830 in conjunction wtih 12031, 12032, 12034, 12035, 12036, 12037, 13100, 13101, 13102, 14000-14001, 14300)

(15831 deleted 2007 edition. To report abdominoplasty with panniculectomy, see 15830 in conjunction with 15847. To report other abdominoplasty, use 17999.)

15832 Excision, excessive skin and subcutaneous tissue (including lipectomy); thigh

15833 leg

15834 hip

15835 buttock

15836 arm

15837 forearm or hand

15838 submental fat pad

15839 other area

(For bilateral procedure, add modifier -50)

15840 Graft for facial nerve paralysis; free fascia graft (including obtaining fascia)

(For bilateral procedure, add modifier -50)

15841 free muscle graft (including obtaining graft)

15842 free muscle flap by microsurgical technique

(Do not report code 69990 in addition to code 15842)

15845 regional muscle transfer

(For intravenous fluorescein examination of blood flow in graft or flap, use 15860)

(For nerve transfers, decompression, or repair, see 64831-64876, 64905, 64907, 69720, 69725, 69740, 69745, 69955)

●+15847 Excision, excessive skin and subcutaneous tissue (includes lipectomy), abdomen (eg, abdominoplasty) (includes umbilical transposition and fascial plication) (List separately in addition to code for primary procedure)

(Use 15847 in conjunction with 15830)

(For abdominal wall hernia repair, see 49491-49587)

(To report other abdominoplasty, use 17999)

15850 Removal of sutures under anesthesia (other than local), same surgeon

15851 Removal of sutures under anesthesia (other than local), other surgeon

15852 Dressing change (for other than burns) under anesthesia (other than local)

15860 Intravenous injection of agent (eg, fluorescein) to test vascular flow in flap or graft

15876 Suction assisted lipectomy; head and neck

15877 trunk

15878 upper extremity

15879 lower extremity

PRESSURE ULCERS (DECUBITUS ULCERS)

15920 Excision, coccygeal pressure ulcer, with coccygectomy; with primary suture

15922 with flap closure

15931 Excision, sacral pressure ulcer, with primary suture;

15933 with ostectomy

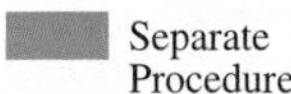
Separate Procedure

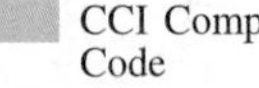
Unlisted Procedure

CCI Comp. Code

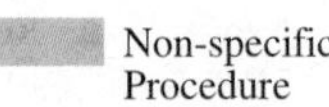
Non-specific Procedure

15934 Excision, sacral pressure ulcer, with skin flap closure;

15935 with ostectomy

15936 Excision, sacral pressure ulcer, in preparation for muscle or myocutaneous flap or skin graft closure;

15937 with ostectomy

(For repair of defect using muscle or myocutaneous flap, use code(s) 15734 and/or 15738 in addition to 15936, 15937. For repair of defect using split skin graft, use codes 15100 and/or 15101 in addition to 15936, 15937)

15940 Excision, ischial pressure ulcer, with primary suture;

15941 with ostectomy (ischiectomy)

15944 Excision, ischial pressure ulcer, with skin flap closure;

15945 with ostectomy

15946 Excision, ischial pressure ulcer, with ostectomy, in preparation for muscle or myocutaneous flap or skin graft closure

(For repair of defect using muscle or myocutaneous flap, use code(s) 15734 and/or 15738 in addition to 15946. For repair of defect using split skin graft, use codes 15100 and/or 15101 in addition to 15946)

15950 Excision, trochanteric pressure ulcer, with primary suture;

15951 with ostectomy

15952 Excision, trochanteric pressure ulcer, with skin flap closure;

15953 with ostectomy

15956 Excision, trochanteric pressure ulcer, in preparation for muscle or myocutaneous flap or skin graft closure;

15958 with ostectomy

(For repair of defect using muscle or myocutaneous flap, use code(s) 15734 and/or 15738 in addition to 15956, 15958. For repair of defect using split skin graft, use codes 15100 and/or 15101 in addition to 15956, 15958)

15999 Unlisted procedure, excision pressure ulcer

(For free skin graft to close ulcer or donor site, see 15002 et seq)

BURNS, LOCAL TREATMENT

Procedures 16000-16036 refer to local treatment of burned surface only. Codes 16020-16030 include the application of materials (*eg, Biobrane®, other dressings*) not described in 15100-15431.

For the application of skin grafts or skin substitutes, see 15100-15650.

16000 Initial treatment, first degree burn, when no more than local treatment is required

(16010 deleted 2006 edition. To report, see 16020-16030)

(16015 deleted 2006 edition. To report, see 16020-16030)

16020 Dressings and/or debridement of partial-thickness burns, initial or subsequent; small (less than 5% total body surface area)

16025 medium (eg, whole face or whole extremity, or 5% to 10% total body surface area)

16030 large (eg, more than one extremity, or greater than 10% total body surface area)

16035 Escharotomy; initial incision

+ **16036** each additional incision (List separately in addition to code for primary procedure)

(Use 16036 in conjunction with code 16035)

(For debridement, curettement of burn wound, see 16020-16030)

DESTRUCTION

(For destruction of lesion(s) in specific anatomic sites, see 40820, 46900-46917, 46924, 54050-54057, 54065, 56501, 56515, 57061, 57065, 67850, 68135)

(For paring or cutting of benign hyperkeratotic lesions (eg, corns or calluses), see 11055-11057)

(For sharp removal or electrosurgical destruction of skin tags and fibrocutaneous tags, see 11200, 11201)

(For cryotherapy of acne, use 17340)

(For initiation or follow-up care of topical chemotherapy (eg, 5-FU or similar agents), see appropriate office visits)

(For shaving of epidermal or dermal lesions, see 11300-11313)

DESTRUCTION, BENIGN OR PREMALIGNANT LESIONS

▲ **17000** Destruction (eg, laser surgery, electrosurgery, cryosurgery, chemosurgery, surgical curettement), premalignant lesions (eg, actinic keratoses); first lesion

+ **17003** second through 14 lesions, each (List separately in addition to code for first lesion)

(Use 17003 in conjunction with 17000)

(For destruction of common or plantar warts, see 17110-17111)

⊘▲**17004** Destruction (eg, laser surgery, electrosurgery, cryosurgery, chemosurgery, surgical curettement), premalignant lesions (eg, actinic keratoses), 15 or more lesions

(Do not report 17004 in conjunction with codes 17000-17003)

17106 Destruction of cutaneous vascular proliferative lesions (eg, laser technique); less than 10 sq cm

17107 10.0 to 50.0 sq cm

17108 over 50.0 sq cm

▲ **17110** Destruction (eg, laser surgery, electrosurgery, cryosurgery, chemosurgery, surgical curettement), of benign lesions other than skin tags or cutaneous vascular lesions; up to 14 lesions

17111 15 or more lesions

17250 Chemical cauterization of granulation tissue (proud flesh, sinus or fistula)

(17250 is not to be used with removal or excision codes for the same lesion)

DESTRUCTION, MALIGNANT LESIONS, ANY METHOD

17260 Destruction, malignant lesion (eg, laser surgery, electrosurgery, cryosurgery, chemosurgery, surgical curettement), trunk, arms or legs; lesion diameter 0.5 cm or less

17261 lesion diameter 0.6 to 1.0 cm

17262 lesion diameter 1.1 to 2.0 cm

17263 lesion diameter 2.1 to 3.0 cm

17264 lesion diameter 3.1 to 4.0 cm

17266 lesion diameter over 4.0 cm

17270 Destruction, malignant lesion (eg, laser surgery, electrosurgery, cryosurgery, chemosurgery, surgical curettement), scalp, neck, hands, feet, genitalia; lesion diameter 0.5 cm or less

17271 lesion diameter 0.6 to 1.0 cm

17272 lesion diameter 1.1 to 2.0 cm

17273 lesion diameter 2.1 to 3.0 cm

17274 lesion diameter 3.1 to 4.0 cm

17276 lesion diameter over 4.0 cm

17280 Destruction, malignant lesion, (eg, laser surgery, electrosurgery, cryosurgery, chemosurgery, surgical curettement), face, ears, eyelids, nose, lips, mucous membrane; lesion diameter 0.5 cm or less

17281 lesion diameter 0.6 to 1.0 cm

17282 lesion diameter 1.1 to 2.0 cm

17283 lesion diameter 2.1 to 3.0 cm

17284 lesion diameter 3.1 to 4.0 cm

17286 lesion diameter over 4.0 cm

MOHS MICROGRAPHIC SURGERY

Mohs micrographic surgery is a technique for the removal of complex or ill-defined skin cancer with histologic examination of 100% of the surgical margins. It requires a single physician to act in two integrated but separate and distinct capacities: surgeon and pathologist. If either of these responsibilities is delegated to another physician who reports the services separately, these codes should not be reported. The Mohs surgeon removes the tumor tissue and maps and divides the tumor specimen into pieces, and each piece is embedded into an individual tissue block for histopathologic examination. Thus a tissue block in Mohs surgery is defined as an individual tissue piece embedded in a mounting medium for sectioning.

(17304 deleted 2007 edition, see 17311)

(17305 deleted 2007 edition, see 17312, 17314)

(17306 deleted 2007 edition, see 17312, 17314)

(17307 deleted 2007 edition, see 17312, 17314)

(17310 deleted 2007 edition, see 17315)

(If additional special pathology procedures, stains or immunostains are required, use 88311-88314, 88342)

(Do not report 88314 in conjunction with 17311-17315 for routine frozen section stain (eg., hematoxylin and eosin, toluidine blue) performed during Mohs surgery. When a nonroutine histochemical stain on frozen tissue is utilized, report 88314 with modifier -59)

(Do not report 88302-88309 on the same specimen as part of the Mohs surgery)

● **17311** Mohs micrographic technique, including removal of all gross tumor, surgical excision of tissue specimens, mapping, color coding of specimens, microscopic examination of specimens by the surgeon, and histopathologic preparation including routine stain(s) (eg, hematoxylin and eosin, toluidine blue), head, neck, hands, feet, genitalia, or any location with surgery directly involving muscle, cartilage, bone, tendon, major nerves, or vessels; first stage, up to 5 tissue blocks

●**+17312** each additional stage after the first stage, up to 5 tissue blocks (List separately in addition to code for primary procedure)

(Use 17312 in conjunction with 17311)

● **17313** Mohs micrographic technique, including removal of all gross tumor, surgical excision of tissue specimens, mapping, color coding of specimens, microscopic examination of specimens by the surgeon, and histopathologic preparation including routine stain(s) (eg, hematoxylin and eosin, toluidine blue), of the trunk, arms, or legs; first stage, up to 5 tissue blocks

●+**17314** each additional stage after the first stage, up to 5 tissue blocks (List separately in addition to code for primary procedure)

(Use 17314 in conjunction with 17313)

●+**17315** Mohs micrographic technique, including removal of all gross tumor, surgical excision of tissue specimens, mapping, color coding of specimens, microscopic examination of specimens by the surgeon, and histopathologic preparation including routine stain(s) (eg, hematoxylin and eosin, toluidine blue), each additional block after the first 5 tissue blocks, any stage (List separately in addition to code for primary procedure)

(Use 17315 in conjunction with 17311-17314)

OTHER PROCEDURES

17340 Cryotherapy (CO_2 slush, liquid N_2) for acne

17360 Chemical exfoliation for acne (eg, acne paste, acid)

17380 Electrolysis epilation, each 1/2 hour

(For actinotherapy, use 96900)

17999 Unlisted procedure, skin, mucous membrane and subcutaneous tissue

BREAST

Fine needle aspiration biopsies, core biopsies, open incisional or excisional biopsies, and related procedures performed to procure tissue from a lesion for which an established diagnosis exists are not to be reported separately at the time of a lesion excision unless performed on a different lesion or on the contralateral breast. However, if a diagnosis is not established, and the decision to perform the excision or mastectomy is dependent on the results of the biopsy, then the biopsy is separately reported. Modifier -58 may be used appropriately to indicate that the biopsy and the excision or mastectomy are staged or planned procedures.

Because excision of lesions occurs in the course of performing a mastectomy, breast excisions are not separately reported from a mastectomy unless performed

to establish the malignant diagnosis before proceeding to the mastectomy. Specifically CPT codes 19110-19126 (breast excision) are in general included in all mastectomy CPT codes 19140-19240 of the same side. However, if the excision is performed to obtain tissue to determine pathologic diagnosis of malignancy prior to proceeding to a mastectomy, the excision is separately reportable with the mastectomy. Modifier û58 should be utilized in this situation.

Use of other integumentary codes for incision and closure are included in the codes describing various breast excision or mastectomy codes. Because of the frequent need to excise lymph node or muscle tissue in conjunction with mastectomies, these procedures have been included in the CPT coding for mastectomy. It would be inappropriate to separately report ipsilateral lymph node excision in conjunction with the appropriate mastectomy codes. However, sentinel lymph node biopsy is separately reported when performed prior to a localized excision of breast or a mastectomy with or without lymphadenectomy.

Open biopsy or excision of sentinel lymph node(s) should be reported as follows: axillary (CPT codes 38500 or 38525), deep cervical (CPT code 38510), internal mammary (CPT code 38530). (CPT code 38740(axillary lymphadenectomy; superficial) should not be reported for a sentinel lymph node biopsy.

Sentinel lymph node biopsy of superficial axillary lymph node(s) is correctly reported as CPT code 38500 (biopsy or excision of lymph node(s), superficial) which includes the removal of one or more discretely identified superficial lymph nodes. By contrast a superficial axillary lymphadenectomy (CPT code 38740) requires removal of all superficial axillary adipose tissue with all lymph nodes in this adipose tissue.)

In the circumstance where a breast lesion is identified and it is determined to be medically necessary to biopsy or excise the contralateral lymph nodes, use of the biopsy or lymph node dissection codes (using the appropriate anatomic modifier, -LT or -RT for left or right) would be acceptable. Additionally, breast reconstruction codes that include the insertion of a prosthetic implant are not to be reported with CPT codes that describe the insertion of a breast prosthesis only.

The CPT coding for breast procedures generally refers to unilateral procedures; when performed bilaterally, modifier -50 would be appropriate. This is identified parenthetically, where appropriate, in the CPT narrative.

INCISION

19000 Puncture aspiration of cyst of breast;

+ **19001** each additional cyst (List separately in addition to code for primary procedure)

(Use 19001 in conjunction with code 19000)

(If imaging guidance is performed, see 76942, 77021, 77031, 77032)

19020 Mastotomy with exploration or drainage of abscess, deep

19030 Injection procedure only for mammary ductogram or galactogram

(For radiological supervision and interpretation, see 77053, 77054)

(For catheter lavage of mammary ducts for collection of cytology specimens, use Category III codes 0046T, 0047T)

EXCISION

(All codes for bilateral procedures have been deleted. To report, add modifier -50)

19100 Biopsy of breast; percutaneous, needle core, not using imaging guidance (separate procedure)

(For fine needle aspiration, use 10021)

(For image guided breast biopsy, see 19102, 19103, 10022)

19101 open, incisional

19102 percutaneous, needle core, using imaging guidance

(For placement of percutaneous localization clip, use 19295)

19103 percutaneous, automated vacuum assisted or rotating biopsy device, using imaging guidance

(For imaging guidance performed in conjunction with 19102, 19103, see 76942, 77012, 77021, 77031, 77032)

(For placement of percutaneous localization clip, use 19295)

● **19105** Ablation, cryosurgical, of fibroadenoma, including ultrasound guidance, each fibroadenoma

(Do not report 19105 in conjunction with 76940, 76942)

(For adjacent lesions treated with one cryoprobe insertion, report once)

19110 Nipple exploration, with or without excision of a solitary lactiferous duct or a papilloma lactiferous duct

19112 Excision of lactiferous duct fistula

▲ **19120** Excision of cyst, fibroadenoma, or other benign or malignant tumor, aberrant breast tissue, duct lesion, nipple or areolar lesion (except 19300), open, male or female, one or more lesions

19125 Excision of breast lesion identified by preoperative placement of radiological marker, open; single lesion

+ **19126** each additional lesion separately identified by a preoperative radiological marker (List separately in addition to code for primary procedure)

(Use 19126 in conjunction with code 19125)

(19140 deleted 2007 edition, see 19300)

(19160 deleted 2007 edition, see 19301)

(19162 deleted 2007 edition, see19302)

(19180 deleted 2007 edition, see 19303)

(19182 deleted 2007 edition, see 19304)

(19200 deleted 2007 edition, see 19305)

(19220 deleted 2007 edition, see 19306)

(19240 deleted 2007 edition, see 19307)

19260 Excision of chest wall tumor including ribs

19271 Excision of chest wall tumor involving ribs, with plastic reconstruction; without mediastinal lymphadenectomy

19272 with mediastinal lymphadenectomy

(Do not report 19260, 19271, 19272 in conjunction with 32002, 32020, 32100, 32503, 32504)

INTRODUCTION

19290 Preoperative placement of needle localization wire, breast;

\+ **19291** each additional lesion (List separately in addition to code for primary procedure)

(Use 19291 in conjunction with code 19290)

(For radiological supervision and interpretation, see 76942, 77031, 77032)

\+ **19295** Image guided placement, metallic localization clip, percutaneous, during breast biopsy (List separately in addition to code for primary procedure)

(Use 19295 in conjunction with codes 19102, 19103)

19296 Placement of radiotherapy afterloading balloon catheter into the breast for interstitial radioelement application following partial mastectomy, includes imaging guidance; on date separate from partial mastectomy

\+ **19297** concurrent with partial mastectomy (List separately in addition to code for primary procedure)

(Use 19297 in conjunction with 19160 or 19162)

⊙ **19298** Placement of radiotherapy afterloading brachytherapy catheters (multiple tube and button type) into the breast for interstitial radioelement application following (at the time of or subsequent to) partial mastectomy, includes imaging guidance

MASTECTOMY PROCEDURES

● **19300** Mastectomy for gynecomastia

● **19301** Mastectomy, partial (eg, lumpectomy, tylectomy, quadrantectomy, segmentectomy);

● **19302** with axillary lymphadenectomy

(For placement of radiotherapy afterloading balloon/brachytherapy catheters, see 19296-19298)

● **19303** Mastectomy, simple, complete

(For immediate or delayed insertion of implant, see 19340, 19342)

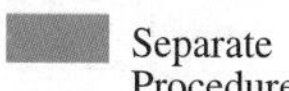 Separate Procedure 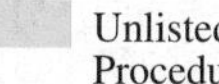 Unlisted Procedure 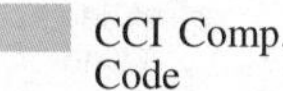 CCI Comp. Code 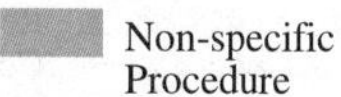 Non-specific Procedure

(For gynecomastia, use 19300)

● **19304** Mastectomy, subcutaneous

(For immediate or delayed insertion of implant, see 19340, 19342)

● **19305** Mastectomy, radical, including pectoral muscles, axillary lymph nodes

(For immediate or delayed insertion of implant, see 19340, 19342)

● **19306** Mastectomy, radical, including pectoral muscles, axillary and internal mammary lymph nodes (Urban type operation)

(For immediate or delayed insertion of implant, see 19340, 19342)

● **19307** Mastectomy, modified radical, including axillary lymph nodes, with or without pectoralis minor muscle, but excluding pectoralis major muscle

(For immediate or delayed insertion of implant, see 19340, 19342)

REPAIR AND/OR RECONSTRUCTION

19316 Mastopexy

19318 Reduction mammaplasty

19324 Mammaplasty, augmentation; without prosthetic implant

19325 with prosthetic implant

(For flap or graft, use also appropriate number)

19328 Removal of intact mammary implant

19330 Removal of mammary implant material

19340 Immediate insertion of breast prosthesis following mastopexy, mastectomy or in reconstruction

19342 Delayed insertion of breast prosthesis following mastopexy, mastectomy or in reconstruction

(For supply of implant, use 99070)

● New Code ▲ Revised Code + Add-On Code ⊘ Modifier -51 Exempt ⊙ Conscious Sedation

(For preparation of custom breast implant, use 19396)

19350 Nipple/areola reconstruction

19355 Correction of inverted nipples

19357 Breast reconstruction, immediate or delayed, with tissue expander, including subsequent expansion

▲ **19361** Breast reconstruction with latissimus dorsi flap, without prosthetic implant

(For insertion of prosthesis, use also 19340)

19364 Breast reconstruction with free flap

(Do not report code 69990 in addition to code 19364)

(19364 includes harvesting of the flap, microvascular transfer, closure of the donor site, and inset shaping the flap into a breast)

19366 Breast reconstruction with other technique

(For operating microscope, use 69990)

(For insertion of prosthesis, use also 19340 or 19342)

19367 Breast reconstruction with transverse rectus abdominis myocutaneous flap (TRAM), single pedicle, including closure of donor site;

19368 with microvascular anastomosis (supercharging)

(Do not report code 69990 in addition to code 19368)

19369 Breast reconstruction with transverse rectus abdominis myocutaneous flap (TRAM), double pedicle, including closure of donor site

19370 Open periprosthetic capsulotomy, breast

19371 Periprosthetic capsulectomy, breast

19380 Revision of reconstructed breast

19396 Preparation of moulage for custom breast implant

OTHER PROCEDURES

(For microwave thermotherapy of the breast, use Category III code 0061T)

19499 Unlisted procedure, breast

MUSCULOSKELETAL SYSTEM

Musculoskeletal procedure codes include the application and removal of the initial cast or traction device. Use codes in range 29000 to 29999 to report subsequent cast or traction-device applications. Review the instructional notes under the "Application of Casts and Strapping" to identify other uses for these codes.

The procedures and services listed in this section of the CPT coding system include the application and removal of the first cast or traction device only. Subsequent replacement of the cast and/or traction device may be coded using the cast and strapping procedure CPT codes appearing at the end of the section.

MISCELLANEOUS CODING RULES

Most bone, cartilage and fascia graft procedures include obtaining of the graft by the operating surgeon. When a surgical associate obtains the graft for the operating surgeon, the additional service should be coded and coded separately using CPT codes from the 20900-20926 range. In addition, a surgical modifier for assistant surgeon or co-surgeon should be included when reporting the associates services.

CPT codes 20100-20103 relate to treatment of wounds resulting from penetrating trauma (e.g., gunshot, stab wound). Use these codes for wound explorations only if the procedure does not require a thoracotomy or laparotomy and/or repairs to major structure(s) or major blood vessels.

The term "complicated" appears in some narratives in the musculoskeletal subsection. This term implies that an infection occurred, treatment was delayed, or the surgery took longer than usual to perform. Send supporting documentation when the codes containing this descriptor are assigned.

An intermediate repair associated with a musculoskeletal surgery is an integral portion of the surgery and should not be coded separately.

Code the injection codes according to the location of the joint injected or aspirated. Example: small joint = fingers, toes; intermediate joint = wrist, elbow; and major joint = shoulder, hip, or knee.

When removing a foreign body or performing soft tissue biopsy, determine the site and whether or not the foreign body/biopsy is superficial or deep.

FRACTURES

Remember to differentiate between the type of fracture and the type of treatment when coding fractures. Review the meanings of open and closed treatment of fractures. Dislocations must also be coded with emphasis on whether the treatment is open or closed.

When coding the re-reduction of a fracture and/or dislocation performed by the primary physician, add modifier -76 to the procedure code. If the re-reduction were performed by another physician, then modifier -77 would be added to the procedure code.

DEFINITIONS

Closed treatment specifically means that the fracture site is not surgically open (exposed to the external environment and directly visualized). This terminology is used to describe procedures that treat fractures by three methods: 1. without manipulation; 2. with manipulation; and 3. with or without traction.

Open treatment is used when the fractured bone is either: 1. surgically opened and the fracture (bone ends) visualized and internal fixation may be used; or 2. the fractured bone is opened remote from the fracture site in order to insert an intramedullary nail across the fracture site (the fracture site is not opened and visualized).

Percutaneous skeletal fixation describes fracture treatment which is neither open nor closed. In this procedure, the fracture fragments are not visualized, but fixation (eg., pins) placed across the fracture site, usually under X-ray imaging.

The type of fracture (open, compound, closed) does not have any coding correlation with the type of treatment (eg., closed, open or percutaneous) provided.

The codes for treatment of fractures and joint injuries (dislocations) are categorized by the type of manipulation (reduction) and stabilization (fixation or immobilization). These codes can apply to either open (compound) or closed fractures or joint injuries.

Skeletal traction is the application of a force (distracting or traction force) to a limb segment through a wire, pin, screw, or clamp that is attached (eg., penetrates) to bone.

Skin traction is the application of a force (longitudinal) to a limb using felt or strapping applied directly to skin only.

External fixation ist he usage of skeletal pins plus an attaching mechanism/device used for temporary or definitive treatment of acute or chronic bony deformity.

(For computer-assisted musculoskeletal surgical navigational orthopedic procedures, report 0054T-0056T)

GENERAL

INCISION

20000 Incision of soft tissue abscess (eg, secondary to osteomyelitis); superficial

20005 deep or complicated

WOUND EXPLORATION—TRAUMA (EG, PENETRATING GUNSHOT, STAB WOUND)

20100 Exploration of penetrating wound (separate procedure); neck

20101 chest

20102 abdomen/flank/back

20103 extremity

EXCISION

20150 Excision of epiphyseal bar, with or without autogenous soft tissue graft obtained through same fascial incision

(For aspiration of bone marrow, use 38220)

20200 Biopsy, muscle; superficial

20205 deep

20206 Biopsy, muscle, percutaneous needle

(If imaging guidance is performed, see 76942, 77012, 77021)

(For fine needle aspiration, use 10021 or 10022)

(For evaluation of fine needle aspirate, see 88172-88173)

(For excision of muscle tumor, deep, see specific anatomic section)

20220 Biopsy, bone, trocar, or needle; superficial (eg, ilium, sternum, spinous process, ribs)

20225 deep (eg, vertebral body, femur)

(For bone marrow biopsy, use 38221)

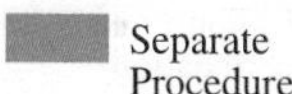
Separate Procedure
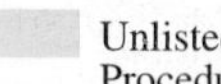
Unlisted Procedure
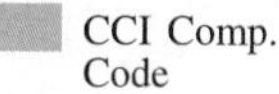
CCI Comp. Code
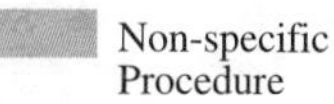
Non-specific Procedure

(For radiologic supervision and interpretation, see 77002, 77012, 77021)

20240 Biopsy, bone, open; superficial (eg, ilium, sternum, spinous process, ribs, trochanter of femur)

20245 deep (eg, humerus, ischium, femur)

20250 Biopsy, vertebral body, open; thoracic

20251 lumbar or cervical

(For sequestrectomy, osteomyelitis or drainage of bone abscess, see anatomical area)

INTRODUCTION OR REMOVAL

(For injection procedure for arthrography, see anatomical area)

20500 Injection of sinus tract; therapeutic (separate procedure)

20501 diagnostic (sinogram)

(For radiological supervision and interpretation, use 76080)

20520 Removal of foreign body in muscle or tendon sheath; simple

20525 deep or complicated

20526 Injection, therapeutic (eg, local anesthetic, corticosteroid), carpal tunnel

20550 Injection(s); single tendon sheath, or ligament, aponeurosis (eg, plantar "fascia")

20551 single tendon origin/insertion

20552 Injection(s); single or multiple trigger point(s), one or two muscle(s)

20553 single or multiple trigger point(s), three or more muscle(s)

(If imaging guidance is performed, see 76942, 77002, 77021)

20600 Arthrocentesis, aspiration and/or injection; small joint or bursa (eg, fingers, toes)

20605 intermediate joint or bursa (eg, temporomandibular, acromioclavicular, wrist, elbow or ankle, olecranon bursa)

20610 major joint or bursa (eg, shoulder, hip, knee joint, subacromial bursa)

(If imaging guidance is performed, see 76942, 77002, 77012, 77021)

20612 Aspiration and/or injection of ganglion cyst(s) any location

(To report multiple ganglion cyst aspirations/injections, use 20612 and append modifier '-59')

20615 Aspiration and injection for treatment of bone cyst

20650 Insertion of wire or pin with application of skeletal traction, including removal (separate procedure)

⃠ **20660** Application of cranial tongs, caliper, or stereotactic frame, including removal (separate procedure)

20661 Application of halo, including removal; cranial

20662 pelvic

20663 femoral

20664 Application of halo, including removal, cranial, 6 or more pins placed, for thin skull osteology (eg, pediatric patients, hydrocephalus, osteogenesis imperfecta), requiring general anesthesia

20665 Removal of tongs or halo applied by another physician

20670 Removal of implant; superficial, (eg, buried wire, pin or rod) (separate procedure)

20680 deep (eg, buried wire, pin, screw, metal band, nail,rod or plate)

⃠ **20690** Application of a uniplane (pins or wires in one plane), unilateral, external fixation system

⃠ **20692** Application of a multiplane (pins or wires in more than one plane), unilateral, external fixation system (eg, Ilizarov, Monticelli type)

20693 Adjustment or revision of external fixation system requiring anesthesia (eg, new pin(s) or wire(s) and/or new ring(s) or bar(s))

20694 Removal, under anesthesia, of external fixation system

REPLANTATION

20802 Replantation, arm (includes surgical neck of humerus through elbow joint), complete amputation

(To report replantation of incomplete arm amputation, see specific code(s) for repair of bone(s), ligament(s), tendon(s), nerve(s), or blood vessel(s) with modifier -52)

20805 Replantation, forearm (includes radius and ulna to radial carpal joint), complete amputation

(To report replantation of incomplete forearm amputation, see specific code(s) for repair of bone(s), ligament(s), tendon(s), nerve(s), or blood vessel(s) with modifier -52)

20808 Replantation, hand (includes hand through metacarpophalangeal joints), complete amputation

(To report replantation of incomplete hand amputation, see specific code(s) for repair of bone(s), ligament(s), tendon(s), nerve(s), or blood vessel(s) with modifier -52)

20816 Replantation, digit, excluding thumb (includes metacarpophalangeal joint to insertion of flexor sublimis tendon), complete amputation

(To report replantation of incomplete digit amputation excluding thumb, see specific code(s) for repair of bone(s), ligament(s), tendon(s), nerve(s), or blood vessel(s) with modifier -52)

20822 Replantation, digit, excluding thumb (includes distal tip to sublimis tendon insertion), complete amputation

(To report replantation of incomplete digit amputation excluding thumb, see specific code(s) for repair of bone(s), ligament(s), tendon(s), nerve(s), or blood vessel(s) with modifier -52)

20824 Replantation, thumb (includes carpometacarpal joint to MP joint), complete amputation

(To report replantation of incomplete thumb amputation, see specific code(s) for repair of bone(s), ligament(s), tendon(s), nerve(s), or blood vessel(s) with modifier -52)

20827 Replantation, thumb (includes distal tip to MP joint), complete amputation

(To report replantation of incomplete thumb amputation, see specific code(s) for repair of bone(s), ligament(s), tendon(s), nerve(s), or blood vessel(s) with modifier -52)

(To report replantation of complete leg amputation see specific code(s) for repair of bone(s), ligament(s), tendon(s), nerve(s), or blood vessel(s) with modifier -52)

(To report replantation of incomplete leg amputation, see specific code(s) for repair of bone(s), ligament(s), tendon(s), nerve(s), or blood vessel(s) with modifier -52)

20838 Replantation, foot, complete amputation

(To report replantation of incomplete foot amputation, see specific code(s) for repair of bone(s), ligament(s), tendon(s), nerve(s), or blood vessel(s) with modifier -52)

GRAFTS (OR IMPLANTS)

(For spinal surgery bone graft(s) see codes 20930-20938)

⊘ **20900** Bone graft, any donor area; minor or small (eg, dowel or button)

⊘ **20902** major or large

⊘ **20910** Cartilage graft; costochondral

⊘ **20912** nasal septum

(For ear cartilage, use 21235)

⊘ **20920** Fascia lata graft; by stripper

⊘ **20922** by incision and area exposure, complex or sheet

⊘ **20924** Tendon graft, from a distance (eg, palmaris, toe extensor, plantaris)

⊘ **20926** Tissue grafts, other (eg, paratenon, fat, dermis)

(Codes 20930-20938 are reported in addition to codes for the definitive procedure(s) without modifier -51)

⊘ **20930** Allograft for spine surgery only; morselized

⊘ **20931** structural

⊘ **20936** Autograft for spine surgery only (includes harvesting the graft); local (eg, ribs, spinous process, or laminar fragments) obtained from same incision

⊘ **20937** morselized (through separate skin or fascial incision)

⊘ **20938** structural, bicortical or tricortical (through separate skin or fascial incision)

(For needle aspiration of bone marrow for the purpose of bone grafting, use 38220)

OTHER PROCEDURES

20950 Monitoring of interstitial fluid pressure (includes insertion of device,eg, wick catheter technique, needle manometer technique) in detection of muscle compartment syndrome

20955 Bone graft with microvascular anastomosis; fibula

20956 iliac crest

20957 metatarsal

20962 other than fibula, iliac crest, or metatarsal

(Do not report code 69990 in addition to codes 20955-20962)

20969 Free osteocutaneous flap with microvascular anastomosis; other than iliac crest, metatarsal, or great toe

20970 iliac crest

20972 metatarsal

20973 great toe with web space

(Do not report code 69990 in addition to codes 20969-20973)

(For great toe, wrap-around procedure, use 26551)

⊘ **20974** Electrical stimulation to aid bone healing; noninvasive (nonoperative)

⊘ **20975** invasive (operative)

20979 Low intensity ultrasound stimulation to aid bone healing, noninvasive (nonoperative)

⊙ **20982** Ablation, bone tumor(s) (eg, osteoid osteoma, metastasis) radiofrequency, percutaneous, including computed tomographic guidance

(Do not report 20982 in conjunction with 77013)

20999 Unlisted procedure, musculoskeletal system, general

HEAD

INCISION

(For drainage of superficial abscess and hematoma, use 20000)

(For removal of embedded foreign body from dentoalveolar structure, see 41805, 41806)

21010 Arthrotomy, temporomandibular joint

(To report bilateral procedures, report 21010 with modifier -50)

EXCISION

21015 Radical resection of tumor (eg, malignant neoplasm), soft tissue of face or scalp

(To report excision of skull tumor for osteomyelitis, use 61501)

21025 Excision of bone (eg, for osteomyelitis or bone abscess); mandible

21026 facial bone(s)

21029 Removal by contouring of benign tumor of facial bone (eg, fibrous dysplasia)

21030 Excision of benign tumor or cyst of maxilla or zygoma by enucleation and curettage

21031 Excision of torus mandibularis

21032 Excision of maxillary torus palatinus

21034 Excision of malignant tumor of maxilla or zygoma

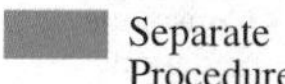 Separate Procedure Unlisted Procedure CCI Comp. Code 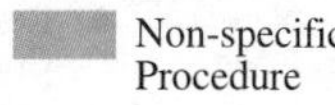 Non-specific Procedure

21040 Excision of benign tumor or cyst of mandible, by enucleation and/or curettage

(For enucleation and/or curettage of benign cysts or tumors of mandible not requiring osteotomy, use 21040)

(For excision of benign tumor or cyst of mandible requiring osteotomy, see 21046-21047)

21044 Excision of malignant tumor of mandible;

21045 radical resection

(For bone graft, use 21215)

21046 Excision of benign tumor or cyst of mandible; requiring intra-oral osteotomy (eg, locally aggressive or destructive lesion(s))

21047 requiring extra-oral osteotomy and partial mandibulectomy (eg, locally aggressive or destructive lesion(s))

21048 Excision of benign tumor or cyst of maxilla; requiring intra-oral osteotomy (eg, locally aggressive or destructive lesion(s))

21049 requiring extra-oral osteotomy and partial maxillectomy (eg, locally aggressive or destructive lesion(s))

21050 Condylectomy, temporomandibular joint (separate procedure)

(For bilateral procedures, report 21050 with modifier -50)

21060 Meniscectomy, partial or complete, temporomandibular joint (separate procedure)

(For bilateral procedures, report 21060 with modifier -50)

21070 Coronoidectomy (separate procedure)

(For bilateral procedures, report 21070 with modifier -50)

HEAD PROSTHESIS

21076 Impression and custom preparation; surgical obturator prosthesis

21077 orbital prosthesis

21079 interim obturator prosthesis

21080 definitive obturator prosthesis

21081 mandibular resection prosthesis

21082 palatal augmentation prosthesis

21083 palatal lift prosthesis

21084 speech aid prosthesis

21085 oral surgical splint

21086 auricular prosthesis

21087 nasal prosthesis

21088 facial prosthesis

Other Procedures

21089 Unlisted maxillofacial prosthetic procedure

INTRODUCTION OR REMOVAL

21100 Application of halo type appliance for maxillofacial fixation, includes removal (separate procedure)

21110 Application of interdental fixation device for conditions other than fracture or dislocation, includes removal

(For removal of interdental fixation by another physician, see 20670-20680)

21116 Injection procedure for temporomandibular joint arthrography

(For radiological supervision and interpretation, use 70332. Do not report 77002 in addition to 70332)

REPAIR, REVISION AND/OR RECONSTRUCTION

(For cranioplasty, see 21179, 21180 and 62116, 62120, 62140-62147)

21120 Genioplasty; augmentation (autograft, allograft, prosthetic material)

21121 sliding osteotomy, single piece

21122 sliding osteotomies, two or more osteotomies (eg, wedge excision or bone wedge reversal for asymmetrical chin)

21123 sliding, augmentation with interpositional bone grafts (includes obtaining autografts)

21125 Augmentation, mandibular body or angle; prosthetic material

21127 with bone graft, onlay or interpositional (includes obtaining autograft)

21137 Reduction forehead; contouring only

21138 contouring and application of prosthetic material or bone graft (includes obtaining autograft)

21139 contouring and setback of anterior frontal sinus wall

21141 Reconstruction midface, LeFort I; single piece, segment movement in any direction (eg, for Long Face Syndrome), without bone graft

21142 two pieces, segment movement in any direction, without bone graft

21143 three or more pieces, segment movement in any direction, without bone graft

21145 single piece, segment movement in any direction, requiring bone grafts (includes obtaining autografts)

21146 two pieces, segment movement in any direction, requiring bone grafts (includes obtaining autografts) (eg, ungrafted unilateral alveolar cleft)

21147 three or more pieces, segment movement in any direction, requiring bone grafts (includes obtaining autografts) (eg, ungrafted bilateral alveolar cleft or multiple osteotomies)

21150 Reconstruction midface, LeFort II; anterior intrusion (eg, Treacher-Collins Syndrome)

21151 any direction, requiring bone grafts (includes obtaining autografts)

21154 Reconstruction midface, LeFort III (extracranial), any type, requiring bone grafts (includes obtaining autografts); without LeFort I

21155 with LeFort I

21159 Reconstruction midface, LeFort III (extra and intracranial) with forehead advancement (eg, mono bloc), requiring bone grafts (includes obtaining autografts); without LeFort I

21160 with LeFort I

21172 Reconstruction superior-lateral orbital rim and lower forehead, advancement or alteration, with or without grafts (includes obtaining autografts)

(For frontal or parietal craniotomy performed for craniosynostosis, use 61556)

21175 Reconstruction, bifrontal, superior-lateral orbital rims and lower forehead, advancement or alteration (eg, plagiocephaly, trigonocephaly, brachycephaly), with or without grafts (includes obtaining autografts)

(For bifrontal craniotomy performed for craniosynostosis, use 61557)

21179 Reconstruction, entire or majority of forehead and/or supraorbital rims; with grafts (allograft or prosthetic material)

21180 with autograft (includes obtaining grafts)

(For extensive craniectomy for multiple suture craniosynostosis, use only 61558 or 61559)

21181 Reconstruction by contouring of benign tumor of cranial bones (eg, fibrous dysplasia), extracranial

21182 Reconstruction of orbital walls, rims, forehead, nasoethmoid complex following intra- and extracranial excision of benign tumor of cranial bone (eg, fibrous dysplasia), with multiple autografts (includes obtaining grafts); total area of bone grafting less than 40 sq cm

21183 total area of bone grafting greater than 40 sq cm but less than 80 sq cm

21184 total area of bone grafting greater than 80 sq cm

Separate Procedure | Unlisted Procedure | CCI Comp. Code | Non-specific Procedure

(For excision of benign tumor of cranial bones, see 61563, 61564)

21188 Reconstruction midface, osteotomies (other than LeFort type) and bone grafts (includes obtaining autografts)

21193 Reconstruction of mandibular rami, horizontal, vertical, C, or L osteotomy; without bone graft

21194 with bone graft (includes obtaining graft)

21195 Reconstruction of mandibular rami and/or body, sagittal split; without internal rigid fixation

21196 with internal rigid fixation

21198 Osteotomy, mandible, segmental;

21199 with genioglossus advancement

(To report total osteotomy of the maxilla, see 21141-21160)

21206 Osteotomy, maxilla, segmental (eg, Wassmund or Schuchard)

21208 Osteoplasty, facial bones; augmentation (autograft, allograft, or prosthetic implant)

21209 reduction

21210 Graft, bone; nasal, maxillary or malar areas (includes obtaining graft)

(For cleft palate repair, see 42200-42225)

21215 mandible (includes obtaining graft)

21230 Graft; rib cartilage, autogenous, to face, chin, nose or ear (includes obtaining graft)

21235 ear cartilage, autogenous, to nose or ear (includes obtaining graft)

(To report graft augmentation of facial bones, use 21208)

21240 Arthroplasty, temporomandibular joint, with or without autograft (includes obtaining graft)

21242 Arthroplasty, temporomandibular joint, with allograft

21243 Arthroplasty, temporomandibular joint, with prosthetic joint replacement

21244 Reconstruction of mandible, extraoral, with transosteal bone plate (eg, mandibular staple bone plate)

21245 Reconstruction of mandible or maxilla, subperiosteal implant; partial

21246 complete

21247 Reconstruction of mandibular condyle with bone and cartilage autografts (includes obtaining grafts) (eg, for hemifacial microsomia)

21248 Reconstruction of mandible or maxilla, endosteal implant (eg, blade, cylinder); partial

21249 complete

(To report midface reconstruction, see 21141-21160)

21255 Reconstruction of zygomatic arch and glenoid fossa with bone and cartilage (includes obtaining autografts)

21256 Reconstruction of orbit with osteotomies (extracranial) and with bone grafts (includes obtaining autografts) (eg, micro-ophthalmia)

21260 Periorbital osteotomies for orbital hypertelorism, with bone grafts; extracranial approach

21261 combined intra- and extracranial approach

21263 with forehead advancement

21267 Orbital repositioning, periorbital osteotomies, unilateral, with bone grafts; extracranial approach

21268 combined intra- and extracranial approach

21270 Malar augmentation, prosthetic material

(For malar augmentation with bone graft, use 21210)

Separate Procedure | Unlisted Procedure | CCI Comp. Code | Non-specific Procedure

21275 Secondary revision of orbitocraniofacial reconstruction

21280 Medial canthopexy (separate procedure)

(For medial canthoplasty, use 67950)

21282 Lateral canthopexy

21295 Reduction of masseter muscle and bone (eg, for treatment of benign masseteric hypertrophy); extraoral approach

21296 intraoral approach

OTHER PROCEDURES

21299 Unlisted craniofacial and maxillofacial procedure

FRACTURE AND/OR DISLOCATION

(21300 deleted 2007 edition)

(For operative repair of skull fracture, see 62000-62010)

(To report closed treatment of skull fracture, use the appropriate Evaluation and Management code)

21310 Closed treatment of nasal bone fracture without manipulation

21315 Closed treatment of nasal bone fracture; without stabilization

21320 with stabilization

21325 Open treatment of nasal fracture; uncomplicated

21330 complicated, with internal and/or external skeletal fixation

21335 with concomitant open treatment of fractured septum

21336 Open treatment of nasal septal fracture, with or without stabilization

21337 Closed treatment of nasal septal fracture, with or without stabilization

21338 Open treatment of nasoethmoid fracture; without external fixation

21339 with external fixation

21340 Percutaneous treatment of nasoethmoid complex fracture, with splint, wire or headcap fixation, including repair of canthal ligaments and/or the nasolacrimal apparatus

21343 Open treatment of depressed frontal sinus fracture

21344 Open treatment of complicated (eg, comminuted or involving posterior wall) frontal sinus fracture, via coronal or multiple approaches

21345 Closed treatment of nasomaxillary complex fracture (LeFort II type), with interdental wire fixation or fixation of denture or splint

21346 Open treatment of nasomaxillary complex fracture (LeFort II type); with wiring and/or local fixation

21347 requiring multiple open approaches

21348 with bone grafting (includes obtaining graft)

21355 Percutaneous treatment of fracture of malar area, including zygomatic arch and malar tripod, with manipulation

21356 Open treatment of depressed zygomatic arch fracture (eg, Gillies approach)

21360 Open treatment of depressed malar fracture, including zygomatic arch and malar tripod

21365 Open treatment of complicated (eg, comminuted or involving cranial nerve foramina) fracture(s) of malar area, including zygomatic arch and malar tripod; with internal fixation and multiple surgical approaches

21366 with bone grafting (includes obtaining graft)

21385 Open treatment of orbital floor blowout fracture; transantral approach (Caldwell-Luc type operation)

21386 periorbital approach

21387 combined approach

21390 periorbital approach, with alloplastic or other implant

21395 periorbital approach with bone graft (includes obtaining graft)

21400 Closed treatment of fracture of orbit, except blowout; without manipulation

21401 with manipulation

21406 Open treatment of fracture of orbit, except blowout; without implant

21407 with implant

21408 with bone grafting (includes obtaining graft)

21421 Closed treatment of palatal or maxillary fracture (LeFort I type), with interdental wire fixation or fixation of denture or splint

21422 Open treatment of palatal or maxillary fracture (LeFort I type);

21423 complicated (comminuted or involving cranial nerve foramina), multiple approaches

21431 Closed treatment of craniofacial separation (LeFort III type) using interdental wire fixation of denture or splint

21432 Open treatment of craniofacial separation (LeFort III type); with wiring and/or internal fixation

21433 complicated (eg, comminuted or involving cranial nerve foramina), multiple surgical approaches

21435 complicated, utilizing internal and/or external fixation techniques (eg, head cap, halo device, and/or intermaxillary fixation)

(For removal of internal or external fixation device, use 20670)

21436 complicated, multiple surgical approaches, internal fixation, with bone grafting (includes obtaining graft)

21440 Closed treatment of mandibular or maxillary alveolar ridge fracture (separate procedure)

21445 Open treatment of mandibular or maxillary alveolar ridge fracture (separate procedure)

21450 Closed treatment of mandibular fracture; without manipulation

21451 with manipulation

21452 Percutaneous treatment of mandibular fracture, with external fixation

21453 Closed treatment of mandibular fracture with interdental fixation

21454 Open treatment of mandibular fracture with external fixation

21461 Open treatment of mandibular fracture; without interdental fixation

21462 with interdental fixation

21465 Open treatment of mandibular condylar fracture

21470 Open treatment of complicated mandibular fracture by multiple surgical approaches including internal fixation, interdental fixation, and/or wiring of dentures or splints

21480 Closed treatment of temporomandibular dislocation; initial or subsequent

21485 complicated (eg, recurrent requiring intermaxillary fixation or splinting), initial or subsequent

21490 Open treatment of temporomandibular dislocation

(For interdental wire fixation, use 21497)

(21493 deleted 2006 edition. To report, use the applicable Evaluation and Management codes)

(21494 deleted 2006 edition. To report, use the applicable Evaluation and Management codes)

21495 Open treatment of hyoid fracture

(For laryngoplasty with open reduction of fracture, use 31584)

(To report treatment of closed fracture of larynx, use the applicable Evaluation and Management codes)

21497 Interdental wiring, for condition other than fracture

OTHER PROCEDURES

21499 Unlisted musculoskeletal procedure, head

(For unlisted craniofacial or maxillofacial procedure, use 21299)

NECK (SOFT TISSUES) AND THORAX

(For cervical spine and back, see 21920 et seq)

(For injection of fracture site or trigger point, use 20550)

INCISION

(For incision and drainage of abscess or hematoma, superficial, see 10060, 10140)

21501 Incision and drainage, deep abscess or hematoma, soft tissues of neck or thorax;

(For posterior spine subfascial incision and drainage, see 22010-22015)

21502 with partial rib ostectomy

21510 Incision, deep, with opening of bone cortex (eg, for osteomyelitis or bone abscess), thorax

EXCISION

(For bone biopsy, see 20220-20251)

21550 Biopsy, soft tissue of neck or thorax

(For needle biopsy of soft tissue, use 20206)

21555 Excision tumor, soft tissue of neck or thorax; subcutaneous

21556 deep, subfascial, intramuscular

21557 Radical resection of tumor (eg, malignant neoplasm), soft tissue of neck or thorax

21600 Excision of rib, partial

● New Code ▲ Revised Code + Add-On Code ⃠ Modifier -51 Exempt ⊙ Conscious Sedation

(For radical resection of chest wall and rib cage for tumor, use 19260)

(For radical debridement of chest wall and rib cage for injury, see 11040-11044)

21610 Costotransversectomy (separate procedure)

21615 Excision first and/or cervical rib;

21616 with sympathectomy

21620 Ostectomy of sternum, partial

21627 Sternal debridement

(For debridement and closure, use 21750)

21630 Radical resection of sternum;

21632 with mediastinal lymphadenectomy

REPAIR, REVISION, AND/OR RECONSTRUCTION

(For superficial wound, see Integumentary System section under Repair, Simple)

21685 Hyoid myotomy and suspension

21700 Division of scalenus anticus; without resection of cervical rib

21705 with resection of cervical rib

21720 Division of sternocleidomastoid for torticollis, open operation; without cast application

(For transection of spinal accessory and cervical nerves, see 63191, 64722)

21725 with cast application

21740 Reconstructive repair of pectus excavatum or carinatum; open

21742 minimally invasive approach (Nuss procedure), without thoracoscopy

21743 minimally invasive approach (Nuss procedure), with thoracoscopy

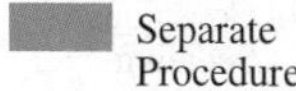
Separate Procedure | Unlisted Procedure | CCI Comp. Code | Non-specific Procedure

21750 Closure of median sternotomy separation with or without debridement (separate procedure)

FRACTURE AND/OR DISLOCATION

21800 Closed treatment of rib fracture, uncomplicated, each

21805 Open treatment of rib fracture without fixation, each

21810 Treatment of rib fracture requiring external fixation (flail chest)

21820 Closed treatment of sternum fracture

21825 Open treatment of sternum fracture with or without skeletal fixation

(For sternoclavicular dislocation, see 23520-23532)

OTHER PROCEDURES

21899 Unlisted procedure, neck or thorax

BACK AND FLANK

EXCISION

21920 Biopsy, soft tissue of back or flank; superficial

21925 deep

(For needle biopsy of soft tissue, use 20206)

21930 Excision, tumor, soft tissue of back or flank

21935 Radical resection of tumor (eg, malignant neoplasm), soft tissue of back or flank

SPINE (VERTEBRAL COLUMN)

(Do not append modifier -62 to bone graft code 20931)

(For injection procedure for myelography, use 62284)

(For injection procedure for discography, see 62290, 62291)

(For injection procedure, chemonucleolysis, single or multiple leveles, use 62292)

(For injection procedure for facet joints, see 64470-64476, 64622-64627)

(For needle or trocar biopsy, see 20220-20225)

INCISION

22010 Incision and drainage, open, of deep abscess (subfascial), posterior spine; cervical, thoracic, or cervicothoracic

22015 lumbar, sacral, or lumbosacral

(Do not report 22015 in conjunction with 22010)

(Do not report 22015 in conjunction with instrumentation removal, 10180, 22850, 22852)

(For incision and drainage of abscess or hematoma, superficial, see 10060, 10140)

EXCISION

(For bone biopsy, see 20220-20251)

(To report soft tissue biopsy of back or flank, see 21920-21925)

(For needle biopsy of soft tissue, use 20206)

(To report excision of soft tissue tumor of back or flank, use 21930)

22100 Partial excision of posterior vertebral component (eg, spinous process, lamina or facet) for intrinsic bony lesion, single vertebral segment; cervical

22101 thoracic

22102 lumbar

+ **22103** each additional segment (List separately in addition to code for primary procedure)

(Use 22103 in conjunction with codes 22100, 22101, 22102)

22110 Partial excision of vertebral body, for intrinsic bony lesion, without decompression of spinal cord or nerve root(s), single vertebral segment; cervical

22112 thoracic

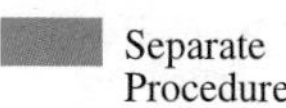
Separate Procedure
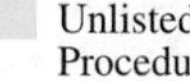
Unlisted Procedure
CCI Comp. Code
Non-specific Procedure

22114 lumbar

+ **22116** each additional vertebral segment (List separately in addition to code for primary procedure)

(Use 22116 in conjunction with codes 22110, 22112, 22114)

(For complete or near complete resection of vertebral body, see vertebral corpectomy, 63081-63091)

(For spinal reconstruction with bone graft (autograft, allograft) and/or methacrylate of cervical vertebral body, use 63081 and 22554 and 20931 or 20938)

(For spinal reconstruction with bone graft (autograft, allograft) and/or methacrylate of thoracic vertebral body, use 63085 or 63087 and 22556 and 20931 or 20938)

(For spinal reconstruction with bone graft (autograft, allograft) and/or methacrylate of lumbar vertebral body, use 63087 or 63090 and 22558 and 20931 or 20938)

(For spinal reconstruction following vertebral body resection, use 63082 or 63086 or 63088 or 63091, and 22585)

(For harvest of bone autograft for vertebral reconstruction, see 20931 or 20938)

(For cervical spinal reconstruction with prosthetic replacement of resected vertebral bodies, see codes 63081 and 22554 and 20931 or 20938 and 22851)

(For thoracic spinal reconstruction with prosthetic replacement of resected vertebral bodies, see codes 63085 or 63087 and 22556 and 20931 or 20938 and 22851)

(For lumbar spinal reconstruction with prosthetic replacement of resected vertebral bodies, see codes 63087 or 63090 and 22558, and 20931 or 20938 and 22851)

(For osteotomy of spine, see 22210-22226)

OSTEOTOMY

22210 Osteotomy of spine, posterior or posterolateral approach, one vertebral segment; cervical

22212 thoracic

22214 lumbar

● New Code ▲ Revised Code + Add-On Code ⊘ Modifier -51 Exempt ⊙ Conscious Sedation

+ **22216** each additional vertebral segment (List separately in addition to primary procedure)

(Use 22216 in conjunction with codes 22210, 22212, 22214)

22220 Osteotomy of spine, including diskectomy, anterior approach, single vertebral segment; cervical

22222 thoracic

22224 lumbar

+ **22226** each additional vertebral segment (List separately in addition to code for primary procedure)

(Use 22226 in conjunction with codes 22220, 22222, 22224)

(For vertebral corpectomy, see 63081-63091)

FRACTURE AND/OR DISLOCATION

22305 Closed treatment of vertebral process fracture(s)

22310 Closed treatment of vertebral body fracture(s), without manipulation, requiring and including casting or bracing

22315 Closed treatment of vertebral fracture(s) and/or dislocation(s) requiring casting or bracing, with and including casting and/or bracing, with or without anesthesia, by manipulation or traction

(For spinal subluxation, use 97140)

22318 Open treatment and/or reduction of odontoid fracture(s) and or dislocation(s) (including os odontoideum), anterior approach, including placement of internal fixation; without grafting

22319 with grafting

22325 Open treatment and/or reduction of vertebral fracture(s) and/or dislocation(s), posterior approach, one fractured vertebrae or dislocated segment; lumbar

22326 cervical

22327 thoracic

+ **22328** each additional fractured vertebrae or dislocated segment (List separately in addition to code for primary procedure)

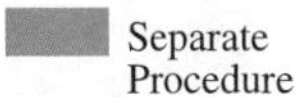
Separate Procedure

Unlisted Procedure

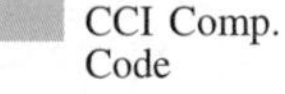
CCI Comp. Code

Non-specific Procedure

(Use 22328 in conjunction with codes 22325, 22326, 22327)

(For treatment of vertebral fracture by the anterior approach, see corpectomy 63081-63091, and appropriate arthrodesis, bone graft and instrument codes)

(For decompression of spine following fracture, see 63001-63091; for arthrodesis of spine following fracture, see 22548-22632)

MANIPULATION

(For spinal manipulation without anesthesia, use 97140)

22505 Manipulation of spine requiring anesthesia, any region

VERTEBRAL BODY, EMBOLIZATION OR INJECTION

22520 Percutaneous vertebroplasty, one vertebral body, unilateral or bilateral injection; thoracic

22521 lumbar

+ **22522** each additional thoracic or lumbar vertebral body (List separately in addition to code for primary procedure)

(Use 22522 in conjunction with codes 22520, 22521 as appropriate)

(For radiological supervision and interpretation, see 72291, 72292)

22523 Percutaneous vertebral augmentation, including cavity creation (fracture reduction and bone biopsy included when performed) using mechanical device, one vertebral body, unilateral or bilateral cannulation (eg, kyphoplasty); thoracic

22524 lumbar

+ **22525** each additional thoracic or lumbar vertebral body (List separately in addition to code for primary procedure)

(Do not report 22525 in conjunction with 20225 when performed at the same level as 22523-22525)

(Use 22525 in conjunction with 22523, 22524)

(For radiological supervision and interpretation, see 72291, 72292)

●⊙22526 Percutaneous intradiscal electrothermal annuloplasty, unilateral or bilateral including fluoroscopic guidance; single level

●+⊙22527 one or more additional levels (List separately in addition to code for primary procedure)

(Do not report codes 22526, 22527 in conjunction with 77002, 77003)

(For percutaneous intradiscal annuloplasty using method other than electrothermal, see 0062T, 0063T)

ARTHRODESIS

To report instrumentation procedures, see 22840-22855. (Codes 22840-22848, 22851 are reported in conjunction with code(s) for the definitive procedure(s) without modifier 51. When instrumentation reinsertion or removal is reported in conjunction with other definitive procedures including arthrodesis, decompression, and exploration of fusion, append modifier 51 to 22849, 22850, 22852, and 22855.) To report exploration of fusion, use 22830. (When exploration is reported in conjunction with other definitive procedures, including arthrodesis and decompression, append modifier 51 to 22830.) Do not append modifier 62 to spinal instrumentation codes 22840-22848 and 22850-22852.

Lateral Extracavitary Approach Technique

22532 Arthrodesis, lateral extracavitary technique, including minimal diskectomy to prepare interspace (other than for decompression); thoracic

22533 lumbar

+ 22534 thoracic or lumbar, each additional vertebral segment (List separately in addition to code for primary procedure)

(Use 22534 in conjunction with 22532 and 22533)

Anterior or Anterolateral Approach Technique

22548 Arthrodesis, anterior transoral or extraoral technique, clivus-C1-C2 (atlas-axis), with or without excision of odontoid process

(For intervertebral disc excision by laminotomy or laminectomy, see 63020-63042)

22554 Arthrodesis, anterior interbody technique, including minimal diskectomy to prepare interspace (other than for decompression); cervical below C2

Separate Procedure | Unlisted Procedure | CCI Comp. Code | Non-specific Procedure

22556 thoracic

22558 lumbar

+ **22585** each additional interspace (List separately in addition to code for primary procedure)

(Use 22585 in conjunction with codes 22554, 22556, 22558)

Posterior, Posterolateral or Lateral Transverse Process Technique

22590 Arthrodesis, posterior technique, craniocervical (occiput-C2)

22595 Arthrodesis, posterior technique, atlas-axis (C1-C2)

22600 Arthrodesis, posterior or posterolateral technique, single level; cervical below C2 segment

22610 thoracic (with or without lateral transverse technique)

22612 lumbar (with or without lateral transverse technique)

+ **22614** each additional vertebral segment (List separately in addition to code for primary procedure)

(Use 22614 in conjunction with codes 22600, 22610, 22612)

22630 Arthrodesis, posterior interbody technique, including laminectomy and/or diskectomy to prepare interspace (other than for decompression), single interspace; lumbar

+ **22632** each additional interspace (List separately in addition to code for primary procedure)

(Use 22632 in conjunction with code 22630)

Spine Deformity (eg, Scoliosis, Kyphosis)

22800 Arthrodesis, posterior, for spinal deformity, with or without cast; up to 6 vertebral segments

22802 7 to 12 vertebral segments

22804 13 or more vertebral segments

22808 Arthrodesis, anterior, for spinal deformity, with or without cast; 2 to 3 vertebral segments

22810 4 to 7 vertebral segments

22812 8 or more vertebral segments

22818 Kyphectomy, circumferential exposure of spine and resection of vertebral segment(s) (including body and posterior elements); single or 2 segments

22819 3 or more segments

(To report arthrodesis, see 22800-22804 and add modifier -51)

EXPLORATION

To report instrumentation procedures, see 22840-22855. (Codes 22840-22848, 22851 are reported in conjunction with code(s) for the definitive procedure(s) without modifier 51. When instrumentation reinsertion or removal is reported in conjunction with other definitive procedures including arthrodesis, decompression, and exploration of fusion, append modifier 51 to 22849, 22850, 22852 and 22855.) To report exploration of fusion, see 22830. (When exploration is reported in conjunction with other definitive procedures, including arthrodesis and decompression, append modifier 51 to 22830.)

(To report bone graft procedures, see 20930-20938)

22830 Exploration of spinal fusion

SPINAL INSTRUMENTATION

List 22840-22855 separately, in conjunction with code(s) for fracture, dislocation, arthrodesis or exploration of fusion of the spine 22325-22328, 22532-22534, 22548-22812, and 22830. Codes 22840-22848, 22851 are reported in conjunction with code(s) for the definitive procedure(s) without modifier -51. Codes 22849, 22850, 22852, and 22855 are subject to modifier -51 if reported with other definitive procedure(s), including arthrodesis, decompression, and exploration of fusion. Code 22849 should not be reported with 22850, 22852, and 22855 at the same spinal levels.

⊘ **22840** Posterior non-segmental instrumentation (eg, Harrington rod technique, pedicle fixation across one interspace, atlantoaxial transarticular screw fixation, sublaminar wiring at C1, facet screw fixation)

⊘ **22841** Internal spinal fixation by wiring of spinous processes

⊘ **22842** Posterior segmental instrumentation (eg, pedicle fixation, dual rods with multiple hooks and sublaminar wires); 3 to 6 vertebral segments

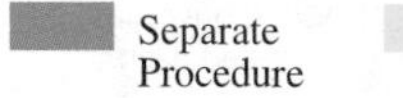

⊘ **22843** 7 to 12 vertebral segments

⊘ **22844** 13 or more vertebral segments

⊘ **22845** Anterior instrumentation; 2 to 3 vertebral segments

⊘ **22846** 4 to 7 vertebral segments

⊘ **22847** 8 or more vertebral segments

⊘ **22848** Pelvic fixation (attachment of caudal end of instrumentation to pelvic bony structures) other than sacrum

22849 Reinsertion of spinal fixation device

22850 Removal of posterior nonsegmental instrumentation (eg, Harrington rod)

⊘ **22851** Application of intervertebral biomechanical device(s) (eg, synthetic cage(s), threaded bone dowel(s), methylmethacrylate) to vertebral defect or interspace

22852 Removal of posterior segmental instrumentation

22855 Removal of anterior instrumentation

● **22857** Total disc arthroplasty (artificial disc), anterior approach, including discectomy to prepare interspace (other than for decompression), lumbar, single interspace

(Do not report 22857 in conjunction with 22558, 22845, 22851, 49010 when performed at the same level)

(For additional interspace, use Category III code 0163T)

● **22862** Revision including replacement of total disc arthroplasty (artificial disc) anterior approach, lumbar, single interspace

(Do not report 22862 in conjunction with 22558, 22845, 22851, 22865, 49010 when performed at the same level)

(For additional interspace, use Category III code 0165T)

● **22865** Removal of total disc arthroplasty (artificial disc), anterior approach, lumbar, single interspace

(Do not report 22865 in conjunction with 49010)

(For additional interspace, use Category III code 0164T)

(22857-22865 include fluoroscopy when performed)

(For decompression, see 63001-63048)

OTHER PROCEDURES

22899 Unlisted procedure, spine

ABDOMEN

EXCISION

22900 Excision, abdominal wall tumor, subfascial (eg, desmoid)

OTHER PROCEDURES

22999 Unlisted procedure, abdomen, musculoskeletal system

SHOULDER

INCISION

23000 Removal of subdeltoid calcareous deposits, open

(For arthroscopic removal of bursal deposits, use 29999)

23020 Capsular contracture release (eg, Sever type procedure)

(For incision and drainage procedures, superficial, see 10040-10160)

23030 Incision and drainage, shoulder area; deep abscess or hematoma

23031 infected bursa

23035 Incision, bone cortex (eg, osteomyelitis or bone abscess), shoulder area

23040 Arthrotomy, glenohumeral joint, including exploration, drainage, or removal of foreign body

23044 Arthrotomy, acromioclavicular, sternoclavicular joint, including exploration, drainage, or removal of foreign body

EXCISION

23065 Biopsy, soft tissue of shoulder area; superficial

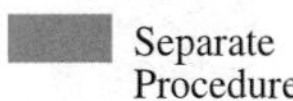
Separate Procedure
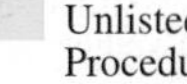
Unlisted Procedure
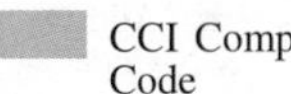
CCI Comp. Code
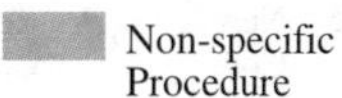
Non-specific Procedure

23066 deep

(For needle biopsy of soft tissue, use 20206)

23075 Excision, soft tissue tumor, shoulder area; subcutaneous

23076 deep, subfascial, or intramuscular

23077 Radical resection of tumor (eg, malignant neoplasm), soft tissue of shoulder area

23100 Arthrotomy, glenohumeral joint, including biopsy

23101 Arthrotomy, acromioclavicular joint or sternoclavicular joint, including biopsy and/or excision of torn cartilage

23105 Arthrotomy; glenohumeral joint, with synovectomy, with or without biopsy

23106 sternoclavicular joint, with synovectomy, with or without biopsy

23107 Arthrotomy, glenohumeral joint, with joint exploration, with or without removal of loose or foreign body

23120 Claviculectomy; partial

(For arthroscopic procedure, use 29824)

23125 total

23130 Acromioplasty or acromionectomy, partial, with or without coracoacromial ligament release

23140 Excision or curettage of bone cyst or benign tumor of clavicle or scapula;

23145 with autograft (includes obtaining graft)

23146 with allograft

23150 Excision or curettage of bone cyst or benign tumor of proximal humerus;

23155 with autograft (includes obtaining graft)

23156 with allograft

23170 Sequestrectomy (eg, for osteomyelitis or bone abscess), clavicle

23172 Sequestrectomy (eg, for osteomyelitis or bone abscess), scapula

23174 Sequestrectomy (eg, for osteomyelitis or bone abscess), humeral head to surgical neck

23180 Partial excision (craterization, saucerization, or diaphysectomy) bone (eg, osteomyelitis), clavicle

23182 Partial excision (craterization, saucerization, or diaphysectomy) bone (eg, osteomyelitis), scapula

23184 Partial excision (craterization, saucerization, or diaphysectomy) bone (eg, osteomyelitis), proximal humerus

23190 Ostectomy of scapula, partial (eg, superior medial angle)

23195 Resection, humeral head

(For replacement with implant, use 23470)

23200 Radical resection for tumor; clavicle

23210 scapula

23220 Radical resection of bone tumor, proximal humerus;

23221 with autograft (includes obtaining graft)

23222 with prosthetic replacement

INTRODUCTION OR REMOVAL

(For arthrocentesis or needling of bursa, use 20610)

(For K-wire or pin insertion or removal, see 20650, 20670, 20680)

23330 Removal of foreign body, shoulder; subcutaneous

23331 deep (eg, Neer hemiarthroplasty removal)

23332 complicated (eg, total shoulder)

23350 Injection procedure for shoulder arthrography or enhanced CT/MRI shoulder arthrography

(For radiographic arthrography, radiological supervision and interpretation, use 73040. Fluoroscopy [77002] is inclusive of radiographic arthrography)

(When fluoroscopic guided injection is performed for enhanced CT arthrography, use 23350, 77002 and 73201 or 73202)

(When fluoroscopic guided injection is performed for enhanced MR arthrography, use codes 23350, 77002, and 73222 or 73223)

(For enhanced CT or enhanced MRI arthrography, use 77002 and either 73201, 73202, 73222 or 73223)

(To report biopsy of the shoulder and joint, see 29805-29826)

REPAIR, REVISION AND/OR RECONSTRUCTION

23395 Muscle transfer, any type, shoulder or upper arm; single

23397 multiple

23400 Scapulopexy (eg, Sprengels deformity or for paralysis)

23405 Tenotomy, shoulder area; single tendon

23406 multiple tendons through same incision

23410 Repair of ruptured musculotendinous cuff (eg, rotator cuff) open; acute

23412 chronic

(For arthroscopic procedure, use 29827)

23415 Coracoacromial ligament release, with or without acromioplasty

(For arthroscopic procedure, use 29826)

23420 Reconstruction of complete shoulder (rotator) cuff avulsion, chronic (includes acromioplasty)

23430 Tenodesis of long tendon of biceps

23440 Resection or transplantation of long tendon of biceps

23450 Capsulorrhaphy, anterior; Putti-Platt procedure or Magnuson type operation

(To report arthroscopic thermal capsulorrhaphy, use 29999)

23455 with labral repair (eg, Bankart procedure)

(For arthroscopic procedure, use 29806)

23460 Capsulorrhaphy, anterior, any type; with bone block

23462 with coracoid process transfer

(To report open thermal capsulorrhaphy, use 23929)

23465 Capsulorrhaphy, glenohumeral joint, posterior, with or without bone block

(For sternoclavicular and acromioclavicular reconstruction, see 23530, 23550)

23466 Capsulorrhaphy, glenohumeral joint, any type multi-directional instability

23470 Arthroplasty, glenohumeral joint; hemiarthroplasty

23472 total shoulder (glenoid and proximal humeral replacement (eg, total shoulder))

(For removal of total shoulder implants, see 23331, 23332)

(For osteotomy, proximal humerus, use 24400)

23480 Osteotomy, clavicle, with or without internal fixation;

23485 with bone graft for nonunion or malunion (includes obtaining graft and/or necessary fixation)

23490 Prophylactic treatment (nailing, pinning, plating or wiring) with or without methylmethacrylate; clavicle

23491 proximal humerus

FRACTURE AND/OR DISLOCATION

23500 Closed treatment of clavicular fracture; without manipulation

23505 with manipulation

23515 Open treatment of clavicular fracture, with or without internal or external fixation

Separate Procedure | Unlisted Procedure | CCI Comp. Code | Non-specific Procedure

23520 Closed treatment of sternoclavicular dislocation; without manipulation

23525 with manipulation

23530 Open treatment of sternoclavicular dislocation, acute or chronic;

23532 with fascial graft (includes obtaining graft)

23540 Closed treatment of acromioclavicular dislocation; without manipulation

23545 with manipulation

23550 Open treatment of acromioclavicular dislocation, acute or chronic;

23552 with fascial graft (includes obtaining graft)

23570 Closed treatment of scapular fracture; without manipulation

23575 with manipulation, with or without skeletal traction (with or without shoulder joint involvement)

23585 Open treatment of scapular fracture (body, glenoid or acromion) with or without internal fixation

23600 Closed treatment of proximal humeral (surgical or anatomical neck) fracture; without manipulation

23605 with manipulation, with or without skeletal traction

23615 Open treatment of proximal humeral (surgical or anatomical neck) fracture, with or without internal or external fixation, with or without repair of tuberosity(-ies);

23616 with proximal humeral prosthetic replacement

23620 Closed treatment of greater humeral tuberosity fracture; without manipulation

23625 with manipulation

23630 Open treatment of greater humeral tuberosity fracture, with or without internal or external fixation

23650 Closed treatment of shoulder dislocation, with manipulation; without anesthesia

23655 requiring anesthesia

23660 Open treatment of acute shoulder dislocation

(Repairs for recurrent dislocations, see 23450-23466)

23665 Closed treatment of shoulder dislocation, with fracture of greater humeral tuberosity, with manipulation

23670 Open treatment of shoulder dislocation, with fracture of greater humeral tuberosity, with or without internal or external fixation

23675 Closed treatment of shoulder dislocation, with surgical or anatomical neck fracture, with manipulation

23680 Open treatment of shoulder dislocation, with surgical or anatomical neck fracture, with or without internal or external fixation

MANIPULATION

23700 Manipulation under anesthesia, shoulder joint, including application of fixation apparatus (dislocation excluded)

ARTHRODESIS

23800 Arthrodesis, glenohumeral joint;

23802 with autogenous graft (includes obtaining graft)

AMPUTATION

23900 Interthoracoscapular amputation (forequarter)

23920 Disarticulation of shoulder;

23921 secondary closure or scar revision

OTHER PROCEDURES

23929 Unlisted procedure, shoulder

HUMERUS (UPPER ARM) AND ELBOW

INCISION

(For incision and drainage procedures, superficial, see 10040-10160)

23930 Incision and drainage, upper arm or elbow area; deep abscess or hematoma

23931 bursa

23935 Incision, deep, with opening of bone cortex (eg, for osteomyelitis or bone abscess), humerus or elbow

24000 Arthrotomy, elbow, including exploration, drainage, or removal of foreign body

24006 Arthrotomy of the elbow, with capsular excision for capsular release (separate procedure)

EXCISION

24065 Biopsy, soft tissue of upper arm or elbow area; superficial

24066 deep (subfascial or intramuscular)

(For needle biopsy of soft tissue, use 20206)

24075 Excision, tumor, soft tissue of upper arm or elbow area; subcutaneous

24076 deep (subfascial or intramuscular)

24077 Radical resection of tumor (eg, malignant neoplasm), soft tissue of upper arm or elbow area

24100 Arthrotomy, elbow; with synovial biopsy only

24101 with joint exploration, with or without biopsy, with or without removal of loose or foreign body

24102 with synovectomy

24105 Excision, olecranon bursa

24110 Excision or curettage of bone cyst or benign tumor, humerus;

● New Code ▲ Revised Code + Add-On Code ⊘ Modifier -51 Exempt ⊙ Conscious Sedation

24115 with autograft (includes obtaining graft)

24116 with allograft

24120 Excision or curettage of bone cyst or benign tumor of head or neck of radius or olecranon process;

24125 with autograft (includes obtaining graft)

24126 with allograft

24130 Excision, radial head

(For replacement with implant, use 24366)

24134 Sequestrectomy (eg, for osteomyelitis or bone abscess), shaft or distal humerus

24136 Sequestrectomy (eg, for osteomyelitis or bone abscess), radial head or neck

24138 Sequestrectomy (eg, for osteomyelitis or bone abscess), olecranon process

24140 Partial excision (craterization, saucerization, or diaphysectomy) bone (eg, osteomyelitis), humerus

24145 Partial excision (craterization, saucerization, or diaphysectomy) bone (eg, osteomyelitis), radial head or neck

24147 Partial excision (craterization, saucerization, or diaphysectomy) bone (eg, osteomyelitis), olecranon process

24149 Radical resection of capsule, soft tissue, and heterotopic bone, elbow, with contracture release (separate procedure)

(For capsular and soft tissue release only, use 24006)

24150 Radical resection for tumor, shaft or distal humerus;

24151 with autograft (includes obtaining graft)

24152 Radical resection for tumor, radial head or neck;

24153 with autograft (includes obtaining graft)

24155 Resection of elbow joint (arthrectomy)

INTRODUCTION OR REMOVAL

(For K-wire or pin insertion or removal, see 20650, 20670, 20680)

(For arthrocentesis or needling of bursa or joint, use 20605)

24160 Implant removal; elbow joint

24164 radial head

24200 Removal of foreign body, upper arm or elbow area; subcutaneous

24201 deep (subfascial or intramuscular)

24220 Injection procedure for elbow arthrography

(For radiological supervision and interpretation, use 73085. Do not report 77002 in addition to 73085)

(For injection of tennis elbow, use 20550)

REPAIR, REVISION, AND/OR RECONSTRUCTION

24300 Manipulation, elbow, under anesthesia

(For application of external fixation, see 20690 or 20692)

24301 Muscle or tendon transfer, any type, upper arm or elbow, single (excluding 24320-24331)

24305 Tendon lengthening, upper arm or elbow, each tendon

24310 Tenotomy, open, elbow to shoulder, each tendon

24320 Tenoplasty, with muscle transfer, with or without free graft, elbow to shoulder, single (Seddon-Brookes type procedure)

24330 Flexor-plasty, elbow (eg, Steindler type advancement);

24331 with extensor advancement

24332 Tenolysis, triceps

24340 Tenodesis of biceps tendon at elbow (separate procedure)

24341 Repair, tendon or muscle, upper arm or elbow, each tendon or muscle, primary or secondary (excludes rotator cuff)

24342 Reinsertion of ruptured biceps or triceps tendon, distal, with or without tendon graft

24343 Repair lateral collateral ligament, elbow, with local tissue

24344 Reconstruction lateral collateral ligament, elbow, with tendon graft (includes harvesting of graft)

24345 Repair medial collateral ligament, elbow, with local tissue

24346 Reconstruction medial collateral ligament, elbow, with tendon graft (includes harvesting of graft)

24350 Fasciotomy, lateral or medial (eg, tennis elbow or epicondylitis);

24351 with extensor origin detachment

24352 with annular ligament resection

24354 with stripping

24356 with partial ostectomy

24360 Arthroplasty, elbow; with membrane (eg, fascial)

24361 with distal humeral prosthetic replacement

24362 with implant and fascia lata ligament reconstruction

24363 with distal humerus and proximal ulnar prosthetic replacement (eg, total elbow)

24365 Arthroplasty, radial head;

24366 with implant

24400 Osteotomy, humerus, with or without internal fixation

24410 Multiple osteotomies with realignment on intramedullary rod, humeral shaft (Sofield type procedure)

24420 Osteoplasty, humerus (eg, shortening or lengthening) (excluding 64876)

Separate Procedure | Unlisted Procedure | CCI Comp. Code | Non-specific Procedure

24430 Repair of nonunion or malunion, humerus; without graft (eg, compression technique)

24435 with iliac or other autograft (includes obtaining graft)

(For proximal radius and/or ulna, see 25400-25420)

24470 Hemiepiphyseal arrest (eg, cubitus varus or valgus, distal humerus)

24495 Decompression fasciotomy, forearm, with brachial artery exploration

24498 Prophylactic treatment (nailing, pinning, plating or wiring), with or without methylmethacrylate, humeral shaft

FRACTURE AND/OR DISLOCATION

24500 Closed treatment of humeral shaft fracture; without manipulation

24505 with manipulation, with or without skeletal traction

24515 Open treatment of humeral shaft fracture with plate/screws, with or without cerclage

24516 Treatment of humeral shaft fracture, with insertion of intramedullary implant, with or without cerclage and/or locking screws

24530 Closed treatment of supracondylar or transcondylar humeral fracture, with or without intercondylar extension; without manipulation

24535 with manipulation, with or without skin or skeletal traction

24538 Percutaneous skeletal fixation of supracondylar or transcondylar humeral fracture, with or without intercondylar extension

24545 Open treatment of humeral supracondylar or transcondylar fracture, with or without internal or external fixation; without intercondylar extension

24546 with intercondylar extension

24560 Closed treatment of humeral epicondylar fracture, medial or lateral; without manipulation

24565 with manipulation

24566 Percutaneous skeletal fixation of humeral epicondylar fracture, medial or lateral, with manipulation

24575 Open treatment of humeral epicondylar fracture, medial or lateral, with or without internal or external fixation

24576 Closed treatment of humeral condylar fracture, medial or lateral; without manipulation

24577 with manipulation

24579 Open treatment of humeral condylar fracture, medial or lateral, with or without internal or external fixation

(To report closed treatment of fractures without manipulation, see 24530, 24560, 24576, 24650, 24670)

(To report closed treatment of fractures with manipulation, see 24535, 24565, 24577, 24675)

24582 Percutaneous skeletal fixation of humeral condylar fracture, medial or lateral, with manipulation

24586 Open treatment of periarticular fracture and/or dislocation of the elbow (fracture distal humerus and proximal ulna and/or proximal radius);

24587 with implant arthroplasty

(See also 24361)

24600 Treatment of closed elbow dislocation; without anesthesia

24605 requiring anesthesia

24615 Open treatment of acute or chronic elbow dislocation

24620 Closed treatment of Monteggia type of fracture dislocation at elbow (fracture proximal end of ulna with dislocation of radial head), with manipulation

24635 Open treatment of Monteggia type of fracture dislocation at elbow (fracture proximal end of ulna with dislocation of radial head), with or without internal or external fixation

24640 Closed treatment of radial head subluxation in child, nursemaid elbow, with manipulation

24650 Closed treatment of radial head or neck fracture; without manipulation

24655 with manipulation

24665 Open treatment of radial head or neck fracture, with or without internal fixation or radial head excision;

24666 with radial head prosthetic replacement

24670 Closed treatment of ulnar fracture, proximal end (olecranon process); without manipulation

24675 with manipulation

24685 Open treatment of ulnar fracture proximal end (olecranon process), with or without internal or external fixation

ARTHRODESIS

24800 Arthrodesis, elbow joint; local

24802 with autogenous graft (includes obtaining graft)

AMPUTATION

24900 Amputation, arm through humerus; with primary closure

24920 open, circular (guillotine)

24925 secondary closure or scar revision

24930 re-amputation

24931 with implant

24935 Stump elongation, upper extremity

24940 Cineplasty, upper extremity, complete procedure

OTHER PROCEDURES

24999 Unlisted procedure, humerus or elbow

FOREARM AND WRIST

INCISION

25000 Incision, extensor tendon sheath, wrist (eg, deQuervains disease)

(For decompression median nerve or for carpal tunnel syndrome, use 64721)

25001 Incision, flexor tendon sheath, wrist (eg, flexor carpi radialis)

25020 Decompression fasciotomy, forearm and/or wrist, flexor OR extensor compartment; without debridement of nonviable muscle and/or nerve

25023 with debridement of nonviable muscle and/or nerve

(For decompression fasciotomy with brachial artery exploration, use 24495)

(For incision and drainage procedures, superficial, see 10040-10160)

(For debridement, see also 11000-11044)

25024 Decompression fasciotomy, forearm and/or wrist, flexor AND extensor compartment; without debridement of nonviable muscle and/or nerve

25025 with debridement of nonviable muscle and/or nerve

25028 Incision and drainage, forearm and/or wrist; deep abscess or hematoma

25031 bursa

25035 Incision, deep, bone cortex, forearm and/or wrist (eg, osteomyelitis or bone abscess)

25040 Arthrotomy, radiocarpal or midcarpal joint, with exploration, drainage, or removal of foreign body

EXCISION

25065 Biopsy, soft tissue of forearm and/or wrist; superficial

25066 deep (subfascial or intramuscular)

Separate Procedure | Unlisted Procedure | CCI Comp. Code | Non-specific Procedure

(For needle biopsy of soft tissue, use 20206)

25075 Excision, tumor, soft tissue of forearm and/or wrist area; subcutaneous

25076 deep (subfascial or intramuscular)

25077 Radical resection of tumor (eg, malignant neoplasm), soft tissue of forearm and/or wrist area

25085 Capsulotomy, wrist (eg, contracture)

25100 Arthrotomy, wrist joint; with biopsy

25101 with joint exploration, with or without biopsy, with or without removal of loose or foreign body

25105 with synovectomy

25107 Arthrotomy, distal radioulnar joint including repair of triangular cartilage, complex

● **25109** Excision of tendon, forearm and/or wrist, flexor or extensor, each

25110 Excision, lesion of tendon sheath, forearm and/or wrist

25111 Excision of ganglion, wrist (dorsal or volar); primary

25112 recurrent

(For hand or finger, use 26160)

25115 Radical excision of bursa, synovia of wrist, or forearm tendon sheaths (eg, tenosynovitis, fungus, Tbc, or other granulomas, rheumatoid arthritis); flexors

25116 extensors, with or without transposition of dorsal retinaculum

(For finger synovectomies, use 26145)

25118 Synovectomy, extensor tendon sheath, wrist, single compartment;

25119 with resection of distal ulna

 ● New Code ▲ Revised Code + Add-On Code ⃠ Modifier -51 Exempt ⊙ Conscious Sedation

25120 Excision or curettage of bone cyst or benign tumor of radius or ulna (excluding head or neck of radius and olecranon process);

(For head or neck of radius or olecranon process, see 24120-24126)

25125 with autograft (includes obtaining graft)

25126 with allograft

25130 Excision or curettage of bone cyst or benign tumor of carpal bones;

25135 with autograft (includes obtaining graft)

25136 with allograft

25145 Sequestrectomy (eg, for osteomyelitis or bone abscess), forearm and/or wrist

25150 Partial excision (craterization, saucerization, or diaphysectomy) of bone (eg, for osteomyelitis); ulna

25151 radius

(For head or neck of radius or olecranon process, see 24145, 24147)

25170 Radical resection for tumor, radius or ulna

25210 Carpectomy; one bone

(For carpectomy with implant, see 25441-25445)

25215 all bones of proximal row

25230 Radial styloidectomy (separate procedure)

25240 Excision distal ulna partial or complete (eg, Darrach type or matched resection)

(For implant replacement, distal ulna, use 25442)

(For obtaining fascia for interposition, see 20920, 20922)

Separate Procedure 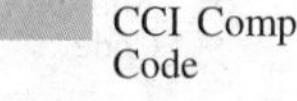 Unlisted Procedure 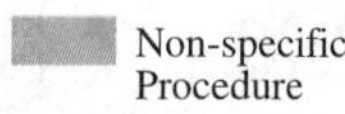 CCI Comp. Code Non-specific Procedure

INTRODUCTION OR REMOVAL

(For K-wire, pin or rod insertion or removal, see 20650, 20670, 20680)

25246 Injection procedure for wrist arthrography

(For radiological supervision and interpretation, use 73115. Do not report 77002 in addition to 73115)

(For foreign body removal, superficial use 20520)

25248 Exploration with removal of deep foreign body, forearm or wrist

25250 Removal of wrist prosthesis; (separate procedure)

25251 complicated, including total wrist

25259 Manipulation, wrist, under anesthesia

(For application of external fixation, see 20690 or 20692)

REPAIR, REVISION, AND/OR RECONSTRUCTION

25260 Repair, tendon or muscle, flexor, forearm and/or wrist; primary, single, each tendon or muscle

25263 secondary, single, each tendon or muscle

25265 secondary, with free graft (includes obtaining graft), each tendon or muscle

25270 Repair, tendon or muscle, extensor, forearm and/or wrist; primary, single, each tendon or muscle

25272 secondary, single, each tendon or muscle

25274 secondary, with free graft (includes obtaining graft), each tendon or muscle

25275 Repair, tendon sheath, extensor, forearm and/or wrist, with free graft (includes obtaining graft) (eg, for extensor carpi ulnaris subluxation)

25280 Lengthening or shortening of flexor or extensor tendon, forearm and/or wrist, single, each tendon

25290 Tenotomy, open, flexor or extensor tendon, forearm and/or wrist, single, each tendon

25295 Tenolysis, flexor or extensor tendon, forearm and/or wrist, single, each tendon

25300 Tenodesis at wrist; flexors of fingers

25301 extensors of fingers

25310 Tendon transplantation or transfer, flexor or extensor, forearm and/or wrist, single; each tendon

25312 with tendon graft(s) (includes obtaining graft), each tendon

25315 Flexor origin slide (eg, for cerebral palsy, Volkmann contracture), forearm and/or wrist;

25316 with tendon(s) transfer

25320 Capsulorrhaphy or reconstruction, wrist, open (eg, capsulodesis, ligament repair, tendon transfer or graft) (includes synovectomy, capsulotomy and open reduction) for carpal instability

25332 Arthroplasty, wrist, with or without interposition, with or without external or internal fixation

(For obtaining fascia for interposition, see 20920, 20922)

(For prosthetic replacement arthroplasty, see 25441-25446)

25335 Centralization of wrist on ulna (eg, radial club hand)

25337 Reconstruction for stabilization of unstable distal ulna or distal radioulnar joint, secondary by soft tissue stabilization (eg, tendon transfer, tendon graft or weave, or tenodesis) with or without open reduction of distal radioulnar joint

(For harvesting of fascia lata graft, see 20920, 20922)

25350 Osteotomy, radius; distal third

25355 middle or proximal third

25360 Osteotomy; ulna

25365 radius AND ulna

25370 Multiple osteotomies, with realignment on intramedullary rod (Sofield type procedure); radius OR ulna

25375 radius AND ulna

25390 Osteoplasty, radius OR ulna; shortening

25391 lengthening with autograft

25392 Osteoplasty, radius AND ulna; shortening (excluding 64876)

25393 lengthening with autograft

25394 Osteoplasty, carpal bone, shortening

25400 Repair of nonunion or malunion, radius OR ulna; without graft (eg, compression technique)

25405 with autograft (includes obtaining graft)

25415 Repair of nonunion or malunion, radius AND ulna; without graft (eg, compression technique)

25420 with autograft (includes obtaining graft)

25425 Repair of defect with autograft; radius OR ulna

25426 radius AND ulna

25430 Insertion of vascular pedicle into carpal bone (eg, Hori procedure)

25431 Repair of nonunion of carpal bone (excluding carpal scaphoid (navicular) (includes obtaining graft and necessary fixation), each bone

25440 Repair of nonunion, scaphoid carpal (navicular) bone, with or without radial styloidectomy (includes obtaining graft and necessary fixation)

25441 Arthroplasty with prosthetic replacement; distal radius

25442 distal ulna

25443 scaphoid carpal (navicular)

● New Code ▲ Revised Code + Add-On Code ⊘ Modifier -51 Exempt ⊙ Conscious Sedation

25444 lunate

25445 trapezium

25446 distal radius and partial or entire carpus (total wrist)

25447 Arthroplasty, interposition, intercarpal or carpometacarpal joints

(For wrist arthroplasty, use 25332)

25449 Revision of arthroplasty, including removal of implant, wrist joint

25450 Epiphyseal arrest by epiphysiodesis or stapling; distal radius OR ulna

25455 distal radius AND ulna

25490 Prophylactic treatment (nailing, pinning, plating or wiring) with or without methylmethacrylate; radius

25491 ulna

25492 radius AND ulna

FRACTURE AND/OR DISLOCATION

(For application of external fixation in addition to internal fixation, use 20690 and the appropriate internal fixation code)

25500 Closed treatment of radial shaft fracture; without manipulation

25505 with manipulation

25515 Open treatment of radial shaft fracture, with or without internal or external fixation

25520 Closed treatment of radial shaft fracture and closed treatment of dislocation of distal radioulnar joint (Galeazzi fracture/dislocation)

25525 Open treatment of radial shaft fracture, with internal and/or external fixation and closed treatment of dislocation of distal radioulnar joint (Galeazzi fracture/dislocation), with or without percutaneous skeletal fixation

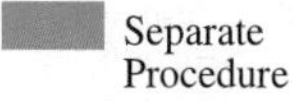 Separate Procedure 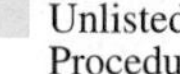 Unlisted Procedure 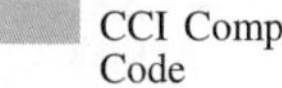 CCI Comp. Code 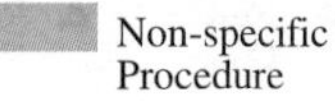 Non-specific Procedure

25526 Open treatment of radial shaft fracture, with internal and/or external fixation and open treatment, with or without internal or external fixation of distal radioulnar joint (Galeazzi fracture/dislocation), includes repair of triangular fibrocartilage complex

25530 Closed treatment of ulnar shaft fracture; without manipulation

25535 with manipulation

25545 Open treatment of ulnar shaft fracture, with or without internal or external fixation

25560 Closed treatment of radial and ulnar shaft fractures; without manipulation

25565 with manipulation

25574 Open treatment of radial AND ulnar shaft fractures, with internal or external fixation; of radius OR ulna

25575 of radius AND ulna

▲ **25600** Closed treatment of distal radial fracture (eg, Colles or Smith type) or epiphyseal separation, includes closed treatment of fracture of ulnar styloid, when performed; without manipulation

25605 with manipulation

(Do not report 25600, 25605 in conjunction with 25650)

● **25606** Percutaneous skeletal fixation of distal radial fracture or epiphyseal separation

(Do not report 25606 in conjunction with 25650)

(For percutaneous treatment of ulnar styloid fracture, use 25651)

(For open treatment of ulnar styloid fracture, use 25652)

● **25607** Open treatment of distal radial extra-articular fracture or epiphyseal separation, with internal fixation

(Do not report 25607 in conjunction with 25650)

(For percutaneous treatment of ulnar styloid fracture, use 25651)

● New Code ▲ Revised Code + Add-On Code ⊘ Modifier -51 Exempt ⊙ Conscious Sedation

(For open treatment of ulnar styloid fracture, use 25652)

● **25608** Open treatment of distal radial intra-articular fracture or epiphyseal separation; with internal fixation of 2 fragments

(Do not report 25608 in conjunction with 25609)

(Do not report 25608 in conjunction with 25650)

● **25609** Open treatment of distal radial intra-articular fracture or epiphyseal separation; with internal fixation of 3 or more fragments

(Do not report 25608, 25609 in conjunction with 25650)

(For percutaneous treatment of ulnar styloid fracture, use 25651)

(For open treatment of ulnar styloid fracture, use 25652)

(25611 deleted 2007 edition, see 25606)

(25620 deleted 2007 edition, see 25607-25609)

25622 Closed treatment of carpal scaphoid (navicular) fracture; without manipulation

25624 with manipulation

25628 Open treatment of carpal scaphoid (navicular) fracture, with or without internal or external fixation

25630 Closed treatment of carpal bone fracture (excluding carpal scaphoid (navicular)); without manipulation, each bone

25635 with manipulation, each bone

25645 Open treatment of carpal bone fracture (other than carpal scaphoid (navicular)), each bone

25650 Closed treatment of ulnar styloid fracture

(Do not report 25650 in conjunction with 25600, 25605, 25607-25609)

25651 Percutaneous skeletal fixation of ulnar styloid fracture

25652 Open treatment of ulnar styloid fracture

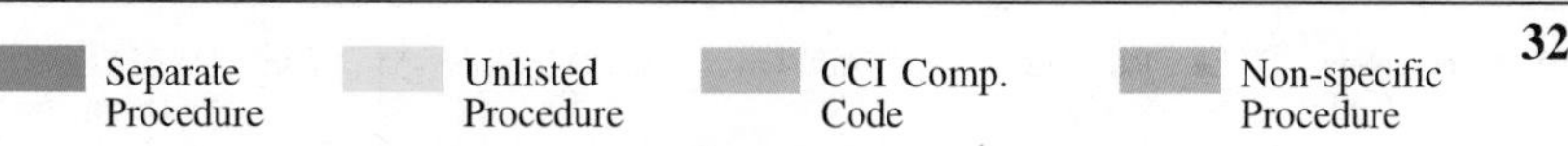

25660 Closed treatment of radiocarpal or intercarpal dislocation, one or more bones, with manipulation

25670 Open treatment of radiocarpal or intercarpal dislocation, one or more bones

25671 Percutaneous skeletal fixation of distal radioulnar dislocation

25675 Closed treatment of distal radioulnar dislocation with manipulation

25676 Open treatment of distal radioulnar dislocation, acute or chronic

25680 Closed treatment of trans-scaphoperilunar type of fracture dislocation, with manipulation

25685 Open treatment of trans-scaphoperilunar type of fracture dislocation

25690 Closed treatment of lunate dislocation, with manipulation

25695 Open treatment of lunate dislocation

ARTHRODESIS

25800 Arthrodesis, wrist; complete, without bone graft (includes radiocarpal and/or intercarpal and/or carpometacarpal joints)

25805 with sliding graft

25810 with iliac or other autograft (includes obtaining graft)

25820 Arthrodesis, wrist; limited, without bone graft (eg, intercarpal or radiocarpal)

25825 with autograft (includes obtaining graft)

25830 Arthrodesis, distal radioulnar joint with segmental resection of ulna, with or without bone graft (eg, Sauve-Kapandji procedure)

AMPUTATION

25900 Amputation, forearm, through radius and ulna;

25905 open, circular (guillotine)

● New Code ▲ Revised Code + Add-On Code ⦸ Modifier -51 Exempt ⊙ Conscious Sedation

25907 secondary closure or scar revision

25909 re-amputation

25915 Krukenberg procedure

25920 Disarticulation through wrist;

25922 secondary closure or scar revision

25924 re-amputation

25927 Transmetacarpal amputation;

25929 secondary closure or scar revision

25931 re-amputation

OTHER PROCEDURES

25999 Unlisted procedure, forearm or wrist

HAND AND FINGERS

INCISION

26010 Drainage of finger abscess; simple

26011 complicated (eg, felon)

26020 Drainage of tendon sheath, digit and/or palm, each

26025 Drainage of palmar bursa; single, bursa

26030 multiple bursa

26034 Incision, bone cortex, hand or finger (eg, osteomyelitis or bone abscess)

26035 Decompression fingers and/or hand, injection injury (eg, grease gun)

26037 Decompressive fasciotomy, hand (excludes 26035)

(For injection injury, use 26035)

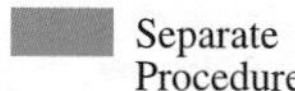
Separate Procedure

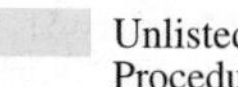
Unlisted Procedure

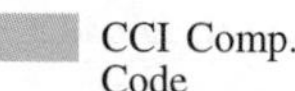
CCI Comp. Code

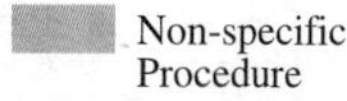
Non-specific Procedure

26040 Fasciotomy, palmar (eg, Dupuytren's contracture); percutaneous

26045 open, partial

(For fasciectomy, see 26121-26125)

26055 Tendon sheath incision (eg, for trigger finger)

26060 Tenotomy, percutaneous, single, each digit

26070 Arthrotomy, with exploration, drainage, or removal of loose or foreign body; carpometacarpal joint

26075 metacarpophalangeal joint, each

26080 interphalangeal joint, each

EXCISION

26100 Arthrotomy with biopsy; carpometacarpal joint, each

26105 metacarpophalangeal joint, each

26110 interphalangeal joint, each

26115 Excision, tumor or vascular malformation, soft tissue of hand or finger; subcutaneous

26116 deep (subfascial or intramuscular)

26117 Radical resection of tumor (eg, malignant neoplasm), soft tissue of hand or finger

26121 Fasciectomy, palm only, with or without Z-plasty, other local tissue rearrangement, or skin grafting (includes obtaining graft)

26123 Fasciectomy, partial palmar with release of single digit including proximal interphalangeal joint, with or without Z-plasty, other local tissue rearrangement, or skin grafting (includes obtaining graft);

\+ **26125** each additional digit (List separately in addition to code for primary procedure)

(Use 26125 in conjunction with code 26123)

(For fasciotomy, see 26040, 26045)

26130 Synovectomy, carpometacarpal joint

26135 Synovectomy, metacarpophalangeal joint including intrinsic release and extensor hood reconstruction, each digit

26140 Synovectomy, proximal interphalangeal joint, including extensor reconstruction, each interphalangeal joint

26145 Synovectomy, tendon sheath, radical (tenosynovectomy), flexor tendon, palm and/or finger, each tendon

(For tendon sheath synovectomies at wrist, see 25115, 25116)

26160 Excision of lesion of tendon sheath or joint capsule (eg, cyst, mucous cyst, or ganglion), hand or finger

(For wrist ganglion, see 25111, 25112)

(For trigger digit, use 26055)

▲ **26170** Excision of tendon, palm, flexor or extensor, single, each tendon

(Do not report 26170 in conjunction with 26390, 26415)

▲ **26180** Excision of tendon, finger, flexor or extensor, each tendon

(Do not report 26180 in conjunction with 26390, 26415)

26185 Sesamoidectomy, thumb or finger (separate procedure)

26200 Excision or curettage of bone cyst or benign tumor of metacarpal;

26205 with autograft (includes obtaining graft)

26210 Excision or curettage of bone cyst or benign tumor of proximal, middle, or distal phalanx of finger;

26215 with autograft (includes obtaining graft)

26230 Partial excision (craterization, saucerization, or diaphysectomy) bone (eg, osteomyelitis); metacarpal

26235 proximal or middle phalanx of finger

26236 distal phalanx of finger

26250 Radical resection, metacarpal (eg, tumor);

26255 with autograft (includes obtaining graft)

26260 Radical resection, proximal or middle phalanx of finger (eg, tumor);

26261 with autograft (includes obtaining graft)

26262 Radical resection, distal phalanx of finger (eg, tumor)

INTRODUCTION OR REMOVAL

26320 Removal of implant from finger or hand

(For removal of foreign body in hand or finger, see 20520, 20525)

REPAIR, REVISION, AND/OR RECONSTRUCTION

26340 Manipulation, finger joint, under anesthesia, each joint

(For application of external fixation, see 20690 or 20692)

26350 Repair or advancement, flexor tendon, not in zone 2 digital flexor tendon sheath (eg, no man's land); primary or secondary without free graft, each tendon

26352 secondary with free graft (includes obtaining graft), each tendon

26356 Repair or advancement, flexor tendon, in zone 2 digital flexor tendon sheath (eg, no man's land); primary, without free graft, each tendon

26357 secondary, without free graft, each tendon

26358 secondary with free graft (includes obtaining graft), each tendon

26370 Repair or advancement of profundus tendon, with intact superficialis tendon; primary, each tendon

26372 secondary with free graft (includes obtaining graft), each tendon

26373 secondary without free graft, each tendon

26390 Excision flexor tendon, with implantation of synthetic rod for delayed tendon graft, hand or finger, each rod

26392 Removal of synthetic rod and insertion of flexor tendon graft, hand or finger (includes obtaining graft), each rod

26410 Repair, extensor tendon, hand, primary or secondary; without free graft, each tendon

26412 with free graft (includes obtaining graft), each tendon

26415 Excision of extensor tendon, with implantation of synthetic rod for delayed tendon graft, hand or finger, each rod

26416 Removal of synthetic rod and insertion of extensor tendon graft (includes obtaining graft), hand or finger, each rod

26418 Repair, extensor tendon, finger, primary or secondary; without free graft, each tendon

26420 with free graft (includes obtaining graft) each tendon

26426 Repair of extensor tendon, central slip, secondary (eg, boutonniere deformity); using local tissue(s), including lateral band(s), each finger

26428 with free graft (includes obtaining graft), each finger

26432 Closed treatment of distal extensor tendon insertion, with or without percutaneous pinning (eg, mallet finger)

26433 Repair of extensor tendon, distal insertion, primary or secondary; without graft (eg, mallet finger)

26434 with free graft (includes obtaining graft)

(For tenovaginotomy for trigger finger, use 26055)

26437 Realignment of extensor tendon, hand, each tendon

26440 Tenolysis, flexor tendon; palm OR finger, each tendon

26442 palm AND finger, each tendon

26445 Tenolysis, extensor tendon, hand or finger; each tendon

26449 Tenolysis, complex, extensor tendon, finger, including forearm, each tendon

26450 Tenotomy, flexor, palm, open, each tendon

26455 Tenotomy, flexor, finger, open, each tendon

26460 Tenotomy, extensor, hand or finger, open, each tendon

26471 Tenodesis; of proximal interphalangeal joint, each joint

26474 of distal joint, each joint

26476 Lengthening of tendon, extensor, hand or finger, each tendon

26477 Shortening of tendon, extensor, hand or finger, each tendon

26478 Lengthening of tendon, flexor, hand or finger, each tendon

26479 Shortening of tendon, flexor, hand or finger, each tendon

26480 Transfer or transplant of tendon, carpometacarpal area or dorsum of hand; without free graft, each tendon

26483 with free tendon graft (includes obtaining graft), each tendon

26485 Transfer or transplant of tendon, palmar; without free tendon graft, each tendon

26489 with free tendon graft (includes obtaining graft), each tendon

26490 Opponensplasty; superficialis tendon transfer type, each tendon

26492 tendon transfer with graft (includes obtaining graft), each tendon

26494 hypothenar muscle transfer

26496 other methods

(For thumb fusion in opposition, use 26820)

26497 Transfer of tendon to restore intrinsic function; ring and small finger

26498 all four fingers

26499 Correction claw finger, other methods

26500 Reconstruction of tendon pulley, each tendon; with local tissues (separate procedure)

26502 with tendon or fascial graft (includes obtaining graft) (separate procedure)

(26504 deleted 2007 edition, see 26390)

26508 Release of thenar muscle(s) (eg, thumb contracture)

26510 Cross intrinsic transfer, each tendon

26516 Capsulodesis, metacarpophalangeal joint; single digit

26517 two digits

26518 three or four digits

26520 Capsulectomy or capsulotomy; metacarpophalangeal joint, each joint

26525 interphalangeal joint, each joint

(To report carpometacarpal joint arthroplasty, use 25447)

26530 Arthroplasty, metacarpophalangeal joint; each joint

26531 with prosthetic implant, each joint

26535 Arthroplasty, interphalangeal joint; each joint

26536 with prosthetic implant, each joint

26540 Repair of collateral ligament, metacarpophalangeal or interphalangeal joint

26541 Reconstruction, collateral ligament, metacarpophalangeal joint, single; with tendon or fascial graft (includes obtaining graft)

26542 with local tissue (eg, adductor advancement)

Separate Procedure 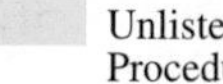 Unlisted Procedure 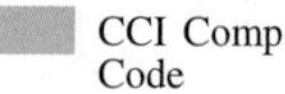 CCI Comp. Code 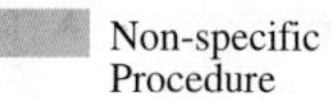 Non-specific Procedure

26545 Reconstruction, collateral ligament, interphalangeal joint, single, including graft, each joint

26546 Repair non-union, metacarpal or phalanx, (includes obtaining bone graft with or without external or internal fixation)

26548 Repair and reconstruction, finger, volar plate, interphalangeal joint

26550 Pollicization of a digit

26551 Transfer, toe-to-hand with microvascular anastomosis; great toe wrap-around with bone graft

(For great toe with web space, use 20973)

26553 other than great toe, single

26554 other than great toe, double

(Do not report code 69990 in addition to codes 26551-26554)

26555 Transfer, finger to another position without microvascular anastomosis

26556 Transfer, free toe joint, with microvascular anastomosis

(Do not report code 69990 in addition to code 26556)

(To report great toe-to-hand transfer, use 20973)

26560 Repair of syndactyly (web finger) each web space; with skin flaps

26561 with skin flaps and grafts

26562 complex (eg, involving bone, nails)

26565 Osteotomy; metacarpal, each

26567 phalanx of finger, each

26568 Osteoplasty, lengthening, metacarpal or phalanx

26580 Repair cleft hand

26587 Reconstruction of polydactylous digit, soft tissue and bone

(For excision of polydactylous digit, soft tissue only, use 11200)

26590 Repair macrodactylia, each digit

26591 Repair, intrinsic muscles of hand, each muscle

26593 Release, intrinsic muscles of hand, each muscle

26596 Excision of constricting ring of finger, with multiple Z-plasties

(To report release of scar contracture or graft repairs, see 11041-11042, 14040-14041, or 15120, 15240)

FRACTURE AND/OR DISLOCATION

26600 Closed treatment of metacarpal fracture, single; without manipulation, each bone

26605 with manipulation, each bone

26607 Closed treatment of metacarpal fracture, with manipulation, with external fixation, each bone

26608 Percutaneous skeletal fixation of metacarpal fracture, each bone

26615 Open treatment of metacarpal fracture, single, with or without internal or external fixation, each bone

26641 Closed treatment of carpometacarpal dislocation, thumb, with manipulation

26645 Closed treatment of carpometacarpal fracture dislocation, thumb (Bennett fracture), with manipulation

26650 Percutaneous skeletal fixation of carpometacarpal fracture dislocation, thumb (Bennett fracture), with manipulation, with or without external fixation

26665 Open treatment of carpometacarpal fracture dislocation, thumb (Bennett fracture), with or without internal or external fixation

26670 Closed treatment of carpometacarpal dislocation, other than thumb, with manipulation, each joint; without anesthesia

26675 requiring anesthesia

26676 Percutaneous skeletal fixation of carpometacarpal dislocation, other than thumb, with manipulation, each joint

26685 Open treatment of carpometacarpal dislocation, other than thumb; with or without internal or external fixation, each joint

26686 complex, multiple or delayed reduction

26700 Closed treatment of metacarpophalangeal dislocation, single, with manipulation; without anesthesia

26705 requiring anesthesia

26706 Percutaneous skeletal fixation of metacarpophalangeal dislocation, single, with manipulation

26715 Open treatment of metacarpophalangeal dislocation, single, with or without internal or external fixation

26720 Closed treatment of phalangeal shaft fracture, proximal or middle phalanx, finger or thumb; without manipulation, each

26725 with manipulation, with or without skin or skeletal traction, each

26727 Percutaneous skeletal fixation of unstable phalangeal shaft fracture, proximal or middle phalanx, finger or thumb, with manipulation, each

26735 Open treatment of phalangeal shaft fracture, proximal or middle phalanx, finger or thumb, with or without internal or external fixation, each

26740 Closed treatment of articular fracture, involving metacarpophalangeal or interphalangeal joint; without manipulation, each

26742 with manipulation, each

26746 Open treatment of articular fracture, involving metacarpophalangeal or interphalangeal joint, with or without internal or external fixation, each

26750 Closed treatment of distal phalangeal fracture, finger or thumb; without manipulation, each

26755 with manipulation, each

● New Code ▲ Revised Code + Add-On Code ⊘ Modifier -51 Exempt ⊙ Conscious Sedation

26756 Percutaneous skeletal fixation of distal phalangeal fracture, finger or thumb, each

26765 Open treatment of distal phalangeal fracture, finger or thumb, with or without internal or external fixation, each

26770 Closed treatment of interphalangeal joint dislocation, single, with manipulation; without anesthesia

26775 requiring anesthesia

26776 Percutaneous skeletal fixation of interphalangeal joint dislocation, single, with manipulation

26785 Open treatment of interphalangeal joint dislocation, with or without internal or external fixation, single

ARTHRODESIS

26820 Fusion in opposition, thumb, with autogenous graft (includes obtaining graft)

26841 Arthrodesis, carpometacarpal joint, thumb, with or without internal fixation;

26842 with autograft (includes obtaining graft)

26843 Arthrodesis, carpometacarpal joint, digit, other than thumb, each;

26844 with autograft (includes obtaining graft)

26850 Arthrodesis, metacarpophalangeal joint, with or without internal fixation;

26852 with autograft (includes obtaining graft)

26860 Arthrodesis, interphalangeal joint, with or without internal fixation;

+ **26861** each additional interphalangeal joint (List separately in addition to code for primary procedure)

(Use 26861 in conjunction with code 26860)

26862 with autograft (includes obtaining graft)

Separate Procedure | Unlisted Procedure | CCI Comp. Code | Non-specific Procedure

+ 26863 with autograft (includes obtaining graft), each additional joint (List separately in addition to code for primary procedure)

(Use 26863 in conjunction with code 26862)

AMPUTATION

(For hand through metacarpal bones, use 25927)

26910 Amputation, metacarpal, with finger or thumb (ray amputation), single, with or without interosseous transfer

(For repositioning see 26550, 26555)

26951 Amputation, finger or thumb, primary or secondary, any joint or phalanx, single, including neurectomies; with direct closure

26952 with local advancement flaps (V-Y, hood)

(For repair of soft tissue defect requiring split or full thickness graft or other pedicle flaps, see 15050-15758)

OTHER PROCEDURES

26989 Unlisted procedure, hands or fingers

PELVIS AND HIP JOINT

INCISION

(For incision and drainage procedures, superficial, see 10040-10160)

26990 Incision and drainage, pelvis or hip joint area; deep abscess or hematoma

26991 infected bursa

26992 Incision, bone cortex, pelvis and/or hip joint (eg, osteomyelitis or bone abscess)

27000 Tenotomy, adductor of hip, percutaneous (separate procedure)

27001 Tenotomy, adductor of hip, open

(To report bilateral procedures, report 27001 with modifier -50)

27003 Tenotomy, adductor, subcutaneous, open, with obturator neurectomy

(To report bilateral procedures, report 27003 with modifier -50)

27005 Tenotomy, hip flexor(s), open (separate procedure)

27006 Tenotomy, abductors and/or extensor(s) of hip, open (separate procedure)

27025 Fasciotomy, hip or thigh, any type

(To report bilateral procedures, report 27025 with modifier -50)

27030 Arthrotomy, hip, with drainage (eg, infection)

27033 Arthrotomy, hip, including exploration or removal of loose or foreign body

27035 Denervation, hip joint, intrapelvic or extrapelvic intra-articular branches of sciatic, femoral, or obturator nerves

(For obturator neurectomy, see 64763, 64766)

27036 Capsulectomy or capsulotomy, hip, with or without excision of heterotopic bone, with release of hip flexor muscles (ie, gluteus medius, gluteus minimus, tensor fascia latae, rectus femoris, sartorius, iliopsoas)

EXCISION

27040 Biopsy, soft tissue of pelvis and hip area; superficial

27041 deep, subfascial or intramuscular

(For needle biopsy of soft tissue, use 20206)

27047 Excision, tumor, pelvis and hip area; subcutaneous tissue

27048 deep, subfascial, intramuscular

27049 Radical resection of tumor, soft tissue of pelvis and hip area (eg, malignant neoplasm)

27050 Arthrotomy, with biopsy; sacroiliac joint

27052 hip joint

Separate Procedure Unlisted Procedure 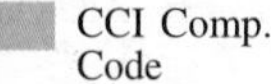 CCI Comp. Code 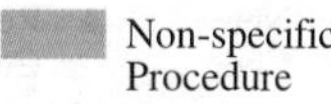 Non-specific Procedure

27054 Arthrotomy with synovectomy, hip joint

27060 Excision; ischial bursa

27062 trochanteric bursa or calcification

(For arthrocentesis or needling of bursa, use 20610)

27065 Excision of bone cyst or benign tumor; superficial (wing of ilium, symphysis pubis, or greater trochanter of femur) with or without autograft

27066 deep, with or without autograft

27067 with autograft requiring separate incision

27070 Partial excision (craterization, saucerization) (eg, osteomyelitis or bone abscess); superficial (eg, wing of ilium, symphysis pubis, or greater trochanter of femur)

27071 deep (subfascial or intramuscular)

27075 Radical resection of tumor or infection; wing of ilium, one pubic or ischial ramus or symphysis pubis

27076 ilium, including acetabulum, both pubic rami, or ischium and acetabulum

27077 innominate bone, total

27078 ischial tuberosity and greater trochanter of femur

27079 ischial tuberosity and greater trochanter of femur, with skin flaps

27080 Coccygectomy, primary

(For pressure (decubitus) ulcer, see 15920, 15922 and 15931-15958)

INTRODUCTION OR REMOVAL

27086 Removal of foreign body, pelvis or hip; subcutaneous tissue

27087 deep (subfascial or intramuscular)

27090 Removal of hip prosthesis; (separate procedure)

● New Code ▲ Revised Code + Add-On Code ⦸ Modifier -51 Exempt ⊙ Conscious Sedation

27091 complicated, including total hip prosthesis, methylmethacrylate with or without insertion of spacer

27093 Injection procedure for hip arthrography; without anesthesia

(For radiological supervision and interpretation, use 73525. Do not report 77002 in conjunction with 73525)

27095 with anesthesia

(For radiological supervision and interpretation, use 73525. Do not report 77002 in conjunction with 73525)

27096 Injection procedure for sacroiliac joint, arthrography and/or anesthetic/steroid

(27096 is to be used only with imaging confirmation of intra-articular needle positioning)

(For radiological supervision and interpretation of sacroiliac joint arthrography, use 73542)

(For fluoroscopic guidance without formal arthrography, use 77003)

(Code 27096 is a unilateral procedure. For bilateral procedure, use modifier -50)

REPAIR, REVISION, AND/OR RECONSTRUCTION

27097 Release or recession, hamstring, proximal

27098 Transfer, adductor to ischium

27100 Transfer external oblique muscle to greater trochanter including fascial or tendon extension (graft)

27105 Transfer paraspinal muscle to hip (includes fascial or tendon extension graft)

27110 Transfer iliopsoas; to greater trochanter of femur

27111 to femoral neck

27120 Acetabuloplasty; (eg, Whitman, Colonna, Haygroves, or cup type)

27122 resection, femoral head (eg, Girdlestone procedure)

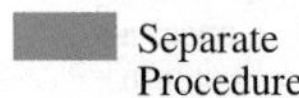 Separate Procedure 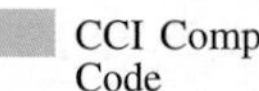 Unlisted Procedure CCI Comp. Code 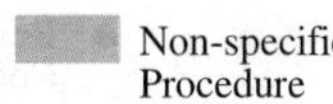 Non-specific Procedure

27125 Hemiarthroplasty, hip, partial (eg, femoral stem prosthesis, bipolar arthroplasty)

(For prosthetic replacement following fracture of the hip, use 27236)

27130 Arthroplasty, acetabular and proximal femoral prosthetic replacement (total hip arthroplasty), with or without autograft or allograft

27132 Conversion of previous hip surgery to total hip arthroplasty, with or without autograft or allograft

27134 Revision of total hip arthroplasty; both components, with or without autograft or allograft

27137 acetabular component only, with or without autograft or allograft

27138 femoral component only, with or without allograft

27140 Osteotomy and transfer of greater trochanter of femur (separate procedure)

27146 Osteotomy, iliac, acetabular or innominate bone;

27147 with open reduction of hip

27151 with femoral osteotomy

27156 with femoral osteotomy and with open reduction of hip

27158 Osteotomy, pelvis, bilateral (eg, congenital malformation)

27161 Osteotomy, femoral neck (separate procedure)

27165 Osteotomy, intertrochanteric or subtrochanteric including internal or external fixation and/or cast

27170 Bone graft, femoral head, neck, intertrochanteric or subtrochanteric area (includes obtaining bone graft)

27175 Treatment of slipped femoral epiphysis; by traction, without reduction

27176 by single or multiple pinning, in situ

27177 Open treatment of slipped femoral epiphysis; single or multiple pinning or bone graft (includes obtaining graft)

27178 closed manipulation with single or multiple pinning

27179 osteoplasty of femoral neck (Heyman type procedure)

27181 osteotomy and internal fixation

27185 Epiphyseal arrest by epiphysiodesis or stapling, greater trochanter of femur

27187 Prophylactic treatment (nailing, pinning, plating or wiring) with or without methylmethacrylate, femoral neck and proximal femur

FRACTURE AND/OR DISLOCATION

27193 Closed treatment of pelvic ring fracture, dislocation, diastasis or subluxation; without manipulation

27194 with manipulation, requiring more than local anesthesia

27200 Closed treatment of coccygeal fracture

27202 Open treatment of coccygeal fracture

27215 Open treatment of iliac spine(s), tuberosity avulsion, or iliac wing fracture(s) (eg, pelvic fracture(s) which do not disrupt the pelvic ring), with internal fixation

27216 Percutaneous skeletal fixation of posterior pelvic ring fracture and/or dislocation (includes ilium, sacroiliac joint and/or sacrum)

27217 Open treatment of anterior ring fracture and/or dislocation with internal fixation (includes pubic symphysis and/or rami)

27218 Open treatment of posterior ring fracture and/or dislocation with internal fixation (includes ilium, sacroiliac joint and/or sacrum)

27220 Closed treatment of acetabulum (hip socket) fracture(s); without manipulation

27222 with manipulation, with or without skeletal traction

27226 Open treatment of posterior or anterior acetabular wall fracture, with internal fixation

27227 Open treatment of acetabular fracture(s) involving anterior or posterior (one) column, or a fracture running transversely across the acetabulum, with internal fixation

27228 Open treatment of acetabular fracture(s) involving anterior and posterior (two) columns, includes T-fracture and both column fracture with complete articular detachment, or single column or transverse fracture with associated acetabular wall fracture, with internal fixation

27230 Closed treatment of femoral fracture, proximal end, neck; without manipulation

27232 with manipulation, with or without skeletal traction

27235 Percutaneous skeletal fixation of femoral fracture, proximal end, neck

27236 Open treatment of femoral fracture, proximal end, neck, internal fixation or prosthetic replacement

27238 Closed treatment of intertrochanteric, pertrochanteric, or subtrochanteric femoral fracture; without manipulation

27240 with manipulation, with or without skin or skeletal traction

27244 Treatment of intertrochanteric, pertrochanteric or subtrochanteric femoral fracture; with plate/screw type implant, with or without cerclage

27245 with intramedullary implant, with or without interlocking screws and/or cerclage

27246 Closed treatment of greater trochanteric fracture, without manipulation

27248 Open treatment of greater trochanteric fracture, with or without internal or external fixation

27250 Closed treatment of hip dislocation, traumatic; without anesthesia

27252 requiring anesthesia

● New Code ▲ Revised Code + Add-On Code ⊘ Modifier -51 Exempt ⊙ Conscious Sedation

27253 Open treatment of hip dislocation, traumatic, without internal fixation

27254 Open treatment of hip dislocation, traumatic, with acetabular wall and femoral head fracture, with or without internal or external fixation

(For treatment of acetabular fracture with fixation, see 27226, 27227)

27256 Treatment of spontaneous hip dislocation (developmental, including congenital or pathological), by abduction, splint or traction; without anesthesia, without manipulation

27257 with manipulation, requiring anesthesia

27258 Open treatment of spontaneous hip dislocation (developmental, including congenital or pathological), replacement of femoral head in acetabulum (including tenotomy, etc);

27259 with femoral shaft shortening

27265 Closed treatment of post hip arthroplasty dislocation; without anesthesia

27266 requiring regional or general anesthesia

MANIPULATION

27275 Manipulation, hip joint, requiring general anesthesia

ARTHRODESIS

27280 Arthrodesis, sacroiliac joint (including obtaining graft)

(To report bilateral procedures, report 27280 with modifier -50)

27282 Arthrodesis, symphysis pubis (including obtaining graft)

27284 Arthrodesis, hip joint (including obtaining graft);

27286 with subtrochanteric osteotomy

AMPUTATION

27290 Interpelviabdominal amputation (hindquarter amputation)

27295 Disarticulation of hip

OTHER PROCEDURES

27299 Unlisted procedure, pelvis or hip joint

FEMUR (THIGH REGION) AND KNEE JOINT

INCISION

(For incision and drainage of abscess or hematoma, superficial, see 10040-10160)

27301 Incision and drainage, deep abscess, bursa, or hematoma, thigh or knee region

27303 Incision, deep, with opening of bone cortex, femur or knee (eg, osteomyelitis or bone abscess)

27305 Fasciotomy, iliotibial (tenotomy), open

(For combined Ober-Yount fasciotomy, use 27025)

27306 Tenotomy, percutaneous, adductor or hamstring; single tendon (separate procedure)

27307 multiple tendons

27310 Arthrotomy, knee, with exploration, drainage, or removal of foreign body(eg, infection)

(27315 deleted 2007 edition, see 27325)

(27320 deleted 2007 edition, see 27326)

EXCISION

27323 Biopsy, soft tissue of thigh or knee area; superficial

27324 deep (subfascial or intramuscular)

(For needle biopsy of soft tissue, use 20206)

● **27325** Neurectomy, hamstring muscle

● **27326** Neurectomy, popliteal (gastrocnemius)

● New Code ▲ Revised Code + Add-On Code ⃠ Modifier -51 Exempt ⊙ Conscious Sedation

27327 Excision, tumor, thigh or knee area; subcutaneous

27328 deep, subfascial, or intramuscular

27329 Radical resection of tumor (eg, malignant neoplasm), soft tissue of thigh or knee area

27330 Arthrotomy, knee; with synovial biopsy only

27331 including joint exploration, biopsy, or removal of loose or foreign bodies

27332 Arthrotomy, with excision of semilunar cartilage (meniscectomy) knee; medial OR lateral

27333 medial AND lateral

27334 Arthrotomy, with synovectomy, knee; anterior OR posterior

27335 anterior AND posterior including popliteal area

27340 Excision, prepatellar bursa

27345 Excision of synovial cyst of popliteal space (eg, Baker's cyst)

27347 Excision of lesion of meniscus or capsule (eg, cyst, ganglion), knee

27350 Patellectomy or hemipatellectomy

27355 Excision or curettage of bone cyst or benign tumor of femur;

27356 with allograft

27357 with autograft (includes obtaining graft)

+ **27358** with internal fixation (List in addition to code for primary procedure)

(Use 27358 in conjunction with codes 27355, 27356 or 27357)

27360 Partial excision (craterization, saucerization, or diaphysectomy) bone, femur, proximal tibia and/or fibula (eg, osteomyelitis or bone abscess)

27365 Radical resection of tumor, bone, femur or knee

Separate Procedure | Unlisted Procedure | CCI Comp. Code | Non-specific Procedure

(For radical resection of tumor, soft tissue, use 27329)

INTRODUCTION OR REMOVAL

27370 Injection procedure for knee arthrography

(For radiological supervision and interpretation, use 73580. Do not report 77002 in conjunction with 73580)

27372 Removal of foreign body, deep, thigh region or knee area

(For removal of knee prosthesis including "total knee," use 27488)

(For surgical arthroscopic knee procedures, see 29870-29887)

REPAIR, REVISION, AND/OR RECONSTRUCTION

27380 Suture of infrapatellar tendon; primary

27381 secondary reconstruction, including fascial or tendon graft

27385 Suture of quadriceps or hamstring muscle rupture; primary

27386 secondary reconstruction, including fascial or tendon graft

27390 Tenotomy, open, hamstring, knee to hip; single tendon

27391 multiple tendons, one leg

27392 multiple tendons, bilateral

27393 Lengthening of hamstring tendon; single tendon

27394 multiple tendons, one leg

27395 multiple tendons, bilateral

27396 Transplant, hamstring tendon to patella; single tendon

27397 multiple tendons

27400 Transfer, tendon or muscle, hamstrings to femur (eg, Egger's type procedure)

27403 Arthrotomy with meniscus repair, knee

(For arthroscopic repair, use 29882)

27405 Repair, primary, torn ligament and/or capsule, knee; collateral

27407 cruciate

(For cruciate ligament reconstruction, use 27427)

27409 collateral and cruciate ligaments

(For ligament reconstruction, see 27427-27429)

27412 Autologous chondrocyte implantation, knee

(Do not report 27412 in conjunction with 20926, 27331, 27570)

(For harvesting of chondrocytes, use 29870)

27415 Osteochondral allograft, knee, open

(For arthroscopic implant of osteochondral allograft, use 29867)

27418 Anterior tibial tubercleplasty (eg, Maquet type procedure)

27420 Reconstruction of dislocating patella; (eg, Hauser type procedure)

27422 with extensor realignment and/or muscle advancement or release (eg, Campbell, Goldwaite type procedure)

27424 with patellectomy

27425 Lateral retinacular release open

(For arthroscopic lateral release, use 29873)

27427 Ligamentous reconstruction (augmentation), knee; extra-articular

27428 intra-articular (open)

27429 intra-articular (open) and extra-articular

(For primary repair of ligament(s) performed in addition to reconstruction, report 27405, 27407 or 27409 in addition to code 27427, 27428 or 27429)

27430 Quadricepsplasty (eg, Bennett or Thompson type)

27435 Capsulotomy, posterior capsular release, knee

27437 Arthroplasty, patella; without prosthesis

27438 with prosthesis

27440 Arthroplasty, knee, tibial plateau;

27441 with debridement and partial synovectomy

27442 Arthroplasty, femoral condyles or tibial plateau(s), knee;

27443 with debridement and partial synovectomy

27445 Arthroplasty, knee, hinge prosthesis (eg, Walldius type)

27446 Arthroplasty, knee, condyle and plateau; medial OR lateral compartment

27447 medial AND lateral compartments with or without patella resurfacing (total knee arthroplasty)

(For revision of total knee arthroplasty, use 27487)

(For removal of total knee prosthesis, use 27488)

27448 Osteotomy, femur, shaft or supracondylar; without fixation

(To report bilateral procedures, report 27448 with modifier -50)

27450 with fixation

(To report bilateral procedures, report 27450 with modifier -50)

27454 Osteotomy, multiple, with realignment on intramedullary rod, femoral shaft (eg, Sofield type procedure)

27455 Osteotomy, proximal tibia, including fibular excision or osteotomy (includes correction of genu varus (bowleg) or genu valgus (knock-knee)); before epiphyseal closure

(To report bilateral procedures, report 27455 with modifier -50)

27457 after epiphyseal closure

(To report bilateral procedures, report 27457 with modifier -50)

27465 Osteoplasty, femur; shortening (excluding 64876)

27466 lengthening

27468 combined, lengthening and shortening with femoral segment transfer

27470 Repair, nonunion or malunion, femur, distal to head and neck; without graft (eg, compression technique)

27472 with iliac or other autogenous bone graft (includes obtaining graft)

27475 Arrest, epiphyseal, any method (eg, epiphysiodesis); distal femur

27477 tibia and fibula, proximal

27479 combined distal femur, proximal tibia and fibula

27485 Arrest, hemiepiphyseal, distal femur or proximal tibia or fibula (eg, genu varus or valgus)

27486 Revision of total knee arthroplasty, with or without allograft; one component

27487 femoral and entire tibial component

27488 Removal of prosthesis, including total knee prosthesis, methylmethacrylate with or without insertion of spacer, knee

27495 Prophylactic treatment (nailing, pinning, plating or wiring) with or without methylmethacrylate, femur

27496 Decompression fasciotomy, thigh and/or knee, one compartment (flexor or extensor or adductor);

27497 with debridement of nonviable muscle and/or nerve

27498 Decompression fasciotomy, thigh and/or knee, multiple compartments;

27499 with debridement of nonviable muscle and/or nerve

FRACTURE AND/OR DISLOCATION

(For arthroscopic treatment of intercondylar spine(s) and tuberosity fracture(s) of the knee, see 29850, 29851)

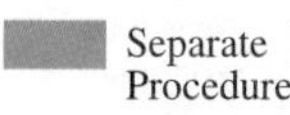
Separate Procedure
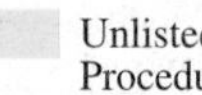
Unlisted Procedure
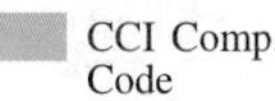
CCI Comp. Code
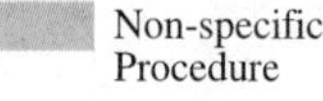
Non-specific Procedure

(For arthroscopic treatment of tibial fracture, see 29855, 29856)

27500 Closed treatment of femoral shaft fracture, without manipulation

27501 Closed treatment of supracondylar or transcondylar femoral fracture with or without intercondylar extension, without manipulation

27502 Closed treatment of femoral shaft fracture, with manipulation, with or without skin or skeletal traction

27503 Closed treatment of supracondylar or transcondylar femoral fracture with or without intercondylar extension, with manipulation, with or without skin or skeletal traction

27506 Open treatment of femoral shaft fracture, with or without external fixation, with insertion of intramedullary implant, with or without cerclage and/or locking screws

27507 Open treatment of femoral shaft fracture with plate/screws, with or without cerclage

27508 Closed treatment of femoral fracture, distal end, medial or lateral condyle, without manipulation

27509 Percutaneous skeletal fixation of femoral fracture, distal end, medial or lateral condyle, or supracondylar or transcondylar, with or without intercondylar extension, or distal femoral epiphyseal separation

27510 Closed treatment of femoral fracture, distal end, medial or lateral condyle, with manipulation

27511 Open treatment of femoral supracondylar or transcondylar fracture without intercondylar extension, with or without internal or external fixation

27513 Open treatment of femoral supracondylar or transcondylar fracture with intercondylar extension, with or without internal or external fixation

27514 Open treatment of femoral fracture, distal end, medial or lateral condyle, with or without internal or external fixation

27516 Closed treatment of distal femoral epiphyseal separation; without manipulation

● New Code 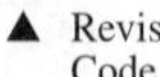 ▲ Revised Code + Add-On Code ⊘ Modifier -51 Exempt ⊙ Conscious Sedation

27517 with manipulation, with or without skin or skeletal traction

27519 Open treatment of distal femoral epiphyseal separation, with or without internal or external fixation

27520 Closed treatment of patellar fracture, without manipulation

27524 Open treatment of patellar fracture, with internal fixation and/or partial or complete patellectomy and soft tissue repair

27530 Closed treatment of tibial fracture, proximal (plateau); without manipulation

27532 with or without manipulation, with skeletal traction

(For arthroscopic treatment, see 29855, 29856)

27535 Open treatment of tibial fracture, proximal (plateau); unicondylar, with or without internal or external fixation

27536 bicondylar, with or without internal fixation

(For arthroscopic treatment, see 29855, 29856)

27538 Closed treatment of intercondylar spine(s) and/or tuberosity fracture(s) of knee, with or without manipulation

(For arthroscopic treatment, see 29850, 29851)

27540 Open treatment of intercondylar spine(s) and/or tuberosity fracture(s) of the knee, with or without internal or external fixation

27550 Closed treatment of knee dislocation; without anesthesia

27552 requiring anesthesia

27556 Open treatment of knee dislocation, with or without internal or external fixation; without primary ligamentous repair or augmentation/reconstruction

27557 with primary ligamentous repair

27558 with primary ligamentous repair, with augmentation/ reconstruction

27560 Closed treatment of patellar dislocation; without anesthesia

Separate Procedure | Unlisted Procedure | CCI Comp. Code | Non-specific Procedure

(For recurrent dislocation, see 27420-27424)

27562 requiring anesthesia

27566 Open treatment of patellar dislocation, with or without partial or total patellectomy

MANIPULATION

27570 Manipulation of knee joint under general anesthesia (includes application of traction or other fixation devices)

ARTHRODESIS

27580 Arthrodesis, knee, any technique

AMPUTATION

27590 Amputation, thigh, through femur, any level;

27591 immediate fitting technique including first cast

27592 open, circular (guillotine)

27594 secondary closure or scar revision

27596 re-amputation

27598 Disarticulation at knee

OTHER PROCEDURES

27599 Unlisted procedure, femur or knee

LEG (TIBIA AND FIBULA) AND ANKLE JOINT

INCISION

27600 Decompression fasciotomy, leg; anterior and/or lateral compartments only

27601 posterior compartment(s) only

27602 anterior and/or lateral, and posterior compartment(s)

(For incision and drainage procedures, superficial, see 10040-10160)

● New Code ▲ Revised Code + Add-On Code ⃠ Modifier -51 Exempt ⊙ Conscious Sedation

(For decompression fasciotomy with debridement, see 27892-27894)

27603 Incision and drainage, leg or ankle; deep abscess or hematoma

27604 infected bursa

27605 Tenotomy, percutaneous, Achilles tendon (separate procedure); local anesthesia

27606 general anesthesia

27607 Incision (eg, osteomyelitis or bone abscess), leg or ankle

27610 Arthrotomy, ankle, including exploration, drainage, or removal of foreign body

27612 Arthrotomy, posterior capsular release, ankle, with or without Achilles tendon lengthening

(See also 27685)

EXCISION

27613 Biopsy, soft tissue of leg or ankle area; superficial

27614 deep (subfascial or intramuscular)

(For needle biopsy of soft tissue, use 20206)

27615 Radical resection of tumor (eg, malignant neoplasm), soft tissue of leg or ankle area

27618 Excision, tumor, leg or ankle area; subcutaneous tissue

27619 deep (subfascial or intramuscular)

27620 Arthrotomy, ankle, with joint exploration, with or without biopsy, with or without removal of loose or foreign body

27625 Arthrotomy, with synovectomy, ankle;

27626 including tenosynovectomy

27630 Excision of lesion of tendon sheath or capsule (eg, cyst or ganglion), leg and/or ankle

27635 Excision or curettage of bone cyst or benign tumor, tibia or fibula;

27637 with autograft (includes obtaining graft)

27638 with allograft

27640 Partial excision (craterization, saucerization, or diaphysectomy) bone (eg, osteomyelitis or exostosis); tibia

27641 fibula

27645 Radical resection of tumor, bone; tibia

27646 fibula

27647 talus or calcaneus

INTRODUCTION OR REMOVAL

27648 Injection procedure for ankle arthrography

(For radiological supervision and interpretation use 73615. Do not report 77002 in addition to 73615)

(For ankle arthroscopy, see 29894-29898)

REPAIR, REVISION, AND/OR RECONSTRUCTION

27650 Repair, primary, open or percutaneous, ruptured Achilles tendon;

27652 with graft (includes obtaining graft)

27654 Repair, secondary, Achilles tendon, with or without graft

27656 Repair, fascial defect of leg

27658 Repair, flexor tendon, leg; primary, without graft, each tendon

27659 secondary, with or without graft, each tendon

27664 Repair, extensor tendon, leg; primary, without graft, each tendon

27665 secondary, with or without graft, each tendon

27675 Repair, dislocating peroneal tendons; without fibular osteotomy

27676 with fibular osteotomy

27680 Tenolysis, flexor or extensor tendon, leg and/or ankle; single, each tendon

27681 multiple tendons (through separate incision(s))

27685 Lengthening or shortening of tendon, leg or ankle; single tendon (separate procedure)

27686 multiple tendons (through same incision), each

27687 Gastrocnemius recession (eg, Strayer procedure)

(Toe extensors are considered as a group to be single tendon when transplanted into midfoot)

27690 Transfer or transplant of single tendon (with muscle redirection or rerouting); superficial (eg, anterior tibial extensors into midfoot)

27691 deep (eg, anterior tibial or posterior tibial through interosseous space, flexor digitorum longus, flexor hallucis longus, or peroneal tendon to midfoot or hind foot)

+ **27692** each additional tendon (List separately in addition to code for primary procedure)

(Use 27692 in conjunction with codes 27690, 27691)

27695 Repair, primary, disrupted ligament, ankle; collateral

27696 both collateral ligaments

27698 Repair, secondary disrupted ligament, ankle, collateral (eg, Watson-Jones procedure)

27700 Arthroplasty, ankle;

27702 with implant (total ankle)

27703 revision, total ankle

27704 Removal of ankle implant

27705 Osteotomy; tibia

27707 fibula

27709 tibia and fibula

27712 multiple, with realignment on intramedullary rod (eg, Sofield type procedure)

(For osteotomy to correct genu varus (bowleg) or genu valgus (knock-knee), see 27455-27457)

27715 Osteoplasty, tibia and fibula, lengthening or shortening

27720 Repair of nonunion or malunion, tibia; without graft, (eg, compression technique)

27722 with sliding graft

27724 with iliac or other autograft (includes obtaining graft)

27725 by synostosis, with fibula, any method

27727 Repair of congenital pseudarthrosis, tibia

27730 Arrest, epiphyseal (epiphysiodesis), open; distal tibia

27732 distal fibula

27734 distal tibia and fibula

27740 Arrest, epiphyseal (epiphysiodesis), any method, combined, proximal and distal tibia and fibula;

27742 and distal femur

(For epiphyseal arrest of proximal tibia and fibula, use 27477)

27745 Prophylactic treatment (nailing, pinning, plating or wiring) with or without methylmethacrylate, tibia

FRACTURE AND/OR DISLOCATION

27750 Closed treatment of tibial shaft fracture (with or without fibular fracture); without manipulation

27752 with manipulation, with or without skeletal traction

27756 Percutaneous skeletal fixation of tibial shaft fracture (with or without fibular fracture) (eg, pins or screws)

27758 Open treatment of tibial shaft fracture, (with or without fibular fracture) with plate/screws, with or without cerclage

27759 Treatment of tibial shaft fracture (with or without fibular fracture) by intramedullary implant, with or without interlocking screws and/or cerclage

27760 Closed treatment of medial malleolus fracture; without manipulation

27762 with manipulation, with or without skin or skeletal traction

27766 Open treatment of medial malleolus fracture, with or without internal or external fixation

27780 Closed treatment of proximal fibula or shaft fracture; without manipulation

27781 with manipulation

27784 Open treatment of proximal fibula or shaft fracture, with or without internal or external fixation

27786 Closed treatment of distal fibular fracture (lateral malleolus); without manipulation

27788 with manipulation

27792 Open treatment of distal fibular fracture (lateral malleolus), with or without internal or external fixation

(For treatment of tibia and fibula shaft fractures, see 27750-27759)

27808 Closed treatment of bimalleolar ankle fracture, (including Potts); without manipulation

27810 with manipulation

27814 Open treatment of bimalleolar ankle fracture, with or without internal or external fixation

27816 Closed treatment of trimalleolar ankle fracture; without manipulation

27818 with manipulation

27822 Open treatment of trimalleolar ankle fracture, with or without internal or external fixation, medial and/or lateral malleolus; without fixation of posterior lip

27823 with fixation of posterior lip

27824 Closed treatment of fracture of weight bearing articular portion of distal tibia (eg, pilon or tibial plafond), with or without anesthesia; without manipulation

27825 with skeletal traction and/or requiring manipulation

27826 Open treatment of fracture of weight bearing articular surface/portion of distal tibia (eg, pilon or tibial plafond), with internal or external fixation; of fibula only

27827 of tibia only

27828 of both tibia and fibula

27829 Open treatment of distal tibiofibular joint (syndesmosis) disruption, with or without internal or external fixation

27830 Closed treatment of proximal tibiofibular joint dislocation; without anesthesia

27831 requiring anesthesia

27832 Open treatment of proximal tibiofibular joint dislocation, with or without internal or external fixation, or with excision of proximal fibula

27840 Closed treatment of ankle dislocation; without anesthesia

27842 requiring anesthesia, with or without percutaneous skeletal fixation

27846 Open treatment of ankle dislocation, with or without percutaneous skeletal fixation; without repair or internal fixation

27848 with repair or internal or external fixation

(For surgical diagnostic arthroscopic procedures, see 29894-29898)

● New Code ▲ Revised Code + Add-On Code ⊘ Modifier -51 Exempt ⊙ Conscious Sedation

MANIPULATION

27860 Manipulation of ankle under general anesthesia (includes application of traction or other fixation apparatus)

ARTHRODESIS

27870 Arthrodesis, ankle, open

(For arthroscopic ankle arthrodesis, use 29899)

27871 Arthrodesis, tibiofibular joint, proximal or distal

AMPUTATION

27880 Amputation, leg, through tibia and fibula;

27881 with immediate fitting technique including application of first cast

27882 open, circular (guillotine)

27884 secondary closure or scar revision

27886 re-amputation

27888 Amputation, ankle, through malleoli of tibia and fibula (eg, Syme, Pirogoff type procedures), with plastic closure and resection of nerves

27889 Ankle disarticulation

OTHER PROCEDURES

27892 Decompression fasciotomy, leg; anterior and/or lateral compartments only, with debridement of nonviable muscle and/or nerve

(For decompression fasciotomy of the leg without debridement, use 27600)

27893 posterior compartment(s) only, with debridement of nonviable muscle and/or nerve

(For decompession fasciotomy of the leg without debridement, use 27601)

27894 anterior and/or lateral, and posterior compartment(s), with debridement of nonviable muscle and/or nerve

(For decompression fasciotomy of the leg without debridement, use 27602)

27899 Unlisted procedure, leg or ankle

FOOT AND TOES

INCISION

(For incision and drainage procedures, superficial, see 10040-10160)

28001 Incision and drainage, bursa, foot

28002 Incision and drainage below fascia, with or without tendon sheath involvement, foot; single bursal space

28003 multiple areas

28005 Incision, bone cortex (eg, osteomyelitis or bone abscess), foot

28008 Fasciotomy, foot and/or toe

(See also 28060, 28062, 28250)

28010 Tenotomy, percutaneous, toe; single tendon

28011 multiple tendons

(For open tenotomy, see 28230-28234)

28020 Arthrotomy, including exploration, drainage, or removal of loose or foreign body; intertarsal or tarsometatarsal joint

28022 metatarsophalangeal joint

28024 interphalangeal joint

(28030 deleted 2007 edition, see 28055)

28035 Release, tarsal tunnel (posterior tibial nerve decompression)

(For other nerve entrapments, see 64704, 64722)

● New Code ▲ Revised Code + Add-On Code ⃠ Modifier -51 Exempt ⊙ Conscious Sedation

EXCISION

28043 Excision, tumor, foot; subcutaneous tissue

28045 deep, subfascial, intramuscular

28046 Radical resection of tumor (eg, malignant neoplasm), soft tissue of foot

28050 Arthrotomy with biopsy; intertarsal or tarsometatarsal joint

28052 metatarsophalangeal joint

28054 interphalangeal joint

● **28055** Neurectomy, intrinsic musculature of foot

28060 Fasciectomy, plantar fascia; partial (separate procedure)

28062 radical (separate procedure)

(For plantar fasciotomy, see 28008, 28250)

28070 Synovectomy; intertarsal or tarsometatarsal joint, each

28072 metatarsophalangeal joint, each

28080 Excision, interdigital (Morton) neuroma, single, each

28086 Synovectomy, tendon sheath, foot; flexor

28088 extensor

28090 Excision of lesion, tendon, tendon sheath, or capsule (including synovectomy) (eg, cyst or ganglion); foot

28092 toe(s), each

28100 Excision or curettage of bone cyst or benign tumor, talus or calcaneus;

28102 with iliac or other autograft (includes obtaining graft)

28103 with allograft

Separate Procedure | Unlisted Procedure | CCI Comp. Code | Non-specific Procedure

28104 Excision or curettage of bone cyst or benign tumor, tarsal or metatarsal, except talus or calcaneus;

28106 with iliac or other autograft (includes obtaining graft)

28107 with allograft

28108 Excision or curettage of bone cyst or benign tumor, phalanges of foot

(For ostectomy, partial (eg, hallux valgus, Silver type procedure), use 28290)

28110 Ostectomy, partial excision, fifth metatarsal head (bunionette) (separate procedure)

28111 Ostectomy, complete excision; first metatarsal head

28112 other metatarsal head (second, third or fourth)

28113 fifth metatarsal head

28114 all metatarsal heads, with partial proximal phalangectomy, excluding first metatarsal (eg, Clayton type procedure)

28116 Ostectomy, excision of tarsal coalition

28118 Ostectomy, calcaneus;

28119 for spur, with or without plantar fascial release

28120 Partial excision (craterization, saucerization, sequestrectomy, or diaphysectomy) bone (eg, osteomyelitis or bossing); talus or calcaneus

28122 tarsal or metatarsal bone, except talus or calcaneus

(For partial excision of talus or calcaneus, use 28120)

(For cheilectomy for hallux rigidus, use 28289)

28124 phalanx of toe

28126 Resection, partial or complete, phalangeal base, each toe

28130 Talectomy (astragalectomy)

● New Code ▲ Revised Code + Add-On Code ⊘ Modifier -51 Exempt ⊙ Conscious Sedation

(For calcanectomy, use 28118)

28140 Metatarsectomy

28150 Phalangectomy, toe, each toe

28153 Resection, condyle(s), distal end of phalanx, each toe

28160 Hemiphalangectomy or interphalangeal joint excision, toe, proximal end of phalanx, each

28171 Radical resection of tumor, bone; tarsal (except talus or calcaneus)

28173 metatarsal

28175 phalanx of toe

(For talus or calcaneus, use 27647)

INTRODUCTION OR REMOVAL

28190 Removal of foreign body, foot; subcutaneous

28192 deep

28193 complicated

REPAIR, REVISION, AND/OR RECONSTRUCTION

28200 Repair, tendon, flexor, foot; primary or secondary, without free graft, each tendon

28202 secondary with free graft, each tendon (includes obtaining graft)

28208 Repair, tendon, extensor, foot; primary or secondary, each tendon

28210 secondary with free graft, each tendon (includes obtaining graft)

28220 Tenolysis, flexor, foot; single tendon

28222 multiple tendons

28225 Tenolysis, extensor, foot; single tendon

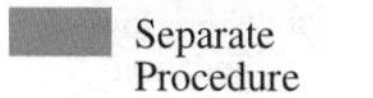
Separate Procedure
Unlisted Procedure
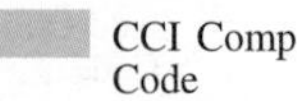
CCI Comp. Code
Non-specific Procedure

28226 multiple tendons

28230 Tenotomy, open, tendon flexor; foot, single or multiple tendon(s) (separate procedure)

28232 toe, single tendon (separate procedure)

28234 Tenotomy, open, extensor, foot or toe, each tendon

(For tendon transfer to midfoot or hindfoot, see 27690, 27691)

28238 Reconstruction (advancement), posterior tibial tendon with excision of accessory tarsal navicular bone (eg, Kidner type procedure)

(For subcutaneous tenotomy, see 28010, 28011)

(For transfer or transplant of tendon with muscle redirection or rerouting, see 27690-27692)

(For extensor hallucis longus transfer with great toe IP fusion (Jones procedure), use 28760)

28240 Tenotomy, lengthening, or release, abductor hallucis muscle

28250 Division of plantar fascia and muscle (eg, Steindler stripping) (separate procedure)

28260 Capsulotomy, midfoot; medial release only (separate procedure)

28261 with tendon lengthening

28262 extensive, including posterior talotibial capsulotomy and tendon(s) lengthening (eg, resistant clubfoot deformity)

28264 Capsulotomy, midtarsal (eg, Heyman type procedure)

28270 Capsulotomy; metatarsophalangeal joint, with or without tenorrhaphy, each joint (separate procedure)

28272 interphalangeal joint, each joint (separate procedure)

28280 Syndactylization, toes (eg, webbing or Kelikian type procedure)

28285 Correction, hammertoe (eg, interphalangeal fusion, partial or total phalangectomy)

● New Code ▲ Revised Code + Add-On Code ⊘ Modifier -51 Exempt ⊙ Conscious Sedation

28286 Correction, cock-up fifth toe, with plastic skin closure (eg, Ruiz-Mora type procedure)

28288 Ostectomy, partial, exostectomy or condylectomy, metatarsal head, each metatarsal head

28289 Hallux rigidus correction with cheilectomy, debridement and capsular release of the first metatarsophalangeal joint

28290 Correction, hallux valgus (bunion), with or without sesamoidectomy; simple exostectomy (eg, Silver type procedure)

28292 Keller, McBride, or Mayo type procedure

28293 resection of joint with implant

28294 with tendon transplants (eg, Joplin type procedure)

28296 with metatarsal osteotomy (eg, Mitchell, Chevron, or concentric type procedures)

28297 Lapidus type procedure

28298 by phalanx osteotomy

28299 by double osteotomy

28300 Osteotomy; calcaneus (eg, Dwyer or Chambers type procedure), with or without internal fixation

28302 talus

28304 Osteotomy, tarsal bones, other than calcaneus or talus;

28305 with autograft (includes obtaining graft) (eg, Fowler type)

28306 Osteotomy, with or without lengthening, shortening or angular correction, metatarsal; first metatarsal

28307 first metatarsal with autograft (other than first toe)

28308 other than first metatarsal, each

28309 multiple (eg, Swanson type cavus foot procedure)

Separate Procedure | Unlisted Procedure | 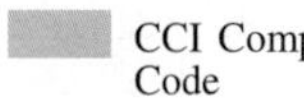 CCI Comp. Code | Non-specific Procedure

28310 Osteotomy, shortening, angular or rotational correction; proximal phalanx, first toe (separate procedure)

28312 other phalanges, any toe

28313 Reconstruction, angular deformity of toe, soft tissue procedures only (eg, overlapping second toe, fifth toe, curly toes)

28315 Sesamoidectomy, first toe (separate procedure)

28320 Repair, nonunion or malunion; tarsal bones

28322 metatarsal, with or without bone graft (includes obtaining graft)

28340 Reconstruction, toe, macrodactyly; soft tissue resection

28341 requiring bone resection

28344 Reconstruction, toe(s); polydactyly

28345 syndactyly, with or without skin graft(s), each web

28360 Reconstruction, cleft foot

FRACTURE AND/OR DISLOCATION

28400 Closed treatment of calcaneal fracture; without manipulation

28405 with manipulation

28406 Percutaneous skeletal fixation of calcaneal fracture, with manipulation

28415 Open treatment of calcaneal fracture, with or without internal or external fixation;

28420 with primary iliac or other autogenous bone graft (includes obtaining graft)

28430 Closed treatment of talus fracture; without manipulation

28435 with manipulation

28436 Percutaneous skeletal fixation of talus fracture, with manipulation

● New Code ▲ Revised Code + Add-On Code ⦸ Modifier -51 Exempt ⊙ Conscious Sedation

28445 Open treatment of talus fracture, with or without internal or external fixation

28450 Treatment of tarsal bone fracture (except talus and calcaneus); without manipulation, each

28455 with manipulation, each

28456 Percutaneous skeletal fixation of tarsal bone fracture (except talus and calcaneus), with manipulation, each

28465 Open treatment of tarsal bone fracture (except talus and calcaneus), with or without internal or external fixation, each

28470 Closed treatment of metatarsal fracture; without manipulation, each

28475 with manipulation, each

28476 Percutaneous skeletal fixation of metatarsal fracture, with manipulation, each

28485 Open treatment of metatarsal fracture, with or without internal or external fixation, each

28490 Closed treatment of fracture great toe, phalanx or phalanges; without manipulation

28495 with manipulation

28496 Percutaneous skeletal fixation of fracture great toe, phalanx or phalanges, with manipulation

28505 Open treatment of fracture great toe, phalanx or phalanges, with or without internal or external fixation

28510 Closed treatment of fracture, phalanx or phalanges, other than great toe; without manipulation, each

28515 with manipulation, each

28525 Open treatment of fracture, phalanx or phalanges, other than great toe, with or without internal or external fixation, each

28530 Closed treatment of sesamoid fracture

28531 Open treatment of sesamoid fracture, with or without internal fixation

28540 Closed treatment of tarsal bone dislocation, other than talotarsal; without anesthesia

28545 requiring anesthesia

28546 Percutaneous skeletal fixation of tarsal bone dislocation, other than talotarsal, with manipulation

28555 Open treatment of tarsal bone dislocation, with or without internal or external fixation

28570 Closed treatment of talotarsal joint dislocation; without anesthesia

28575 requiring anesthesia

28576 Percutaneous skeletal fixation of talotarsal joint dislocation, with manipulation

28585 Open treatment of talotarsal joint dislocation, with or without internal or external fixation

28600 Closed treatment of tarsometatarsal joint dislocation; without anesthesia

28605 requiring anesthesia

28606 Percutaneous skeletal fixation of tarsometatarsal joint dislocation, with manipulation

28615 Open treatment of tarsometatarsal joint dislocation, with or without internal or external fixation

28630 Closed treatment of metatarsophalangeal joint dislocation; without anesthesia

28635 requiring anesthesia

28636 Percutaneous skeletal fixation of metatarsophalangeal joint dislocation, with manipulation

28645 Open treatment of metatarsophalangeal joint dislocation, with or without internal or external fixation

28660 Closed treatment of interphalangeal joint dislocation; without anesthesia

28665 requiring anesthesia

28666 Percutaneous skeletal fixation of interphalangeal joint dislocation, with manipulation

28675 Open treatment of interphalangeal joint dislocation, with or without internal or external fixation

ARTHRODESIS

28705 Arthrodesis; pantalar

28715 triple

28725 subtalar

28730 Arthrodesis, midtarsal or tarsometatarsal, multiple or transverse;

28735 with osteotomy (eg, flatfoot correction)

28737 Arthrodesis, with tendon lengthening and advancement, midtarsal, tarsal navicular-cuneiform (eg, Miller type procedure)

28740 Arthrodesis, midtarsal or tarsometatarsal, single joint

28750 Arthrodesis, great toe; metatarsophalangeal joint

28755 interphalangeal joint

28760 Arthrodesis, with extensor hallucis longus transfer to first metatarsal neck, great toe, interphalangeal joint (eg, Jones type procedure)

(For hammertoe operation or interphalangeal fusion, use 28285)

AMPUTATION

28800 Amputation, foot; midtarsal (eg, Chopart type procedure)

28805 transmetatarsal

28810 Amputation, metatarsal, with toe, single

Separate Procedure | Unlisted Procedure | CCI Comp. Code | Non-specific Procedure

28820 Amputation, toe; metatarsophalangeal joint

28825 interphalangeal joint

(For amputation of tuft of distal phalanx, use 11752)

OTHER PROCEDURES

28890 Extracorporeal shock wave, high energy, performed by a physician, requiring anesthesia other than local, including ultrasound guidance, involving the plantar fascia

(For extracorporeal shock wave therapy involving musculoskeletal system, not otherwise specified, see Category III codes 0019T, 0101T, 0102T)

28899 Unlisted procedure, foot or toes

APPLICATION OF CASTS AND STRAPPING

CPT codes in this section are used only when the cast application or strapping is a replacement procedure performed during or after the period of follow-up care. An additional evaluation and management service code, dependent on location, is reportable only if significant identifiable other services are provided at the time of the cast application or strapping.

For coding cast or strap application in situations not involving surgery, for example, casting of a sprained ankle or knee, use the appropriate level of evaluation and management services code plus code 99070 or equivalent HCPCS Level II code to report casting materials.

(For orthotics management and training, see 97760-97762)

BODY AND UPPER EXTREMITY

Casts

29000 Application of halo type body cast (see 20661-20663 for insertion)

29010 Application of Risser jacket, localizer, body; only

29015 including head

29020 Application of turnbuckle jacket, body; only

29025 including head

29035 Application of body cast, shoulder to hips;

29040 including head, Minerva type

29044 including one thigh

29046 including both thighs

29049 Application, cast; figure-of-eight

29055 shoulder spica

29058 plaster Velpeau

29065 shoulder to hand (long arm)

29075 elbow to finger (short arm)

29085 hand and lower forearm (gauntlet)

29086 finger (eg, contracture)

Splints

29105 Application of long arm splint (shoulder to hand)

29125 Application of short arm splint (forearm to hand); static

29126 dynamic

29130 Application of finger splint; static

29131 dynamic

Strapping - Any Age

29200 Strapping; thorax

29220 low back

29240 shoulder (eg, Velpeau)

29260 elbow or wrist

29280 hand or finger

LOWER EXTREMITY

Casts

29305 Application of hip spica cast; one leg

29325 one and one-half spica or both legs

(For hip spica (body) cast, including thighs only, use 29046)

29345 Application of long leg cast (thigh to toes);

29355 walker or ambulatory type

29358 Application of long leg cast brace

29365 Application of cylinder cast (thigh to ankle)

29405 Application of short leg cast (below knee to toes);

29425 walking or ambulatory type

29435 Application of patellar tendon bearing (PTB) cast

29440 Adding walker to previously applied cast

29445 Application of rigid total contact leg cast

29450 Application of clubfoot cast with molding or manipulation, long or short leg

(To report bilateral procedures, use 29450 with modifier -50)

Splints

29505 Application of long leg splint (thigh to ankle or toes)

29515 Application of short leg splint (calf to foot)

Strapping - Any Age

29520 Strapping; hip

29530 knee

29540 ankle and/or foot

29550 toes

29580 Unna boot

29590 Denis-Browne splint strapping

REMOVAL OR REPAIR

29700 Removal or bivalving; gauntlet, boot or body cast

29705 full arm or full leg cast

29710 shoulder or hip spica, Minerva, or Risser jacket, etc.

29715 turnbuckle jacket

29720 Repair of spica, body cast or jacket

29730 Windowing of cast

29740 Wedging of cast (except clubfoot casts)

29750 Wedging of clubfoot cast

(To report bilateral procedures, use 29750 with modifier -50)

OTHER PROCEDURES

29799 Unlisted procedure, casting or strapping

ENDOSCOPY/ARTHROSCOPY

Surgical endoscopy/arthroscopy always includes a diagnostic endoscopy/ arthroscopy and is therefore never reported in addition to the surgical procedure. However, there are several arthroscopy procedures defined as separate procedures, indicating that the codes may be reported if the diagnostic arthroscopy is the only procedure performed.

When arthroscopy is performed in conjunction with arthrotomy, add modifier -51.

29800 Arthroscopy, temporomandibular joint, diagnostic, with or without synovial biopsy (separate procedure)

29804 Arthroscopy, temporomandibular joint, surgical

(For open procedure, use 21010)

29805 Arthroscopy, shoulder, diagnostic, with or without synovial biopsy (separate procedure)

(For open procedure, see 23065-23066, 23100-23101)

29806 Arthroscopy, shoulder, surgical; capsulorrhaphy

(For open procedure, see 23450-23466)

(To report thermal capsulorrhaphy, use 29999)

29807 repair of slap lesion

29819 with removal of loose body or foreign body

(For open procedure, see 23040-23044, 23107)

29820 synovectomy, partial

(For open procedure, see 23105)

29821 synovectomy, complete

(For open procedure, see 23105)

29822 debridement, limited

(For open procedure, see specific open shoulder procedure performed)

29823 debridement, extensive

(For open procedure, see specific open shoulder procedure performed)

29824 distal claviculectomy including distal articular surface (Mumford procedure)

(For open procedure, use 23120)

29825 with lysis and resection of adhesions, with or without manipulation

(For open procedure, see specific open shoulder procedure performed)

29826 decompression of subacromial space with partial acromioplasty, with or without coracoacromial release

(For open procedure, use 23130 or 23415)

29827 with rotator cuff repair

(For open or mini-open rotator cuff repair, use 23412)

(When arthroscopic subacromial decompression is performed at the same setting, use 29826 and append modifier '-51')

(When arthroscopic distal clavicle resection is performed at the same setting, use 29824 and append modifier '-51')

29830 Arthroscopy, elbow, diagnostic, with or without synovial biopsy (separate procedure)

29834 Arthroscopy, elbow, surgical; with removal of loose body or foreign body

29835 synovectomy, partial

29836 synovectomy, complete

29837 debridement, limited

29838 debridement, extensive

29840 Arthroscopy, wrist, diagnostic, with or without synovial biopsy (separate procedure)

29843 Arthroscopy, wrist, surgical; for infection, lavage and drainage

29844 synovectomy, partial

29845 synovectomy, complete

29846 excision and/or repair of triangular fibrocartilage and/or joint debridement

29847 internal fixation for fracture or instability

29848 Endoscopy, wrist, surgical, with release of transverse carpal ligament

(For open procedure, use 64721)

29850 Arthroscopically aided treatment of intercondylar spine(s) and/or tuberosity fracture(s) of the knee, with or without manipulation; without internal or external fixation (includes arthroscopy)

Separate Procedure | Unlisted Procedure | CCI Comp. Code | Non-specific Procedure

29851 with internal or external fixation (includes arthroscopy)

(For bone graft, use 20900, 20902)

29855 Arthroscopically aided treatment of tibial fracture, proximal (plateau); nicondylar, with or without internal or external fixation (includes arthroscopy)

29856 bicondylar, with or without internal or external fixation (includes arthroscopy)

(For bone graft, use 20900, 20902)

29860 Arthroscopy, hip, diagnostic with or without synovial biopsy (separate procedure)

29861 Arthroscopy, hip, surgical; with removal of loose body or foreign body

29862 with debridement/shaving of articular cartilage (chondroplasty), abrasion arthroplasty, and/or resection of labrum

29863 with synovectomy

29866 Arthroscopy, knee, surgical; osteochondral autograft(s) (eg, mosaicplasty) (includes harvesting of the autograft)

(Do not report 29866 in conjunction with 29870, 29871, 29875, 29884 when performed at the same session and/or 29874, 29877, 29879, 29885-29887 when performed in the same compartment)

29867 osteochondral allograft (eg, mosaicplasty)

(Do not report 29867 in conjunction with 27570, 29870, 29871, 29875, 29884 when performed at the same session and/or 29874, 29877, 29879, 29885-29887 when performed in the same compartment)

(Do not report 29867 in conjunction with 27415)

29868 meniscal transplantation (includes arthrotomy for meniscal insertion), medial or lateral

(Do not report 29868 in conjunction with 29870, 29871, 29875, 29880, 29883, 29884 when performed at the same session or 29874, 29877, 29881, 29882 when performed in the same compartment)

29870 Arthroscopy, knee, diagnostic, with or without synovial biopsy (separate procedure)

(For open autologous chondrocyte implantation of the knee, use 27412)

29871 Arthroscopy, knee, surgical; for infection, lavage and drainage

(For implantation of osteochondral graft for treatment of articular surface defect, see 27412, 27415, 29866, 29867)

29873 with lateral release

(For open lateral release, use 27425)

29874 for removal of loose body or foreign body (eg, osteochondritis dissecans fragmentation, chondral fragmentation)

29875 synovectomy, limited (eg, plica or shelf resection) (separate procedure)

29876 synovectomy, major, two or more compartments (eg, medial or lateral)

29877 debridement/shaving of articular cartilage (chondroplasty)

29879 abrasion arthroplasty (includes chondroplasty where necessary) or multiple drilling or microfracture

29880 with meniscectomy (medial AND lateral, including any meniscal shaving)

29881 with meniscectomy (medial OR lateral, including any meniscal shaving)

29882 with meniscus repair (medial OR lateral)

29883 with meniscus repair (medial AND lateral)

(For meniscal transplantation, medial or lateral, knee, use 29868)

29884 with lysis of adhesions, with or without manipulation (separate procedure)

Separate Procedure 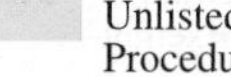 Unlisted Procedure 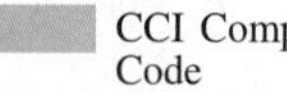 CCI Comp. Code 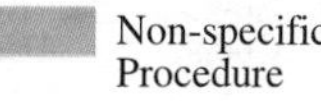 Non-specific Procedure

29885 drilling for osteochondritis dissecans with bone grafting, with or without internal fixation (including debridement of base of lesion)

29886 drilling for intact osteochondritis dissecans lesion

29887 drilling for intact osteochondritis dissecans lesion with internal fixation

29888 Arthroscopically aided anterior cruciate ligament repair/augmentation or reconstruction

29889 Arthroscopically aided posterior cruciate ligament repair/augmentation or reconstruction

(Procedures 29888 and 29889 should not be used with reconstruction procedures 27427-27429)

29891 Arthroscopy, ankle, surgical, excision of osteochondral defect of talus and/or tibia, including drilling of the defect

29892 Arthroscopically aided repair of large osteochondritis dissecans lesion, talar dome fracture, or tibial plafond fracture, with or without internal fixation (includes arthroscopy)

29893 Endoscopic plantar fasciotomy

29894 Arthroscopy, ankle (tibiotalar and fibulotalar joints), surgical; with removal of loose body or foreign body

29895 synovectomy, partial

29897 debridement, limited

29898 debridement, extensive

29899 with ankle arthrodesis

(For open ankle arthrodesis, use 27870)

29900 Arthroscopy, metacarpophalangeal joint, diagnostic, includes synovial biopsy

(Do not report 29900 with 29901, 29902)

29901 Arthroscopy, metacarpophalangeal joint, surgical; with debridement

● New Code ▲ Revised Code + Add-On Code ⃠ Modifier -51 Exempt ⊙ Conscious Sedation

29902 with reduction of displaced ulnar collateral ligament (eg, Stenar lesion)

29999 Unlisted procedure, arthroscopy

This page intentionally left blank.

RESPIRATORY SYSTEM

CPT codes from this section of the CPT coding system are used to report invasive and surgical procedures performed on the nose, sinuses, larynx, trachea and bronchi, and the lungs and pleura.

MISCELLANEOUS CODING RULES

Functional Endoscopic Sinus Surgery (FESS) codes are coded based on the procedures described in the operative report or on the nasal sinus endoscopy report. Each FESS code represents a unilateral procedure. To express that a procedure was performed bilaterally requires the application of the modifier -50, bilateral procedure.

Indirect laryngoscopy involves the visualization of the larynx using a warm laryngeal mirror positioned at the back of the throat. Direct laryngoscopy involves the visualization using a rigid or fiberoptic endoscope. Operative direct laryngoscopy involves an endoscopic examination under general anesthesia.

To code nasal hemorrhages appropriately, documentation needs to substantiate whether the hemorrhage is anterior or posterior and how the hemorrhage is controlled. Control of anterior nasal hemorrhage typically involves the insertion of gauze packing, or anterior packing or performance of cauterization. Control of posterior nasal hemorrhage most likely requires the insertion of nasal stents, tampons, balloon catheters, or posterior packing.

NOSE

INCISION

30000 Drainage abscess or hematoma, nasal, internal approach

(For external approach, see 10060, 10140)

30020 Drainage abscess or hematoma, nasal septum

(For lateral rhinotomy, see specific application (eg, 30118, 30320))

EXCISION

30100 Biopsy, intranasal

(For biopsy skin of nose, see 11100, 11101)

30110 Excision, nasal polyp(s), simple

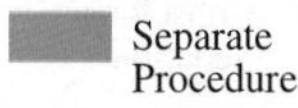 Separate Procedure 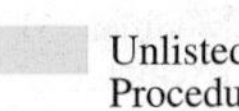 Unlisted Procedure 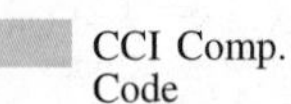 CCI Comp. Code 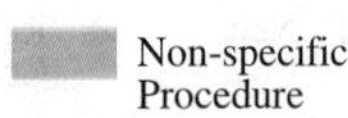 Non-specific Procedure

(30110 would normally be completed in an office setting)

(To report bilateral procedure, use 30110 with modifier -50)

30115 Excision, nasal polyp(s), extensive

(30115 would normally require the facilities available in a hospital setting)

(To report bilateral procedure, use 30115 with modifier -50)

30117 Excision or destruction (eg, laser), intranasal lesion; internal approach

30118 external approach (lateral rhinotomy)

30120 Excision or surgical planing of skin of nose for rhinophyma

30124 Excision dermoid cyst, nose; simple, skin, subcutaneous

30125 complex, under bone or cartilage

30130 Excision inferior turbinate, partial or complete, any method

(For excision of superior or middle turbinate, use 30999)

30140 Submucous resection inferior turbinate, partial or complete, any method

(Do not report 30130 or 30140 in conjunction with 30801, 30802, 30930)

(For submucous resection of superior or middle turbinate, use 30999)

(For endoscopic resection of concha bullosa of middle turbinate, use 31240)

(For submucous resection of nasal septum, use 30520)

(For reduction of turbinates, use 30140 with modifier -52)

30150 Rhinectomy; partial

30160 total

(For closure and/or reconstruction, primary or delayed, see Integumentary System, 13150-13160, 14060-14300, 15120, 15121, 15260, 15261, 15760, 20900-20912)

INTRODUCTION

30200 Injection into turbinate(s), therapeutic

30210 Displacement therapy (Proetz type)

30220 Insertion, nasal septal prosthesis (button)

REMOVAL OF FOREIGN BODY

30300 Removal foreign body, intranasal; office type procedure

30310 requiring general anesthesia

30320 by lateral rhinotomy

REPAIR

(For obtaining tissues for graft, see 20900-20926, 21210)

30400 Rhinoplasty, primary; lateral and alar cartilages and/or elevation of nasal tip

(For columellar reconstruction, see 13150 et seq)

30410 complete, external parts including bony pyramid, lateral and alar cartilages, and/or elevation of nasal tip

30420 including major septal repair

30430 Rhinoplasty, secondary; minor revision (small amount of nasal tip work)

30435 intermediate revision (bony work with osteotomies)

30450 major revision (nasal tip work and osteotomies)

30460 Rhinoplasty for nasal deformity secondary to congenital cleft lip and/or palate, including columellar lengthening; tip only

30462 tip, septum, osteotomies

30465 Repair of nasal vestibular stenosis (eg, spreader grafting, lateral nasal wall reconstruction)

(30465 excludes obtaining graft. For graft procedure, see 20900-20926, 21210)

Separate Procedure | Unlisted Procedure | CCI Comp. Code | Non-specific Procedure

(30465 is used to report a bilateral procedure. For unilateral procedure, use modifier -52)

30520 Septoplasty or submucous resection, with or without cartilage scoring, contouring or replacement with graft

(For submucous resection of turbinates, use 30140)

30540 Repair choanal atresia; intranasal

30545 transpalatine

(Do not report modifier '-63' in conjunction with 30540, 30545)

30560 Lysis intranasal synechia

30580 Repair fistula; oromaxillary (combine with 31030 if antrotomy is included)

30600 oronasal

30620 Septal or other intranasal dermatoplasty (does not include obtaining graft)

30630 Repair nasal septal perforations

DESTRUCTION

30801 Cautery and/or ablation, mucosa of inferior turbinates, unilateral or bilateral, any method; superficial

(For cautery and ablation of superior or middle turbinates, use 30999)

30802 intramural

(Do not report 30801, 30802, 30930 in conjunction with 30130 or 30140)

(For cautery performed for control of nasal hemorrhage, see 30901-30906)

OTHER PROCEDURES

30901 Control nasal hemorrhage, anterior, simple (limited cautery and/or packing) any method

(To report bilateral procedure, use 30901 with modifier -50)

30903 Control nasal hemorrhage, anterior, complex (extensive cautery and/or packing) any method

(To report bilateral procedure, use 30903 with modifier -50)

30905 Control nasal hemorrhage, posterior, with posterior nasal packs and/or cautery, any method; initial

30906 subsequent

30915 Ligation arteries; ethmoidal

30920 internal maxillary artery, transantral

(For ligation external carotid artery, use 37600)

30930 Fracture nasal inferior turbinate(s), therapeutic

(Do not report 30801, 30802, 30930 in conjunction with 30130 or 30140)

(For fracture of superior or middle turbinate(s), use 30999)

30999 Unlisted procedure, nose

ACCESSORY SINUSES

INCISION

31000 Lavage by cannulation; maxillary sinus (antrum puncture or natural ostium)

(To report bilateral procedure, use 31000 with modifier -50)

31002 sphenoid sinus

31020 Sinusotomy, maxillary (antrotomy); intranasal

(To report bilateral procedure, use 31020 with modifier -50)

31030 radical (Caldwell-Luc) without removal of antrochoanal polyps

(To report bilateral procedure, use 31030 with modifier -50)

31032 radical (Caldwell-Luc) with removal of antrochoanal polyps

(To report bilateral procedure, use 31032 with modifier -50)

Separate Procedure | Unlisted Procedure | CCI Comp. Code | Non-specific Procedure

31040 Pterygomaxillary fossa surgery, any approach

(For transantral ligation of internal maxillary artery, use 30920)

31050 Sinusotomy, sphenoid, with or without biopsy;

31051 with mucosal stripping or removal of polyp(s)

31070 Sinusotomy frontal; external, simple (trephine operation)

(For frontal intranasal sinusotomy, use 31276)

31075 transorbital, unilateral (for mucocele or osteoma, Lynch type)

31080 obliterative without osteoplastic flap, brow incision (includes ablation)

31081 obliterative, without osteoplastic flap, coronal incision (includes ablation)

31084 obliterative, with osteoplastic flap, brow incision

31085 obliterative, with osteoplastic flap, coronal incision

31086 nonobliterative, with osteoplastic flap, brow incision

31087 nonobliterative, with osteoplastic flap, coronal incision

31090 Sinusotomy, unilateral, three or more paranasal sinuses (frontal, maxillary, ethmoid, sphenoid)

EXCISION

31200 Ethmoidectomy; intranasal, anterior

31201 intranasal, total

31205 extranasal, total

31225 Maxillectomy; without orbital exenteration

31230 with orbital exenteration (en bloc)

(For orbital exenteration only, see 65110 et seq)

(For skin graft, see 15120 et seq)

ENDOSCOPY

31231 Nasal endoscopy, diagnostic, unilateral or bilateral (separate procedure)

31233 Nasal/sinus endoscopy, diagnostic with maxillary sinusoscopy (via inferior meatus or canine fossa puncture)

31235 Nasal/sinus endoscopy, diagnostic with sphenoid sinusoscopy (via puncture of sphenoidal face or cannulation of ostium)

31237 Nasal/sinus endoscopy, surgical; with biopsy, polypectomy or debridement (separate procedure)

31238 with control of nasal hemorrhage

31239 with dacryocystorhinostomy

31240 with concha bullosa resection

(For endoscopic osteomeatal complex (OMC) resection with antrostomy and/or anterior ethmoidectomy, with or without removal of polyp(s), use 31254 and 31256)

(For endoscopic osteomeatal complex (OMC) resection with antrostomy, removal of antral mucosal disease, and/or anterior ethmoidectomy, with or without removal of polyp(s), use 31254 and 31257)

(For endoscopic frontal sinus exploration, osteomeatal complex (OMC) resection and./or anterior ethmoidecomy, with or without removal of polyp(s), use 31254 and 31276)

(For endoscopic frontal sinus exploration, osteomeatal complex (OMC) resection, antrostomy, and./or anterior ethmoidecomy, with or without removal of polyp(s), use 31254, 31256 and 31276)

(For endoscopic nasal diagnostic endoscopy, see 31231-31235)

(For endoscopic osteomeatal complex (OMC) resection, frontal sinus exploration, antrostomy, removal of antral mucosal disease, and/or anterior ethmoidecomy, with or without removal of polyp(s), use 31254, 31267, and 31276)

31254 Nasal/sinus endoscopy, surgical; with ethmoidectomy, partial (anterior)

31255 with ethmoidectomy, total (anterior andposterior)

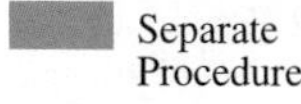
Separate Procedure
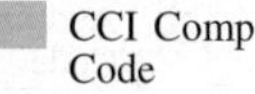
Unlisted Procedure
CCI Comp. Code
Non-specific Procedure

31256 Nasal/sinus endoscopy, surgical, with maxillary antrostomy;

(For endoscopic anterior and posterior ethmoidectomy (APE) and antrostomy, with or without removal of polyp(s), use 31255 and 31256)

(For endoscopic anterior and posterior ethmoidectomy (APE), antrostomy and removal of antral mucosal disease, with or without removal of polyp(s), use 31255 and 31267)

(For endoscopic anterior and posterior ethmoidectomy (APE) and frontal sinus exploration, with or without removal of polyp(s), use 31255 and 31276)

31267 with removal of tissue from maxillary sinus

(For endoscopic anterior and posterior ethmoidectomy (APE) and frontal sinus exploration and antrostomy, with or without removal of polyp(s), use 31255, 31256, and 31276)

(For endoscopic anterior and posterior ethmoidectomy (APE), frontal sinus exploration, antrostomy, and removal of antral mucosal disease, with or without removal of polyp(s), use 31255, 31267, and 31276)

31276 Nasal/sinus endoscopy, surgical with frontal sinus exploration, with or without removal of tissue from frontal sinus

(For endoscopic anterior and posterior ethmoidectomy and sphenoidotomy (APS), with or without removal of polyp(s), use 31255, 31287 or 31288)

(For endoscopic anterior and posterior ethmoidectomy and sphenoidotomy (APS), and antrostomy, with or without removal of polyp(s), use 31255, 31256, and 31287 or 31288)

(For endoscopic anterior and posterior ethmoidectomy and sphenoidotomy (APS), antrostomy and removal of antral mucosal disease, with or without removal of polyp(s), use 31255, 31267, and 31287 or 31288)

(For endoscopic anterior and posterior ethmoidectomy and sphenoidotomy (APS), and frontal sinus exploration, with or without removal of polyp(s), use 31255, 31287 or 31288, and 31276)

(For endoscopic anterior and posterior ethmoidectomy and sphenoidotomy (APS), with or without removal of polyp(s), with frontal sinus exploration and antrostomy, use 31255, 31256, 31287 or 31288, and 31276)

(For unilateral endoscopy of two or more sinuses, see 31231-31235)

(For endoscopic anterior and posterior ethmoidectomy and sphenoidotomy (APS), frontal sinus exploration, antrostomy and removal of antral mucosal disease, with or without the removal of polyp(s), see 31255, 31267, 31287 or 31288, and 31276)

31287 Nasal/sinus endoscopy, surgical, with sphenoidotomy;

31288 with removal of tissue from the sphenoid sinus

31290 Nasal/sinus endoscopy, surgical, with repair of cerebrospinal fluid leak; ethmoid region

31291 sphenoid region

31292 Nasal/sinus endoscopy, surgical; with medial or inferior orbital wall decompression

31293 with medial orbital wall and inferior orbital wall decompression

31294 with optic nerve decompression

OTHER PROCEDURES

(For hypophysectomy, transantral or transeptal approach, use 61548)

(For transcranial hypophysectomy, use 61546)

31299 Unlisted procedure, accessory sinuses

LARYNX

EXCISION

31300 Laryngotomy (thyrotomy, laryngofissure); with removal of tumor or laryngocele, cordectomy

31320 diagnostic

31360 Laryngectomy; total, without radical neck dissection

31365 total, with radical neck dissection

31367 subtotal supraglottic, without radical neck dissection

31368 subtotal supraglottic, with radical neck dissection

31370 Partial laryngectomy (hemilaryngectomy); horizontal

31375 laterovertical

31380 anterovertical

31382 antero-latero-vertical

31390 Pharyngolaryngectomy, with radical neck dissection; without reconstruction

31395 with reconstruction

31400 Arytenoidectomy or arytenoidopexy, external approach

(For endoscopic arytenoidecomy, use 31560)

31420 Epiglottidectomy

INTRODUCTION

⃠ **31500** Intubation, endotracheal, emergency procedure

(For injection procedure for segmental bronchography, see 31656)

31502 Tracheotomy tube change prior to establishment of fistula tract

ENDOSCOPY

31505 Laryngoscopy, indirect; diagnostic (separate procedure)

31510 with biopsy

31511 with removal of foreign body

31512 with removal of lesion

31513 with vocal cord injection

31515 Laryngoscopy direct, with or without tracheoscopy; for aspiration

31520 diagnostic, newborn

● New Code ▲ Revised Code + Add-On Code ⃠ Modifier -51 Exempt ⊙ Conscious Sedation

(Do not report modifier '-63' in conjunction with 31520)

31525 diagnostic, except newborn

31526 diagnostic, with operating microscope or telescope

(Do not report code 69990 in addition to code 31526)

31527 with insertion of obturator

31528 with dilation, initial

31529 with dilation, subsequent

31530 Laryngoscopy, direct, operative, with foreign body removal;

31531 with operating microscope or telescope

(Do not report code 69990 in addition to code 31531)

31535 Laryngoscopy, direct, operative, with biopsy;

31536 with operating microscope or telescope

(Do not report code 69990 in addition to code 31536)

31540 Laryngoscopy, direct, operative, with excision of tumor and/or stripping of vocal cords or epiglottis;

31541 with operating microscope or telescope

(Do not report code 69990 in addition to code 31541)

31545 Laryngoscopy, direct, operative, with operating microscope or telescope, with submucosal removal of non-neoplastic lesion(s) of vocal cord; reconstruction with local tissue flap(s)

31546 reconstruction with graft(s) (includes obtaining autograft)

(Do not report 31546 in addition to 20926 for graft harvest)

(For reconstruction of vocal cord with allograft, use 31599)

(Do not report 31545 or 31546 in conjunction with 31540, 31541, 69990)

31560 Laryngoscopy, direct, operative, with arytenoidectomy;

Separate Procedure | Unlisted Procedure | CCI Comp. Code | Non-specific Procedure

31561 with operating microscope or telescope

(Do not report code 69990 in addition to code 31561)

31570 Laryngoscopy, direct, with injection into vocal cord(s), therapeutic;

31571 with operating microscope or telescope

(Do not report code 69990 in addition to code 31571)

31575 Laryngoscopy, flexible fiberoptic; diagnostic

31576 with biopsy

31577 with removal of foreign body

31578 with removal of lesion

(To report flexible fiberoptic endoscopic evaluation of swallowing, see 92612-92613)

(To report flexible fiberoptic endoscopic evaluation with sensory testing, see 92614-92615)

(To report flexible fiberoptic endoscopic evaluation of swallowing with sensory testing, see 92616-92617)

(For flexible fiberoptic laryngoscopy as part of flexible fiberoptic endoscopic evaluation of swallowing and/or laryngeal sensory testing by cine or video recording, see 92612-92617)

31579 Laryngoscopy, flexible or rigid fiberoptic, with stroboscopy

REPAIR

31580 Laryngoplasty; for laryngeal web, two stage, with keel insertion and removal

31582 for laryngeal stenosis, with graft or core mold, including tracheotomy

31584 with open reduction of fracture

(31585 deleted 2006 edition. To report, use the appropriate Evaluation and Management codes)

(31586 deleted 2006 edition. To report, use the appropriate Evaluation and Management codes)

● New Code ▲ Revised Code + Add-On Code ⃠ Modifier -51 Exempt ⊙ Conscious Sedation

31587 Laryngoplasty, cricoid split

31588 Laryngoplasty, not otherwise specified (eg, for burns, reconstruction after partial laryngectomy)

31590 Laryngeal reinnervation by neuromuscular pedicle

DESTRUCTION

31595 Section recurrent laryngeal nerve, therapeutic (separate procedure), unilateral

OTHER PROCEDURES

31599 Unlisted procedure, larynx

TRACHEA AND BRONCHI

INCISION

31600 Tracheostomy, planned (separate procedure);

31601 under two years

31603 Tracheostomy, emergency procedure; transtracheal

31605 cricothyroid membrane

31610 Tracheostomy, fenestration procedure with skin flaps

(For endotracheal intubation, use 31500)

(For tracheal aspiration under direct vision, use 31515)

31611 Construction of tracheoesophageal fistula and subsequent insertion of an alaryngeal speech prosthesis (eg, voice button, Blom-Singer prosthesis)

31612 Tracheal puncture, percutaneous with transtracheal aspiration and/or injection

31613 Tracheostoma revision; simple, without flap rotation

31614 complex, with flap rotation

Separate Procedure

Unlisted Procedure

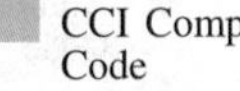
CCI Comp. Code

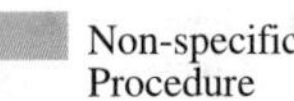
Non-specific Procedure

ENDOSCOPY

(For tracheoscopy, see laryngoscopy codes 31515-31578)

⊙ **31615** Tracheobronchoscopy through established tracheostomy incision

⊙+**31620** Endobronchial ultrasound (EBUS) during bronchoscopic diagnostic or therapeutic intervention(s) (List separately in addition to code for primary procedure(s))

(Use 31620 in conjunction with 31622-31646)

⊙ **31622** Bronchoscopy, rigid or flexible, with or without fluoroscopic guidance; diagnostic, with or without cell washing (separate procedure)

⊙ **31623** with brushing or protected brushings

⊙ **31624** with bronchial alveolar lavage

⊙ **31625** with bronchial or endobronchial biopsy(s), single or multiple sites

⊙ **31628** with transbronchial lung biopsy(s), single lobe

(31628 should be reported only once regardless of how many transbronchial lung biopsies are performed in a lobe)

(To report transbronchial lung biopsies performed on additional lobe, use 31632)

⊙ **31629** with transbronchial needle aspiration biopsy(s), trachea, main stem and/or lobar bronchus(i)

(31629 should be reported only once for upper airway biopsies regardless of how many transbronchial needle aspiration biopsies are performed in the upper airway or in a lobe)

(To report transbronchial needle aspiration biopsies performed on additional lobe(s), use 31633)

31630 with tracheal/bronchial dilation or closed reduction of fracture

31631 with placement of tracheal stent(s) (includes tracheal/ bronchial dilation as required)

(For placement of bronchial stent, see 31636, 31637)

(For revision of tracheal/bronchial stent, use 31638)

+ **31632** with transbronchial lung biopsy(s), each additional lobe (List separately in addition to code for primary procedure)

(Use 31632 in conjunction with 31628)

(31632 should be reported only once regardless of how many transbronchial lung biopsies are performed in a lobe)

+ **31633** with transbronchial needle aspiration biopsy(s), each additional lobe (List separately in addition to code for primary procedure)

(Use 31633 in conjunction with 31629)

(31633 should be reported only once regardless of how many transbronchial needle aspiration biopsies are performed in the trachea or the additional lobe)

⊙ **31635** with removal of foreign body

31636 with placement of bronchial stent(s) (includes tracheal/bronchial dilation as required), initial bronchus

+ **31637** each additional major bronchus stented (List separately in addition to code for primary procedure)

(Use 31637 in conjunction with 31636)

31638 with revision of tracheal or bronchial stent inserted at previous session (includes tracheal/bronchial dilation as required)

31640 with excision of tumor

31641 Bronchoscopy, (rigid or flexible); with destruction of tumor or relief of stenosis by any method other than excision (eg, laser therapy, cryotherapy)

(For bronchoscopic photodynamic therapy, report 31641 in addition to 96570, 96571 as appropriate)

31643 with placement of catheter(s) for intracavitary radioelement application

(For intracavitary radioelement application, see 77761-77763, 77781-77784)

⊙ **31645** with therapeutic aspiration of tracheobronchial tree, initial (eg, drainage of lung abscess)

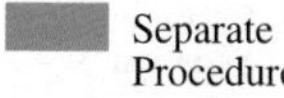
Separate Procedure
Unlisted Procedure
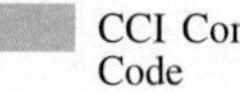
CCI Comp. Code
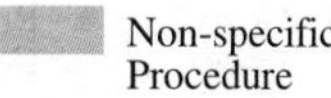
Non-specific Procedure

⊙ **31646** with therapeutic aspiration of tracheobronchial tree, subsequent

(For catheter aspiration of tracheobronchial tree at bedside, use 31725)

⊙ **31656** with injection of contrast material for segmental bronchography (fiberscope only)

(For radiological supervision and interpretation, see 71040, 71060)

INTRODUCTION

(For endotracheal intubation, use 31500)

(For tracheal aspiration under direct vision, see 31515)

(31700 deleted 2007 edition)

(31708 deleted 2007 edition)

(31710 deleted 2007 edition)

31715 Transtracheal injection for bronchography

(For radiological supervision and interpretation, see 71040, 71060)

(For prolonged services, see 99354-99360)

31717 Catheterization with bronchial brush biopsy

31720 Catheter aspiration (separate procedure); nasotracheal

⊙ **31725** tracheobronchial with fiberscope, bedside

31730 Transtracheal (percutaneous) introduction of needle wire dilator/stent or indwelling tube for oxygen therapy

EXCISION, REPAIR

31750 Tracheoplasty; cervical

31755 tracheopharyngeal fistulization, each stage

31760 intrathoracic

31766 Carinal reconstruction

● New Code ▲ Revised Code + Add-On Code ⊘ Modifier -51 Exempt ⊙ Conscious Sedation

31770 Bronchoplasty; graft repair

31775 excision stenosis and anastomosis

(For lobectomy and bronchoplasty, use 32501)

31780 Excision tracheal stenosis and anastomosis; cervical

31781 cervicothoracic

31785 Excision of tracheal tumor or carcinoma; cervical

31786 thoracic

31800 Suture of tracheal wound or injury; cervical

31805 intrathoracic

31820 Surgical closure tracheostomy or fistula; without plastic repair

31825 with plastic repair

(For repair tracheoesophageal fistula, see 43305, 43312)

31830 Revision of tracheostomy scar

OTHER PROCEDURES

31899 Unlisted procedure, trachea, bronchi

LUNGS AND PLEURA

INCISION

⊘ **32000** Thoracentesis, puncture of pleural cavity for aspiration, initial or subsequent

(If imaging guidance is performed, see 76942, 77002, 77012)

(For total lung lavage, use 32997)

⊘ **32002** Thoracentesis with insertion of tube with or without water seal (eg, for pneumothorax) (separate procedure)

(Do not report 32002 in conjunction with 19260, 19271, 19272, 32503, 32504)

(If imaging guidance is performed, see 76942, 77002, 77012)

 Separate Procedure 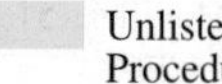 Unlisted Procedure 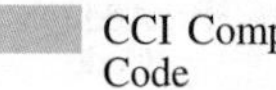 CCI Comp. Code 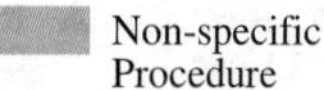 Non-specific Procedure

32005 Chemical pleurodesis (eg, for recurrent or persistent pneumothorax)

⊙ **32019** Insertion of indwelling tunneled pleural catheter with cuff

(Do not report 32019 in conjunction with 32000-32005, 32020, 36000, 36410, 62318, 62319, 64450, 64470, 64475)

(If imaging guidance is performed, use 75989)

⃠⊙ **32020** Tube thoracostomy with or without water seal (eg, for abscess, hemothorax, empyema) (separate procedure)

(Do not report 32020 in conjunction with 19260, 19271, 19272, 32503, 32504)

(If imaging guidance is performed, use 75989)

32035 Thoracostomy; with rib resection for empyema

32036 with open flap drainage for empyema

32095 Thoracotomy, limited, for biopsy of lung or pleura

(To report wound exploration due to penetrating trauma without thoractomy, use 20102)

32100 Thoracotomy, major; with exploration and biopsy

(Do not report 32100 in conjunction with 19260, 19271, 19272, 32503, 32504)

32110 with control of traumatic hemorrhage and/or repair of lung tear

32120 for postoperative complications

32124 with open intrapleural pneumonolysis

32140 with cyst(s) removal, with or without a pleural procedure

32141 with excision-plication of bullae, with or without any pleural procedure

(For lung volume reduction, use 32491)

32150 with removal of intrapleural foreign body or fibrin deposit

32151 with removal of intrapulmonary foreign body

● New Code ▲ Revised Code + Add-On Code ⃠ Modifier -51 Exempt ⊙ Conscious Sedation

32160 with cardiac massage

(For segmental or other resections of lung, see 32480-32504)

32200 Pneumonostomy; with open drainage of abscess or cyst

⊙ **32201** with percutaneous drainage of abscess or cyst

(For radiological supervision and interpretation, use 75989)

32215 Pleural scarification for repeat pneumothorax

32220 Decortication, pulmonary (separate procedure); total

32225 partial

EXCISION

32310 Pleurectomy, parietal (separate procedure)

32320 Decortication and parietal pleurectomy

32400 Biopsy, pleura; percutaneous needle

(If imaging guidance is performed, see 76942, 77002, 77012, 77021)

(For fine needle aspiration, use 10021 or 10022)

(For evaluation of fine needle aspirate, see 88172, 88173)

32402 open

32405 Biopsy, lung or mediastinum, percutaneous needle

(For radiological supervision and interpretation, see 76942, 77002, 77012, 77021)

(For fine needle aspiration, use 10022)

(For evaluation of fine needle aspirate, see 88172, 88173)

REMOVAL

32420 Pneumocentesis, puncture of lung for aspiration

32440 Removal of lung, total pneumonectomy;

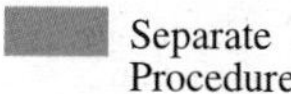 Separate Procedure 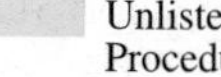 Unlisted Procedure 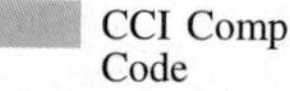 CCI Comp. Code 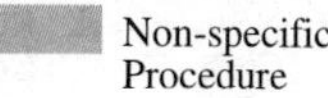 Non-specific Procedure

32442 with resection of segment of trachea followed by broncho-tracheal anastomosis (sleeve pneumonectomy)

32445 extrapleural

(For extrapleural pneumonectomy, with empyemectomy, use 32445 and 32540)

(If lung resection is performed with chest wall tumor resection, report the appropriate chest wall tumor resection code, 19260-19272, in addition to lung resection code 32440-32445)

32480 Removal of lung, other than total pneumonectomy; single lobe (lobectomy)

32482 two lobes (bilobectomy)

32484 single segment (segmentectomy)

(For removal of lung with bronchoplasty, use 32501)

32486 with circumferential resection of segment of bronchus followed by broncho-bronchial anastomosis (sleeve lobectomy)

32488 all remaining lung following previous removal of a portion of lung (completion pneumonectomy)

(For total or segmental lobectomy, with concomitant decortication, use 32320 and the appropriate removal of lung code)

32491 excision-plication of emphysematous lung(s) (bullous or non-bullous) for lung volume reduction, sternal split or transthoracic approach, with or without any pleural procedure

32500 wedge resection, single or multiple

(If lung resection is performed with chest wall tumor resection, report the appropriate chest wall tumor resection code, 19260-19272, in addition to lung resection code 32480-32500)

+ 32501 Resection and repair of portion of bronchus (bronchoplasty) when performed at time of lobectomy or segmentectomy (List separately in addition to code for primary procedure)

(Use 32501 in conjunction with codes 32480, 32482, 32484)

(32501 is to be used when a portion of the bronchus to preserved lung is removed and requires plastic closure to preserve function of that preserved lung. It is not to be used for closure for the proximal end of a resected bronchus.)

32503 Resection of apical lung tumor (eg, Pancoast tumor), including chest wall resection, rib(s) resection(s), neurovascular dissection, when performed; without chest wall reconstruction(s)

32504 with chest wall reconstruction

(Do not report 32503, 32504 in conjunction with 19260, 19271, 19272, 32002, 32020, 32100)

(For performance of lung resection in conjunction with chest wall resection, see 19260, 19271, 19272 and 32480-32500, 32503, 32504)

(32520 deleted 2006 edition.)

(32522 deleted 2006 edition.)

(32525 deleted 2006 edition.)

32540 Extrapleural enucleation of empyema (empyemectomy)

(For extrapleural enucleation of empyema (empyemectomy) with lobectomy, use 32540 and the appropriate removal of lung code)

ENDOSCOPY

32601 Thoracoscopy, diagnostic (separate procedure); lungs and pleural space, without biopsy

32602 lungs and pleural space, with biopsy

32603 pericardial sac, without biopsy

32604 pericardial sac, with biopsy

32605 mediastinal space, without biopsy

32606 mediastinal space, with biopsy

(Surgical thoracoscopy always includes diagnostic thoracoscopy)

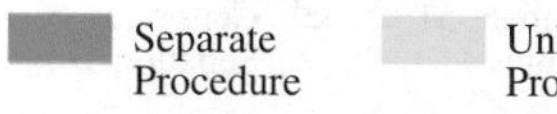
Separate Procedure
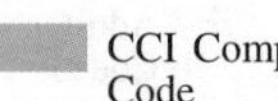
Unlisted Procedure
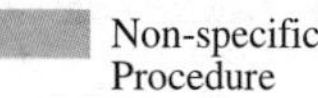
CCI Comp. Code
Non-specific Procedure

32650 Thoracoscopy, surgical; with pleurodesis (eg, mechanical or chemical)

32651 with partial pulmonary decortication

32652 with total pulmonary decortication, including intrapleural pneumonolysis

32653 with removal of intrapleural foreign body or fibrin deposit

32654 with control of traumatic hemorrhage

32655 with excision-plication of bullae, including any pleural procedure

32656 with parietal pleurectomy

32657 with wedge resection of lung, single or multiple

32658 with removal of clot or foreign body from pericardial sac

32659 with creation of pericardial window or partial resection of pericardial sac for drainage

32660 with total pericardiectomy

32661 with excision of pericardial cyst, tumor, or mass

32662 with excision of mediastinal cyst, tumor, or mass

32663 with lobectomy, total or segmental

32664 with thoracic sympathectomy

32665 with esophagomyotomy (Heller type)

(For exploratory thoracoscopy, and exploratory throacoscopy with biopsy, see 32601-32606)

REPAIR

32800 Repair lung hernia through chest wall

32810 Closure of chest wall following open flap drainage for empyema (Clagett type procedure)

32815 Open closure of major bronchial fistula

32820 Major reconstruction, chest wall (posttraumatic)

LUNG TRANSPLANTATION

Lung allotransplantation involves three distinct components of physician work:

1) **Cadaver donor pneumonectomy(s)**, which include(s) harvesting the allograft and cold preservation of the allograft (perfusing with cold preservation solution and cold maintenance) (use 32850).

2) **Backbench work:**

Preparation of a cadaver donor single lung allograft prior to transplantation, including dissection of the allograft from surrounding soft tissues to prepare the pulmonary venous/atrial cuff, pulmonary artery, and bronchus unilaterally (use 32855).

Preparation of a cadaver donor double lung allograft prior to transplantation, including dissection of the allograft from surrounding soft tissues to prepare the pulmonary venous/atrial cuff, pulmonary artery, and bronchus bilaterally (use 32856).

3) **Recipient lung allotransplantation**, which includes transplantation of a single or double lung allograft and care of the recipient (see 32851-32854).

32850 Donor pneumonectomy (including cold preservation), from cadaver donor

32851 Lung transplant, single; without cardiopulmonary bypass

32852 with cardiopulmonary bypass

32853 Lung transplant, double (bilateral sequential or en bloc); without cardiopulmonary bypass

32854 with cardiopulmonary bypass

32855 Backbench standard preparation of cadaver donor lung allograft prior to transplantation, including dissection of allograft from surrounding soft tissues to prepare pulmonary venous/atrial cuff, pulmonary artery, and bronchus; unilateral

32856 bilateral

(For repair or resection procedures on the donor lung, see 32491, 32500, 35216, or 35276)

SURGICAL COLLAPSE THERAPY; THORACOPLASTY

(See also 32503, 32504)

32900 Resection of ribs, extrapleural, all stages

32905 Thoracoplasty, Schede type or extrapleural (all stages);

32906 with closure of bronchopleural fistula

(For open closure of major bronchial fistula, use 32815)

(For resection of first rib for thoracic outlet compression, see 21615, 21616)

32940 Pneumonolysis, extraperiosteal, including filling or packing procedures

32960 Pneumothorax, therapeutic, intrapleural injection of air

OTHER PROCEDURES

32997 Total lung lavage (unilateral)

(For bronchoscopic bronchial alveolar lavage, use 31624)

● **32998** Ablation therapy for reduction or eradication of one or more pulmonary tumor(s) including pleura or chest wall when involved by tumor extension, percutaneous, radiofrequency, unilateral

(For imaging guidance and monitoring, see 76940, 77013, 77022)

32999 Unlisted procedure, lungs and pleura

● New Code ▲ Revised Code + Add-On Code ⃠ Modifier -51 Exempt ⊙ Conscious Sedation

CARDIOVASCULAR SYSTEM

CPT codes from this section of the CPT coding system are used to report invasive and surgical procedures performed on the heart and pericardium, including pacemakers or defibrillators; cardiac valves; coronary arteries; aorta; and arteries and veins.

For coding services such as monitoring, operation of pump and other non-surgical services performed during cardiovascular surgery, see the Special Services CPT codes 99150, 99151, 99160-99162 or CPT codes 99291-99292 and 99190-99192 from the evaluation and management section of the CPT coding system.

MISCELLANEOUS CODING RULES

A pacemaker system includes a pulse generator containing electronics, a battery, and one or more electrodes (leads) inserted one of several ways. Pulse generators may be placed in a subcutaneous "pocket" created in either a subclavicular or intra-abdominal site. Electrodes may be inserted through a vein (transvenous) or on the surface of the heart (epicardial). A single chamber system includes a pulse generator, one electrode inserted into either the atrium or ventricle. A dual chamber system includes a pulse generator, one electrode inserted in the atrium, and one electrode inserted in the ventricle.

Assign two CPT codes when a pacemaker or cardioverter-defibrillator "battery"/pulse generator is replaced. One code should describe the removal of the old pulse generator and the other should describe the insertion of the new pulse generator.

Cardiac catheterization codes are classified in the Medicine Section of the CPT coding system. Insertion of a dilator into a vein prior to the placement of a catheter should not be separately coded.

(For monitoring, operation of pump and other nonsurgical services, see 99190-99192, 99291, 99292, 99354-99360)

(For other medical or laboratory related services, see appropriate section)

(For radiological supervision and interpretation, see 75600-75978)

HEART AND PERICARDIUM

PERICARDIUM

⊙ **33010** Pericardiocentesis; initial

(For radiological supervision and interpretation, use 76930)

Separate Procedure | Unlisted Procedure | CCI Comp. Code | Non-specific Procedure

⊙ **33011** subsequent

(For radiological supervision and interpretation, use 76930)

33015 Tube pericardiostomy

33020 Pericardiotomy for removal of clot or foreign body (primary procedure)

33025 Creation of pericardial window or partial resection for drainage

33030 Pericardiectomy, subtotal or complete; without cardiopulmonary bypass

33031 with cardiopulmonary bypass

33050 Excision of pericardial cyst or tumor

CARDIAC TUMOR

33120 Excision of intracardiac tumor, resection with cardiopulmonary bypass

33130 Resection of external cardiac tumor

TRANSMYOCARDIAL REVASCULARIZATION

33140 Transmyocardial laser revascularization, by thoracotomy (separate procedure)

\+ **33141** performed at the time of other open cardiac procedure(s) (List separately in addition to code for primary procedure)

(Use 33141 in conjunction with codes 33400-33496, 33510-33536, 33542)

PACEMAKER OR PACING CARDIOVERTER-DEFIBRILLATOR

A pacemaker generally has two parts; a generator and the leads. The generator is where the battery and the information to regulate the heartbeat are stored. The leads are wires that go from the generator through a large vein to the heart, where the wires are anchored. The leads send the electrical impulses to the heart to tell it to beat. The battery can last anywhere from 7-8 years on average and will be routinely monitored by your health care professional and replaced when necessary.

A pacemaker can usually sense if the heartbeat is above a certain level, at which point it will automatically turn off. Likewise, the pacemaker can sense when the heartbeat slows down too much, and will automatically turn back on in order to

● New Code ▲ Revised Code + Add-On Code ⊘ Modifier -51 Exempt ⊙ Conscious Sedation

start pacing again. A pacemaker is often the treatment of choice for bradycardia. Less commonly, pacemakers may also be used to terminate tachycardia. The pacemaker can sense the abnormally fast heart rate and take control of it by first speeding up, then slowing down to normal.

In most cases, the procedure for inserting a pacemaker takes about one hour. The patient is awake for the procedure, and pain medication is given throughout the procedure. A small incision is made traditionally in the left side of the chest, and a small "pocket" is created underneath the skin. After the leads have been positioned in the heart under X-ray guidance, they are then connected to the generator. The generator is then placed into the pocket, and the pocket is closed with sutures. Most patients are able to go home within 1 day of the procedure, if there are no other medical issues requiring further hospitalization.

IMPLANTABLE CARDIOVERTER DEFIBRILLATOR

An implantable cardioverter defibrillator is used in patients at risk for recurrent, sustained ventricular tachycardia or fibrillation.

The device is connected to leads positioned inside the heart or on its surface. These leads are used to deliver electrical shocks, sense the cardiac rhythm and sometimes pace the heart, as needed. The various leads are tunneled to a pulse generator, which is implanted in a pouch beneath the skin of the chest or abdomen. These generators are typically a little larger than a wallet and have electronics that automatically monitor and treat heart rhythms recognized as abnormal. Newer devices are smaller and have simpler lead systems. They can be installed through blood vessels, eliminating the need for open chest surgery.

When an implantable cardioverter defibrillator detects ventricular tachycardia or fibrillation, it shocks the heart to restore the normal rhythm. New devices also provide overdrive pacing to electrically convert a sustained ventricular tachycardia, and "backup" pacing if bradycardia occurs. They also offer a host of other sophisticated functions (such as storage of detected arrhythmic events and the ability to do "noninvasive" electrophysiologic testing).

(For electronic, telephonic analysis of internal pacemaker system, see 93731-93736)

(For radiological supervision and interpretation with insertion of pacemaker, use 71090)

(33200 deleted 2007 edition)

(33201 deleted 2007 edition)

● **33202** Insertion of epicardial electrode(s); open incision (eg, thoracotomy, median sternotomy, subxiphoid approach)

● **33203** Insertion of epicardial electrode(s); endoscopic approach (eg, thoracoscopy, pericardioscopy)

(When epicardial lead placement is performed by the same physician at the same session as insertion of the generator, report 33202, 33203 in conjunction with 33212, 33213 as appropriate)

⊙ **33206** Insertion or replacement of permanent pacemaker with transvenous electrode(s); atrial

⊙ **33207** ventricular

⊙ **33208** atrial and ventricular

(Codes 33206-33208 include subcutaneous insertion of the pulse generator and transvenous placement of electrode(s))

⊙ **33210** Insertion or replacement of temporary transvenous single chamber cardiac electrode or pacemaker catheter (separate procedure)

⊙ **33211** Insertion or replacement of temporary transvenous dual chamber pacing electrodes (separate procedure)

⊙ **33212** Insertion or replacement of pacemaker pulse generator only; single chamber, atrial or ventricular

⊙ **33213** dual chamber

(Use 33212, 33213, as appropriate, in conjunction with the epicardial lead placement codes 33202, 33203 to report the insertion of the generator when done by the same physician during the same session)

⊙ **33214** Upgrade of implanted pacemaker system, conversion of single chamber system to dual chamber system (includes removal of previously placed pulse generator, testing of existing lead, insertion of new lead, insertion of new pulse generator)

(When epicardial electrode placement is performed, report 33214 in conjunction with 33202, 33203)

33215 Repositioning of previously implanted transvenous pacemaker or pacing cardioverter-defibillator (right atrial or right ventricular) electrode

● New Code ▲ Revised Code + Add-On Code ⃠ Modifier -51 Exempt ⊙ Conscious Sedation

⊙ **33216** Insertion of a transvenous electrode; single chamber (one electrode) permanent pacemaker or single chamber pacing cardioverter-defibrillator

⊙ **33217** dual chamber (two electrodes) permanent pacemaker or dual chamber pacing cardioverter-defibrillator

(Do not report 33216-33217 in conjunction with code 33214)

⊙ **33218** Repair of single transvenous electrode for a single chamber, permanent pacemaker or single chamber pacing cardioverter-defibrillator

(For atrial or ventricular single chamber repair of pacemaker electrode(s) with replacement of pulse generator, see 33212 or 33213 and 33218 or 33220)

⊙ **33220** Repair of two transvenous electrodes for a dual chamber permanent pacemaker or dual chamber pacing cardioverter-defibrillator

⊙ **33222** Revision or relocation of skin pocket for pacemaker

⊙ **33223** Revision of skin pocket for single or dual chamber pacing cardioverter-defibrillator

33224 Insertion of pacing electrode, cardiac venous system, for left ventricular pacing, with attachment to previously placed pacemaker or pacing cardioverter-defibrillator pulse generator (including revision of pocket, removal, insertion and/or replacement of generator)

(When epicardial electrode placement is performed, report 33224 in conjunction with 33202, 33203)

\+ **33225** Insertion of pacing electrode, cardiac venous system, for left ventricular pacing, at time of insertion of pacing cardioverter-defibrillator or pacemaker pulse generator (including upgrade to dual chamber system) (List separately in addition to code for primary procedure)

(Use 33225 in conjunction with 33206, 33207, 33208, 33212, 33213, 33214, 33216, 33217, 33222, 33233, 33234, 33235, 33240, 33249)

33226 Repositioning of previously implanted cardiac venous system (left ventricular) electrode (including removal, insertion and/or replacement of generator)

⊙ **33233** Removal of permanent pacemaker pulse generator

⊙ **33234** Removal of transvenous pacemaker electrode(s); single lead system, atrial or ventricular

⊙ **33235** dual lead system

33236 Removal of permanent epicardial pacemaker and electrodes by thoracotomy; single lead system, atrial or ventricular

33237 dual lead system

33238 Removal of permanent transvenous electrode(s) by thoracotomy

⊙ **33240** Insertion of single or dual chamber pacing cardioverter-defibrillator pulse generator

(Use 33240, as appropriate, in addition to the epicardial lead placement codes to report the insertion of the generator when done by the same physician during the same session)

⊙ **33241** Subcutaneous removal of single or dual chamber pacing cardioverter-defibrillator pulse generator

(For removal of electrode(s) by thoracotomy, use 33243 in conjunction with code 33241)

(For removal of electrode(s) by transvenous extraction, use 33244 in conjunction with code 33241)

(For removal and reinsertion of a pacing cardioverter-defibrillator system (pulse generator and electrodes), report 33241 and 33243 or 33244 and 33249)

(For repair of implantable cardioverter-defibrillator pulse generator and/or leads, see 33218, 33220)

33243 Removal of single or dual chamber pacing cardioverter-defibrillator electrode(s); by thoracotomy

⊙ **33244** by transvenous extraction

(For subcutaneous removal of the pulse generator, use 33241 in conjunction with code 33243 or 33244)

(33245 deleted 2007 edition)

(33246 deleted 2007 edition)

● New Code ▲ Revised Code + Add-On Code ⊘ Modifier -51 Exempt ⊙ Conscious Sedation

⊙ **33249** Insertion or repositioning of electrode lead(s) for single or dual chamber pacing cardioverter-defibrillator and insertion of pulse generator

(For removal and reinsertion of a pacing cardioverter-defibrillator system (pulse generator and electrodes), report 33241 and 33243 or 33244 and 33249)

(For insertion of implantable cardioverter-defibrillator lead(s), without thoracotomy, use 33216)

ELECTROPHYSIOLOGIC OPERATIVE PROCEDURES

Incision

33250 Operative ablation of supraventricular arrhythmogenic focus or pathway (eg, Wolff-Parkinson-White, atrioventricular node re-entry), tract(s) and/or focus (foci); without cardiopulmonary bypass

33251 with cardiopulmonary bypass

(33253 deleted 2007 edition, see 33254-33256)

● **33254** Operative tissue ablation and reconstruction of atria, limited (eg, modified maze procedure)

● **33255** Operative tissue ablation and reconstruction of atria, extensive (eg, maze procedure); without cardiopulmonary bypass

● **33256** with cardiopulmonary bypass

(Do not report 33254-33256 in conjunction with 32020, 32100, 33120, 33130, 33210, 33211, 33400-33507, 33510-33523, 33533-33548, 33600-33853, 33860-33863, 33910-33920)

33261 Operative ablation of ventricular arrhythmogenic focus with cardiopulmonary bypass

Endoscopy

● **33265** Endoscopy, surgical; operative tissue ablation and reconstruction of atria, limited (eg, modified maze procedure), without cardiopulmonary bypass

● **33266** Endoscopy, surgical; operative tissue ablation and reconstruction of atria, extensive (eg, maze procedure), without cardiopulmonary bypass

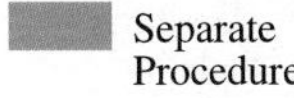
Separate Procedure | Unlisted Procedure | CCI Comp. Code | Non-specific Procedure

(Do not report 33265-33266 in conjunction with 32020, 33210, 33211)

PATIENT-ACTIVATED EVENT RECORDER

33282 Implantation of patient-activated cardiac event recorder

(Initial implantation includes programming. For subsequent electronic analysis and/or reprogramming, use 93727)

33284 Removal of an implantable, patient-activated cardiac event recorder

WOUNDS OF THE HEART AND GREAT VESSELS

33300 Repair of cardiac wound; without bypass

33305 with cardiopulmonary bypass

33310 Cardiotomy, exploratory (includes removal of foreign body, atrial or ventricular thrombus); without bypass

33315 with cardiopulmonary bypass

(Do not report removal of thrombus (33310-33315) in conjunction with other cardiac procedures unless a separate incision in the heart is required to remove the atrial or ventricular thrombus)

(If removal of thrombus with coronary bypass (33315) is reported in conjunction with 33120, 33130, 33420-33430, 33460-33468, 33496, 33542, 33545, 33641-33647, 33670, 33681, 33975-33980 which requires a separate heart incision, report 33315 with modifier '-59')

33320 Suture repair of aorta or great vessels; without shunt or cardiopulmonary bypass

33321 with shunt bypass

33322 with cardiopulmonary bypass

33330 Insertion of graft, aorta or great vessels; without shunt, or cardiopulmonary bypass

33332 with shunt bypass

33335 with cardiopulmonary bypass

● New Code ▲ Revised Code + Add-On Code ⦸ Modifier -51 Exempt ⊙ Conscious Sedation

CARDIAC VALVES

(For multiple valve procedures, see 33400-33478 and add modifier -51 to the secondary valve procedure code)

Aortic Valve

33400 Valvuloplasty, aortic valve; open, with cardiopulmonary bypass

33401 open, with inflow occlusion

33403 using transventricular dilation, with cardiopulmonary bypass

(Do not report modifier '-63' in conjunction with 33401, 33403)

33404 Construction of apical-aortic conduit

33405 Replacement, aortic valve, with cardiopulmonary bypass; with prosthetic valve other than homograft or stentless valve

33406 with allograft valve (freehand)

(For aortic valve valvotomy, (commissurotomy) with inflow occlusion, use 33401)

(For aortic valve valvotomy, (commissurotomy) with cardiopulmonary bypass, use 33403)

33410 with stentless tissue valve

33411 Replacement, aortic valve; with aortic annulus enlargement, noncoronary cusp

33412 with transventricular aortic annulus enlargement (Konno procedure)

33413 by translocation of autologous pulmonary valve with allograft replacement of pulmonary valve (Ross procedure)

33414 Repair of left ventricular outflow tract obstruction by patch enlargement of the outflow tract

33415 Resection or incision of subvalvular tissue for discrete subvalvular aortic stenosis

33416 Ventriculomyotomy (-myectomy) for idiopathic hypertrophic subaortic stenosis (eg, asymmetric septal hypertrophy)

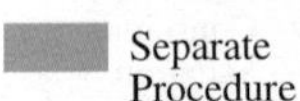 Separate Procedure 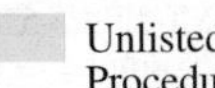 Unlisted Procedure 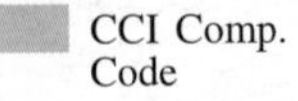 CCI Comp. Code 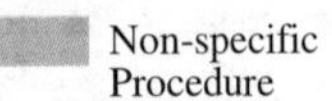 Non-specific Procedure

33417 Aortoplasty (gusset) for supravalvular stenosis

Mitral Valve

33420 Valvotomy, mitral valve; closed heart

33422 open heart, with cardiopulmonary bypass

33425 Valvuloplasty, mitral valve, with cardiopulmonary bypass;

33426 with prosthetic ring

33427 radical reconstruction, with or without ring

33430 Replacement, mitral valve, with cardiopulmonary bypass

Tricuspid Valve

33460 Valvectomy, tricuspid valve, with cardiopulmonary bypass

33463 Valvuloplasty, tricuspid valve; without ring insertion

33464 with ring insertion

33465 Replacement, tricuspid valve, with cardiopulmonary bypass

33468 Tricuspid valve repositioning and plication for Ebstein anomaly

Pulmonary Valve

33470 Valvotomy, pulmonary valve, closed heart; transventricular

(Do not report modifier '-63' in conjunction with 33470)

33471 via pulmonary artery

(To report percutaneous valvuloplasty of pulmonary valve, use 92990)

33472 Valvotomy, pulmonary valve, open heart; with inflow occlusion

(Do not report modifier '-63' in conjunction with 33472)

33474 with cardiopulmonary bypass

33475 Replacement, pulmonary valve

● New Code ▲ Revised Code + Add-On Code ⦸ Modifier -51 Exempt ⊙ Conscious Sedation

33476 Right ventricular resection for infundibular stenosis, with or without commissurotomy

33478 Outflow tract augmentation (gusset), with or without commissurotomy or infundibular resection

(Use 33478 in conjunction with 33768 when a cavopulmonary anastomosis to a second superior vena cava is performed)

OTHER VALVULAR PROCEDURES

33496 Repair of non-structural prosthetic valve dysfunction with cardiopulmonary bypass (separate procedure)

(For reoperation, use 33530 in addition to 33496)

CORONARY ARTERY ANOMALIES

33500 Repair of coronary arteriovenous or arteriocardiac chamber fistula; with cardiopulmonary bypass

33501 without cardiopulmonary bypass

33502 Repair of anomalous coronary artery from pulmonary artery origin; by ligation

33503 by graft, without cardiopulmonary bypass

(Do not report modifier '-63' in conjunction with 33502, 33503)

33504 by graft, with cardiopulmonary bypass

33505 with construction of intrapulmonary artery tunnel (Takeuchi procedure)

33506 by translocation from pulmonary artery to aorta

(Do not report modifier '-63' in conjunction with 33505, 33506)

33507 Repair of anomalous (eg, intramural) aortic origin of coronary artery by unroofing or translocation

ENDOSCOPY

(Surgical vascular endoscopy always includes diagnostic endoscopy)

+ **33508** Endoscopy, surgical, including video-assisted harvest of vein(s) for coronary artery bypass procedure (List separately in addition to code for primary procedure)

(Use 33508 in conjunction with code 33510-33523)

(For open harvest of upper extremity vein procedure, use 35500)

VENOUS GRAFTING ONLY FOR CORONARY ARTERY BYPASS

33510 Coronary artery bypass, vein only; single coronary venous graft

33511 two coronary venous grafts

33512 three coronary venous grafts

33513 four coronary venous grafts

33514 five coronary venous grafts

33516 six or more coronary venous grafts

COMBINED ARTERIAL-VENOUS GRAFTING FOR CORONARY BYPASS

⊘ **33517** Coronary artery bypass, using venous graft(s) and arterial graft(s); single vein graft (List separately in addition to code for arterial graft)

⊘ **33518** two venous grafts (List separately in addition to code for arterial graft)

⊘ **33519** three venous grafts (List separately in addition to code for arterial graft)

⊘ **33521** four venous grafts (List separately in addition to code for arterial graft)

⊘ **33522** five venous grafts (List separately in addition to code for arterial graft)

⊘ **33523** six or more venous grafts (List separately in addition to code for arterial graft)

+ **33530** Reoperation, coronary artery bypass procedure or valve procedure, more than one month after original operation (List separately in addition to code for primary procedure)

(Use 33530 in conjunction with codes 33400-33496; 33510-33536, 33863)

ARTERIAL GRAFTING FOR CORONARY ARTERY BYPASS

33533 Coronary artery bypass, using arterial graft(s); single arterial graft

33534 two coronary arterial grafts

33535 three coronary arterial grafts

33536 four or more coronary arterial grafts

33542 Myocardial resection (eg, ventricular aneurysmectomy)

33545 Repair of postinfarction ventricular septal defect, with or without myocardial resection

33548 Surgical ventricular restoration procedure, includes prosthetic patch, when performed (eg, ventricular remodeling, SVR, SAVER, DOR procedures)

(Do not report 33548 in conjunction with 32020, 33210, 33211, 33310, 33315)

(For Batista procedure or pachopexy, use 33999)

CORONARY ENDARTERECTOMY

+ **33572** Coronary endarterectomy, open, any method, of left anterior descending, circumflex, or right coronary artery performed in conjunction with coronary artery bypass graft procedure, each vessel (List separately in addition to primary procedure)

(Use 33572 in conjunction with 33510-33516, 33533-33536)

SINGLE VENTRICLE AND OTHER COMPLEX CARDIAC ANOMALIES

33600 Closure of atrioventricular valve (mitral or tricuspid) by suture or patch

33602 Closure of semilunar valve (aortic or pulmonary) by suture or patch

33606 Anastomosis of pulmonary artery to aorta (Damus-Kaye-Stansel procedure)

33608 Repair of complex cardiac anomaly other than pulmonary atresia with ventricular septal defect by construction or replacement of conduit from right or left ventricle to pulmonary artery

(For repair of pulmonary artery arborization anomalies by unifocalization, see 33925-33926)

33610 Repair of complex cardiac anomalies (eg, single ventricle with subaortic obstruction) by surgical enlargement of ventricular septal defect

(Do not report modifier '-63' in conjunction with 33610)

33611 Repair of double outlet right ventricle with intraventricular tunnel repair;

(Do not report modifier '-63' in conjunction with 33611)

33612 with repair of right ventricular outflow tract obstruction

33615 Repair of complex cardiac anomalies (eg, tricuspid atresia) by closure of atrial septal defect and anastomosis of atria or vena cava to pulmonary artery (simple Fontan procedure)

33617 Repair of complex cardiac anomalies (eg, single ventricle) by modified Fontan procedure

(Use 33617 in conjunction with 33768 when a cavopulmonary anastomosis to a second superior vena cava is performed)

33619 Repair of single ventricle with aortic outflow obstruction and aortic arch hypoplasia (hypoplastic left heart syndrome) (eg, Norwood procedure)

(Do not report modifier '-63' in conjunction with 33619)

SEPTAL DEFECT

33641 Repair atrial septal defect, secundum, with cardiopulmonary bypass, with or without patch

33645 Direct or patch closure, sinus venosus, with or without anomalous pulmonary venous drainage

(Do not report 33645 in conjunction with 33724, 33726)

● New Code ▲ Revised Code + Add-On Code ⊘ Modifier -51 Exempt ⊙ Conscious Sedation

33647 Repair of atrial septal defect and ventricular septal defect, with direct or patch closure

(Do not report modifier -63 in conjunction with 33647)

(For repair of tricuspid atresia (eg., Fontan, Gago procedures), use 33615)

33660 Repair of incomplete or partial atrioventricular canal (ostium primum atrial septal defect), with or without atrioventricular valve repair

33665 Repair of intermediate or transitional atrioventricular canal, with or without atrioventricular valve repair

33670 Repair of complete atrioventricular canal, with or without prosthetic valve

(Do not report modifier -63 in conjunction with 33670)

● **33675** Closure of multiple ventricular septal defects;

● **33676** with pulmonary valvotomy or infundibular resection (acyanotic)

● **33677** with removal of pulmonary artery band, with or without gusset

(Do not report 33675-33677 in conjunction with 32002, 32020, 32100, 33210, 33681, 33684, 33688)

(For transmyocardial closure, see Category III codes 0166T and 0167T)

(For percutaneous closure, use 93581)

▲ **33681** Closure of single ventricular septal defect, with or without patch;

33684 with pulmonary valvotomy or infundibular resection (acyanotic)

33688 with removal of pulmonary artery band, with or without gusset

(For pulmonary vein repair requiring creation of atrial septal defect, use 33724)

33690 Banding of pulmonary artery

(Do not report modifier -63 in conjunction with 33690)

33692 Complete repair tetralogy of Fallot without pulmonary atresia;

33694 with transannular patch

(Do not report modifier -63 in conjunction with 33694)

(For ligation and takedown of a systematic-to-pulmonary artery shunt, performed in conjunction with a congenital heart procedure, see 33924)

33697 Complete repair tetralogy of Fallot with pulmonary atresia including construction of conduit from right ventricle to pulmonary artery and closure of ventricular septal defect

(For ligation and takedown of a systemic-to-pulmonary artery shunt, performed in conjunction with a congenital heart procedure, see 33924)

SINUS OF VALSALVA

33702 Repair sinus of Valsalva fistula, with cardiopulmonary bypass;

33710 with repair of ventricular septal defect

33720 Repair sinus of Valsalva aneurysm, with cardiopulmonary bypass

33722 Closure of aortico-left ventricular tunnel

VENOUS ANOMALIES

● **33724** Repair of isolated partial anomalous pulmonary venous return (eg, Scimitar Syndrome)

(Do not report 33724 in conjunction with 32020, 33210, 33211)

● **33726** Repair of pulmonary venous stenosis

(Do not report 33726 in conjunction with 32020, 33210, 33211)

33730 Complete repair of anomalous venous return (supracardiac, intracardiac, or infracardiac types)

(Do not report modifier '-63' in conjunction with 33730)

(For partial anomalous pulmonary venous return, use 33724; for repair of pulmonary venous stenosis, use 33726)

● New Code ▲ Revised Code + Add-On Code ⦸ Modifier -51 Exempt ⊙ Conscious Sedation

33732 Repair of cor triatriatum or supravalvular mitral ring by resection of left atrial membrane

(Do not report modifier -63 in conjunction with 33732)

SHUNTING PROCEDURES

33735 Atrial septectomy or septostomy; closed heart (Blalock-Hanlon type operation)

33736 open heart with cardiopulmonary bypass

(Do not report modifier '-63' in conjunction with 33735, 33736)

33737 open heart, with inflow occlusion

(For transvenous method cadiac catheterization balloon atrial septectomy or septostomy (Rashkind type), use 92992)

(For blade method cardiac catheterization atrial septectomy or septostomy (Sang-Park septostomy), use 92993)

33750 Shunt; subclavian to pulmonary artery (Blalock-Taussig type operation)

33755 ascending aorta to pulmonary artery (Waterston type operation)

33762 descending aorta to pulmonary artery (Potts-Smith type operation)

(Do not report modifier -63 in conjunction with 33750, 33755, 33762)

33764 central, with prosthetic graft

33766 superior vena cava to pulmonary artery for flow to one lung (classical Glenn procedure)

33767 superior vena cava to pulmonary artery for flow to both lungs (bidirectional Glenn procedure)

+ **33768** Anastomosis, cavopulmonary, second superior vena cava (List separately in addition to primary procedure)

(Use 33768 in conjunction with 33478, 33617, 33767)

(Do not report 33768 in conjunction with 32020, 33210, 33211)

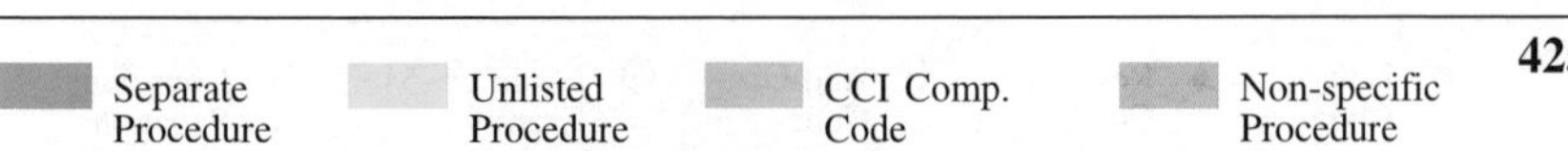

TRANSPOSITION OF THE GREAT VESSELS

33770 Repair of transposition of the great arteries with ventricular septal defect and subpulmonary stenosis; without surgical enlargement of ventricular septal defect

33771 with surgical enlargement of ventricular septal defect

33774 Repair of transposition of the great arteries, atrial baffle procedure (eg, Mustard or Senning type) with cardiopulmonary bypass;

33775 with removal of pulmonary band

33776 with closure of ventricular septal defect

33777 with repair of subpulmonic obstruction

33778 Repair of transposition of the great arteries, aortic pulmonary artery reconstruction (eg, Jatene type);

(Do not report modifier '-63' in conjunction with 33778)

33779 with removal of pulmonary band

33780 with closure of ventricular septal defect

33781 with repair of subpulmonic obstruction

TRUNCUS ARTERIOSUS

33786 Total repair, truncus arteriosus (Rastelli type operation)

(Do not report modifier '-63' in conjunction with 33786)

33788 Reimplantation of an anomalous pulmonary artery

(For pulmonary artery band, use 33690)

AORTIC ANOMALIES

33800 Aortic suspension (aortopexy) for tracheal decompression (eg, for tracheomalacia) (separate procedure)

33802 Division of aberrant vessel (vascular ring);

33803 with reanastomosis

● New Code ▲ Revised Code + Add-On Code ⃠ Modifier -51 Exempt ⊙ Conscious Sedation

33813 Obliteration of aortopulmonary septal defect; without cardiopulmonary bypass

33814 with cardiopulmonary bypass

33820 Repair of patent ductus arteriosus; by ligation

33822 by division, under 18 years

33824 by division, 18 years and older

33840 Excision of coarctation of aorta, with or without associated patent ductus arteriosus; with direct anastomosis

33845 with graft

33851 repair using either left subclavian artery or prosthetic material as gusset for enlargement

33852 Repair of hypoplastic or interrupted aortic arch using autogenous or prosthetic material; without cardiopulmonary bypass

33853 with cardiopulmonary bypass

(For repair of hypoplastic left heart syndrome (eg., Norwood type), via excision of coarctation of aorta, use 33619)

THORACIC AORTIC ANEURYSM

33860 Ascending aorta graft, with cardiopulmonary bypass, with or without valve suspension;

33861 with coronary reconstruction

33863 with aortic root replacement using composite prosthesis and coronary reconstruction

(For grafting of ascending aorta, with cardiopulmonary bypass and valve replacement, with or without coronary implant or valve suspension; use 33860 or 33861 and 33405 or 33406)

33870 Transverse arch graft, with cardiopulmonary bypass

33875 Descending thoracic aorta graft, with or without bypass

Separate Procedure  Unlisted Procedure 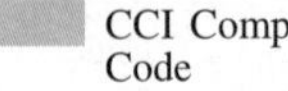 CCI Comp. Code 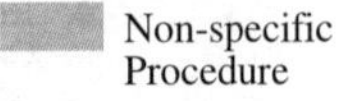 Non-specific Procedure

33877 Repair of thoracoabdominal aortic aneurysm with graft, with or without cardiopulmonary bypass

ENDOVASCULAR REPAIR OF DESCENDING THORACIC AORTA

33880 Endovascular repair of descending thoracic aorta (eg, aneurysm, pseudoaneurysm, dissection, penetrating ulcer, intramural hematoma, or traumatic disruption); involving coverage of left subclavian artery origin, initial endoprosthesis plus descending thoracic aortic extension(s), if required, to level of celiac artery origin

(For radiological supervision and interpretation, use 75956 in conjunction with 33880)

33881 not involving coverage of left subclavian artery origin, initial endoprosthesis plus descending thoracic aortic extension(s), if required, to level of celiac artery origin

(For radiological supervision and interpretation, use 75957 in conjunction with 33881)

33883 Placement of proximal extension prosthesis for endovascular repair of descending thoracic aorta (eg, aneurysm, pseudoaneurysm, dissection, penetrating ulcer, intramural hematoma, or traumatic disruption); initial extension

(For radiological supervision and interpretation, use 75958 in conjunction with 33883)

(Do not report 33881, 33883 when extension placement converts repair to cover left subclavian origin. Use only 33880)

+ 33884 each additional proximal extension (List separately in addition to code for primary procedure)

(Use 33884 in conjunction with 33883)

(For radiological supervision and interpretation, use 75958 in conjunction with 33884)

33886 Placement of distal extension prosthesis(es) delayed after endovascular repair of descending thoracic aorta

(Do not report 33886 in conjunction with 33880, 33881)

(Report 33886 once, regardless of number of modules deployed)

(For radiological supervision and interpretation, use 75959 in conjunction with 33886)

33889 Open subclavian to carotid artery transposition performed in conjunction with endovascular repair of descending thoracic aorta, by neck incision, unilateral

(Do not report 33889 in conjunction with 35694)

33891 Bypass graft, with other than vein, transcervical retropharyngeal carotid-carotid, performed in conjunction with endovascular repair of descending thoracic aorta, by neck incision

(Do not report 33891 in conjunction with 35509, 35601)

PULMONARY ARTERY

33910 Pulmonary artery embolectomy; with cardiopulmonary bypass

33915 without cardiopulmonary bypass

33916 Pulmonary endarterectomy, with or without embolectomy, with cardiopulmonary bypass

33917 Repair of pulmonary artery stenosis by reconstruction with patch or graft

(33918 deleted 2006 edition. To report, see 33925, 33926)

(33919 deleted 2006 edition. To report, see 33925, 33926)

33920 Repair of pulmonary atresia with ventricular septal defect, by construction or replacement of conduit from right or left ventricle to pulmonary artery

(For repair of other complex cardiac anomalies by construction or replacement of right or left ventricle to pulmonary artery conduit, use 33608)

33922 Transection of pulmonary artery with cardiopulmonary bypass

(Do not report modifier '-63' in conjunction with 33922)

\+ **33924** Ligation and takedown of a systemic-to-pulmonary artery shunt, performed in conjunction with a congenital heart procedure (List separately in addition to code for primary procedure)

(Use 33924 in conjunction with 33470-33475, 33600-33619, 33684-33688, 33692-33697, 33735-33767, 33770-33781, 33786, 33920-33922)

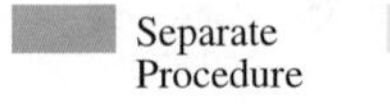

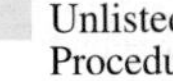

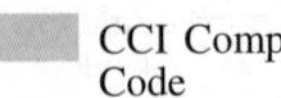

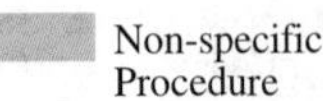

33925 Repair of pulmonary artery arborization anomalies by unifocalization; without cardiopulmonary bypass

33926 with cardiopulmonary bypass

HEART/LUNG TRANSPLANTATION

Heart with or without lung allotransplantation involves three distinct components of physician work:

1) **Cadaver donor cardiectomy with or without pneumonectomy**, which includes harvesting the allograft and cold preservation of the allograft (perfusing with cold preservation solution and cold maintenance) (see 33930, 33940).

2) **Backbench work**:

Preparation of a cadaver donor heart and lung allograft prior to transplantation, including dissection of the allograft from surrounding soft tissues to prepare the aorta, superior vena cava, inferior vena cava, and trachea for implantation (use 33933).

Preparation of a cadaver donor heart allograft prior to transplantation, including dissection of the allograft from surrounding soft tissues to prepare aorta, superior vena cava, inferior vena cava, pulmonary artery, and left atrium for implantation (use 33944).

3) **Recipient heart with or without lung allotransplantation**, which includes transplantation of allograft and care of the recipient (see 33935, 33945).

(For implantation of a total replacement heart system (artificial heart) with recipient cardiectomy or heart replacement system components, see Category III codes 0051T-0053T)

33930 Donor cardiectomy-pneumonectomy (including cold preservation)

33933 Backbench standard preparation of cadaver donor heart/lung allograft prior to transplantation, including dissection of allograft from surrounding soft tissues to prepare aorta, superior vena cava, inferior vena cava, and trachea for implantation

33935 Heart-lung transplant with recipient cardiectomy-pneumonectomy

33940 Donor cardiectomy (including cold preservation)

33944 Backbench standard preparation of cadaver donor heart allograft prior to transplantation, including dissection of allograft from surrounding soft tissues to prepare aorta, superior vena cava, inferior vena cava, pulmonary artery, and left atrium for implantation

(For repair or resection procedures on the donor heart, see 33300, 33310, 33320, 33400, 33463, 33464, 33510, 33641, 35216, 35276 or 35685)

33945 Heart transplant, with or without recipient cardiectomy

CARDIAC ASSIST

(For percutaneous implantation of extracorporeal ventricular assist device or for removal of percutaneously implanted extracorporeal ventricular assist device, see Category III codes 0048T-0050T)

33960 Prolonged extracorporeal circulation for cardiopulmonary insufficiency; initial 24 hours

+ **33961** each additional 24 hours (List separately in addition to code for primary procedure)

(Do not report modifier '-63' in conjunction with 33960, 33961)

(Use 33961 in conjunction with code 33960)

(For insertion of cannula for prolonged extracorporeal circulation, use 36822)

33967 Insertion of intra-aortic balloon assist device, percutaneous

33968 Removal of intra-aortic balloon assist device, percutaneous

33970 Insertion of intra-aortic balloon assist device through the femoral artery, open approach

33971 Removal of intra-aortic balloon assist device including repair of femoral artery, with or without graft

33973 Insertion of intra-aortic balloon assist device through the ascending aorta

33974 Removal of intra-aortic balloon assist device from the ascending aorta, including repair of the ascending aorta, with or without graft

33975 Insertion of ventricular assist device; extracorporeal, single ventricle

33976 extracorporeal, biventricular

33977 Removal of ventricular assist device; extracorporeal, single ventricle

33978 extracorporeal, biventricular

33979 Insertion of ventricular assist device, implantable intracorporeal, single ventricle

33980 Removal of ventricular assist device, implantable intracorporeal, single ventricle

OTHER PROCEDURES, CARDIAC SURGERY

33999 Unlisted procedure, cardiac surgery

ARTERIES AND VEINS

EMBOLECTOMY/THROMBECTOMY

Arterial, With or Without Catheter

34001 Embolectomy or thrombectomy, with or without catheter; carotid, subclavian or innominate artery, by neck incision

34051 innominate, subclavian artery, by thoracic incision

34101 axillary, brachial, innominate, subclavian artery, by arm incision

34111 radial or ulnar artery, by arm incision

34151 renal, celiac, mesentery, aortoiliac artery, by abdominal incision

34201 femoropopliteal, aortoiliac artery, by leg incision

34203 popliteal-tibio-peroneal artery, by leg incision

Venous, Direct or With Catheter

34401 Thrombectomy, direct or with catheter; vena cava, iliac vein, by abdominal incision

34421 vena cava, iliac, femoropopliteal vein, by leg incision

34451 vena cava, iliac, femoropopliteal vein, by abdominal and leg incision

34471 subclavian vein, by neck incision

34490 axillary and subclavian vein, by arm incision

VENOUS RECONSTRUCTION

34501 Valvuloplasty, femoral vein

34502 Reconstruction of vena cava, any method

34510 Venous valve transposition, any vein donor

34520 Cross-over vein graft to venous system

34530 Saphenopopliteal vein anastomosis

ENDOVASCULAR REPAIR OF ABDOMINAL AORTIC ANEURYSM

34800 Endovascular repair of infrarenal abdominal aortic aneurysm or dissection; using aorto-aortic tube prosthesis

34802 using modular bifurcated prosthesis (one docking limb)

34803 using modular bifurcated prosthesis (two docking limbs)

(For endovascular repair of abdominal aortic aneurysm or dissection involving visceral vessels using a fenestrated modular bifurcated prosthesis (two docking limbs), use Category III codes 0078T, 0079T)

34804 using unibody bifurcated prosthesis

34805 using aorto-uniiliac or aorto-unifemoral prosthesis

+ 34808 Endovascular placement of iliac artery occlusion device (List separately in addition to code for primary procedure)

(Use 34808 in conjunction with codes 34800, 34805, 34813, 34825, 34826)

(For radiological supervision and interpretation, use 75952 in conjunction with 34800-34808)

 Separate Procedure

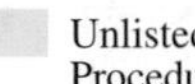 Unlisted Procedure

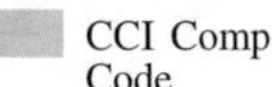 CCI Comp. Code

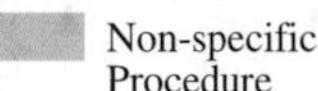 Non-specific Procedure

(For open arterial exposure, report codes 34812, 34820, 34833, 34834 as appropriate, in addition to codes 34800-34808)

34812 Open femoral artery exposure for delivery of endovascular prosthesis, by groin incision, unilateral

(For bilateral procedure, use modifier -50)

+ **34813** Placement of femoral-femoral prosthetic graft during endovascular aortic aneurysm repair (List separately in addition to code for primary procedure)

(Use 34813 in conjunction with code 34812)

(For femoral artery grafting, see 35521, 35533, 35539, 35540, 35551-35558, 35566, 35621, 35646, 35651-35661, 35666, 35700)

34820 Open iliac artery exposure for delivery of endovascular prosthesis or iliac occlusion during endovascular therapy, by abdominal or retroperitoneal incision, unilateral

(For bilateral procedure, use modifier -50)

34825 Placement of proximal or distal extension prosthesis for endovascular repair of infrarenal abdominal aortic or iliac aneurysm, false aneurysm, or dissection; initial vessel

+ **34826** each additional vessel (List separately in addition to code for primary procedure)

(Use 34826 in conjunction with code 34825)

(Use 34825, 34826 in addition to codes 34800-34808, 34900 as appropriate)

(For staged procedure, use modifier -58)

(For radiological supervision and interpretation, use 75953)

34830 Open repair of infrarenal aortic aneurysm or dissection, plus repair of associated arterial trauma, following unsuccessful endovascular repair; tube prosthesis

34831 aorto-bi-iliac prosthesis

34832 aorto-bifemoral prosthesis

34833 Open iliac artery exposure with creation of conduit for delivery of aortic or iliac endovascular prosthesis, by abdominal or retroperitoneal incision, unilateral

(For bilateral procedure, use modifier -50)

(Do not report 34833 in addition to 34820)

34834 Open brachial artery exposure to assist in the deployment of aortic or iliac endovascular prosthesis by arm incision, unilateral

(For bilateral procedure, use modifier -50)

ENDOVASCULAR REPAIR OF ILIAC ANEURYSM

34900 Endovascular graft replacement for repair of iliac artery (eg, aneurysm, pseudoaneurysm, arteriovenous malformation, trauma)

(For radiological supervision and interpretation, use 75954)

(For placement of extension prosthesis during endovascular iliac artery repair, use 34825)

(For bilateral procedure, use modifier '-50')

DIRECT REPAIR OF ANEURYSM OR EXCISION (PARTIAL OR TOTAL) AND GRAFT INSERTION FOR ANEURYSM, PSEUDOANEURYSM, RUPTURED ANEURYSM, AND ASSOCIATED OCCLUSIVE DISEASE

(For direct repairs associated with occlusive disease only, see 35201-35286)

(For intracranial aneurysm, see 61700 et seq)

(For endovascular repair of abdominal aortic aneurysm, see 34800-34826)

(For endovascular repair of iliac artery aneurysm, see 34900)

(For thoracic aortic aneurysm, see 33860-33875)

(For endovascular repair of descending thoracic aorta, involving coverage of left subclavian artery origin, use 33880)

35001 Direct repair of aneurysm, pseudoaneurysm, or excision (partial or total) and graft insertion, with or without patch graft; for aneurysm and associated occlusive disease, carotid, subclavian artery, by neck incision

35002 for ruptured aneurysm, carotid, subclavian artery, by neck incision

35005 for aneurysm, pseudoaneurysm, and associated occlusive disease, vertebral artery

35011 for aneurysm and associated occlusive disease, axillary-brachial artery, by arm incision

35013 for ruptured aneurysm, axillary-brachial artery, by arm incision

35021 for aneurysm, pseudoaneurysm, and associated occlusive disease, innominate, subclavian artery, by thoracic incision

35022 for ruptured aneurysm, innominate, subclavian artery, by thoracic incision

35045 for aneurysm, pseudoaneurysm, and associated occlusive disease, radial or ulnar artery

35081 for aneurysm, pseudoaneurysm, and associated occlusive disease, abdominal aorta

35082 for ruptured aneurysm, abdominal aorta

35091 for aneurysm, pseudoaneurysm, and associated occlusive disease, abdominal aorta involving visceral vessels (mesenteric, celiac, renal)

35092 for ruptured aneurysm, abdominal aorta involving visceral vessels (mesenteric, celiac, renal)

35102 for aneurysm, pseudoaneurysm, and associated occlusive disease, abdominal aorta involving iliac vessels (common, hypogastric, external)

35103 for ruptured aneurysm, abdominal aorta involving iliac vessels (common, hypogastric, external)

35111 for aneurysm, pseudoaneurysm, and associated occlusive disease, splenic artery

35112 for ruptured aneurysm, splenic artery

35121 for aneurysm, pseudoaneurysm, and associated occlusive disease, hepatic, celiac, renal, or mesenteric artery

35122 for ruptured aneurysm, hepatic, celiac, renal, or mesenteric artery

35131 for aneurysm, pseudoaneurysm, and associated occlusive disease, iliac artery (common, hypogastric, external)

35132 for ruptured aneurysm, iliac artery (common, hypogastric, external)

35141 for aneurysm, pseudoaneurysm, and associated occlusive disease, common femoral artery (profunda femoris, superficial femoral)

35142 for ruptured aneurysm, common femoral artery (profunda femoris, superficial femoral)

35151 for aneurysm, pseudoaneurysm, and associated occlusive disease, popliteal artery

35152 for ruptured aneurysm, popliteal artery

(35161 deleted 2005 edition. To report, use 37799)

(35162 deleted 2005 edition. To report, use 37799)

REPAIR ARTERIOVENOUS FISTULA

35180 Repair, congenital arteriovenous fistula; head and neck

35182 thorax and abdomen

35184 extremities

35188 Repair, acquired or traumatic arteriovenous fistula; head and neck

35189 thorax and abdomen

35190 extremities

REPAIR BLOOD VESSEL OTHER THAN FOR FISTULA, WITH OR WITHOUT PATCH ANGIOPLASTY

(For AV fistula repair, see 35180-35190)

35201 Repair blood vessel, direct; neck

35206 upper extremity

35207 hand, finger

35211 intrathoracic, with bypass

35216 intrathoracic, without bypass

35221 intra-abdominal

35226 lower extremity

35231 Repair blood vessel with vein graft; neck

35236 upper extremity

35241 intrathoracic, with bypass

35246 intrathoracic, without bypass

35251 intra-abdominal

35256 lower extremity

35261 Repair blood vessel with graft other than vein; neck

35266 upper extremity

35271 intrathoracic, with bypass

35276 intrathoracic, without bypass

35281 intra-abdominal

35286 lower extremity

THROMBOENDARTERECTOMY

(For coronary artery, see 33510-33536 and 33572)

(35301-35372 include harvest of saphenous or upper extremity vein when performed)

▲ **35301** Thromboendarterectomy, including patch graft, if performed; carotid, vertebral, subclavian, by neck incision

● **35302** superficial femoral artery

● **35303** popliteal artery

(Do not report 35302, 35303 in conjunction with 35483, 35500)

● **35304** tibioperoneal trunk artery

● New Code ▲ Revised Code + Add-On Code ⃠ Modifier -51 Exempt ⊙ Conscious Sedation

● **35305** tibial or peroneal artery, initial vessel

●+**35306** each additional tibial or peroneal artery (List separately in addition to code for primary procedure)

(Use 35306 in conjunction with 35305)

(Do not report 35304, 35305, 35306 in conjunction with 35485, 35500)

35311 subclavian, innominate, by thoracic incision

35321 axillary-brachial

35331 abdominal aorta

35341 mesenteric, celiac, or renal

35351 iliac

35355 iliofemoral

35361 combined aortoiliac

35363 combined aortoiliofemoral

35371 common femoral

35372 deep (profunda) femoral

(35381 deleted 2007 edition. For thromboendarterectomy of the superficial femoral artery, use 35302; of the popliteal artery, use 35303; of the tibioperoneal trunk, use 35304; of the tibial or peroneal artery, see 35305, 35306)

+ **35390** Reoperation, carotid, thromboendarterectomy, more than one month after original operation (List separately in addition to code for primary procedure)

(Use 35390 in conjunction with code 35301)

ANGIOSCOPY

+ **35400** Angioscopy (non-coronary vessels or grafts) during therapeutic intervention (List separately in addition to code for primary procedure)

TRANSLUMINAL ANGIOPLASTY

(For radiological supervision and interpretation, see 75962-75968 and 75978)

Open

35450 Transluminal balloon angioplasty, open; renal or other visceral artery

35452 aortic

35454 iliac

35456 femoral-popliteal

35458 brachiocephalic trunk or branches, each vessel

35459 tibioperoneal trunk and branches

35460 venous

Percutaneous

⊙ **35470** Transluminal balloon angioplasty, percutaneous; tibioperoneal trunk or branches, each vessel

⊙ **35471** renal or visceral artery

⊙ **35472** aortic

⊙ **35473** iliac

⊙ **35474** femoral-popliteal

⊙ **35475** brachiocephalic trunk or branches, each vessel

⊙ **35476** venous

(For radiological supervision and interpretation, use 75978)

TRANSLUMINAL ATHERECTOMY

(For radiological supervision and interpretation, see 75992-75996)

Open

35480 Transluminal peripheral atherectomy, open; renal or other visceral artery

35481 aortic

35482 iliac

35483 femoral-popliteal

35484 brachiocephalic trunk or branches, each vessel

35485 tibioperoneal trunk and branches

Percutaneous

35490 Transluminal peripheral atherectomy, percutaneous; renal or other visceral artery

35491 aortic

35492 iliac

35493 femoral-popliteal

35494 brachiocephalic trunk or branches, each vessel

35495 tibioperoneal trunk and branches

BYPASS GRAFT

Peripheral vascular bypass CPT codes describe bypass procedures using venous grafts (CPT codes 35501-35587) and using other types of bypass procedures (arterial reconstruction, composite). Because, at a given site of obstruction, only one type of bypass is performed, these groups of codes are mutually exclusive. When different sites are treated with different bypass procedures in the same operative session, the different bypass procedures may be separately reported, using an anatomic modifier or modifier -59.

Vein

+ **35500** Harvest of upper extremity vein, one segment, for lower extremity or coronary artery bypass procedure (List separately in addition to code for primary procedure)

(Use 35500 in conjunction with codes 33510-33536, 35556, 35566, 35571, 35583-35587)

(For harvest of more than one vein segment, see 35682, 35683)

(For endoscopic procedure, use 33508)

▲ **35501** Bypass graft, with vein; common carotid-ipsilateral internal carotid

▲ **35506** carotid-subclavian or subclavian-carotid

(35507 deleted 2007 edition, see 35506)

35508 carotid-vertebral

▲ **35509** carotid-contralateral carotid

35510 carotid-brachial

35511 subclavian-subclavian

35512 subclavian-brachial

35515 subclavian-vertebral

35516 subclavian-axillary

35518 axillary-axillary

35521 axillary-femoral

(For bypass graft performed with synthetic graft, use 35621)

35522 axillary-brachial

35525 brachial-brachial

35526 aortosubclavian or carotid

(For bypass graft performed with synthetic graft, use 35626)

35531 aortoceliac or aortomesenteric

35533 axillary-femoral-femoral

(For bypass graft performed with synthetic graft, use 35654)

35536 splenorenal

● 35537 Bypass graft, with vein; aortoiliac

(For bypass graft performed with synthetic graft, use 35637)

(Do not report 35537 in conjunction with 35538)

● 35538 aortobi-iliac

(For bypass graft performed with synthetic graft, use 35638)

(Do not report 35538 in conjunction with 35537)

● 35539 aortofemoral

(For bypass graft performed with synthetic graft, use 35647)

(Do not report 35539 in conjunction with 35540)

● 35540 aortobifemoral

(For bypass graft performed with synthetic graft, use 35646)

(Do not report 35540 in conjunction with 35539)

(35541 deleted 2007 edition. For aortoiliac graft with vein, use 35537. For aortobi-iliac graft with vein, use 35538)

(35546 deleted 2007 edition. For aortofemoral graft with vein, use 35539. For aortobifemoral graft with vein, use 35540)

35548 aortoiliofemoral, unilateral

(For bypass graft performed with synthetic graft, use 37799)

35549 aortoiliofemoral, bilateral

(For bypass graft performed with synthetic graft, use 37799)

35551 aortofemoral-popliteal

35556 femoral-popliteal

35558 femoral-femoral

35560 aortorenal

35563 ilioiliac

35565 iliofemoral

35566 femoral-anterior tibial, posterior tibial, peroneal artery or other distal vessels

35571 popliteal-tibial, -peroneal artery or other distal vessels

+ **35572** Harvest of femoropopliteal vein, one segment, for vascular reconstruction procedure (eg, aortic, vena caval, coronary, peripheral artery) (List separately in addition to code for primary procedure)

(Use 35572 in conjunction with codes 33510-33516, 33517-33523, 33533-33536, 34502, 34520, 35001, 35002, 35011-35022, 35102, 35103, 35121-35152, 35231-35256, 35501-35587, 35879-35907)

(For bilateral procedure, use modifier '-50')

In-Situ Vein

(35582 deleted 2005 edition)

(To report aortobifemoral bypass using synthetic conduit, and femoral-popliteal bypass with vein conduit in situ, use 35646 and 35583. To report aorto(uni)femoral bypass with synthetic conduit, and femoral-popliteal bypass with vein conduit in-situ, use 35647 and 35583. To report aortofemoral bypass using vein conduit, and femoral-popliteal bypass with vein conduit in situ, use 35539 and 35583)

35583 In-situ vein bypass; femoral-popliteal

35585 femoral-anterior tibial, posterior tibial, or peroneal artery

35587 popliteal-tibial, peroneal

Other Than Vein

(For aterial transposition and/or reimplantation, see 35691-35695)

⊘ 35600 Harvest of upper extremity artery, one segment, for coronary artery bypass procedure

▲ 35601 Bypass graft, with other than vein; common carotid-ipsilateral internal carotid

35606 carotid-subclavian

(For open transcervical common carotid-common carotid bypass performed in conjunction with endovascular repair of descending thoracic aorta, use 33891)

(For open subclavian to carotid artery transposition performed in conjunction with endovascular thoracic aneurysm repair by neck incision, use 33889)

35612 subclavian-subclavian

35616 subclavian-axillary

35621 axillary-femoral

35623 axillary-popliteal or -tibial

35626 aortosubclavian or carotid

35631 aortoceliac, aortomesenteric, aortorenal

35636 splenorenal (splenic to renal arterial anastomosis)

● 35637 aortoiliac

(Do not report 35637 in conjunction with 35638, 35646)

● 35638 aortobi-iliac

(Do not report 35638 in conjunction with 35637, 35646)

(35641 deleted 2007 edition. For aortoiliac graft constructed with conduit other than vein, use 35637. For aortobi-iliac graft with othre than vein, use 35638)

(For open placement of aorto-bi-iliac prosthesis following unsuccessful endovascular repair, use 34831)

Separate Procedure | Unlisted Procedure | CCI Comp. Code | Non-specific Procedure

35642 carotid-vertebral

35645 subclavian-vertebral

35646 aortobifemoral

(For bypass graft performed with vein graft, use 35540)

(For open placement of aortobifemoral prosthesis following unsuccessful endovascular repair, use 34832)

35647 aortofemoral

(For bypass graft performed with vein graft, use 35539)

35650 axillary-axillary

35651 aortofemoral-popliteal

35654 axillary-femoral-femoral

35656 femoral-popliteal

35661 femoral-femoral

35663 ilioiliac

35665 iliofemoral

35666 femoral-anterior tibial, posterior tibial, or peroneal artery

35671 popliteal-tibial or -peroneal artery

COMPOSITE GRAFTS

+ **35681** Bypass graft; composite, prosthetic and vein (List separately in addition to code for primary procedure)

(Do not report 35681 in addition to 35682, 35683)

+ **35682** autogenous composite, two segments of veins from two locations (List separately in addition to code for primary procedure)

(Do not report 35682 in addition to 35681, 35683)

+ **35683** autogenous composite, three or more segments of vein from two or more locations (List separately in addition to code for primary procedure)

(Do not report 35683 in addition to 35681, 35682)

ADJUVANT TECHNIQUES

(For composite graft(s), see 35681-35683)

+ **35685** Placement of vein patch or cuff at distal anastomosis of bypass graft, synthetic conduit (List separately in addition to code for primary procedure)

(Use 35685 in conjunction with codes 35656, 35666 or 35671)

+ **35686** Creation of distal arteriovenous fistula during lower extremity bypass surgery (non-hemodialysis) (List separately in addition to code for primary procedure)

(Use 35686 in conjunction with codes 35556, 35566, 35571, 35583-35587, 35623, 35656, 35666, 35671)

ARTERIAL TRANSPOSITION

35691 Transposition and/or reimplantation; vertebral to carotid artery

35693 vertebral to subclavian artery

35694 subclavian to carotid artery

(For open subclavian to carotid artery transposition performed in conjunction with endovascular repair of descending thoracic aorta, use 33889)

35695 carotid to subclavian artery

+ **35697** Reimplantation, visceral artery to infrarenal aortic prosthesis, each artery (List separately in addition to code for primary procedure)

(Do not report 35697 in conjunction with 33877)

EXCISION, EXPLORATION, REPAIR, REVISION

+ **35700** Reoperation, femoral-popliteal or femoral (popliteal)-anterior tibial, posterior tibial, peroneal artery or other distal vessels, more than one month after original operation (List separately in addition to code for primary procedure)

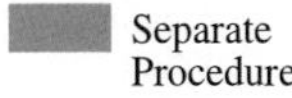 Separate Procedure
Unlisted Procedure
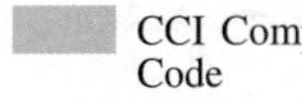 CCI Comp. Code
Non-specific Procedure

(Use 35700 in conjunction with codes 35556, 35566, 35571, 35583, 35585, 35587, 35656, 35666, 35671)

35701 Exploration (not followed by surgical repair), with or without lysis of artery; carotid artery

35721 femoral artery

35741 popliteal artery

35761 other vessels

35800 Exploration for postoperative hemorrhage, thrombosis or infection; neck

35820 chest

35840 abdomen

35860 extremity

35870 Repair of graft-enteric fistula

35875 Thrombectomy of arterial or venous graft (other than hemodialysis graft or fistula);

35876 with revision of arterial or venous graft

(For thrombectomy of hemodialysis graft or fistula, see 36831, 36833)

35879 Revision, lower extremity arterial bypass, without thrombectomy, open; with vein patch angioplasty

35881 with segmental vein interposition

(For revision or femoral anastomosis of sythetic arterial bypass graft, see 35883, 35884)

(For excision of infected graft, see 35901-35907 and appropriate revascularization code)

● **35883** Revision, femoral anastomosis of synthetic arterial bypass graft in groin, open; with nonautogenous patch graft (eg, Dacron, ePTFE, bovine pericardium)

(For bilateral procedure, use modifier 50)

● New Code ▲ Revised Code + Add-On Code ⦸ Modifier -51 Exempt ⊙ Conscious Sedation

(Do not report 35883 in conjunction with 35700, 35875, 35876, 35884)

● **35884** with autogenous vein patch graft

(For bilateral procedure, use modifier -50)

(Do not report 35884 in conjunction with 35700, 35875, 35876, 35883)

35901 Excision of infected graft; neck

35903 extremity

35905 thorax

35907 abdomen

VASCULAR INJECTION PROCEDURES

When using CPT codes from this section, note that the listed procedures include local anesthesia, introduction of needles or catheter, injection of contrast medium with or without automatic power injection, and pre- and post-injection care specifically related to the injection procedure.

Note that catheters, drugs and contrast media are not included in CPT codes listed in this section. These should be coded using CPT code 99070 or the appropriate HCPCS Level II code for Medicare patients.

CPT codes listed in this section do not cover radiological vascular injections, injection procedures for cardiac catheterization or chemotherapy. Refer to the RADIOLOGY or MEDICINE sections of CPT for the appropriate CPT codes for these procedures.

(For radiological supervision and interpretation, see RADIOLOGY)

(For injection procedures in conjunction with cardiac catheterization, see 93541-93545)

(For chemotherapy of malignant disease, see 96400-96549)

Intravenous

36000 Introduction of needle or intracatheter, vein

36002 Injection procedures (eg, thrombin) for percutaneous treatment of extremity pseudoaneurysm

Separate Procedure 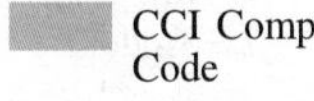 Unlisted Procedure CCI Comp. Code 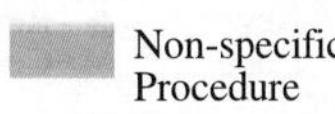 Non-specific Procedure

(For imaging guidance, see 76942, 77002, 77012, 77021)

(For ultrasound guided compression repair of pseudoaneurysms, use 76936)

(Do not report 36002 for vascular sealant of an arteriotomy site)

36005 Injection procedure for extremity venography (including introduction of needle or intracatheter)

(For radiological supervision and interpretation, see 75820, 75822)

36010 Introduction of catheter, superior or inferior vena cava

36011 Selective catheter placement, venous system; first order branch (eg, renal vein, jugular vein)

36012 second order, or more selective, branch (eg, left adrenal vein, petrosal sinus)

36013 Introduction of catheter, right heart or main pulmonary artery

36014 Selective catheter placement, left or right pulmonary artery

36015 Selective catheter placement, segmental or subsegmental pulmonary artery

(For insertion of flow directed catheter (eg, Swan-Ganz), use 93503)

(For venous catheterization for selective organ blood sampling, use 36500)

Intra-Arterial/Intra-Aortic

(For radiological supervision and interpretation, see RADIOLOGY)

36100 Introduction of needle or intracatheter, carotid or vertebral artery

(For bilateral procedure, report 36100 with modifier -50)

36120 Introduction of needle or intracatheter; retrograde brachial artery

36140 extremity artery

36145 arteriovenous shunt created for dialysis (cannula, fistula, or graft)

(For insertion of arteriovenous cannula, see 36810-36821)

36160 Introduction of needle or intracatheter, aortic, translumbar

36200 Introduction of catheter, aorta

36215 Selective catheter placement, arterial system; each first order thoracic or brachiocephalic branch, within a vascular family

(For catheter placement for coronary angiography, use 93508)

36216 initial second order thoracic or brachiocephalic branch, within a vascular family

36217 initial third order or more selective thoracic or brachiocephalic branch, within a vascular family

+ **36218** additional second order, third order, and beyond, thoracic or brachiocephalic branch, within a vascular family (List in addition to code for initial second or third order vessel as appropriate)

(Use 36218 in conjunction with codes 36216, 36217)

(For angiography, see 75600-75790)

(For angioplasty, see 35470-35475)

(For transcatheter therapies, see 37200-37208, 61624, 61626)

(When coronary artery, arterial conduit (eg., internal mammary, inferior epicastric or free radical artery) or venous bypass graft angiography is performed in conjunction with cardiac catheterization, see the appropriate cardiac catheterization, injection procedure, and imaging supervision code(s) (93501-93556) in the Medicine section of CPT. When coronary artery, arterial coronary conduit or venous bypass graft angiography is performed wihtout concomitant left heart cardiac catheterization, use 93508. When internal mammary artery angiography only is performed without a concomitant left heart cardiac catheterization, use 36216 or 36217 as appropriate.)

36245 Selective catheter placement, arterial system; each first order abdominal, pelvic, or lower extremity artery branch, within a vascular family

36246 initial second order abdominal, pelvic, or lower extremity artery branch, within a vascular family

36247 initial third order or more selective abdominal, pelvic, or lower extremity artery branch, within a vascular family

+ **36248** additional second order, third order, and beyond, abdominal, pelvic, or lower extremity artery branch, within a vascular family (List in addition to code for initial second or third order vessel as appropriate)

(Use 36248 in conjunction with codes 36246, 36247)

36260 Insertion of implantable intra-arterial infusion pump (eg, for chemotherapy of liver)

36261 Revision of implanted intra-arterial infusion pump

36262 Removal of implanted intra-arterial infusion pump

36299 Unlisted procedure, vascular injection

Venous

36400 Venipuncture, under age 3 years, necessitating physician's skill, not to be used for routine venipuncture; femoral or jugular vein

36405 scalp vein

36406 other vein

36410 Venipuncture, age 3 years or older, necessitating physician's skill (separate procedure), for diagnostic or therapeutic purposes (not to be used for routine venipuncture)

36415 Collection of venous blood by venipuncture

(Do not report modifier '-63' in conjunction with 36415)

36416 Collection of capillary blood specimen (eg, finger, heel, ear stick)

36420 Venipuncture, cutdown; under age 1 year

(Do not report modifier '-63' in conjunction with 36420)

36425 age 1 or over

● New Code ▲ Revised Code + Add-On Code ⊘ Modifier -51 Exempt ⊙ Conscious Sedation

36430 Transfusion, blood or blood components

36440 Push transfusion, blood, 2 years or under

36450 Exchange transfusion, blood; newborn

(Do not report modifier '-63' in conjunction with 36450)

36455 other than newborn

36460 Transfusion, intrauterine, fetal

(Do not report modifier '-63' in conjunction with 36460)

(For radiological supervision and interpretation, use 76941)

36468 Single or multiple injections of sclerosing solutions, spider veins (telangiectasia); limb or trunk

36469 face

36470 Injection of sclerosing solution; single vein

36471 multiple veins, same leg

36475 Endovenous ablation therapy of incompetent vein, extremity, inclusive of all imaging guidance and monitoring, percutaneous, radiofrequency; first vein treated

+ **36476** second and subsequent veins treated in a single extremity, each through separate access sites (list separately in addition to code for primary procedure)

(Use 36476 in conjunction with 36475)

(Do not report 36475, 36476 in conjunction with 36000-36005, 36410, 36425, 36478, 36479, 37204, 75894, 76000, 76001, 76937, 76942, 77002, 93970, 93971)

36478 Endovenous ablation therapy of incompetent vein, extremity, inclusive of all imaging guidance and monitoring, percutaneous, laser; first vein treated

+ **36479** second and subsequent veins treated in a single extremity, each through separate access sites (List separately in addition to code for primary procedure)

(Use 36479 in conjunction with 36478)

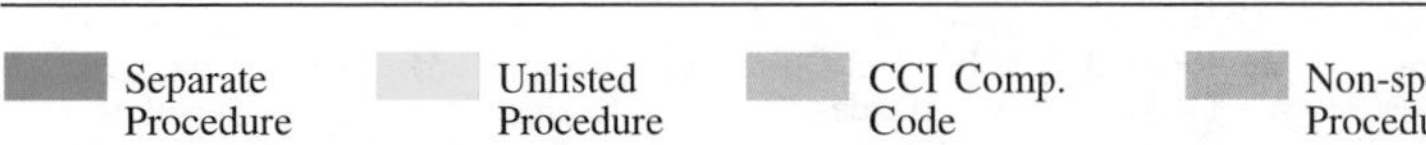

(Do not report 36478, 36479 in conjunction with 36000-36005, 36410, 36425, 36475, 36476, 37204, 75894, 76000, 76001, 76937, 76942, 77002, 93970, 93971)

36481 Percutaneous portal vein catheterization by any method

(For radiological supervision and interpretation, see 75885, 75887)

(36488 deleted 2004 edition. To report, see 36555-36556, 36568-36569, 36580, 36584)

(36489 deleted 2004 edition. To report, see 36555-36556, 36568-36569, 36580, 36584)

(36490 deleted 2004 edition. To report, see 36555-36556, 36568-36569, 36580, 36584)

(36491 deleted 2004 edition. To report, see 36555-36556, 36568-36569, 36580, 36584)

(36493 deleted 2004 edition. To report, use 36597)

36500 Venous catheterization for selective organ blood sampling

(For catheterization in superior or inferior vena cava, use 36010)

(For radiological supervision and interpretation, use 75893)

36510 Catheterization of umbilical vein for diagnosis or therapy, newborn

(Do not report modifier '-63' in conjunction with 36510)

36511 Therapeutic apheresis; for white blood cells

36512 for red blood cells

36513 for platelets

36514 for plasma pheresis

36515 with extracorporeal immunoadsorption and plasma reinfusion

36516 with extracorporeal selective adsorption or selective filtration and plasma reinfusion

(for physician evaluation, use modifier -26)

36522 Photopheresis, extracorporeal

(36530 deleted 2004 edition. To report, use 36563)

(36531 deleted 2004 edition. To report, see 36575-36576, 36578, 36581-36582, 36584-36585)

(36532 deleted 2004 edition. To report, use 36590)

(36533 deleted 2004 edition. To report, see 36557-36561, 36565-36566, 36570-36571)

(36534 deleted 2004 edition. To report, see 36575-36578, 36581-36583, 36585)

(36535 deleted 2004 edition. To report, use 36589)

(36536 deleted 2004 edition. To report, use 36595)

(36537 deleted 2004 edition. To report, use 36596)

36540 Collection of blood specimen from a completely implantable venous access device

(Do not report 36540 in conjunction with 36415, 36416)

(For collection of venous blood specimen by venipuncture, use 36415)

(For collection of capillary blood specimen, use 36416)

36550 Declotting by thrombolytic agent of implanted vascular access device or catheter

Central Venous Access Procedures

(For refilling and maintenance of an implantable pump or reservoir for intravenous or intra-arterial drug delivery, use 96530)

Insertion of Central Venous Access Device

⊙ **36555** Insertion of non-tunneled centrally inserted central venous catheter; under 5 years of age

(For peripherally inserted non-tunneled central venous catheter, under 5 years of age, use 36568)

36556 age 5 years or older

(For peripherally inserted non-tunneled central venous catheter, age 5 years or older, use 36569)

⊙ **36557** Insertion of tunneled centrally inserted central venous catheter, without subcutaneous port or pump; under 5 years of age

⊙ **36558** age 5 years or older

(For peripherally inserted central venous catheter with port, age 5 years or older, use 36571)

⊙ **36560** Insertion of tunneled centrally inserted central venous access device, with subcutaneous port; under 5 years of age

(For peripherally inserted central venous access device with subcutaneous port, under 5 years of age, use 36570)

⊙ **36561** age 5 years or older

(For peripherally inserted central venous catheter with subcutaneous port, 5 years or older, use 36571)

⊙ **36563** Insertion of tunneled centrally inserted central venous access device with subcutaneous pump

⊙ **36565** Insertion of tunneled centrally inserted central venous access device, requiring two catheters via two separate venous access sites; without subcutaneous port or pump (eg, Tesio type catheter)

⊙ **36566** with subcutaneous port(s)

⊙ **36568** Insertion of peripherally inserted central venous catheter (PICC), without subcutaneous port or pump; under 5 years of age

(For placement of centrally inserted non-tunneled central venous catheter, without subcutaneous port or pump, under 5 years of age, use 36555)

36569 age 5 years or older

(For placement of centrally inserted non-tunneled central venous catheter, without subcutaneous port or pump, age 5 years or older, use 36556)

⊙ **36570** Insertion of peripherally inserted central venous access device, with subcutaneous port; under 5 years of age

● New Code ▲ Revised Code + Add-On Code ⊘ Modifier -51 Exempt ⊙ Conscious Sedation

(For insertion of tunneled centrally inserted central venous access device with subcutaneous port, under 5 years of age, use 36560)

⊙ **36571** age 5 years or older

(For insertion of tunneled centrally inserted central venous access device with subcutaneous port, age 5 years or older, use 36561)

Repair of Central Venous Access Device

(For mechanical removal of pericatheter obstructive material, use 36595)

(For mechancial removal of intracatheter obstructive material, use 36596)

36575 Repair of tunneled or non-tunneled central venous access catheter, without subcutaneous port or pump, central or peripheral insertion site

⊙ **36576** Repair of central venous access device, with subcutaneous port or pump, central or peripheral insertion site

Partial Replacement of Central Venous Access Device (Catheter Only)

⊙ **36578** Replacement, catheter only, of central venous access device, with subcutaneous port or pump, central or peripheral insertion site

(For complete replacement of entire device through same venous access, use 36582 or 36583)

Complete Replacement of Central Venous Access Device Through Same Venous Access Site

36580 Replacement, complete, of a non-tunneled centrally inserted central venous catheter, without subcutaneous port or pump, through same venous access

⊙ **36581** Replacement, complete, of a tunneled centrally inserted central venous catheter, without subcutaneous port or pump, through same venous access

⊙ **36582** Replacement, complete, of a tunneled centrally inserted central venous access device, with subcutaneous port, through same venous access

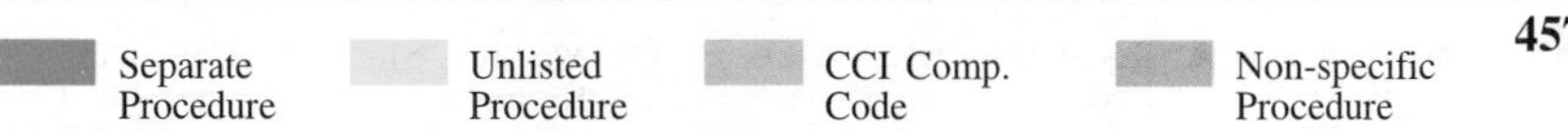

⊙ **36583** Replacement, complete, of a tunneled centrally inserted central venous access device, with subcutaneous pump, through same venous access

36584 Replacement, complete, of a peripherally inserted central venous catheter (PICC), without subcutaneous port or pump, through same venous access

⊙ **36585** Replacement, complete, of a peripherally inserted central venous access device, with subcutaneous port, through same venous access

Removal of Central Venous Access Device

36589 Removal of tunneled central venous catheter, without subcutaneous port or pump

⊙ **36590** Removal of tunneled central venous access device, with subcutaneous port or pump, central or peripheral insertion

(Do not report 36589 or 36590 for removal of non-tunneled central venous catheters)

Mechanical Removal of Obstructive Material

36595 Mechanical removal of pericatheter obstructive material (eg, fibrin sheath) from central venous device via separate venous access

(Do not report 36550 in addition to 36595)

(For venous catheterization, see 36010-36012)

(For radiological supervision and interpretation, use 75901)

36596 Mechanical removal of intraluminal (intracatheter) obstructive material from central venous device through device lumen

(Do not report 36550 in addition to 36596)

(For venous catheterization, see 36010-36012)

(For radiological supervision and interpretation, use 75902)

Other Central Venous Access Procedures

36597 Repositioning of previously placed central venous catheter under fluoroscopic guidance

(For fluoroscopic guidance, use 76000)

● New Code ▲ Revised Code + Add-On Code ⊘ Modifier -51 Exempt ⊙ Conscious Sedation

36598 Contrast injection(s) for radiologic evaluation of existing central venous access device, including fluoroscopy, image documentation and report

(Do not report 36598 in conjunction with 76000)

(Do not report 36598 in conjunction with 36595, 36596)

(For complete diagnostic studies, see 75820, 75825, 75827)

ARTERIAL

36600 Arterial puncture, withdrawal of blood for diagnosis

⊘ **36620** Arterial catheterization or cannulation for sampling, monitoring or transfusion (separate procedure); percutaneous

36625 cutdown

36640 Arterial catheterization for prolonged infusion therapy (chemotherapy), cutdown

(See also 96420-96425)

(For arterial catheterization for occlusion therapy, see 75894)

⊘ **36660** Catheterization, umbilical artery, newborn, for diagnosis or therapy

(Do not report modifier '-63' in conjunction with 36660)

INTRAOSSEOUS

36680 Placement of needle for intraosseous infusion

HEMODIALYSIS ACCESS, INTERVASCULAR CANNULIZATION FOR EXTRACORPOREAL CIRCULATION, OR SHUNT INSERTION

36800 Insertion of cannula for hemodialysis, other purpose (separate procedure); vein to vein

36810 arteriovenous, external (Scribner type)

36815 arteriovenous, external revision, or closure

36818 Arteriovenous anastomosis, open; by upper arm cephalic vein transposition

(Do not report 36818 in conjunction with 36819, 36820, 36821, 36830 during a unilateral upper extremity procedure. For

Separate Procedure | Unlisted Procedure | CCI Comp. Code | Non-specific Procedure

bilateral upper extremity open arteriovenous anastomoses performed at the same operative session, use modifier 50 or 59 as appropriate)

36819 by upper arm basilic vein transposition

(Do not report 36819 in conjunction with 36818, 36820, 36821, 36830 during a unilateral upper extremity procedure. For bilateral upper extremity open arteriovenous anastomoses performed at the same operative session, use modifier 50 or 59 as appropriate)

36820 by forearm vein transposition

36821 direct, any site (eg, Cimino type) (separate procedure)

36822 Insertion of cannula(s) for prolonged extracorporeal circulation for cardiopulmonary insufficiency (ECMO) (separate procedure)

(For maintenance of prolonged extracorporeal circulation, use 33960, 33961)

36823 Insertion of arterial and venous cannula(s) for isolated extracorporeal circulation including regional chemotherapy perfusion to an extremity, with or without hyperthermia, with removal of cannula(s) and repair of arteriotomy and venotomy sites

(36823 includes chemotherapy perfusion supported by a membrane oxygenator/perfusion pump. Do not report 96408-96425 in conjunction with 36823)

36825 Creation of arteriovenous fistula by other than direct arteriovenous anastomosis (separate procedure); autogenous graft

(For direct arteriovenous anastomosis, use 36821)

36830 nonautogenous graft (eg, biological collagen, thermoplastic graft)

(For direct arteriovenous anastomosis, use 36821)

36831 Thrombectomy, open, arteriovenous fistula without revision, autogenous or nonautogenous dialysis graft (separate procedure)

36832 Revision, open, arteriovenous fistula; without thrombectomy, autogenous or nonautogenous dialysis graft (separate procedure)

36833 with thrombectomy, autogenous or nonautogenous dialysis graft (separate procedure)

36834 Plastic repair of arteriovenous aneurysm (separate procedure)

36835 Insertion of Thomas shunt (separate procedure)

36838 Distal revascularization and interval ligation (DRIL), upper extremity hemodialysis access (steal syndrome)

(Do not report 36838 in conjunction with 35512, 35522, 36832, 37607, 37618)

36860 External cannula declotting (separate procedure); without balloon catheter

36861 with balloon catheter

(If imaging guidance is performed, use 76000)

⊙ **36870** Thrombectomy, percutaneous, arteriovenous fistula, autogenous or nonautogenous graft (includes mechanical thrombus extraction and intra-graft thrombolysis)

(Do not report 36550 in conjunction with code 36870)

(For catheterization, use 36145)

(For radiological supervision and interpretation, use 75790)

PORTAL DECOMPRESSION PROCEDURES

37140 Venous anastomosis, open; portocaval

(For peritoneal-venous shunt, use 49425)

37145 renoportal

37160 caval-mesenteric

37180 splenorenal, proximal

37181 splenorenal, distal (selective decompression of esophagogastric varices, any technique)

(For percutaneous procedure, use 37182)

37182 Insertion of transvenous intrahepatic portosystemic shunt(s) (TIPS) (includes venous access, hepatic and portal vein catheterization, portography with hemodynamic evaluation, intrahepatic tract formation/dilatation, stent placement and all associated imaging guidance and documentation)

Separate Procedure | Unlisted Procedure | CCI Comp. Code | Non-specific Procedure

(Do not report 75885 or 75887 in conjunction with code 37182)

(For open procedure, use 37140)

37183 Revision of transvenous intrahepatic portosystemic shunt(s) (TIPS) (includes venous access, hepatic and portal vein catheterization, portography with hemodynamic evaluation, intrahepatic tract recanulization/dilatation, stent placement and all associated imaging guidance and documentation)

(Do not report 75885 or 75887 in conjunction with code 37183)

(For repair of arteriovenous aneurysm, use 36834)

TRANSCATHETER PROCEDURES

Arterial Mechanical Thrombectomy

⊙ **37184** Primary percutaneous transluminal mechanical thrombectomy, noncoronary, arterial or arterial bypass graft, including fluoroscopic guidance and intraprocedural pharmacological thrombolytic injection(s); initial vessel

(Do not report 37184 in conjunction with 76000, 76001, 90774, 99143-99150)

⊙+**37185** second and all subsequent vessel(s) within the same vascular family (List separately in addition to code for primary mechanical thrombectomy procedure)

(Do not report 37185 in conjunction with 76000, 76001, 90775)

⊙+**37186** Secondary percutaneous transluminal thrombectomy (eg, nonprimary mechanical, snare basket, suction technique), noncoronary, arterial or arterial bypass graft, including fluoroscopic guidance and intraprocedural pharmacological thrombolytic injections, provided in conjunction with another percutaneous intervention other than primary mechanical thrombectomy (List separately in addition to code for primary procedure)

(Do not report 37186 in conjunction with 76000, 76001, 90775)

Venous Mechanical Thrombectomy

⊙ **37187** Percutaneous transluminal mechanical thrombectomy, vein(s), including intraprocedural pharmacological thrombolytic injections and fluoroscopic guidance

● New Code ▲ Revised Code + Add-On Code ⃠ Modifier -51 Exempt ⊙ Conscious Sedation

(Do not report 37187 in conjunction with 76000, 76001, 90775)

⊙ **37188** Percutaneous transluminal mechanical thrombectomy, vein(s), including intraprocedural pharmacological thrombolytic injections and fluoroscopic guidance, repeat treatment on subsequent day during course of thrombolytic therapy

(Do not report 37188 in conjunction with 76000, 76001, 90775)

Other Procedures

37195 Thrombolysis, cerebral, by intravenous infusion

37200 Transcatheter biopsy

(For radiological supervision and interpretation, use 75970)

37201 Transcatheter therapy, infusion for thrombolysis other than coronary

(For radiological supervision and interpretation, use 75896)

37202 Transcatheter therapy, infusion other than for thrombolysis, any type (eg, spasmolytic, vasoconstrictive)

(For thrombolysis of coronary vessels, see 92975, 92977)

(For radiological supervision and interpretation, use 75896)

⊙ **37203** Transcatheter retrieval, percutaneous, of intravascular foreign body (eg, fractured venous or arterial catheter)

(For radiological supervision and interpretation, use 75961)

37204 Transcatheter occlusion or embolization (eg, for tumor destruction, to achieve hemostasis, to occlude a vascular malformation), percutaneous, any method, non-central nervous system, non-head or neck

(See also 61624, 61626)

(For radiological supervision and interpretation, use 75894)

(For uterine fibroid embolization [uterine artery embolization performed to treat uterine fibroids], use 37210)

(For obstetrical and gynecological embolization procedures other than uterine fibroid embolization (eg., embolization to treat obstetrical or postpartum hemorrhage), use 37204)

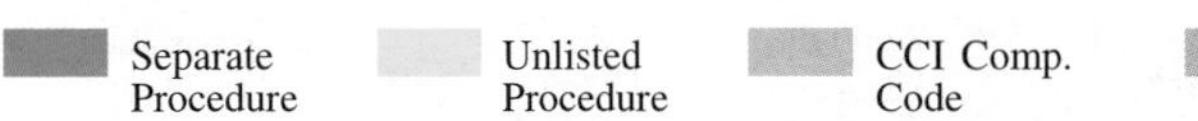

37205 Transcatheter placement of an intravascular stent(s), (except coronary, carotid, and vertebral vessel), percutaneous; initial vessel

(For radiological supervision and interpretation, use 75960)

(For coronary stent placement, see 92980, 92981; intracranial, use 61635)

+ **37206** each additional vessel (List separately in addition to code for primary procedure)

(Use 37206 in conjunction with 37205)

(For transcatheter placement of intravascular cervical carotid artery stent(s), see 37215, 37216)

(For transcatheter placement of extracranial vertebral or intrathoracic carotid artery stent(s), see Category III codes 0075T, 0076T)

(For radiological supervision and interpretation, use 75960)

37207 Transcatheter placement of an intravascular stent(s), (non-coronary vessel), open; initial vessel

+ **37208** each additional vessel (List separately in addition to code for primary procedure)

(Use 37208 in conjunction with 37207)

(For radiological supervision and interpretation, use 75960)

(For catheterizations, see 36215-36248)

(For transcatheter placement of intracoronary stent(s), see 92980, 92981)

37209 Exchange of a previously placed intravascular catheter during thrombolytic therapy

(For radiological supervision and interpretation, use 75900)

●⊙**37210** Uterine fibroid embolization (UFE, embolization of the uterine arteries to treat uterine fibroids, leiomyomata), percutaneous approach inclusive of vascular access, vessel selection, embolization, and all radiological supervision and interpretation, intraprocedural roadmapping, and imaging guidance necessary to complete the procedure

(37210 includes all catheterization and intraprocedural imaging required for a UFE procedure to confirm the presence of

● New Code ▲ Revised Code + Add-On Code ⃠ Modifier -51 Exempt ⊙ Conscious Sedation

previously known fibroids and to roadmap vascular anatomy to enable appropriate therapy)

(Do not report 37210 in conjunction with 36200, 36245-36248, 37204, 75894, 75898)

(For all othre non-central nervous system (CNS) embolization procedures, use 37204)

⊙ **37215** Transcatheter placement of intravascular stent(s), cervical carotid artery, percutaneous; with distal embolic protection

⊙ **37216** without distal embolic protection

(37215 and 37216 include all ipsilateral selective carotid catheterization, all diagnostic imaging for ipsilateral, cervical and cerebral carotid arteriography, and all related radiological supervision and interpretation. When ipsilateral carotid arteriogram (including imaging and selective catheterization) confirms the need for carotid stenting, 37215 and 37216 are inclusive of these services. If carotid stenting is not indicated, then the appropriate codes for carotid catheterization and imaging should be reported in lieu of 37215 and 37216)

(Do not report 37215, 37216 in conjunction with 75671, 75680)

(For transcatheter placement of extracranial vertebral or intrathoracic carotid artery stent(s), see Category III codes 0075T, 0076T)

(For percutaneous transcatheter placement of intravascular stents other than coronary, carotid, or vertebral, see 37205, 37206)

INTRAVASCULAR ULTRASOUND SERVICES

+ **37250** Intravascular ultrasound (non-coronary vessel) during diagnostic evaluation and/or therapeutic intervention; initial vessel (List separately in addition to code for primary procedure)

+ **37251** each additional vessel (List separately in addition to code for primary procedure)

(Use 37251 in conjunction with 37250)

(For catheterizations, see 36215-36248)

(For transcatheter therapies, see 37200-37208, 61624, 61626)

(For radiological supervision and interpretation, see 75945, 75946)

ENDOSCOPY

37500 Vascular endoscopy, surgical, with ligation or perforator veins, subfascial (SEPS)

(For open procedure, use 37760)

37501 Unlisted vascular endoscopy procedure

LIGATION

(For phleborraphy and arteriorraphy, see 35201-35286)

37565 Ligation, internal jugular vein

37600 Ligation; external carotid artery

37605 internal or common carotid artery

37606 internal or common carotid artery, with gradual occlusion, as with Selverstone or Crutchfield clamp

(For transcatheter permanent arterial occlusion or embolization, see 61624-61626)

(For endovascular temporary arterial balloon occlusion, use 61623)

(For ligation treatment of intracranial aneurysm, use 61703)

37607 Ligation or banding of angioaccess arteriovenous fistula

37609 Ligation or biopsy, temporal artery

37615 Ligation, major artery (eg, post-traumatic, rupture); neck

37616 chest

37617 abdomen

37618 extremity

37620 Interruption, partial or complete, of inferior vena cava by suture, ligation, plication, clip, extravascular, intravascular (umbrella device)

(For radiological supervision and interpretation, use 75940)

37650 Ligation of femoral vein

(For bilateral procedure, report 37650 with modifier -50)

37660 Ligation of common iliac vein

37700 Ligation and division of long saphenous vein at saphenofemoral junction, or distal interruptions

(Do not report 37700 in conjunction with 37718, 37722)

(For bilateral procedure, report 37700 with modifier -50)

37718 Ligation, division, and stripping, short saphenous vein

(For bilateral procedure, use modifier 50)

(Do not report 37718 in conjunction with 37735, 37780)

(37720 deleted 2006 edition.)

37722 Ligation, division, and stripping, long (greater) saphenous veins from saphenofemoral junction to knee or below

(For ligation and stripping of the short saphenous vein, use 37718)

(For bilateral procedure, report 37722 with modifier 50)

(Do not report 37722 in conjunction with 37700, 37735)

(37730 deleted 2006 edition. For ligation, division, and stripping of the greater saphenous vein, use 37722. For ligation, division, and stripping of the short saphenous vein, use 37718)

37735 Ligation and division and complete stripping of long or short saphenous veins with radical excision of ulcer and skin graft and/or interruption of communicating veins of lower leg, with excision of deep fascia

(Do not report 37735 in conjunction with 37700, 37718, 37722, 37780)

(For bilateral procedure, report 37735 with modifier -50)

37760 Ligation of perforator veins, subfascial, radical (Linton type), with or without skin graft, open

(For endoscopic procedure, use 37500)

37765 Stab phlebectomy of varicose veins, one extremity; 10-20 stab incisions

(For less than 10 incisions, use 37799)

(For more than 20 incisions, use 37766)

37766 more than 20 incisions

37780 Ligation and division of short saphenous vein at saphenopopliteal junction (separate procedure)

(For bilateral procedure, report 37780 with modifier -50)

37785 Ligation, division, and/or excision of varicose vein cluster(s), one leg

(For bilateral procedure, report 37785 with modifier -50)

OTHER PROCEDURES

37788 Penile revascularization, artery, with or without vein graft

37790 Penile venous occlusive procedure

37799 Unlisted procedure, vascular surgery

HEMIC AND LYMPHATIC SYSTEMS

CPT codes from this section of CPT are used to report invasive and surgical procedures performed on the spleen and lymph nodes. Bone marrow transplants are reported using CPT codes 38230-38241 from this section.

When bone marrow aspiration is performed alone, the appropriate code to report is CPT code 38220. When a bone marrow biopsy is performed, the appropriate code is CPT code 38221 (bone marrow biopsy). This code cannot be reported with CPT code 20220 (bone biopsy). CPT codes 38220 and 38221 may only be reported together if the two procedures are performed at separate sites or at separate patient encounters. Separate sites include bone marrow aspiration and biopsy in different bones or two separate skin incisions over the same bone.

When both a bone marrow biopsy (CPT code 38221) and bone marrow aspiration (CPT code 38220) are performed at the same site through the same skin incision, do not report the bone marrow aspiration, CPT code 38220, in addition to the bone marrow biopsy (CPT code 38221). HCPCS/CPT code G0364 may be reported to describe the bone marrow aspiration performed with bone marrow biopsy through the same skin incision on the same date of service.

SPLEEN

EXCISION

38100 Splenectomy; total (separate procedure)

38101 partial (separate procedure)

+ **38102** total, en bloc for extensive disease, in conjunction with other procedure (List in addition to code for primary procedure)

REPAIR

38115 Repair of ruptured spleen (splenorrhaphy) with or without partial splenectomy

LAPAROSCOPY

38120 Laparoscopy, surgical, splenectomy

38129 Unlisted laparoscopy procedure, spleen

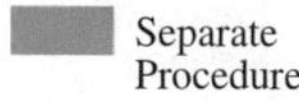
Separate Procedure
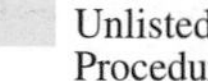
Unlisted Procedure
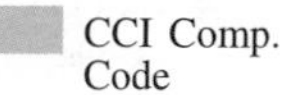
CCI Comp. Code
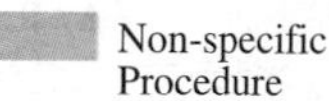
Non-specific Procedure

INTRODUCTION

38200 Injection procedure for splenoportography

(For radiological supervision and interpretation, use 75810)

GENERAL

BONE MARROW OR STEM CELL SERVICES/PROCEDURES

CPT codes 38207-38215 may be reported once a day, regardless of the number of cells manipulated.

38204 Management of recipient hematopoietic progenitor cell donor search and cell acquisition

38205 Blood-derived hematopoietic progenitor cell harvesting for transplantation, per collection; allogenic

38206 autologous

38207 Transplant preparation of hematopoietic progenitor cells; cryopreservation and storage

(For diagnostic cryopreservation and storage, see 88240)

38208 thawing of previously frozen harvest, without washing

(For diagnostic thawing and expansion of frozen cells, see 88241)

38209 thawing of previuosly frozen harvest, with washing

38210 specific cell depletion within harvest, T-cell depletion

38211 tumor cell depletion

38212 red blood cell removal

38213 platelet depletion

38214 plasma (volume) depletion

38215 cell concentration in plasma, mononuclear, or buffy coat layer

(Do not report 38207-38215 in conjunction with 88182, 88184-88189)

38220 Bone marrow; aspiration only

38221 biopsy, needle or trocar

(For bone marrow biopsy interpretation, use 88305)

38230 Bone marrow harvesting for transplantation

(For autologous and allogenic blood-derived peripheral stem cell harvesting for transplantation, see 38205-38206)

38240 Bone marrow or blood-derived peripheral stem cell transplantation; allogenic

38241 autologous

38242 allogeneic donor lymphocyte infusions

(For bone marrow aspiration, use 38220)

(For modification, treatment, and processing of bone marrow or blood-derived stem cell specimens for transplantation, see 38210-38213)

(For cryopreservation, freezing and storage of blood-derived stem cells for transplantation, use 88240)

(For thawing and expansion of blood-derived stem cells for transplantation, use 88241)

(For compatibility studies, see 86812-86822)

LYMPH NODES AND LYMPHATIC CHANNELS

INCISION

38300 Drainage of lymph node abscess or lymphadenitis; simple

38305 extensive

38308 Lymphangiotomy or other operations on lymphatic channels

38380 Suture and/or ligation of thoracic duct; cervical approach

38381 thoracic approach

38382 abdominal approach

EXCISION

(For injection for sentinel node identification, use 38792)

38500 Biopsy or excision of lymph node(s); open, superficial

(Do not report 38500 with 38700-38780)

38505 by needle, superficial (eg, cervical, inguinal, axillary)

(If imaging guidance is performed, see 76942, 77012, 77021)

(For fine needle aspiration, use 10021 or 10022)

(For evaluation of fine needle aspirate, see 88172, 88173)

38510 open, deep cervical node(s)

38520 open, deep cervical node(s) with excision scalene fat pad

38525 open, deep axillary node(s)

38530 open, internal mammary node(s)

(Do not report 38530 with 38720-38746)

(For percutaneous needle biopsy, retroperitoneal lymph node or mass, use 49180. For fine needle aspiration, use 10022)

38542 Dissection, deep jugular node(s)

(For radical cervical neck dissection, use 38720)

38550 Excision of cystic hygroma, axillary or cervical; without deep neurovascular dissection

38555 with deep neurovascular dissection

LIMITED LYMPHADENECTOMY FOR STAGING

38562 Limited lymphadenectomy for staging (separate procedure); pelvic and para-aortic

(When combined with prostatectomy, use 55812 or 55842)

(When combined with insertion of radioactive substance into prostate, use 55862)

38564 retroperitoneal (aortic and/or splenic)

LAPAROSCOPY

38570 Laparoscopy, surgical; with retroperitoneal lymph node sampling (biopsy), single or multiple

38571 with bilateral total pelvic lymphadenectomy

38572 with bilateral total pelvic lymphadenectomy and peri-aortic lymph node sampling (biopsy), single or multiple

(For drainage of lymphocele to peritoneal cavity, use 49323)

38589 Unlisted laparoscopy procedure, lymphatic system

RADICAL LYMPHADENECTOMY (RADICAL RESECTION OF LYMPH NODES)

(For limited pelvic and retroperitoneal lymphadenectomies, see 38562, 38564)

38700 Suprahyoid lymphadenectomy

(For bilateral procedure, report 38700 with modifier -50)

38720 Cervical lymphadenectomy (complete)

(For bilateral procedure, report 38720 with modifier -50)

38724 Cervical lymphadenectomy (modified radical neck dissection)

38740 Axillary lymphadenectomy; superficial

38745 complete

+ **38746** Thoracic lymphadenectomy, regional, including mediastinal and peritracheal nodes (List separately in addition to code for primary procedure)

+ **38747** Abdominal lymphadenectomy, regional, including celiac, gastric, portal, peripancreatic, with or without para-aortic and vena caval nodes (List separately in addition to code for primary procedure)

38760 Inguinofemoral lymphadenectomy, superficial, including Cloquets node (separate procedure)

(For bilateral procedure, report 38760 with modifier -50)

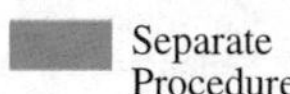 Separate Procedure 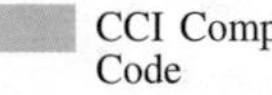 Unlisted Procedure CCI Comp. Code 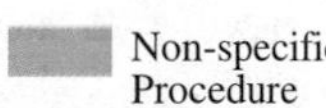 Non-specific Procedure

38765 Inguinofemoral lymphadenectomy, superficial, in continuity with pelvic lymphadenectomy, including external iliac, hypogastric, and obturator nodes (separate procedure)

(For bilateral procedure, report 38765 with modifier -50)

38770 Pelvic lymphadenectomy, including external iliac, hypogastric, and obturator nodes (separate procedure)

(For bilateral procedure, report 38770 with modifier -50)

38780 Retroperitoneal transabdominal lymphadenectomy, extensive, including pelvic, aortic, and renal nodes (separate procedure)

(For excision and repair of lymphedematous skin and subcutaneous tissue, see 15004-15005, 15570-15650)

INTRODUCTION

38790 Injection procedure; lymphangiography

(For bilateral procedure, report 38790 with modifier -50)

(For radiological supervision and interpretation, see 75801-75807)

⊘ **38792** for identification of sentinel node

(For excision of sentinel node, see 38500-38542)

(For nuclear medicine lymphatics and lymph gland imaging, use 78195)

38794 Cannulation, thoracic duct

OTHER PROCEDURES

38999 Unlisted procedure, hemic or lymphatic system

● New Code ▲ Revised Code + Add-On Code ⊘ Modifier -51 Exempt ⊙ Conscious Sedation

MEDIASTINUM AND DIAPHRAGM

CPT codes from this section of CPT are used to report invasive and surgical procedures performed on the mediastinum and the diaphragm.

MEDIASTINUM

INCISION

39000 Mediastinotomy with exploration, drainage, removal of foreign body, or biopsy; cervical approach

39010 transthoracic approach, including either transthoracic or median sternotomy

EXCISION

39200 Excision of mediastinal cyst

39220 Excision of mediastinal tumor

(For substernal thyroidectomy, use 60270)

(For thymectomy, use 60520)

ENDOSCOPY

39400 Mediastinoscopy, with or without biopsy

OTHER PROCEDURES

39499 Unlisted procedure, mediastinum

DIAPHRAGM

REPAIR

(For transabdominal repair of diaphragmatic (esophageal hiatal) hernia, see 43324, 43325)

39501 Repair, laceration of diaphragm, any approach

39502 Repair, paraesophageal hiatus hernia, transabdominal, with or without fundoplasty, vagotomy, and/or pyloroplasty, except neonatal

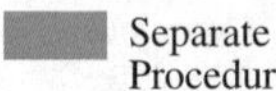
Separate Procedure

Unlisted Procedure

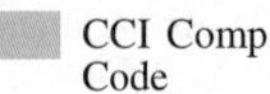
CCI Comp. Code

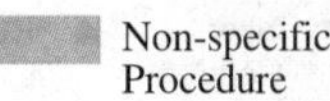
Non-specific Procedure

39503 Repair, neonatal diaphragmatic hernia, with or without chest tube insertion and with or without creation of ventral hernia

(Do not report modifier '-63' in conjunction with 39503)

39520 Repair, diaphragmatic hernia (esophageal hiatal); transthoracic

39530 combined, thoracoabdominal

39531 combined, thoracoabdominal, with dilation of stricture (with or without gastroplasty)

39540 Repair, diaphragmatic hernia (other than neonatal), traumatic; acute

39541 chronic

39545 Imbrication of diaphragm for eventration, transthoracic or transabdominal, paralytic or nonparalytic

39560 Resection, diaphragm; with simple repair (eg, primary suture)

39561 with complex repair (eg, prosthetic material, local muscle flap)

OTHER PROCEDURES

39599 Unlisted procedure, diaphragm

● New Code ▲ Revised Code + Add-On Code ⊘ Modifier -51 Exempt ⊙ Conscious Sedation

DIGESTIVE SYSTEM

CPT codes from this section of the CPT coding system are used to report invasive and surgical procedures performed on the lips; mouth; tongue; dentoalveolar structures; palate; salivary gland; pharynx, adenoids and tonsils; esophagus; stomach; intestines; rectum; anus; liver; biliary tract; pancreas; and the abdomen, peritoneum, and omentum.

MISCELLANEOUS CODING RULES

Gastrointestinal endoscopy codes should be assigned based on the extent of visualization performed. CMS's official guidelines for excision or destruction of a lesion are:

1. *use only the biopsy code if a single lesion is biopsied but not excised;*
2. *code only for the excision if a lesion is biopsied and the remaining portion is excised;*
3. *use the biopsy code once even if multiple biopsies are performed and none are excised; and*
4. *use both a biopsy and excision code if each lesion is taken from different sites.*

If the phrase "with or without biopsy" appears in the excision code's narrative, do not use a separate biopsy code. Diagnostic endoscopies are included in surgical endoscopies.

For upper gastrointestinal endoscopies, choose the appropriate code from documentation indicating whether the procedure was a simple exam, a diagnostic procedure or surgical procedure. Remember that code selection is based on the procedure(s) performed and the anatomical sites through which the scope passes. For example, if the scope is passed to the esophagus only, the code would be chosen from endoscopy codes beginning with 43200. If the scope is passed through the esophagus to the stomach, duodenum and/or the jejunum, the code selection would begin at 43235.

HERNIA REPAIR

Review the patient's age, the kind of hernia, the clinical presentation of the hernia, and method of repair documented in the medical record before assigning a hernia repair code.

APPENDECTOMY

To code appendectomies appropriately, review the documentation for an indicated purpose for the removal. If there is none, then it is probably incidental to a more serious surgery and should not be coded.

LIPS

(For procedures on skin of lips, see 10040 et seq)

EXCISION

40490 Biopsy of lip

40500 Vermilionectomy (lip shave), with mucosal advancement

40510 Excision of lip; transverse wedge excision with primary closure

40520 V-excision with primary direct linear closure

(For excision of mucous lesions, see 40810-40816)

40525 full thickness, reconstruction with local flap (eg, Estlander or fan)

40527 full thickness, reconstruction with cross lip flap (Abbe-Estlander)

40530 Resection of lip, more than one-fourth, without reconstruction

(For reconstruction, see 13131 et seq)

REPAIR (CHEILOPLASTY)

40650 Repair lip, full thickness; vermilion only

40652 up to half vertical height

40654 over one-half vertical height, or complex

40700 Plastic repair of cleft lip/nasal deformity; primary, partial or complete, unilateral

40701 primary bilateral, one stage procedure

40702 primary bilateral, one of two stages

40720 secondary, by recreation of defect and reclosure

(For bilateral procedure, report 40720 with modifier -50)

(To report rhinoplasty only for nasal deformity secondary to congenital cleft lip, see 30460, 30462)

(For repair of cleft lip, with cross lip pedicle flap (Abbe-Estlander type), use 40527)

40761 with cross lip pedicle flap (Abbe-Estlander type), including sectioning and inserting of pedicle

(For repair cleft palate, see 42200 et seq)

(For other reconstructive procedures, see 14060, 14061, 15120-15261, 15574, 15576, 15630)

OTHER PROCEDURES

40799 Unlisted procedure, lips

VESTIBULE OF MOUTH

INCISION

40800 Drainage of abscess, cyst, hematoma, vestibule of mouth; simple

40801 complicated

40804 Removal of embedded foreign body, vestibule of mouth; simple

40805 complicated

40806 Incision of labial frenum (frenotomy)

EXCISION, DESTRUCTION

40808 Biopsy, vestibule of mouth

40810 Excision of lesion of mucosa and submucosa, vestibule of mouth; without repair

40812 with simple repair

40814 with complex repair

Separate Procedure | Unlisted Procedure | CCI Comp. Code | Non-specific Procedure

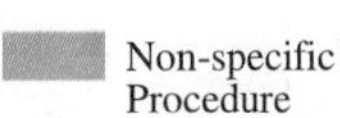

40816 complex, with excision of underlying muscle

40818 Excision of mucosa of vestibule of mouth as donor graft

40819 Excision of frenum, labial or buccal (frenumectomy, frenulectomy, frenectomy)

40820 Destruction of lesion or scar of vestibule of mouth by physical methods (eg, laser, thermal, cryo, chemical)

REPAIR

40830 Closure of laceration, vestibule of mouth; 2.5 cm or less

40831 over 2.5 cm or complex

40840 Vestibuloplasty; anterior

40842 posterior, unilateral

40843 posterior, bilateral

40844 entire arch

40845 complex (including ridge extension, muscle repositioning)

(For skin grafts, see 15002 et seq)

OTHER PROCEDURES

40899 Unlisted procedure, vestibule of mouth

TONGUE AND FLOOR OF MOUTH

INCISION

41000 Intraoral incision and drainage of abscess, cyst, or hematoma of tongue or floor of mouth; lingual

41005 sublingual, superficial

41006 sublingual, deep, supramylohyoid

41007 submental space

41008 submandibular space

● New Code ▲ Revised Code + Add-On Code ⊘ Modifier -51 Exempt ⊙ Conscious Sedation

41009 masticator space

41010 Incision of lingual frenum (frenotomy)

41015 Extraoral incision and drainage of abscess, cyst, or hematoma of floor of mouth; sublingual

41016 submental

41017 submandibular

41018 masticator space

(For frenoplasty, use 41520)

EXCISION

41100 Biopsy of tongue; anterior two-thirds

41105 posterior one-third

41108 Biopsy of floor of mouth

41110 Excision of lesion of tongue without closure

41112 Excision of lesion of tongue with closure; anterior two-thirds

41113 posterior one-third

41114 with local tongue flap

(List 41114 in addition to code 41112 or 41113)

41115 Excision of lingual frenum (frenectomy)

41116 Excision, lesion of floor of mouth

41120 Glossectomy; less than one-half tongue

41130 hemiglossectomy

41135 partial, with unilateral radical neck dissection

41140 complete or total, with or without tracheostomy, without radical neck dissection

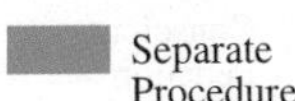 Separate Procedure 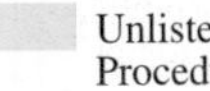 Unlisted Procedure 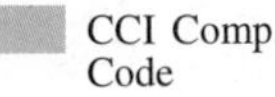 CCI Comp. Code 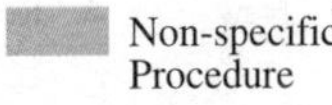 Non-specific Procedure

41145 complete or total, with or without tracheostomy, with unilateral radical neck dissection

41150 composite procedure with resection floor of mouth and mandibular resection, without radical neck dissection

41153 composite procedure with resection floor of mouth, with suprahyoid neck dissection

41155 composite procedure with resection floor of mouth, mandibular resection, and radical neck dissection (Commando type)

REPAIR

41250 Repair of laceration 2.5 cm or less; floor of mouth and/or anterior two-thirds of tongue

41251 posterior one-third of tongue

41252 Repair of laceration of tongue, floor of mouth, over 2.6 cm or complex

OTHER PROCEDURES

41500 Fixation of tongue, mechanical, other than suture (eg, K-wire)

41510 Suture of tongue to lip for micrognathia (Douglas type procedure)

41520 Frenoplasty (surgical revision of frenum, eg, with Z-plasty)

(For frenotomy, see 40806, 41010)

41599 Unlisted procedure, tongue, floor of mouth

DENTOALVEOLAR STRUCTURES

INCISION

41800 Drainage of abscess, cyst, hematoma from dentoalveolar structures

41805 Removal of embedded foreign body from dentoalveolar structures; soft tissues

41806 bone

EXCISION, DESTRUCTION

41820 Gingivectomy, excision gingiva, each quadrant

41821 Operculectomy, excision pericoronal tissues

41822 Excision of fibrous tuberosities, dentoalveolar structures

41823 Excision of osseous tuberosities, dentoalveolar structures

41825 Excision of lesion or tumor (except listed above), dentoalveolar structures; without repair

41826 with simple repair

41827 with complex repair

(For nonexcisional destruction, use 41850)

41828 Excision of hyperplastic alveolar mucosa, each quadrant (specify)

41830 Alveolectomy, including curettage of osteitis or sequestrectomy

41850 Destruction of lesion (except excision), dentoalveolar structures

OTHER PROCEDURES

41870 Periodontal mucosal grafting

41872 Gingivoplasty, each quadrant (specify)

41874 Alveoloplasty, each quadrant (specify)

(For closure of lacerations, see 40830, 40831)

(For segmental osteotomy, use 21206)

(For reduction of fractures, see 21421-21490)

41899 Unlisted procedure, dentoalveolar structures

PALATE AND UVULA

INCISION

42000 Drainage of abscess of palate, uvula

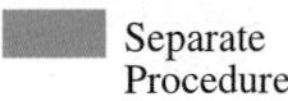
Separate Procedure

Unlisted Procedure

CCI Comp. Code

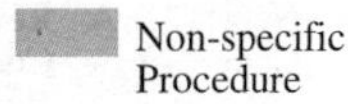
Non-specific Procedure

EXCISION, DESTRUCTION

42100 Biopsy of palate, uvula

42104 Excision, lesion of palate, uvula; without closure

42106 with simple primary closure

42107 with local flap closure

(For skin graft, see 14040-14300)

(For mucosal graft, use 40818)

42120 Resection of palate or extensive resection of lesion

(For reconstruction of palate with extraoral tissue, see 14040-14300, 15050, 15120, 15240, 15576)

42140 Uvulectomy, excision of uvula

42145 Palatopharyngoplasty (eg, uvulopalatopharyngoplasty, uvulopharyngoplasty)

(For removal of exostosis of the bony palate, see 21031, 21032)

42160 Destruction of lesion, palate or uvula (thermal, cryo or chemical)

REPAIR

42180 Repair, laceration of palate; up to 2 cm

42182 over 2 cm or complex

42200 Palatoplasty for cleft palate, soft and/or hard palate only

42205 Palatoplasty for cleft palate, with closure of alveolar ridge; soft tissue only

42210 with bone graft to alveolar ridge (includes obtaining graft)

42215 Palatoplasty for cleft palate; major revision

42220 secondary lengthening procedure

42225 attachment pharyngeal flap

42226 Lengthening of palate, and pharyngeal flap

42227 Lengthening of palate, with island flap

42235 Repair of anterior palate, including vomer flap

(For repair of oronasal fistula, use 30600)

42260 Repair of nasolabial fistula

(For repair of cleft lip, see 40700 et seq)

42280 Maxillary impression for palatal prosthesis

42281 Insertion of pin-retained palatal prosthesis

OTHER PROCEDURES

42299 Unlisted procedure, palate, uvula

SALIVARY GLAND AND DUCTS

INCISION

42300 Drainage of abscess; parotid, simple

42305 parotid, complicated

42310 submaxillary or sublingual, intraoral

42320 submaxillary, external

(42325 deleted 2006 edition.)

(42326 deleted 2006 edition.)

42330 Sialolithotomy; submandibular (submaxillary), sublingual or parotid, uncomplicated, intraoral

42335 submandibular (submaxillary), complicated, intraoral

42340 parotid, extraoral or complicated intraoral

EXCISION

42400 Biopsy of salivary gland; needle

(For fine needle aspiration, see 10021, 10022)

(For evaluation of fine needle aspirate, see 88172, 88173)

(If imaging guidance, is performed, see 76942, 77002, 77012, 77021)

42405 incisional

(If imaging guidance is performed, see 76942, 77002, 77012, 77021)

42408 Excision of sublingual salivary cyst (ranula)

42409 Marsupialization of sublingual salivary cyst (ranula)

42410 Excision of parotid tumor or parotid gland; lateral lobe, without nerve dissection

42415 lateral lobe, with dissection and preservation of facial nerve

42420 total, with dissection and preservation of facial nerve

42425 total, en bloc removal with sacrifice of facial nerve

42426 total, with unilateral radical neck dissection

(For suture or grafting of facial nerve, see 64864, 64865, 69740, 69745)

42440 Excision of submandibular (submaxillary) gland

42450 Excision of sublingual gland

REPAIR

42500 Plastic repair of salivary duct, sialodochoplasty; primary or simple

42505 secondary or complicated

42507 Parotid duct diversion, bilateral (Wilke type procedure);

42508 with excision of one submandibular gland

● New Code ▲ Revised Code + Add-On Code ⊘ Modifier -51 Exempt ⊙ Conscious Sedation

42509 with excision of both submandibular glands

42510 with ligation of both submandibular (Wharton's) ducts

OTHER PROCEDURES

42550 Injection procedure for sialography

(For radiological supervision and interpretation, use 70390)

42600 Closure salivary fistula

42650 Dilation salivary duct

42660 Dilation and catheterization of salivary duct, with or without injection

42665 Ligation salivary duct, intraoral

42699 Unlisted procedure, salivary glands or ducts

PHARYNX, ADENOIDS, AND TONSILS

INCISION

42700 Incision and drainage abscess; peritonsillar

42720 retropharyngeal or parapharyngeal, intraoral approach

42725 retropharyngeal or parapharyngeal, external approach

EXCISION, DESTRUCTION

42800 Biopsy; oropharynx

42802 hypopharynx

42804 nasopharynx, visible lesion, simple

42806 nasopharynx, survey for unknown primary lesion

(For laryngoscopic biopsy, see 31510, 31535, 31536)

42808 Excision or destruction of lesion of pharynx, any method

42809 Removal of foreign body from pharynx

Separate Procedure | Unlisted Procedure | CCI Comp. Code | Non-specific Procedure

42810 Excision branchial cleft cyst or vestige, confined to skin and subcutaneous tissues

42815 Excision branchial cleft cyst, vestige, or fistula, extending beneath subcutaneous tissues and/or into pharynx

42820 Tonsillectomy and adenoidectomy; under age 12

42821 age 12 or over

42825 Tonsillectomy, primary or secondary; under age 12

42826 age 12 or over

42830 Adenoidectomy, primary; under age 12

42831 age 12 or over

42835 Adenoidectomy, secondary; under age 12

42836 age 12 or over

42842 Radical resection of tonsil, tonsillar pillars, and/or retromolar trigone; without closure

42844 closure with local flap (eg, tongue, buccal)

42845 closure with other flap

(For closure with other flap(s), use appropriate number for flap(s))

(When combined with radical neck dissection, use also 38720)

42860 Excision of tonsil tags

42870 Excision or destruction lingual tonsil, any method (separate procedure)

(For resection of the nasopharynx (eg., juvenile angiofibroma) by bicoronal and/or transzygomatic approach, see 61586 and 61600)

42890 Limited pharyngectomy

● New Code ▲ Revised Code + Add-On Code ⃠ Modifier -51 Exempt ⊙ Conscious Sedation

42892 Resection of lateral pharyngeal wall or pyriform sinus, direct closure by advancement of lateral and posterior pharyngeal walls

(When combined with radical neck dissection, use also 38720)

42894 Resection of pharyngeal wall requiring closure with myocutaneous flap

(When combined with radical neck dissection, use also 38720)

(For limited pharyngectomy with radical neck dissection, use 38720 with 42890)

REPAIR

42900 Suture pharynx for wound or injury

42950 Pharyngoplasty (plastic or reconstructive operation on pharynx)

(For pharyngeal flap, use 42225)

42953 Pharyngoesophageal repair

(For closure with myocutaneous or other flap, use appropriate number in addition)

OTHER PROCEDURES

42955 Pharyngostomy (fistulization of pharynx, external for feeding)

42960 Control oropharyngeal hemorrhage, primary or secondary (eg, post-tonsillectomy); simple

42961 complicated, requiring hospitalization

42962 with secondary surgical intervention

42970 Control of nasopharyngeal hemorrhage, primary or secondary (eg, postadenoidectomy); simple, with posterior nasal packs, with or without anterior packs and/or cautery

42971 complicated, requiring hospitalization

42972 with secondary surgical intervention

42999 Unlisted procedure, pharynx, adenoids, or tonsils

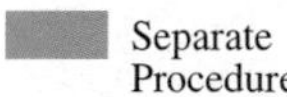

Separate Procedure | Unlisted Procedure | CCI Comp. Code | Non-specific Procedure

ESOPHAGUS

INCISION

(For esophageal intubation with laparotomy, use 43510)

43020 Esophagotomy, cervical approach, with removal of foreign body

43030 Cricopharyngeal myotomy

43045 Esophagotomy, thoracic approach, with removal of foreign body

EXCISION

(For gastrointestinal reconstruction for previous esophagectomy, see 43360, 43361)

43100 Excision of lesion, esophagus, with primary repair; cervical approach

43101 thoracic or abdominal approach

(For wide excision of malignant lesion of cervical esophagus, with total laryngectomy without radical neck dissection, see 43107, 43116, 43124 and 31360)

(For wide excision of malignant lesion of cervical esophagus, with total laryngectomy with radical neck dissection, see 43107, 43116, 43124, and 31365)

43107 Total or near total esophagectomy, without thoracotomy; with pharyngogastrostomy or cervical esophagogastrostomy, with or without pyloroplasty (transhiatal)

43108 with colon interposition or small intestine reconstruction, including intestine mobilization, preparation and anastomosis(es)

43112 Total or near total esophagectomy, with thoracotomy; with pharyngogastrostomy or cervical esophagogastrostomy, with or without pyloroplasty

43113 with colon interposition or small intestine reconstruction, including intestine mobilization, preparation, and anastomosis(es)

43116 Partial esophagectomy, cervical, with free intestinal graft, including microvascular anastomosis, obtaining the graft and intestinal reconstruction

(Do not report 43116 in conjunction with 69990)

(Report 43116 with the modifier -52 appended if intestinal or free jejunal graft with microvascular anastomosis is performed by another physician)

(For free jejunal graft with microvascular anastomosis performed by another physician, use 43496)

43117 Partial esophagectomy, distal two-thirds, with thoracotomy and separate abdominal incision, with or without proximal gastrectomy; with thoracic esophagogastrostomy, with or without pyloroplasty (Ivor Lewis)

43118 with colon interposition or small intestine reconstruction, including intestine mobilization, preparation, and anastomosis(es)

(For total esophagectomy with gastropharyngostomy, see 43107, 43124)

(For esophagogastrectomy (lower third) and vagotomy, use 43122)

43121 Partial esophagectomy, distal two-thirds, with thoracotomy only, with or without proximal gastrectomy, with thoracic esophagogastrostomy, with or without pyloroplasty

43122 Partial esophagectomy, thoracoabdominal or abdominal approach, with or without proximal gastrectomy; with esophagogastrostomy, with or without pyloroplasty

43123 with colon interposition or small intestine reconstruction, including intestine mobilization, preparation, and anastomosis(es)

43124 Total or partial esophagectomy, without reconstruction (any approach), with cervical esophagostomy

43130 Diverticulectomy of hypopharynx or esophagus, with or without myotomy; cervical approach

43135 thoracic approach

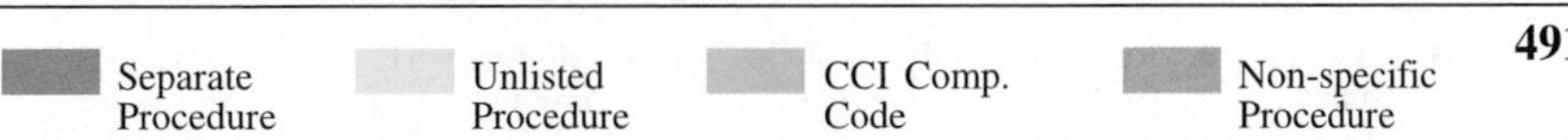

ENDOSCOPY

⊙ **43200** Esophagoscopy, rigid or flexible; diagnostic, with or without collection of specimen(s) by brushing or washing (separate procedure)

⊙ **43201** with directed submucosal injection(s), any substance

(For injection sclerosis of esophageal varices, use 43204)

⊙ **43202** with biopsy, single or multiple

⊙ **43204** with injection sclerosis of esophageal varices

⊙ **43205** with band ligation of esophageal varices

⊙ **43215** with removal of foreign body

(For radiological supervision and interpretation, use 74235)

⊙ **43216** with removal of tumor(s), polyp(s), or other lesion(s) by hot biopsy forceps or bipolar cautery

⊙ **43217** with removal of tumor(s), polyp(s), or other lesion(s) by snare technique

⊙ **43219** with insertion of plastic tube or stent

⊙ **43220** with balloon dilation (less than 30 mm diameter)

(If imaging guidance is performed, use 74360)

(For endoscopic dilation with balloon 30 mm diameter or larger, use 43458)

(For dilation without visualization, see 43450-43453)

(For diagnostic fiberoptic esophagogastroscopy, use 43200, 43235)

(For fiberoptic esophagogastroscopy with biopsy or collection of specimen, use 43200, 43202, 43235, 43239)

(For fiberoptic esophagogastroscopy with removal of foreign body, use 43215, 43247)

(For fiberoptic esophagogastroscopy with removal of polyp(s), use 43217, 43251)

⊙ **43226** with insertion of guide wire followed by dilation over guide wire

● New Code ▲ Revised Code + Add-On Code ⊘ Modifier -51 Exempt ⊙ Conscious Sedation

(For radiological supervision and interpretation, use 74360)

⊙ **43227** with control of bleeding (eg, injection, bipolar cautery, unipolar cautery, laser, heater probe, stapler, plasma coagulator)

⊙ **43228** with ablation of tumor(s), polyp(s), or other lesion(s), not amenable to removal by hot biopsy forceps, bipolar cautery or snare technique

(For esophagoscopic photodynamic therapy, report 43228 in addition to 96570, 96571 as appropriate)

⊙ **43231** with endoscopic ultrasound examination

(Do not report 43231 in conjunction with 76975)

⊙ **43232** with transendoscopic ultrasound-guided intramural or transmural fine needle aspiration/biopsy(s)

(Do not report 43232 in conjunction with 76942, 76975)

(For interpretation of specimen, see 88172-88173)

⊙ **43234** Upper gastrointestinal endoscopy, simple primary examination (eg, with small diameter flexible endoscope) (separate procedure)

⊙ **43235** Upper gastrointestinal endoscopy including esophagus, stomach, and either the duodenum and/or jejunum as appropriate; diagnostic, with or without collection of specimen(s) by brushing or washing (separate procedure)

⊙ **43236** with directed submucosal injection(s), any substance

(For injection sclerosis of esophageal and/or gastric varices, use 43243)

⊙ **43237** with endoscopic ultrasound examination limited to the esophagus

(Do not report 43237 in conjunction with 76975)

⊙ **43238** with transendoscopic ultrasound-guided intramural or transmural fine needle aspiration/biopsy(s), esophagus (includes endoscopic ultrasound examination limited to the esophagus)

(Do not report 43238 in conjunction with 76942 or 76975)

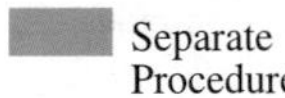

Separate Procedure | Unlisted Procedure | CCI Comp. Code | Non-specific Procedure

⊙ **43239** with biopsy, single or multiple

(For upper gastrointestinal endoscopy with suturing of the esophagogastric junction, use Category III code 0008T)

(For upper gastrointestinal endoscopy with injection of implant material into and along the muscle of the lower esophageal sphincter, use Category III code 0133T)

⊙ **43240** with transmural drainage of pseudocyst

⊙ **43241** with transendoscopic intraluminal tube or catheter placement

⊙ **43242** with transendoscopic ultrasound-guided intramural or transmural fine needle aspiration/biopsy(s) (includes endoscopic ultrasound examination of the esophagus, stomach, and either the duodenum and/or jejunum as appropriate

(Do not report 43242 in conjunction with 76942 or 76975)

(For transendoscopic fine needle aspiration/biopsy limited to esophagus, use 43238)

(For interpretation of specimen, see 88172-88173)

⊙ **43243** with injection sclerosis of esophageal and/or gastric varices

⊙ **43244** with band ligation of esophageal and/or gastric varices

⊙ **43245** with dilation of gastric outlet for obstruction (eg, balloon, guide wire, bougie)

(Do not report 43245 in conjunction with 43256)

⊙ **43246** with directed placement of percutaneous gastrostomy tube

(For radiological supervision and interpretation, use 74350)

⊙ **43247** with removal of foreign body

(For radiological supervision and interpretation, use 74235)

⊙ **43248** with insertion of guide wire followed by dilation of esophagus over guide wire

⊙ **43249** with balloon dilation of esophagus (less than 30 mm diameter)

⊙ **43250** with removal of tumor(s), polyp(s), or other lesion(s) by hot biopsy forceps or bipolar cautery

⊙ **43251** with removal of tumor(s), polyp(s), or other lesion(s) by snare technique

⊙ **43255** with control of bleeding, any method

⊙ **43256** with transendoscopic stent placement (includes predilation)

⊙ **43257** with delivery of thermal energy to the muscle of lower esophageal sphincter and/or gastric cardia, for treatment of gastroesophageal reflux disease

⊙ **43258** with ablation of tumor(s), polyp(s), or other lesion(s) not amenable to removal by hot biopsy forceps, bipolar cautery or snare technique

(For injection sclerosis of esophageal varices, use 43204 or 43243)

⊙ **43259** with endoscopic ultrasound examination, including the esophagus, stomach, and either the duodenum and/or jejunum as appropriate

(Do not report 43259 in conjunction with 76975)

⊙ **43260** Endoscopic retrograde cholangiopancreatography (ERCP); diagnostic, with or without collection of specimen(s) by brushing or washing (separate procedure)

(For radiological supervision and interpretation, see 74328, 74329, 74330)

⊙ **43261** with biopsy, single or multiple

(For radiological supervision and interpretation, see 74328, 74329, 74330)

⊙ **43262** with sphincterotomy/papillotomy

(For radiological supervision and interpretation, see 74328, 74329, 74330)

⊙ **43263** with pressure measurement of sphincter of Oddi (pancreatic duct or common bile duct)

(For radiological supervision and interpretation, see 74328, 74329, 74330)

⊙ **43264** with endoscopic retrograde removal of calculus/calculi from biliary and/or pancreatic ducts

(When done with sphincterotomy, also use 43262)

(For radiological supervision and interpretation, see 74328, 74329, 74330)

⊙ **43265** with endoscopic retrograde destruction, lithotripsy of calculus/calculi, any method

(When done with sphincterotomy, also use 43262)

(For radiological supervision and interpretation, see 74328, 74329, 74330)

⊙ **43267** with endoscopic retrograde insertion of nasobiliary or nasopancreatic drainage tube

(When done with sphincterotomy, also use 43262)

(For radiological supervision and interpretation, see 74328, 74329, 74330)

⊙ **43268** with endoscopic retrograde insertion of tube or stent into bile or pancreatic duct

(When done with sphincterotomy, also use 43262)

(For radiological supervision and interpretation, see 74328, 74329, 74330)

⊙ **43269** with endoscopic retrograde removal of foreign body and/or change of tube or stent

(When done with sphincterotomy, also use 43262)

(For radiological supervision and interpretation, see 74328, 74329, 74330)

⊙ **43271** with endoscopic retrograde balloon dilation of ampulla, biliary and/or pancreatic duct(s)

(When done with sphincterotomy, also use 43262)

(For radiological supervision and interpretation, see 74328, 74329, 74330)

⊙ **43272** with ablation of tumor(s), polyp(s), or other lesion(s) not amenable to removal by hot biopsy forceps, bipolar cautery or snare technique

(For radiological supervision and interpretation, see 74328, 74329, 74330)

LAPAROSCOPY

43280 Laparoscopy, surgical, esophagogastric fundoplasty (eg, Nissen, Toupet procedures)

(For open approach, use 43324)

43289 Unlisted laparoscopy procedure, esophagus

REPAIR

43300 Esophagoplasty, (plastic repair or reconstruction), cervical approach; without repair of tracheoesophageal fistula

43305 with repair of tracheoesophageal fistula

43310 Esophagoplasty, (plastic repair or reconstruction), thoracic approach; without repair of tracheoesophageal fistula

43312 with repair of tracheoesophageal fistula

43313 Esophagoplasty for congenital defect, (plastic repair or reconstruction), thoracic approach; without repair of congenital tracheoesophageal fistula

43314 with repair of congenital tracheoesophageal fistula

(Do not report modifier '-63' in conjunction with 43313, 43314)

43320 Esophagogastrostomy (cardioplasty), with or without vagotomy and pyloroplasty, transabdominal or transthoracic approach

43324 Esophagogastric fundoplasty (eg, Nissen, Belsey IV, Hill procedures)

(For laparoscopic procedure, use 43280)

43325 Esophagogastric fundoplasty; with fundic patch (Thal-Nissen procedure)

(For cricopharyngeal myotomy, use 43030)

43326 with gastroplasty (eg, Collis)

43330 Esophagomyotomy (Heller type); abdominal approach

43331 thoracic approach

(For thoracoscopic esophagomyotomy, use 32665)

43340 Esophagojejunostomy (without total gastrectomy); abdominal approach

43341 thoracic approach

43350 Esophagostomy, fistulization of esophagus, external; abdominal approach

43351 thoracic approach

43352 cervical approach

43360 Gastrointestinal reconstruction for previous esophagectomy, for obstructing esophageal lesion or fistula, or for previous esophageal exclusion; with stomach, with or without pyloroplasty

43361 with colon interposition or small intestine reconstruction, including intestine mobilization, preparation, and anastomosis(es)

43400 Ligation, direct, esophageal varices

43401 Transection of esophagus with repair, for esophageal varices

43405 Ligation or stapling at gastroesophageal junction for pre-existing esophageal perforation

43410 Suture of esophageal wound or injury; cervical approach

43415 transthoracic or transabdominal approach

43420 Closure of esophagostomy or fistula; cervical approach

43425 transthoracic or transabdominal approach

(For repair of esophageal hiatal hernia, see 39520 et seq)

● New Code ▲ Revised Code + Add-On Code ⊘ Modifier -51 Exempt ⊙ Conscious Sedation

MANIPULATION

(For associated esophagogram, use 74220)

43450 Dilation of esophagus, by unguided sound or bougie, single or multiple passes

(For radiological supervision and interpretation, use 74360)

⊙ **43453** Dilation of esophagus, over guide wire

(For dilation with direct visualization, use 43220)

(For dilation of esophagus, by balloon or dilator, see 43220, 43458, and 74360)

(For radiological supervision and interpretation, use 74360)

⊙ **43456** Dilation of esophagus, by balloon or dilator, retrograde

(For radiological supervision and interpretation, use 74360)

⊙ **43458** Dilation of esophagus with balloon (30 mm diameter or larger) for achalasia

(For dilation with balloon less than 30 mm diameter, use 43220)

(For radiological supervision and interpretation, use 74360)

43460 Esophagogastric tamponade, with balloon (Sengstaaken type)

(For removal of esophageal foreign body by balloon catheter, see 43215, 43247, 74235)

OTHER PROCEDURES

43496 Free jejunum transfer with microvascular anastomosis

(Do not report code 69990 in addition to code 43496)

43499 Unlisted procedure, esophagus

STOMACH

INCISION

43500 Gastrotomy; with exploration or foreign body removal

43501 with suture repair of bleeding ulcer

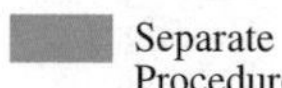

43502 with suture repair of pre-existing esophagogastric laceration (eg, Mallory-Weiss)

43510 with esophageal dilation and insertion of permanent intraluminal tube (eg, Celestin or Mousseaux-Barbin)

43520 Pyloromyotomy, cutting of pyloric muscle (Fredet-Ramstedt type operation)

(Do not report modifier '-63' in conjunction with 43520)

EXCISION

43600 Biopsy of stomach; by capsule, tube, peroral (one or more specimens)

43605 by laparotomy

43610 Excision, local; ulcer or benign tumor of stomach

43611 malignant tumor of stomach

43620 Gastrectomy, total; with esophagoenterostomy

43621 with Roux-en-Y reconstruction

43622 with formation of intestinal pouch, any type

43631 Gastrectomy, partial, distal; with gastroduodenostomy

43632 with gastrojejunostomy

43633 with Roux-en-Y reconstruction

43634 with formation of intestinal pouch

\+ **43635** Vagotomy when performed with partial distal gastrectomy (List separately in addition to code(s) for primary procedure)

(Use 43635 in conjunction with codes 43631, 43632, 43633, 43634)

(43638 deleted 2006 edition.)

(43639 deleted 2006 edition.)

43640 Vagotomy including pyloroplasty, with or without gastrostomy; truncal or selective

(For pyloroplasty, use 43800)

(For vagotomy, see 64752-64760)

43641 parietal cell (highly selective)

(For upper gastrointestinal endoscopy, see 43234-43259)

LAPAROSCOPY

(For upper gastrointestinal endoscopy including esophagus, stomach, and either the duodenum and/or jejunum, see 43235-43259)

43644 Laparoscopy, surgical, gastric restrictive procedure; with gastric bypass and Roux-en-Y gastroenterostomy (Roux limb 150 cm or less)

(Do not report 43644 in conjunction with 43846, 49320)

(Esophagogastroduodenoscopy (EGD) performed for a separate condition should be reported with modifier 59)

(For greater than 150 cm, use 43645)

(For open procedure, use 43846)

43645 with gastric bypass and small intestine reconstruction to limit absorption

(Do not report 43645 in conjunction with 49320, 43847)

● **43647** Laparoscopy, surgical; implantation or replacement of gastric neurostimulator electrodes, antrum

● **43648** Laparoscopy, surgical; revision or removal of gastric neurostimulator electrodes, antrum

(For open approach, see 43881, 43882)

(For insertion of gastric neruostimulator pulse generator, use 64590)

(For revision or removal of gastric neurostimulator pulse generator, use 64595)

(For electrical analaysis and programming of gastric neurostimulator pulse generator, use 95999)

(For laparoscopic implantation, revision, or removal of gastric neurostimulator electrodes, lesser curvature (morbid obesity), see Category III codes 0155T, 0156T)

(For electronic analysis, programming, and reprogramming of gastric neurostimulator pulse generator, lesser curvature (morbid obesity), use Category III code 0162T)

43651 Laparoscopy, surgical; transection of vagus nerves, truncal

43652 transection of vagus nerves, selective or highly selective

43653 gastrostomy, without construction of gastric tube (eg, Stamm procedure) (separate procedure)

43659 Unlisted laparoscopy procedure, stomach

INTRODUCTION

43750 Percutaneous placement of gastrostomy tube

(For radiological supervision and interpretation, use 74350)

43752 Naso- or oro-gastric tube placement, requiring physician's skill and fluoroscopic guidance (includes fluoroscopy, image documentation and report)

(For enteric tube placement, see 44500, 74340)

(Do not report 43752 in conjunction with critical care codes 99291-99292, neonatal critical care codes 99295-99296, pediatric critical care codes 99293-99294 or low birth weight intensive care service codes 99298-99299)

43760 Change of gastrostomy tube

(For endoscopic placement of gastrostomy tube, use 43246)

(For radiological supervision and interpretation, use 75984)

43761 Repositioning of the gastric feeding tube, any method, through the duodenum for enteric nutrition

(If imaging guidance is performed, use 75984)

BARIATRIC SURGERY

43770 Laparoscopy, surgical, gastric restrictive procedure; placement of adjustable gastric band (gastric band and subcutaneous port components)

(For individual component placement, report 43770 with modifier 52)

43771 revision of adjustable gastric band component only

43772 removal of adjustable gastric band component only

43773 removal and replacement of adjustable gastric band component only

(Do not report 43773 in conjunction with 43772)

43774 removal of adjustable gastric band and subcutaneous port components

(For removal and replacement of both gastric band and subcutaneous port components, use 43659)

OTHER PROCEDURES

43800 Pyloroplasty

(For pyloroplasty and vagotomy, use 43640)

43810 Gastroduodenostomy

43820 Gastrojejunostomy; without vagotomy

43825 with vagotomy, any type

43830 Gastrostomy, open; without construction of gastric tube (eg, Stamm procedure) (separate procedure)

43831 neonatal, for feeding

(For change of gastrostomy tube, use 43760)

(Do not report modifier '-63' in conjunction with 43831)

43832 with construction of gastric tube (eg, Janeway procedure)

(For percutaneous endoscopic gastrostomy, use 43246)

43840 Gastrorrhaphy, suture of perforated duodenal or gastric ulcer, wound, or injury

43842 Gastric restrictive procedure, without gastric bypass, for morbid obesity; vertical-banded gastroplasty

43843 other than vertical-banded gastroplasty

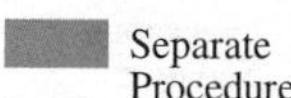 Separate Procedure 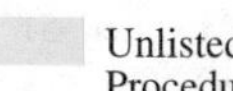 Unlisted Procedure 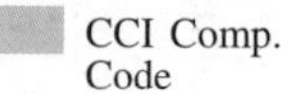 CCI Comp. Code 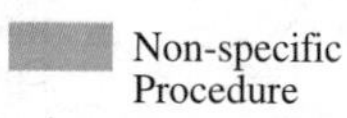 Non-specific Procedure

43845 Gastric restrictive procedure with partial gastrectomy, pylorus-preserving duodenoileostomy and ileoileostomy (50 to 100 cm common channel) to limit absorption (biliopancreatic diversion with duodenal switch)

(Do not report 43845 in conjunction with 43633, 43847, 44130, 49000)

43846 Gastric restrictive procedure, with gastric bypass for morbid obesity; with short limb (150 cm or less) Roux-en-Y gastroenterostomy

(For greater than 150 cm, use 43847)

(For laparoscopic procedure, use 43644)

43847 with small intestine reconstruction to limit absorption

43848 Revision, open, of gastric restrictive procedure for morbid obesity, other than adjustable gastric band (separate procedure)

(For adjustable gastric band procedures, see 43770-43774, 43886-43888)

43850 Revision of gastroduodenal anastomosis (gastroduodenostomy) with reconstruction; without vagotomy

43855 with vagotomy

43860 Revision of gastrojejunal anastomosis (gastrojejunostomy) with reconstruction, with or without partial gastrectomy or intestine resection; without vagotomy

43865 with vagotomy

43870 Closure of gastrostomy, surgical

43880 Closure of gastrocolic fistula

● **43881** Implantation or replacement of gastric neurostimulator electrodes, antrum, open

● **43882** Revision or removal of gastric neurostimulator electrodes, antrum, open

(For laparoscopic approach, see 43647, 43648)

(For insertion of gastric neurostimulator pulse generator, use 64590)

(For revision or removal of gastric neurostimulator pulse generator, use 64595)

(For electronic analysis and programming of gastric neurostimulator pulse generator, use 95999)

(For open implantation, revision, or removal of gastric neurostimulator electrodes, lesser curvature [morbid obesity], see Category III codes 0157T, 0158T)

(For electronic analysis, programming, and reprogramming of gastric neurostimulator pulse generator, lesser curvature [morbid obesity], use Category III code 0162T)

43886 Gastric restrictive procedure, open; revision of subcutaneous port component only

43887 removal of subcutaneous port component only

43888 removal and replacement of subcutaneous port component only

(Do not report 43888 in conjunction with 43774, 43887)

(For laparoscopic removal of both gastric band and subcutaneous port components, use 43774)

(For removal and replacement of both gastric band and subcutaneous port components, use 43659)

43999 Unlisted procedure, stomach

INTESTINES (EXCEPT RECTUM)

INCISION

44005 Enterolysis (freeing of intestinal adhesion) (separate procedure)

(Do not report 44005 in addition to 45136)

(For laparoscopic approach, use 44180)

44010 Duodenotomy, for exploration, biopsy(s), or foreign body removal

+ **44015** Tube or needle catheter jejunostomy for enteral alimentation, intraoperative, any method (List separately in addition to primary procedure)

Separate Procedure | Unlisted Procedure | CCI Comp. Code | Non-specific Procedure

44020 Enterotomy, small intestine, other than duodenum; for exploration, biopsy(s), or foreign body removal

44021 for decompression (eg, Baker tube)

44025 Colotomy, for exploration, biopsy(s), or foreign body removal

(For exteriorization of intestine (Mikulicz resection with crushing of spur), see 44602-44605)

44050 Reduction of volvulus, intussusception, internal hernia, by laparotomy

44055 Correction of malrotation by lysis of duodenal bands and/or reduction of midgut volvulus (eg, Ladd procedure)

(Do not report modifier '-63' in conjunction with 44055)

EXCISION

Intestinal allotransplantation involves three distinct components of physician work:

1) **Cadaver donor enterectomy**, which includes harvesting the intestine graft and cold preservation of the graft (perfusing with cold preservation solution and cold maintenance) (use 44132). **Living donor enterectomy**, which includes harvesting the intestine graft, cold preservation of the graft (perfusing with cold preservation solution and cold maintenance), and care of the donor (use 44133).

2) **Backbench work**:

Standard preparation of an intestine allograft prior to transplantation includes mobilization and fashioning of the superior mesenteric artery and vein (see 44715).

Additional reconstruction of an intestine allograft prior to transplantation may include venous and/or arterial anastomosis(es) (see 44720-44721).

3) **Recipient intestinal allotransplantation with or without recipient enterectomy**, which includes transplantation of allograft and care of the recipient (see 44135, 44136)

44100 Biopsy of intestine by capsule, tube, peroral (one or more specimens)

44110 Excision of one or more lesions of small or large intestine not requiring anastomosis, exteriorization, or fistulization; single enterotomy

44111 multiple enterotomies

 ● New Code ▲ Revised Code + Add-On Code ⦸ Modifier -51 Exempt ⊙ Conscious Sedation

44120 Enterectomy, resection of small intestine; single resection and anastomosis

(Do not report 44120 in addition to 45136)

+ **44121** each additional resection and anastomosis (List separately in addition to code for primary procedure)

(Use 44121 in conjunction with code 44120)

44125 with enterostomy

44126 Enterectomy, resection of small intestine for congenital atresia, single resection and anastomosis of proximal segment of intestine; without tapering

44127 with tapering

+ **44128** each additional resection and anastomosis (List separately in addition to code for primary procedure)

(Use 44128 in conjunction with codes 44126, 44127)

(Do not report modifier '-63' in conjunction with 44126, 44127, 44128)

44130 Enteroenterostomy, anastomosis of intestine, with or without cutaneous enterostomy (separate procedure)

44132 Donor enterectomy (including cold preservation), open; from cadaver donor

44133 partial, from living donor

(For backbench intestinal graft preparation or reconstruction, see 44715, 44720, 44721)

44135 Intestinal allotransplantation; from cadaver donor

44136 from living donor

44137 Removal of transplanted intestinal allograft, complete

(For partial removal of transplant allograft, see 44120, 44121, 44140)

+ **44139** Mobilization (take-down) of splenic flexure performed in conjunction with partial colectomy (List separately in addition to primary procedure)

Separate Procedure | Unlisted Procedure | CCI Comp. Code | Non-specific Procedure

(Use 44139 in conjunction with codes 44140-44147)

44140 Colectomy, partial; with anastomosis

(For laparoscopic procedure, use 44204)

44141 with skin level cecostomy or colostomy

44143 with end colostomy and closure of distal segment (Hartmann type procedure)

(For laparoscopic procedure, use 44206)

44144 with resection, with colostomy or ileostomy and creation of mucofistula

44145 with coloproctostomy (low pelvic anastomosis)

(For laparoscopic procedure, use 44207)

44146 with coloproctostomy (low pelvic anastomosis), with colostomy

(For laparoscopic procedure, use 44208)

44147 abdominal and transanal approach

44150 Colectomy, total, abdominal, without proctectomy; with ileostomy or ileoproctostomy

(For laparoscopic procedure, use 44210)

44151 with continent ileostomy

(44152 deleted 2007 edition, see 44799)

(44153 deleted 2007 edition, see 44799)

44155 Colectomy, total, abdominal, with proctectomy; with ileostomy

(For laparoscopic procedure, use 44212)

44156 with continent ileostomy

● **44157** Colectomy, total, abdominal, with proctectomy; with ileoanal anastomosis, includes loop ileostomy, and rectal mucosectomy, when performed

● **44158** Colectomy, total, abdominal, with proctectomy; with ileoanal anastomosis, creation of ileal reservoir (S or J), includes loop ileostomy, and rectal mucosectomy, when performed

(For laparoscopic procedure, use 44211)

44160 Colectomy, partial, with removal of terminal ileum and ileocolostomy

(For laparoscopic procedure, use 44205)

LAPAROSCOPY

Incision

44180 Laparoscopy, surgical, enterolysis (freeing of intestinal adhesion) (separate procedure)

(For laparoscopy with salpingolysis, ovariolysis, use 58660)

Enterostomy—External Fistulization of Intestines

44186 Laparoscopy, surgical; jejunostomy (eg, for decompression or feeding)

44187 ileostomy or jejunostomy, non-tube

(For open procedure, use 44310)

44188 Laparoscopy, surgical, colostomy or skin level cecostomy

(For open procedure, use 44320)

(Do not report 44188 in conjunction with 44970)

(44200 deleted 2006 edition. To report, use 44180)

(44201 deleted 2006 edition. To report, use 44186)

Excision

44202 Laparoscopy, surgical; enterectomy, resection of small intestine, single resection and anastomosis

\+ **44203** each additional small intestine resection and anastomosis (List separately in addition to code for primary procedure)

(Use 44203 in conjunction with code 44202)

(For open procedure, see 44120, 44121)

44204 colectomy, partial, with anastomosis

(For open procedure, use 44140)

44205 colectomy, partial, with removal of terminal ileum with ileocolostomy

(For open procedure, use 44160)

44206 colectomy, partial, with end colostomy and closure of distal segment (Hartmann type procedure)

(For open procedure, use 44143)

44207 colectomy, partial, with anastomosis, with coloproctostomy (low pelvic anastomosis)

(For open procedure, use 44145)

44208 colectomy, partial, with anastomosis, with coloproctostomy (low pelvic anastomosis) with colostomy

(For open procedure, use 44146)

44210 colectomy, total, abdominal, without proctectomy, with ileostomy or ileoproctostomy

(For open procedure, use 44150)

▲ **44211** colectomy, total, abdominal, with proctectomy, with ileoanal anastomosis, creation of ileal reservoir (S or J), with loop ileostomy, includes rectal mucosectomy, when performed

(For open procedure, see 44157, 44158)

44212 colectomy, total, abdominal, with proctectomy, with ileostomy

(For open procedure, use 44155)

+ **44213** Laparoscopy, surgical, mobilization (take-down) of splenic flexure performed in conjunction with partial colectomy (List separately in addition to primary procedure)

(Use 44213 in conjunction with 44204-44208)

(For open procedure, use 44139)

Repair

44227 Laparoscopy, surgical, closure of enterostomy, large or small intestine, with resection and anastomosis

(For open procedure, see 44625, 44626)

Other Procedures

44238 Unlisted laparoscopy procedure, intestine (except rectum)

(44239 deleted 2006 edition. To report, use 45499)

ENTEROSTOMY—EXTERNAL FISTULIZATION OF INTESTINES

44300 Enterostomy or cecostomy, tube (eg, for decompression or feeding) (separate procedure)

44310 Ileostomy or jejunostomy, non-tube

(For laparoscopic procedure, use 44187)

(Do not report 44310 in conjunction with 44144, 44150-44153, 44155, 44156, 45113, 45119, 45136)

44312 Revision of ileostomy; simple (release of superficial scar) (separate procedure)

44314 complicated (reconstruction in-depth) (separate procedure)

44316 Continent ileostomy (Kock procedure) (separate procedure)

(For fiberoptic evaluation, use 44385)

44320 Colostomy or skin level cecostomy

(For laparoscopic procedure, use 44188)

(Do not report 44320 in conjunction with 44141, 44144, 44146, 44605, 45110, 45119, 45126, 45563, 45805, 45825, 50810, 51597, 57307, or 58240)

44322 with multiple biopsies (eg, for congenital megacolon) (separate procedure)

44340 Revision of colostomy; simple (release of superficial scar) (separate procedure)

44345 complicated (reconstruction in-depth) (separate procedure)

Separate Procedure | Unlisted Procedure | CCI Comp. Code | Non-specific Procedure

44346 with repair of paracolostomy hernia (separate procedure)

ENDOSCOPY, SMALL INTESTINE AND STOMAL

(For upper gastrointestinal endoscopy, see 43234-43258)

⊙ **44360** Small intestinal endoscopy, enteroscopy beyond second portion of duodenum, not including ileum; diagnostic, with or without collection of specimen(s) by brushing or washing (separate procedure)

⊙ **44361** with biopsy, single or multiple

⊙ **44363** with removal of foreign body

⊙ **44364** with removal of tumor(s), polyp(s), or other lesion(s) by snare technique

⊙ **44365** with removal of tumor(s), polyp(s), or other lesion(s) by hot biopsy forceps or bipolar cautery

⊙ **44366** with control of bleeding (eg, injection, bipolar cautery, unipolar cautery, laser, heater probe, stapler, plasma coagulator)

⊙ **44369** with ablation of tumor(s), polyp(s), or other lesion(s) not amenable to removal by hot biopsy forceps, bipolar cautery or snare technique

⊙ **44370** with transendoscopic stent placement (includes predilation)

⊙ **44372** with placement of percutaneous jejunostomy tube

⊙ **44373** with conversion of percutaneous gastrostomy tube to percutaneous jejunostomy tube

(For fiberoptic jejunostomy through stoma, use 43235)

⊙ **44376** Small intestinal endoscopy, enteroscopy beyond second portion of duodenum, including ileum; diagnostic, with or without collection of specimen(s) by brushing or washing (separate procedure)

⊙ **44377** with biopsy, single or multiple

⊙ **44378** with control of bleeding (eg, injection, bipolar cautery, unipolar cautery, laser, heater probe, stapler, plasma coagulator)

⊙ **44379** with transendoscopic stent placement (includes predilation)

⊙ **44380** Ileoscopy, through stoma; diagnostic, with or without collection of specimen(s) by brushing or washing (separate procedure)

⊙ **44382** with biopsy, single or multiple

⊙ **44383** with transendoscopic stent placement (includes predilation)

⊙ **44385** Endoscopic evaluation of small intestinal (abdominal or pelvic) pouch; diagnostic, with or without collection of specimen(s) by brushing or washing (separate procedure)

⊙ **44386** with biopsy, single or multiple

⊙ **44388** Colonoscopy through stoma; diagnostic, with or without collection of specimen(s) by brushing or washing (separate procedure)

⊙ **44389** with biopsy, single or multiple

⊙ **44390** with removal of foreign body

⊙ **44391** with control of bleeding (eg, injection, bipolar cautery, unipolar cautery, laser, heater probe, stapler, plasma coagulator)

⊙ **44392** with removal of tumor(s), polyp(s), or other lesion(s) by hot biopsy forceps or bipolar cautery

⊙ **44393** with ablation of tumor(s), polyp(s), or other lesion(s) not amenable to removal by hot biopsy forceps, bipolar cautery or snare technique

⊙ **44394** with removal of tumor(s), polyp(s), or other lesion(s) by snare technique

(For colonoscopy per rectum, see 45330-45385)

⊙ **44397** with transendoscopic stent placement (includes predilation)

INTRODUCTION

⊘ ⊙**44500** Introduction of long gastrointestinal tube (eg, Miller-Abbott) (separate procedure)

(For radiological supervision and interpretation, use 74340)

(For naso- or oro-gastric tube placement, use 43752)

Separate Procedure | Unlisted Procedure | CCI Comp. Code | Non-specific Procedure

REPAIR

44602 Suture of small intestine (enterorrhaphy) for perforated ulcer, diverticulum, wound, injury or rupture; single perforation

44603 multiple perforations

44604 Suture of large intestine (colorrhaphy) for perforated ulcer, diverticulum, wound, injury, or rupture (single or multiple perforations); without colostomy

44605 with colostomy

44615 Intestinal stricturoplasty (enterotomy and enterorrhaphy) with or without dilation, for intestinal obstruction

44620 Closure of enterostomy, large or small intestine;

44625 with resection and anastomosis other than colorectal

44626 with resection and colorectal anastomosis (eg, closure of Hartmann type procedure)

(For laparoscopic procedure, use 44227)

44640 Closure of intestinal cutaneous fistula

44650 Closure of enteroenteric or enterocolic fistula

44660 Closure of enterovesical fistula; without intestinal or bladder resection

44661 with intestine and/or bladder resection

(For closure of renocolic fistula, see 50525, 50526)

(For closure of gastrocolic fistula, use 43880)

(For closure of rectovesical fistula, see 45800, 45805)

44680 Intestinal plication (separate procedure)

OTHER PROCEDURES

44700 Exclusion of small intestine from pelvis by mesh or other prosthesis, or native tissue (eg, bladder or omentum)

● New Code ▲ Revised Code + Add-On Code ⃠ Modifier -51 Exempt ⊙ Conscious Sedation

(For therapeutic radiation clinical treatment, see Radiation Oncology section)

+ **44701** Intraoperative colonic lavage (List separately in addition to code for primary procedure)

(Use 44701 in conjunction with codes 44140, 44145, 44150, or 44604 as appropriate)

(Do not report 44701 in conjunction with 44300, 44950-44960)

44715 Backbench standard preparation of cadaver or living donor intestine allograft prior to transplantation, including mobilization and fashioning of the superior mesenteric artery and vein

44720 Backbench reconstruction of cadaver or living donor intestine allograft prior to transplantation; venous anastomosis, each

44721 arterial anastomosis, each

44799 Unlisted procedure, intestine

(For unlisted laparoscopic procedure, intestine except rectum, use 44238)

MECKEL'S DIVERTICULUM AND THE MESENTERY

EXCISION

44800 Excision of Meckel's diverticulum (diverticulectomy) or omphalomesenteric duct

44820 Excision of lesion of mesentery (separate procedure)

(With intestine resection, see 44120 or 44140 et seq)

SUTURE

44850 Suture of mesentery (separate procedure)

(For reduction and repair of internal hernia, use 44050)

OTHER PROCEDURES

44899 Unlisted procedure, Meckel's diverticulum and the mesentery

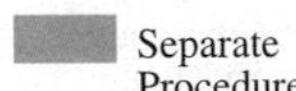 Separate Procedure 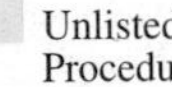 Unlisted Procedure 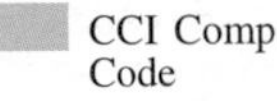 CCI Comp. Code 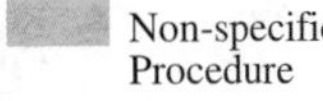 Non-specific Procedure

APPENDIX

INCISION

44900 Incision and drainage of appendiceal abscess; open

⊙ **44901** percutaneous

(For radiological supervision and interpretation, use 75989)

EXCISION

44950 Appendectomy;

(Incidental appendectomy during intra-abdominal surgery does not usually warrant a separate identification. If necessary to report, add modifier -52)

+ **44955** when done for indicated purpose at time of other major procedure (not as separate procedure) (List separately in addition to code for primary procedure)

44960 for ruptured appendix with abscess or generalized peritonitis

LAPAROSCOPY

44970 Laparoscopy, surgical, appendectomy

44979 Unlisted laparoscopy procedure, appendix

RECTUM

INCISION

45000 Transrectal drainage of pelvic abscess

45005 Incision and drainage of submucosal abscess, rectum

45020 Incision and drainage of deep supralevator, pelvirectal, or retrorectal abscess

(See also 46050, 46060)

EXCISION

45100 Biopsy of anorectal wall, anal approach (eg, congenital megacolon)

(For endoscopic biopsy, use 45305)

45108 Anorectal myomectomy

45110 Proctectomy; complete, combined abdominoperineal, with colostomy

(For laparoscopic procedure, use 45395)

45111 partial resection of rectum, transabdominal approach

45112 Proctectomy, combined abdominoperineal, pull-through procedure (eg, colo-anal anastomosis)

(For colo-anal anastomosis with colonic reservoir or pouch, use 45119)

45113 Proctectomy, partial, with rectal mucosectomy, ileoanal anastomosis, creation of ileal reservoir (S or J), with or without loop ileostomy

45114 Proctectomy, partial, with anastomosis; abdominal and transsacral approach

45116 transsacral approach only (Kraske type)

45119 Proctectomy, combined abdominoperineal pull-through procedure (eg, colo-anal anastomosis), with creation of colonic reservoir (eg, J-pouch), with diverting enterostomy when performed

(For laparoscopic procedure, use 45397)

45120 Proctectomy, complete (for congenital megacolon), abdominal and perineal approach; with pull-through procedure and anastomosis (eg, Swenson, Duhamel, or Soave type operation)

45121 with subtotal or total colectomy, with multiple biopsies

45123 Proctectomy, partial, without anastomosis, perineal approach

45126 Pelvic exenteration for colorectal malignancy, with proctectomy (with or without colostomy), with removal of bladder and ureteral transplantations, and/or hysterectomy, or cervicectomy, with or without removal of tube(s), with or without removal of ovary(s), or any combination thereof

45130 Excision of rectal procidentia, with anastomosis; perineal approach

Separate Procedure | Unlisted Procedure | CCI Comp. Code | Non-specific Procedure

45135 abdominal and perineal approach

45136 Excision of ileoanal reservoir with ileostomy

(Do not report 45136 in addition to 44005, 44120, 44310)

45150 Division of stricture of rectum

45160 Excision of rectal tumor by proctotomy, transsacral or transcoccygeal approach

45170 Excision of rectal tumor, transanal approach

DESTRUCTION

45190 Destruction of rectal tumor (eg, electrodessiccation, electrosurgery, laser ablation, laser resection, cryosurgery) transanal approach

ENDOSCOPY

45300 Proctosigmoidoscopy, rigid; diagnostic, with or without collection of specimen(s) by brushing or washing (separate procedure)

⊙ **45303** with dilation (eg, balloon, guide wire, bougie)

(For radiological supervision and interpretation, use 74360)

⊙ **45305** with biopsy, single or multiple

⊙ **45307** with removal of foreign body

⊙ **45308** with removal of single tumor, polyp, or other lesion by hot biopsy forceps or bipolar cautery

⊙ **45309** with removal of single tumor, polyp, or other lesion by snare technique

⊙ **45315** with removal of multiple tumors, polyps, or other lesions by hot biopsy forceps, bipolar cautery or snare technique

⊙ **45317** with control of bleeding (eg, injection, bipolar cautery, unipolar cautery, laser, heater probe, stapler, plasma coagulator)

⊙ **45320** with ablation of tumor(s), polyp(s), or other lesion(s) not amenable to removal by hot biopsy forceps, bipolar cautery or snare technique (eg, laser)

⊙ **45321** with decompression of volvulus

⊙ **45327** with transendoscopic stent placement (includes predilation)

45330 Sigmoidoscopy, flexible; diagnostic, with or without collection of specimen(s) by brushing or washing (separate procedure)

45331 with biopsy, single or multiple

⊙ **45332** with removal of foreign body

⊙ **45333** with removal of tumor(s), polyp(s), or other lesion(s) by hot biopsy forceps or bipolar cautery

⊙ **45334** with control of bleeding (eg, injection, bipolar cautery, unipolar cautery, laser, heater probe, stapler, plasma coagulator)

⊙ **45335** with directed submucosal injection(s), any substance

⊙ **45337** with decompression of volvulus, any method

⊙ **45338** with removal of tumor(s), polyp(s), or other lesion(s) by snare technique

⊙ **45339** with ablation of tumor(s), polyp(s), or other lesion(s) not amenable to removal by hot biopsy forceps, bipolar cautery or snare technique

⊙ **45340** with dilation by balloon, 1 or more strictures

(Do not report 45340 in conjunction with 45345)

⊙ **45341** with endoscopic ultrasound examination

⊙ **45342** with transendoscopic ultrasound guided intramural or transmural fine needle aspiration/biopsy(s)

(Do not report 45341, 45342 in conjunction with 76942, 76975)

(For interpretation of specimen, see 88172-88173)

(For transrectal ultrasound utilizing rigid probe device, use 76872)

Separate Procedure  Unlisted Procedure 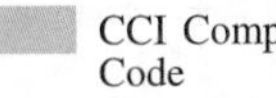 CCI Comp. Code 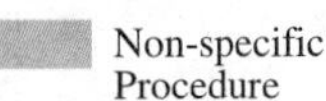 Non-specific Procedure

⊙ **45345** with transendoscopic stent placement (includes predilation)

⊙ **45355** Colonoscopy, rigid or flexible, transabdominal via colotomy, single or multiple

(For fiberoptic colonoscopy beyond 25 cm to splenic flexure, see 45330-45345)

⊙ **45378** Colonoscopy, flexible, proximal to splenic flexure; diagnostic, with or without collection of specimen(s) by brushing or washing, with or without colon decompression (separate procedure)

⊙ **45379** with removal of foreign body

⊙ **45380** with biopsy, single or multiple

⊙ **45381** with directed submucosal injection(s), any substance

⊙ **45382** with control of bleeding (eg, injection, bipolar cautery, unipolar cautery, laser, heater probe, stapler, plasma coagulator)

⊙ **45383** with ablation of tumor(s), polyp(s), or other lesion(s) not amenable to removal by hot biopsy forceps, bipolar cautery or snare technique

⊙ **45384** with removal of tumor(s), polyp(s), or other lesion(s) by hot biopsy forceps or bipolar cautery

⊙ **45385** with removal of tumor(s), polyp(s), or other lesion(s) by snare technique

(For small intestine and stomal endoscopy, see 44360-44393)

⊙ **45386** with dilation by balloon, 1 or more strictures

(Do not report 45386 in conjunction with 45387)

⊙ **45387** with transendoscopic stent placement (includes predilation)

⊙ **45391** with endoscopic ultrasound examination

(Do not report 45391 in conjunction with 45330, 45341, 45342, 45378, 76872)

⊙ **45392** with transendoscopic ultrasound guided intramural or transmural fine needle aspiration/biopsy(s)

(Do not report 45392 in conjunction with 45330, 45341, 45342, 45378, 76872)

LAPAROSCOPY

Excision

45395 Laparoscopy, surgical; proctectomy, complete, combined abdominoperineal, with colostomy

(For open procedure, use 45110)

45397 proctectomy, combined abdominoperineal pull-through procedure (eg, colo-anal anastomosis), with creation of colonic reservoir (eg, J-pouch), with diverting enterostomy, when performed

(For open procedure, use 45119)

Repair

45400 Laparoscopy, surgical; proctopexy (for prolapse)

(For open procedure, use 45540, 45541)

45402 proctopexy (for prolapse), with sigmoid resection

(For open procedure, use 45550)

45499 Unlisted laparoscopy procedure, rectum

REPAIR

45500 Proctoplasty; for stenosis

45505 for prolapse of mucous membrane

45520 Perirectal injection of sclerosing solution for prolapse

45540 Proctopexy (eg, for prolapse); abdominal approach

(For laparoscopic procedure, use 45400)

45541 perineal approach

45550 with sigmoid resection, abdominal approach

(For laparoscopic procedure, use 45402)

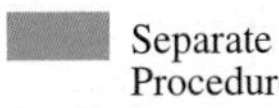 Separate Procedure 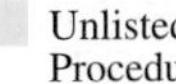 Unlisted Procedure 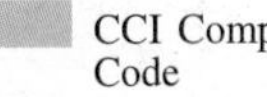 CCI Comp. Code 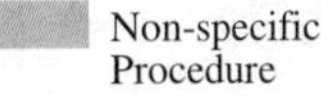 Non-specific Procedure

45560 Repair of rectocele (separate procedure)

(For repair of rectocele with posterior colporrhaphy, use 57250)

45562 Exploration, repair, and presacral drainage for rectal injury;

45563 with colostomy

45800 Closure of rectovesical fistula;

45805 with colostomy

45820 Closure of rectourethral fistula;

45825 with colostomy

(For rectovaginal fistula closure, see 57300-57308)

MANIPULATION

45900 Reduction of procidentia (separate procedure) under anesthesia

45905 Dilation of anal sphincter (separate procedure) under anesthesia other than local

45910 Dilation of rectal stricture (separate procedure) under anesthesia other than local

45915 Removal of fecal impaction or foreign body (separate procedure) under anesthesia

OTHER PROCEDURES

45990 Anorectal exam, surgical, requiring anesthesia (general, spinal, or epidural), diagnostic

(Do not report 45990 in conjunction with 45300-45327, 46600, 57410, 99170)

45999 Unlisted procedure, rectum

(For unlisted laparoscopic procedure, rectum, use 45499)

ANUS

INCISION

(For subcutaneous fistulotomy, use 46270)

46020 Placement of seton

(Do not report 46020 in addition to 46060, 46280, 46600)

46030 Removal of anal seton, other marker

46040 Incision and drainage of ischiorectal and/or perirectal abscess (separate procedure)

46045 Incision and drainage of intramural, intramuscular, or submucosal abscess, transanal, under anesthesia

46050 Incision and drainage, perianal abscess, superficial

(See also 45020, 46060)

46060 Incision and drainage of ischiorectal or intramural abscess, with fistulectomy or fistulotomy, submuscular, with or without placement of seton

(Do not report 46060 in addition to 46020)

(See also 45020)

46070 Incision, anal septum (infant)

(For anoplasty, see 46700-46705)

(Do not report modifier '-63' in conjunction with 46070)

46080 Sphincterotomy, anal, division of sphincter (separate procedure)

46083 Incision of thrombosed hemorrhoid, external

EXCISION

46200 Fissurectomy, with or without sphincterotomy

46210 Cryptectomy; single

46211 multiple (separate procedure)

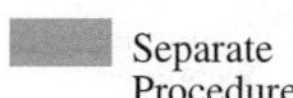

Separate Procedure | Unlisted Procedure | CCI Comp. Code | Non-specific Procedure

46220 Papillectomy or excision of single tag, anus (separate procedure)

46221 Hemorrhoidectomy, by simple ligature (eg, rubber band)

46230 Excision of external hemorrhoid tags and/or multiple papillae

46250 Hemorrhoidectomy, external, complete

46255 Hemorrhoidectomy, internal and external, simple;

46257 with fissurectomy

46258 with fistulectomy, with or without fissurectomy

46260 Hemorrhoidectomy, internal and external, complex or extensive;

46261 with fissurectomy

46262 with fistulectomy, with or without fissurectomy

(For injection of hemorrhoids, use 46500; for destruction, see 46934-46936; for ligation, see 46945, 46946; for hemorrhoidopexy, use 46947)

46270 Surgical treatment of anal fistula (fistulectomy/fistulotomy); subcutaneous

46275 submuscular

46280 complex or multiple, with or without placement of seton

(Do not report 46280 in addition to 46020)

46285 second stage

46288 Closure of anal fistula with rectal advancement flap

46320 Enucleation or excision of external thrombotic hemorrhoid

INTRODUCTION

46500 Injection of sclerosing solution, hemorrhoids

(For excision of hemorrhoids, see 46250-46262; for destruction, see 46934-46936; for ligation, see 46945, 46946; for hemorrhoidopexy, use 46947)

● New Code ▲ Revised Code + Add-On Code ⊘ Modifier -51 Exempt ⊙ Conscious Sedation

46505 Chemodenervation of internal anal sphincter

(For chemodenervation of other muscles, see 64612-64614, 64640)

(Report the specific service in conjunction with the specific substance(s) or drug(s) provided)

ENDOSCOPY

46600 Anoscopy; diagnostic, with or without collection of specimen(s) by brushing or washing (separate procedure)

(Do not report 46600 in addition to 46020)

46604 with dilation (eg, balloon, guide wire, bougie)

46606 with biopsy, single or multiple

46608 with removal of foreign body

46610 with removal of single tumor, polyp, or other lesion by hot biopsy forceps or bipolar cautery

46611 with removal of single tumor, polyp, or other lesion by snare technique

46612 with removal of multiple tumors, polyps, or other lesions by hot biopsy forceps, bipolar cautery or snare technique

46614 with control of bleeding (eg, injection, bipolar cautery, unipolar cautery, laser, heater probe, stapler, plasma coagulator)

46615 with ablation of tumor(s), polyp(s), or other lesion(s) not amenable to removal by hot biopsy forceps, bipolar cautery or snare technique

REPAIR

46700 Anoplasty, plastic operation for stricture; adult

46705 infant

(For simple incision of anal septum, use 46070)

(Do not report modifier '-63' in conjunction with 46705)

46706 Repair of anal fistula with fibrin glue

46710 Repair of ileoanal pouch fistula/sinus (eg, perineal or vaginal), pouch advancement; transperineal approach

46712 combined transperineal and transabdominal approach

46715 Repair of low imperforate anus; with anoperineal fistula (cut-back procedure)

46716 with transposition of anoperineal or anovestibular fistula

(Do not report modifier '-63' in conjunction with 46715, 46716)

46730 Repair of high imperforate anus without fistula; perineal or sacroperineal approach

46735 combined transabdominal and sacroperineal approaches

(Do not report modifier '-63' in conjunction with 46730, 46735)

46740 Repair of high imperforate anus with rectourethral or rectovaginal fistula; perineal or sacroperineal approach

46742 combined transabdominal and sacroperineal approaches

(Do not report modifier '-63' in conjunction with 46740, 46742)

46744 Repair of cloacal anomaly by anorectovaginoplasty and urethroplasty, sacroperineal approach

(Do not report modifier '-63' in conjunction with 46744)

46746 Repair of cloacal anomaly by anorectovaginoplasty and urethroplasty, combined abdominal and sacroperineal approach;

46748 with vaginal lengthening by intestinal graft or pedicle flaps

46750 Sphincteroplasty, anal, for incontinence or prolapse; adult

46751 child

46753 Graft (Thiersch operation) for rectal incontinence and/or prolapse

46754 Removal of Thiersch wire or suture, anal canal

46760 Sphincteroplasty, anal, for incontinence, adult; muscle transplant

46761 levator muscle imbrication (Park posterior anal repair)

46762 implantation artificial sphincter

DESTRUCTION

46900 Destruction of lesion(s), anus (eg, condyloma, papilloma, molluscum contagiosum, herpetic vesicle), simple; chemical

46910 electrodesiccation

46916 cryosurgery

46917 laser surgery

46922 surgical excision

46924 Destruction of lesion(s), anus (eg, condyloma, papilloma, molluscum contagiosum, herpetic vesicle), extensive (eg, laser surgery, electrosurgery, cryosurgery, chemosurgery)

46934 Destruction of hemorrhoids, any method; internal

46935 external

46936 internal and external

(For excision of hemorrhoids, see 46250-46262; for injection, use 46500; for ligation, see 46945, 46946; for hemorrhoidopexy, use 46947)

46937 Cryosurgery of rectal tumor; benign

46938 malignant

46940 Curettage or cautery of anal fissure, including dilation of anal sphincter (separate procedure); initial

46942 subsequent

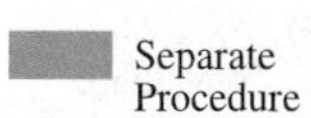 Separate Procedure 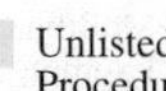 Unlisted Procedure 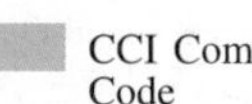 CCI Comp. Code 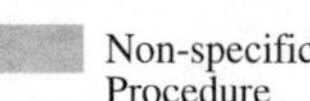 Non-specific Procedure

SUTURE

46945 Ligation of internal hemorrhoids; single procedure

46946 multiple procedures

46947 Hemorrhoidopexy (eg, for prolapsing internal hemorrhoids) by stapling

(For excision of hemorrhoids, see 46250-46262; for injection, use 46500; for destruction, see 46934-46936)

OTHER PROCEDURES

46999 Unlisted procedure, anus

LIVER

INCISION

47000 Biopsy of liver, needle; percutaneous

(If imaging guidance is performed, see 76942, 77002, 77012, 77021)

+ **47001** when done for indicated purpose at time of other major procedure (List separately in addition to code for primary procedure)

(If imaging guidance is performed, see 76942, 77002)

(For fine needle aspiration in conjunction with 47000, 47001, see 10021, 10022)

(For evaluation of fine needle aspirate in conjunction with 47000, 47001, see 88172, 88173)

47010 Hepatotomy; for open drainage of abscess or cyst, one or two stages

⊙ **47011** for percutaneous drainage of abscess or cyst, one or two stages

(For radiological supervision and interpretation, use 75989)

47015 Laparotomy, with aspiration and/or injection of hepatic parasitic (eg, amoebic or echinococcal) cyst(s) or abscess(es)

EXCISION

47100 Biopsy of liver, wedge

47120 Hepatectomy, resection of liver; partial lobectomy

47122 trisegmentectomy

47125 total left lobectomy

47130 total right lobectomy

LIVER TRANSPLANTATION

Liver allotransplantation involves three distinct components of physician work:

1) **Cadaver donor hepatectomy**, which includes harvesting the graft and cold preservation of the graft (perfusing with cold preservation solution and cold maintenance) (use 47133). **Living donor hepatectomy**, which includes harvesting the graft, cold preservation of the graft (perfusing with cold preservation solution and cold maintenance), and care of the donor (see 47140-47142).

2) **Backbench work**:

Standard preparation of the whole liver graft will include one of the following:

Preparation of whole liver graft (including cholecystectomy, if necessary, and dissection and removal of surrounding soft tissues to prepare vena cava, portal vein, hepatic artery, and common bile duct for implantation) (use 47143).

Preparation as described for whole liver graft, plus trisegment split into two partial grafts (use 47144).

Preparation as described for whole liver graft, plus lobe split into two partial grafts (use 47145).

Additional reconstruction of the liver graft may include venous and/or arterial anastomosis(es) (see 47146, 47147).

3) **Recipient liver allotransplantation**, which includes recipient hepatectomy (partial or whole), transplantation of the allograft (partial or whole), and care of the recipient (see 47135, 47136).

47133 Donor hepatectomy (including cold preservation), from cadaver donor

47135 Liver allotransplantation; orthotopic, partial or whole, from cadaver or living donor, any age

Separate Procedure | Unlisted Procedure | CCI Comp. Code | Non-specific Procedure

47136 heterotopic, partial or whole, from cadaver or living donor, any age

47140 Donor hepatectomy (including cold preservation), from living donor; left lateral segment only (segments II and III)

47141 total left lobectomy (segments II, III, and IV)

47142 total right lobectomy (segments V, VI, VII, and VIII)

47143 Backbench standard preparation of cadaver donor whole liver graft prior to allotransplantation, including cholecystectomy, if necessary, and dissection and removal of surrounding soft tissues to prepare the vena cava, portal vein, hepatic artery, and common bile duct for implantation; without trisegment or lobe split

47144 with trisegment split of whole liver graft into two partial liver grafts (ie, left lateral segment (segments II and III) and right trisegment (segments I and IV through VIII))

47145 with lobe split of whole liver graft into two partial liver grafts (ie, left lobe (segments II, III, and IV) and right lobe (segments I and V through VIII))

47146 Backbench reconstruction of cadaver or living donor liver graft prior to allotransplantation; venous anastomosis, each

47147 arterial anastomosis, each

(Do not report 47143-47147 in conjunction with 47120-47125, 47600, 47610)

REPAIR

47300 Marsupialization of cyst or abscess of liver

47350 Management of liver hemorrhage; simple suture of liver wound or injury

47360 complex suture of liver wound or injury, with or without hepatic artery ligation

47361 exploration of hepatic wound, extensive debridement, coagulation and/or suture, with or without packing of liver

47362 re-exploration of hepatic wound for removal of packing

LAPAROSCOPY

47370 Laparoscopy, surgical, ablation of one or more liver tumor(s); radiofrequency

(For imaging guidance, use 76490)

47371 cryosurgical

(For imaging guidance, use 76490)

47379 Unlisted laparoscopic procedure, liver

OTHER PROCEDURES

47380 Ablation, open, of one or more liver tumor(s); radiofrequency

(For imaging guidance, use 76490)

47381 cryosurgical

(For imaging guidance, use 76490)

47382 Ablation, one or more liver tumor(s), percutaneous, radiofrequency

(For imaging guidance and monitoring, see 76490, 77013, 77022)

47399 Unlisted procedure, liver

BILIARY TRACT

INCISION

47400 Hepaticotomy or hepaticostomy with exploration, drainage, or removal of calculus

47420 Choledochotomy or choledochostomy with exploration, drainage, or removal of calculus, with or without cholecystotomy; without transduodenal sphincterotomy or sphincteroplasty

47425 with transduodenal sphincterotomy or sphincteroplasty

47460 Transduodenal sphincterotomy or sphincteroplasty, with or without transduodenal extraction of calculus (separate procedure)

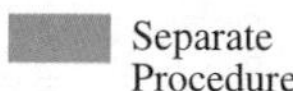 Separate Procedure 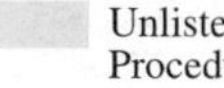 Unlisted Procedure 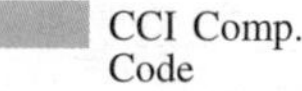 CCI Comp. Code 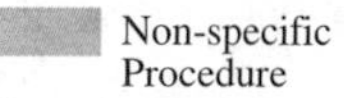 Non-specific Procedure

47480 Cholecystotomy or cholecystostomy with exploration, drainage, or removal of calculus (separate procedure)

47490 Percutaneous cholecystostomy

(For radiological supervision and interpretation, use 75989)

INTRODUCTION

47500 Injection procedure for percutaneous transhepatic cholangiography

(For radiological supervision and interpretation, use 74320)

47505 Injection procedure for cholangiography through an existing catheter (eg, percutaneous transhepatic or T-tube)

(For radiological supervision and interpretation, use 74305)

47510 Introduction of percutaneous transhepatic catheter for biliary drainage

(For radiological supervision and interpretation, use 75980)

47511 Introduction of percutaneous transhepatic stent for internal and external biliary drainage

(For radiological supervision and interpretation, use 75982)

47525 Change of percutaneous biliary drainage catheter

(For radiological supervision and interpretation, use 75984)

47530 Revision and/or reinsertion of transhepatic tube

(For radiological supervision and interpretation, use 75984)

ENDOSCOPY

+ **47550** Biliary endoscopy, intraoperative (choledochoscopy) (List separately in addition to code for primary procedure)

47552 Biliary endoscopy, percutaneous via T-tube or other tract; diagnostic, with or without collection of specimen(s) by brushing and/or washing (separate procedure)

47553 with biopsy, single or multiple

47554 with removal of calculus/calculi

47555 with dilation of biliary duct stricture(s) without stent

47556 with dilation of biliary duct stricture(s) with stent

(For ERCP, see 43260-43272, 74363)

(If imaging guidance is performed, see 74363, 75982)

LAPAROSCOPY

47560 Laparoscopy, surgical; with guided transhepatic cholangiography, without biopsy

47561 with guided transhepatic cholangiography with biopsy

47562 cholecystectomy

47563 cholecystectomy with cholangiography

47564 cholecystectomy with exploration of common duct

47570 cholecystoenterostomy

47579 Unlisted laparoscopy procedure, biliary tract

EXCISION

47600 Cholecystectomy;

47605 with cholangiography

(For laparoscopic approach, see 47562-47564)

47610 Cholecystectomy with exploration of common duct;

(For cholecystectomy with exploration of common duct with biliary endoscopy, use 47610 with 47550)

47612 with choledochoenterostomy

47620 with transduodenal sphincterotomy or sphincteroplasty, with or without cholangiography

47630 Biliary duct stone extraction, percutaneous via T-tube tract, basket, or snare (eg, Burhenne technique)

(For radiological supervision and interpretation, use 74327)

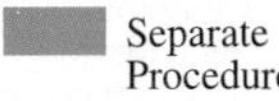 Separate Procedure 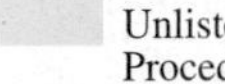 Unlisted Procedure 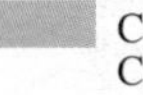 CCI Comp. Code 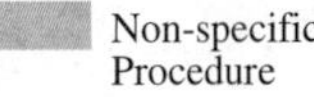 Non-specific Procedure

47700 Exploration for congenital atresia of bile ducts, without repair, with or without liver biopsy, with or without cholangiography

(Do not report modifier -63 in conjunction with 47700)

47701 Portoenterostomy (eg, Kasai procedure)

(Do not report modifier -63 in conjunction with 47701)

47711 Excision of bile duct tumor, with or without primary repair of bile duct; extrahepatic

47712 intrahepatic

(For anastomosis, see 47760-47800)

47715 Excision of choledochal cyst

(47716 deleted 2007 edition, see 47719)

REPAIR

● **47719** Anastomosis, choledochal cyst, without excision

47720 Cholecystoenterostomy; direct

(For laparoscopic approach, use 47570)

47721 with gastroenterostomy

47740 Roux-en-Y

47741 Roux-en-Y with gastroenterostomy

47760 Anastomosis, of extrahepatic biliary ducts and gastrointestinal tract

47765 Anastomosis, of intrahepatic ducts and gastrointestinal tract

47780 Anastomosis, Roux-en-Y, of extrahepatic biliary ducts and gastrointestinal tract

47785 Anastomosis, Roux-en-Y, of intrahepatic biliary ducts and gastrointestinal tract

47800 Reconstruction, plastic, of extrahepatic biliary ducts with end-to-end anastomosis

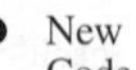

47801 Placement of choledochal stent

47802 U-tube hepaticoenterostomy

47900 Suture of extrahepatic biliary duct for pre-existing injury (separate procedure)

OTHER PROCEDURES

47999 Unlisted procedure, biliary tract

PANCREAS

(For peroral pancreatic endoscopic procedures, see 43260-43272)

INCISION

48000 Placement of drains, peripancreatic, for acute pancreatitis;

48001 with cholecystostomy, gastrostomy, and jejunostomy

(48005 deleted 2007 edition, see 48105)

48020 Removal of pancreatic calculus

EXCISION

48100 Biopsy of pancreas, open (eg, fine needle aspiration, needle core biopsy, wedge biopsy)

48102 Biopsy of pancreas, percutaneous needle

(For radiological supervision and interpretation, see 76942, 77002, 77012, 77021)

(For fine needle aspiration, use 10022)

(For evaluation of fine needle aspirate, see 88172, 88173)

● **48105** Resection or debridement of pancreas and peripancreatic tissue for acute necrotizing pancreatitis

48120 Excision of lesion of pancreas (eg, cyst, adenoma)

48140 Pancreatectomy, distal subtotal, with or without splenectomy; without pancreaticojejunostomy

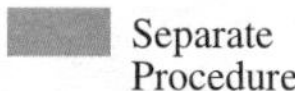 Separate Procedure 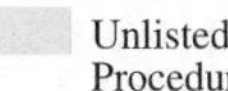 Unlisted Procedure 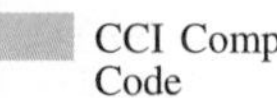 CCI Comp. Code 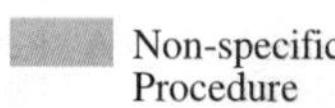 Non-specific Procedure

48145 with pancreaticojejunostomy

48146 Pancreatectomy, distal, near-total with preservation of duodenum (Child-type procedure)

48148 Excision of ampulla of Vater

48150 Pancreatectomy, proximal subtotal with total duodenectomy, partial gastrectomy, choledochoenterostomy and gastrojejunostomy (Whipple-type procedure); with pancreatojejunostomy

48152 without pancreatojejunostomy

48153 Pancreatectomy, proximal subtotal with near-total duodenectomy, choledochoenterostomy, and duodenojejunostomy (pylorus-sparing, whipple-type procedure); with pancreatojejunostomy

48154 without pancreatojejunostomy

48155 Pancreatectomy, total

48160 Pancreatectomy, total or subtotal, with autologous transplantation of pancreas or pancreatic islet cells

(48180 deleted 2007 edition, see 48548)

INTRODUCTION

\+ **48400** Injection procedure for intraoperative pancreatography (List separately in addition to code for primary procedure)

(For radiological supervision and interpretation, see 74300-74305)

REPAIR

48500 Marsupialization of pancreatic cyst

48510 External drainage, pseudocyst of pancreas; open

⊙ **48511** percutaneous

(For radiological supervision and interpretation, use 75989)

48520 Internal anastomosis of pancreatic cyst to gastrointestinal tract; direct

48540 Roux-en-Y

48545 Pancreatorrhaphy for injury

48547 Duodenal exclusion with gastrojejunostomy for pancreatic injury

● **48548** Pancreaticojejunostomy, side-to-side anastomosis (Puestow-type operation)

PANCREAS TRANSPLANTATION

Pancreas allotransplantation involves three distinct components of physician work:

1) **Cadaver donor pancreatectomy**, which includes harvesting the pancreas graft, with or without duodenal segment, and cold preservation of the graft (perfusing with cold preservation solution and cold maintenance) (use 48550).

2) **Backbench work**:

Standard preparation of a cadaver donor pancreas allograft prior to transplantation includes dissection of the allograft from surrounding soft tissues, splenectomy, duodenotomy, ligation of bile duct, ligation of mesenteric vessels, and Y-graft arterial anastomoses from the iliac artery to the superior mesenteric artery and to the splenic artery (use 48551).

Additional reconstruction of a cadaver donor pancreas allograft prior to transplantation may include venous anastomosis(es) (use 48552).

3) **Recipient pancreas allotransplantation**, which includes transplantation of allograft, and care of the recipient (use 48554).

48550 Donor pancreatectomy (including cold preservation), with or without duodenal segment for transplantation

48551 Backbench standard preparation of cadaver donor pancreas allograft prior to transplantation, including dissection of allograft from surrounding soft tissues, splenectomy, duodenotomy, ligation of bile duct, ligation of mesenteric vessels, and Y-graft arterial anastomoses from iliac artery to superior mesenteric artery and to splenic artery

48552 Backbench reconstruction of cadaver donor pancreas allograft prior to transplantation, venous anastomosis, each

(Do not report 48551 and 48552 in conjunction with 35531, 35563, 35685, 38100-38102, 44010, 44820, 44850, 47460, 47505-47525, 47550-47556, 48100-48120, 48545)

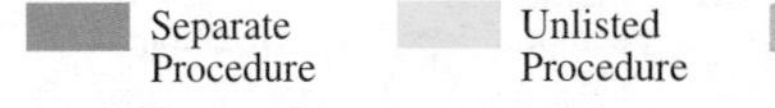
Separate Procedure

Unlisted Procedure

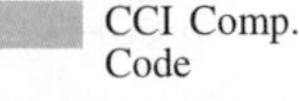
CCI Comp. Code

Non-specific Procedure

48554 Transplantation of pancreatic allograft

48556 Removal of transplanted pancreatic allograft

OTHER PROCEDURES

48999 Unlisted procedure, pancreas

ABDOMEN, PERITONEUM, AND OMENTUM

INCISION

49000 Exploratory laparotomy, exploratory celiotomy with or without biopsy(s) (separate procedure)

(To report wound exploration due to penetrating trauma without laparatomy, use 20102)

49002 Reopening of recent laparotomy

(To report re-exploration of hepatic wound for removal of packing, use 47362)

49010 Exploration, retroperitoneal area with or without biopsy(s) (separate procedure)

(To report wound exploration due to penetrating trauma without laparotomy, use 20102)

49020 Drainage of peritoneal abscess or localized peritonitis, exclusive of appendiceal abscess; open

(For appendiceal abscess, use 44900)

⊙ **49021** percutaneous

(For radiological supervision and interpretation, use 75989)

49040 Drainage of subdiaphragmatic or subphrenic abscess; open

⊙ **49041** percutaneous

(For radiological supervision and interpretation, use 75989)

49060 Drainage of retroperitoneal abscess; open

⊙ **49061** percutaneous

(For laparoscopic drainage, use 49323)

● New Code ▲ Revised Code + Add-On Code ⃠ Modifier -51 Exempt ⊙ Conscious Sedation

(For radiological supervision and interpretation, use 75989)

49062 Drainage of extraperitoneal lymphocele to peritoneal cavity, open

49080 Peritoneocentesis, abdominal paracentesis, or peritoneal lavage (diagnostic or therapeutic); initial

49081 subsequent

(If imaging guidance is performed, see 76942, 77012)

(49085 deleted 2007 edition, see 49402)

EXCISION, DESTRUCTION

(For lysis of intestinal adhesions, use 44005)

49180 Biopsy, abdominal or retroperitoneal mass, percutaneous needle

(If imaging guidance is performed, see 76942, 77002, 77012, 77021)

(For fine needle aspiration, use 10021 or 10022)

(For evaluation of fine needle aspirate, see 88172, 88173)

49200 Excision or destruction, open, intra-abdominal or retroperitoneal tumors or cysts or endometriomas;

49201 extensive

(For resection of recurrent ovarian, tubal, primary peritoneal, or uterine malignancy, see 58957, 58958)

(For open cryoablation of renal tumor, use 50250)

(For percutaneous cryotherapy ablation of renal tumors, use Category III code 0135T)

49215 Excision of presacral or sacrococcygeal tumor

(Do not report modifier '-63' in conjunction with 49215)

49220 Staging laparotomy for Hodgkins disease or lymphoma (includes splenectomy, needle or open biopsies of both liver lobes, possibly also removal of abdominal nodes, abdominal node and/or bone marrow biopsies, ovarian repositioning)

49250 Umbilectomy, omphalectomy, excision of umbilicus (separate procedure)

49255 Omentectomy, epiploectomy, resection of omentum (separate procedure)

LAPAROSCOPY

49320 Laparoscopy, abdomen, peritoneum, and omentum; diagnostic, with or without collection of specimen(s) by brushing or washing (separate procedure)

49321 Laparoscopy, surgical; with biopsy (single or multiple)

49322 with aspiration of cavity or cyst (eg, ovarian cyst) (single or multiple)

49323 with drainage of lymphocele to peritoneal cavity

(For percutaneous or open drainage, see 49060, 49061)

● **49324** Laparoscopy, surgical; with insertion of intraperitoneal cannula or catheter, permanent

(For subcutaneous extension of intraperitoneal catheter with remote chest exit site, use 49435 in conjunction with 49324)

(For open insertion of permanent intraperitoneal cannula or catheter, use 49421)

● **49325** with revision of previously placed intraperitoneal cannula or catheter, with removal of intraluminal obstructive material if performed

●+**49326** with omentopexy (omental tacking procedure) (List separately in addition to code for primary procedure)

(Use 49326 in conjunction with 49324, 49325)

49329 Unlisted laparoscopy procedure, abdomen, peritoneum and omentum

INTRODUCTION, REVISION, REMOVAL

49400 Injection of air or contrast into peritoneal cavity (separate procedure)

(For radiological supervision and interpretation, use 74190)

● New Code ▲ Revised Code + Add-On Code ⊘ Modifier -51 Exempt ⊙ Conscious Sedation

● **49402** Removal of peritoneal foreign body from peritoneal cavity

(For lysis of intestinal adhesions, use 44005)

49419 Insertion of intraperitoneal cannula or catheter, with subcutaneous reservoir, permanent (ie, totally implantable)

(For removal, use 49422)

49420 Insertion of intraperitoneal cannula or catheter for drainage or dialysis; temporary

49421 permanent

(For laparoscopic insertion of permanent intraperitoneal cannula or catheter, use 49324)

(For subcutaneous extension of intraperitoneal catheter with remote chest exit site, use 49435 in conjunction with 49421)

49422 Removal of permanent intraperitoneal cannula or catheter

(For removal of a temporary catheter/cannula, use appropriate E/M code)

49423 Exchange of previously placed abscess or cyst drainage catheter under radiological guidance (separate procedure)

(For radiological supervision and interpretation, use 75984)

49424 Contrast injection for assessment of abscess or cyst via previously placed drainage catheter or tube (separate procedure)

(For radiological supervision and interpretation, use 76080)

49425 Insertion of peritoneal-venous shunt

49426 Revision of peritoneal-venous shunt

(For shunt patency test, use 78291)

49427 Injection procedure (eg, contrast media) for evaluation of previously placed peritoneal-venous shunt

(For radiological supervision and interpretation, see 75809, 78291)

49428 Ligation of peritoneal-venous shunt

49429 Removal of peritoneal-venous shunt

●+**49435** Insertion of subcutaneous extension to intraperitoneal cannula or catheter with remote chest exit site (List separately in addition to code for primary procedure)

(Use 49435 in conjunction with 49324, 49421)

● **49436** Delayed creation of exit site from embedded subcutaneous segment of intraperitoneal cannula or catheter

REPAIR

Hernioplasty, Herniorrhaphy, Herniotomy

(For reduction and repair of intra-abdominal hernia, use 44050)

(For debridement of abdominal wall, see 11042, 11043)

(Codes 49491-49651 are unilateral procedures. To report bilateral procedures, report modifier -50 with the appropriate procedure code)

49491 Repair, initial inguinal hernia, preterm infant (less than 37 weeks gestation at birth), performed from birth up to 50 weeks postconception age, with or without hydrocelectomy; reducible

49492 incarcerated or strangulated

(Do not report modifier -63 in conjunction with 49491, 49492)

(Post-conception age equals gestational age at birth plus age of infant in weeks at the time of the hernia repair. Initial inguinal hernia repairs that are performed on preterm infants who are over 50 weeks postconceptual age and under age 6 months at the time of surgery, should be reported using codes 49495, 49496)

49495 Repair, initial inguinal hernia, full term infant under age 6 months, or preterm infant over 50 weeks postconception age and under age 6 months at the time of surgery, with or without hydrocelectomy; reducible

49496 incarcerated or strangulated

(Do not report modifier -63 in conjunction with 49491, 49492)

(Post-conception age equals gestational age at birth plus age in weeks at the time of the hernia repair. Initial inguinal hernia repairs that are performed on preterm infants who are under or up to 50 weeks postconceptual age but under 6 months of age since birth, should be reported using codes 49491, 49492. Inguinal hernia repairs on infants age 6 months to under 5 years should be reported using codes 49500-49501)

49500 Repair initial inguinal hernia, age 6 months to under 5 years, with or without hydrocelectomy; reducible

49501 incarcerated or strangulated

49505 Repair initial inguinal hernia, age 5 years or over; reducible

49507 incarcerated or strangulated

(For inguinal hernia repair, with simple orchiectomy, see 49505 or 49507 and 54520)

(For inguinal hernia repair, with excision of hydrocele or spermatocele, see 49505 or 49507 and 54840 or 55040)

49520 Repair recurrent inguinal hernia, any age; reducible

49521 incarcerated or strangulated

49525 Repair inguinal hernia, sliding, any age

(For incarcerated or strangulated inguinal hernia repair, see 49496, 49501, 49507, 49521)

49540 Repair lumbar hernia

49550 Repair initial femoral hernia, any age; reducible

49553 incarcerated or strangulated

49555 Repair recurrent femoral hernia; reducible

49557 incarcerated or strangulated

49560 Repair initial incisional or ventral hernia; reducible

49561 incarcerated or strangulated

49565 Repair recurrent incisional or ventral hernia; reducible

49566 incarcerated or strangulated

+ **49568** Implantation of mesh or other prosthesis for incisional or ventral hernia repair (List separately in addition to code for the incisional or ventral hernia repair)

49570 Repair epigastric hernia (eg, preperitoneal fat); reducible (separate procedure)

49572 incarcerated or strangulated

49580 Repair umbilical hernia, under age 5 years; reducible

49582 incarcerated or strangulated

49585 Repair umbilical hernia, age 5 years or over; reducible

49587 incarcerated or strangulated

49590 Repair spigelian hernia

49600 Repair of small omphalocele, with primary closure

(Do not report modifier -63 in conjunction with 49600)

49605 Repair of large omphalocele or gastroschisis; with or without prosthesis

49606 with removal of prosthesis, final reduction and closure, in operating room

(Do not report modifier -63 in conjunction with 49605, 49606)

49610 Repair of omphalocele (Gross type operation); first stage

49611 second stage

(Do not report modifier -63 in conjunction with 49610, 49611)

(For diaphragmatic or hiatal hernia repair, see 39502-39541)

(For surgical repair of omentum, use 49999)

LAPAROSCOPY

49650 Laparoscopy, surgical; repair initial inguinal hernia

49651 repair recurrent inguinal hernia

49659 Unlisted laparoscopy procedure, hernioplasty, herniorrhaphy, herniotomy

SUTURE

49900 Suture, secondary, of abdominal wall for evisceration or dehiscence

(For suture of ruptured diaphragm, see 39540, 39541)

(For debridement of abdominal wall, see 11042, 11043)

OTHER PROCEDURES

49904 Omental flap, extra-abdominal (eg, for reconstruction of sternal and chest wall defects)

(Code 49904 includes harvest and transfer. If a second surgeon harvests the omental flap, then the two surgeons should code 49904 as co-surgeons, using modifier -62)

+ **49905** Omental flap, intra-abdominal (List separately in addition to code for primary procedure)

(Do not report 49905 in conjunction with 44700)

49906 Free omental flap with microvascular anastomosis

(Do not report code 69990 in addition to code 49906)

49999 Unlisted procedure, abdomen, peritoneum and omentum

This page intentionally left blank.

URINARY SYSTEM

CPT codes from this section are used to report invasive and surgical procedures performed on the kidney; ureter; bladder; prostate (resection); and urethra.

URODYNAMICS

CPT codes in this section may be used separately or in various combinations. When multiple procedures are performed in the same session, modifier -51 should be added to the second and all subsequent CPT codes. Procedures in this section are performed by, or under the direct supervision of, a physician.

In addition, all materials and supplies, used in the provision of these services, such as instruments, equipment, fluids, gases, probes, catheters, technician's fees, medications, gloves, trays, tubing and other sterile supplies are considered to be included in the base code. Use modifier -26 to code and report interpretation of results or operation of equipment only.

CYSTOSCOPY, URETHROSCOPY, and CYSTOURETHROSCOPY

The descriptions of CPT codes in this section are listed so that the main procedure can be identified without having to list all of the minor related procedures performed at the same time. For example:

52601 Transurethral electrosurgical resection of prostate, including control of postoperative bleeding, complete (vasectomy, meatotomy, cystourethroscopy, urethral calibration and/or dilation, and internal urethrotomy are included)

All of the secondary procedures are included in the single code 52601. If any of the secondary procedures requires significant additional time and effort, to the point of making the procedure "unusual", modifier -22 should be added with an appropriate increase in fee and a report explaining what made the procedure unusual.

(For provision of chemotherapeutic agents, report both the specific service in addition to code(s) for the specific substance(s) or drug(s) provided)

KIDNEY

INCISION

(For retroperitoneal exploration, abscess, tumor, or cyst, see 49010, 49060, 49200, 49201)

50010 Renal exploration, not necessitating other specific procedures

(For laparoscopic ablation of renal mass lesion(s), use 50542)

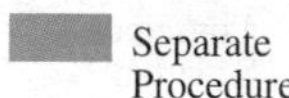

Separate Procedure | Unlisted Procedure | CCI Comp. Code | Non-specific Procedure

50020 Drainage of perirenal or renal abscess; open

⊙ **50021** percutaneous

(For radiological supervision and interpretation, use 75989)

50040 Nephrostomy, nephrotomy with drainage

50045 Nephrotomy, with exploration

(For renal endoscopy performed in conjunction with this procedure, see 50570-50580)

50060 Nephrolithotomy; removal of calculus

50065 secondary surgical operation for calculus

50070 complicated by congenital kidney abnormality

50075 removal of large staghorn calculus filling renal pelvis and calyces (including anatrophic pyelolithotomy)

50080 Percutaneous nephrostolithotomy or pyelostolithotomy, with or without dilation, endoscopy, lithotripsy, stenting, or basket extraction; up to 2 cm

50081 over 2cm

(For establishment of nephrostomy without nephrostolithotomy, see 50040, 50395, 52334)

(For fluoroscopic guidance, see 76000, 76001)

50100 Transection or repositioning of aberrant renal vessels (separate procedure)

50120 Pyelotomy; with exploration

(For renal endoscopy performed in conjunction with this procedure, see 50570-50580)

50125 with drainage, pyelostomy

50130 with removal of calculus (pyelolithotomy, pelviolithotomy, including coagulum pyelolithotomy)

50135 complicated (eg, secondary operation, congenital kidney abnormality)

(For supply of anticarcinogenic agents, use 99070 in addition to code for primary procedure)

EXCISION

(For excision of retroperitoneal tumor or cyst, see 49200, 49201)

(For laparoscopic ablation of renal mass lesion(s), use 50542)

50200 Renal biopsy; percutaneous, by trocar or needle

(For radiological supervision and interpretation, see 76942, 77002, 77012, 77021)

(For fine needle aspiration, use 10022)

(For evaluation of fine needle aspirate, see 88172, 88173)

50205 by surgical exposure of kidney

50220 Nephrectomy, including partial ureterectomy, any open approach including rib resection;

50225 complicated because of previous surgery on same kidney

50230 radical, with regional lymphadenectomy and/or vena caval thrombectomy

(When vena caval resection with reconstruction is necessary, use 37799)

50234 Nephrectomy with total ureterectomy and bladder cuff; through same incision

50236 through separate incision

50240 Nephrectomy, partial

(For laparoscopic partial nephrectomy, use 50543)

50250 Ablation, open, one or more renal mass lesion(s), cryosurgical, including intraoperative ultrasound, if performed

(For laparoscopic ablation of renal mass lesions, use 50542)

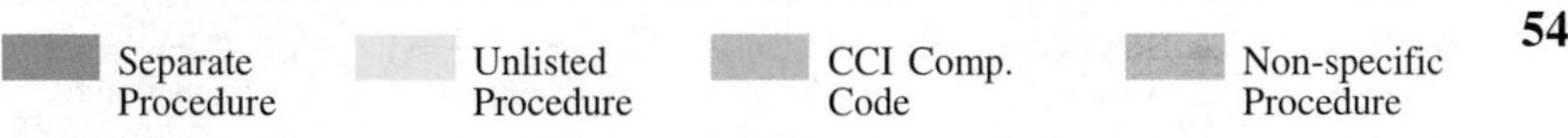

(For percutaneous cryotherapy ablation of renal tumors, use 0135T)

50280 Excision or unroofing of cyst(s) of kidney

(For laparoscopic ablation of renal cysts, use 50541)

50290 Excision of perinephric cyst

RENAL TRANSPLANTATION

Kidney transplantation or renal transplantation is the organ transplant of a kidney in a patient with chronic renal failure or some renal tumors. The main types are deceased and living donor transplant. In the former, the kidney originates from a deceased person. In the latter, the kidney is being donated by a living organ donor.

Occasionally, the kidney is transplanted together with the pancreas. This is done in patients with diabetes mellitus type I, in whom the diabetes is due to destruction of the beta cells of the pancreas and in whom the diabetes has caused renal failure (diabetic nephropathy). This is almost always a deceased donor transplant. Only a few living donor (partial) pancreas transplants have been done. For individuals with diabetes and renal failure, the advantages of earlier transplant from a living donor are approximately equal to the risks of continued dialysis until a combined kidney and pancreas are available from a deceased donor.

The donor and recipient must be ABO blood group compatible, and should ideally share as many HLA and "minor antigens" as possible. This decreases the risk of transplant rejection and need for dialysis and a further transplant. The risk of rejection after transplant may be reduced if the donor and recipient share as many HLA antigens as possible, if the recipient is not already sensitized to potential donor HLA antigens, and if immunosuppressant levels are kept in an appropriate range. In the United States, up to 17% of all deceased donor kidney transplants have no HLA mismatch.

Problems after a transplant may include:

- *Transplant rejection (hyperacute, acute or chronic)*
- *Infections and sepsis due to the immunosuppressant drugs that are required to decrease risk of rejection*
- *Post-transplant lymphoproliferative disorder (a form of lymphoma due to the immune suppressants)*
- *Imbalances in electrolytes including Calcium and Phosphate which can lead to bone problems amongst other things*

Other side effects of medications including gastrointestinal inflammation and ulceration of the stomach and esophagus, hirsutism (excessive hair growth in a male-pattern distribution), hair loss, obesity, acne, diabetes mellitus (type 2), hypercholesterolemia and others.

There are two types of renal transplantation. Renal autotransplantation is the process of transplanting tissue from one part of the body to another. The transplanted tissue is called an autograft. Renal allotransplantation is the transfer of an organ or tissue between genetically different individuals of the same species.

The renal allotransplantation may be between a living donor and a recipient or a cadaver donor and a recipient. The allotransplantation is divided into three separate components:

1) Cadaver donor or living donor nephrectomy

2) Backbench work consisting of preparing the allograft for transplantation

3) Transplantation of the allograft into the recipient

(For dialysis, see 90935-90999)

(For laparoscopic donor nephrectomy, use 50547)

(For laparoscopic drainage of lymphocele to peritoneal cavity, use 49323)

50300 Donor nephrectomy (including cold preservation); from cadaver donor, unilateral or bilateral

50320 open, from living donor

50323 Backbench standard preparation of cadaver donor renal allograft prior to transplantation, including dissection and removal of perinephric fat, diaphragmatic and retroperitoneal attachments, excision of adrenal gland, and preparation of ureter(s), renal vein(s), and renal artery(s), ligating branches, as necessary

(Do not report 50323 in conjunction with 60540, 60545)

50325 Backbench standard preparation of living donor renal allograft (open or laparoscopic) prior to transplantation, including dissection and removal of perinephric fat and preparation of ureter(s), renal vein(s), and renal artery(s), ligating branches, as necessary

50327 Backbench reconstruction of cadaver or living donor renal allograft prior to transplantation; venous anastomosis, each

50328 arterial anastomosis, each

50329 ureteral anastomosis, each

50340 Recipient nephrectomy (separate procedure)

(For bilateral procedure, report 50340 with modifier -50)

50360 Renal allotransplantation, implantation of graft; without recipient nephrectomy

50365 with recipient nephrectomy

(For bilateral procedure, report 50365 with modifier -50)

50370 Removal of transplanted renal allograft

50380 Renal autotransplantation, reimplantation of kidney

(For renal autotransplantation extra-corporeal (bench) surgery, use autotransplantation as the primary procedure and report secondary procedure(s) (eg, partial nephrectomy, nephrolithotomy) with modifier -51)

INTRODUCTION

Renal Pelvis Catheter Procedures

Internally Dwelling

⊙ **50382** Removal (via snare/capture) and replacement of internally dwelling ureteral stent via percutaneous approach, including radiological supervision and interpretation

(For bilateral procedure, use modifier 50)

⊙ **50384** Removal (via snare/capture) of internally dwelling ureteral stent via percutaneous approach, including radiological supervision and interpretation

(For bilateral procedure, use modifier 50)

(Do not report 50382, 50384 in conjunction with 50395)

Externally Accessible

⊙ **50387** Removal and replacement of externally accessible transnephric ureteral stent (eg, external/internal stent) requiring fluoroscopic guidance, including radiological supervision and interpretation

● New Code ▲ Revised Code + Add-On Code ⊘ Modifier -51 Exempt ⊙ Conscious Sedation

(For bilateral procedure, use modifier 50)

(For removal and replacement of externally accessible ureteral stent via ureterostomy or ileal conduit, use 50688)

(For removal without replacement of an externally accessible ureteral stent not requiring fluoroscopic guidance, see Evaluation and Management services codes)

50389 Removal of nephrostomy tube, requiring fluoroscopic guidance (eg, with concurrent indwelling ureteral stent)

(Removal of nephrostomy tube not requiring fluoroscopic guidance is considered inherent to E/M services. Report the appropriate level of E/M service provided)

Other Introduction Procedures

50390 Aspiration and/or injection of renal cyst or pelvis by needle, percutaneous

(For radiological supervision and interpretation, see 74425, 74470, 76942, 77002, 77012, 77021)

(For evaluation of fine needle aspirate, see 88172, 88173)

50391 Instillation(s) of therapeutic agent into renal pelvis and/or ureter through established nephrostomy, pyelostomy or ureterostomy tube (eg, anticarcinogenic or antifungal agent)

50392 Introduction of intracatheter or catheter into renal pelvis for drainage and/or injection, percutaneous

(For radiological supervision and interpretation, see 74475, 76942, 77012)

50393 Introduction of ureteral catheter or stent into ureter through renal pelvis for drainage and/or injection, percutaneous

(For radiological supervision and interpretation, see 74480, 76942, 77002, 77012)

50394 Injection procedure for pyelography (as nephrostogram, pyelostogram, antegrade pyeloureterograms) through nephrostomy or pyelostomy tube, or indwelling ureteral catheter

(For radiological supervision and interpretation, use 74425)

50395 Introduction of guide into renal pelvis and/or ureter with dilation to establish nephrostomy tract, percutaneous

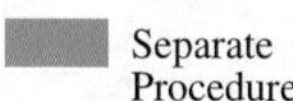 Separate Procedure 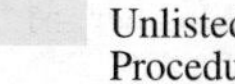 Unlisted Procedure 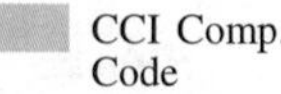 CCI Comp. Code 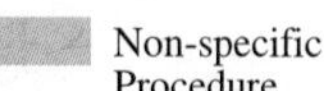 Non-specific Procedure

(For radiological supervision and interpretation, see 74475, 74480, 74485)

(For nephrostolithotomy, see 50080, 50081)

(For retrograde percutaneous nephrostomy, use 52334)

(For endoscopic surgery, see 50551-50561)

50396 Manometric studies through nephrostomy or pyelostomy tube, or indwelling ureteral catheter

(For radiological supervision and interpretation, see 74425, 74475, 74480)

50398 Change of nephrostomy or pyelostomy tube

(For radiological supervision and interpretation, use 75984)

REPAIR

50400 Pyeloplasty (Foley Y-pyeloplasty), plastic operation on renal pelvis, with or without plastic operation on ureter, nephropexy, nephrostomy, pyelostomy, or ureteral splinting; simple

50405 complicated (congenital kidney abnormality, secondary pyeloplasty, solitary kidney, calycoplasty)

(For laparoscopic approach, use 50544)

50500 Nephrorrhaphy, suture of kidney wound or injury

50520 Closure of nephrocutaneous or pyelocutaneous fistula

50525 Closure of nephrovisceral fistula (eg, renocolic), including visceral repair; abdominal approach

50526 thoracic approach

50540 Symphysiotomy for horseshoe kidney with or without pyeloplasty and/or other plastic procedure, unilateral or bilateral (one operation)

LAPAROSCOPY

50541 Laparoscopy, surgical; ablation of renal cysts

50542 ablation of renal mass lesion(s)

(For open procedure, see 50220-50240)

(For open cryosurgical ablation, use 50250)

(For percutaneous cryotherapy ablation of renal tumors, use 0135T)

50543 partial nephrectomy

(For open procedure, use 50240)

50544 pyeloplasty

50545 radical nephrectomy (includes removal of Gerota's fascia and surrounding fatty tissue, removal of regional lymph nodes, and adrenalectomy

(For open procedure, use 50230)

50546 nephrectomy including partial ureterectomy

50547 donor nephrectomy (including cold preservation), from living donor

(For open procedure, use 50320)

(For backbench renal allograft standard preparation prior to transplantation, use 50325)

(For backbench renal allograft reconstruction prior to transplantation, see 50327-50329)

50548 nephrectomy with total ureterectomy

(For open procedure, see 50234, 50236)

50549 Unlisted laparoscopy procedure, renal

(For laparoscopic drainage of lymphocele to peritoneal cavity, use 49323)

ENDOSCOPY

(For supplies and materials, use 99070)

50551 Renal endoscopy through established nephrostomy or pyelostomy, with or without irrigation, instillation, or ureteropyelography, exclusive of radiologic service;

50553 with ureteral catheterization, with or without dilation of ureter

50555 with biopsy

50557 with fulguration and/or incision, with or without biopsy

(50559 deleted 2005 edition)

50561 with removal of foreign body or calculus

50562 with resection of tumor

(When procedures 50570-50580 provide a significant identifiable service, they may be added to 50045 and 50120)

50570 Renal endoscopy through nephrotomy or pyelotomy, with or without irrigation, instillation, or ureteropyelography, exclusive of radiologic service;

(For nephrotomy, use 50045)

(For pyelotomy, use 50120)

50572 with ureteral catheterization, with or without dilation of ureter

50574 with biopsy

50575 with endopyelotomy (includes cystoscopy, ureteroscopy, dilation of ureter and ureteral pelvic junction, incision of ureteral pelvic junction and insertion of endopyelotomy stent)

50576 with fulguration and/or incision, with or without biopsy

(50578 deleted 2005 edition)

50580 with removal of foreign body or calculus

OTHER PROCEDURES

50590 Lithotripsy, extracorporeal shock wave

⊙ **50592** Ablation, one or more renal tumor(s), percutaneous, unilateral, radiofrequency

(50592 is a unilateral procedure. For bilateral procedure, report 50592 with modifier 50)

(For imaging guidance and monitoring, see 76940, 77013, 77022)

(For percutaneous cryotherapy ablation of renal tumors, use 0135T)

URETER

INCISION

50600 Ureterotomy with exploration or drainage (separate procedure)

(For ureteral endoscopy performed in conjunction with this procedure, see 50970-50980)

50605 Ureterotomy for insertion of indwelling stent, all types

50610 Ureterolithotomy; upper one-third of ureter

50620 middle one-third of ureter

50630 lower one-third of ureter

(For laparoscopic approach, use 50945)

(For transvesical ureterolithotomy, use 51060)

(For cystotomy with stone basket extraction of ureteral calculus, use 51065)

(For endoscopic extraction or manipulation of ureteral calculus, see 50080, 50081, 50561, 50961, 50980, 52320-52330, 52352, 52353)

EXCISION

(For ureterocele, see 51535, 52300)

50650 Ureterectomy, with bladder cuff (separate procedure)

50660 Ureterectomy, total, ectopic ureter, combination abdominal, vaginal and/or perineal approach

INTRODUCTION

50684 Injection procedure for ureterography or ureteropyelography through ureterostomy or indwelling ureteral catheter

(For radiological supervision and interpretation, use 74425)

50686 Manometric studies through ureterostomy or indwelling ureteral catheter

Separate Procedure | Unlisted Procedure | CCI Comp. Code | Non-specific Procedure

50688 Change of ureterostomy tube or externally accessible ureteral stent via ileal conduit

(If imaging guidance is performed, use 75984)

50690 Injection procedure for visualization of ileal conduit and/or ureteropyelography, exclusive of radiologic service

(For radiological supervision and interpretation, use 74425)

REPAIR

50700 Ureteroplasty, plastic operation on ureter (eg, stricture)

50715 Ureterolysis, with or without repositioning of ureter for retroperitoneal fibrosis

(For bilateral procedure, report 50715 with modifier -50)

50722 Ureterolysis for ovarian vein syndrome

50725 Ureterolysis for retrocaval ureter, with reanastomosis of upper urinary tract or vena cava

50727 Revision of urinary-cutaneous anastomosis (any type urostomy);

50728 with repair of fascial defect and hernia

50740 Ureteropyelostomy, anastomosis of ureter and renal pelvis

50750 Ureterocalycostomy, anastomosis of ureter to renal calyx

50760 Ureteroureterostomy

50770 Transureteroureterostomy, anastomosis of ureter to contralateral ureter

(Codes 50780-50785 include minor procedures to prevent vesicoureteral reflux)

50780 Ureteroneocystostomy; anastomosis of single ureter to bladder

(For bilateral procedure, report 50780 with modifier -50)

(When combined with cystourethroplasty or vesical neck revision, use 51820)

50782 anastomosis of duplicated ureter to bladder

● New Code ▲ Revised Code + Add-On Code ⃠ Modifier -51 Exempt ⊙ Conscious Sedation

50783 with extensive ureteral tailoring

50785 with vesico-psoas hitch or bladder flap

(For bilateral procedure, report 50785 with modifier -50)

50800 Ureteroenterostomy, direct anastomosis of ureter to intestine

(For bilateral procedure, report 50800 with modifier -50)

50810 Ureterosigmoidostomy, with creation of sigmoid bladder and establishment of abdominal or perineal colostomy, including intestine anastomosis

50815 Ureterocolon conduit, including intestine anastomosis

(For bilateral procedure, report 50815 with modifier -50)

50820 Ureteroileal conduit (ileal bladder), including intestine anastomosis (Bricker operation)

(For bilateral procedure, report 50820 with modifier -50)

(For combination of 50800-50820 with cystectomy, see 51580-51595)

50825 Continent diversion, including intestine anastomosis using any segment of small and/or large intestine (Kock pouch or Camey enterocystoplasty)

50830 Urinary undiversion (eg, taking down of ureteroileal conduit, ureterosigmoidostomy or ureteroenterostomy with ureteroureterostomy or ureteroneocystostomy)

50840 Replacement of all or part of ureter by intestine segment, including intestine anastomosis

(For bilateral procedure, report 50840 with modifier -50)

50845 Cutaneous appendico-vesicostomy

50860 Ureterostomy, transplantation of ureter to skin

(For bilateral procedure, report 50860 with modifier -50)

50900 Ureterorrhaphy, suture of ureter (separate procedure)

50920 Closure of ureterocutaneous fistula

50930 Closure of ureterovisceral fistula (including visceral repair)

50940 Deligation of ureter

(For ureteroplasty, ureterolysis, see 50700-50860)

LAPAROSCOPY

50945 Laparoscopy, surgical; ureterolithotomy

50947 ureteroneocystostomy with cystoscopy and ureteral stent placement

50948 ureteroneocystostomy without cystoscopy and ureteral stent placement

(For open ureteroneocystostomy, see 50780-50785)

50949 Unlisted laparoscopy procedure, ureter

ENDOSCOPY

50951 Ureteral endoscopy through established ureterostomy, with or without irrigation, instillation, or ureteropyelography, exclusive of radiologic service;

50953 with ureteral catheterization, with or without dilation of ureter

50955 with biopsy

50957 with fulguration and/or incision, with or without biopsy

(50959 deleted 2005 edition)

50961 with removal of foreign body or calculus

(When procedures 50970-50980 provide a significant identifiable service, they may be added to 50600)

50970 Ureteral endoscopy through ureterotomy, with or without irrigation, instillation, or ureteropyelography, exclusive of radiologic service;

(For ureterotomy, use 50600)

50972 with ureteral catheterization, with or without dilation of ureter

50974 with biopsy

50976 with fulguration and/or incision, with or without biopsy

(50978 deleted 2005 edition)

50980 with removal of foreign body or calculus

BLADDER

INCISION

51000 Aspiration of bladder by needle

51005 Aspiration of bladder; by trocar or intracatheter

51010 with insertion of suprapubic catheter

(If imaging guidance is performed, see 76942, 77002, 77012)

51020 Cystotomy or cystostomy; with fulguration and/or insertion of radioactive material

51030 with cryosurgical destruction of intravesical lesion

51040 Cystostomy, cystotomy with drainage

51045 Cystotomy, with insertion of ureteral catheter or stent (separate procedure)

51050 Cystolithotomy, cystotomy with removal of calculus, without vesical neck resection

51060 Transvesical ureterolithotomy

51065 Cystotomy, with calculus basket extraction and/or ultrasonic or electrohydraulic fragmentation of ureteral calculus

51080 Drainage of perivesical or prevesical space abscess

EXCISION

51500 Excision of urachal cyst or sinus, with or without umbilical hernia repair

Separate Procedure 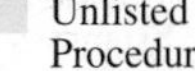 Unlisted Procedure 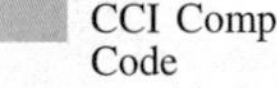 CCI Comp. Code 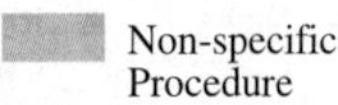 Non-specific Procedure

51520 Cystotomy; for simple excision of vesical neck (separate procedure)

51525 for excision of bladder diverticulum, single or multiple (separate procedure)

51530 for excision of bladder tumor

(For transurethral resection, see 52234-52240, 52305)

51535 Cystotomy for excision, incision, or repair of ureterocele

(For bilateral procedure, report 51535 with modifier -50)

(For transurethral excision, use 52300)

51550 Cystectomy, partial; simple

51555 complicated (eg, postradiation, previous surgery, difficult location)

51565 Cystectomy, partial, with reimplantation of ureter(s) into bladder (ureteroneocystostomy)

51570 Cystectomy, complete; (separate procedure)

51575 with bilateral pelvic lymphadenectomy, including external iliac, hypogastric, and obturator nodes

51580 Cystectomy, complete, with ureterosigmoidostomy or ureterocutaneous transplantations;

51585 with bilateral pelvic lymphadenectomy, including external iliac, hypogastric, and obturator nodes

51590 Cystectomy, complete, with ureteroileal conduit or sigmoid bladder, including intestine anastomosis;

51595 with bilateral pelvic lymphadenectomy, including external iliac, hypogastric, and obturator nodes

51596 Cystectomy, complete, with continent diversion, any open technique, using any segment of small and/or large intestine to construct neobladder

● New Code ▲ Revised Code + Add-On Code ⊘ Modifier -51 Exempt ⊙ Conscious Sedation

51597 Pelvic exenteration, complete, for vesical, prostatic or urethral malignancy, with removal of bladder and ureteral transplantations, with or without hysterectomy and/or abdominoperineal resection of rectum and colon and colostomy, or any combination thereof

(For pelvic exenteration for gynecologic malignancy, use 58240)

INTRODUCTION

51600 Injection procedure for cystography or voiding urethrocystography

(For radiological supervision and interpretation, see 74430, 74455)

51605 Injection procedure and placement of chain for contrast and/or chain urethrocystography

(For radiological supervision and interpretation, use 74430)

51610 Injection procedure for retrograde urethrocystography

(For radiological supervision and interpretation, use 74450)

51700 Bladder irrigation, simple, lavage and/or instillation

(Codes 51701-51702 are reported only when performed independently. Do not report 51701-51702 when catheter insertion is an inclusive component of another procedure.)

51701 Insertion of non-indwelling bladder catheter (eg, straight catheterization of residual urine)

51702 Insertion of temporary indwelling bladder catheter; simple (eg, Foley)

51703 complicated (eg, altered anatomy, fractured catheter/balloon)

51705 Change of cystostomy tube; simple

51710 complicated

(If imaging guidance is performed, use 75984)

51715 Endoscopic injection of implant material into the submucosal tissues of the urethra and/or bladder neck

 Separate Procedure 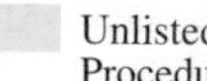 Unlisted Procedure 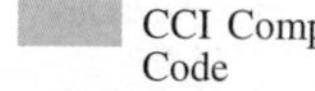 CCI Comp. Code 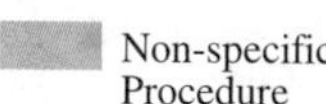 Non-specific Procedure

▲ **51720** Bladder instillation of anticarcinogenic agent (including retention time)

URODYNAMICS

51725 Simple cystometrogram (CMG) (eg, spinal manometer)

51726 Complex cystometrogram (eg, calibrated electronic equipment)

51736 Simple uroflowmetry (UFR) (eg, stop-watch flow rate, mechanical uroflowmeter)

51741 Complex uroflowmetry (eg, calibrated electronic equipment)

51772 Urethral pressure profile studies (UPP) (urethral closure pressure profile), any technique

51784 Electromyography studies (EMG) of anal or urethral sphincter, other than needle, any technique

51785 Needle electromyography studies (EMG) of anal or urethral sphincter, any technique

51792 Stimulus evoked response (eg, measurement of bulbocavernosus reflex latency time)

51795 Voiding pressure studies (VP); bladder voiding pressure, any technique

51797 intra-abdominal voiding pressure (AP) (rectal, gastric, intraperitoneal)

51798 Measurement of post-voiding residual urine and/or bladder capacity by ultrasound, non-imaging

REPAIR

51800 Cystoplasty or cystourethroplasty, plastic operation on bladder and/or vesical neck (anterior Y-plasty, vesical fundus resection), any procedure, with or without wedge resection of posterior vesical neck

51820 Cystourethroplasty with unilateral or bilateral ureteroneocystostomy

51840 Anterior vesicourethropexy, or urethropexy (eg, Marshall-Marchetti-Krantz, Burch); simple

● New Code ▲ Revised Code + Add-On Code ⊘ Modifier -51 Exempt ⊙ Conscious Sedation

51841 complicated (eg, secondary repair)

(For urethropexy (Pereyra type), use 57289)

51845 Abdomino-vaginal vesical neck suspension, with or without endoscopic control (eg, Stamey, Raz, modified Pereyra)

51860 Cystorrhaphy, suture of bladder wound, injury or rupture; simple

51865 complicated

51880 Closure of cystostomy (separate procedure)

51900 Closure of vesicovaginal fistula, abdominal approach

(For vaginal approach, see 57320-57330)

51920 Closure of vesicouterine fistula;

51925 with hysterectomy

(For closure of vesicoenteric fistula, see 44660, 44661)

(For closure of rectovesical fistula, see 45800-45805)

51940 Closure, exstrophy of bladder

(See also 54390)

51960 Enterocystoplasty, including intestinal anastomosis

51980 Cutaneous vesicostomy

LAPAROSCOPY

51990 Laparoscopy, surgical; urethral suspension for stress incontinence

51992 sling operation for stress incontinence (eg, fascia or synthetic)

(For open sling operation for stress incontinence, use 57288)

(For reversal or removal of sling operation for stress incontinence, use 57287)

51999 Unlisted laparoscopy procedure, bladder

ENDOSCOPY—CYSTOSCOPY, URETHROSCOPY, CYSTOURETHROSCOPY

52000 Cystourethroscopy (separate procedure)

52001 Cystourethroscopy with irrigation and evacuation of multiple obstructing clots

(Do not report 52001 in addition to 52000)

52005 Cystourethroscopy, with ureteral catheterization, with or without irrigation, instillation, or ureteropyelography, exclusive of radiologic service;

52007 with brush biopsy of ureter and/or renal pelvis

52010 Cystourethroscopy, with ejaculatory duct catheterization, with or without irrigation, instillation, or duct radiography, exclusive of radiologic service

(For radiological supervision and interpretation, use 74440)

TRANSURETHRAL SURGERY

Urethra and Bladder

▲ **52204** Cystourethroscopy, with biopsy(s)

52214 Cystourethroscopy, with fulguration (including cryosurgery or laser surgery) of trigone, bladder neck, prostatic fossa, urethra, or periurethral glands

52224 Cystourethroscopy, with fulguration (including cryosurgery or laser surgery) or treatment of MINOR (less than 0.5 cm) lesion(s) with or without biopsy

52234 Cystourethroscopy, with fulguration (including cryosurgery or laser surgery) and/or resection of; SMALL bladder tumor(s) (0.5 up to 2.0 cm)

52235 MEDIUM bladder tumor(s) (2.0 to 5.0 cm)

52240 LARGE bladder tumor(s)

52250 Cystourethroscopy with insertion of radioactive substance, with or without biopsy or fulguration

52260 Cystourethroscopy, with dilation of bladder for interstitial cystitis; general or conduction (spinal) anesthesia

52265 local anesthesia

52270 Cystourethroscopy, with internal urethrotomy; female

52275 male

52276 Cystourethroscopy with direct vision internal urethrotomy

52277 Cystourethroscopy, with resection of external sphincter (sphincterotomy)

52281 Cystourethroscopy, with calibration and/or dilation of urethral stricture or stenosis, with or without meatotomy, with or without injection procedure for cystography, male or female

52282 Cystourethroscopy, with insertion of urethral stent

52283 Cystourethroscopy, with steroid injection into stricture

52285 Cystourethroscopy for treatment of the female urethral syndrome with any or all of the following: urethral meatotomy, urethral dilation, internal urethrotomy, lysis of urethrovaginal septal fibrosis, lateral incisions of the bladder neck, and fulguration of polyp(s) of urethra, bladder neck, and/or trigone

52290 Cystourethroscopy; with ureteral meatotomy, unilateral or bilateral

52300 with resection or fulguration of orthotopic ureterocele(s), unilateral or bilateral

52301 with resection or fulguration of ectopic ureterocele(s), unilateral or bilateral

52305 with incision or resection of orifice of bladder diverticulum, single or multiple

52310 Cystourethroscopy, with removal of foreign body, calculus, or ureteral stent from urethra or bladder (separate procedure); simple

52315 complicated

52317 Litholapaxy: crushing or fragmentation of calculus by any means in bladder and removal of fragments; simple or small (less than 2.5 cm)

52318 complicated or large (over 2.5 cm)

URETER AND PELVIS

(To report a diagnostic cystourethroscopy, use 52000)

(To report a diagnostic cystourethroscopy with ureteroscopy and/or pyeloscopy, use 52351)

(Do not report 52000 in conjunction with 52320-52343)

(Do not report 52351 in conjunction with 52344-52346, 52352-52355)

(The insertion and removal of a temporary ureteral catheter (52005) during diagnostic or therapeutic cystourethroscopic with ureteroscopy and/or pyeloscopy is included in 52320-52355 and should not be reported separately)

(To report insertion of a self-retaining, indwelling stent performed during diagnostic or therapeutic cystourethroscopy with ureteroscopy and/or pyeloscopy, report 52332 in addition to primary procedure(s) performed (52320-52355) andappend modifier -51)

(52332 is used to report a unilateral procedure unless otherwise specified)

(To report cystourethroscopic removal of a self-retaining indwelling ureteral stent, see 52310, 52315, and append modifier -58 if appropriate)

52320 Cystourethroscopy (including ureteral catheterization); with removal of ureteral calculus

52325 with fragmentation of ureteral calculus (eg, ultrasonic or electro-hydraulic technique)

52327 with subureteric injection of implant material

52330 with manipulation, without removal of ureteral calculus

52332 Cystourethroscopy, with insertion of indwelling ureteral stent (eg, Gibbons or double-J type)

52334 Cystourethroscopy with insertion of ureteral guide wire through kidney to establish a percutaneous nephrostomy, retrograde

(For percutaneous nephrostolithotomy, see 50080, 50081; for establishment of nephrostomy tract only, use 50395)

(For cystourethroscopy, with ureteroscopy and/or pyeloscopy, see 52351-52355)

(For cystourethroscopy with incision, fulguration, or resection of congential posterior urethral valves or obstructive hypertrophic mucosal folds, use 52400)

52341 Cystourethroscopy; with treatment of ureteral stricture (eg, balloon dilation, laser, electrocautery, and incision)

52342 with treatment of ureteropelvic junction stricture (eg, balloon dilation, laser, electrocautery, and incision)

52343 with treatment of intra-renal stricture (eg, balloon dilation, laser, electrocautery, and incision)

52344 Cystourethroscopy with ureteroscopy; with treatment of ureteral stricture (eg, balloon dilation, laser, electrocautery, and incision)

52345 with treatment of ureteropelvic junction stricture (eg, balloon dilation, laser, electrocautery, and incision)

52346 with treatment of intra-renal stricture (eg, balloon dilation, laser, electrocautery, and incision)

(52347 deleted 2005 edition)

(For transurethral resection or incision of ejaculatory ducts, use 52402)

52351 Cystourethroscopy, with ureteroscopy and/or pyeloscopy; diagnostic

(For radiological supervision and interpretation, use 74485)

(Do not report 52351 in conjunction with 52341-52346, 52352-52355)

52352 with removal or manipulation of calculus (ureteral catheterization is included)

52353 with lithotripsy (ureteral catheterization is included)

Separate Procedure | Unlisted Procedure | CCI Comp. Code | 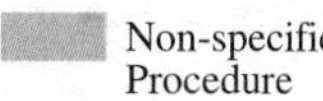 Non-specific Procedure

52354 with biopsy and/or fulguration of ureteral or renal pelvic lesion

52355 with resection of ureteral or renal pelvic tumor

VESICAL NECK AND PROSTATE

52400 Cystourethroscopy with incision, fulguration, or resection of congenital posterior urethral valves, or congenital obstructive hypertrophic mucosal folds

52402 Cystourethroscopy with transurethral resection or incision of ejaculatory ducts

52450 Transurethral incision of prostate

52500 Transurethral resection of bladder neck (separate procedure)

52510 Transurethral balloon dilation of the prostatic urethra

52601 Transurethral electrosurgical resection of prostate, including control of postoperative bleeding, complete (vasectomy, meatotomy, cystourethroscopy, urethral calibration and/or dilation, and internal urethrotomy are included)

(For other approaches, see 55801-55845)

52606 Transurethral fulguration for postoperative bleeding occurring after the usual follow-up time

52612 Transurethral resection of prostate; first stage of two-stage resection (partial resection)

52614 second stage of two-stage resection (resection completed)

52620 Transurethral resection; of residual obstructive tissue after 90 days postoperative

52630 of regrowth of obstructive tissue longer than one year postoperative

52640 of postoperative bladder neck contracture

52647 Laser coagulation of prostate, including control of postoperative bleeding, complete (vasectomy, meatotomy, cystourethroscopy, urethral calibration and/or dilation, and internal urethrotomy are included if performed)

52648 Laser vaporization of prostate, including control of postoperative bleeding, complete (vasectomy, meatotomy, cystourethroscopy, urethral calibration and/or dilation, internal urethrotomy and transurethral resection of prostate are included if performed)

52700 Transurethral drainage of prostatic abscess

(For litholapaxy, use 52317, 52318)

URETHRA

(For endoscopy, see cystoscopy, urethroscopy, cystourethroscopy, 52000-52700)

(For injection procedure for urethrocystography, see 51600-51610)

INCISION

53000 Urethrotomy or urethrostomy, external (separate procedure); pendulous urethra

53010 perineal urethra, external

53020 Meatotomy, cutting of meatus (separate procedure); except infant

53025 infant

(Do not report modifier '-63' in conjunction with 53025)

53040 Drainage of deep periurethral abscess

(For subcutaneous abscess, see 10060, 10061)

53060 Drainage of Skene's gland abscess or cyst

53080 Drainage of perineal urinary extravasation; uncomplicated (separate procedure)

53085 complicated

Separate Procedure

Unlisted Procedure

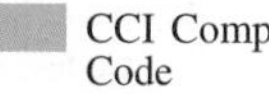
CCI Comp. Code

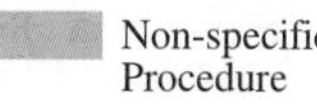
Non-specific Procedure

EXCISION

53200 Biopsy of urethra

53210 Urethrectomy, total, including cystostomy; female

53215 male

53220 Excision or fulguration of carcinoma of urethra

53230 Excision of urethral diverticulum (separate procedure); female

53235 male

53240 Marsupialization of urethral diverticulum, male or female

53250 Excision of bulbourethral gland (Cowper's gland)

53260 Excision or fulguration; urethral polyp(s), distal urethra

(For endoscopic approach, see 52214, 52224)

53265 urethral caruncle

53270 Skene's glands

53275 urethral prolapse

REPAIR

(For hypospadias, see 54300-54352)

53400 Urethroplasty; first stage, for fistula, diverticulum, or stricture (eg, Johannsen type)

53405 second stage (formation of urethra), including urinary diversion

53410 Urethroplasty, one-stage reconstruction of male anterior urethra

53415 Urethroplasty, transpubic or perineal, one stage, for reconstruction or repair of prostatic or membranous urethra

53420 Urethroplasty, two-stage reconstruction or repair of prostatic or membranous urethra; first stage

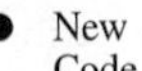
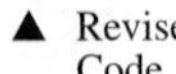
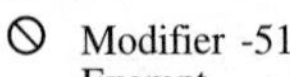

53425 second stage

53430 Urethroplasty, reconstruction of female urethra

53431 Urethroplasty with tubularization of posterior urethra and/or lower bladder for incontinence (eg, Tenago, Leadbetter procedure)

53440 Sling operation for correction of male urinary incontinence (eg, fascia or synthetic)

53442 Removal or revision of sling for male urinary incontinence (eg, fascia or synthetic)

53444 Insertion of tandem cuff (dual cuff)

53445 Insertion of inflatable urethral/bladder neck sphincter, including placement of pump, reservoir, and cuff

53446 Removal of inflatable urethral/bladder neck sphincter, including pump, reservoir, and cuff

53447 Removal and replacement of inflatable urethral/bladder neck sphincter including pump, reservoir, and cuff at the same operative session

53448 Removal and replacement of inflatable urethral/bladder neck sphincter including pump, reservoir, and cuff through an infected field at the same operative session including irrigation and debridement of infected tissue

(Do not report 11040-11043 in addition to 53448)

53449 Repair of inflatable urethral/bladder neck sphincter, including pump, reservoir, and cuff

53450 Urethromeatoplasty, with mucosal advancement

(For meatotomy, see 53020, 53025)

53460 Urethromeatoplasty, with partial excision of distal urethral segment (Richardson type procedure)

53500 Urethrolysis, transvaginal, secondary, open, including cystourethroscopy (eg, postsurgical obstruction, scarring)

(For urethrolysis by retropubic approach, use 53899)

(Do not report 53500 in conjunction with 52000)

53502 Urethrorrhaphy, suture of urethral wound or injury; female

53505 penile

53510 perineal

53515 prostatomembranous

53520 Closure of urethrostomy or urethrocutaneous fistula, male (separate procedure)

(For closure of urethrovaginal fistula, use 57310)

(For closure of urethrorectal fistula, see 45820, 45825)

MANIPULATION

(For radiological supervision and interpretation, use 74485)

53600 Dilation of urethral stricture by passage of sound or urethral dilator, male; initial

53601 subsequent

53605 Dilation of urethral stricture or vesical neck by passage of sound or urethral dilator, male, general or conduction (spinal) anesthesia

53620 Dilation of urethral stricture by passage of filiform and follower, male; initial

53621 subsequent

53660 Dilation of female urethra including suppository and/or instillation; initial

53661 subsequent

53665 Dilation of female urethra, general or conduction (spinal) anesthesia

(For urethral catheterization, see 51701-51703)

OTHER PROCEDURES

(For two or three glass urinalysis, use 81020)

53850 Transurethral destruction of prostate tissue; by microwave thermotherapy

53852 by radiofrequency thermotherapy

53853 by water-induced thermotherapy

53899 Unlisted procedure, urinary system

This page intentionally left blank.

● New Code ▲ Revised Code + Add-On Code ⊘ Modifier -51 Exempt ⊙ Conscious Sedation

MALE GENITAL SYSTEM

CPT codes from this section of CPT are used to report invasive and surgical procedures performed on the penis; testis; epididymis; scrotum; spermatic cord and prostate.

Transurethral drainage of a prostatic abscess (e.g. CPT code 52700) is included in male transurethral prostatic procedures and is not reported separately.

Urethral catheterization (e.g. CPT codes 51701, 51702, and 51703), when medically necessary to successfully accomplish a procedure, should not be separately reported.

The puncture aspiration of a hydrocele (e.g. CPT code 55000) is included in services involving the tunica vaginalis and proximate anatomy (scrotum, vas deferens) and in inguinal hernia repairs.

A number of codes describe surgical procedures of a progressively more comprehensive nature or with different approaches to accomplish similar services. In general, these groups of codes are not to be reported together (see mutually exclusive policy). While a number of these groups of codes exist in CPT, a specific example includes the series of codes describing prostate procedures (CPT codes 55801-55845). In addition, all prostatectomy procedures (e.g. CPT codes 52601-52648 and 55801- 55845) are also mutually exclusive of one another.

PENIS

INCISION

(For abdominal perineal gangrene debridement, see 11004-11006)

54000 Slitting of prepuce, dorsal or lateral (separate procedure); newborn

(Do not report modifier '-63' in conjunction with 54000)

54001 except newborn

54015 Incision and drainage of penis, deep

(For skin and subcutaneous abscess, see 10060-10160)

DESTRUCTION

54050 Destruction of lesion(s), penis (eg, condyloma, papilloma, molluscum contagiosum, herpetic vesicle), simple; chemical

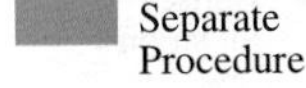

Separate Procedure | Unlisted Procedure | CCI Comp. Code | Non-specific Procedure

54055 electrodesiccation

54056 cryosurgery

54057 laser surgery

54060 surgical excision

54065 Destruction of lesion(s), penis (eg, condyloma, papilloma, molluscum contagiosum, herpetic vesicle), extensive (eg, laser surgery, electosurgery, cryosurgery, chemosurgery)

(For destruction or excision of other lesions, see Integumentary System)

EXCISION

54100 Biopsy of penis; (separate procedure)

54105 deep structures

54110 Excision of penile plaque (Peyronie disease);

54111 with graft to 5 cm in length

54112 with graft greater than 5 cm in length

54115 Removal foreign body from deep penile tissue (eg, plastic implant)

54120 Amputation of penis; partial

54125 complete

54130 Amputation of penis, radical; with bilateral inguinofemoral lymphadenectomy

54135 in continuity with bilateral pelvic lymphadenectomy, including external iliac, hypogastric and obturator nodes

(For lymphadenectomy (separate procedure) see 38760-38770)

▲ **54150** Circumcision, using clamp or other device with regional dorsal penile or ring block

(Do not report modifier -63 in conjunction with 54150)

● New Code ▲ Revised Code + Add-On Code ⊘ Modifier -51 Exempt ⊙ Conscious Sedation

(Report 54150 with modifier 52 when performed without dorsal penile or ring block)

(54152 deleted 2007 edition, see 54150)

▲ **54160** Circumcision, surgical excision other than clamp, device or dorsal slit; neonate (28 days of age or less)

(Do not report modifier -63 in conjunction with 54160)

▲ **54161** older than 28 days of age

54162 Lysis or excision of penile post-circumcision adhesions

54163 Repair incomplete circumcision

54164 Frenulotomy of penis

(Do not report with circumcision codes 54150-54161, 54162, 54163)

INTRODUCTION

54200 Injection procedure for Peyronie disease;

54205 with surgical exposure of plaque

54220 Irrigation of corpora cavernosa for priapism

54230 Injection procedure for corpora cavernosography

(For radiological supervision and interpretation, use 74445)

54231 Dynamic cavernosometry, including intracavernosal injection of vasoactive drugs (eg, papaverine, phentolamine)

54235 Injection of corpora cavernosa with pharmacologic agent(s) (eg, papaverine, phentolamine)

54240 Penile plethysmography

54250 Nocturnal penile tumescence and/or rigidity test

Separate Procedure 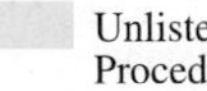 Unlisted Procedure 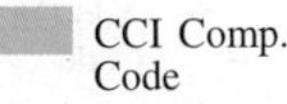 CCI Comp. Code 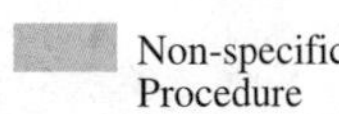 Non-specific Procedure

REPAIR

(For other urethroplasties, see 53400-53430)

(For penile revascularization, use 37788)

54300 Plastic operation of penis for straightening of chordee (eg, hypospadias), with or without mobilization of urethra

54304 Plastic operation on penis for correction of chordee or for first stage hypospadias repair with or without transplantation of prepuce and/or skin flaps

54308 Urethroplasty for second stage hypospadias repair (including urinary diversion); less than 3 cm

54312 greater than 3 cm

54316 Urethroplasty for second stage hypospadias repair (including urinary diversion) with free skin graft obtained from site other than genitalia

54318 Urethroplasty for third stage hypospadias repair to release penis from scrotum (eg, third stage Cecil repair)

54322 One stage distal hypospadias repair (with or without chordee or circumcision); with simple meatal advancement (eg, Magpi, V-flap)

54324 with urethroplasty by local skin flaps (eg, flip-flap, prepucial flap)

54326 with urethroplasty by local skin flaps and mobilization of urethra

54328 with extensive dissection to correct chordee and urethroplasty with local skin flaps, skin graft patch, and/or island flap

(For urethroplasty and straightening of chordee, use 54308)

54332 One stage proximal penile or penoscrotal hypospadias repair requiring extensive dissection to correct chordee and urethroplasty by use of skin graft tube and/or island flap

54336 One stage perineal hypospadias repair requiring extensive dissection to correct chordee and urethroplasty by use of skin graft tube and/or island flap

54340 Repair of hypospadias complications (ie, fistula, stricture, diverticula); by closure, incision, or excision, simple

54344 requiring mobilization of skin flaps and urethroplasty with flap or patch graft

54348 requiring extensive dissection and urethroplasty with flap, patch or tubed graft (includes urinary diversion)

54352 Repair of hypospadias cripple requiring extensive dissection and excision of previously constructed structures including re-release of chordee and reconstruction of urethra and penis by use of local skin as grafts and island flaps and skin brought in as flaps or grafts

54360 Plastic operation on penis to correct angulation

54380 Plastic operation on penis for epispadias distal to external sphincter;

54385 with incontinence

54390 with exstrophy of bladder

54400 Insertion of penile prosthesis; non-inflatable (semi-rigid)

54401 inflatable (self-contained)

(For removal or replacement of penile prosthesis, see 54415, 54416)

54405 Insertion of multi-component inflatable penile prosthesis, including placement of pump, cylinders, and reservoir

(For reduced services, report 54405 with modifier -52)

54406 Removal of all components of a multi-component inflatable penile prosthesis without replacement of prosthesis

(For reduced services, report 54406 with modifier -52)

54408 Repair of component(s) of a multi-component, inflatable penile prosthesis

54410 Removal and replacement of all component(s) of a multi-component inflatable penile prosthesis at the same operative session

Separate Procedure 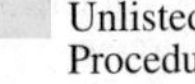 Unlisted Procedure 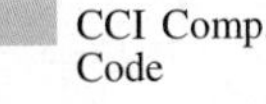 CCI Comp. Code 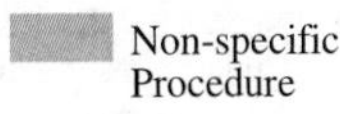 Non-specific Procedure

54411 Removal and replacement of all components of a multi-component inflatable penile prosthesis through an infected field at the same operative session, including irrigation and debridement of infected tissue

(For reduced services, report 54411 with modifier -52)

(Do not report 11040-11043 in addition to 54411)

54415 Removal of non-inflatable (semi-rigid) or inflatable (self-contained) penile prosthesis, without replacement of prosthesis

54416 Removal and replacement of non-inflatable (semi-rigid) or inflatable (self-contained) penile prosthesis at the same operative session

54417 Removal and replacement of non-inflatable (semi-rigid) or inflatable (self-contained) penile prosthesis through an infected field at the same operative session, including irrigation and debridement of infected tissue

(Do not report 11040-11043 in addition to 54417)

54420 Corpora cavernosa-saphenous vein shunt (priapism operation), unilateral or bilateral

54430 Corpora cavernosa-corpus spongiosum shunt (priapism operation), unilateral or bilateral

54435 Corpora cavernosa-glans penis fistulization (eg, biopsy needle, Winter procedure, rongeur, or punch) for priapism

54440 Plastic operation of penis for injury

MANIPULATION

54450 Foreskin manipulation including lysis of preputial adhesions and stretching

TESTIS

EXCISION

(For abdominal perineal gangrene debridement, see 11004-11006)

54500 Biopsy of testis, needle (separate procedure)

(For fine needle aspiration, see 10021, 10022)

(For evaluation of fine needle aspirate, see 88172, 88173)

54505 Biopsy of testis, incisional (separate procedure)

(For bilateral procedure, report 54505 with modifier -50)

(When combined with vasogram, seminal vesiculogram, or epididymogram, use 55300)

54512 Excision of extraparenchymal lesion of testis

54520 Orchiectomy, simple (including subcapsular), with or without testicular prosthesis, scrotal or inguinal approach

(For bilateral procedure, report 54520 with modifier -50)

54522 Orchiectomy, partial

54530 Orchiectomy, radical, for tumor; inguinal approach

54535 with abdominal exploration

(For orchiectomy with repair of hernia, see 49505 or 49507 and 54520)

(For radical retroperitoneal lymphadenectomy, use 38780)

EXPLORATION

54550 Exploration for undescended testis (inguinal or scrotal area)

(For bilateral procedure, report 54550 with modifier -50)

54560 Exploration for undescended testis with abdominal exploration

(For bilateral procedure, report 54560 with modifier -50)

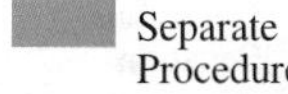 Separate Procedure  Unlisted Procedure 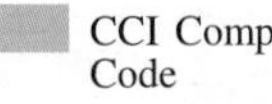 CCI Comp. Code 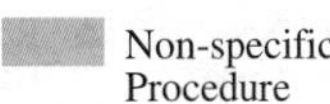 Non-specific Procedure

REPAIR

54600 Reduction of torsion of testis, surgical, with or without fixation of contralateral testis

54620 Fixation of contralateral testis (separate procedure)

54640 Orchiopexy, inguinal approach, with or without hernia repair

(For bilateral procedure, report 54640 with modifier -50)

(For inguinal hernia repair performed in conjunction with inguinal orchiopexy, see 49495-49525)

54650 Orchiopexy, abdominal approach, for intra-abdominal testis (eg, Fowler-Stephens)

(For laparoscopic approach, use 54692)

54660 Insertion of testicular prosthesis (separate procedure)

(For bilateral procedure, report 54660 with modifier -50)

54670 Suture or repair of testicular injury

54680 Transplantation of testis(es) to thigh (because of scrotal destruction)

LAPAROSCOPY

54690 Laparoscopy, surgical; orchiectomy

54692 orchiopexy for intra-abdominal testis

54699 Unlisted laparoscopy procedure, testis

EPIDIDYMIS

INCISION

54700 Incision and drainage of epididymis, testis and/or scrotal space (eg, abscess or hematoma)

EXCISION

54800 Biopsy of epididymis, needle

(For fine needle aspiration, see 10021, 10022)

(For evaluation of fine needle aspirate, see 88172, 88173)

(54820 deleted 2007 edition, see 54865)

54830 Excision of local lesion of epididymis

54840 Excision of spermatocele, with or without epididymectomy

54860 Epididymectomy; unilateral

54861 bilateral

EXPLORATION

● **54865** Exploration of epididymis, with or without biopsy

REPAIR

54900 Epididymovasostomy, anastomosis of epididymis to vas deferens; unilateral

54901 bilateral

(For operating microscope, use 69990)

TUNICA VAGINALIS

INCISION

55000 Puncture aspiration of hydrocele, tunica vaginalis, with or without injection of medication

EXCISION

55040 Excision of hydrocele; unilateral

55041 bilateral

(With hernia repair, see 49495-49501)

REPAIR

55060 Repair of tunica vaginalis hydrocele (Bottle type)

Separate Procedure | Unlisted Procedure | CCI Comp. Code 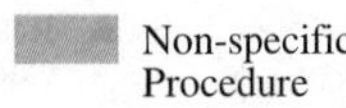 Non-specific Procedure

SCROTUM

INCISION

55100 Drainage of scrotal wall abscess

(See also 54700)

55110 Scrotal exploration

55120 Removal of foreign body in scrotum

EXCISION

(For excision of local lesion of skin of scrotum, see Integumentary System)

55150 Resection of scrotum

REPAIR

55175 Scrotoplasty; simple

55180 complicated

VAS DEFERENS

INCISION

55200 Vasotomy, cannulization with or without incision of vas, unilateral or bilateral (separate procedure)

EXCISION

55250 Vasectomy, unilateral or bilateral (separate procedure), including postoperative semen examination(s)

INTRODUCTION

55300 Vasotomy for vasograms, seminal vesiculograms, or epididymograms, unilateral or bilateral

(For radiological supervision and interpretation, use 74440)

(When combined with biopsy of testis, see 54505 and use modifier -51)

● New Code ▲ Revised Code + Add-On Code ⃠ Modifier -51 Exempt ⊙ Conscious Sedation

REPAIR

55400 Vasovasostomy, vasovasorrhaphy

(For operating microscope, use 69990)

SUTURE

55450 Ligation (percutaneous) of vas deferens, unilateral or bilateral (separate procedure)

SPERMATIC CORD

EXCISION

55500 Excision of hydrocele of spermatic cord, unilateral (separate procedure)

55520 Excision of lesion of spermatic cord (separate procedure)

55530 Excision of varicocele or ligation of spermatic veins for varicocele; (separate procedure)

55535 abdominal approach

55540 with hernia repair

LAPAROSCOPY

55550 Laparoscopy, surgical, with ligation of spermatic veins for varicocele

55559 Unlisted laparoscopy procedure, spermatic cord

SEMINAL VESICLES

INCISION

55600 Vesiculotomy;

(For bilateral procedure, report 55600 with modifier -50)

55605 complicated

EXCISION

55650 Vesiculectomy, any approach

(For bilateral procedure, report 55650 with modifier -50)

55680 Excision of Mullerian duct cyst

(For injection procedure, see 52010, 55300)

PROSTATE

INCISION

55700 Biopsy, prostate; needle or punch, single or multiple, any approach

(For prostate needle biopsy saturation sampling for prostate mapping, use Category III code 0137T)

(If imaging guidance is performed, use 76942)

(For fine needle aspiration, see 10021, 10022)

(For evaluation of fine needle aspirate, see 88172, 88173)

55705 incisional, any approach

55720 Prostatotomy, external drainage of prostatic abscess, any approach; simple

55725 complicated

(For transurethral drainage, use 52700)

EXCISION

(For transurethral removal of prostate, see 52601-52640)

(For transurethral destruction of prostate, see 53850-53852)

(For limited pelvic lymphadenectomy for staging (separate procedure), use 38562)

(For independent node dissection, see 38770-38780)

55801 Prostatectomy, perineal, subtotal (including control of postoperative bleeding, vasectomy, meatotomy, urethral calibration and/or dilation, and internal urethrotomy)

55810 Prostatectomy, perineal radical;

55812 with lymph node biopsy(s) (limited pelvic lymphadenectomy)

55815 with bilateral pelvic lymphadenectomy, including external iliac, hypogastric and obturator nodes

(If 55815 is carried out on separate days, use 38770 with modifier -50 and 55810)

55821 Prostatectomy (including control of postoperative bleeding, vasectomy, meatotomy, urethral calibration and/or dilation, and internal urethrotomy); suprapubic, subtotal, one or two stages

55831 retropubic, subtotal

55840 Prostatectomy, retropubic radical, with or without nerve sparing;

55842 with lymph node biopsy(s) (limited pelvic lymphadenectomy)

55845 with bilateral pelvic lymphadenectomy, including external iliac, hypogastric, and obturator nodes

(If 55845 is carried out on separate days, use 38770 with modifier -50 and 55840)

(For laparoscopic retropubic radical prostatectomy, use 55866)

(55859 deleted 2007 edition, see 55875)

55860 Exposure of prostate, any approach, for insertion of radioactive substance;

(For application of interstitial radioelement, see 77776-77778)

55862 with lymph node biopsy(s) (limited pelvic lymphadenectomy)

55865 with bilateral pelvic lymphadenectomy, including external iliac, hypogastric and obturator nodes

LAPAROSCOPY

55866 Laparoscopy, surgical prostatectomy, retropubic radical, including nerve sparing

(For open procedure, use 55840)

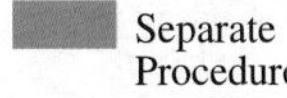 Separate Procedure  Unlisted Procedure 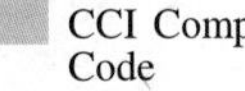 CCI Comp. Code 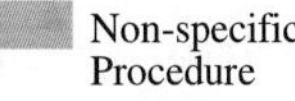 Non-specific Procedure

OTHER PROCEDURES

(For artificial insemination, see 58321, 58322)

55870 Electroejaculation

55873 Cryosurgical ablation of the prostate (includes ultrasonic guidance for interstitial cryosurgical probe placement)

● **55875** Transperineal placement of needles or catheters into prostate for interstitial radioelement application, with or without cystoscopy

(For interstitial radioelement application, see 77776-77784)

(For ultrasonic guidance for interstitial radioelement application, use 76965)

● **55876** Placement of interstitial device(s) for radiation therapy guidance (eg, fiducial markers, dosimeter), prostate (via needle, any approach), single or multiple

(Report supply of device separately)

(For imaging guidance, see 76942, 77002, 77012, 77021)

55899 Unlisted procedure, male genital system

INTERSEX SURGERY

55970 Intersex surgery; male to female

55980 female to male

Separate Procedure | Unlisted Procedure | CCI Comp. Code | Non-specific Procedure

This page intentionally left blank

FEMALE GENITAL SYSTEM

When a pelvic examination is performed in conjunction with a gynecologic procedure, either as a necessary part of the procedure or as a confirmatory examination, the pelvic examination is not separately reported. A diagnostic pelvic examination may be performed for the purposes of deciding to perform a procedure; however, this examination is included in the evaluation and management service at the time the decision to perform the procedure is made.

All surgical laparoscopic, hysteroscopic or peritoneoscopic procedures include diagnostic procedures. Therefore, CPT code 49320 is included in 38120, 38570-38572, 43280, 43651-43653, 44200- 44202, 44970, 47560-47570, 49321- 49323, 49650-49651, 54690-54692, 55550, 58545-58554, 58660-58673, 60650; and 58555 is included in 58558- 58563.

Lysis of adhesions (CPT code 58660) is not to be reported separately when done in conjunction with other surgical laparoscopic procedures.

Pelvic exam under anesthesia indicated by CPT code 57410, is included in all major and most minor gynecological procedures and is not to be reported separately. This procedure represents routine evaluation of the surgical field.

Dilation of vagina or cervix (CPT codes 57400 or 57800), when done in conjunction with vaginal approach procedures, is not to be reported separately unless the CPT code descriptor states "without cervical dilation." 6. Administration of anesthesia, when necessary, is included in every surgical procedure code, when performed by the surgeon.

Colposcopy (CPT codes 56820, 57420, 57452) should not be reported separately when performed as a "scout" procedure to confirm the lesion or to assess the surgical field prior to a surgical procedure. A diagnostic colposcopy resulting in the decision to perform a non-colposcopic procedure may be reported with modifier - 58. Diagnostic colposcopies (56820, 57420, 57452) are not separately reported with other colposcopic procedures.

(For pelvic laparotomy, use 49000)

(For excision or destruction of endometriomas, open method, see 49200, 49201)

(For paracentesis, see 49080, 49081)

(For secondary closure of abdominal wall evisceration or disruption, use 49900)

(For fulguration or excision of lesions, laparoscopic approach, use 58662)

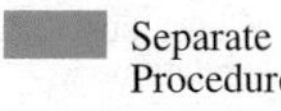

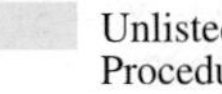

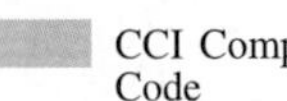

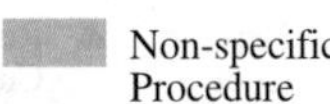

(For chemotherapy, see 96401-96549)

VULVA, PERINEUM AND INTROITUS

INCISION

(For incision and drainage of sebaceous cyst, furuncle, or abscess, see 10040, 10060, 10061)

56405 Incision and drainage of vulva or perineal abscess

56420 Incision and drainage of Bartholin's gland abscess

(For incision and drainage of Skene's gland abscess or cyst, use 53060)

56440 Marsupialization of Bartholin's gland cyst

56441 Lysis of labial adhesions

● **56442** Hymenotomy, simple incision

DESTRUCTION

56501 Destruction of lesion(s), vulva; simple (eg, laser surgery, electrosurgery, cryosurgery, chemosurgery)

56515 extensive (eg, laser surgery, electrosurgery, cryosurgery, chemosurgery)

(For destruction of Skene's gland cyst or abscess, use 53270)

(For cautery destruction of urethral caruncle, use 53265)

EXCISION

56605 Biopsy of vulva or perineum (separate procedure); one lesion

+ **56606** each separate additional lesion (List separately in addition to code for primary procedure)

(Use 56606 in conjunction with code 56605)

(For excision of local lesion, see 11420-11426, 11620-11626)

56620 Vulvectomy simple; partial

56625 complete

(For skin graft, see 15002 et seq)

56630 Vulvectomy, radical, partial;

(For skin graft, if used, see 15004-15005, 15120, 15121, 15240, 15241)

56631 with unilateral inguinofemoral lymphadenectomy

56632 with bilateral inguinofemoral lymphadenectomy

56633 Vulvectomy, radical, complete;

56634 with unilateral inguinofemoral lymphadenectomy

56637 with bilateral inguinofemoral lymphadenectomy

56640 Vulvectomy, radical, complete, with inguinofemoral, iliac, and pelvic lymphadenectomy

(For bilateral procedure, report 56640 with modifier -50)

(For lymphadenectomy, see 38760-38780)

56700 Partial hymenectomy or revision of hymenal ring

(56720 deleted 2007 edition, see 56442)

56740 Excision of Bartholin's gland or cyst

(For excision of Skene's gland, use 53270)

(For excision of urethral caruncle, use 53265)

(For excision or fulguration of urethral carcinoma, use 53220)

(For excision or marsupialization of urethral diverticulum, see 53230, 53240)

REPAIR

(For repair of urethra for mucosal prolapse, use 53275)

56800 Plastic repair of introitus

56805 Clitoroplasty for intersex state

56810 Perineoplasty, repair of perineum, nonobstetrical (separate procedure)

(See also 56800)

(For repair of wounds to genitalia, see 12001-12007, 12041-12047, 13131-13133)

(For repair of recent injury of vagina and perineum, nonobstetrical, use 57210)

(For anal sphincteroplasty, see 46750, 46751)

(For episiorrhaphy, episioperineorrhaphy for recent injury of vulva and/or perineum, nonobstetrical, use 57210)

ENDOSCOPY

56820 Colposcopy of the vulva

56821 with biopsy(s)

(For colposcopic examinations/procedures involving the vagina, see 57420, 57421; cervix, see 57452-57461)

VAGINA

INCISION

57000 Colpotomy; with exploration

57010 with drainage of pelvic abscess

57020 Colpocentesis (separate procedure)

57022 Incision and drainage of vaginal hematoma; obstetrical/postpartum

57023 non-obstetrical (eg, post-trauma, spontaneous bleeding)

DESTRUCTION

57061 Destruction of vaginal lesion(s); simple (eg, laser surgery, electrosurgery, cryosurgery, chemosurgery)

57065 extensive (eg, laser surgery, electrosurgery, cryosurgery, chemosurgery)

EXCISION

57100 Biopsy of vaginal mucosa; simple (separate procedure)

57105 extensive, requiring suture (including cysts)

57106 Vaginectomy, partial removal of vaginal wall;

57107 with removal of paravaginal tissue (radical vaginectomy)

57109 with removal of paravaginal tissue (radical vaginectomy) with bilateral total pelvic lymphadenectomy and para-aortic lymph node sampling (biopsy)

57110 Vaginectomy, complete removal of vaginal wall;

57111 with removal of paravaginal tissue (radical vaginectomy)

57112 with removal of paravaginal tissue (radical vaginectomy) with bilateral total pelvic lymphadenectomy and para-aortic lymph node sampling (biopsy)

57120 Colpocleisis (Le Fort type)

57130 Excision of vaginal septum

57135 Excision of vaginal cyst or tumor

INTRODUCTION

57150 Irrigation of vagina and/or application of medicament for treatment of bacterial, parasitic, or fungoid disease

57155 Insertion of uterine tandems and/or vaginal ovoids for clinical brachytherapy

(For insertion of radioelement sources or ribbons, see 77761-77763, 77781-77784)

57160 Fitting and insertion of pessary or other intravaginal support device

57170 Diaphragm or cervical cap fitting with instructions

57180 Introduction of any hemostatic agent or pack for spontaneous or traumatic nonobstetrical vaginal hemorrhage (separate procedure)

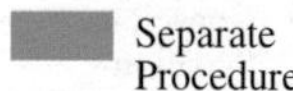 Separate Procedure

Unlisted Procedure

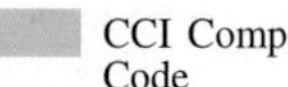 CCI Comp. Code

Non-specific Procedure

REPAIR

(For urethral suspension, Marshall-Marchetti-Krantz type, abdominal approach, see 51840, 51841)

(For laparoscopic suspension, use 51990)

57200 Colporrhaphy, suture of injury of vagina (nonobstetrical)

57210 Colpoperineorrhaphy, suture of injury of vagina and/or perineum (nonobstetrical)

57220 Plastic operation on urethral sphincter, vaginal approach (eg, Kelly urethral plication)

57230 Plastic repair of urethrocele

57240 Anterior colporrhaphy, repair of cystocele with or without repair of urethrocele

57250 Posterior colporrhaphy, repair of rectocele with or without perineorrhaphy

(For repair of rectocele (separate procedure) without posterior colporrhaphy, use 45560)

57260 Combined anteroposterior colporrhaphy;

57265 with enterocele repair

+ **57267** Insertion of mesh or other prosthesis for repair of pelvic floor defect, each site (anterior, posterior compartment), vaginal approach (List separately in addition to code for primary procedure)

(Use 57267 in addition to 45560, 57240-57265)

57268 Repair of enterocele, vaginal approach (separate procedure)

57270 Repair of enterocele, abdominal approach (separate procedure)

57280 Colpopexy, abdominal approach

57282 Colpopexy, vaginal; extra-peritoneal approach (sacrospinous, iliococcygeus)

57283 intra-peritoneal approach (uterosacral, levator myorrhaphy)

57284 Paravaginal defect repair (including repair of cystocele, stress urinary incontinence, and/or incomplete vaginal prolapse)

57287 Removal or revision of sling for stress incontinence (eg, fascia or synthetic)

57288 Sling operation for stress incontinence (eg, fascia or synthetic)

(For laparoscopic approach, use 51992)

57289 Pereyra procedure, including anterior colporrhaphy

57291 Construction of artificial vagina; without graft

57292 with graft

57295 Revision (including removal) of prosthetic vaginal graft, vaginal approach

● **57296** open abdominal approach

57300 Closure of rectovaginal fistula; vaginal or transanal approach

57305 abdominal approach

57307 abdominal approach, with concomitant colostomy

57308 transperineal approach, with perineal body reconstruction, with or without levator plication

57310 Closure of urethrovaginal fistula;

57311 with bulbocavernosus transplant

57320 Closure of vesicovaginal fistula; vaginal approach

(For concomitant cystostomy, see 51005-51040)

57330 transvesical and vaginal approach

(For abdominal approach, use 51900)

57335 Vaginoplasty for intersex state

MANIPULATION

57400 Dilation of vagina under anesthesia

57410 Pelvic examination under anesthesia

57415 Removal of impacted vaginal foreign body (separate procedure) under anesthesia

(For removal without anesthesia of an impacted vaginal foreign body, use the appropriate E/M code)

ENDOSCOPY

(For speculoscopy, see Category III codes 0030T, 0031T)

57420 Colposcopy of the entire vagina, with cervix if present;

57421 with biopsy(s) of vagina/cervix

(For colposcopic visualization of cervix and adjacent upper vagina, use 57452)

(When reporting colposcopies of multiple sites, use modifier -51 as appropriate. For colposcopic examinations/procedures involving the vulva, see 56820, 56821; cervix, see 57452-57461)

(For endometrial sampling (biopsy) performed in conjunction with colposcopy, use 58110)

57425 Laparoscopy, surgical, colpopexy (suspension of vaginal apex)

CERVIX UTERI

(For cervicography, see Category III code 0003T)

ENDOSCOPY

(For colposcopic examinations/procedures involving the vulva, see 56820, 56821; vagina, see 57420, 57421)

57452 Colposcopy of the cervix including upper/adjacent vagina

(Do not report 57452 in addition to 57454-57461)

57454 with biopsy(s) of the cervix and endocervical curettage

57455 with biopsy(s) of the cervix

57456 with endocervical curettage

57460 with loop electrode biopsy(s) of the cervix

 ● New Code ▲ Revised Code + Add-On Code ⊘ Modifier -51 Exempt ⊙ Conscious Sedation

57461 with loop electrode conization of the cervix

(Do not report 57456 in addition to 57461)

(For endometrial sampling (biopsy) performed in conjunction with colposcopy, use 58110)

EXCISION

(For radical surgical procedures, see 58200-58240)

57500 Biopsy, single or multiple, or local excision of lesion, with or without fulguration (separate procedure)

57505 Endocervical curettage (not done as part of a dilation and curettage)

57510 Cautery of cervix; electro or thermal

57511 cryocautery, initial or repeat

57513 laser ablation

57520 Conization of cervix, with or without fulguration, with or without dilation and curettage, with or without repair; cold knife or laser

(See also 58120)

57522 loop electrode excision

57530 Trachelectomy (cervicectomy), amputation of cervix (separate procedure)

57531 Radical trachelectomy, with bilateral total pelvic lymphadenectomy and para-aortic lymph node sampling biopsy, with or without removal of tube(s), with or without removal of ovary(s)

(For radical abdominal hysterectomy, use 58210)

57540 Excision of cervical stump, abdominal approach;

57545 with pelvic floor repair

57550 Excision of cervical stump, vaginal approach;

57555 with anterior and/or posterior repair

57556 with repair of enterocele

(For insertion of intrauterine device, use 58300)

(For insertion of any hemostatic agent or pack for control of spontaneous non-obstetrical hemorrhage, see 57180)

● **57558** Dilation and curettage of cervical stump

REPAIR

57700 Cerclage of uterine cervix, nonobstetrical

57720 Trachelorrhaphy, plastic repair of uterine cervix, vaginal approach

MANIPULATION

57800 Dilation of cervical canal, instrumental (separate procedure)

(57820 deleted 2007 edition, see 57558)

CORPUS UTERI

EXCISION

58100 Endometrial sampling (biopsy) with or without endocervical sampling (biopsy), without cervical dilation, any method (separate procedure)

(For endocervical curettage only, use 57505)

(For endometrial sampling (biopsy) performed in conjunction with colposcopy (57420, 57421, 57452-57461), use 58110)

+ **58110** Endometrial sampling (biopsy) performed in conjunction with colposcopy (List separately in addition to code for primary procedure)

(Use 58110 in conjunction with 57420, 57421, 57452-57461)

58120 Dilation and curettage, diagnostic and/or therapeutic (nonobstetrical)

(For postpartum hemorrhage, use 59160)

58140 Myomectomy, excision of fibroid tumor(s) of uterus, 1 to 4 intramural myoma(s) with total weight of 250 grams or less and/or removal of surface myomas; abdominal approach

58145 vaginal approach

58146 Myomectomy, excision of fibroid tumor(s) of uterus, 5 or more intramural myomas and/or intramural myomas with total weight greater than 250 grams, abdominal approach

(Do not report 58146 in addition to 58140-58145, 58150-58240)

Hysterectomy Procedures

58150 Total abdominal hysterectomy (corpus and cervix), with or without removal of tube(s), with or without removal of ovary(s);

58152 with colpo-urethrocystopexy (eg, Marshall-Marchetti-Krantz, Burch)

(For urethrocystopexy without hysterectomy, see 51840, 51841)

58180 Supracervical abdominal hysterectomy (subtotal hysterectomy), with or without removal of tube(s), with or without removal of ovary(s)

58200 Total abdominal hysterectomy, including partial vaginectomy, with para-aortic and pelvic lymph node sampling, with or without removal of tube(s), with or without removal of ovary(s)

58210 Radical abdominal hysterectomy, with bilateral total pelvic lymphadenectomy and para-aortic lymph node sampling (biopsy), with or without removal of tube(s), with or without removal of ovary(s)

(For radical hysterectomy with ovarian transposition, use also 58825)

58240 Pelvic exenteration for gynecologic malignancy, with total abdominal hysterectomy or cervicectomy, with or without removal of tube(s), with or without removal of ovary(s), with removal of bladder and ureteral transplantations, and/or abdominoperineal resection of rectum and colon and colostomy, or any combination thereof

(For pelvic exenteration for lower urinary tract or male genital malignancy, use 51597)

58260 Vaginal hysterectomy, for uterus 250 grams or less;

58262 with removal of tube(s), and/or ovary(s)

Separate Procedure | Unlisted Procedure | CCI Comp. Code | Non-specific Procedure

58263 with removal of tube(s), and/or ovary(s), with repair of enterocele

(Do not report 58263 in addition to 57283)

58267 with colpo-urethrocystopexy (Marshall-Marchetti-Krantz type, Pereyra type) with or without endoscopic control

58270 with repair of enterocele

(For repair of enterocele with removal of tubes and/or ovaries, use 58263)

58275 Vaginal hysterectomy, with total or partial vaginectomy;

58280 with repair of enterocele

58285 Vaginal hysterectomy, radical (Schauta type operation)

58290 Vaginal hysterectomy, for uterus greater than 250 grams;

58291 with removal of tube(s) and/or ovary(s)

58292 with removal of tube(s) and/or ovary(s), with repair of enterocele

58293 with colpo-urethrocystopexy (Marshall-Marchetti-Krantz type, Pereyra type) with or without endoscopic control

58294 with repair of enterocele

INTRODUCTION

(For insertion/removal of implantable contraceptive capsules, see 11975, 11976, 11977)

58300 Insertion of intrauterine device (IUD)

58301 Removal of intrauterine device (IUD)

58321 Artificial insemination; intra-cervical

58322 intra-uterine

58323 Sperm washing for artificial insemination

● New Code ▲ Revised Code 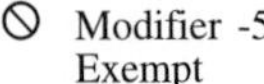 + Add-On Code ⊘ Modifier -51 Exempt 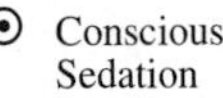 ⊙ Conscious Sedation

58340 Catheterization and introduction of saline or contrast material for saline infusion sonohysterography (SIS) or hysterosalpingography

(For radiological supervision and interpretation of saline infusion sonohysterography, use 76831)

(For radiological supervision and interpretation of hysterosalpingography, use 74740)

58345 Transcervical introduction of fallopian tube catheter for diagnosis and/or re-establishing patency (any method), with or without hysterosalpingography

(For radiological supervision and interpretation, use 74742)

58346 Insertion of Heyman capsules for clinical brachytherapy

(For insertion of radioelement sources or ribbons, see 77761-77763, 77781-77784)

58350 Chromotubation of oviduct, including materials

(For materials supplied by physician, use 99070)

58353 Endometrial ablation, thermal, without hysteroscopic guidance

(For hysteroscopic procedure, use 58563)

58356 Endometrial cryoablation with ultrasonic guidance, including endometrial curettage, when performed

(Do not report 58356 in conjunction with 58100, 58120, 58340, 76700, 76856)

REPAIR

58400 Uterine suspension, with or without shortening of round ligaments, with or without shortening of sacrouterine ligaments; (separate procedure)

58410 with presacral sympathectomy

(For anastomosis of tubes to uterus, use 58752)

58520 Hysterorrhaphy, repair of ruptured uterus (nonobstetrical)

58540 Hysteroplasty, repair of uterine anomaly (Strassman type)

(For closure of vesicouterine fistula, use 51920)

Separate Procedure | Unlisted Procedure | CCI Comp. Code | Non-specific Procedure

LAPAROSCOPY-HYSTEROSCOPY

● **58541** Laparoscopy, surgical, supracervical hysterectomy, for uterus 250 g or less;

● **58542** with removal of tube(s) and/or ovary(s)

(Do not report 58541, 58542 in conjunction with 49320, 57410, 58140, 58150, 58661, 58670, 58671)

● **58543** Laparoscopy, surgical, supracervical hysterectomy, for uterus greater than 250 g;

● **58544** with removal of tube(s) and/or ovary(s)

(Do not report 58544, 58544 in conjunction with 49320, 57410, 58140, 58150, 58661, 58670, 58671)

58545 Laparoscopy, surgical, myomectomy, excision; 1 to 4 intramural myomas with total weight of 250 g or less and/or removal of surface myomas

58546 5 or more intramural myomas and/or intramural myomas with total weight greater than 250 g

● **58548** Laparoscopy, surgical, with radical hysterectomy, with bilateral total pelvic lymphadenectomy and para-aortic lymph node sampling (biopsy), with removal of tube(s) and ovary(s), if performed

(Do not report 58548 in conjunction with 38570-38572, 58210 58285, 58550-58554)

58550 Laparoscopy, surgical with vaginal hysterectomy, for uterus 250 grams or less;

58552 with removal of tube(s) and/or ovary(s)

58553 Laparoscopy, surgical, with vaginal hysterectomy, for uterus greater than 250 grams;

58554 with removal of tube(s) and/or ovary(s)

58555 Hysteroscopy, diagnostic (separate procedure)

58558 Hysteroscopy, surgical; with sampling (biopsy) of endometrium and/or polypectomy, with or without D & C

● New Code ▲ Revised Code + Add-On Code ⃠ Modifier -51 Exempt ⊙ Conscious Sedation

58559 with lysis of intrauterine adhesions (any method)

58560 with division or resection of intrauterine septum (any method)

58561 with removal of leiomyomata

58562 with removal of impacted foreign body

58563 with endometrial ablation (eg, endometrial resection, electrosurgical ablation, thermoablation)

58565 with bilateral fallopian tube cannulation to induce occlusion by placement of permanent implants

(Do not report 58565 in conjunction with 58555 or 57800)

(For unilateral procedure, use modifier 52)

58578 Unlisted laparoscopy procedure, uterus

58579 Unlisted hysteroscopy procedure, uterus

OVIDUCT/OVARY

INCISION

58600 Ligation or transection of fallopian tube(s), abdominal or vaginal approach, unilateral or bilateral

58605 Ligation or transection of fallopian tube(s), abdominal or vaginal approach, postpartum, unilateral or bilateral, during same hospitalization (separate procedure)

(For laparoscopic procedures, use 58670, 58671)

+ **58611** Ligation or transection of fallopian tube(s) when done at the time of cesarean delivery or intra-abdominal surgery (not a separate procedure) (List separately in addition to code for primary procedure)

58615 Occlusion of fallopian tube(s) by device (eg, band, clip, Falope ring) vaginal or suprapubic approach

(For laparoscopic approach, use 58671)

(For lysis of adnexal adhesions, use 58740)

Separate Procedure | Unlisted Procedure | CCI Comp. Code | Non-specific Procedure

LAPAROSCOPY

58660 Laparoscopy, surgical; with lysis of adhesions (salpingolysis, ovariolysis) (separate procedure)

58661 with removal of adnexal structures (partial or total oophorectomy and/or salpingectomy)

58662 with fulguration or excision of lesions of the ovary, pelvic viscera, or peritoneal surface by any method

58670 with fulguration of oviducts (with or without transection)

58671 with occlusion of oviducts by device (eg, band, clip, or Falope ring)

58672 with fimbrioplasty

58673 with salpingostomy (salpingoneostomy)

(Codes 58672 and 58673 are used to report unilateral procedures. For bilateral procedure, use modifier -50)

58679 Unlisted laparoscopy procedure, oviduct, ovary

(For laparoscopic aspiration of ovarian cyst, use 49322)

(For laparoscopic biopsy of the ovary or fallopian tube, use 49321)

EXCISION

58700 Salpingectomy, complete or partial, unilateral or bilateral (separate procedure)

58720 Salpingo-oophorectomy, complete or partial, unilateral or bilateral (separate procedure)

REPAIR

58740 Lysis of adhesions (salpingolysis, ovariolysis)

(For laparoscopic approach, use 58660)

(For excision or destruction of endometriomas, open method, see 49200, 49201)

(For fulguration or excision of lesions, laparscopic approach, use 58662)

58750 Tubotubal anastomosis

58752 Tubouterine implantation

58760 Fimbrioplasty

(For laparoscopic approach, use 58672)

58770 Salpingostomy (salpingoneostomy)

(For laparscopic approach, use 58673)

OVARY

INCISION

58800 Drainage of ovarian cyst(s), unilateral or bilateral, (separate procedure); vaginal approach

58805 abdominal approach

58820 Drainage of ovarian abscess; vaginal approach, open

58822 abdominal approach

⊙ **58823** Drainage of pelvic abscess, transvaginal or transrectal approach, percutaneous (eg, ovarian, pericolic)

(For radiological supervision and interpretation, use 75989)

58825 Transposition, ovary(s)

EXCISION

58900 Biopsy of ovary, unilateral or bilateral (separate procedure)

(For laparoscopic biopsy of the ovary or fallopian tube, use 49321)

58920 Wedge resection or bisection of ovary, unilateral or bilateral

58925 Ovarian cystectomy, unilateral or bilateral

58940 Oophorectomy, partial or total, unilateral or bilateral;

(For oophorectomy with concomitant debulking for ovarian malignancy, use 58592)

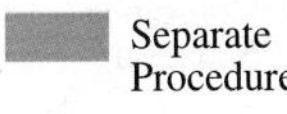
Separate Procedure
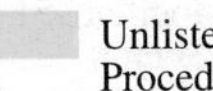
Unlisted Procedure
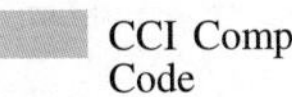
CCI Comp. Code
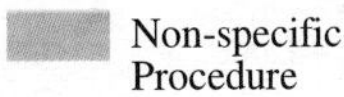
Non-specific Procedure

58943 for ovarian, tubal or primary peritoneal malignancy, with para-aortic and pelvic lymph node biopsies, peritoneal washings, peritoneal biopsies, diaphragmatic assessments, with or without salpingectomy(s), with or without omentectomy

▲ **58950** Resection (initial) of ovarian, tubal or primary peritoneal malignancy with bilateral salpingo-oophorectomy and omentectomy;

58951 with total abdominal hysterectomy, pelvic and limited para-aortic lymphadenectomy

58952 with radical dissection for debulking (ie, radical excision or destruction, intra-abdominal or retroperitoneal tumors)

(For resection of recurrent ovarian, tubal, primary peritoneal, or uterine malignancy, see 58597, 58958)

58953 Bilateral salpingo-oophorectomy with omentectomy, total abdominal hysterectomy and radical dissection for debulking;

58954 with pelvic lymphadenectomy and limited para-aortic lymphadenectomy

58956 Bilateral salpingo-oophorectomy with total omentectomy, total abdominal hysterectomy for malignancy

(Do not report 58956 in conjunction with 49255, 58150, 58180, 58262, 58263, 58550, 58661, 58700, 58720, 58900, 58925, 58940, 58957, 58958)

● **58957** Resection (tumor debulking) of recurrent ovarian, tubal, primary peritoneal, uterine malignancy (intra-abdominal, retroperitoneal tumors), with omentectomy, if performed;

● **58958** Resection (tumor debulking) of recurrent ovarian, tubal, primary peritoneal, uterine malignancy (intra-abdominal, retroperitoneal tumors), with omentectomy, if performed; with pelvic lymphadenectomy and limited para-aortic lymphadenectomy

(Do not report 58957, 58958 in conjunction with 38770, 38780, 44005, 49000, 49200-49215, 49255, 58900-58960)

58960 Laparotomy, for staging or restaging of ovarian, tubal or primary peritoneal malignancy (second look), with or without omentectomy, peritoneal washing, biopsy of abdominal and pelvic peritoneum, diaphragmatic assessment with pelvic and limited para-aortic lymphadenectomy

(Do not report 58960 in conjunction with 58957, 58958)

IN VITRO FERTILIZATION

58970 Follicle puncture for oocyte retrieval, any method

(For radiological supervision and interpretation, use 76948)

58974 Embryo transfer, intrauterine

58976 Gamete, zygote, or embryo intrafallopian transfer, any method

(For laparoscopic adnexal procedures, see 58660-58673)

OTHER PROCEDURES

58999 Unlisted procedure, female genital system (nonobstetrical)

This page intentionally left blank.

● New Code ▲ Revised Code + Add-On Code ⃠ Modifier -51 Exempt ⊙ Conscious Sedation

MATERNITY CARE AND DELIVERY

CPT codes from this section are used to report routine maternity care and invasive and surgical procedures performed as part of prenatal, delivery and post-partum care. The services normally provided in uncomplicated maternity cases include antepartum care, delivery, and postpartum care.

ANTEPARTUM CARE

The definition of antepartum care for coding purposes includes the initial and subsequent history, physical examinations, recording of weight, blood pressures, fetal heart tones, routine chemical urinalysis, and routine visits. Routine antepartum visits are defined as:

- *Monthly visits up to 28 weeks gestation*
- *Biweekly visits up to 36 weeks gestation, and*
- *Weekly visits until delivery*

Any other visits or services provided within this time period should be coded separately. Using 6 to 8 weeks gestation as the typical starting point, the above definition translates into between 9 and 11 routine visits per patient.

DELIVERY

Delivery services are defined as including hospital admission, the admission history and physical examination, management of uncomplicated labor, and vaginal or cesarean delivery.

- *The definition of delivery services includes the hospital admission, and admission history and physical.*
- *Resuscitation of newborn infants when necessary, defined in previous editions, is not included in the delivery services. If the delivering physician has to resuscitate the newborn infant, he/she may code this service as a separate procedure.*
- *Medical problems "complicating labor and delivery management" may require additional resources and should be reported using evaluation and management service codes.*

POSTPARTUM CARE

Postpartum care is defined as hospital and office visits following vaginal or cesarean delivery. No number of visits is defined by CPT; however, the typical fee for total obstetrical care includes a single office follow-up visit six weeks postpartum.

COMPLICATIONS OF PREGNANCY

The services defined previously are for normal, uncomplicated maternity care. For medical complications of pregnancy, for example, cardiac problems, neurological problems, diabetes, hypertension, toxemia, hyperemesis, pre-term labor and premature rupture of membranes, use evaluation and management service codes.

For surgical complications of pregnancy, such as appendectomy, hernia, ovarian cyst, Bartholin cysts, etc., use CPT codes from the SURGERY section of CPT. Note that in either case, complications are not considered to be part of routine maternity care and should be coded and reported in addition to maternity CPT codes.

PARTIAL MATERNITY SERVICES

Occasionally a physician may provide all or part of the antepartum and/or postpartum care but does not perform the actual delivery due to termination of the pregnancy by abortion, or referral to another physician for delivery. In this circumstance, the physician has the option of using the inclusive CPT codes 59420 or 59430 from the Maternity Care and Delivery section reporting each visit using evaluation and management service codes 99201-99215.

MISCELLANEOUS CODING RULES

The majority of procedures in this section (CPT codes 59000-59899) include only what is described by the code in the CPT definition. Additional procedures performed on the same day would be reported separately.

The few exceptions to this rule consist of: CPT codes 59050 and 59051(fetal monitoring during labor), 59300 (episiotomy) and 59414 (delivery of placenta) are included in CPT codes 59400 (routine obstetric care, vaginal delivery), 59409 (vaginal delivery only), 59410 (vaginal delivery and postpartum care), 59510 (routine obstetric care, cesarean delivery), 59514 (cesarean delivery only), 59515 (cesarean delivery and postpartum care), 59610 (routine obstetric care, vaginal delivery, after previous cesarean delivery), 59612 (vaginal delivery only after previous cesarean delivery), 59614 (vaginal delivery and postpartum care after previous cesarean delivery), 59618 (routine obstetric care, cesarean delivery, after previous cesarean delivery), 59620 (cesarean delivery only after previous cesarean delivery), and 59622 (cesarean delivery and postpartum care after previous cesarean delivery). They are not to be separately reported.

The total obstetrical packages (e.g. CPT codes 59400 and 59510) include antepartum care, the delivery, and postpartum care. They do not include among other services, ultrasound, amniocentesis, special screening tests for genetic conditions, visits for unrelated conditions (incidental to pregnancy) or additional and frequent visits due to high risk conditions.

Obstetric care can be coded as a global package or can be broken down when necessary into antepartum, delivery and postpartum care.

Complicated pregnancies and deliveries need to be coded appropriately to indicate the increased work on the physician's part during the patient's care. There are several options for recording these circumstances.

(For circumcision of newborn, see 54150, 54160)

ANTEPARTUM SERVICES

(For insertion of transcervical or transvaginal fetal oximetry sensor, use Category III code 0021T)

59000 Amniocentesis, diagnostic

(For radiological supervision and interpretation, use 76946)

59001 therapeutic amniotic fluid reduction (includes ultrasound guidance)

59012 Cordocentesis (intrauterine), any method

(For radiological supervision and interpretation, use 76941)

59015 Chorionic villus sampling, any method

(For radiological supervision and interpretation, use 76945)

59020 Fetal contraction stress test

59025 Fetal non-stress test

59030 Fetal scalp blood sampling

(For repeat fetal scalp blood sampling, use 59030 and see modifiers -76 and -77)

59050 Fetal monitoring during labor by consulting physician (ie, non-attending physician) with written report; supervision and interpretation

59051 interpretation only

59070 Transabdominal amnioinfusion, including ultrasound guidance

59072 Fetal umbilical cord occlusion, including ultrasound guidance

59074 Fetal fluid drainage (eg, vesicocentesis, thoracocentesis, paracentesis), including ultrasound guidance

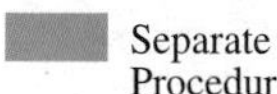
Separate Procedure

Unlisted Procedure

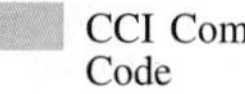
CCI Comp. Code

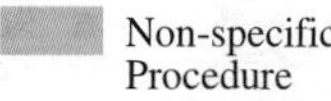
Non-specific Procedure

59076 Fetal shunt placement, including ultrasound guidance

(For unlisted fetal invasive procedure, use 59897)

EXCISION

59100 Hysterotomy, abdominal (eg, for hydatidiform mole, abortion)

(When tubal ligation is performed at the same time as hysterotomy, use 58611 in addition to 59100)

59120 Surgical treatment of ectopic pregnancy; tubal or ovarian, requiring salpingectomy and/or oophorectomy, abdominal or vaginal approach

59121 tubal or ovarian, without salpingectomy and/or oophorectomy

59130 abdominal pregnancy

59135 interstitial, uterine pregnancy requiring total hysterectomy

59136 interstitial, uterine pregnancy with partial resection of uterus

59140 cervical, with evacuation

59150 Laparoscopic treatment of ectopic pregnancy; without salpingectomy and/or oophorectomy

59151 with salpingectomy and/or oophorectomy

59160 Curettage, postpartum

INTRODUCTION

(For intrauterine fetal transfusion, use 36460)

(For introduction of hypertonic solution and/or prostaglandins to initiate labor, see 59850-59857)

59200 Insertion of cervical dilator (eg, laminaria, prostaglandin) (separate procedure)

REPAIR

(For tracheoplasty, use 57700)

59300 Episiotomy or vaginal repair, by other than attending physician

59320 Cerclage of cervix, during pregnancy; vaginal

59325 abdominal

59350 Hysterorrhaphy of ruptured uterus

VAGINAL DELIVERY, ANTEPARTUM AND POSTPARTUM CARE

(For insertion of transcervical or transvaginal fetal oximetry sensor, use Category III code 0021T)

59400 Routine obstetric care including antepartum care, vaginal delivery (with or without episiotomy, and/or forceps) and postpartum care

59409 Vaginal delivery only (with or without episiotomy and/or forceps);

59410 including postpartum care

59412 External cephalic version, with or without tocolysis

(Use 59412 in addition to code(s) for delivery)

59414 Delivery of placenta (separate procedure)

(For antepartum care only, see 59425, 59426 or appropriate E/M code(s))

(For 1-3 antepartum care visits, see appropriate E/M code(s))

59425 Antepartum care only; 4-6 visits

59426 7 or more visits

59430 Postpartum care only (separate procedure)

CESAREAN DELIVERY

(For standby attendance for infant, use 99360)

(For insertion of transcervical or transvaginal fetal oximetry sensor, use Category III code 0021T)

(For low cervical cesarean section, see 59510, 59515, 59525)

Separate Procedure 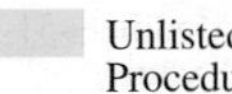 Unlisted Procedure 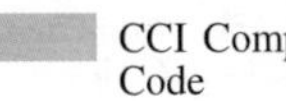 CCI Comp. Code 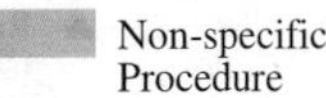 Non-specific Procedure

59510 Routine obstetric care including antepartum care, cesarean delivery, and postpartum care

59514 Cesarean delivery only;

59515 including postpartum care

(For classic cesarean section, see 59510, 59515, 59525)

+ **59525** Subtotal or total hysterectomy after cesarean delivery (List separately in addition to code for primary procedure)

(Use 59525 in conjunction with codes 59510, 59514, 59515, 59618, 59620, 59622)

(For extraperitoneal cesarean section, or cesarean section with subtotal or total hysterectomy, see 59510, 59515, 59525)

DELIVERY AFTER PREVIOUS CESAREAN DELIVERY

(For insertion of transcervical or transvaginal fetal oximetry sensor, use Category III code 0021T)

59610 Routine obstetric care including antepartum care, vaginal delivery (with or without episiotomy, and/or forceps) and postpartum care, after previous cesarean delivery

59612 Vaginal delivery only, after previous cesarean delivery (with or without episiotomy and/or forceps);

59614 including postpartum care

59618 Routine obstetric care including antepartum care, cesarean delivery, and postpartum care, following attempted vaginal delivery after previous cesarean delivery

59620 Cesarean delivery only, following attempted vaginal delivery after previous cesarean delivery;

59622 including postpartum care

ABORTION

(For medical treatment of spontaneous complete abortion, any trimester, use E/M codes 99201-99233)

(For surgical treatment of spontaneous abortion, use 59812)

59812 Treatment of incomplete abortion, any trimester, completed surgically

59820 Treatment of missed abortion, completed surgically; first trimester

59821 second trimester

59830 Treatment of septic abortion, completed surgically

59840 Induced abortion, by dilation and curettage

59841 Induced abortion, by dilation and evacuation

59850 Induced abortion, by one or more intra-amniotic injections (amniocentesis-injections), including hospital admission and visits, delivery of fetus and secundines;

59851 with dilation and curettage and/or evacuation

59852 with hysterotomy (failed intra-amniotic injection)

(For insertion of cervical dilator, use 59200)

59855 Induced abortion, by one or more vaginal suppositories (eg, prostaglandin) with or without cervical dilation (eg, laminaria), including hospital admission and visits, delivery of fetus and secundines;

59856 with dilation and curettage and/or evacuation

59857 with hysterotomy (failed medical evacuation)

OTHER PROCEDURES

59866 Multifetal pregnancy reduction(s) (MPR)

59870 Uterine evacuation and curettage for hydatidiform mole

59871 Removal of cerclage suture under anesthesia (other than local)

59897 Unlisted fetal invasive procedure, including ultrasound guidance

59898 Unlisted laparoscopy procedure, maternity care and delivery

59899 Unlisted procedure, maternity care and delivery

Separate Procedure | Unlisted Procedure | CCI Comp. Code | Non-specific Procedure

This page intentionally left blank.

ENDOCRINE SYSTEM

CPT codes from this section of CPT are used to report invasive and surgical procedures performed on the thyroid gland, parathyroid, thymus, adrenal glands and carotid body.

(For pituitary and pineal surgery, see Nervous System)

THYROID GLAND

INCISION

60000 Incision and drainage of thyroglossal duct cyst, infected

EXCISION

60001 Aspiration and/or injection, thyroid cyst

(For fine needle aspiration, see 10021, 10022)

(If imaging guidance is performed, see 76942, 77012)

60100 Biopsy thyroid, percutaneous core needle

(If imaging guidance is performed, see 76942, 77002, 77012, 77021)

(For fine needle aspiration, use 10021 or 10022)

(For evaluation of fine needle aspirate, see 88172, 88173)

60200 Excision of cyst or adenoma of thyroid, or transection of isthmus

60210 Partial thyroid lobectomy, unilateral; with or without isthmusectomy

60212 with contralateral subtotal lobectomy, including isthmusectomy

60220 Total thyroid lobectomy, unilateral; with or without isthmusectomy

60225 with contralateral subtotal lobectomy, including isthmusectomy

60240 Thyroidectomy, total or complete

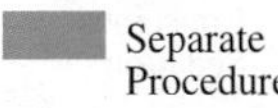 Separate Procedure 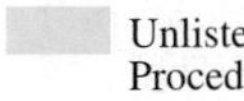 Unlisted Procedure 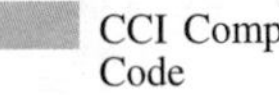 CCI Comp. Code 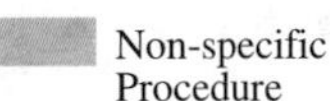 Non-specific Procedure

(For thyroidectomy, subtotal or partial, use 60271)

60252 Thyroidectomy, total or subtotal for malignancy; with limited neck dissection

60254 with radical neck dissection

60260 Thyroidectomy, removal of all remaining thyroid tissue following previous removal of a portion of thyroid

(For bilateral procedure, report 60260 with modifier -50)

60270 Thyroidectomy, including substernal thyroid; sternal split or transthoracic approach

60271 cervical approach

60280 Excision of thyroglossal duct cyst or sinus;

60281 recurrent

(For thyroid ultrasonography, use 76536)

PARATHYROID, THYMUS, ADRENAL GLANDS, PANCREAS, AND CAROTID BODY

EXCISION

(For pituitary and pineal surgery, see Nervous System)

60500 Parathyroidectomy or exploration of parathyroid(s);

60502 re-exploration

60505 with mediastinal exploration, sternal split or transthoracic approach

+ **60512** Parathyroid autotransplantation (List separately in addition to code for primary procedure)

(Use 60512 in conjunction with codes 60500, 60502, 60505, 60212, 60225, 60240, 60252, 60254, 60260, 60270, 60271)

60520 Thymectomy, partial or total; transcervical approach (separate procedure)

60521 sternal split or transthoracic approach, without radical mediastinal dissection (separate procedure)

● New Code ▲ Revised Code + Add-On Code ⊘ Modifier -51 Exempt ⊙ Conscious Sedation

60522 sternal split or transthoracic approach, with radical mediastinal dissection (separate procedure)

60540 Adrenalectomy, partial or complete, or exploration of adrenal gland with or without biopsy, transabdominal, lumbar or dorsal (separate procedure);

60545 with excision of adjacent retroperitoneal tumor

(Do not report 60540, 60545 in conjunction with 50323)

(For bilateral procedure, report 60540 with modifier 50)

(For excision of remote or disseminated pheochromocytoma, see 49200, 49201)

(For laparoscopic approach, use 56321)

60600 Excision of carotid body tumor; without excision of carotid artery

60605 with excision of carotid artery

LAPAROSCOPY

60650 Laparoscopy, surgical, with adrenalectomy, partial or complete, or exploration of adrenal gland with or without biopsy, transabdominal, lumbar or dorsal

60659 Unlisted laparoscopy procedure, endocrine system

OTHER PROCEDURES

60699 Unlisted procedure, endocrine system

Separate Procedure 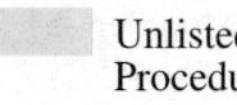 Unlisted Procedure 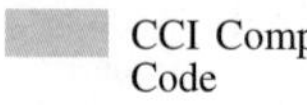 CCI Comp. Code 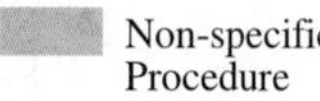 Non-specific Procedure

This page intentionally left blank.

NERVOUS SYSTEM

CPT codes from this section of the CPT coding system are used to report invasive and surgical procedures on the skull; meninges and brain; spine and spinal cord; and the extracranial nerves, peripheral nerves and autonomic nervous system.

There are numerous codes for spinal injections found in this section. Review documentation for whether the injection is a single one, differential one or continuous. Also determine the number of levels involved when a regional block is administered.

SKULL, MENINGES, AND BRAIN

(For injection procedure for cerebral angiography, see 36100-36218)

(For injection procedure for ventriculography, see 61026, 61120, 61130)

(For injection procedure for pneumoencephalography, use 61055)

INJECTION, DRAINAGE OR ASPIRATION

61000 Subdural tap through fontanelle, or suture, infant, unilateral or bilateral; initial

61001 subsequent taps

61020 Ventricular puncture through previous burr hole, fontanelle, suture, or implanted ventricular catheter/reservoir; without injection

61026 with injection of medication or other substance for diagnosis or treatment

61050 Cisternal or lateral cervical (C1-C2) puncture; without injection (separate procedure)

61055 with injection of medication or other substance for diagnosis or treatment (eg, C1-C2)

(For radiological supervision and interpretation, see Radiology)

61070 Puncture of shunt tubing or reservoir for aspiration or injection procedure

(For radiological supervision and interpretation, use 75809)

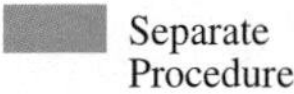 Separate Procedure   Unlisted Procedure   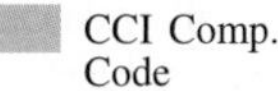 CCI Comp. Code   Non-specific Procedure

TWIST DRILL, BURR HOLE(S), OR TREPHINE

61105 Twist drill hole(s) for subdural or ventricular puncture;

⊘▲**61107** Twist drill hole(s) for subdural, intracerebral or ventricular puncture; for implanting ventricular catheter, pressure recording device, or other intracerebral monitoring device

(For intracranial neuroendoscopic ventricular catheter placement, use 62160)

(For twist drill or burr hole performed to place thermal perfusion probe, use Category III code 0077T)

61108 for evacuation and/or drainage of subdural hematoma

61120 Burr hole(s) for ventricular puncture (including injection of gas, contrast media, dye, or radioactive material)

61140 Burr hole(s) or trephine; with biopsy of brain or intracranial lesion

61150 with drainage of brain abscess or cyst

61151 with subsequent tapping (aspiration) of intracranial abscess or cyst

61154 Burr hole(s) with evacuation and/or drainage of hematoma, extradural or subdural

(For bilateral procedure, report 61154 with modifier -50)

61156 Burr hole(s); with aspiration of hematoma or cyst, intracerebral

⊘▲**61210** for implanting ventricular catheter, reservoir, EEG electrode(s), pressure recording device, or other cerebral monitoring device (separate procedure)

(For intracranial neuroendoscopic ventricular catheter placement, use 62160)

61215 Insertion of subcutaneous reservoir, pump or continuous infusion system for connection to ventricular catheter

(For refilling and maintenance of an implantable infusion pump for spinal or brain drug therapy, use 95990)

(For chemotherapy, use 96450)

61250 Burr hole(s) or trephine, supratentorial, exploratory, not followed by other surgery

(For bilateral procedure, report 61250 with modifier -50)

61253 Burr hole(s) or trephine, infratentorial, unilateral or bilateral

(If burr hole(s) or trephine are followed by craniotomy at same operative session, use 61304-61321; do not use 61250 or 61253)

CRANIECTOMY OR CRANIOTOMY

61304 Craniectomy or craniotomy, exploratory; supratentorial

61305 infratentorial (posterior fossa)

61312 Craniectomy or craniotomy for evacuation of hematoma, supratentorial; extradural or subdural

61313 intracerebral

61314 Craniectomy or craniotomy for evacuation of hematoma, infratentorial; extradural or subdural

61315 intracerebellar

+ **61316** Incision and subcutaneous placement of cranial bone graft (List separately in addition to code for primary procedure)

(Use 61316 in conjunction with codes 61304, 61312, 61313, 61322, 61323, 61340, 61570, 61571, 61680-61705)

61320 Craniectomy or craniotomy, drainage of intracranial abscess; supratentorial

61321 infratentorial

61322 Craniectomy or craniotomy, decompressive, with or without duraplasty, for treatment of intracranial hypertension, without evacuation of associated intraparenchymal hematoma; without lobectomy

(Do not report 61313 in addition to 61322)

(For subtemporal decompression, use 61340)

61323 with lobectomy

(Do not report 61313 in addition to 61323)

(For subtemporal decompression, use 61340)

61330 Decompression of orbit only, transcranial approach

(For bilateral procedure, report 61330 with modifier -50)

61332 Exploration of orbit (transcranial approach); with biopsy

61333 with removal of lesion

61334 with removal of foreign body

61340 Subtemporal cranial decompression (pseudotumor cerebri, slit ventricle syndrome)

(For bilateral procedure, report 61340 with modifier -50)

(For decompressive craniotomy or craniectomy for intracranial hypertension, without hematoma evacuation, see 61322, 61323)

61343 Craniectomy, suboccipital with cervical laminectomy for decompression of medulla and spinal cord, with or without dural graft (eg, Arnold-Chiari malformation)

61345 Other cranial decompression, posterior fossa

(For orbital decompression by lateral wall approach, Kroenlein type, use 67445)

61440 Craniotomy for section of tentorium cerebelli (separate procedure)

61450 Craniectomy, subtemporal, for section, compression, or decompression of sensory root of gasserian ganglion

61458 Craniectomy, suboccipital; for exploration or decompression of cranial nerves

61460 for section of one or more cranial nerves

61470 for medullary tractotomy

61480 for mesencephalic tractotomy or pedunculotomy

61490 Craniotomy for lobotomy, including cingulotomy

(For bilateral procedure, report 61490 with modifier -50)

61500 Craniectomy; with excision of tumor or other bone lesion of skull

61501 for osteomyelitis

61510 Craniectomy, trephination, bone flap craniotomy; for excision of brain tumor, supratentorial, except meningioma

61512 for excision of meningioma, supratentorial

61514 for excision of brain abscess, supratentorial

61516 for excision or fenestration of cyst, supratentorial

(For excision of pituitary tumor or craniopharyngioma, see 61545, 61546, 61548)

+ **61517** Implantation of brain intracavitary chemotherapy agent (List separately in addition to code for primary procedure)

(Use 61517 only in conjunction with codes 61510 or 61518)

(Do not report 61517 for brachytherapy insertion. For intracavitary insertion of radioelement sources or ribbons, see 77781-77784)

61518 Craniectomy for excision of brain tumor, infratentorial or posterior fossa; except meningioma, cerebellopontine angle tumor, or midline tumor at base of skull

61519 meningioma

61520 cerebellopontine angle tumor

61521 midline tumor at base of skull

61522 Craniectomy, infratentorial or posterior fossa; for excision of brain abscess

61524 for excision or fenestration of cyst

61526 Craniectomy, bone flap craniotomy, transtemporal (mastoid) for excision of cerebellopontine angle tumor;

 Separate Procedure 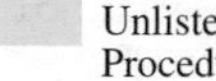 Unlisted Procedure 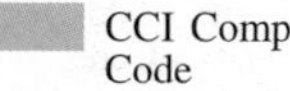 CCI Comp. Code 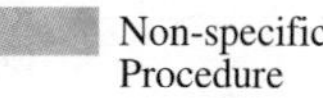 Non-specific Procedure

61530 combined with middle/posterior fossa craniotomy/craniectomy

61531 Subdural implantation of strip electrodes through one or more burr or trephine hole(s) for long term seizure monitoring

(For stereotactic implantation of electrodes, use 61760)

(For craniotomy for excision of intracranial arteriovenous malformation, see 61680-61692)

61533 Craniotomy with elevation of bone flap; for subdural implantation of an electrode array, for long term seizure monitoring

(For continuous EEG monitoring, see 95950-95954)

61534 for excision of epileptogenic focus without electrocorticography during surgery

61535 for removal of epidural or subdural electrode array, without excision of cerebral tissue (separate procedure)

61536 for excision of cerebral epileptogenic focus, with electrocorticography during surgery (includes removal of electrode array)

61537 for lobectomy, temporal lobe, without electrocorticography during surgery

61538 for lobectomy, temporal lobe, with electrocorticography during surgery

61539 for lobectomy, other than temporal lobe, partial or total, with electrocorticography during surgery

61540 for lobectomy, other than temporal lobe, partial or total, without electrocorticography during surgery

61541 for transection of corpus callosum

61542 for total hemispherectomy

61543 for partial or subtotal (functional) hemispherectomy

61544 for excision or coagulation of choroid plexus

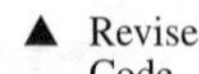

● New Code ▲ Revised Code + Add-On Code ⊘ Modifier -51 Exempt ⊙ Conscious Sedation

61545 for excision of craniopharyngioma

(For craniotomy for selective amygdalohippocampectomy, use 61566)

(For craniotomy for multiple subpial transections during surgery, use 61567)

61546 Craniotomy for hypophysectomy or excision of pituitary tumor, intracranial approach

61548 Hypophysectomy or excision of pituitary tumor, transnasal or transseptal approach, nonstereotactic

(Do not report code 69990 in addition to code 61548)

61550 Craniectomy for craniosynostosis; single cranial suture

61552 multiple cranial sutures

(For cranial reconstruction for orbital hypertelorism, see 21260-21263)

(For reconstruction, see 21172-21180)

61556 Craniotomy for craniosynostosis; frontal or parietal bone flap

61557 bifrontal bone flap

61558 Extensive craniectomy for multiple cranial suture craniosynostosis (eg, cloverleaf skull); not requiring bone grafts

61559 recontouring with multiple osteotomies and bone autografts (eg, barrel-stave procedure) (includes obtaining grafts)

(For reconstruction, see 21172-21180)

61563 Excision, intra and extracranial, benign tumor of cranial bone (eg, fibrous dysplasia); without optic nerve decompression

61564 with optic nerve decompression

(For reconstruction, see 21181-21183)

61566 Craniotomy with elevation of bone flap; for selective amygdalohippocampectomy

61567 for multiple subpial transections, with electrocorticography during surgery

61570 Craniectomy or craniotomy; with excision of foreign body from brain

61571 with treatment of penetrating wound of brain

(For sequestrectomy for osteomyelitis, use 61501)

61575 Transoral approach to skull base, brain stem or upper spinal cord for biopsy, decompression or excision of lesion;

61576 requiring splitting of tongue and/or mandible (including tracheostomy)

(For arthrodesis, use 22548)

SURGERY OF SKULL BASE

APPROACH PROCEDURES

Anterior Cranial Fossa

61580 Craniofacial approach to anterior cranial fossa; extradural, including lateral rhinotomy, ethmoidectomy, sphenoidectomy, without maxillectomy or orbital exenteration

61581 extradural, including lateral rhinotomy, orbital exenteration, ethmoidectomy, sphenoidectomy and/or maxillectomy

61582 extradural, including unilateral or bifrontal craniotomy, elevation of frontal lobe(s), osteotomy of base of anterior cranial fossa

61583 intradural, including unilateral or bifrontal craniotomy, elevation or resection of frontal lobe, osteotomy of base of anterior cranial fossa

61584 Orbitocranial approach to anterior cranial fossa, extradural, including supraorbital ridge osteotomy and elevation of frontal and/or temporal lobe(s); without orbital exenteration

61585 with orbital exenteration

61586 Bicoronal, transzygomatic and/or LeFort I osteotomy approach to anterior cranial fossa with or without internal fixation, without bone graft

Middle Cranial Fossa

61590 Infratemporal pre-auricular approach to middle cranial fossa (parapharyngeal space, infratemporal and midline skull base, nasopharynx), with or without disarticulation of the mandible, including parotidectomy, craniotomy, decompression and/or mobilization of the facial nerve and/or petrous carotid artery

61591 Infratemporal post-auricular approach to middle cranial fossa (internal auditory meatus, petrous apex, tentorium, cavernous sinus, parasellar area, infratemporal fossa) including mastoidectomy, resection of sigmoid sinus, with or without decompression and/or mobilization of contents of auditory canal or petrous carotid artery

61592 Orbitocranial zygomatic approach to middle cranial fossa (cavernous sinus and carotid artery, clivus, basilar artery or petrous apex) including osteotomy of zygoma, craniotomy, extra- or intradural elevation of temporal lobe

Posterior Cranial Fossa

61595 Transtemporal approach to posterior cranial fossa, jugular foramen or midline skull base, including mastoidectomy, decompression of sigmoid sinus and/or facial nerve, with or without mobilization

61596 Transcochlear approach to posterior cranial fossa, jugular foramen or midline skull base, including labyrinthectomy, decompression, with or without mobilization of facial nerve and/or petrous carotid artery

61597 Transcondylar (far lateral) approach to posterior cranial fossa, jugular foramen or midline skull base, including occipital condylectomy, mastoidectomy, resection of C1-C3 vertebral body(s), decompression of vertebral artery, with or without mobilization

61598 Transpetrosal approach to posterior cranial fossa, clivus or foramen magnum, including ligation of superior petrosal sinus and/or sigmoid sinus

DEFINITIVE PROCEDURES

Base of Anterior Cranial Fossa

61600 Resection or excision of neoplastic, vascular or infectious lesion of base of anterior cranial fossa; extradural

61601 intradural, including dural repair, with or without graft

Base of Middle Cranial Fossa

61605 Resection or excision of neoplastic, vascular or infectious lesion of infratemporal fossa, parapharyngeal space, petrous apex; extradural

61606 intradural, including dural repair, with or without graft

61607 Resection or excision of neoplastic, vascular or infectious lesion of parasellar area, cavernous sinus, clivus or midline skull base; extradural

61608 intradural, including dural repair, with or without graft

(Codes 61609-61612 are reported in addition to code(s) for primary procedure(s) 61605-61608. Report only one transection or ligation of carotid artery code per operative session.)

+ **61609** Transection or ligation, carotid artery in cavernous sinus; without repair (List separately in addition to code for primary procedure)

+ **61610** with repair by anastomosis or graft (List separately in addition to code for primary procedure)

+ **61611** Transection or ligation, carotid artery in petrous canal; without repair (List separately in addition to code for primary procedure)

+ **61612** with repair by anastomosis or graft (List separately in addition to code for primary procedure)

61613 Obliteration of carotid aneurysm, arteriovenous malformation, or carotid-cavernous fistula by dissection within cavernous sinus

Base of Posterior Cranial Fossa

61615 Resection or excision of neoplastic, vascular or infectious lesion of base of posterior cranial fossa, jugular foramen, foramen magnum, or C1-C3 vertebral bodies; extradural

61616 intradural, including dural repair, with or without graft

REPAIR AND/OR RECONSTRUCTION OF SURGICAL DEFECTS OF SKULL BASE

61618 Secondary repair of dura for cerebrospinal fluid leak, anterior, middle or posterior cranial fossa following surgery of the skull base; by free tissue graft (eg, pericranium, fascia, tensor fascia lata, adipose tissue, homologous or synthetic grafts)

61619 by local or regionalized vascularized pedicle flap or myocutaneous flap (including galea, temporalis, frontalis or occipitalis muscle)

ENDOVASCULAR THERAPY

61623 Endovascular temporary balloon arterial occlusion, head or neck (extracranial/intracranial) including selective catheterization of vessel to be occluded, positioning and inflation of occlusion balloon, concomitant neurological monitoring, and radiologic supervision and interpretation of all angiography required for balloon occlusion and to exclude vascular injury post occlusion

(If selective catheterization and angiography of arteries other than artery to be occluded is performed, use appropriate catheterization and radiologic supervision and interpretation codes)

(If complete diagnostic angiography of the artery to be occluded is performed immediately prior to temporary occlusion, use appropriate radiologic supervision and interpretation codes only)

61624 Transcatheter permanent occlusion or embolization (eg, for tumor destruction, to achieve hemostasis, to occlude a vascular malformation), percutaneous, any method; central nervous system (intracranial, spinal cord)

(See also 37204)

(For radiological supervision and interpretation, use 75894)

61626 non-central nervous system, head or neck (extracranial, brachiocephalic branch)

(See also 37204)

(For radiological supervision and interpretation, use 75894)

61630 Balloon angioplasty, intracranial (eg, atherosclerotic stenosis), percutaneous

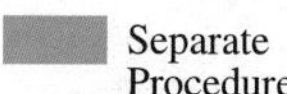

61635 Transcatheter placement of intravascular stent(s), intracranial (eg, atherosclerotic stenosis), including balloon angioplasty, if performed

(61630 and 61635 include all selective vascular catheterization of the target vascular family, all diagnostic imaging for arteriography of the target vascular family, and all related radiological supervision and interpretation. When diagnostic arteriogram (including imaging and selective catheterization) confirms the need for angioplasty or stent placement, 61630 and 61635 are inclusive of these services. If angioplasty or stenting are not indicated, then the appropriate codes for selective catheterization and imaging should be reported in lieu of 61630 and 61635)

61640 Balloon dilatation of intracranial vasospasm, percutaneous; initial vessel

+ **61641** each additional vessel in same vascular family (List separately in addition to code for primary procedure)

+ **61642** each additional vessel in different vascular family (List separately in addition to code for primary procedure)

(Use 61641 and 61642 in conjunction with 61640)

(61640, 61641, 61642 include all selective vascular catheterization of the target vessel, contrast injection(s), vessel measurement, roadmapping, postdilatation angiography, and fluoroscopic guidance for the balloon dilatation)

SURGERY FOR ANEURYSM, ARTERIOVENOUS MALFORMATION OR VASCULAR DISEASE

61680 Surgery of intracranial arteriovenous malformation; supratentorial, simple

61682 supratentorial, complex

61684 infratentorial, simple

61686 infratentorial, complex

61690 dural, simple

61692 dural, complex

61697 Surgery of complex intracranial aneurysm, intracranial approach; carotid circulation

61698 vertebrobasilar circulation

(61697, 61698 involve aneurysms that are larger than 15 mm or with calcification of the aneurysm neck, or with incorporation of normal vessels into the aneurysm neck, or a procedure requiring temporary vessel occlusion, trapping or cardiopulmonary bypass to successfully treat the aneurysm)

61700 Surgery of simple intracranial aneurysm, intracranial approach; carotid circulation

61702 vertebrobasilar circulation

61703 Surgery of intracranial aneurysm, cervical approach by application of occluding clamp to cervical carotid artery (Selverstone-Crutchfield type)

(For cervical approach for direct ligation of carotid artery, see 37600-37606)

61705 Surgery of aneurysm, vascular malformation or carotid-cavernous fistula; by intracranial and cervical occlusion of carotid artery

61708 by intracranial electrothrombosis

(For ligation or gradual occlusion of internal/common carotid artery, see 37605, 37606)

61710 by intra-arterial embolization, injection procedure, or balloon catheter

61711 Anastomosis, arterial, extracranial-intracranial (eg, middle cerebral/cortical) arteries

(For carotid or vertebral thromboendarterectomy, use 35301)

(Use 69990 when the surgical microscope is employed for the microsurgical procedure. Do not use 69990 for visualization with magnifying loupes or corrected vision)

STEREOTAXIS

61720 Creation of lesion by stereotactic method, including burr hole(s) and localizing and recording techniques, single or multiple stages; globus pallidus or thalamus

61735 subcortical structure(s) other than globus pallidus or thalamus

61750 Stereotactic biopsy, aspiration, or excision, including burr hole(s), for intracranial lesion;

61751 with computed tomography and/or magnetic resonance guidance

(For radiological supervision and interpretation of computerized tomography, see 70450, 70460, or 70470 as appropriate)

(For radiological supervision and interpretation of magnetic resonance imaging, see 70551, 70552, or 70553 as appropriate)

61760 Stereotactic implantation of depth electrodes into the cerebrum for long term seizure monitoring

61770 Stereotactic localization, including burr hole(s), with insertion of catheter(s) or probe(s) for placement of radiation source

61790 Creation of lesion by stereotactic method, percutaneous, by neurolytic agent (eg, alcohol, thermal, electrical, radiofrequency); gasserian ganglion

61791 trigeminal medullary tract

61793 Stereotactic radiosurgery (particle beam, gamma ray or linear accelerator), one or more sessions

(For intensity modulated beam delivery plan and treatment, see 77301, 77418)

\+ **61795** Stereotactic computer assisted volumetric (navigational) procedure, intracranial, extracranial, or spinal (List separately in addition to code for primary procedure)

NEUROSTIMULATORS (INTRACRANIAL)

61850 Twist drill or burr hole(s) for implantation of neurostimulator electrodes, cortical

61860 Craniectomy or craniotomy for implantation of neurostimulator electrodes, cerebral, cortical

(61862 deleted 2004 edition. To report, see 61867, 61868)

61863 Twist drill, burr hole, craniotomy, or craniectomy with stereotactic implantation of neurostimulator electrode array in subcortical site (eg, thalamus, globus pallidus, subthalamic nucleus, periventricular, periaqueductal gray), without use of intraoperative microelectrode recording; first array

+ **61864** each additional array (List separately in addition to primary procedure)

(Use 61864 in conjunction with 61863)

61867 Twist drill, burr hole, craniotomy, or craniectomy with stereotactic implantation of neurostimulator electrode array in subcortical site (eg, thalamus, globus pallidus, subthalamic nucleus, periventricular, periaqueductal gray), with use of intraoperative microelectrode recording; first array

+ **61868** each additional array (List separately in addition to primary procedure)

(Use 61868 in conjunction with 61867)

61870 Craniectomy for implantation of neurostimulator electrodes, cerebellar; cortical

61875 subcortical

61880 Revision or removal of intracranial neurostimulator electrodes

61885 Insertion or replacement of cranial neurostimulator pulse generator or receiver, direct or inductive coupling; with connection to a single electrode array

61886 with connection to two or more electrode arrays

(For open placement of cranial nerve (eg, vagal, trigeminal) neurostimulator electrode(s), use 64573)

(For percutaneous placement of cranial nerve (eg, vagal, trigeminal) neurostimulator electrode(s), use 64553)

(For revision or removal of cranial nerve (eg, vagal, trigeminal) neurostimulator electrode(s), use 64585)

61888 Revision or removal of cranial neurostimulator pulse generator or receiver

(Do not report 61888 in conjunction with 61885 or 61886 for the same pulse generator)

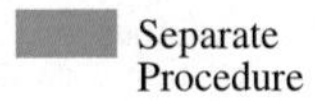

REPAIR

62000 Elevation of depressed skull fracture; simple, extradural

62005 compound or comminuted, extradural

62010 with repair of dura and/or debridement of brain

62100 Craniotomy for repair of dural/cerebrospinal fluid leak, including surgery for rhinorrhea/otorrhea

(For repair of spinal dural/CSF leak, see 63707, 63709)

62115 Reduction of craniomegalic skull (eg, treated hydrocephalus); not requiring bone grafts or cranioplasty

62116 with simple cranioplasty

62117 requiring craniotomy and reconstruction with or without bone graft (includes obtaining grafts)

62120 Repair of encephalocele, skull vault, including cranioplasty

62121 Craniotomy for repair of encephalocele, skull base

62140 Cranioplasty for skull defect; up to 5 cm diameter

62141 larger than 5 cm diameter

62142 Removal of bone flap or prosthetic plate of skull

62143 Replacement of bone flap or prosthetic plate of skull

62145 Cranioplasty for skull defect with reparative brain surgery

62146 Cranioplasty with autograft (includes obtaining bone grafts); up to 5 cm diameter

62147 larger than 5 cm diameter

\+ **62148** Incision and retrieval of subcutaneous cranial bone graft for cranioplasty (List separately in addition to code for primary procedure)

(Use 62148 in conjunction with codes 62140-62147)

● New Code ▲ Revised Code + Add-On Code ⊘ Modifier -51 Exempt ⊙ Conscious Sedation

NEUROENDOSCOPY

(Surgical endoscopy always includes diagnostic endoscopy)

+ **62160** Neuroendoscopy, intracranial, for placement or replacement of ventricular catheter and attachment to shunt system or external drainage (List separately in addition to code for primary procedure)

(Use 62160 only in conjunction with codes 61107, 61210, 62220-62230, 62258)

62161 Neuroendoscopy, intracranial; with dissection of adhesions, fenestration of septum pellucidum or intraventricular cysts (including placement, replacement, or removal of ventricular catheter)

62162 with fenestration or excision of colloid cyst, including placement of external ventricular catheter for drainage

62163 with retrieval of foreign body

62164 with excision of brain tumor, including placement of external ventricular catheter for drainage

62165 with excision of pituitary tumor, transnasal or transsphenoidal approach

CEREBROSPINAL FLUID (CSF) SHUNT

62180 Ventriculocisternostomy (Torkildsen type operation)

62190 Creation of shunt; subarachnoid/subdural-atrial, -jugular, -auricular

62192 subarachnoid/subdural-peritoneal, -pleural, other terminus

62194 Replacement or irrigation, subarachnoid/subdural catheter

62200 Ventriculocisternostomy, third ventricle;

62201 stereotactic, neuroendoscopic method

(For intracranial neuroendoscopic procedures, see 62161-62165)

62220 Creation of shunt; ventriculo-atrial, -jugular, -auricular

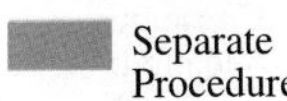 Separate Procedure 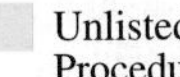 Unlisted Procedure 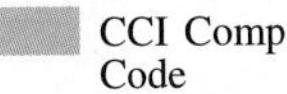 CCI Comp. Code Non-specific Procedure

(For intracranial neuroendoscopic ventricular catheter placement, use 62160)

62223 ventriculo-peritoneal, -pleural, other terminus

(For intracranial neuroendoscopic ventricular catheter placement, use 62160)

62225 Replacement or irrigation, ventricular catheter

(For intracranial neuroendoscopic ventricular catheter placement, use 62160)

62230 Replacement or revision of cerebrospinal fluid shunt, obstructed valve, or distal catheter in shunt system

(For intracranial neuroendoscopic ventricular catheter placement, use 62160)

62252 Reprogramming of programmable cerebrospinal shunt

62256 Removal of complete cerebrospinal fluid shunt system; without replacement

62258 with replacement by similar or other shunt at same operation

(For percutaneous irrigation or aspiration of shunt reservoir, use 61070)

(For reprogramming of programmable CSF shunt, use 62252)

(For intracranial neuroendoscopic ventricular catheter placement, use 62160)

SPINE AND SPINAL CORD

(For application of caliper or tongs, use 20660)

(For treatment of fracture or dislocation of spine, see 22305-22327)

INJECTION, DRAINAGE, OR ASPIRATION

(Report 01996 for daily hospital management of continuous epidural or subarachnoid drug administration performed in conjunction with 62318-62319)

(For endoscopic lysis of epidural adhesions, use Category III code 0027T)

62263 Percutaneous lysis of epidural adhesions using solution injection (eg, hypertonic saline, enzyme) or mechanical means (eg, catheter) including radiologic localization (includes contrast when administered), multiple adhesiolysis sessions; 2 or more days

(62263 includes codes 72275 and 77003)

62264 1 day

(Do not report 62264 with 62263)

(62264 includes codes 72275 and 77003)

62268 Percutaneous aspiration, spinal cord cyst or syrinx

(For radiological supervision and interpretation, see 76942, 77002, 77012)

62269 Biopsy of spinal cord, percutaneous needle

(For radiological supervision and interpretation, see 76942, 77002, 77012)

(For fine needle aspiration, see 10021, 10022)

(For evaluation of fine needle aspirate, see 88172, 88173)

62270 Spinal puncture, lumbar, diagnostic

62272 Spinal puncture, therapeutic, for drainage of cerebrospinal fluid (by needle or catheter)

62273 Injection, epidural, of blood or clot patch

(For injection of diagnostic or therapeutic substance(s), see 62310, 62311, 62318, 62319)

62280 Injection/infusion of neurolytic substance (eg, alcohol, phenol, iced saline solutions), with or without other therapeutic substance; subarachnoid

62281 epidural, cervical or thoracic

62282 epidural, lumbar, sacral (caudal)

⊘ **62284** Injection procedure for myelography and/or computed tomography, spinal (other than C1-C2 and posterior fossa)

(For injection procedure at C1-C2, use 61055)

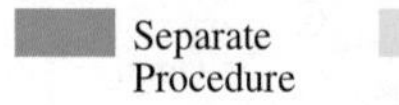

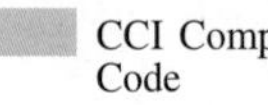

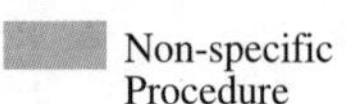

(For radiological supervision and interpretation, see Radiology)

62287 Aspiration or decompression procedure, percutaneous, of nucleus pulposus of intervertebral disk, any method, single or multiple levels, lumbar (eg, manual or automated percutaneous diskectomy, percutaneous laser diskectomy)

(For fluoroscopic guidance, use 77002)

(For injection of non-neurolytic diagnostic or therapeutic substance(s), see 62310, 62311)

62290 Injection procedure for diskography, each level; lumbar

62291 cervical or thoracic

(For radiological supervision or interpretation, see 72285, 72295)

62292 Injection procedure for chemonucleolysis, including diskography, intervertebral disk, single or multiple levels, lumbar

62294 Injection procedure, arterial, for occlusion of arteriovenous malformation, spinal

62310 Injection, single (not via indwelling catheter), not including neurolytic substances, with or without contrast (for either localization or epidurography), of diagnostic or therapeutic substance(s) (including anesthetic, antispasmodic, opioid, steroid, other solution), epidural or subarachnoid; cervical or thoracic

62311 lumbar, sacral (caudal)

62318 Injection, including catheter placement, continuous infusion with intermittent bolus not including neurolytic substances, with or without contrast (for either localization or epidurography), of diagnostic or therapeutic substance(s) (including anesthetic, antispasmodic, opioid, steroid, other solution), epidural or subarachnoid; cervical or thoracic

62319 lumbar, sacral (caudal)

(For transforaminal epidural injection, see 64479-64484)

(Report 01996 for daily hospital management of continuous epidural or subarachnoid drug administration performed in conjunction with codes 62318-62319)

CATHETER IMPLANTATION

(For percutaneous placement of intrathecal or epidural catheter, see codes 62270-62273, 62280-62284, 62310-62319)

62350 Implantation, revision or repositioning of tunneled intrathecal or epidural catheter, for long-term medication administration via an external pump or implantable reservoir/infusion pump; without laminectomy

62351 with laminectomy

(For refilling and maintenance of an implantable infusion pump for spinal or brain drug therapy, use 95990)

62355 Removal of previously implanted intrathecal or epidural catheter

RESERVOIR/PUMP IMPLANTATION

62360 Implantation or replacement of device for intrathecal or epidural drug infusion; subcutaneous reservoir

62361 non-programmable pump

62362 programmable pump, including preparation of pump, with or without programming

62365 Removal of subcutaneous reservoir or pump, previously implanted for intrathecal or epidural infusion

62367 Electronic analysis of programmable, implanted pump for intrathecal or epidural drug infusion (includes evaluation of reservoir status, alarm status, drug prescription status); without reprogramming

62368 with reprogramming

(For refilling and maintenance of an implantable infusion pump for spinal or brain drug therapy, use 95990)

POSTERIOR EXTRADURAL LAMINOTOMY OR LAMINECTOMY FOR EXPLORATION/DECOMPRESSION OF NEURAL ELEMENTS OR EXCISION OF HERNIATED INTERVERTEBRAL DISKS

(When 63001-63048 are followed by arthrodesis, see 22590-22614)

63001 Laminectomy with exploration and/or decompression of spinal cord and/or cauda equina, without facetectomy, foraminotomy or diskectomy, (eg, spinal stenosis), one or two vertebral segments; cervical

63003 thoracic

63005 lumbar, except for spondylolisthesis

63011 sacral

63012 Laminectomy with removal of abnormal facets and/or pars inter-articularis with decompression of cauda equina and nerve roots for spondylolisthesis, lumbar (Gill type procedure)

63015 Laminectomy with exploration and/or decompression of spinal cord and/or cauda equina, without facetectomy, foraminotomy or diskectomy, (eg, spinal stenosis), more than 2 vertebral segments; cervical

63016 thoracic

63017 lumbar

63020 Laminotomy (hemilaminectomy), with decompression of nerve root(s), including partial facetectomy, foraminotomy and/or excision of herniated intervertebral disk; one interspace, cervical

(For bilateral procedure, report 63020 with modifier -50)

63030 one interspace, lumbar (including open or endoscopically assisted approach)

(For bilateral procedure, report 63030 with modifier -50)

+ **63035** each additional interspace, cervical or lumbar (List separately in addition to code for primary procedure)

(Use 63035 in conjunction with codes 63020-63030)

(For bilateral procedures, report 63035 with modifier -50)

63040 Laminotomy (hemilaminectomy), with decompression of nerve root(s), including partial facetectomy, foraminotomy and/or excision of herniated intervertebral disk, reexploration, single interspace; cervical

(For bilateral procedure, report 63040 with modifier -50)

63042 lumbar

(For bilateral procedure, report 63042 with modifier -50)

+ **63043** each additional cervical interspace (List separately in addition to code for primary procedure)

(Use 63043 in conjunction with code 63040)

(For bilateral procedure, report 63043 with modifier -50)

+ **63044** each additional lumbar interspace (List separately in addition to code for primary procedure)

(Use 63044 in conjunction with code 63042)

(For bilateral procedure, report 63044 with modifier -50)

63045 Laminectomy, facetectomy and foraminotomy (unilateral or bilateral with decompression of spinal cord, cauda equina and/or nerve root(s), (eg, spinal or lateral recess stenosis)), single vertebral segment; cervical

63046 thoracic

63047 lumbar

+ **63048** each additional segment, cervical, thoracic, or lumbar (List separately in addition to code for primary procedure)

(Use 63048 in conjunction with codes 63045-63047)

63050 Laminoplasty, cervical, with decompression of the spinal cord, two or more vertebral segments;

63051 with reconstruction of the posterior bony elements (including the application of bridging bone graft and non-segmental fixation devices (eg, wire, suture, mini-plates), when performed)

(Do not report 63050 or 63051 in conjunction with 22600, 22614, 22840-22842, 63001, 63015, 63045, 63048, 63295 for the same vertebral segment(s))

TRANSPEDICULAR OR COSTOVERTEBRAL APPROACH FOR POSTEROLATERAL EXTRADURAL EXPLORATION/ DECOMPRESSION

63055 Transpedicular approach with decompression of spinal cord, equina and/or nerve root(s) (eg, herniated intervertebral disk), single segment; thoracic

63056 lumbar (including transfacet, or lateral extraforaminal approach) (eg, far lateral herniated intervertebral disk)

+ **63057** each additional segment, thoracic or lumbar (List separately in addition to code for primary procedure)

(Use 63057 in conjunction with codes 63055, 63056)

63064 Costovertebral approach with decompression of spinal cord or nerve root(s), (eg, herniated intervertebral disk), thoracic; single segment

+ **63066** each additional segment (List separately in addition to code for primary procedure)

(Use 63066 in conjunction with code 63064)

(For excision of thoracic intraspinal lesions by laminectomy, see 63266, 63271, 63276, 63281, 63286)

ANTERIOR OR ANTEROLATERAL APPROACH FOR EXTRADURAL EXPLORATION/DECOMPRESSION

63075 Diskectomy, anterior, with decompression of spinal cord and/or nerve root(s), including osteophytectomy; cervical, single interspace

+ **63076** cervical, each additional interspace (List separately in addition to code for primary procedure)

(Use 63076 in conjunction with code 63075)

63077 thoracic, single interspace

+ **63078** thoracic, each additional interspace (List separately in addition to code for primary procedure)

(Use 63078 in conjunction with code 63077)

(Do not report code 69990 in addition to codes 63075-63078)

● New Code ▲ Revised Code + Add-On Code ⊘ Modifier -51 Exempt ⊙ Conscious Sedation

63081 Vertebral corpectomy (vertebral body resection), partial or complete, anterior approach with decompression of spinal cord and/or nerve root(s); cervical, single segment

+ **63082** cervical, each additional segment (List separately in addition to code for primary procedure)

(Use 63082 in conjunction with code 63081)

(For transoral approach, see 61575, 61576)

63085 Vertebral corpectomy (vertebral body resection), partial or complete, transthoracic approach with decompression of spinal cord and/or nerve root(s); thoracic, single segment

+ **63086** thoracic, each additional segment (List separately in addition to code for primary procedure)

(Use 63086 in conjunction with code 63085)

63087 Vertebral corpectomy (vertebral body resection), partial or complete, combined thoracolumbar approach with decompression of spinal cord, cauda equina or nerve root(s), lower thoracic or lumbar; single segment

+ **63088** each additional segment (List separately in addition to code for primary procedure)

(Use 63088 in conjunction with code 63087)

63090 Vertebral corpectomy (vertebral body resection), partial or complete, transperitoneal or retroperitoneal approach with decompression of spinal cord, cauda equina or nerve root(s), lower thoracic, lumbar, or sacral; single segment

+ **63091** each additional segment (List separately in addition to code for primary procedure)

(Use 63091 in conjunction with code 63090)

(Procedures 63081-63091 include diskectomy above and/or below vertebral segment)

(If followed by arthrodesis, see 22548-22812)

(For reconstruction of spine, use appropriate vertebral corpectomy codes 63081-63091, bone graft codes 20930-20938, arthrodesis codes 22548-22812, and spinal instrumentation codes 22840-22855)

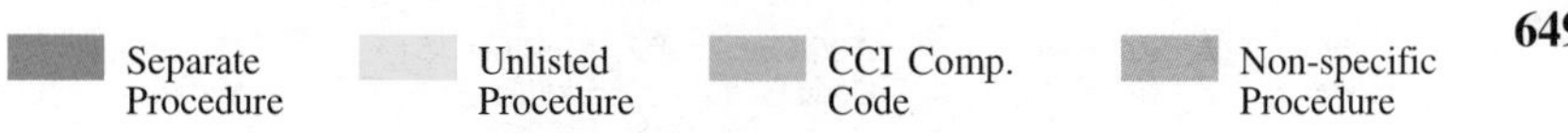

LATERAL EXTRACAVITARY APPROACH FOR EXTRADURAL EXPLORATION/DECOMPRESSION

63101 Vertebral corpectomy (vertebral body resection), partial or complete, lateral extracavitary approach with decompression of spinal cord and/or nerve root(s) (eg, for tumor or retropulsed bone fragments); thoracic, single segment

63102 lumbar, single segment

+ **63103** thoracic or lumbar, each additional segment (List separately in addition to code for primary procedure)

(Use 63103 in conjunction with 63101 and 63102)

INCISION

63170 Laminectomy with myelotomy (eg, Bischof or DREZ type), cervical, thoracic, or thoracolumbar

63172 Laminectomy with drainage of intramedullary cyst/syrinx; to subarachnoid space

63173 to peritoneal or pleural space

63180 Laminectomy and section of dentate ligaments, with or without dural graft, cervical; one or two segments

63182 more than two segments

63185 Laminectomy with rhizotomy; one or two segments

63190 more than two segments

63191 Laminectomy with section of spinal accessory nerve

(For bilateral procedure, report 63191 with modifier -50)

(For resection of sternocleidomastoid muscle, use 21720)

63194 Laminectomy with cordotomy, with section of one spinothalamic tract, one stage; cervical

63195 thoracic

63196 Laminectomy with cordotomy, with section of both spinothalamic tracts, one stage; cervical

63197 thoracic

63198 Laminectomy with cordotomy with section of both spinothalamic tracts, two stages within 14 days; cervical

63199 thoracic

63200 Laminectomy, with release of tethered spinal cord, lumbar

EXCISION BY LAMINECTOMY OF LESION OTHER THAN HERNIATED DISK

63250 Laminectomy for excision or occlusion of arteriovenous malformation of spinal cord; cervical

63251 thoracic

63252 thoracolumbar

63265 Laminectomy for excision or evacuation of intraspinal lesion other than neoplasm, extradural; cervical

63266 thoracic

63267 lumbar

63268 sacral

63270 Laminectomy for excision of intraspinal lesion other than neoplasm, intradural; cervical

63271 thoracic

63272 lumbar

63273 sacral

63275 Laminectomy for biopsy/excision of intraspinal neoplasm; extradural, cervical

63276 extradural, thoracic

63277 extradural, lumbar

63278 extradural, sacral

63280 intradural, extramedullary, cervical

63281 intradural, extramedullary, thoracic

63282 intradural, extramedullary, lumbar

63283 intradural, sacral

63285 intradural, intramedullary, cervical

63286 intradural, intramedullary, thoracic

63287 intradural, intramedullary, thoracolumbar

63290 combined extradural-intradural lesion, any level

(For drainage of intramedullary cyst/syrinx, use 63172, 63173)

+ **63295** Osteoplastic reconstruction of dorsal spinal elements, following primary intraspinal procedure (List separately in addition to code for primary procedure)

(Use 63295 in conjunction with 63172, 63173, 63185, 63190, 63200-63290)

(Do not report 63295 in conjunction with 22590-22614, 22840-22844, 63050, 63051 for the same vertebral segment(s))

EXCISION, ANTERIOR OR ANTEROLATERAL APPROACH, INTRASPINAL LESION

(For arthrodesis, see 22548-22585)

(For reconstruction of spine, see 20930-20938)

63300 Vertebral corpectomy (vertebral body resection), partial or complete, for excision of intraspinal lesion, single segment; extradural, cervical

63301 extradural, thoracic by transthoracic approach

63302 extradural, thoracic by thoracolumbar approach

63303 extradural, lumbar or sacral by transperitoneal or retroperitoneal approach

63304 intradural, cervical

63305 intradural, thoracic by transthoracic approach

63306 intradural, thoracic by thoracolumbar approach

63307 intradural, lumbar or sacral by transperitoneal or retroperitoneal approach

+ **63308** each additional segment (List separately in addition to codes for single segment)

(Use 63308 in conjunction with codes 63300-63307)

STEREOTAXIS

63600 Creation of lesion of spinal cord by stereotactic method, percutaneous, any modality (including stimulation and/or recording)

63610 Stereotactic stimulation of spinal cord, percutaneous, separate procedure not followed by other surgery

63615 Stereotactic biopsy, aspiration, or excision of lesion, spinal cord

NEUROSTIMULATORS (SPINAL)

63650 Percutaneous implantation of neurostimulator electrode array, epidural

63655 Laminectomy for implantation of neurostimulator electrodes, plate/paddle, epidural

63660 Revision or removal of spinal neurostimulator electrode percutaneous array(s) or plate/paddle(s)

63685 Insertion or replacement of spinal neurostimulator pulse generator or receiver, direct or inductive coupling

(Do not report 63685 in conjunction with 63688 for the same pulse generator or receiver)

63688 Revision or removal of implanted spinal neurostimulator pulse generator or receiver

(For electronic analysis of implanted neurostimulator pulse generator system, see 95970-95975)

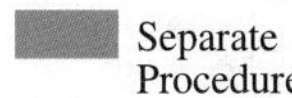
Separate Procedure

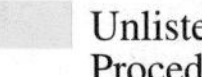
Unlisted Procedure

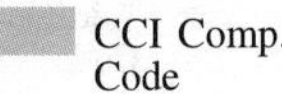
CCI Comp. Code

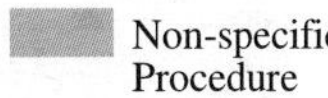
Non-specific Procedure

REPAIR

63700 Repair of meningocele; less than 5 cm diameter

63702 larger than 5 cm diameter

(Do not use modifier -63 in conjunction with 63700, 63702)

63704 Repair of myelomeningocele; less than 5 cm diameter

63706 larger than 5 cm diameter

(Do not use modifier -63 in conjunction with 63704, 63706)

(For complex skin closure, see Integumentary System)

63707 Repair of dural/cerebrospinal fluid leak, not requiring laminectomy

63709 Repair of dural/cerebrospinal fluid leak or pseudomeningocele, with laminectomy

63710 Dural graft, spinal

(For laminectomy and section of dentate ligaments, with or without dural graft, cervical, see 63180, 63182)

SHUNT, SPINAL CSF

63740 Creation of shunt, lumbar, subarachnoid-peritoneal, -pleural, or other; including laminectomy

63741 percutaneous, not requiring laminectomy

63744 Replacement, irrigation or revision of lumbosubarachnoid shunt

63746 Removal of entire lumbosubarachnoid shunt system without replacement

(For insertion of subarachnoid catheter with reservoir and/or pump for intermittent or continuous infusion of drug including laminectomy, see 62351 and 62360, 62361 or 62362)

(For insertion or replacement of subarachnoid or epidural catheter, with reservoir and/or pump for drug infusion without laminectomy, see 62350 and 62360, 62361 or 62362)

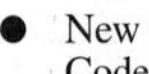

● New Code ▲ Revised Code + Add-On Code ⦸ Modifier -51 Exempt ⊙ Conscious Sedation

EXTRACRANIAL NERVES, PERIPHERAL NERVES, AND AUTONOMIC NERVOUS SYSTEM

(For intracranial surgery on cranial nerves, see 61450, 61460, 61790)

INTRODUCTION/INJECTION OF ANESTHETIC AGENT (NERVE BLOCK), DIAGNOSTIC OR THERAPEUTIC

Somatic Nerves

64400 Injection, anesthetic agent; trigeminal nerve, any division or branch

64402 facial nerve

64405 greater occipital nerve

64408 vagus nerve

64410 phrenic nerve

64412 spinal accessory nerve

64413 cervical plexus

64415 brachial plexus, single

64416 brachial plexus, continuous infusion by catheter (including catheter placement) including daily management for anesthetic agent administration

(Do not report 01996 in addition to 64416)

64417 axillary nerve

64418 suprascapular nerve

64420 intercostal nerve, single

64421 intercostal nerves, multiple, regional block

64425 ilioinguinal, iliohypogastric nerves

64430 pudendal nerve

64435 paracervical (uterine) nerve

64445 sciatic nerve, single

64446 sciatic nerve, continuous infusion by catheter, (including catheter placement) including daily management for anesthetic agent administration

(Do not report 64446 in conjuction with 01996)

64447 femoral nerve, single

(Do not report 64447 in conjunction with 01996)

64448 femoral nerve, continuous infusion by catheter (including catheter placement) including daily management for anesthetic agent administration

(Do not report 64448 in conjunction with 01996)

64449 lumbar plexus, posterior approach, continuous infusion by catheter (including catheter placement) including daily managemnt for anesthetic agent administration

(Do not report 64449 in conjunction with 01996)

64450 other peripheral nerve or branch

(For phenol destruction, see 64622-64627)

(For subarachnoid or subdural injection, see 62280, 62310-62319)

(For epidural or caudal injection, see 62273, 62281-62282, 62310-62319)

(Codes 64470-64484 are unilateral procedures. For bilateral procedures, use modifier -50)

(For fluoroscopic guidance and localization for needle placement and injection in conjunction with codes 64470-64484, use code 77003)

64470 Injection, anesthetic agent and/or steroid, paravertebral facet joint or facet joint nerve; cervical or thoracic, single level

+ **64472** cervical or thoracic, each additional level (List separately in addition to code for primary procedure)

(Use code 64472 in conjunction with code 64470)

64475 lumbar or sacral, single level

● New Code ▲ Revised Code + Add-On Code ⃠ Modifier -51 Exempt ⊙ Conscious Sedation

+ **64476** lumbar or sacral, each additional level (List separately in addition to code for primary procedure)

(Use code 64476 in conjunction with code 64475)

64479 Injection, anesthetic agent and/or steroid, transforaminal epidural; cervical or thoracic, single level

+ **64480** cervical or thoracic, each additional level (List separately in addition to code for primary procedure)

(Use code 64480 in conjunction with code 64479)

64483 lumbar or sacral, single level

+ **64484** lumbar or sacral, each additional level (List separately in addition to code for primary procedure)

(Use code 64484 in conjunction with code 64483)

Sympathetic Nerves

64505 Injection, anesthetic agent; sphenopalatine ganglion

64508 carotid sinus (separate procedure)

64510 stellate ganglion (cervical sympathetic)

64517 superior hypogastric plexus

64520 lumbar or thoracic (paravertebral sympathetic)

64530 celiac plexus, with or without radiologic monitoring

NEUROSTIMULATORS (PERIPHERAL NERVE)

64550 Application of surface (transcutaneous) neurostimulator

64553 Percutaneous implantation of neurostimulator electrodes; cranial nerve

(For open placement of cranial nerve (eg, vagal, trigeminal) neurostimulator pulse generator or receiver, see 61885, 61886, as appropriate)

64555 peripheral nerve (excludes sacral nerve)

64560 autonomic nerve

64561 sacral nerve (transforaminal placement)

64565 neuromuscular

64573 Incision for implantation of neurostimulator electrodes; cranial nerve

(For open placement of cranial nerve (eg, vagal, trigeminal) neurostimulator pulse generator or receiver, see 61885, 61886, as appropriate)

(For revision or removal of cranial nerve (eg, vagal, trigeminal) neurostimulator pulse generator or receiver, use 61888)

64575 peripheral nerve (excludes sacral nerve)

64577 autonomic nerve

64580 neuromuscular

64581 sacral nerve (transforaminal placement)

64585 Revision or removal of peripheral neurostimulator electrodes

▲ **64590** Insertion or replacement of peripheral or gastric neurostimulator pulse generator or receiver, direct or inductive coupling

(Do not report 64590 in conjunction with 64595)

▲ **64595** Revision or removal of peripheral or gastric neurostimulator pulse generator or receiver

DESTRUCTION BY NEUROLYTIC AGENT (eg, CHEMICAL, THERMAL, ELECTRICAL, OR RADIOFREQUENCY)

Somatic Nerves

64600 Destruction by neurolytic agent, trigeminal nerve; supraorbital, infraorbital, mental, or inferior alveolar branch

64605 second and third division branches at foramen ovale

64610 second and third division branches at foramen ovale under radiologic monitoring

64612 Chemodenervation of muscle(s); muscle(s) innervated by facial nerve (eg, for blepharospasm, hemifacial spasm)

64613 neck muscle(s) (eg, for spasmodic torticollis, spasmodic dysphonia)

64614 extremity(s) and/or trunk muscle(s) (eg, for dystonia, cerebral palsy, multiple sclerosis)

(For chemodenervation guided by needle electromyography or muscle electrical stimulation, see 95873, 95874)

(For chemodenervation for strabismus involving the extraocular muscles, use 67345)

(For chemodenervation of internal anal sphincter, use 46505)

64620 Destruction by neurolytic agent, intercostal nerve

(For fluoroscopic guidance and localization for needle placement and neurolysis in conjunction with codes 64622-64627, use 77003)

64622 Destruction by neurolytic agent, paravertebral facet joint nerve; lumbar or sacral, single level

(For bilateral procedure, report 64622 with modifier -50)

+ **64623** lumbar or sacral, each additional level (List separately in addition to code for primary procedure)

(Use 64623 in conjunction with code 64622)

(For bilateral procedure, report 64623 with modifier -50)

64626 cervical or thoracic, single level

(For bilateral procedure, report 64626 with modifier -50)

+ **64627** cervical or thoracic, each additional level (List separately in addition to code for primary procedure)

(Use 64627 in conjunction with code 64626)

(For bilateral procedure, report 64627 with modifier -50)

64630 Destruction by neurolytic agent; pudendal nerve

64640 other peripheral nerve or branch

Sympathetic Nerves

64650 Chemodenervation of eccrine glands; both axillae

64653 other area(s) (eg, scalp, face, neck), per day

(Report the specific service in conjunction with code(s) for the specific substance(s) or drug(s) provided)

(For chemodenervation of extremities (eg, hands or feet), use 64999)

64680 Destruction by neurolytic agent, with or without radiologic monitoring; celiac plexus

64681 superior hypogastric plexus

NEUROPLASTY (EXPLORATION, NEUROLYSIS OR NERVE DECOMPRESSION)

(For internal neurolysis requiring use of operating microscope, use 64727)

(For facial nerve decompression, use 69720)

64702 Neuroplasty; digital, one or both, same digit

64704 nerve of hand or foot

64708 Neuroplasty, major peripheral nerve, arm or leg; other than specified

64712 sciatic nerve

64713 brachial plexus

64714 lumbar plexus

64716 Neuroplasty and/or transposition; cranial nerve (specify)

64718 ulnar nerve at elbow

64719 ulnar nerve at wrist

64721 median nerve at carpal tunnel

(For arthroscopic procedure, use 29848)

64722 Decompression; unspecified nerve(s) (specify)

64726 plantar digital nerve

● New Code ▲ Revised Code + Add-On Code ⊘ Modifier -51 Exempt ⊙ Conscious Sedation

+ **64727** Internal neurolysis, requiring use of operating microscope (List separately in addition to code for neuroplasty) (Neuroplasty includes external neurolysis)

(Do not report code 69990 in addition to code 64727)

TRANSECTION OR AVULSION

(For stereotactic lesion of gasserian ganglion, use 61790)

64732 Transection or avulsion of; supraorbital nerve

64734 infraorbital nerve

64736 mental nerve

64738 inferior alveolar nerve by osteotomy

64740 lingual nerve

64742 facial nerve, differential or complete

64744 greater occipital nerve

64746 phrenic nerve

(For section of recurrent laryngeal nerve, use 31595)

64752 vagus nerve (vagotomy), transthoracic

64755 vagus nerves limited to proximal stomach (selective proximal vagotomy, proximal gastric vagotomy, parietal cell vagotomy, supra- or highly selective vagotomy)

(For laparoscopic approach, use 43652)

64760 vagus nerve (vagotomy), abdominal

(For laparoscopic approach, use 43651)

64761 pudendal nerve

(For bilateral procedure, report 64761 with modifier -50)

64763 Transection or avulsion of obturator nerve, extrapelvic, with or without adductor tenotomy

(For bilateral procedure, report 64763 with modifier -50)

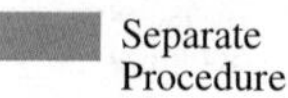
Separate Procedure

Unlisted Procedure

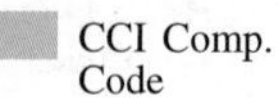
CCI Comp. Code

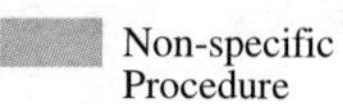
Non-specific Procedure

64766 Transection or avulsion of obturator nerve, intrapelvic, with or without adductor tenotomy

(For bilateral procedure, report 64766 with modifier -50)

64771 Transection or avulsion of other cranial nerve, extradural

64772 Transection or avulsion of other spinal nerve, extradural

(For excision of tender scar, skin and subcutaneous tissue, with or without tiny neuroma, see 11400-11446, 13100-13153)

EXCISION

Somatic Nerves

(For Morton neurectomy, use 28080)

64774 Excision of neuroma; cutaneous nerve, surgically identifiable

64776 digital nerve, one or both, same digit

+ **64778** digital nerve, each additional digit (List separately in addition to code for primary procedure)

(Use 64778 in conjunction with code 64776)

64782 hand or foot, except digital nerve

+ **64783** hand or foot, each additional nerve, except same digit (List separately in addition to code for primary procedure)

(Use 64783 in conjunction with code 64782)

64784 major peripheral nerve, except sciatic

64786 sciatic nerve

+ **64787** Implantation of nerve end into bone or muscle (List separately in addition to neuroma excision)

(Use 64787 in conjunction with codes 64774-64786)

64788 Excision of neurofibroma or neurolemmoma; cutaneous nerve

64790 major peripheral nerve

64792 extensive (including malignant type)

64795 Biopsy of nerve

Sympathetic Nerves

64802 Sympathectomy, cervical

(For bilateral procedure, report 64802 with modifier -50)

64804 Sympathectomy, cervicothoracic

(For bilateral procedure, report 64804 with modifier -50)

64809 Sympathectomy, thoracolumbar

(For bilateral procedure, report 64809 with modifier -50)

64818 Sympathectomy, lumbar

(For bilateral procedure, report 64818 with modifier -50)

64820 Sympathectomy; digital arteries, each digit

(Do not report 69990 in addition to code 64820)

64821 radial artery

(Do not report 69990 in addition to code 64821)

64822 ulnar artery

(Do not report 69990 in addition to code 64822)

64823 superficial palmar arch

(Do not report 69990 in addition to code 64823)

NEURORRHAPHY

64831 Suture of digital nerve, hand or foot; one nerve

+ **64832** each additional digital nerve (List separately in addition to code for primary procedure)

(Use 64832 in conjunction with code 64831)

64834 Suture of one nerve, hand or foot; common sensory nerve

64835 median motor thenar

64836 ulnar motor

+ **64837** Suture of each additional nerve, hand or foot (List separately in addition to code for primary procedure)

(Use 64837 in conjunction with codes 64834-64836)

64840 Suture of posterior tibial nerve

64856 Suture of major peripheral nerve, arm or leg, except sciatic; including transposition

64857 without transposition

64858 Suture of sciatic nerve

+ **64859** Suture of each additional major peripheral nerve (List separately in addition to code for primary procedure)

(Use 64859 in conjunction with codes 64856, 64857)

64861 Suture of; brachial plexus

64862 lumbar plexus

64864 Suture of facial nerve; extracranial

64865 infratemporal, with or without grafting

64866 Anastomosis; facial-spinal accessory

64868 facial-hypoglossal

64870 facial-phrenic

+ **64872** Suture of nerve; requiring secondary or delayed suture (List separately in addition to code for primary neurorrhaphy)

(Use 64872 in conjunction with codes 64831-64865)

+ **64874** requiring extensive mobilization, or transposition of nerve (List separately in addition to code for nerve suture)

(Use 64874 in conjunction with codes 64831-64865)

+ **64876** requiring shortening of bone of extremity (List separately in addition to code for nerve suture)

(Use 64876 in conjunction with codes 64831-64865)

NEURORRHAPHY WITH NERVE GRAFT, VEIN GRAFT, OR CONDUIT

64885 Nerve graft (includes obtaining graft), head or neck; up to 4 cm in length

64886 more than 4 cm length

64890 Nerve graft (includes obtaining graft), single strand, hand or foot; up to 4 cm length

64891 more than 4 cm length

64892 Nerve graft (includes obtaining graft), single strand, arm or leg; up to 4 cm length

64893 more than 4 cm length

64895 Nerve graft (includes obtaining graft), multiple strands (cable), hand or foot; up to 4 cm length

64896 more than 4 cm length

64897 Nerve graft (includes obtaining graft), multiple strands (cable), arm or leg; up to 4 cm length

64898 more than 4 cm length

+ **64901** Nerve graft, each additional nerve; single strand (List separately in addition to code for primary procedure)

(Use 64901 in conjunction with codes 64885-64893)

+ **64902** multiple strands (cable) (List separately in addition to code for primary procedure)

(Use 64902 in conjunction with codes 64885, 64886, 64895-64898)

64905 Nerve pedicle transfer; first stage

64907 second stage

● **64910** Nerve repair; with synthetic conduit or vein allograft (eg, nerve tube), each nerve

Separate Procedure | Unlisted Procedure | CCI Comp. Code | Non-specific Procedure

● **64911** Nerve repair; with autogenous vein graft (includes harvest of vein graft), each nerve

(Do not report 69990 in addition to 64910, 64911)

OTHER PROCEDURES

64999 Unlisted procedure, nervous system

EYE AND OCULAR ADNEXA

CPT codes from this section of the CPT coding system are used to report surgical procedures on the eye and ocular adnexa. Diagnostic services and medical treatment of the eye are defined in the Medicine Section of the CPT manual.

If surgical procedures are performed only on the eyelid, code from the Integumentary System subsection of the CPT coding system. Cataract codes are selected on the type of procedure performed. Whenever injections are performed during cataract surgery, do not report them separately.

When a subconjunctival injection (e.g. CPT code 68200) with a local anesthetic is performed as part of a more extensive anesthetic procedure (e.g. peribulbar or retrobulbar block), a separate service for this procedure is not to be reported. This is a routine part of the anesthetic procedure and does not represent a separate service.

Iridectomy, trabeculectomy, and anterior vitrectomy may be performed in conjunction with cataract removal. When an iridectomy is performed in order to accomplish the cataract extraction, it is an integral part of the procedure; it does not represent a separate service, and is not separately reported. Similarly, the minimal vitreous loss occurring during routine cataract extraction does not represent a vitrectomy and is not to be separately reported unless it is medically necessary for a different diagnosis.

While a trabeculectomy is not performed as a part of a cataract extraction, it may be performed to control glaucoma at the same time as a cataract extraction. If the procedure is medically necessary at the same time as a cataract extraction, it can be reported under a different diagnosis (e.g. glaucoma). The codes describing iridectomies, trabeculectomies, and anterior vitrectomies, when performed with a cataract extraction under a separate diagnosis, must be reported with modifier -59. This indicates that the procedure was performed as a different service for a separate situation. The medical record should reflect the medical necessity of the service if separately reported.

For example, if a patient presents with a cataract and has evidence of glaucoma, (i.e. elevated intraocular pressure preoperatively) and a trabeculectomy represents the appropriate treatment for the glaucoma, a separate service for the trabeculectomy would be separately reported. Performance of a trabeculectomy as a preventative service for an expected transient increase in intraocular pressure postoperatively, without other evidence for glaucoma, is not to be separately reported.

The various approaches to removing a cataract are mutually exclusive of one another when performed on the same eye.

Some retinal detachment repair procedures include some vitreous procedures (e.g. CPT code 67108 includes 67015, 67025, 67028, 67031, 67036, 67039, and 67040). Certain retinal detachment repairs are mutually exclusive to anterior procedures such as focal endolaser photocoagulation (e.g. CPT codes 67110 and 67112 are mutually exclusive to CPT code 67108).

CPT codes 68020-68200 (incision, drainage, excision of the conjunctiva) are included in all conjunctivoplasties (CPT codes 68320-68362).

CPT code 67950 (canthoplasty) is included in repair procedures such as blepharoplasties (CPT codes 67917, 67924, 67961, 67966).

Correction of lid retraction (CPT code 67911) includes full thickness graft (e.g. CPT code 15260) as part of the total service performed.

In the circumstance that it is medically necessary and reasonable to inject sclerosing agents in the same session as surgery to correct glaucoma, the service is included in the glaucoma surgery. Accordingly, codes such as CPT codes 67500, 67515, and 68200 for injection of sclerosing agents (e.g. 5-FU, HCPCS/CPT code J9190) should not be reported with other pressure- reducing or glaucoma procedures.

(For diagnostic and treatment ophthalmological services, see Medicine, Ophthalmology, and 92002 et seq)

(Do not report code 69990 in addition to codes 65091-68850)

EYEBALL

REMOVAL OF EYE

65091 Evisceration of ocular contents; without implant

65093 with implant

65101 Enucleation of eye; without implant

65103 with implant, muscles not attached to implant

65105 with implant, muscles attached to implant

(For conjunctivoplasty after enucleation, see 68320 et seq)

65110 Exenteration of orbit (does not include skin graft), removal of orbital contents; only

65112 with therapeutic removal of bone

● New Code ▲ Revised Code + Add-On Code ⃠ Modifier -51 Exempt ⊙ Conscious Sedation

65114 with muscle or myocutaneous flap

(For skin graft to orbit (split skin), see 15120, 15121; free, full thickness, see 15260, 15261)

(For eyelid repair involving more than skin, see 67930 et seq)

SECONDARY IMPLANT(S) PROCEDURES

65125 Modification of ocular implant with placement or replacement of pegs (eg, drilling receptacle for prosthesis appendage) (separate procedure)

65130 Insertion of ocular implant secondary; after evisceration, in scleral shell

65135 after enucleation, muscles not attached to implant

65140 after enucleation, muscles attached to implant

65150 Reinsertion of ocular implant; with or without conjunctival graft

65155 with use of foreign material for reinforcement and/or attachment of muscles to implant

65175 Removal of ocular implant

(For orbital implant (implant outside muscle cone) insertion, use 67550; removal, use 67560)

REMOVAL OF FOREIGN BODY

(For removal of implanted material: ocular implant, use 65175; anterior segment implant, use 65920; posterior segment implant, use 67120; orbital implant, use 67560)

(For diagnostic x-ray for foreign body, use 70030)

(For diagnostic echography for foreign body, use 76529)

(For removal of foreign body from orbit: frontal approach, use 67413; lateral approach, use 67430; transcranial approach, use 61334)

(For removal of foreign body from eyelid, embedded, use 67938)

(For removal of foreign body from lacrimal system, use 68530)

65205 Removal of foreign body, external eye; conjunctival superficial

Separate Procedure | Unlisted Procedure | CCI Comp. Code | Non-specific Procedure

65210 conjunctival embedded (includes concretions), subconjunctival, or scleral nonperforating

65220 corneal, without slit lamp

65222 corneal, with slit lamp

(For repair of corneal laceration with foreign body, use 65275)

65235 Removal of foreign body, intraocular; from anterior chamber of eye or lens

(For removal of implanted material from anterior segment, use 65920)

65260 from posterior segment, magnetic extraction, anterior or posterior route

65265 from posterior segment, nonmagnetic extraction

(For removal of implanted material from posterior segment, use 67120)

REPAIR OF LACERATION

(For fracture of orbit, see 21385 et seq)

(For repair of wound of eyelid, skin, linear, simple, see 12011-12018; intermediate, layered closure, see 12051-12057; linear, complex, see 13150-13160; other, see 67930, 67935)

(For repair of wound of lacrimal system, use 68700)

(For repair of operative wound, use 66250)

65270 Repair of laceration; conjunctiva, with or without nonperforating laceration sclera, direct closure

65272 conjunctiva, by mobilization and rearrangement, without hospitalization

65273 conjunctiva, by mobilization and rearrangement, with hospitalization

65275 cornea, nonperforating, with or without removal foreign body

65280 cornea and/or sclera, perforating, not involving uveal tissue

65285 cornea and/or sclera, perforating, with reposition or resection of uveal tissue

65286 application of tissue glue, wounds of cornea and/or sclera

(Repair of laceration includes use of conjunctival flap and restoration of anterior chamber, by air or saline injection when indicated)

(For repair of iris or ciliary body, use 66680)

65290 Repair of wound, extraocular muscle, tendon and/or Tenon's capsule

ANTERIOR SEGMENT

CORNEA

Excision

65400 Excision of lesion, cornea (keratectomy, lamellar, partial), except pterygium

65410 Biopsy of cornea

65420 Excision or transposition of pterygium; without graft

65426 with graft

Removal or Destruction

65430 Scraping of cornea, diagnostic, for smear and/or culture

65435 Removal of corneal epithelium; with or without chemocauterization (abrasion, curettage)

65436 with application of chelating agent (eg, EDTA)

65450 Destruction of lesion of cornea by cryotherapy, photocoagulation or thermocauterization

65600 Multiple punctures of anterior cornea (eg, for corneal erosion, tattoo)

Keratoplasty

(Keratoplasty excludes refractive keratoplasty procedures, 65760, 65765, and 65767)

65710 Keratoplasty (corneal transplant); lamellar

65730 penetrating (except in aphakia)

65750 penetrating (in aphakia)

65755 penetrating (in pseudophakia)

Other Procedures

65760 Keratomileusis

65765 Keratophakia

65767 Epikeratoplasty

65770 Keratoprosthesis

65771 Radial keratotomy

65772 Corneal relaxing incision for correction of surgically induced astigmatism

65775 Corneal wedge resection for correction of surgically induced astigmatism

(For fitting of contact lens for treatment of disease, use 92070)

(For unlisted procedures on cornea, use 66999)

65780 Ocular surface reconstruction; amniotic membrane transplantation

65781 limbal stem cell allograft (eg, cadaveric or living donor)

65782 limbal conjunctival autograft (includes obtaining graft)

(For harvesting conjunctival allograft, living donor, use 68371)

ANTERIOR CHAMBER

Incision

65800 Paracentesis of anterior chamber of eye (separate procedure); with diagnostic aspiration of aqueous

65805 with therapeutic release of aqueous

65810 with removal of vitreous and/or discission of anterior hyaloid membrane, with or without air injection

65815 with removal of blood, with or without irrigation and/or air injection

(For injection, see 66020-66030)

(For removal of blood clot, use 65930)

65820 Goniotomy

(Do not report modifier -63 in conjunction with 65820)

(For use of ophthalmic endoscope with 65820, use 66990)

65850 Trabeculotomy ab externo

65855 Trabeculoplasty by laser surgery, one or more sessions (defined treatment series)

(If re-treatment is necessary after several months because of disease progression, a new treatment or treatment series should be reported with a modifier, if necessary, to indicate lesser or greater complexity)

(For trabeculectomy, use 66170)

65860 Severing adhesions of anterior segment, laser technique (separate procedure)

Other Procedures

65865 Severing adhesions of anterior segment of eye, incisional technique (with or without injection of air or liquid) (separate procedure); goniosynechiae

(For trabeculoplasty by laser surgery, use 65855)

65870 anterior synechiae, except goniosynechiae

65875 posterior synechiae

(For use of ophthalmic endoscope with 65875, use 66990)

65880 corneovitreal adhesions

(For laser surgery, use 66821)

65900 Removal of epithelial downgrowth, anterior chamber of eye

65920 Removal of implanted material, anterior segment of eye

(For use of ophthalmic endoscope with 65920, use 66990)

65930 Removal of blood clot, anterior segment of eye

66020 Injection, anterior chamber of eye (separate procedure); air or liquid

66030 medication

(For unlisted procedures on anterior segment, use 66999)

ANTERIOR SCLERA

Excision

(For removal of intraocular foreign body, use 65235)

(For operations on posterior sclera, use 67250, 67255)

66130 Excision of lesion, sclera

66150 Fistulization of sclera for glaucoma; trephination with iridectomy

66155 thermocauterization with iridectomy

66160 sclerectomy with punch or scissors, with iridectomy

66165 iridencleisis or iridotasis

66170 trabeculectomy ab externo in absence of previous surgery

(For trabeculotomy ab externo, use 65850)

(For repair of operative wound, use 66250)

66172 trabeculectomy ab externo with scarring from previous ocular surgery or trauma (includes injection of antifibrotic agents)

(For transciliary body sclera fistulization, use Category III code 0123T)

Aqueous Shunt

66180 Aqueous shunt to extraocular reservoir (eg, Molteno, Schocket, Denver-Krupin)

66185 Revision of aqueous shunt to extraocular reservoir

(For removal of implanted shunt, use 67120)

Repair or Revision

(For scleral procedures in retinal surgery, see 67101 et seq)

66220 Repair of scleral staphyloma; without graft

66225 with graft

(For scleral reinforcement, see 67250, 67255)

66250 Revision or repair of operative wound of anterior segment, any type, early or late, major or minor procedure

(For unlisted procedures on anterior sclera, use 66999)

IRIS, CILIARY BODY

Incision

66500 Iridotomy by stab incision (separate procedure); except transfixion

66505 with transfixion as for iris bombe

(For iridotomy by photocoagulation, use 66761)

Excision

66600 Iridectomy, with corneoscleral or corneal section; for removal of lesion

66605 with cyclectomy

Separate Procedure

Unlisted Procedure

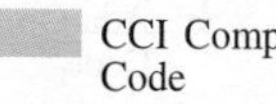
CCI Comp. Code

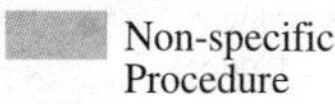
Non-specific Procedure

66625 peripheral for glaucoma (separate procedure)

66630 sector for glaucoma (separate procedure)

66635 optical (separate procedure)

(For coreoplasty by photocoagulation, use 66762)

Repair

66680 Repair of iris, ciliary body (as for iridodialysis)

(For reposition or resection of uveal tissue with perforating wound of cornea or sclera, use 65285)

66682 Suture of iris, ciliary body (separate procedure) with retrieval of suture through small incision (eg, McCannel suture)

Destruction

66700 Ciliary body destruction; diathermy

66710 cyclophotocoagulation, transscleral

66711 cyclophotocoagulation, endoscopic

(Do not report 66711 in conjunction with 66990)

⊙ **66720** cryotherapy

66740 cyclodialysis

66761 Iridotomy/iridectomy by laser surgery (eg, for glaucoma) (one or more sessions)

66762 Iridoplasty by photocoagulation (one or more sessions) (eg, for improvement of vision, for widening of anterior chamber angle)

66770 Destruction of cyst or lesion iris or ciliary body (nonexcisional procedure)

(For excision lesion iris, ciliary body, see 66600, 66605; for removal of epithelial downgrowth, use 65900)

(For unlisted procedures on iris, ciliary body, use 66999)

LENS

Incision

66820 Discission of secondary membranous cataract (opacified posterior lens capsule and/or anterior hyaloid); stab incision technique (Ziegler or Wheeler knife)

66821 laser surgery (eg, YAG laser) (one or more stages)

66825 Repositioning of intraocular lens prosthesis, requiring an incision (separate procedure)

Removal Cataract

66830 Removal of secondary membranous cataract (opacified posterior lens capsule and/or anterior hyaloid) with corneo-scleral section, with or without iridectomy (iridocapsulotomy, iridocapsulectomy)

66840 Removal of lens material; aspiration technique, one or more stages

66850 phacofragmentation technique (mechanical or ultrasonic) (eg, phacoemulsification), with aspiration

66852 pars plana approach, with or without vitrectomy

66920 intracapsular

66930 intracapsular, for dislocated lens

66940 extracapsular (other than 66840, 66850, 66852)

(For removal of intralenticular foreign body without lens extraction, use 65235)

(For repair of operative wound, use 66250)

66982 Extracapsular cataract removal with insertion of intraocular lens prosthesis (one stage procedure), manual or mechanical technique (eg, irrigation and aspiration or phacoemulsification), complex, requiring devices or techniques not generally used in routine cataract surgery (eg, iris expansion device, suture support for intraocular lens, or primary posterior capsulorrhexis) or performed on patients in the amblyogenic developmental stage

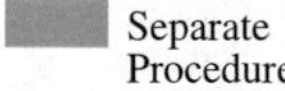

Separate Procedure | Unlisted Procedure | CCI Comp. Code | Non-specific Procedure

66983 Intracapsular cataract extraction with insertion of intraocular lens prosthesis (one stage procedure)

66984 Extracapsular cataract removal with insertion of intraocular lens prosthesis (one stage procedure), manual or mechanical technique (eg, irrigation and aspiration or phacoemulsification)

(For complex extracapsular cataract removal, use 66982)

66985 Insertion of intraocular lens prosthesis (secondary implant), not associated with concurrent cataract removal

(To code implant at time of concurrent cataract surgery, see 66982, 66983, 66984)

(For intraocular lens prosthesis supplied by physician, use 99070)

(For ultrasonic determination of intraocular lens power, use 76519)

(For removal of implanted material from anterior segment, use 65920)

(For secondary fixation (separate procedure), use 66682)

(For use of ophthalmic endoscope with 66985, use 66990)

66986 Exchange of intraocular lens

(For use of ophthalmic endoscope with 66986, use 66990)

+ **66990** Use of ophthalmic endoscope (List separately in addition to code for primary procedure)

(66990 may be used only with codes 65820, 65875, 65920, 66985, 66986, 67036, 67038, 67039, 67040, 67112)

OTHER PROCEDURES

66999 Unlisted procedure, anterior segment of eye

POSTERIOR SEGMENT

VITREOUS

67005 Removal of vitreous, anterior approach (open sky technique or limbal incision); partial removal

67010 subtotal removal with mechanical vitrectomy

(For removal of vitreous by paracentesis of anterior chamber, use 65810)

(For removal of corneovitreal adhesions, use 65880)

67015 Aspiration or release of vitreous, subretinal or choroidal fluid, pars plana approach (posterior sclerotomy)

67025 Injection of vitreous substitute, pars plana or limbal approach, (fluid-gas exchange), with or without aspiration (separate procedure)

67027 Implantation of intravitreal drug delivery system (eg, ganciclovir implant), includes concomitant removal of vitreous

(For removal, use 67121)

67028 Intravitreal injection of a pharmacologic agent (separate procedure)

67030 Discission of vitreous strands (without removal), pars plana approach

67031 Severing of vitreous strands, vitreous face adhesions, sheets, membranes or opacities, laser surgery (one or more stages)

67036 Vitrectomy, mechanical, pars plana approach;

67038 with epiretinal membrane stripping

67039 with focal endolaser photocoagulation

67040 with endolaser panretinal photocoagulation

(For use of ophthalmic endoscope with 67036, 67038, 67039, 67040, use 66990)

(For associated lensectomy, use 66850)

(For use of vitrectomy in retinal detachment surgery, use 67108)

(For associated removal of foreign body, see 65260, 65265)

(For unlisted procedures on vitreous, use 67299)

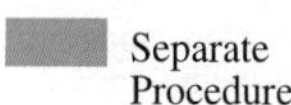 Separate Procedure  Unlisted Procedure CCI Comp. Code 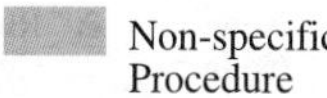 Non-specific Procedure

RETINA OR CHOROID

Repair

(If diathermy, cryotherapy and/or photocoagulation are combined, report under principal modality used)

67101 Repair of retinal detachment, one or more sessions; cryotherapy or diathermy, with or without drainage of subretinal fluid

67105 photocoagulation, with or without drainage of subretinal fluid

67107 Repair of retinal detachment; scleral buckling (such as lamellar scleral dissection, imbrication or encircling procedure), with or without implant, with or without cryotherapy, photocoagulation, and drainage of subretinal fluid

67108 with vitrectomy, any method, with or without air or gas tamponade, focal endolaser photocoagulation, cryotherapy, drainage of subretinal fluid, scleral buckling, and/or removal of lens by same technique

67110 by injection of air or other gas (eg, pneumatic retinopexy)

67112 by scleral buckling or vitrectomy, on patient having previous ipsilateral retinal detachment repair(s) using scleral buckling or vitrectomy techniques

(For aspiration of drainage of subretinal or subchoroidal fluid, use 67015)

(For use of ophthalmic endoscope with 67112, use 66990)

67115 Release of encircling material (posterior segment)

67120 Removal of implanted material, posterior segment; extraocular

67121 intraocular

(For removal from anterior segment, use 65920)

(For removal of foreign body, see 65260, 65265)

Prophylaxis

67141 Prophylaxis of retinal detachment (eg, retinal break, lattice degeneration) without drainage, one or more sessions; cryotherapy, diathermy

67145 photocoagulation (laser or xenon arc)

Destruction

67208 Destruction of localized lesion of retina (eg, macular edema, tumors), one or more sessions; cryotherapy, diathermy

67210 photocoagulation

67218 radiation by implantation of source (includes removal of source)

67220 Destruction of localized lesion of choroid (eg, choroidal neovascularization); photocoagulation (eg, laser), one or more sessions

(For destruction of macular drusen, photocoagulation, use Category III code 0017T)

(For destruction of localized lesion of choroid by transpupillary thermotherapy, use Category III code 0016T)

67221 photodynamic therapy (includes intravenous infusion)

+ 67225 photodynamic therapy, second eye, at single session (List separately in addition to code for primary eye treatment)

(Use 67225 in conjunction with code 67221)

67227 Destruction of extensive or progressive retinopathy (eg, diabetic retinopathy), one or more sessions; cryotherapy, diathermy

67228 photocoagulation (laser or xenon arc)

(For unlisted procedures on retina, use 67299)

POSTERIOR SCLERA

Repair

(For excision lesion sclera, use 66130)

67250 Scleral reinforcement (separate procedure); without graft

67255 with graft

(For repair scleral staphyloma, see 66220, 66225)

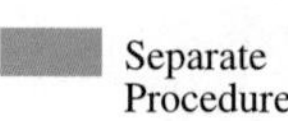 Separate Procedure 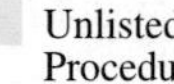 Unlisted Procedure 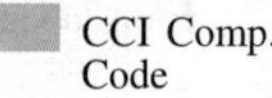 CCI Comp. Code 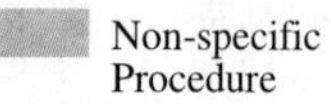 Non-specific Procedure

OTHER PROCEDURES

67299 Unlisted procedure, posterior segment

OCULAR ADNEXA

EXTRAOCULAR MUSCLES

67311 Strabismus surgery, recession or resection procedure; one horizontal muscle

67312 two horizontal muscles

67314 one vertical muscle (excluding superior oblique)

67316 two or more vertical muscles (excluding superior oblique)

(For adjustable sutures, use 67335 in addition to codes 67311-67334 for primary procedure reflecting number of muscles operated on)

67318 Strabismus surgery, any procedure, superior oblique muscle

+ **67320** Transposition procedure (eg, for paretic extraocular muscle), any extraocular muscle (specify) (List separately in addition to code for primary procedure)

(Use 67320 in conjunction with codes 67311-67318)

+ **67331** Strabismus surgery on patient with previous eye surgery or injury that did not involve the extraocular muscles (List separately in addition to code for primary procedure)

(Use 67331 in conjunction with codes 67311-67318)

+ **67332** Strabismus surgery on patient with scarring of extraocular muscles (eg, prior ocular injury, strabismus or retinal detachment surgery) or restrictive myopathy (eg, dysthyroid ophthalmopathy) (List separately in addition to code for primary procedure)

(Use 67332 in conjunction with codes 67311-67318)

+ **67334** Strabismus surgery by posterior fixation suture technique, with or without muscle recession (List separately in addition to code for primary procedure)

(Use 67334 in conjunction with codes 67311-67318)

+ **67335** Placement of adjustable suture(s) during strabismus surgery, including postoperative adjustment(s) of suture(s) (List separately in addition to code for specific strabismus surgery)

(Use 67335 in conjunction with codes 67311-67334)

+ **67340** Strabismus surgery involving exploration and/or repair of detached extraocular muscle(s) (List separately in addition to code for primary procedure)

(Use 67340 in conjunction with codes 67311-67334)

67343 Release of extensive scar tissue without detaching extraocular muscle (separate procedure)

(Use 67343 in conjunction with codes 67311-67340, when such procedures are performed other than on the affected muscle)

67345 Chemodenervation of extraocular muscle

(For chemodenervation for blepharospasm and other neurological disorders, see 64612 and 64613)

● **67346** Biopsy of extraocular muscle

(For repair of wound, extraocular muscle, tendon or Tenon's capsule, use 65290)

Other Procedures

(67350 deleted 2007 edition, see 67346)

67399 Unlisted procedure, ocular muscle

ORBIT

Exploration, Excision, Decompression

67400 Orbitotomy without bone flap (frontal or transconjunctival approach); for exploration, with or without biopsy

67405 with drainage only

67412 with removal of lesion

67413 with removal of foreign body

67414 with removal of bone for decompression

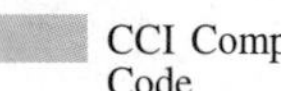

Separate Procedure | Unlisted Procedure | CCI Comp. Code | Non-specific Procedure

67415 Fine needle aspiration of orbital contents

(For exenteration, enucleation, and repair, see 65101 et seq; for optic nerve decompression, use 67570)

67420 Orbitotomy with bone flap or window, lateral approach (eg, Kroenlein); with removal of lesion

67430 with removal of foreign body

67440 with drainage

67445 with removal of bone for decompression

(For optic nerve sheath decompression, use 67570)

67450 for exploration, with or without biopsy

(For orbitotomy, transcranial approach, see 61330-61334)

(For orbital implant, see 67550, 67560)

(For removal of eyeball or for repair after removal, see 65091-65175)

Other Procedures

67500 Retrobulbar injection; medication (separate procedure, does not include supply of medication)

67505 alcohol

67515 Injection of medication or other substance into Tenon's capsule

(For subconjunctival injection, use 68200)

67550 Orbital implant (implant outside muscle cone); insertion

67560 removal or revision

(For ocular implant (implant inside muscle cone), see 65093-65105, 65130-65175)

(For treatment of fractures of malar area, orbit, see 21355 et seq)

67570 Optic nerve decompression (eg, incision or fenestration of optic nerve sheath)

● New Code ▲ Revised Code + Add-On Code ⊘ Modifier -51 Exempt ⊙ Conscious Sedation

67599 Unlisted procedure, orbit

EYELIDS

Incision

67700 Blepharotomy, drainage of abscess, eyelid

67710 Severing of tarsorrhaphy

67715 Canthotomy (separate procedure)

(For canthoplasty, use 67950)

(For division of symblepharon, use 68340)

Excision, Destruction

(For removal of lesion, involving mainly skin of eyelid, see 11310-11313; 11440-11446, 11640-11646; 17000-17004)

(For repair of wounds, blepharoplasty, grafts, reconstructive surgery, see 67930-67975)

67800 Excision of chalazion; single

67801 multiple, same lid

67805 multiple, different lids

67808 under general anesthesia and/or requiring hospitalization, single or multiple

67810 Biopsy of eyelid

67820 Correction of trichiasis; epilation, by forceps only

67825 epilation by other than forceps (eg, by electrosurgery, cryotherapy, laser surgery)

67830 incision of lid margin

67835 incision of lid margin, with free mucous membrane graft

67840 Excision of lesion of eyelid (except chalazion) without closure or with simple direct closure

Separate Procedure | Unlisted Procedure | CCI Comp. Code | Non-specific Procedure

(For excision and repair of eyelid by reconstructive surgery, see 67961, 67966)

67850 Destruction of lesion of lid margin (up to 1 cm)

(For Mohs micrographic surgery, see 17311-17315)

(For initiation or follow-up care of topical chemotherapy (eg, 5-FU or similar agents), see appropriate office visits)

Tarsorrhaphy

67875 Temporary closure of eyelids by suture (eg, Frost suture)

67880 Construction of intermarginal adhesions, median tarsorrhaphy, or canthorrhaphy;

67882 with transposition of tarsal plate

(For severing of tarsorrhaphy, use 67710)

(For canthoplasty, reconstruction canthus, use 67950)

(For canthotomy, use 67715)

Repair (Brow Ptosis, Blepharoptosis, Lid Retraction, Ectropion, Entropion)

67900 Repair of brow ptosis (supraciliary, mid-forehead or coronal approach)

(For forehead rhytidectomy, use 15824)

67901 Repair of blepharoptosis; frontalis muscle technique with suture or other material (eg, banked fascia)

67902 frontalis muscle technique with autologous fascial sling (includes obtaining fascia)

67903 (tarso) levator resection or advancement, internal approach

67904 (tarso) levator resection or advancement, external approach

67906 superior rectus technique with fascial sling (includes obtaining fascia)

67908 conjunctivo-tarso-Muller's muscle-levator resection (eg, Fasanella-Servat type)

● New Code ▲ Revised Code + Add-On Code ⊘ Modifier -51 Exempt ⊙ Conscious Sedation

67909 Reduction of overcorrection of ptosis

67911 Correction of lid retraction

(For obtaining autogenous graft materials, see 20920, 20922, or 20926)

(For correction of trichiasis by mucous membrane graft, use 67835)

67912 Correction of lagophthalmos, with implantation of upper eyelid load (eg, gold weight)

67914 Repair of ectropion; suture

67915 thermocauterization

67916 excision tarsal wedge

67917 extensive (eg, tarsal strip operations)

(For correction of everted punctum, use 68705)

67921 Repair of entropion; suture

67922 thermocauterization

67923 excision tarsal wedge

67924 extensive (eg, tarsal strip or capsulopalpebral fascia repairs operation)

(For repair of cicatricial ectropion or entropion requiring scar excision or skin graft, see also 67961 et seq)

Reconstruction

67930 Suture of recent wound, eyelid, involving lid margin, tarsus, and/or palpebral conjunctiva direct closure; partial thickness

67935 full thickness

67938 Removal of embedded foreign body, eyelid

(For repair of skin of eyelid, see 12011-12018; 12051-12057; 13150-13153)

(For tarsorrhaphy, canthorrhaphy, see 67880, 67882)

(For repair of blepharoptosis and lid retraction, see 67901-67911)

(For blepharoplasty for entropion, ectropion, see 67916, 67917, 67923, 67924)

(For correction of blepharochalasis (blepharorhytidectomy), see 15820-15823)

(For repair of skin of eyelid, adjacent tissue transfer, see 14060, 14061; preparation for graft, use 15004; free graft, see 15120, 15121, 15260, 15261)

(For excision of lesion of eyelid, use 67800 et seq)

(For repair of lacrimal canaliculi, use 68700)

67950 Canthoplasty (reconstruction of canthus)

67961 Excision and repair of eyelid, involving lid margin, tarsus, conjunctiva, canthus, or full thickness, may include preparation for skin graft or pedicle flap with adjacent tissue transfer or rearrangement; up to one-fourth of lid margin

67966 over one-fourth of lid margin

(For canthoplasty, use 67950)

(For free skin grafts, see 15120, 15121, 15260, 15261)

(For tubed pedicle flap preparation, use 15576; for delay, use 15630; for attachment, use 15650)

67971 Reconstruction of eyelid, full thickness by transfer of tarsoconjunctival flap from opposing eyelid; up to two-thirds of eyelid, one stage or first stage

67973 total eyelid, lower, one stage or first stage

67974 total eyelid, upper, one stage or first stage

67975 second stage

Other Procedures

67999 Unlisted procedure, eyelids

CONJUNCTIVA

(For removal of foreign body, see 65205 et seq)

INCISION AND DRAINAGE

68020 Incision of conjunctiva, drainage of cyst

68040 Expression of conjunctival follicles (eg, for trachoma)

EXCISION AND/OR DESTRUCTION

68100 Biopsy of conjunctiva

68110 Excision of lesion, conjunctiva; up to 1 cm

68115 over 1 cm

68130 with adjacent sclera

68135 Destruction of lesion, conjunctiva

INJECTION

(For injection into Tenon's capsule or retrobulbar injection, see 67500-67515)

68200 Subconjunctival injection

CONJUNCTIVOPLASTY

(For wound repair, see 65270-65273)

68320 Conjunctivoplasty; with conjunctival graft or extensive rearrangement

68325 with buccal mucous membrane graft (includes obtaining graft)

68326 Conjunctivoplasty, reconstruction cul-de-sac; with conjunctival graft or extensive rearrangement

68328 with buccal mucous membrane graft (includes obtaining graft)

68330 Repair of symblepharon; conjunctivoplasty, without graft

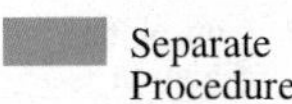 Separate Procedure 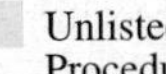 Unlisted Procedure 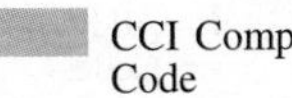 CCI Comp. Code 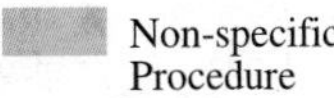 Non-specific Procedure

68335 with free graft conjunctiva or buccal mucous membrane (includes obtaining graft)

68340 division of symblepharon, with or without insertion of conformer or contact lens

OTHER PROCEDURES

68360 Conjunctival flap; bridge or partial (separate procedure)

68362 total (such as Gunderson thin flap or purse string flap)

(For conjunctival flap for perforating injury, see 65280, 65285)

(For repair of operative wound, use 66250)

(For removal of conjunctival foreign body, see 65205, 65210)

68371 Harvesting conjunctival allograft, living donor

68399 Unlisted procedure, conjunctiva

LACRIMAL SYSTEM

Incision

68400 Incision, drainage of lacrimal gland

68420 Incision, drainage of lacrimal sac (dacryocystotomy or dacryocystostomy)

68440 Snip incision of lacrimal punctum

Excision

68500 Excision of lacrimal gland (dacryoadenectomy), except for tumor; total

68505 partial

68510 Biopsy of lacrimal gland

68520 Excision of lacrimal sac (dacryocystectomy)

68525 Biopsy of lacrimal sac

68530 Removal of foreign body or dacryolith, lacrimal passages

68540 Excision of lacrimal gland tumor; frontal approach

68550 involving osteotomy

Repair

68700 Plastic repair of canaliculi

68705 Correction of everted punctum, cautery

68720 Dacryocystorhinostomy (fistulization of lacrimal sac to nasal cavity)

68745 Conjunctivorhinostomy (fistulization of conjunctiva to nasal cavity); without tube

68750 with insertion of tube or stent

68760 Closure of the lacrimal punctum; by thermocauterization, ligation, or laser surgery

68761 by plug, each

68770 Closure of lacrimal fistula (separate procedure)

Probing and/or Related Procedures

68801 Dilation of lacrimal punctum, with or without irrigation

(To report a bilateral procedure, use 68801 with modifier -50)

68810 Probing of nasolacrimal duct, with or without irrigation;

(For bilateral procedure, report 68810 with modifier -50)

68811 requiring general anesthesia

(For bilateral procedure, report 68811 with modifier -50)

68815 with insertion of tube or stent

(See also 92018)

(For bilateral procedure, report 68815 with modifier -50)

68840 Probing of lacrimal canaliculi, with or without irrigation

68850 Injection of contrast medium for dacryocystography

Separate Procedure | Unlisted Procedure | CCI Comp. Code | Non-specific Procedure

(For radiological supervision and interpretation, see 70170, 78660)

Other Procedures

68899 Unlisted procedure, lacrimal system

● New Code ▲ Revised Code + Add-On Code ⃠ Modifier -51 Exempt ⊙ Conscious Sedation

AUDITORY SYSTEM

CPT codes from this subsection of the CPT coding system are used to report invasive and surgical procedures performed on the external ear; middle ear; inner ear and temporal bone. Includes procedures performed on the inner, outer and middle ear and to the temporal bone.

Diagnostic services, such as otoscopy under general anesthesia, audiometry and vestibular tests, are defined in the Medicine Section of the CPT manual.

Wound repairs to the external ear are located in the Integumentary Subsection of the CPT coding system.

When a mastoidectomy is included in the description of an auditory procedure (e.g. CPT codes 69530, 69802, 69910), separate codes describing mastoidectomy are not reported.

Myringotomies (e.g. CPT codes 69420 and 69421) are included in tympanoplasties and tympanostomies.

(For diagnostic services (eg, audiometry, vestibular tests), see 92502 et seq)

EXTERNAL EAR

INCISION

69000 Drainage external ear, abscess or hematoma; simple

69005 complicated

69020 Drainage external auditory canal, abscess

69090 Ear piercing

EXCISION

69100 Biopsy external ear

69105 Biopsy external auditory canal

69110 Excision external ear; partial, simple repair

69120 complete amputation

(For reconstruction of ear, see 15120 et seq)

Separate Procedure | Unlisted Procedure | CCI Comp. Code | Non-specific Procedure

69140 Excision exostosis(es), external auditory canal

69145 Excision soft tissue lesion, external auditory canal

69150 Radical excision external auditory canal lesion; without neck dissection

69155 with neck dissection

(For resection of temporal bone, use 69535)

(For skin grafting, see 15004-15261)

REMOVAL

69200 Removal foreign body from external auditory canal; without general anesthesia

69205 with general anesthesia

69210 Removal impacted cerumen (separate procedure), one or both ears

69220 Debridement, mastoidectomy cavity, simple (eg, routine cleaning)

(For bilateral procedure, report 9220 with modifier -50)

69222 Debridement, mastoidectomy cavity, complex (eg, with anesthesia or more than routine cleaning)

(For bilateral procedure, report 69222 with modifier -50)

REPAIR

(For suture of wound or injury of external ear, see 12011-14300)

⊙ **69300** Otoplasty, protruding ear, with or without size reduction

(For bilateral procedure, report 69300 with modifier -50)

69310 Reconstruction of external auditory canal (meatoplasty) (eg, for stenosis due to injury, infection) (separate procedure)

69320 Reconstruction external auditory canal for congenital atresia, single stage

● New Code ▲ Revised Code + Add-On Code ⊘ Modifier -51 Exempt ⊙ Conscious Sedation

(For combination with middle ear reconstruction, see 69631, 69641)

(For other reconstructive procedures with grafts (eg, skin, cartilage, bone), see 13150-15760, 21230-21235)

OTHER PROCEDURES

(For otoscopy under general anesthesia, use 92502)

69399 Unlisted procedure, external ear

MIDDLE EAR

INTRODUCTION

69400 Eustachian tube inflation, transnasal; with catheterization

69401 without catheterization

69405 Eustachian tube catheterization, transtympanic

(69410 deleted 2006 edition.)

INCISION

69420 Myringotomy including aspiration and/or eustachian tube inflation

69421 Myringotomy including aspiration and/or eustachian tube inflation requiring general anesthesia

69424 Ventilating tube removal requiring general anesthesia

(For bilateral procedure, report 69424 with modifier -50)

(Do not report code 69424 in conjunction with codes 69205, 69210, 69420, 69421, 69433-69676, 69710-69745, 69801-69930)

69433 Tympanostomy (requiring insertion of ventilating tube), local or topical anesthesia

(For bilateral procedure, report 69433 with modifier -50)

69436 Tympanostomy (requiring insertion of ventilating tube), general anesthesia

(For bilateral procedure, report 69436 with modifier -50)

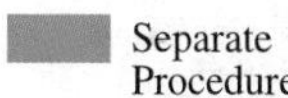
Separate Procedure

Unlisted Procedure

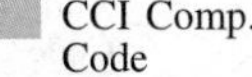
CCI Comp. Code

Non-specific Procedure

69440 Middle ear exploration through postauricular or ear canal incision

(For atticotomy, see 69601 et seq)

69450 Tympanolysis, transcanal

EXCISION

69501 Transmastoid antrotomy (simple mastoidectomy)

69502 Mastoidectomy; complete

69505 modified radical

69511 radical

(For skin graft, see 15004 et seq)

(For mastoidectomy cavity debridement, see 69220, 69222)

69530 Petrous apicectomy including radical mastoidectomy

69535 Resection temporal bone, external approach

(For middle fossa approach, see 69950-69970)

69540 Excision aural polyp

69550 Excision aural glomus tumor; transcanal

69552 transmastoid

69554 extended (extratemporal)

REPAIR

69601 Revision mastoidectomy; resulting in complete mastoidectomy

69602 resulting in modified radical mastoidectomy

69603 resulting in radical mastoidectomy

69604 resulting in tympanoplasty

(For planned secondary tympanoplasty after mastoidectomy, see 69631, 69632)

69605 with apicectomy

(For skin graft, see 15120, 15121, 15260, 15261)

69610 Tympanic membrane repair, with or without site preparation or perforation for closure, with or without patch

69620 Myringoplasty (surgery confined to drumhead and donor area)

69631 Tympanoplasty without mastoidectomy (including canalplasty, atticotomy and/or middle ear surgery), initial or revision; without ossicular chain reconstruction

69632 with ossicular chain reconstruction (eg, postfenestration)

69633 with ossicular chain reconstruction and synthetic prosthesis (eg, partial ossicular replacement prosthesis (PORP), total ossicular replacement prosthesis (TORP))

69635 Tympanoplasty with antrotomy or mastoidotomy (including canalplasty, atticotomy, middle ear surgery, and/or tympanic membrane repair); without ossicular chain reconstruction

69636 with ossicular chain reconstruction

69637 with ossicular chain reconstruction and synthetic prosthesis (eg, partial ossicular replacement prosthesis (PORP), total ossicular replacement prosthesis (TORP))

69641 Tympanoplasty with mastoidectomy (including canalplasty, middle ear surgery, tympanic membrane repair); without ossicular chain reconstruction

69642 with ossicular chain reconstruction

69643 with intact or reconstructed wall, without ossicular chain reconstruction

69644 with intact or reconstructed canal wall, with ossicular chain reconstruction

69645 radical or complete, without ossicular chain reconstruction

69646 radical or complete, with ossicular chain reconstruction

69650 Stapes mobilization

Separate Procedure | Unlisted Procedure | CCI Comp. Code | Non-specific Procedure

69660 Stapedectomy or stapedotomy with reestablishment of ossicular continuity, with or without use of foreign material;

69661 with footplate drill out

69662 Revision of stapedectomy or stapedotomy

69666 Repair oval window fistula

69667 Repair round window fistula

69670 Mastoid obliteration (separate procedure)

69676 Tympanic neurectomy

(For bilateral procedure, report 69676 with modifier -50)

OTHER PROCEDURES

69700 Closure postauricular fistula, mastoid (separate procedure)

69710 Implantation or replacement of electromagnetic bone conduction hearing device in temporal bone

(Replacement procedure includes removal of old device)

69711 Removal or repair of electromagnetic bone conduction hearing device in temporal bone

69714 Implantation, osseointegrated implant, temporal bone, with percutaneous attachment to external speech processor/cochlear stimulator; without mastoidectomy

69715 with mastoidectomy

69717 Replacement (including removal of existing device), osseointegrated implant, temporal bone, with percutaneous attachment to external speech processor/cochlear stimulator; without mastoidectomy

69718 with mastoidectomy

69720 Decompression facial nerve, intratemporal; lateral to geniculate ganglion

69725 including medial to geniculate ganglion

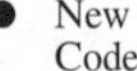

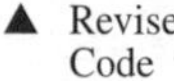

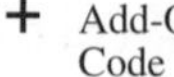

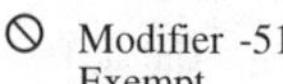

⊙ Conscious Sedation

69740 Suture facial nerve, intratemporal, with or without graft or decompression; lateral to geniculate ganglion

69745 including medial to geniculate ganglion

(For extracranial suture of facial nerve, use 64864)

69799 Unlisted procedure, middle ear

INNER EAR

INCISION AND/OR DESTRUCTION

69801 Labyrinthotomy, with or without cryosurgery including other nonexcisional destructive procedures or perfusion of vestibuloactive drugs (single or multiple perfusions); transcanal

(69801 includes all required infusions performed on initial and subsequent days of treatment)

69802 with mastoidectomy

69805 Endolymphatic sac operation; without shunt

69806 with shunt

69820 Fenestration semicircular canal

69840 Revision fenestration operation

EXCISION

69905 Labyrinthectomy; transcanal

69910 with mastoidectomy

69915 Vestibular nerve section, translabyrinthine approach

(For transcranial approach, use 69950)

INTRODUCTION

69930 Cochlear device implantation, with or without mastoidectomy

OTHER PROCEDURES

69949 Unlisted procedure, inner ear

TEMPORAL BONE, MIDDLE FOSSA APPROACH

(For external approach, use 69535)

69950 Vestibular nerve section, transcranial approach

69955 Total facial nerve decompression and/or repair (may include graft)

69960 Decompression internal auditory canal

69970 Removal of tumor, temporal bone

OTHER PROCEDURES

69979 Unlisted procedure, temporal bone, middle fossa approach

OPERATING MICROSCOPE

Medicare limits the reporting of use of an operating microscope (CPT code 69990) to procedures described by CPT codes 61304-61546, 61550-61711, 62010-62100, 63081-63308, 63704- 63710, 64831, 64834-64836, 64840- 64858, 64861-64870, 64885-64898 and 64905-64907. CPT code 69990 should not be reported with other procedures even if an operating microscope is utilized. CMS guidelines for payment of CPT code 69990 differ from CPT code book instructions following CPT code 69990.

\+ **69990** Microsurgical techniques, requiring use of operating microscope (List separately in addition to code for primary procedure)

This page intentionally left blank.

● New Code ▲ Revised Code + Add-On Code ⊘ Modifier -51 Exempt ⊙ Conscious Sedation

RADIOLOGY

RADIOLOGY SECTION OVERVIEW

The fourth section of the CPT coding system is the radiology section, which includes diagnostic and therapeutic radiology, nuclear medicine and diagnostic ultrasound services. Within each subsection, the CPT codes are arranged by anatomical site.

Diagnostic radiology uses all modalities of radiant energy in medical diagnosis and therapeutic procedures requiring radiologic guidance. This includes imaging techniques and methodologies using radiation emitted by x-ray tubes, radionuclides, ultrasonographic devices, and radiofrequency electromagnetic radiation.

RADIOLOGY SUBSECTIONS

The RADIOLOGY section of the CPT coding system is divided into 7 subsections; namely:

Diagnostic Radiology (Diagnostic Imaging)	70010-76499
Diagnostic Ultrasound	76506-76999
Radiologic Guidance	77001-77032
Breast, Mammography	77051-77059
Bone/Joint Studies	77071-77084
Radiation Oncology	77261-77799
Nuclear Medicine	78000-79999

COMPLETE PROCEDURES

Interventional radiologic procedures or diagnostic studies involving injection of contrast media include all usual preinjection and postinjection services, for example, necessary local anesthesia, placement of needle or catheter, injection of contrast media, supervision of the study, and interpretation of results. When one of these procedures is performed in full by a single physician, it is designated as a "complete procedure."

SUPERVISION AND INTERPRETATION ONLY

When a procedure is performed by a radiologist-clinician team, it is designated as "supervision and interpretation only" and the separate injection procedure is listed in the appropriate section of the SURGERY section of the CPT coding system. These CPT codes are used only when a procedure is performed by more than one physician, for example, a radiologist-clinician team.

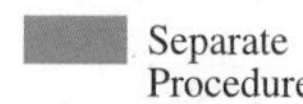
Separate Procedure

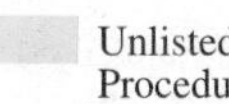
Unlisted Procedure

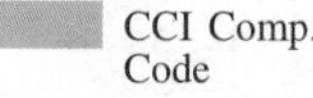
CCI Comp. Code

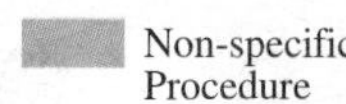
Non-specific Procedure

RADIOLOGY SERVICE MODIFIERS

Listed surgical services and procedures may be modified under certain circumstances. When applicable, the modifying circumstance is identified by adding the appropriate two digit modifier to the base procedure code(s). Modifiers commonly used to report RADIOLOGY services include:

-22 Unusual services

-26 Professional component

-32 Mandated services

-51 Multiple procedures

-52 Reduced services

-62 Two surgeons

-66 Surgical team

-76 Repeat procedure by same physician

-77 Repeat procedure by another physician

-78 Return to the operating room for a related procedure during the postoperative period

-79 Unrelated procedure or service by the same physician during the postoperative period

-80 Assistant surgeon

-90 Reference (outside) laboratory

-99 Multiple modifiers

-LT Left side of body

-RT Right side of body

BILATERAL PROCEDURE CODES

The RADIOLOGY section includes some CPT codes which include the term "bilateral" in the definition. When reporting these services, do not add the modifier -50, because the procedure is already defined as "bilateral."

RADIOLOGY SERVICES MEDICARE CONSIDERATIONS

Most of the CPT codes in this section are subject to Medicare Purchased Diagnostic Services guidelines. Coding and reporting should be as instructed by your local Medicare carrier.

This page intentionally left blank.

RADIOLOGY CODES

DIAGNOSTIC RADIOLOGY (DIAGNOSTIC IMAGING)

HEAD AND NECK

70010 Myelography, posterior fossa, radiological supervision and interpretation

70015 Cisternography, positive contrast, radiological supervision and interpretation

70030 Radiologic examination, eye, for detection of foreign body

70100 Radiologic examination, mandible; partial, less than four views

70110 complete, minimum of four views

70120 Radiologic examination, mastoids; less than three views per side

70130 complete, minimum of three views per side

70134 Radiologic examination, internal auditory meati, complete

70140 Radiologic examination, facial bones; less than three views

70150 complete, minimum of three views

70160 Radiologic examination, nasal bones, complete, minimum of three views

70170 Dacryocystography, nasolacrimal duct, radiological supervision and interpretation

70190 Radiologic examination; optic foramina

70200 orbits, complete, minimum of four views

70210 Radiologic examination, sinuses, paranasal, less than three views

70220 Radiologic examination, sinuses, paranasal, complete, minimum of three views

70240 Radiologic examination, sella turcica

70250 Radiologic examination, skull; less than four views

70260 complete, minimum of four views

70300 Radiologic examination, teeth; single view

70310 partial examination, less than full mouth

70320 complete, full mouth

70328 Radiologic examination, temporomandibular joint, open and closed mouth; unilateral

70330 bilateral

70332 Temporomandibular joint arthrography, radiological supervision and interpretation

(Do not report 70332 in conjunction with 77002)

70336 Magnetic resonance (eg, proton) imaging, temporomandibular joint(s)

70350 Cephalogram, orthodontic

70355 Orthopantogram

70360 Radiologic examination; neck, soft tissue

70370 pharynx or larynx, including fluoroscopy and/or magnification technique

70371 Complex dynamic pharyngeal and speech evaluation by cine or video recording

70373 Laryngography, contrast, radiological supervision and interpretation

70380 Radiologic examination, salivary gland for calculus

70390 Sialography, radiological supervision and interpretation

70450 Computed tomography, head or brain; without contrast material

● New Code ▲ Revised Code + Add-On Code ⃠ Modifier -51 Exempt ⊙ Conscious Sedation

70460 with contrast material(s)

70470 without contrast material, followed by contrast material(s) and further sections

(To report 3D rendering, see 76376, 76377)

70480 Computed tomography, orbit, sella, or posterior fossa or outer, middle, or inner ear; without contrast material

70481 with contrast material(s)

70482 without contrast material, followed by contrast material(s) and further sections

(To report 3D rendering, see 76376, 76377)

70486 Computed tomography, maxillofacial area; without contrast material

70487 with contrast material(s)

70488 without contrast material, followed by contrast material(s) and further sections

(To report 3D rendering, see 76376, 76377)

70490 Computed tomography, soft tissue neck; without contrast material

70491 with contrast material(s)

70492 without contrast material followed by contrast material(s) and further sections

(To report 3D rendering, see 76376, 76377)

(For cervical spine, see 72125, 72126)

70496 Computed tomographic angiography, head, without contrast material(s), followed by contrast material(s) and further sections, including image post-processing

70498 Computed tomographic angiography, neck, without contrast material(s), followed by contrast material(s) and further sections, including image post-processing

▲ **70540** Magnetic resonance (eg, proton) imaging, orbit, face, and/or neck; without contrast material(s)

(For head or neck magnetic resonance angiography studies, see 70544-70546, 70547-70549)

70542 with contrast material(s)

70543 without contrast material(s), followed by contrast material(s) and further sequences

(Report 70540-70543 once per imaging session)

70544 Magnetic resonance angiography, head; without contrast materials

70545 with contrast materials

70546 without contrast material(s), followed by contrast material(s) and further sequences

70547 Magnetic resonance angiography, neck; without contrast materials

70548 with contrast materials

70549 without contrast material(s), followed by contrast material(s) and further sequences

70551 Magnetic resonance (eg, proton) imaging, brain (including brain stem); without contrast material

70552 with contrast material(s)

70553 without contrast material, followed by contrast material(s) and further sequences

(For magnetic spectroscopy, use 76390)

● **70554** Magnetic resonance imaging, brain, functional MRI; including test selection and administration of repetitive body part movement and/or visual stimulation, not requiring physician or psychologist administration

(Do not report 70554 in conjunction with 96020)

● **70555** Magnetic resonance imaging, brain, functional MRI; requiring physician or psychologist administration of entire neurofunctional testing

(Do not report 70555 unless 96020 is performed)

(Do not report 70554, 70555 in conjunction with 70551-70553 unless a separate diagnostic MRI is performed)

70557 Magnetic resonance (eg, proton) imaging, brain (including brain stem and skull base), during open intracranial procedure (eg, to assess for residual tumor or residual vascular malformation); without contrast material

70558 with contrast material(s)

70559 without contrast material(s), followed by contrast material(s) and further sequences

(For stereotactic biopsy of intracranial lesion with magnetic resonance guidance, use 61751. 70557, 70558 or 70559 may be reported only if a separate report is generated. Report only one of the above codes once per operative session. Do not use these codes in conjunction with 61751, 77021, 77022)

CHEST

(For fluoroscopic or ultrasonic guidance for needle placement procedures (eg., biopsy, aspiration, injection, localization device) of the thorax, see 76942, 77002)

71010 Radiologic examination, chest; single view, frontal

71015 stereo, frontal

71020 Radiologic examination, chest, two views, frontal and lateral;

71021 with apical lordotic procedure

71022 with oblique projections

71023 with fluoroscopy

71030 Radiologic examination, chest, complete, minimum of four views;

71034 with fluoroscopy

(For separate chest fluoroscopy, use 76000)

71035 Radiologic examination, chest, special views (eg, lateral decubitus, Bucky studies)

71040 Bronchography, unilateral, radiological supervision and interpretation

71060 Bronchography, bilateral, radiological supervision and interpretation

71090 Insertion pacemaker, fluoroscopy and radiography, radiological supervision and interpretation

(For procedure, see appropriate organ or site)

71100 Radiologic examination, ribs, unilateral; two views

71101 including posteroanterior chest, minimum of three views

71110 Radiologic examination, ribs, bilateral; three views

71111 including posteroanterior chest, minimum of four views

71120 Radiologic examination; sternum, minimum of two views

71130 sternoclavicular joint or joints, minimum of three views

71250 Computed tomography, thorax; without contrast material

71260 with contrast material(s)

71270 without contrast material, followed by contrast material(s) and further sections

(For cardiac computed tomography of the heart, see Category III codes 0144T-0151T)

(To report 3D rendering, see 76376, 76377)

▲ **71275** Computed tomographic angiography, chest (noncoronary), without contrast material(s), followed by contrast material(s) and further sections, including image post-processing

(For coronary artery computed tomographic angiography including calcification score and/or cardiac morphology, see Category III codes 0146T-0149T)

71550 Magnetic resonance (eg, proton) imaging, chest (eg, for evaluation of hilar and mediastinal lymphadenopathy); without contrast material(s)

71551 with contrast material(s)

71552 without contrast material(s), followed by contrast material(s) and further sequences

(For breast MRI, see 77058, 77059)

71555 Magnetic resonance angiography, chest (excluding myocardium), with or without contrast material(s)

SPINE AND PELVIS

72010 Radiologic examination, spine, entire, survey study, anteroposterior and lateral

72020 Radiologic examination, spine, single view, specify level

72040 Radiologic examination, spine, cervical; two or three views

72050 minimum of four views

72052 complete, including oblique and flexion and/or extension studies

72069 Radiologic examination, spine, thoracolumbar, standing (scoliosis)

72070 Radiologic examination, spine; thoracic, two views

72072 thoracic, three views

72074 thoracic, minimum of four views

72080 thoracolumbar, two views

72090 scoliosis study, including supine and erect studies

72100 Radiologic examination, spine, lumbosacral; two or three views

72110 minimum of four views

72114 complete, including bending views

72120 Radiologic examination, spine, lumbosacral, bending views only, minimum of four views

(Contrast material in CT of spine is either by intrathecal or intravenous injection. For intrathecal injection, use also 61055 or 62284. IV injection of contrast material is part of the CT procedure)

72125 Computed tomography, cervical spine; without contrast material

72126 with contrast material

72127 without contrast material, followed by contrast material(s) and further sections

(For intrathecal injection procedure, see 61055, 62284)

72128 Computed tomography, thoracic spine; without contrast material

72129 with contrast material

(For intrathecal injection procedure, see 61055, 62284)

72130 without contrast material, followed by contrast material(s) and further sections

(For intrathecal injection procedure, see 61055, 62284)

72131 Computed tomography, lumbar spine; without contrast material

72132 with contrast material

72133 without contrast material, followed by contrast material(s) and further sections

(For intrathecal injection procedure, see 61055, 62284)

(To report 3D rendering, see 76376, 76377)

72141 Magnetic resonance (eg, proton) imaging, spinal canal and contents, cervical; without contrast material

72142 with contrast material(s)

(For cervical spinal canal imaging without contrast material followed by contrast material, use 72156)

72146 Magnetic resonance (eg, proton) imaging, spinal canal and contents, thoracic; without contrast material

72147 with contrast material(s)

(For thoracic spinal canal imaging without contrast material followed by contrast material, use 72157)

72148 Magnetic resonance (eg, proton) imaging, spinal canal and contents, lumbar; without contrast material

72149 with contrast material(s)

(For lumbar spinal canal imaging without contrast material followed by contrast material, use 72158)

72156 Magnetic resonance (eg, proton) imaging, spinal canal and contents, without contrast material, followed by contrast material(s) and further sequences; cervical

72157 thoracic

72158 lumbar

72159 Magnetic resonance angiography, spinal canal and contents, with or without contrast material(s)

72170 Radiologic examination, pelvis; one or two views

72190 complete, minimum of three views

(For pelvimetry, use 74710)

72191 Computed tomographic angiography, pelvis; without contrast material(s), followed by contrast material(s) and further sections, including image post-processing

(For CTA aorto-iliofemoral runoff, use 75635)

72192 Computed tomography, pelvis; without contrast material

72193 with contrast material(s)

72194 without contrast material, followed by contrast material(s) and further sections

(To report 3D rendering, see 76376, 76377)

(For computed tomographic colonography, see Category III codes 0066T, 0067T. Do not report 72192-72194 in conjunction with 0066T, 0067T)

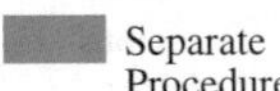
Separate Procedure

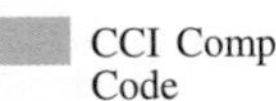
Unlisted Procedure
CCI Comp. Code

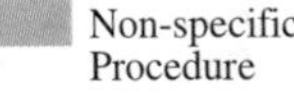
Non-specific Procedure

72195 Magnetic resonance (eg, proton) imaging, pelvis; without contrast material(s)

72196 with contrast material(s)

72197 without contrast material(s), followed by contrast material(s) and further sequences

72198 Magnetic resonance angiography, pelvis, with or without contrast material(s)

72200 Radiologic examination, sacroiliac joints; less than three views

72202 three or more views

72220 Radiologic examination, sacrum and coccyx, minimum of two views

72240 Myelography, cervical, radiological supervision and interpretation

(For complete cervical myelography, see 61055, 62284, 72240)

72255 Myelography, thoracic, radiological supervision and interpretation

(For complete thoracic myelography, see 61055, 62284, 72255)

72265 Myelography, lumbosacral, radiological supervision and interpretation

(For complete lumbosacral myelography, see 61055, 62284, 72265)

72270 Myelography, two or more regions (eg, lumbar/thoracic, cervical/thoracic, lumbar/cervical, lumbar/thoracic/cervical), radiological supervision and interpretation

(For complete myelography of entire spinal canal, see 61055, 62284, 72270)

72275 Epidurography, radiological supervision and interpretation

(72275 includes 77003)

(For injection procedure, see 62280-62282, 62310-62319, 64479-64484, 0027T)

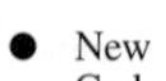

● New Code ▲ Revised Code + Add-On Code ⃠ Modifier -51 Exempt ⊙ Conscious Sedation

(Use 72275 only when an epidurogram is performed, images documented, and a formal radiologic report is issued)

72285 Diskography, cervical or thoracic, radiological supervision and interpretation

● **72291** Radiological supervision and interpretation, percutaneous vertebroplasty or vertebral augmentation including cavity creation, per vertebral body; under fluoroscopic guidance

● **72292** Radiological supervision and interpretation, percutaneous vertebroplasty or vertebral augmentation including cavity creation, per vertebral body; under CT guidance

(For procedure, see 22520-22525)

72295 Diskography, lumbar, radiological supervision and interpretation

UPPER EXTREMITIES

(For stress views, any joint, use 77071)

73000 Radiologic examination; clavicle, complete

73010 scapula, complete

73020 Radiologic examination, shoulder; one view

73030 complete, minimum of two views

73040 Radiologic examination, shoulder, arthrography, radiological supervision and interpretation

(Do not report 77002 in conjunction with 73040)

73050 Radiologic examination; acromioclavicular joints, bilateral, with or without weighted distraction

73060 humerus, minimum of two views

73070 Radiologic examination, elbow; two views

73080 complete, minimum of three views

73085 Radiologic examination, elbow, arthrography, radiological supervision and interpretation

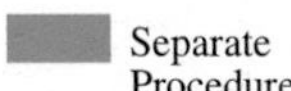

Separate Procedure | Unlisted Procedure | CCI Comp. Code | Non-specific Procedure

(Do not report 77002 in conjunction with 73085)

73090 Radiologic examination; forearm, two views

73092 upper extremity, infant, minimum of two views

73100 Radiologic examination, wrist; two views

73110 complete, minimum of three views

73115 Radiologic examination, wrist, arthrography, radiological supervision and interpretation

(Do not report 77002 in conjunction with 73115)

73120 Radiologic examination, hand; two views

73130 minimum of three views

73140 Radiologic examination, finger(s), minimum of two views

73200 Computed tomography, upper extremity; without contrast material

73201 with contrast material(s)

73202 without contrast material, followed by contrast material(s) and further sections

(To report 3D rendering, see 76376, 76377)

73206 Computed tomographic angiography, upper extremity, without contrast material(s), followed by contrast material(s) and further sections, including image post-processing

73218 Magnetic resonance (eg, proton) imaging, upper extremity, other than joint; without contrast material(s)

73219 with contrast material(s)

73220 without contrast material(s), followed by contrast material(s) and further sequences

73221 Magnetic resonance (eg, proton) imaging, any joint of upper extremity; without contrast material(s)

73222 with contrast material(s)

● New Code ▲ Revised Code + Add-On Code ⊘ Modifier -51 Exempt ⊙ Conscious Sedation

73223 without contrast material(s), followed by contrast material(s) and further sequences

73225 Magnetic resonance angiography, upper extremity, with or without contrast material(s)

LOWER EXTREMITIES

(For stress views, any joint, use 77071)

73500 Radiologic examination, hip, unilateral; one view

73510 complete, minimum of two views

73520 Radiologic examination, hips, bilateral, minimum of two views of each hip, including anteroposterior view of pelvis

73525 Radiologic examination, hip, arthrography, radiological supervision and interpretation

(Do not report 73525 in conjunction with 77002)

73530 Radiologic examination, hip, during operative procedure

73540 Radiologic examination, pelvis and hips, infant or child, minimum of two views

73542 Radiological examination, sacroiliac joint arthrography, radiological supervision and interpretation

(Do not report 73542 in conjunction with 77002)

(For procedure, use 27096. If formal arthrography is not performed, recorded, and a formal radiologic report is not issued, use 77003 for fluoroscopic guidance for sacroiliac joint injections)

73550 Radiologic examination, femur, two views

73560 Radiologic examination, knee; one or two views

73562 three views

73564 complete, four or more views

73565 both knees, standing, anteroposterior

73580 Radiologic examination, knee, arthrography, radiological supervision and interpretation

(Do not report 73580 in conjunction with 77002)

73590 Radiologic examination; tibia and fibula, two views

73592 lower extremity, infant, minimum of two views

73600 Radiologic examination, ankle; two views

73610 complete, minimum of three views

73615 Radiologic examination, ankle, arthrography, radiological supervision and interpretation

(Do not report 73615 in conjunction with 77002)

73620 Radiologic examination, foot; two views

73630 complete, minimum of three views

73650 Radiologic examination; calcaneus, minimum of two views

73660 toe(s), minimum of two views

73700 Computed tomography, lower extremity; without contrast material

73701 with contrast material(s)

73702 without contrast material, followed by contrast material(s) and further sections

(To report 3D rendering, see 76376, 76377)

73706 Computed tomographic angiography, lower extremity, without contrast material(s), followed by contrast material(s) and further sections, including image post-processing

(For CTA aorto-iliofemoral runoff, use 75635)

73718 Magnetic resonance (eg, proton) imaging, lower extremity, other than joint; without contrast material(s)

73719 with contrast material(s)

73720 without contrast material(s), followed by contrast material(s) and further sequences

73721 Magnetic resonance (eg, proton) imaging, any joint of lower extremity; without contrast material

73722 with contrast material

73723 without contrast material followed by contrast material(s) and further sequences

73725 Magnetic resonance angiography, lower extremity, with or without contrast material(s)

ABDOMEN

74000 Radiologic examination, abdomen; single anteroposterior view

74010 anteroposterior and additional oblique and cone views

74020 complete, including decubitus and/or erect views

74022 complete acute abdomen series, including supine, erect, and/or decubitus views, single view chest

74150 Computed tomography, abdomen; without contrast material

74160 with contrast material(s)

74170 without contrast material, followed by contrast material(s) and further sections

(To report 3D rendering, see 76376, 76377)

(For computed tomographic colonography, see Category III codes 0066T, 0067T. Do not report 74150-74170 in conjunction with 0066T, 0067T)

74175 Computed tomographic angiography, abdomen, without contrast material(s), followed by contrast material(s) and further sections, including image post-processing

(For CTA aorto-iliofemoral runoff, use 75635)

74181 Magnetic resonance (eg, proton) imaging, abdomen; without contrast material(s)

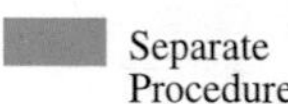 Separate Procedure  Unlisted Procedure 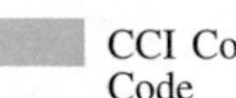 CCI Comp. Code 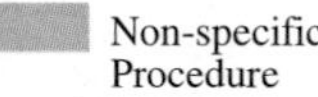 Non-specific Procedure

74182 with contrast material(s)

74183 without contrast material, followed by contrast material(s) and further sequences

74185 Magnetic resonance angiography, abdomen, with or without contrast material(s)

74190 Peritoneogram (eg, after injection of air or contrast), radiological supervision and interpretation

(For procedure, use 49400)

(For computerized axial tomography, see 72192 or 74150)

GASTROINTESTINAL TRACT

(For percutaneous placement of gastrostomy tube, use 43750)

74210 Radiologic examination; pharynx and/or cervical esophagus

74220 esophagus

74230 Swallowing function, with cineradiography/videoradiography

74235 Removal of foreign body(s), esophageal, with use of balloon catheter, radiological supervision and interpretation

(For procedure, see 43215, 43247)

74240 Radiologic examination, gastrointestinal tract, upper; with or without delayed films, without KUB

74241 with or without delayed films, with KUB

74245 with small intestine, includes multiple serial films

74246 Radiological examination, gastrointestinal tract, upper, air contrast, with specific high density barium, effervescent agent, with or without glucagon; with or without delayed films, without KUB

74247 with or without delayed films, with KUB

74249 with small intestine follow-through

74250 Radiologic examination, small intestine, includes multiple serial films;

74251 via enteroclysis tube

74260 Duodenography, hypotonic

74270 Radiologic examination, colon; barium enema, with or without KUB

74280 air contrast with specific high density barium, with or without glucagon

74283 Therapeutic enema, contrast or air, for reduction of intussusception or other intraluminal obstruction (eg, meconium ileus)

74290 Cholecystography, oral contrast;

74291 additional or repeat examination or multiple day examination

74300 Cholangiography and/or pancreatography; intraoperative, radiological supervision and interpretation

+ **74301** additional set intraoperative, radiological supervision and interpretation (List separately in addition to code for primary procedure)

(Use 74301 in conjunction with code 74300)

74305 through existing catheter, radiological supervision and interpretation

(For procedure, see 47505, 48400, 47560-47561, 47563)

(For biliary duct stone extraction, percutaneous, see 47630, 74327)

74320 Cholangiography, percutaneous, transhepatic, radiological supervision and interpretation

74327 Postoperative biliary duct calculus removal, percutaneous via T-tube tract, basket, or snare (eg, Burhenne technique), radiological supervision and interpretation

(For procedure, use 47630)

74328 Endoscopic catheterization of the biliary ductal system, radiological supervision and interpretation

(For procedure, see 43260-43272 as appropriate)

74329 Endoscopic catheterization of the pancreatic ductal system, radiological supervision and interpretation

(For procedure, see 43260-43272 as appropriate)

74330 Combined endoscopic catheterization of the biliary and pancreatic ductal systems, radiological supervision and interpretation

(For procedure, see 43260-43272 as appropriate)

74340 Introduction of long gastrointestinal tube (eg, Miller-Abbott), including multiple fluoroscopies and films, radiological supervision and interpretation

(For tube placement, use 44500)

74350 Percutaneous placement of gastrostomy tube, radiological supervision and interpretation

74355 Percutaneous placement of enteroclysis tube, radiological supervision and interpretation

74360 Intraluminal dilation of strictures and/or obstructions (eg, esophagus), radiological supervision and interpretation

74363 Percutaneous transhepatic dilation of biliary duct stricture with or without placement of stent, radiological supervision and interpretation

(For procedure, see 47510, 47511, 47555, 47556)

URINARY TRACT

74400 Urography (pyelography), intravenous, with or without KUB, with or without tomography

74410 Urography, infusion, drip technique and/or bolus technique;

74415 with nephrotomography

74420 Urography, retrograde, with or without KUB

74425 Urography, antegrade, (pyelostogram, nephrostogram, loopogram), radiological supervision and interpretation

74430 Cystography, minimum of three views, radiological supervision and interpretation

74440 Vasography, vesiculography, or epididymography, radiological supervision and interpretation

74445 Corpora cavernosography, radiological supervision and interpretation

74450 Urethrocystography, retrograde, radiological supervision and interpretation

74455 Urethrocystography, voiding, radiological supervision and interpretation

74470 Radiologic examination, renal cyst study, translumbar, contrast visualization, radiological supervision and interpretation

74475 Introduction of intracatheter or catheter into renal pelvis for drainage and/or injection, percutaneous, radiological supervision and interpretation

74480 Introduction of ureteral catheter or stent into ureter through renal pelvis for drainage and/or injection, percutaneous, radiological supervision and interpretation

(For transurethral surgery (ureter and pelvis), see 52320-52355)

74485 Dilation of nephrostomy, ureters, or urethra, radiological supervision and interpretation

(For dilation of ureter without radiologic guidance, use 52341, 52344)

(For change of nephrostomy or pyelostomy tube, use 50398)

GYNECOLOGICAL AND OBSTETRICAL

(For abdomen and pelvis, see 72170-72190, 74000-74170)

74710 Pelvimetry, with or without placental localization

74740 Hysterosalpingography, radiological supervision and interpretation

(For introduction of saline or contrast for hysterosalpingography, see 58340)

74742 Transcervical catheterization of fallopian tube, radiological supervision and interpretation

(For procedure, use 58345)

74775 Perineogram (eg, vaginogram, for sex determination or extent of anomalies)

HEART

(For separate injection procedures for vascular radiology, see Surgery section, 36000-36299)

(For cardiac catheterization procedures, see 93501-93556)

75552 Cardiac magnetic resonance imaging for morphology; without contrast material

75553 with contrast material

75554 Cardiac magnetic resonance imaging for function, with or without morphology; complete study

75555 limited study

75556 Cardiac magnetic resonance imaging for velocity flow mapping

VASCULAR PROCEDURES

AORTA AND ARTERIES

(For intravenous procedure, see 36000-36013, 36400-36425 and 36100-36248 for intra-arterial procedure)

(For radiological supervision and interpretation, see 75600-75978)

75600 Aortography, thoracic, without serialography, radiological supervision and interpretation

(For injection procedure, use 93544)

75605 Aortography, thoracic, by serialography, radiological supervision and interpretation

(For injection procedure, use 93544)

75625 Aortography, abdominal, by serialography, radiological supervision and interpretation

(For injection procedure, use 93544)

75630 Aortography, abdominal plus bilateral iliofemoral lower extremity, catheter, by serialography, radiological supervision and interpretation

75635 Computed tomographic angiography, abdominal aorta and bilateral iliofemoral lower extremity runoff, radiological supervision and interpretation, without contrast material(s), followed by contrast material(s) and further sections, including image post-processing

75650 Angiography, cervicocerebral, catheter, including vessel origin, radiological supervision and interpretation

75658 Angiography, brachial, retrograde, radiological supervision and interpretation

75660 Angiography, external carotid, unilateral, selective, radiological supervision and interpretation

75662 Angiography, external carotid, bilateral, selective, radiological supervision and interpretation

75665 Angiography, carotid, cerebral, unilateral, radiological supervision and interpretation

75671 Angiography, carotid, cerebral, bilateral, radiological supervision and interpretation

75676 Angiography, carotid, cervical, unilateral, radiological supervision and interpretation

75680 Angiography, carotid, cervical, bilateral, radiological supervision and interpretation

75685 Angiography, vertebral, cervical, and/or intracranial, radiological supervision and interpretation

75705 Angiography, spinal, selective, radiological supervision and interpretation

75710 Angiography, extremity, unilateral, radiological supervision and interpretation

75716 Angiography, extremity, bilateral, radiological supervision and interpretation

75722 Angiography, renal, unilateral, selective (including flush aortogram), radiological supervision and interpretation

75724 Angiography, renal, bilateral, selective (including flush aortogram), radiological supervision and interpretation

75726 Angiography, visceral, selective or supraselective, (with or without flush aortogram), radiological supervision and interpretation

(For selective angiography, each additional visceral vessel studied after basic examination, use 75774)

75731 Angiography, adrenal, unilateral, selective, radiological supervision and interpretation

75733 Angiography, adrenal, bilateral, selective, radiological supervision and interpretation

75736 Angiography, pelvic, selective or supraselective, radiological supervision and interpretation

75741 Angiography, pulmonary, unilateral, selective, radiological supervision and interpretation

(For injection procedure, use 93541)

75743 Angiography, pulmonary, bilateral, selective, radiological supervision and interpretation

(For injection procedure, use 93541)

75746 Angiography, pulmonary, by nonselective catheter or venous injection, radiological supervision and interpretation

(For injection procedure, use 93541)

(For introduction of catheter, injection procedure, see 93501-93533, 93539, 93540, 93545, 93556)

75756 Angiography, internal mammary, radiological supervision and interpretation

(For introduction of catheter, injection procedure, see 93501-93533, 93545, 93556)

+ **75774** Angiography, selective, each additional vessel studied after basic examination, radiological supervision and interpretation (List separately in addition to code for primary procedure)

(Use 75774 in addition to code for specific initial vessel studied)

(For angiography, see codes 75600-75790)

(For catheterizations, see codes 36215-36248)

(For introduction of catheter, injection procedure, see 93501-93533, 93545, 93555, 93556)

75790 Angiography, arteriovenous shunt (eg, dialysis patient), radiological supervision and interpretation

(For introduction of catheter, use 36140, 36145, 36215-36217, 36245-36247)

VEINS AND LYMPHATICS

(For injection procedure for venous system, see 36000-36015, 36400-36510)

(For injection procedure for lymphatic system, use 38790)

75801 Lymphangiography, extremity only, unilateral, radiological supervision and interpretation

75803 Lymphangiography, extremity only, bilateral, radiological supervision and interpretation

75805 Lymphangiography, pelvic/abdominal, unilateral, radiological supervision and interpretation

75807 Lymphangiography, pelvic/abdominal, bilateral, radiological supervision and interpretation

75809 Shuntogram for investigation of previously placed indwelling nonvascular shunt (eg, LeVeen shunt, ventriculoperitoneal shunt, indwelling infusion pump), radiological supervision and interpretation

(For procedure, see 49427 or 61070)

75810 Splenoportography, radiological supervision and interpretation

75820 Venography, extremity, unilateral, radiological supervision and interpretation

75822 Venography, extremity, bilateral, radiological supervision and interpretation

75825 Venography, caval, inferior, with serialography, radiological supervision and interpretation

75827 Venography, caval, superior, with serialography, radiological supervision and interpretation

75831 Venography, renal, unilateral, selective, radiological supervision and interpretation

75833 Venography, renal, bilateral, selective, radiological supervision and interpretation

75840 Venography, adrenal, unilateral, selective, radiological supervision and interpretation

75842 Venography, adrenal, bilateral, selective, radiological supervision and interpretation

75860 Venography, venous sinus (eg, petrosal and inferior sagittal) or jugular, catheter, radiological supervision and interpretation

75870 Venography, superior sagittal sinus, radiological supervision and interpretation

75872 Venography, epidural, radiological supervision and interpretation

75880 Venography, orbital, radiological supervision and interpretation

75885 Percutaneous transhepatic portography with hemodynamic evaluation, radiological supervision and interpretation

75887 Percutaneous transhepatic portography without hemodynamic evaluation, radiological supervision and interpretation

75889 Hepatic venography, wedged or free, with hemodynamic evaluation, radiological supervision and interpretation

75891 Hepatic venography, wedged or free, without hemodynamic evaluation, radiological supervision and interpretation

75893 Venous sampling through catheter, with or without angiography (eg, for parathyroid hormone, renin), radiological supervision and interpretation

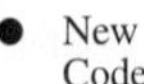

▲ Revised Code + Add-On Code ⦸ Modifier -51 Exempt ⊙ Conscious Sedation

(For procedure, use 36500)

TRANSCATHETER PROCEDURES

75894 Transcatheter therapy, embolization, any method, radiological supervision and interpretation

(For uterine fibroid embolization [uterine artery embolization performed to treat uterine fibroids], use 37210)

(For obstetrical and gynecological embolization procedures other than uterine fibroid embolization [eg., embolization to treat obstetrical or postpartum hemorrhage], use 37204)

75896 Transcatheter therapy, infusion, any method (eg, thrombolysis other than coronary), radiological supervision and interpretation

(For infusion for coronary disease, see 92975, 92977)

75898 Angiography through existing catheter for follow-up study for transcatheter therapy, embolization or infusion

75900 Exchange of a previously placed intravascular catheter during thrombolytic therapy with contrast monitoring, radiological supervision and interpretation

(For procedure, use 37209)

75901 Mechanical removal of pericatheter obstructive material (eg., fibrin sheath) from central venous device via separate venous access, radiologic supervision and interpretation

(For procedure, use 36595)

(For venous catheterization, see 36010-36012)

75902 Mechanical removal of intraluminal (intracatheter) obstructive material from central venous device through device lumen, radiologic supervision and interpretation

(For procedure, use 36596)

(For venous catheterization, see 36010-36012)

75940 Percutaneous placement of IVC filter, radiological supervision and interpretation

75945 Intravascular ultrasound (non-coronary vessel), radiological supervision and interpretation; initial vessel

+ **75946** each additional non-coronary vessel (List separately in addition to code for primary procedure)

(Use 75946 in conjunction with code 75945)

(For catheterizations, see codes 36215-36248)

(For transcatheter therapies, see codes 37200-37208, 61624, 61626)

(For procedure, see 37250, 37251)

75952 Endovascular repair of infrarenal abdominal aortic aneurysm or dissection, radiological supervision and interpretation

(For implantation of endovascular grafts, see 34800-34808)

(For radiologic supervision and interpretation of endovascular repair of abdominal aortic aneurysm involving visceral vessels, see Category III codes 0078T-0081T)

75953 Placement of proximal or distal extension prosthesis for endovascular repair of infrarenal aortic or iliac artery aneurysm, pseudoaneurysm, or dissection, radiological supervision and interpretation

(For implantation of endovascular extension prostheses, see 34825, 34826)

75954 Endovascular repair of iliac artery aneurysm, psuedoaneurysm, arteriovenous malformation, or trauma, radiological supervision and interpretation

(For implantation of endovascular graft, see 34900)

75956 Endovascular repair of descending thoracic aorta (eg, aneurysm, pseudoaneurysm, dissection, penetrating ulcer, intramural hematoma, or traumatic disruption); involving coverage of left subclavian artery origin, initial endoprosthesis plus descending thoracic aortic extension(s), if required, to level of celiac artery origin, radiological supervision and interpretation

(For implantation of endovascular graft, use 33880)

75957 not involving coverage of left subclavian artery origin, initial endoprosthesis plus descending thoracic aortic extension(s), if required, to level of celiac artery origin, radiological supervision and interpretation

(For implantation of endovascular graft, use 33881)

75958 Placement of proximal extension prosthesis for endovascular repair of descending thoracic aorta (eg, aneurysm, pseudoaneurysm, dissection, penetrating ulcer, intramural hematoma, or traumatic disruption), radiological supervision and interpretation

(Report 75958 for each proximal extension)

(For implantation of proximal endovascular extension, see 33883, 33884)

75959 Placement of distal extension prosthesis(es) (delayed) after endovascular repair of descending thoracic aorta, as needed, to level of celiac origin, radiological supervision and interpretation

(Do not report 75959 in conjunction with 75956, 75957)

(Report 75959 once, regardless of number of modules deployed)

(For implantation of distal endovascular extension, use 33886)

75960 Transcatheter introduction of intravascular stent(s), (except coronary, carotid, and vertebral vessel), percutaneous and/or open, radiological supervision and interpretation, each vessel

(For procedure, see 37205-37208)

(For radiologic supervision and interpretation for transcatheter placement of extracranial vertebral or intrathoracic carotid artery stent(s), see Category III codes 0075T, 0076T)

75961 Transcatheter retrieval, percutaneous, of intravascular foreign body (eg, fractured venous or arterial catheter), radiological supervision and interpretation

(For procedure, use 37203)

75962 Transluminal balloon angioplasty, peripheral artery, radiological supervision and interpretation

\+ **75964** Transluminal balloon angioplasty, each additional peripheral artery, radiological supervision and interpretation (List separately in addition to code for primary procedure)

(Use 75964 in conjunction with code 75962)

75966 Transluminal balloon angioplasty, renal or other visceral artery, radiological supervision and interpretation

+ **75968** Transluminal balloon angioplasty, each additional visceral artery, radiological supervision and interpretation (List separately in addition to code for primary procedure)

(Use 75968 in conjunction with code 75966)

(For percutaneous transluminal coronary angioplasty, see 92982-92984)

75970 Transcatheter biopsy, radiological supervision and interpretation

(For injection procedure only for transcatheter therapy or biopsy, see 36100-36299)

(For transcatheter renal and ureteral biopsy, use 52007)

(For percutaneous needle biopsy of pancreas, use 48102; of retroperitoneal lymph node or mass, use 49180)

75978 Transluminal balloon angioplasty, venous (eg, subclavian stenosis), radiological supervision and interpretation

75980 Percutaneous transhepatic biliary drainage with contrast monitoring, radiological supervision and interpretation

75982 Percutaneous placement of drainage catheter for combined internal and external biliary drainage or of a drainage stent for internal biliary drainage in patients with an inoperable mechanical biliary obstruction, radiological supervision and interpretation

75984 Change of percutaneous tube or drainage catheter with contrast monitoring (eg, gastrointestinal system, genitourinary system, abscess), radiological supervision and interpretation

(For change of nephrostomy or pyelostomy tube only, use 50398)

(For introduction procedure only for percutaneous biliary drainage, see 47510, 47511)

(For percutaneous choloecystostomy, use 47490)

(For change of percutaneous biliary drainage catheter only, use 47525)

(For percutaneous nephrostolithotomy or pyelostolithotomy, see 50080, 50081)

75989 Radiological guidance (ie, fluoroscopy, ultrasound, or computed tomography), for percutaneous drainage (eg., abscess, specimen collection), with placement of catheter, radiological supervision and interpretation

TRANSLUMINAL ATHERECTOMY

75992 Transluminal atherectomy, peripheral artery, radiological supervision and interpretation

(For procedure, see 35481-35485, 35491-35495)

+ **75993** Transluminal atherectomy, each additional peripheral artery, radiological supervision and interpretation (List separately in addition to code for primary procedure)

(Use 75993 in conjunction with code 75992)

(For procedure, see 35481-35485, 35491-35495)

75994 Transluminal atherectomy, renal, radiological supervision and interpretation

(For procedure, see 35480, 35490)

75995 Transluminal atherectomy, visceral, radiological supervision and interpretation

(For procedure, see 35480, 35490)

+ **75996** Transluminal atherectomy, each additional visceral artery, radiological supervision and interpretation (List separately in addition to code for primary procedure)

(Use 75996 in conjunction with code 75995)

(For procedure, see 35480, 35490)

OTHER PROCEDURES

(For computed tomography cerebral perfusion analysis, see Category III code 0042T)

(For arthrography of shoulder, use 73040; elbow, use 73085; wrist, use 73115; hip, use 73525; knee, use 73580; ankle, use 73615)

(75998 deleted 2007 edition, see 77001)

76000 Fluoroscopy (separate procedure), up to one hour physician time, other than 71023 or 71034 (eg, cardiac fluoroscopy)

76001 Fluoroscopy, physician time more than one hour, assisting a non-radiologic physician (eg, nephrostolithotomy, ERCP, bronchoscopy, transbronchial biopsy)

(76003 deleted 2007 edition, see 77002)

(76005 deleted 2007 edition, see 77003)

(76006 deleted 2007 edition, see 77071

76010 Radiologic examination from nose to rectum for foreign body, single view, child

(76012 deleted 2007 edition, see 72291)

(76013 deleted 2007 edition, see 72292)

(76020 deleted 2007 edition, see 77072)

(76040 deleted 2007 edition, see 77073)

(76061 deleted 2007 edition, see 77074)

(76062 deleted 2007 edition, see 77075)

(76065 deleted 2007 edition, see 77076)

(76066 deleted 2007 edition, see 77077)

(76070 deleted 2007 edition, see 77078)

(76071 deleted 2007 edition, see 77079)

(76075 deleted 2007 edition, see 77080)

(76076 deleted 2007 edition, see 77081)

(76077 deleted 2007 edition, see 77082)

(76078 deleted 2007 edition, see 77083)

76080 Radiologic examination, abscess, fistula or sinus tract study, radiological supervision and interpretation

(76082 deleted 2007 edition, see 77051)

(76083 deleted 2007 edition, see 77052)

(76085 deleted. To report, see 76082, 76083)

(76086 deleted 2007 edition, see 77053)

(76088 deleted 2007 edition, see 77054)

(76090 deleted 2007 edition, see 77055)

(76091 deleted 2007 edition, see 77056)

(76092 deleted 2007 edition, see 77057)

(76093 deleted 2007 edition, see 77058)

(76094 deleted 2007 edition, see 77059)

(76095 deleted 2007 edition, see 77031)

(76096 deleted 2007 edition, see 77032)

76098 Radiological examination, surgical specimen

76100 Radiologic examination, single plane body section (eg, tomography), other than with urography

76101 Radiologic examination, complex motion (ie, hypercycloidal) body section (eg, mastoid polytomography), other than with urography; unilateral

76102 bilateral

(For nephrotomography, use 74415)

76120 Cineradiography/videoradiography, except where specifically included

+ **76125** Cineradiography/videoradiography to complement routine examination (List separately in addition to code for primary procedure)

76140 Consultation on x-ray examination made elsewhere, written report

76150 Xeroradiography

Separate Procedure | Unlisted Procedure | CCI Comp. Code | Non-specific Procedure

(76150 is to be used for non-mammographic studies only)

76350 Subtraction in conjunction with contrast studies

(76355 deleted 2007 edition, see 77011)

(76360 deleted 2007 edition, see 77012)

(76362 deleted 2007 edition, see 77013)

(76370 deleted 2007 edition, see 77014)

(76375 deleted 2006 edition.)

(2D reformatting is no longer separately reported. To report 3D rendering, see 76376, 76377)

(Codes 76376, 76377 require concurrent physician supervision of image postprocessing 3D manipulation of volumetric data set and image rendering)

76376 3D rendering with interpretation and reporting of computed tomography, magnetic resonance imaging, ultrasound, or other tomographic modality; not requiring image postprocessing on an independent workstation

(Use 76376 in conjunction with code(s) for base imaging procedure(s))

(Do not report 76376 in conjunction with 70496, 70498, 70544-70549, 71275, 71555, 72159, 72191, 72198, 73206, 73225, 73706, 73725, 74175, 74185, 75635, 76377, 78000-78999, 0066T, 0067T, 0144T-0151T)

76377 requiring image postprocessing on an independent workstation

(Use 76377 in conjunction with code(s) for base imaging procedure(s))

(Do not report 76377 in conjunction with 70496, 70498, 70544-70549, 71275, 71555, 72159, 72191, 72198, 73206, 73225, 73225, 73706, 73725, 74175, 74185, 75635, 76376, 78000-78999, 0066T, 0067T, 0144T-0151T)

76380 Computed tomography, limited or localized follow-up study

76390 Magnetic resonance spectroscopy

(For magnetic resonance imaging, use appropriate MRI body site code)

(76393 deleted 2007 edition, see 77021)

(76394 deleted 2007 edition, see 77022)

(76400 deleted 2007 edition, see 77084)

(76490 deleted 2004 edition. To report, use 76940)

76496 Unlisted fluoroscopic procedure (eg., diagnostic, interventional)

76497 Unlisted computed tomography procedure (eg., diagnostic, interventional)

76498 Unlisted magnetic resonance procedure (eg., diagnostic, interventional)

76499 Unlisted diagnostic radiographic procedure

DIAGNOSTIC ULTRASOUND

Diagnostic ultrasound is a non-invasive medical imaging technology that uses high frequency sound waves to form an image of body tissues. Information obtained from these images can be utilized along with other patient data in order to arrive at a medical diagnosis. Ultrasound, when compared to other imaging modalities like MRI (Magnetic Resonance Imaging) and CT (Computed Tomography), is a relatively low cost non-invasive procedure that does not utilize either magnetic fields or ionizing radiation (x-rays).

ULTRASOUND MODES

A-mode *Now obsolete in medical imaging. Wave spikes are represented when a single beam passes through objects of different consistency and hardness. The distance between these spikes (for example A and B) can be measured accurately by dividing the speed of sound in tissue (1540 m/sec) by half the sound travel time.*

B-mode *Same as A-mode, but one-dimensional graphical display, with brightness corresponding to amplitude of reflected sound.*

M-mode *A single beam in an ultrasound scan can be used to produce an M-mode picture, where movement of a structure such as a heart valve can be depicted in a wave-like manner. Because of its high sampling frequency (up to 1000 pulses per second), this is useful in assessing rates and motion and is still used extensively in cardiac and fetal cardiac imaging.*

2D-real time *Most modern ultrasound devices are 2D-real time imaging systems. Multiple crystals (linear, curved or phased-array) or moving crystal. Sequential B-mode pulses sweeping across a plane to display the image in either a linear or 'sector' format. Displayed as real time imaging with up to 100 images per second.*

Abdominal ultrasound examinations (CPT codes 76700-76775) and abdominal duplex examinations (CPT codes 93975, 93976) are generally performed for different clinical scenarios although there are some instances where both types of procedures are medically reasonable and necessary. In the latter case, the abdominal ultrasound procedure CPT code should be reported with an NCCI associated modifier.

(To report diagnostic vascular ultrasound studies, see 93875-93990)

(For focused ultrasound ablation treatment of uterine leiomyomata, see Category III codes 0071T, 0072T)

HEAD AND NECK

▲ **76506** Echoencephalography, real time with image documentation (gray scale) (for determination of ventricular size, delineation of cerebral contents and detection of fluid masses or other intracranial abnormalities), including A-mode encephalography as secondary component where indicated

76510 Ophthalmic ultrasound, diagnostic; B-scan and quantitative A-scan performed during the same patient encounter

76511 Ophthalmic ultrasound, diagnostic; quantitative A-scan only

76512 B-scan (with or without superimposed non-quantitative A-scan)

76513 anterior segment ultrasound, immersion (water bath) B-scan or high resolution biomicroscopy

76514 corneal pachymetry, unilateral or bilateral (determination of corneal thickness)

76516 Ophthalmic biometry by ultrasound echography, A-scan;

76519 with intraocular lens power calculation

(For partial coherence interferometry, use 92136)

76529 Ophthalmic ultrasonic foreign body localization

▲ **76536** Ultrasound, soft tissues of head and neck (eg, thyroid, parathyroid, parotid), real time with image documentation

CHEST

▲ **76604** Ultrasound, chest, (includes mediastinum) real time with image documentation

▲ **76645** Ultrasound, breast(s) (unilateral or bilateral), real time with image documentation

ABDOMEN AND PERITONEUM

▲ **76700** Ultrasound, abdominal, real time with image documentation; complete

76705 limited (eg, single organ, quadrant, follow-up)

▲ **76770** Ultrasound, retroperitoneal (eg, renal, aorta, nodes), real time with image documentation; complete

76775 limited

● **76776** Ultrasound, transplanted kidney, real time and duplex Doppler with image documentation

(For ultrasound or transplanted kidney without duplex Doppler, use 76775)

(Do not report 76776 in conjunction with 93975, 93976)

(76778 deleted 2007 edition, see 76775, 76776)

SPINAL CANAL

76800 Ultrasound, spinal canal and contents

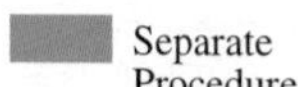
Separate Procedure

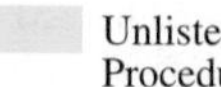
Unlisted Procedure

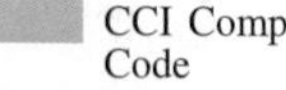
CCI Comp. Code

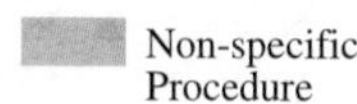
Non-specific Procedure

PELVIS

OBSTETRICAL

76801 Ultrasound, pregnant uterus, real time with image documentation, fetal and maternal evaluation, first trimester (>14 weeks 0 days), transabdominal approach; single or first gestation

(To report first trimester fetal nuchal translucency measurement, use 76813)

+ **76802** each additional gestation (List separately in addition to code for primary procedure)

(Use 76802 in conjunction with code 76801)

(To report first trimester fetal nuchal translucency measurement, use 76814)

76805 Ultrasound, pregnant uterus, real time with image documentation, fetal and maternal evaluation, after first trimester (>or = 14 weeks 0 days), transabdominal approach; single or first gestation

+ **76810** each additional gestation (List separately in addition to code for primary procedure)

(Use 76810 in conjunction with code 76805)

76811 Ultrasound, pregnant uterus, real time with image documentation, fetal and maternal evaluation plus detailed fetal anatomic examination, transabdominal approach; single or first gestation

+ **76812** each additional gestation (List separately in addition to code for primary procedure)

(Use 76812 in conjunction with code 76811)

● **76813** Ultrasound, pregnant uterus, real time with image documentation, first trimester fetal nuchal translucency measurement, transabdominal or transvaginal approach; single or first gestation

●+**76814** each additional gestation (List separately in addition to code for primary procedure)

(Use 76814 in conjunction with 76813)

76815 Ultrasound, pregnant uterus, real time with image documentation, limited (eg., fetal heart beat, placental location, fetal position, and/or qualitative amniotic fluid volume), one or more fetuses

(Use 76815 only once per exam and not per element)

(To report first trimester fetal nuchal translucency measurement, see 76813, 76814)

76816 Ultrasound, pregnant uterus, real time with image documentation, follow-up (eg., re-evaluation of fetal size by measuring standard growth parameters and amniotic fluid volume, re-evaluation of organ system(s) suspected or confirmed to be abnormal on a previous scan), transabdominal approach, per fetus

(Report 76816 with modifier -59 for each additional fetus examined in a multiple pregnancy)

76817 Ultrasound, pregnant uterus, real time with image documentation, transvaginal

(For non-obstetrical transvaginal ultrasound, use 76830)

(If transvaginal examination is done in addition to transabdominal obstetrical ultrasound exam, use 76817 in addition to appropriate transabdominal exam code)

76818 Fetal biophysical profile; with non-stress testing

76819 without non-stress testing

(Fetal biophysical profile assessments for the second and any additional fetuses, should be reported separately by code 76818 or 76819 with the modifier -59 appended)

(For amniotic fluid index without non-stress test, use 76815)

76820 Doppler velocimetry, fetal; umbilical artery

76821 middle cerebral artery

76825 Echocardiography, fetal, cardiovascular system, real time with image documentation (2D), with or without M-mode recording;

76826 follow-up or repeat study

76827 Doppler echocardiography, fetal, pulsed wave and/or continuous wave with spectral display; complete

76828 follow-up or repeat study

(To report the use of color mapping, use 93325)

NON-OBSTETRICAL

76830 Ultrasound, transvaginal

(For obstetrical transvaginal ultrasound, use 76817)

(If transvaginal examination is done in addition to transabdominal non-obstetrical ultrasound exam, use 76830 in addition to appropriate transabdominal exam code)

76831 Saline infusion sonohysterography (SIS), including color flow Doppler, when performed

(For introduction of saline for saline infusion sonohysterography, use 58340)

▲ **76856** Ultrasound, pelvic (nonobstetric), real time with image documentation; complete

76857 limited or follow-up (eg, for follicles)

GENITALIA

76870 Ultrasound, scrotum and contents

76872 Ultrasound, transrectal;

76873 prostate volume study for brachytherapy treatment planning (separate procedure)

EXTREMITIES

▲ **76880** Ultrasound, extremity, non-vascular, real time with image documentation

76885 Ultrasound of infant hips, real time with imaging documentation; dynamic (requiring physician manipulation)

76886 limited, static (not requiring physician manipulation)

ULTRASONIC GUIDANCE PROCEDURES

76930 Ultrasonic guidance for pericardiocentesis, imaging supervision and interpretation

76932 Ultrasonic guidance for endomyocardial biopsy, imaging supervision and interpretation

76936 Ultrasound guided compression repair of arterial pseudoaneurysm or arteriovenous fistulae (includes diagnostic ultrasound evaluation, compression of lesion and imaging)

+ **76937** Ultrasound guidance for vascular access requiring ultrasound evaluation of potential access sites, documentation of selected vessel patency, concurrent realtime ultrasound visualization of vascular needle entry, with permanent recording and reporting (List separately in addition to code for primary procedure)

(Do not use 76937 in conjunction with 76942)

(If extremity venous non-invasive vascular diagnostic study is performed separate from venous access guidance, use 93965, 93970, or 93971)

▲ **76940** Ultrasound guidance for, and monitoring of, parenchymal tissue ablation

(Do not report 76940 in conjunction with 76998)

(For ablation, see 32998, 47370-47382, 50592)

(For percutaneous cryotherapy ablation of renal tumors, use 0135T)

76941 Ultrasonic guidance for intrauterine fetal transfusion or cordocentesis, imaging supervision and interpretation

(For procedure, see 36460, 59012)

76942 Ultrasonic guidance for needle placement (eg, biopsy, aspiration, injection, localization device) imaging supervision and interpretation

(Do not report 76942 in conjunction with 43232, 43237, 43242, 45341, 45342, or 76975)

(For microwave thermotherapy of the breast, use Category III code 0061T)

Separate Procedure | Unlisted Procedure | CCI Comp. Code | Non-specific Procedure

76945 Ultrasonic guidance for chorionic villus sampling, imaging supervision and interpretation

(For procedure, use 59015)

76946 Ultrasonic guidance for amniocentesis, imaging supervision and interpretation

76948 Ultrasonic guidance for aspiration of ova, imaging supervision and interpretation

76950 Ultrasonic guidance for placement of radiation therapy fields

76965 Ultrasonic guidance for interstitial radioelement application

OTHER PROCEDURES

76970 Ultrasound study follow-up (specify)

76975 Gastrointestinal endoscopic ultrasound, imaging supervision and interpretation

(Do not report 76975 in conjunction with 43231, 43232, 43237, 43238, 43242, 43259, 45341, 45342, or 76942)

76977 Ultrasound bone density measurement and interpretation, peripheral site(s), any method

(76986 deleted 2007 edition, see 76998)

● **76998** Ultrasonic guidance, intraoperative

(Do not report 76998 in conjunction with 47370-47382)

(For ultrasound guidance for open and laparoscopic radiofrequency tissue ablation, use 76940)

76999 Unlisted ultrasound procedure (eg., diagnostic, interventional)

RADIOLOGIC GUIDANCE

FLUOROSCOPIC GUIDANCE

●**+77001** Fluoroscopic guidance for central venous access device placement, replacement (catheter only or complete), or removal (includes fluoroscopic guidance for vascular access and catheter manipulation, any necessary contrast injections through access site or catheter with related venography radiologic supervision and interpretation, and radiographic documentation of final catheter position) (List separately in addition to code for primary procedure)

(Do not use 77001 in conjunction with 77002)

(If formal extremity venography is performed from separate venous access and separately interpreted, use 36005 and 75820, 75822, 75825 or 75827)

● **77002** Fluoroscopic guidance for needle placement (eg, biopsy, aspiration, injection, localization device)

(See appropriate surgical code for procedure and anatomic location)

(77002 includes all radiographic arthrography with the exception of supervision and interpretation for CT and MR arthrography)

(Do not report 77002 in addition to 70332, 73040, 73085, 73115, 73525, 73580, 73615)

(77002 is included in the organ/anatomic specific radiological supervision and interpretation procedures 74320, 74350, 74355, 74445, 74470, 74475, 75809, 75810, 75885, 75887, 75980, 75982, 75989)

● **77003** Fluoroscopic guidance and localization of needle or catheter tip for spine or paraspinous diagnostic or therapeutic injection procedures (epidural, transforaminal epidural, subarachnoid, paravertebral facet joint, paravertebral facet joint nerve, or sacroiliac joint), including neurolytic agent destruction

(Injection of contrast during fluoroscopic guidance and localization [77003] is included in 2526, 22527, 62263, 62264, 62270-62282, 62310-62319, 0027T)

(Fluoroscopic guidance for subarachnoid puncture for diagnostic radiographic myelography is included in supervision and interpretation codes 72240-72270)

(For epidural or subarachnoid needle or catheter placement andinjection, see 62270-62282. 62310-62319)

(For sacroiliac joint arthrography, see 27096, 73542. If formal arthrography is not performed and recorded, and a formal radiographic report is not issued, use 77003 for fluoroscopic guidance for sacroiliac joint injections)

(For paravertebral facet joint injection, see 64470-64476. For transforaminal epidural needle placement and injection, see 64479-64484)

(For destruction by neurolytic agent, see 64600-64680)

(For percutaneous or endoscopic lysis of epidural adhesions, 62263, 62264, 0027T include fluoroscopic guidance and localization)

COMPUTED TOMOGRAPHY GUIDANCE

● **77011** Computed tomography guidance for stereotactic localization

● **77012** Computed tomography guidance for needle placement (eg, biopsy, aspiration, injection, localization device), radiological supervision and interpretation

● **77013** Computerized tomography guidance for, and monitoring of, parenchymal tissue ablation

(Do not report 77013 in conjunction with 20982)

(For percutaneous cryotherapy ablation of renal tumors, use 0135T)

(For percutaneous radiofrequency ablation, see 32998, 47382, 50592)

● **77014** Computed tomography guidance for placement of radiation therapy fields

MAGNETIC RESONANCE GUIDANCE

● **77021** Magnetic resonance guidance for needle placement (eg, for biopsy, needle aspiration, injection, or placement of localization device) radiological supervision and interpretation

(For procedure, see appropriate organ or site)

● **77022** Magnetic resonance guidance for, and monitoring of, parenchymal tissue ablation

(For percutaneous radiofrequency ablation, see 32998, 47382, 50592)

(For focused ultrasound ablation treatment of uterine leiomyomata, see Category III codes 0071T, 0072T)

(For percutaneous cryotherapy ablation of renal tumors, use 0135T)

OTHER RADIOLOGIC GUIDANCE

● **77031** Stereotactic localization guidance for breast biopsy or needle placement (eg, for wire localization or for injection), each lesion, radiological supervision and interpretation

(For procedure, see 10022, 19000-19103, 19290, 19291)

(For injection for sentinel node localization without lymphoscintigraphy, use 38792)

● **77032** Mammographic guidance for needle placement, breast (eg, for wire localization or for injection), each lesion, radiological supervision and interpretation

(For procedure, see 10022, 19000, 19102, 19103, 19290, 19291)

(For injection for sentinel node localization without lymphoscintigraphy, use 38792)

BREAST, MAMMOGRAPHY

(For mammographic guidance for needle placement of breast lesion, use 77032)

●**+77051** Computer-aided detection (computer algorithm analysis of digital image data for lesion detection) with further physician review for interpretation, with or without digitization of film radiographic images; diagnostic mammography (List separately in addition to code for primary procedure)

(Use 77051 in conjunction with 77055, 77056)

●**+77052** Computer-aided detection (computer algorithm analysis of digital image data for lesion detection) with further physician review for interpretation, with or without digitization of film radiographic images; screening mammography (List separately in addition to code for primary procedure)

(Use 77052 in conjunction with 77057)

● **77053** Mammary ductogram or galactogram, single duct, radiological supervision and interpretation

(For mammry ductogram or galactogram injection, use 19030)

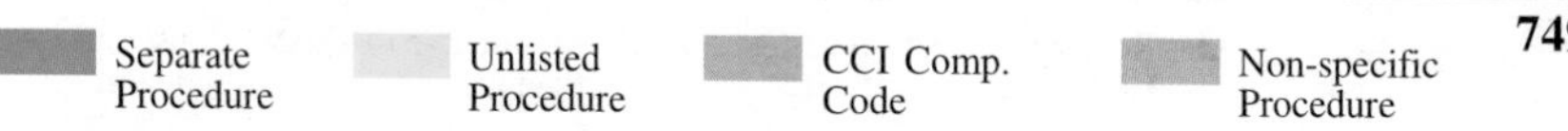

● **77054** Mammary ductogram or galactogram, multiple ducts, radiological supervision and interpretation

● **77055** Mammography; unilateral

● **77056** Mammography; bilateral

(Use 77055, 77056 in conjunction with 77051 for computer-aided detection applied to a diagnostic mammogram)

● **77057** Screening mammography, bilateral (2-view film study of each breast)

(Use 77057 in conjunction with 77052 for computer-aided detection applied to a screening mammogram)

(To report electrical impedance scan of the breast, bilateral, use Category III code 0060T)

● **77058** Magnetic resonance imaging, breast, without and/or with contrast material(s); unilateral

● **77059** bilateral

BONE/JOINT STUDIES

● **77071** Manual application of stress performed by physician for joint radiography, including contralateral joint if indicated

(For radiographic interpretation of stressed images, see appropriate anatomic site and number of views)

● **77072** Bone age studies

● **77073** Bone length studies (orthoroentgenogram, scanogram)

● **77074** Radiologic examination, osseous survey; limited (eg, for metastases)

● **77075** complete (axial and appendicular skeleton)

● **77076** Radiologic examination, osseous survey, infant

● **77077** Joint survey, single view, 2 or more joints (specify)

● **77078** Computed tomography, bone mineral density study, 1 or more sites; axial skeleton (eg, hips, pelvis, spine)

● **77079** appendicular skeleton (peripheral) (eg, radius, wrist, heel)

● **77080** Dual-energy X-ray absorptiometry (DXA), bone density study, 1 or more sites; axial skeleton (eg, hips, pelvis, spine)

● **77081** appendicular skeleton (peripheral) (eg, radius, wrist, heel)

● **77082** vertebral fracture assessment

(To report dual-energy X-ray absorptiometry [DXA] body composition study, 1 or more sites, use Category III code 0028T)

● **77083** Radiographic absorptiometry (eg, photodensitometry, radiogrammetry), 1 or more sites

● **77084** Magnetic resonance (eg, proton) imaging, bone marrow blood supply

RADIATION ONCOLOGY

Radiation therapy is the use of high level radiation to destroy cancer cells. Both tumor cells and healthy cells may be affected by this radiation. The radiation injures the cancer cells so they can no longer continue to divide or multiply. With each treatment, more of the cells die and the tumor shrinks. The dead cells are broken down, carried away by the blood and excreted by the body. Most of the healthy cells are able to recover from this injury. However, the damage to the healthy cells is the reason for the side effects of radiation therapy.

The dose of radiation is determined by the size, extent, type and grade of tumor along with its response to radiation therapy. Complex calculations are done to determine the dose and timing of radiation in treatment planning. Often, the treatment is given over several different angles in order to deliver the maximum amount of radiation to the tumor and the minimum amount to normal tissues.

Services defined in this section of the CPT book coding system teletherapy and brachytherapy. To report Radiation Oncology services, the following must be performed and documented:

- *The initial consultation*
- *Clinical treatment planning with/without simulation*
- *Medical radiation physics, dosimetry, treatment devices and special services*
- *Clinical treatment management procedures*
- *Normal follow-up care during treatment and for three months following completion of treatment*

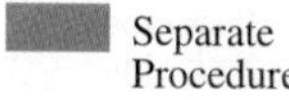 Separate Procedure 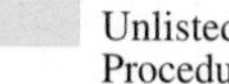 Unlisted Procedure 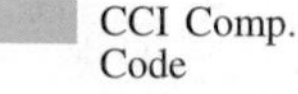 CCI Comp. Code 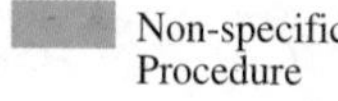 Non-specific Procedure

Continuing medical physics consultation (CPT code 77336) is reported per week of therapy. It may be reported after every five radiation treatments. (It may also be reported if the total number of radiation treatments in a course of radiation therapy is less than five.) Since radiation planning procedures (CPT codes 77261-77334) are generally performed before radiation treatment commences, the NCCI contains edits preventing payment of CPT code 77336 with CPT codes 77261- 77295, 77301-77328, and 77332-77334. Because radiation planning procedures may occasionally be repeated during a course of radiation treatment, the edits allow modifier - 59 to be appended to CPT code 77336 when the radiation planning procedure and continuing medical physics consultation occur on the same date of service.

CONSULTATION OR CLINICAL MANAGEMENT

All consultations, pre-treatment patient evaluations, and/or medical care services are coded using evaluation and management service codes

CLINICAL TREATMENT PLANNING

Clinical treatment planning includes test interpretation, localization of tumor(s), treatment determination, and choice of treatment modality and treatment devices. Clinical treatment planning may be simple, intermediate or complex.

77261 Therapeutic radiology treatment planning; simple

77262 intermediate

77263 complex

77280 Therapeutic radiology simulation-aided field setting; simple

77285 intermediate

77290 complex

77295 three-dimensional

77299 Unlisted procedure, therapeutic radiology clinical treatment planning

MEDICAL RADIATION PHYSICS, DOSIMETRY, TREATMENT DEVICES, AND SPECIAL SERVICES

77300 Basic radiation dosimetry calculation, central axis depth dose calculation, TDF, NSD, gap calculation, off axis factor, tissue inhomogeneity factors, calculation of non-ionizing radiation surface and depth dose, as required during course of treatment, only when prescribed by the treating physician

77301 Intensity modulated radiotherapy plan, including dose-volume histograms for target and critical structure partial tolerance specifications

(Dose plan is optimized using inverse or forward planning technique for modulated beam delivery (eg, binary, dynamic MLC) to create highly conformal dose distribution. Computer plan distribution must be verified for positional accuracy based on dosimetric verification of the intensity map with verification of treatment set up and interpretation of verification methodology)

77305 Teletherapy, isodose plan (whether hand or computer calculated); simple (one or two parallel opposed unmodified ports directed to a single area of interest)

77310 intermediate (three or more treatment ports directed to a single area of interest)

77315 complex (mantle or inverted Y, tangential ports, the use of wedges, compensators, complex blocking, rotational beam, or special beam considerations)

(Only one teletherapy isodose plan may be reported for a given course of therapy to a specific treatment area)

77321 Special teletherapy port plan, particles, hemibody, total body

77326 Brachytherapy isodose plan; simple (calculation made from single plane, one to four sources/ribbon application, remote afterloading brachytherapy, 1 to 8 sources)

(For definition of source/ribbon, see Clinical Brachytherapy)

77327 intermediate (multiplane dosage calculations, application involving 5 to 10 sources/ribbons, remote afterloading brachytherapy, 9 to 12 sources)

77328 complex (multiplane isodose plan, volume implant calculations, over 10 sources/ribbons used, special spatial reconstruction, remote afterloading brachytherapy, over 12 sources)

77331 Special dosimetry (eg, TLD, microdosimetry) (specify), only when prescribed by the treating physician

77332 Treatment devices, design and construction; simple (simple block, simple bolus)

77333 intermediate (multiple blocks, stents, bite blocks, special bolus)

77334 complex (irregular blocks, special shields, compensators, wedges, molds or casts)

77336 Continuing medical physics consultation, including assessment of treatment parameters, quality assurance of dose delivery, and review of patient treatment documentation in support of the radiation oncologist, reported per week of therapy

77370 Special medical radiation physics consultation

STEREOTACTIC RADIATION TREATMENT DELIVERY

● **77371** Radiation treatment delivery, stereotactic radiosurgery (SRS), complete course of treatment of cerebral lesion(s) consisting of 1 session; multi-source Cobalt 60 based

● **77372** linear accelerator based

(For radiation treatment management, use 77432)

● **77373** Stereotactic body radiation therapy, treatment delivery, per fraction to 1 or more lesions, including image guidance, entire course not to exceed 5 fractions

(Do not report 77373 in conjunction with 77401-77416, 77418)

(For single fraction cranial lesions(s), see 77371, 77372)

OTHER PROCEDURES

77399 Unlisted procedure, medical radiation physics, dosimetry and treatment devices, and special services

RADIATION TREATMENT DELIVERY

(Radiation treatment delivery (77401-77416) recognizes the technical component and the various energy levels.)

77401 Radiation treatment delivery, superficial and/or ortho voltage

77402 Radiation treatment delivery, single treatment area, single port or parallel opposed ports, simple blocks or no blocks; up to 5 MeV

77403 6-10 MeV

77404 11-19 MeV

77406 20 MeV or greater

77407 Radiation treatment delivery, two separate treatment areas, three or more ports on a single treatment area, use of multiple blocks; up to 5 MeV

77408 6-10 MeV

77409 11-19 MeV

77411 20 MeV or greater

77412 Radiation treatment delivery, three or more separate treatment areas, custom blocking, tangential ports, wedges, rotational beam, compensators, electron beam; up to 5 MeV

77413 6-10 MeV

77414 11-19 MeV

77416 20 MeV or greater

77417 Therapeutic radiology port film(s)

77418 Intensity modulated treatment delivery, single or multiple fields/arcs, via narrow spatially and temporally modulated beams, binary, dynamic MLC, per treatment session

(For intensity modulated treatment planning, use 77301)

(For compensator-based beam modulation treatment delivery, use Category III code 0073T)

77421 Stereoscopic x-ray guidance for localization of target volume for the delivery of radiation therapy

(Do not report 77421 in conjunction with 77432, 77435)

(For placement of interstitial device(s) for radiation therapy guidance, prostate, use 55876)

NEUTRON BEAM TREATMENT DELIVERY

77422 High energy neutron radiation treatment delivery; single treatment area using a single port or parallel-opposed ports with no blocks or simple blocking

77423 1 or more isocenter(s) with coplanar or non-coplanar geometry with blocking and/or wedge, and/or compensator(s)

RADIATION TREATMENT MANAGEMENT

CPT codes in this section presume treatment on a daily basis (4 or 5 fractions per week) with the use of megavoltage photon or high energy particle sources. Daily and weekly clinical treatment management are mutually exclusive for the same dates. CPT defines three distinct levels of clinical treatment management: simple, intermediate and complex. Review this section of CPT for detailed definitions of these levels of service.

77427 Radiation treatment management, five treatments

77431 Radiation therapy management with complete course of therapy consisting of one or two fractions only

(77431 is not to be used to fill in the last week of a long course of therapy)

77432 Stereotactic radiation treatment management of cerebral lesion(s) (complete course of treatment consisting of one session)

● **77435** Stereotactic body radiation therapy, treatment management, per treatment course, to one or more lesions, including image guidance, entire course not to exceed 5 fractions

(Do not report 77435 in conjunction with 77427-77432)

(When stereotactic radiation therapy is performed jointly by a surgeon and a radiation oncologist (eg., spinal or cranial) the surgeon reports radiosurgery with 61793)

77470 Special treatment procedure (eg, total body irradiation, hemibody irradiation, per oral, endocavitary or vaginal cone irradiation)

(77470 assumes that the procedure is performed one or more times during the course of therapy, in addition to daily or weekly patient management)

77499 Unlisted procedure, therapeutic radiology treatment management

PROTON BEAM TREATMENT DELIVERY

77520 Proton treatment delivery; simple, without compensation

77522 simple, with compensation

77523 intermediate

77525 complex

HYPERTHERMIA

⊙ **77600** Hyperthermia, externally generated; superficial (ie, heating to a depth of 4 cm or less)

⊙ **77605** deep (ie, heating to depths greater than 4 cm)

⊙ **77610** Hyperthermia generated by interstitial probe(s); 5 or fewer interstitial applicators

⊙ **77615** more than 5 interstitial applicators

CLINICAL INTRACAVITARY HYPERTHERMIA

77620 Hyperthermia generated by intracavitary probe(s)

CLINICAL BRACHYTHERAPY

77750 Infusion or instillation of radioelement solution (includes three months follow-up care)

(For administration of radiolabeled monoclonal antibodies, use 79403)

(For non-antibody radiopharmaceutical therapy by intravenous administration only, not including three month follow-up care, use 79101)

77761 Intracavitary radiation source application; simple

77762 intermediate

77763 complex

77776 Interstitial radiation source application; simple

77777 intermediate

77778 complex

77781 Remote afterloading high intensity brachytherapy; 1-4 source positions or catheters

77782 5-8 source positions or catheters

77783 9-12 source positions or catheters

77784 over 12 source positions or catheters

77789 Surface application of radiation source

77790 Supervision, handling, loading of radiation source

77799 Unlisted procedure, clinical brachytherapy

NUCLEAR MEDICINE

Nuclear medicine is used in the diagnosis, management, treatment, and prevention of serious disease. Nuclear medicine imaging procedures often identify abnormalities very early in the progression of a disease. This early detection allows a disease to be treated early in its course when there may be a more successful prognosis.

Nuclear medicine uses very small amounts of radioactive materials or radiopharmaceuticals to diagnose and treat disease. Radiopharmaceuticals are substances that are attracted to specific organs, bones, or tissues. The radiopharmaceuticals used in nuclear medicine emit gamma rays that can be detected externally by special types of cameras: gamma or PET cameras. These cameras work in conjunction with computers used to form images that provide data and information about the area of body being imaged. The amount of radiation from a nuclear medicine procedure is comparable to that received during a diagnostic x-ray.

Nuclear medicine procedures may be performed independently or in the course of overall medical care. If the physician providing nuclear medicine services is also responsible for the diagnostic work-up and/or follow-up care of the patient, evaluation and management service codes should be coded in addition to the nuclear medicine procedures.

Radioimmunoassay tests are located in the Clinical Pathology section (codes 82000-84999). These CPT codes can be appropriately used by any specialist performing such tests in a laboratory licensed and/or certified for radioimmunoassays. The reporting of these tests is not confined to clinical pathology laboratories alone.

The injection of a radiopharmaceutical is included as an inherent component of the procedure. Separate vascular access and injection codes (e.g. 36000, 90783 (90773 in 2006), G0345-G0354 (90760-90772, 90774-90775 in 2006) should not be reported. However, the services do not include the actual radiopharmaceutical or drug used. Diagnostic and therapeutic radiopharmaceuticals and drugs supplied by the physician should be reported separately using the appropriate supply code(s), in addition to the procedure code.

Single photon emission computed tomography (SPECT) studies represent an enhanced methodology over standard planar nuclear imaging. When a limited anatomic area is studied, there is no additional information procured by obtaining both planar and SPECT studies. While both represent medically acceptable imaging studies, when a SPECT study of a limited area is performed, a planar study is not to be separately reported. When vascular flow studies are obtained using planar technology in addition to SPECT studies, the appropriate CPT code for the vascular flow study should be reported, not the flow, planar and SPECT studies. In cases where planar images must be procured because of the extent of the scanned area (e.g. bone imaging), both planar and SPECT scans may be necessary and reported separately.

Myocardial perfusion imaging (CPT codes 78460-78465) are not reportable with cardiac blood pool imaging by gated equilibrium (CPT codes 78472-78473) because the two types of tests utilize different radiopharmaceuticals.

CPT codes 76375 (76376, 76377 in 2006) (3-D rendering) are not separately reportable for nuclear medicine procedures (CPT codes 78000-78999). However, CPT code 76375 (76376, 76377 in 2006) may be separately reported with modifier - 59 on the same date of service as a nuclear medicine procedure if the 3D rendering procedure is performed in association with a third procedure (other than nuclear medicine) for which 3D rendering is appropriately reported.

DIAGNOSTIC NUCLEAR MEDICINE

ENDOCRINE SYSTEM

78000 Thyroid uptake; single determination

78001 multiple determinations

78003 stimulation, suppression or discharge (not including initial uptake studies)

78006 Thyroid imaging, with uptake; single determination

78007 multiple determinations

78010 Thyroid imaging; only

78011 with vascular flow

78015 Thyroid carcinoma metastases imaging; limited area (eg, neck and chest only)

78016 with additional studies (eg, urinary recovery)

78018 whole body

+ **78020** Thyroid carcinoma metastases uptake (List separately in addition to code for primary procedure)

(Use 78020 in conjunction with code 78018 only)

78070 Parathyroid imaging

78075 Adrenal imaging, cortex and/or medulla

78099 Unlisted endocrine procedure, diagnostic nuclear medicine

(For chemical analysis, see Chemistry section)

HEMATOPOIETIC, RETICULOENDOTHELIAL AND LYMPHATIC SYSTEM

78102 Bone marrow imaging; limited area

78103 multiple areas

78104 whole body

● New Code ▲ Revised Code + Add-On Code ⊘ Modifier -51 Exempt ⊙ Conscious Sedation

78110 Plasma volume, radiopharmaceutical volume-dilution technique (separate procedure); single sampling

78111 multiple samplings

78120 Red cell volume determination (separate procedure); single sampling

78121 multiple samplings

78122 Whole blood volume determination, including separate measurement of plasma volume and red cell volume (radiopharmaceutical volume-dilution technique)

78130 Red cell survival study;

78135 differential organ/tissue kinetics, (eg, splenic and/or hepatic sequestration)

78140 Labeled red cell sequestration, differential organ/tissue, (eg, splenic and/or hepatic)

(78160 deleted 2006 edition.)

(78162 deleted 2006 edition.)

(78170 deleted 2006 edition.)

(78172 deleted 2006 edition.)

78185 Spleen imaging only, with or without vascular flow

(If combined with liver study, use procedures 78215 and 78216)

78190 Kinetics, study of platelet survival, with or without differential organ/tissue localization

78191 Platelet survival study

78195 Lymphatics and lymph nodes imaging

(For sentinel node identification without scintigraphy imaging, use 38792)

(For sentinal node excision, see 38500-38542)

Separate Procedure | Unlisted Procedure | CCI Comp. Code | Non-specific Procedure

78199 Unlisted hematopoietic, reticuloendothelial and lymphatic procedure, diagnostic nuclear medicine

(For chemical analysis, see Chemistry section)

GASTROINTESTINAL SYSTEM

78201 Liver imaging; static only

78202 with vascular flow

(For spleen imaging only, use 78185)

78205 Liver imaging (SPECT);

78206 with vascular flow

78215 Liver and spleen imaging; static only

78216 with vascular flow

78220 Liver function study with hepatobiliary agents, with serial images

78223 Hepatobiliary ductal system imaging, including gallbladder, with or without pharmacologic intervention, with or without quantitative measurement of gallbladder function

78230 Salivary gland imaging;

78231 with serial images

78232 Salivary gland function study

78258 Esophageal motility

78261 Gastric mucosa imaging

78262 Gastroesophageal reflux study

78264 Gastric emptying study

78267 Urea breath test, C-14 (isotopic); acquisition for analysis

78268 analysis

● New Code ▲ Revised Code + Add-On Code ⃠ Modifier -51 Exempt ⊙ Conscious Sedation

78270 Vitamin B-12 absorption study (eg, Schilling test); without intrinsic factor

78271 with intrinsic factor

78272 Vitamin B-12 absorption studies combined, with and without intrinsic factor

78278 Acute gastrointestinal blood loss imaging

78282 Gastrointestinal protein loss

78290 Intestine imaging (eg, ectopic gastric mucosa, Meckels localization, volvulus)

78291 Peritoneal-venous shunt patency test (eg, for LeVeen, Denver shunt)

(For injection procedure, use 49427)

78299 Unlisted gastrointestinal procedure, diagnostic nuclear medicine

MUSCULOSKELETAL SYSTEM

78300 Bone and/or joint imaging; limited area

78305 multiple areas

78306 whole body

78315 three phase study

78320 tomographic (SPECT)

78350 Bone density (bone mineral content) study, one or more sites; single photon absorptiometry

78351 dual photon absorptiometry, one or more sites

(For radiographic bone density (photodensitometry), use 77083)

78399 Unlisted musculoskeletal procedure, diagnostic nuclear medicine

CARDIOVASCULAR SYSTEM

78414 Determination of central c-v hemodynamics (non-imaging) (eg, ejection fraction with probe technique) with or without pharmacologic intervention or exercise, single or multiple determinations

78428 Cardiac shunt detection

78445 Non-cardiac vascular flow imaging (ie, angiography, venography)

(78455 deleted 2006 edition.)

78456 Acute venous thrombosis imaging, peptide

78457 Venous thrombosis imaging, venogram; unilateral

78458 bilateral

78459 Myocardial imaging, positron emission tomography (PET), metabolic evaluation

(For myocardial perfusion study, see 78491-78492)

78460 Myocardial perfusion imaging; (planar) single study, at rest or stress (exercise and/or pharmacologic), with or without quantification

78461 multiple studies, (planar) at rest and/or stress (exercise and/or pharmacologic), and redistribution and/or rest injection, with or without quantification

78464 tomographic (SPECT), single study (including attenuation correction when performed), at rest or stress (exercise and/or pharmacologic), with or without quantification

78465 tomographic (SPECT), multiple studies (including attenuation correction when performed), at rest and/or stress (exercise and/or pharmacologic) and redistribution and/or rest injection, with or without quantification

78466 Myocardial imaging, infarct avid, planar; qualitative or quantitative

78468 with ejection fraction by first pass technique

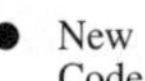

● New Code ▲ Revised Code + Add-On Code ⊘ Modifier -51 Exempt ⊙ Conscious Sedation

78469 tomographic SPECT with or without quantification

78472 Cardiac blood pool imaging, gated equilibrium; planar, single study at rest or stress (exercise and/or pharmacologic), wall motion study plus ejection fraction, with or without additional quantitative processing

(For assessment of right ventricular ejection fraction by first pass technique, use 78496)

78473 multiple studies, wall motion study plus ejection fraction, at rest and stress (exercise and/or pharmacologic), with or without additional quantification

+ **78478** Myocardial perfusion study with wall motion, qualitative or quantitative study (List separately in addition to code for primary procedure)

(Use 78478 in conjunction with codes 78460, 78461, 78464, 78465)

+ **78480** Myocardial perfusion study with ejection fraction (List separately in addition to code for primary procedure)

(Use 78480 in conjunction with codes 78460, 78461, 78464, 78465)

78481 Cardiac blood pool imaging, (planar), first pass technique; single study, at rest or with stress (exercise and/or pharmacologic), wall motion study plus ejection fraction, with or without quantification

78483 multiple studies, at rest and with stress (exercise and/or pharmacologic), wall motion study plus ejection fraction, with or without quantification

(For cerebral blood flow study, use 78615)

78491 Myocardial imaging, positron emission tomography (PET), perfusion; single study at rest or stress

78492 multiple studies at rest and/or stress

78494 Cardiac blood pool imaging, gated equilibrium, SPECT, at rest, wall motion study plus ejection fraction, with or without quantitative processing

+ **78496** Cardiac blood pool imaging, gated equilibrium, single study, at rest, with right ventricular ejection fraction by first pass technique (List separately in addition to code for primary procedure)

(Use 78496 in conjunction with code 78472)

78499 Unlisted cardiovascular procedure, diagnostic nuclear medicine

RESPIRATORY SYSTEM

78580 Pulmonary perfusion imaging, particulate

78584 Pulmonary perfusion imaging, particulate, with ventilation; single breath

78585 rebreathing and washout, with or without single breath

78586 Pulmonary ventilation imaging, aerosol; single projection

78587 multiple projections (eg, anterior, posterior, lateral views)

78588 Pulmonary perfusion imaging, particulate, with ventilation imaging, aerosol, one or multiple projections

78591 Pulmonary ventilation imaging, gaseous, single breath, single projection

78593 Pulmonary ventilation imaging, gaseous, with rebreathing and washout with or without single breath; single projection

78594 multiple projections (eg, anterior, posterior, lateral views)

78596 Pulmonary quantitative differential function (ventilation/perfusion) study

78599 Unlisted respiratory procedure, diagnostic nuclear medicine

NERVOUS SYSTEM

78600 Brain imaging, limited procedure; static

78601 with vascular flow

78605 Brain imaging, complete study; static

78606 with vascular flow

● New Code ▲ Revised Code + Add-On Code ⃠ Modifier -51 Exempt ⊙ Conscious Sedation

78607 tomographic (SPECT)

78608 Brain imaging, positron emission tomography (PET); metabolic evaluation

78609 perfusion evaluation

78610 Brain imaging, vascular flow only

78615 Cerebral vascular flow

78630 Cerebrospinal fluid flow, imaging (not including introduction of material); cisternography

(For injection procedure, see 61000-61070, 62270-62319)

78635 ventriculography

(For injection procedure, see 61000-61070, 62270-62294)

78645 shunt evaluation

(For injection procedure, see 61000-61070, 62270-62294)

78647 tomographic (SPECT)

78650 Cerebrospinal fluid leakage detection and localization

(For injection procedure, see 61000-61070, 62270-62294)

78660 Radiopharmaceutical dacryocystography

78699 Unlisted nervous system procedure, diagnostic nuclear medicine

GENITOURINARY SYSTEM

▲ 78700 Kidney imaging morphology;

78701 with vascular flow

(78704 deleted 2007 edition, see 78707-78709)

▲ 78707 with vascular flow and function, single study without pharmacological intervention

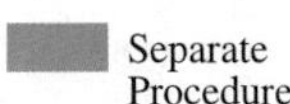 Separate Procedure 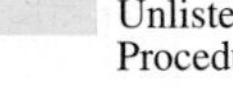 Unlisted Procedure 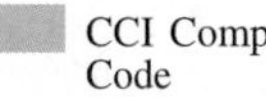 CCI Comp. Code 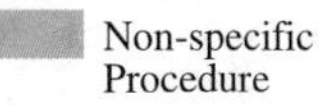 Non-specific Procedure

▲ **78708** with vascular flow and function, single study, with pharmacological intervention (eg, angiotensin converting enzyme inhibitor and/or diuretic)

▲ **78709** with vascular flow and function, multiple studies, with and without pharmacological intervention (eg, angiotensin converting enzyme inhibitor and/or diuretic)

(For introduction of radioactive substance in association with renal endoscopy, see 77776-77778)

▲ **78710** tomographic (SPECT)

(78715 deleted 2007 edition, see 78701-78709)

78725 Kidney function study, non-imaging radioisotopic study

▲**+78730** Urinary bladder residual study (List separately in addition to code for primary procedure)

(Use 78730 in conjunction with 78740)

(For measurement of postvoid residual urine and/or bladder capacity by ultrasound, nonimaging, use 51798)

(For ultrasound imaging of the bladder only, with measurement of postvoid residual urine when performed, use 76857)

78740 Ureteral reflux study (radiopharmaceutical voiding cystogram)

(Use 78740 in conjunction with 78730 for urinary bladder residual study)

(For catheterization, see 51701-51703)

(78760 deleted 2007 edition, see 78761)

▲ **78761** Testicular imaging with vascular flow

78799 Unlisted genitourinary procedure, diagnostic nuclear medicine

(For chemical analysis, see Chemistry section)

OTHER PROCEDURES

(For specific organ, see appropriate heading)

(For radiophosphorus tumor identification, ocular, see 78800)

78800 Radiopharmaceutical localization of tumor or distribution of radiopharmaceutical agent(s); limited area

(For specific organ, see appropriate heading)

78801 multiple areas

78802 whole body, single day imaging

78803 tomographic (SPECT)

78804 whole body, requiring two or more days imaging

78805 Radiopharmaceutical localization of inflammatory process; limited area

78806 whole body

78807 tomographic (SPECT)

(For imaging bone infectious or inflammatory disease with a bone imaging radiopharmaceutical, see 78300, 78305, 78306)

(78810 deleted 2005 edition. To report, see 78811-78813)

(For PET of brain, see 78608, 78609)

(For PET myocardial imaging, see 78459, 78491, 78492)

78811 Tumor imaging, positron emission tomography (PET); limited area (eg, chest, head/neck)

78812 skull base to mid-thigh

78813 whole body

78814 Tumor imaging, positron emission tomography (PET) with concurrently acquired computed tomography (CT) for attenuation correction and anatomical localization; limited area (eg, chest, head/neck)

78815 skull base to mid-thigh

78816 whole body

(Report 78811-78816 only once per imaging session)

(Computed tomography (CT) performed for other than attenuation correction and anatomical localization is reported using the appropriate site specific CT code with modifier 59)

78890 Generation of automated data: interactive process involving nuclear physician and/or allied health professional personnel; simple manipulations and interpretation, not to exceed 30 minutes

78891 complex manipulations and interpretation, exceeding 30 minutes

(Use 78890 or 78891 in addition to primary procedure)

(78990 deleted 2005 edition)

78999 Unlisted miscellaneous procedure, diagnostic nuclear medicine

THERAPEUTIC

(79000 deleted 2005 edition. To report, use 79005)

(79001 deleted 2005 edition. To report, use 79005)

79005 Radiopharmaceutical therapy, by oral administration

(79020 deleted 2005 edition. To report, use 79005)

(79030 deleted 2005 edition. To report, use 79005)

(79035 deleted 2005 edition. To report, use 79005)

(79100 deleted 2005 edition. To report, use 79101)

(For monoclonal antibody therapy, use 79403)

79101 Radiopharmaceutical therapy, by intravenous administration

(Do not report 79101 in conjunction with 36400, 36410, 79403, 90780, 90784, 96408)

(For radiolabeled monoclonal antibody by intravenous infusion, use 79403)

(For infusion or instillation of non-antibody radioelement solution that includes three months follow-up care, use 77750)

79200 Radiopharmaceutical therapy, by intracavitary administration

79300 Radiopharmaceutical therapy, by interstitial radioactive colloid administration

(79400 deleted 2005 edition. To report, use 79101)

79403 Radiopharmaceutical therapy, radiolabeled monoclonal antibody by intravenous infusion

(For pre-treatment imaging, see 78802, 78804)

(Do not report 79403 in conjunction with 79101)

(79420 deleted 2005 edition. To report, use 79445)

79440 Radiopharmaceutical therapy, by intra-articular administration

79445 Radiopharmaceutical therapy, by intra-arterial particulate administration

(Do not report 79445 in conjunction with 90783, 96420)

(Use appropriate procedural and radiological supervision and interpretation codes for the angiographic and interventional procedures provided pre-requisite to intra-arterial radiopharmaceutical therapy)

(79900 deleted 2005 edition)

79999 Radiopharmaceutical therapy, unlisted procedure

This page intentionally left blank.

PATHOLOGY/ LABORATORY

LABORATORY SECTION OVERVIEW

The fifth section of the CPT coding system is the laboratory section, which includes codes for pathology and laboratory services. Within each subsection, the CPT codes are arranged by the type of testing or service.

LABORATORY SUBSECTIONS

The PATHOLOGY AND LABORATORY section of CPT is divided into the following subsections:

Organ or Disease Oriented Panels	80048-80076
Drug Testing	80100-80103
Therapeutic Drug Assays	80150-80299
Evocative/Suppression Testing	80400-80440
Consultations (Clinical Pathology)	80500-80502
Urinalysis	81000-81099
Chemistry	82000-84999
Hematology and Coagulation	85002-85999
Immunology	86000-86849
Transfusion Medicine	86850-86999
Microbiology	87001-87999
Anatomic Pathology	88000-88099
Cytopathology	88104-88199
Cytogenetic Studies	88230-88299
Surgical Pathology	88300-88399
Transcutaneous Procedures	88400
Other Procedures	89049-89240
Reproductive Medicine Procedures	89250-89356

LAB 80000

LABORATORY SERVICE MODIFIERS

Pathology and laboratory services and procedures may be modified under certain circumstances. When applicable, the modifying circumstances should be identified by adding the appropriate modifier to the basic service code. The addition of modifier -22 requires a special report. Modifiers commonly used to report PATHOLOGY and LABORATORY procedures include:

-22 unusual services

-26 professional component

-32 mandated services

-52 reduced services

-90 reference (outside) laboratory

PATHOLOGY

Pathology is that discipline of the practice of medicine that deals with the causes and nature of disease. It contributes to diagnosis, prognosis, and treatment through knowledge gained by the laboratory application of the biologic, chemical, and physical sciences to man, or materials obtained from man. Pathologists diagnose, exclude, and monitor disease by means of information gathered from the microscopic examination of tissue specimens, cells, and body fluids, and from clinical laboratory tests on body fluids and secretions. Pathologists are involved with the management of laboratories and in data processing and with new developments in high technology.

CLINICAL PATHOLOGY

Clinical Pathology focuses on microbiology (including bacteriology, mycology, parasitology, and virology), immunopathology, blood banking/transfusion medicine, chemical pathology, cytogenetics, hematology, coagulation, toxicology, medical microscopy (including urinalysis), molecular biologic techniques, and other advanced diagnostic techniques as they become available.

PATHOLOGY AND LABORATORY CODES

ORGAN OR DISEASE ORIENTED PANELS

CPT codes for organ or disease oriented panels were included in CPT due to the increased use of general screening programs by physicians, clinics, hospitals, and other health care facilities. Other codes in this section define profiles that combine laboratory tests together under a problem oriented classification. There is a list of specific laboratory tests under each of the panel CPT codes which define the components of each panel. However, each laboratory typically establishes its own profile and provides a listing of the components of that panel performed by the laboratory with test results.

The CPT coding system assigns CPT codes to organ or disease oriented panels consisting of a group of specified tests. If all tests of a CPT defined panel are performed, the provider may bill the panel code or the individual component test codes. The panel codes may be used when the tests are ordered as that panel or if the individual component tests of a panel are ordered separately. For example, if the individually ordered tests are cholesterol (CPT code 82465), triglycerides (CPT code 84478), and HDL cholesterol (CPT code 83718), the service could be billed as a lipid panel (CPT code 80061).

80048 Basic metabolic panel

This panel must include the following:
Calcium (82310)
Carbon dioxide (82374)
Chloride (82435)
Creatinine (82565)
Glucose (82947)
Potassium (84132)
Sodium (84295)
Urea Nitrogen (BUN) (84520)

(Do not use 80048 in addition to 80053)

80050 General health panel

This panel must include the following:
Comprehensive metabolic panel (80053)
Blood count, complete (CBC), automated and automated differential WBC count (85025 or 85027 and 85004)
OR
Blood count, complete (CBC), automated (85027) and appropriate manual differential WBC count (85007 or 85009)
Thyroid stimulating hormone (TSH) (84443)

Separate Procedure | Unlisted Procedure | CCI Comp. Code | Non-specific Procedure

80051 Electrolyte panel

This panel must include the following:
Carbon dioxide (82374)
Chloride (82435)
Potassium (84132)
Sodium (84295)

80053 Comprehensive metabolic panel

This panel must include the following:
Albumin (82040)
Bilirubin, total (82247)
Calcium (82310)
Carbon dioxide (bicarbonate) (82374)
Chloride (82435)
Creatinine (82565)
Glucose (82947)
Phosphatase, alkaline (84075)
Potassium (84132)
Protein, total (84155)
Sodium (84295)
Transferase, alanine amino (ALT) (SGPT) (84460)
Transferase, aspartate amino (AST) (SGOT) (84450)
Urea Nitrogen (BUN) (84520)

(Do not use 80053 in addition to 80048, 80076)

80055 Obstetric panel

This panel must include the following:
Blood count, complete (CBC), automated and automated differential WBC count (85025 or 85027 and 85004)
OR
Blood count, complete (CBC), automated (85027) and appropriate manual differential WBC count (85007 or 85009)
Hepatitis B surface antigen (HBsAg) (87340)
Antibody, rubella (86762)
Syphilis test, qualitative (eg, VDRL, RPR, ART) (86592)
Antibody screen, RBC, each serum technique (86850)
Blood typing, ABO (86900) AND
Blood typing, Rh (D) (86901)

80061 Lipid panel

This panel must include the following:
Cholesterol, serum, total (82465)
Lipoprotein, direct measurement, high density cholesterol (HDL cholesterol) (83718)
Triglycerides (84478)

80069 Renal function panel

This panel must include the following:
Albumin (82040)
Calcium (82310)
Carbon dioxide (bicarbonate) (82374)
Chloride (82435)
Creatinine (82565)
Glucose (82947)
Phosphorus inorganic (phosphate) (84100)
Potassium (84132)
Sodium (84295)
Urea nitrogen (BUN) (84520)

80074 Acute hepatitis panel

This panel must include the following:
Hepatitis A antibody (HAAb), IgM antibody (86709)
Hepatitis B core antibody (HbcAb), IgM antibody (86705)
Hepatitis B surface antigen (HbsAg) (87340)
Hepatitis C antibody (86803)

80076 Hepatic function panel

This panel must include the following:
Albumin (82040)
Bilirubin, total (82247)
Bilirubin, direct (82248)
Phosphatase, alkaline (84075)
Protein, total (84155)
Transferase, alanine amino (ALT) (SGPT) (84460)
Transferase, aspartate amino (AST) (SGOT) (84450)

(Do not use 80076 in addition to 80053)

DRUG TESTING

80100 Drug screen, qualitative; multiple drug classes, chromatographic method, each procedure

80101 single drug class method (eg, immunoassay, enzyme assay), each drug class

80102 Drug, confirmation, each procedure

80103 Tissue preparation for drug analysis

 Separate Procedure 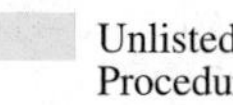 Unlisted Procedure 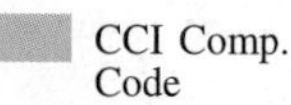 CCI Comp. Code 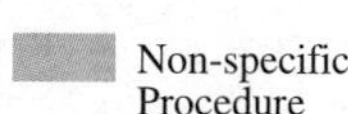 Non-specific Procedure

THERAPEUTIC DRUG ASSAYS

80150 Amikacin

80152 Amitriptyline

80154 Benzodiazepines

80156 Carbamazepine; total

80157 free

80158 Cyclosporine

80160 Desipramine

80162 Digoxin

80164 Dipropylacetic acid (valproic acid)

80166 Doxepin

80168 Ethosuximide

80170 Gentamicin

80172 Gold

80173 Haloperidol

80174 Imipramine

80176 Lidocaine

80178 Lithium

80182 Nortriptyline

80184 Phenobarbital

80185 Phenytoin; total

80186 free

80188 Primidone

80190 Procainamide;

80192 with metabolites (eg, n-acetyl procainamide)

80194 Quinidine

80195 Sirolimus

80196 Salicylate

80197 Tacrolimus

80198 Theophylline

80200 Tobramycin

80201 Topiramate

80202 Vancomycin

80299 Quantitation of drug, not elsewhere specified

EVOCATIVE/SUPPRESSION TESTING

Evocative/suppression testing involves administration of agents to determine a patient's response to those agents (CPT codes 80400-80440 are to be used for reporting the laboratory components of the testing). When the test requires physician administration of the evocative/suppression agent as described by HCPCS/CPT codes 90760-90775, G0345-G0354 (therapeutic or diagnostic injections/infusions), these codes can be separately reported. However, when physician attendance is not required, and the agent is administered by ancillary personnel, these codes are not to be separately reported.

In the inpatient setting, these codes are only reported if the physician performs the service personally. In the office setting, the service can be reported when performed by office personnel if the physician is directly supervising the service. While supplies necessary to perform the testing are included in the testing, the appropriate HCPCS J codes for the drugs can be separately reported for the diagnostic agents. Separate evaluation and management services are not to be reported, including prolonged services (in the case of prolonged infusions) unless a significant, separately identifiable service is provided and documented.

80400 ACTH stimulation panel; for adrenal insufficiency

This panel must include the following:
Cortisol (82533 x 2)

80402 for 21 hydroxylase deficiency

This panel must include the following:
Cortisol (82533 x 2)
17 hydroxyprogesterone (83498 x 2)

80406 for 3 beta-hydroxydehydrogenase deficiency

This panel must include the following:
Cortisol (82533 x 2)
17 hydroxypregnenolone (84143 x 2)

80408 Aldosterone suppression evaluation panel (eg, saline infusion)

This panel must include the following:
Aldosterone (82088 x 2)
Renin (84244 x 2)

80410 Calcitonin stimulation panel (eg, calcium, pentagastrin)

This panel must include the following:
Calcitonin (82308 x 3)

80412 Corticotropic releasing hormone (CRH) stimulation panel

This panel must include the following:
Cortisol (82533 x 6)
Adrenocorticotropic hormone (ACTH) (82024 x 6)

80414 Chorionic gonadotropin stimulation panel; testosterone response.

This panel must include the following:
Testosterone (84403 x 2 on three pooled blood samples)

80415 estradiol response.

This panel must include the following:
Estradiol (82670 x 2 on three pooled blood samples)

80416 Renal vein renin stimulation panel (eg, captopril)

This panel must include the following:
Renin (84244 x 6)

80417 Peripheral vein renin stimulation panel (eg, captopril)

This panel must include the following:
Renin (84244 x 2)

80418 Combined rapid anterior pituitary evaluation panel

This panel must include the following:
Adrenocorticotropic hormone (ACTH) (82024 x 4)
Luteinizing hormone (LH) (83002 x 4)
Follicle stimulating hormone (FSH) (83001 x 4)
Prolactin (84146 x 4)
Human growth hormone (HGH)(83003 x 4)
Cortisol (82533 x 4)
Thyroid stimulating hormone (TSH) (84443 x 4)

80420 Dexamethasone suppression panel, 48 hour

This panel must include the following:
Free cortisol, urine (82530 x 2)
Cortisol (82533 x 2)
Volume measurement for timed collection (81050 x 2)

(For single dose dexamethasone, use 82533)

80422 Glucagon tolerance panel; for insulinoma

This panel must include the following:
Glucose (82947 x 3)
Insulin (83525 x 3)

80424 for pheochromocytoma.

This panel must include the following:
Catecholamines, fractionated (82384 x 2)

80426 Gonadotropin releasing hormone stimulation panel

This panel must include the following:
Follicle stimulating hormone (FSH) (83001 x 4)
Luteinizing hormone (LH)(83002 x 4)

80428 Growth hormone stimulation panel (eg, arginine infusion, l-dopa administration)

This panel must include the following:
Human growth hormone (HGH)(83003 x 4)

80430 Growth hormone suppression panel (glucose administration)

This panel must include the following:
Glucose (82947 x 3)
Human growth hormone (HGH)(83003 x 4)

80432 Insulin-induced C-peptide suppression panel

This panel must include the following:
Insulin (83525)
C-peptide (84681 x 5)
Glucose (82947 x 5)

80434 Insulin tolerance panel; for ACTH insufficiency

This panel must include the following:
Cortisol (82533 x 5)
Glucose (82947 x 5)

80435 for growth hormone deficiency

This panel must include the following:
Glucose (82947 x 5)
Human growth hormone (HGH) (83003 x 5)

80436 Metyrapone panel

This panel must include the following:
Cortisol (82533 x 2)
11 deoxycortisol (82634 x 2)

80438 Thyrotropin releasing hormone (TRH) stimulation panel; one hour

This panel must include the following:
Thyroid stimulating hormone (TSH) (84443 x 3)

80439 two hour

This panel must include the following:
Thyroid stimulating hormone (TSH) (84443 x 4)

80440 for hyperprolactinemia

This panel must include the following:
Prolactin (84146 x 3)

CONSULTATIONS (CLINICAL PATHOLOGY)

80500 Clinical pathology consultation; limited, without review of patients history and medical records

80502 comprehensive, for a complex diagnostic problem, with review of patients history and medical records

(These codes may also be used for pharmacokinetic consultations)

(For consultations involving the examination and evaluation of the patient, see 99241-99275)

URINALYSIS

(For urinalysis, infectious agent detection, semi-quantitative analysis of volatile compounds, use Category III code 0041T)

81000 Urinalysis, by dip stick or tablet reagent for bilirubin, glucose, hemoglobin, ketones, leukocytes, nitrite, pH, protein, specific gravity,urobilinogen, any number of these constituents; non-automated, with microscopy

81001 automated, with microscopy

81002 non-automated, without microscopy

81003 automated, without microscopy

81005 Urinalysis; qualitative or semiquantitative, except immunoassays

(For non-immunoassay reagent strip urinalysis, see 81000, 81002)

(For immunoassay, qualitative or semiquantitative, use 83518)

(For microalbumin, see 82043, 82044)

81007 bacteriuria screen, except by culture or dipstick

(For culture, see 87086-87088)

(For dipstick, use 81000 or 81002)

81015 microscopic only

81020 two or three glass test

Separate Procedure | Unlisted Procedure | CCI Comp. Code | Non-specific Procedure

81025 Urine pregnancy test, by visual color comparison methods

81050 Volume measurement for timed collection, each

81099 Unlisted urinalysis procedure

CHEMISTRY

82000 Acetaldehyde, blood

82003 Acetaminophen

82009 Acetone or other ketone bodies, serum; qualitative

82010 quantitative

82013 Acetylcholinesterase

(Acid, gastric, see gastric acid, 82926, 82928)

(Acid phosphatase, see 84060-84066)

82016 Acylcarnitines; qualitative, each specimen

82017 quantitative, each specimen

(For carnitine, use 82379)

82024 Adrenocorticotropic hormone (ACTH)

82030 Adenosine, 5-monophosphate, cyclic (cyclic AMP)

82040 Albumin; serum

82042 urine, quantitative, each specimen

82043 urine, microalbumin, quantitative

82044 urine, microalbumin, semiquantitative (eg, reagent strip assay)

(For prealbumin, use 84134)

82045 ischemia modified

82055 Alcohol (ethanol); any specimen except breath

● New Code ▲ Revised Code + Add-On Code ⊘ Modifier -51 Exempt ⊙ Conscious Sedation

(For other volatiles, alcohol, use 84600)

82075 breath

82085 Aldolase

82088 Aldosterone

(Alkaline phosphatase, see 84075, 84080)

82101 Alkaloids, urine, quantitative

(Alphaketoglutarate, see 82009, 82010)

(Alpha tocopherol (Vitamin E), use 84446)

82103 Alpha-1-antitrypsin; total

82104 phenotype

82105 Alpha-fetoprotein; serum

82106 amniotic fluid

● **82107** Alpha-fetoprotein (AFP); AFP-L3 fraction isoform and total AFP (including ratio)

82108 Aluminum

82120 Amines, vaginal fluid, qualitative

(For combined pH and amines test for vaginitis, use 82120 and 83986)

82127 Amino acids; single, qualitative, each specimen

82128 multiple, qualitative, each specimen

82131 single, quantitative, each specimen

82135 Aminolevulinic acid, delta (ALA)

82136 Amino acids, 2 to 5 amino acids, quantitative, each specimen

82139 Amino acids, 6 or more amino acids, quantitative, each specimen

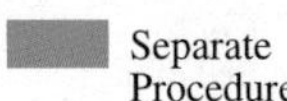

Separate Procedure | Unlisted Procedure | CCI Comp. Code | Non-specific Procedure

82140 Ammonia

82143 Amniotic fluid scan (spectrophotometric)

(For L/S ratio, use 83661)

(Amobarbital, see 80100-80103 for qualitative analysis, 82205 for quantitative analysis)

82145 Amphetamine or methamphetamine

(For qualitative analysis, see 80100-80103)

82150 Amylase

82154 Androstanediol glucuronide

82157 Androstenedione

82160 Androsterone

82163 Angiotensin II

82164 Angiotensin I - converting enzyme (ACE)

(Antidiuretic hormone (ADH), use 84588)

(Antimony, use 83015)

(Antitrypsin, alph-1-, see 82103, 82104)

82172 Apolipoprotein, each

82175 Arsenic

(For heavy metal screening, use 83015)

82180 Ascorbic acid (Vitamin C), blood

(Aspirin, see acetylsalicylic acid, 80196)

(Atherogenic index, blood, ultracentrifugation, quantitative, use 83717)

82190 Atomic absorption spectroscopy, each analyte

82205 Barbiturates, not elsewhere specified

(For qualitative analysis, see 80100-80103)

(For B-Natriuretic peptide, use 83880)

82232 Beta-2 microglobulin

(Bicarbonate, use 82374)

82239 Bile acids; total

82240 cholylglycine

(For bile pigments, urine, see 81000-81005)

82247 Bilirubin; total

82248 direct

82252 feces, qualitative

82261 Biotinidase, each specimen

82270 Blood, occult, by peroxidase activity (eg, guaiac), qualitative; feces, consecutive collected specimens with single determination, for colorectal neoplasm screening (ie, patient was provided three cards or single triple card for consecutive collection)

82271 other sources

82272 Blood, occult, by peroxidase activity (eg, guaiac), qualitative, feces, single specimen (eg, from digital rectal exam)

(Blood urea nitrogen (BUN), see 84520, 84525)

(82273 deleted 2006 edition. To report, use 82271)

82274 Blood, occult, by fecal hemoglobin determination by immunoassay, qualitative, feces, 1-3 simultaneous determinations

82286 Bradykinin

82300 Cadmium

82306 Calcifediol (25-OH Vitamin D-3)

82307 Calciferol (Vitamin D)

(For 1,25-Dihydroxyvitamin D, use 82652)

82308 Calcitonin

82310 Calcium; total

82330 ionized

82331 after calcium infusion test

82340 urine quantitative, timed specimen

82355 Calculus; qualitative analysis

82360 quantitative analysis, chemical

82365 infrared spectroscopy

82370 x-ray diffraction

(Carbamates, see individual listings)

82373 Carbohydrate deficient transferrin

82374 Carbon dioxide (bicarbonate)

(See also 82803)

82375 Carbon monoxide, (carboxyhemoglobin); quantitative

82376 qualitative

(To report end-tidal carbon monoxide, use Category III code 0043T)

82378 Carcinoembryonic antigen (CEA)

82379 Carnitine (total and free), quantitative, each specimen

(For acylcarnitine, see 82016, 82017)

82380 Carotene

82382 Catecholamines; total urine

82383 blood

82384 fractionated

 New Code ▲ Revised Code + Add-On Code 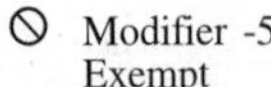 Modifier -51 Exempt ⊙ Conscious Sedation

(For urine metabolites, see 83835, 84585)

82387 Cathepsin-D

82390 Ceruloplasmin

82397 Chemiluminescent assay

82415 Chloramphenicol

82435 Chloride; blood

82436 urine

82438 other source

(For sweat collection by iontophoresis, use 89230)

82441 Chlorinated hydrocarbons, screen

(Chlorpromazine, use 84022)

(Cholecalciferol (Vitamin D), use 82307)

82465 Cholesterol, serum or whole blood, total

(For high density lipoprotein (HDL), use 83718)

82480 Cholinesterase; serum

82482 RBC

82485 Chondroitin B sulfate, quantitative

(Chorionic gonadotropin, see gonadotropin, 84702, 84703)

82486 Chromatography, qualitative; column (eg, gas liquid or HPLC), analyte not elsewhere specified

82487 paper, 1-dimensional, analyte not elsewhere specified

82488 paper, 2-dimensional, analyte not elsewhere specified

82489 thin layer, analyte not elsewhere specified

82491 Chromatography, quantitative, column (eg, gas liquid or HPLC); single analyte not elsewhere specified, single stationary and mobile phase

82492 multiple analytes, single stationary and mobile phase

82495 Chromium

82507 Citrate

82520 Cocaine or metabolite

(Cocaine, qualitative analysis, see 80100-80103)

(Codeine, qualitative analysis, see 80100-80103)

(Codeine, quantitative analysis, see 82101)

(Complement, see 86160-86162)

82523 Collagen cross links, any method

82525 Copper

(Coproporphyrin, see 84119, 84120)

(Corticosteroids, use 83491)

82528 Corticosterone

82530 Cortisol; free

82533 total

(C-peptide, use 84681)

82540 Creatine

82541 Column chromatography/mass spectrometry (eg, GC/MS, or HPLC/MS), analyte not elsewhere specified; qualitative, single stationary and mobile phase

82542 quantitative, single stationary and mobile phase

82543 stable isotope dilution, single analyte, quantitative, single stationary and mobile phase

82544 stable isotope dilution, multiple analytes, quantitative, single stationary and mobile phase

82550 Creatine kinase (CK), (CPK); total

82552 isoenzymes

82553 MB fraction only

82554 isoforms

82565 Creatinine; blood

82570 other source

82575 clearance

82585 Cryofibrinogen

82595 Cryoglobulin, qualitative or semi-quantitative (eg,cryocrit)

(For quantitative, cryoglobulin, see 82784, 82785)

(Crystals, pyrophosphate vs. urate, use 89060)

82600 Cyanide

82607 Cyanocobalamin (Vitamin B-12);

82608 unsaturated binding capacity

(Cyclic AMP, use 82030)

(Cyclic GMP, use 83008)

(Cyclosporine, use 80158)

82615 Cystine and homocystine, urine, qualitative

82626 Dehydroepiandrosterone (DHEA)

82627 Dehydroepiandrosterone-sulfate (DHEA-S)

(Delta-aminolevulinic acid (ALA), use 82135)

82633 Desoxycorticosterone, 11-

82634 Deoxycortisol, 11-

(Dexamethasone suppression test, use 80420)

(Diastase, urine, use 82150)

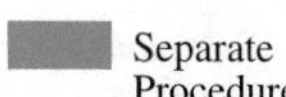
Separate Procedure

Unlisted Procedure
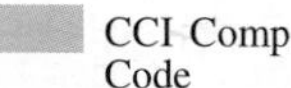
CCI Comp. Code
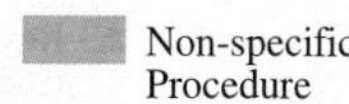
Non-specific Procedure

82638 Dibucaine number

(Dichloroethane, use 84600)

(Dichloromethane, use 84600)

(Diethylether, use 84600)

82646 Dihydrocodeinone

(For qualitative analysis, see 80100-80103)

82649 Dihydromorphinone

(For qualitative analysis, see 80100-80103)

82651 Dihydrotestosterone (DHT)

82652 Dihydroxyvitamin D, 1,25-

82654 Dimethadione

(For qualitative analysis, see 80100-80103)

(Diphenylhydantoin, use 80185)

(Dipropylacetic acid, use 80164)

(Dopamine, see 82382-82384)

(Duodenal contents, see individual enzymes; for intubation and collection, use 89100)

82656 Elastase, pancreatic (EL-1), fecal, qualitative or semi-quantitative

82657 Enzyme activity in blood cells, cultured cells, or tissue, not elsewhere specified; nonradioactive substrate, each specimen

82658 radioactive substrate, each specimen

82664 Electrophoretic technique, not elsewhere specified

(Endocrine receptor assays, see 84233-84235)`

82666 Epiandrosterone

(Epinephrine, see 82382-82384)

82668 Erythropoietin

● New Code ▲ Revised Code + Add-On Code ⊘ Modifier -51 Exempt ⊙ Conscious Sedation

82670 Estradiol

82671 Estrogens; fractionated

82672 total

(Estrogen receptor assay, use 84233)

82677 Estriol

82679 Estrone

(Ethanol, see 82055 and 82075)

82690 Ethchlorvynol

(Ethyl alcohol, see 82055 and 82075)

82693 Ethylene glycol

82696 Etiocholanolone

(For fractionation of ketosteroids, use 83593)

82705 Fat or lipids, feces; qualitative

82710 quantitative

82715 Fat differential, feces, quantitative

82725 Fatty acids, nonesterified

82726 Very long chain fatty acids

(For long-chain (C20-22) omega-3 fatty acids in red blood cell (RBC) membranes, use Category III code 0111T)

82728 Ferritin

(Fetal hemoglobin, see hemoglobin 83030, 83033, and 85460)

(Fetoprotein, alpha-1, see 82105, 82106)

82731 Fetal fibronectin, cervicovaginal secretions, semi-quantitative

82735 Fluoride

82742 Flurazepam

(For qualitative analysis, see 80100-80103)

(Foam stability test, use 83662)

82746 Folic acid; serum

82747 RBC

(Follicle stimulating hormone (FSH), use 83001)

82757 Fructose, semen

(Fructosamine, use 82985)

(Fructose, TLC screen, use 84375)

82759 Galactokinase, RBC

82760 Galactose

82775 Galactose-1-phosphate uridyl transferase; quantitative

82776 screen

82784 Gammaglobulin; IgA, IgD, IgG, IgM, each

82785 IgE

(For allergen specific IgE, see 86003, 86005)

82787 immunoglobulin subclasses, (IgG1, 2, 3, or 4), each

(Gamma-glutamyltransferase (GGT), use 82977)

82800 Gases, blood, pH only

82803 Gases, blood, any combination of pH, pCO_2, pO_2, CO_2, HCO_3 (including calculated O_2 saturation);

(Use 82803 for two or more of the above listed analytes)

82805 with O_2 saturation, by direct measurement, except pulse oximetry

82810 Gases, blood, O_2 saturation only, by direct measurement, except pulse oximetry

(For pulse oximetry, use 94760)

82820 Hemoglobin-oxygen affinity (pO_2 for 50% hemoglobin saturation with oxygen)

82926 Gastric acid, free and total, each specimen

82928 Gastric acid, free or total, each specimen

82938 Gastrin after secretin stimulation

82941 Gastrin

(Gentamicin, use 80170)

(GGT, use 82977)

(GLC, gas liquid chromatography, use 82486)

82943 Glucagon

82945 Glucose, body fluid, other than blood

82946 Glucagon tolerance test

82947 Glucose; quantitative, blood, (except reagent strip)

82948 blood, reagent strip

82950 post glucose dose (includes glucose)

82951 tolerance test (GTT), three specimens (includes glucose)

82952 tolerance test, each additional beyond three specimens

82953 tolbutamide tolerance test

(For insulin tolerance test, see 80434, 80435)

(For leucine tolerance test, use 80428)

(For semiquantitative urine glucose, see 81000, 81002, 81005, 81099)

82955 Glucose-6-phosphate dehydrogenase (G6PD); quantitative

82960 screen

(For glucose tolerance test with medication, use 90774 in addition)

82962 Glucose, blood by glucose monitoring device(s) cleared by the FDA specifically for home use

82963 Glucosidase, beta

82965 Glutamate dehydrogenase

82975 Glutamine (glutamic acid amide)

82977 Glutamyltransferase, gamma (GGT)

82978 Glutathione

82979 Glutathione reductase, RBC

82980 Glutethimide

(Glycohemoglobin, use 83036)

82985 Glycated protein

(Gonadotropin, chorionic, see 84702, 84703)

83001 Gonadotropin; follicle stimulating hormone (FSH)

83002 luteinizing hormone (LH)

(For luteinizing releasing factor (LRH), use 83727)

83003 Growth hormone, human (HGH) (somatotropin)

(For antibody to human growth hormone, use 86277)

83008 Guanosine monophosphate (GMP), cyclic

83009 Helicobacter pylori, blood test analysis for urease activity, non-radioactive isotope (eg, C-13)

(For H. pylori, breath test analysis for urease activity, see 83013, 83014)

83010 Haptoglobin; quantitative

83012 phenotypes

83013 Helicobacter pylori; breath test analysis for urease activity, non-radioactive isotope (eg, C-13)

83014 drug administration

(For H. pylori, stool, use 87338. For H. pylori, liquid scintillation counter, see 78267, 78268. For H. pylori, enzyme immunoassay, use 87339)

(For H. pylori, blood test analysis for urease activity, use 83009)

83015 Heavy metal (eg, arsenic, barium, beryllium, bismuth, antimony, mercury); screen

83018 quantitative, each

83020 Hemoglobin fractionation and quantitation; electrophoresis (eg, A2, S, C, and/or F)

83021 chromotography (eg, A2, S, C,and/or F)

83026 Hemoglobin; by copper sulfate method, non-automated

83030 F (fetal), chemical

83033 F (fetal), qualitative

83036 glycosylated (A1C)

(For fecal hemoglobin detection by immunoassay, use 82274)

83037 glycosylated (A1C) by device cleared by FDA for home use

83045 methemoglobin, qualitative

83050 methemoglobin, quantitative

83051 plasma

83055 sulfhemoglobin, qualitative

83060 sulfhemoglobin, quantitative

83065 thermolabile

83068 unstable, screen

83069 urine

Separate Procedure | Unlisted Procedure | CCI Comp. Code | Non-specific Procedure

83070 Hemosiderin; qualitative

83071 quantitative

(Heroin, see 80100-80103)

(HIAA, use 83497)

(High performance liquid chromatography (HPLC), use 82486)

83080 b-Hexosaminidase, each assay

83088 Histamine

(Hollander test, use 91052)

83090 Homocystine

83150 Homovanillic acid (HVA)

(Hormones, see individual alphabetic listings in Chemistry section)

(Hydrogen breath test, use 91065)

83491 Hydroxycorticosteroids, 17- (17-OHCS)

(For cortisol, see 82530, 82533. For deoxycortisol, use 82634)

83497 Hydroxyindolacetic acid, 5-(HIAA)

(For urine qualitative test, use 81005)

(5-Hydroxytryptamine, use 84260)

83498 Hydroxyprogesterone, 17-d

83499 Hydroxyprogesterone, 20-

83500 Hydroxyproline; free

83505 total

83516 Immunoassay for analyte other than infectious agent antibody or infectious agent antigen, qualitative or semiquantitative; multiple step method

83518 single step method (eg, reagent strip)

● New Code ▲ Revised Code + Add-On Code ⃠ Modifier -51 Exempt ⊙ Conscious Sedation

83519 Immunoassay, analyte, quantitative; by radiopharmaceutical technique (eg, RIA)

83520 not otherwise specified

(For immunoassays for antibodies to infectious agent antigens, see analyte and method specific codes in the Immunology section)

(For immunoassay of tumor antigen not elsewhere specified, use 86316)

(Immunoglobulins, see 82784, 82785)

83525 Insulin; total

(For proinsulin, use 84206)

83527 free

83528 Intrinsic factor

(For intrinsic factor antibodies, use 86340)

83540 Iron

83550 Iron binding capacity

83570 Isocitric dehydrogenase (IDH)

(Isonicotinic acid hydrazide, INH, see code for specific method)

(Isopropyl alcohol, use 84600)

83582 Ketogenic steroids, fractionation

(Ketone bodies, for serum, see 82009, 82010; for urine, see 81000-81003)

83586 Ketosteroids, 17- (17-KS); total

83593 fractionation

83605 Lactate (lactic acid)

83615 Lactate dehydrogenase (LD), (LDH);

83625 isoenzymes, separation and quantitation

Separate Procedure | Unlisted Procedure | CCI Comp. Code | Non-specific Procedure

83630 Lactoferrin, fecal; qualitative

83631 quantitative

83632 Lactogen, human placental (HPL) human chorionic somatomammotropin

83633 Lactose, urine; qualitative

83634 quantitative

(For tolerance, see 82951, 82952)

(For breath hydrogen test for lactase deficiency, use 91065)

83655 Lead

83661 Fetal lung maturity assessment; lecithin-sphingomyelin ratio (L/S ratio)

83662 foam stability test

83663 fluorescence polarization

83664 lamellar body density

(For phosphatidylglycerol, use 84081)

83670 Leucine aminopeptidase (LAP)

83690 Lipase

83695 Lipoprotein (a)

● **83698** Lipoprotein-associated phospholipase A_2, (Lp-PLA_2)

83700 Lipoprotein, blood; electrophoretic separation and quantitation

83701 high resolution fractionation and quantitation of lipoproteins including lipoprotein subclasses when performed (eg, electrophoresis, ultracentrifugation)

83704 quantitation of lipoprotein particle numbers and lipoprotein particle subclasses (eg, by nuclear magnetic resonance spectroscopy)

(83715 deleted 2006 edition. To report, use 83700, 83701)

(83716 deleted 2006 edition. To report, use 83700, 83701)

83718 Lipoprotein, direct measurement; high density cholesterol (HDL cholesterol)

83719 direct measurement, VLDL cholesterol

83721 direct measurement, LDL cholesterol

(For fractionation by high resolution electrophoresis or ultracentrifugation, use 83701)

(For lipoprotein particle numbers and subclasses analysis by nuclear magnetic resonance spectroscopy, use 83695)

(To report direct measurement, intermediate density lipoproteins (remnant lipoproteins), use Category III code 0026T)

83727 Luteinizing releasing factor (LRH)

(Luteinizing hormone (LH), use 83002)

(For qualitative analysis, see 80100-80103)

(Macroglobulins, alpha-2, use 86329)

83735 Magnesium

83775 Malate dehydrogenase

(Maltose tolerance, see 82951, 82952)

(Mammotropin, use 84146)

83785 Manganese

(Marijuana, see 80100-80103)

83788 Mass spectrometry and tandem mass spectrometry (MS, MS/MS), analyte not elsewhere specified; qualitative, each specimen

83789 quantitative, each specimen

83805 Meprobamate

(For qualitative analysis, see 80100-80103)

83825 Mercury, quantitative

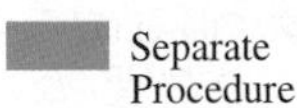 Separate Procedure 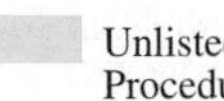 Unlisted Procedure 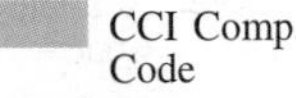 CCI Comp. Code 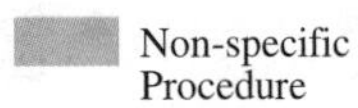 Non-specific Procedure

(Mercury screen, use 83015)

83835 Metanephrines

(For catecholamines, see 82382-82384)

83840 Methadone

(For methadone qualitative analysis, see 80100-80103)

(Methamphetamine, see 80100-80103, 82145)

(Methanol, use 84600)

83857 Methemalbumin

(Methemoglobin, see hemoglobin 83045, 83050)

83858 Methsuximide

(Methyl alcohol, use 84600)

(Microalbumin, see 82043 for quantitative, see 82044 for semiquantitative)

(Microglobulin, beta-2, use 82232)

83864 Mucopolysaccharides, acid; quantitative

83866 screen

83872 Mucin, synovial fluid (Ropes test)

83873 Myelin basic protein, cerebrospinal fluid

(For oligoclonal bands, use 83916)

83874 Myoglobin

(Nalorphine, use 83925)

83880 Natriuretic peptide

83883 Nephelometry, each analyte not elsewhere specified

83885 Nickel

83887 Nicotine

● New Code ▲ Revised Code + Add-On Code ⊘ Modifier -51 Exempt ⊙ Conscious Sedation

Codes 83890-83914 are intended for use with molecular diagnostic techniques for analysis of nucleic acids.

Codes 83890-83914 are coded by procedure rather than analyte.

When molecular diagnostic procedures are performed to test for oncology, hematology, neurology or inherited disorder, use the appropriate modifier to specify probe type or condition tested.

(For microbial identification, see 87470-87801)

(For array technology using more than 10 probes, see 88384-88386)

83890 Molecular diagnostics; molecular isolation or extraction

83891 isolation or extraction of highly purified nucleic acid

83892 enzymatic digestion

83893 dot/slot blot production

83894 separation by gel electrophoresis (eg, agarose, polyacrylamide)

83896 nucleic acid probe, each

83897 nucleic acid transfer (eg, Southern, Northern)

83898 amplification of patient nucleic acid, each nucleic acid sequence

83900 amplification of patient nucleic acid, multiplex, first two nucleic acid sequences

+ **83901** amplification of patient nucleic acid, multiplex, each additional nucleic acid sequence (List separately in addition to code for primary procedure)

(Use 83901 in conjunction with 83900)

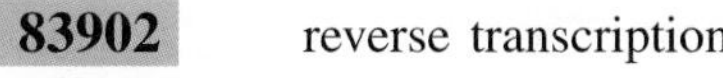

83902 reverse transcription

83903 mutation scanning, by physical properties (eg, single strand conformational polymorphisms (SSCP), heteroduplex, denaturing gradient gel electrophoresis (DGGE), RNA'ase A), single segment, each

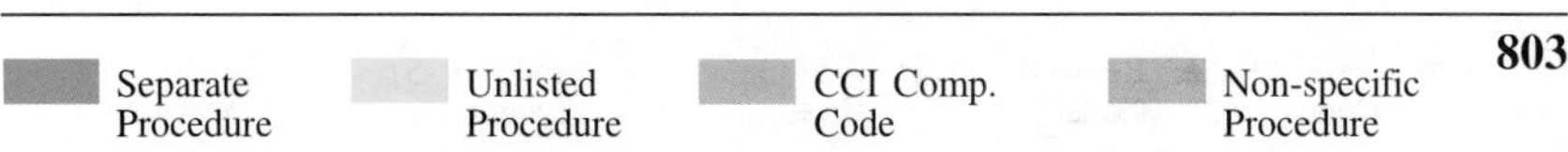

83904 mutation identification by sequencing, single segment, each segment

83905 mutation identification by allele specific transcription, single segment, each segment

83906 mutation identification by allele specific translation, single segment, each segment

83907 lysis of cells prior to nucleic acid extraction (eg, stool specimens, paraffin embedded tissue)

83908 signal amplification of patient nucleic acid, each nucleic acid sequence

(For multiplex amplification, see 83900, 83901)

83909 separation and identification by high resolution technique (eg, capillary electrophoresis)

83912 interpretation and report

● **83913** Molecular diagnostics; RNA stabilization

83914 Mutation identification by enzymatic ligation or primer extension, single segment, each segment (eg, oligonucleotide ligation assay (OLA), single base chain extension (SBCE), or allele-specific primer extension (ASPE))

83915 Nucleotidase 5-

83916 Oligoclonal immune (oligoclonal bands)

83918 Organic acids; total, quantitative, each specimen

83919 qualitative, each specimen

83921 Organic acid, single; quantitative

83925 Opiates, (eg, morphine, meperidine)

83930 Osmolality; blood

83935 urine

83937 Osteocalcin (bone g1a protein)

83945 Oxalate

83950 Oncoprotein, HER-2/neu

(For tissue, see 88342, 88365)

83970 Parathormone (parathyroid hormone)

(Pesticide, quantitative, see code for specific method. For screen for chlorinated hydrocarbons, use 82441)

83986 pH, body fluid, except blood

(For blood pH, see 82800, 82803)

83992 Phencyclidine (PCP)

(For qualitative analysis, see 80100-80103)

(Phenobarbital, use 80184)

84022 Phenothiazine

(For qualitative analysis, see 80100, 80101)

84030 Phenylalanine (PKU), blood

(Phenylalanine-tyrosine ratio, see 84030, 84510)

84035 Phenylketones, qualitative

84060 Phosphatase, acid; total

84061 forensic examination

84066 prostatic

84075 Phosphatase, alkaline;

84078 heat stable (total not included)

84080 isoenzymes

84081 Phosphatidylglycerol

(Phosphates inorganic, use 84100)

(Phosphates, organic, see code for specific method. For cholinesterase, see 82480, 82482)

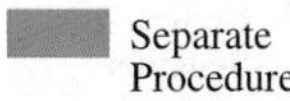
Separate Procedure
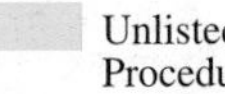
Unlisted Procedure
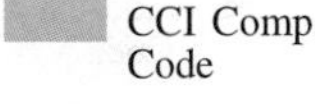
CCI Comp. Code
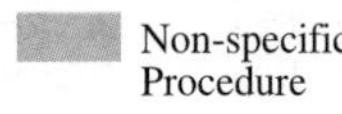
Non-specific Procedure

84085 Phosphogluconate, 6-, dehydrogenase, RBC

84087 Phosphohexose isomerase

84100 Phosphorus inorganic (phosphate);

84105 urine

(Pituitary gonadotropins, see 83001-83002)

(PKU, see 84030, 84035)

84106 Porphobilinogen, urine; qualitative

84110 quantitative

84119 Porphyrins, urine; qualitative

84120 quantitation and fractionation

84126 Porphyrins, feces; quantitative

84127 qualitative

(Porphyrin precursors, see 82135, 84106, 84110)

(For protoporphyrin, RBC, see 84202, 84203)

84132 Potassium; serum

84133 urine

84134 Prealbumin

(For microalbumin, see 82043, 82044)

84135 Pregnanediol

84138 Pregnanetriol

84140 Pregnenolone

84143 17-hydroxypregnenolone

84144 Progesterone

(Progesterone receptor assay, use 84234)

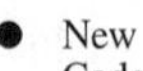
New Code

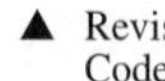
Revised Code

+ Add-On Code

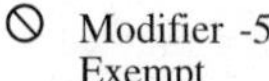
Modifier -51 Exempt

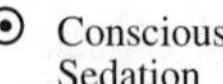
Conscious Sedation

(For proinsulin, use 84206)

84146 Prolactin

84150 Prostaglandin, each

84152 Prostate specific antigen (PSA); complexed (direct measurement)

84153 total

84154 free

84155 Protein, total, except by refractometry; serum

84156 urine

84157 other source (eg, synovial fluid, cerebrospinal fluid)

84160 Protein, total, by refractometry, any source

(For urine total protein by dipstick method, use 81000-81003)

84163 Pregnancy-associated plasma protein-A (PAPP-A)

84165 Protein; electrophoretic fractionation and quantitation, serum

84166 electrophoretic fractionation and quantitation, other fluids with concentration (eg, urine, CSF)

84181 Western Blot, with interpretation and report, blood or other body fluid

84182 Western Blot, with interpretation and report, blood or other body fluid, immunological probe for band identification, each

(For Western Blot tissue analysis, use 88371)

84202 Protoporphyrin, RBC; quantitative

84203 screen

84206 Proinsulin

(Pseudocholinesterase, use 82480)

84207 Pyridoxal phosphate (Vitamin B-6)

84210 Pyruvate

84220 Pyruvate kinase

84228 Quinine

84233 Receptor assay; estrogen

84234 progesterone

84235 endocrine, other than estrogen or progesterone (specify hormone)

84238 non-endocrine (specify receptor)

84244 Renin

84252 Riboflavin (Vitamin B-2)

(Salicylates, use 80196)

(Secretin test, see 99070, 89100 and appropriate analyses)

84255 Selenium

84260 Serotonin

(For urine metabolites (HIAA), use 83497)

84270 Sex hormone binding globulin (SHBG)

84275 Sialic acid

(Sickle hemoglobin, use 85660)

84285 Silica

84295 Sodium; serum

84300 urine

84302 other source

(Somatomammotropin, use 83632)

(Somatotropin, use 83003)

● New Code ▲ Revised Code + Add-On Code ⃠ Modifier -51 Exempt ⊙ Conscious Sedation

84305 Somatomedin

84307 Somatostatin

84311 Spectrophotometry, analyte not elsewhere specified

84315 Specific gravity (except urine)

(For specific gravity, urine, see 81000-81003)

(Stone analysis, see 82355-82370)

84375 Sugars, chromatographic, TLC or paper chromatography

84376 Sugars (mono, di, and oligosaccharides); single qualitative, each specimen

84377 multiple qualitative, each specimen

84378 single quantitative, each specimen

84379 multiple quantitative, each specimen

84392 Sulfate, urine

(Sulfhemoglobin, see hemoglobin, 83055, 83060)

(T-3, see 84479-84481)

(T-4, see 84436-84439)

84402 Testosterone; free

84403 total

84425 Thiamine (Vitamin B-1)

84430 Thiocyanate

84432 Thyroglobulin

(Thyroglobulin, antibody, use 86800)

(Thyrotropin releasing hormone (TRH) test, see 80438, 80439)

84436 Thyroxine; total

84437 requiring elution (eg, neonatal)

Separate Procedure | Unlisted Procedure | CCI Comp. Code | Non-specific Procedure

84439 free

84442 Thyroxine binding globulin (TBG)

84443 Thyroid stimulating hormone (TSH)

84445 Thyroid stimulating immune globulins (TSI)

(Tobramycin, use 80200)

84446 Tocopherol alpha (Vitamin E)

(Tolbutamide tolerance, use 82953)

84449 Transcortin (cortisol binding globulin)

84450 Transferase; aspartate amino (AST) (SGOT)

84460 alanine amino (ALT) (SGPT)

84466 Transferrin

(Iron binding capacity, use 83550)

84478 Triglycerides

84479 Thyroid hormone (T3 or T4) uptake or thyroid hormone binding ratio (THBR)

84480 Triiodothyronine T3; total (TT-3)

84481 free

84482 reverse

84484 Troponin, quantitative

(For Troponin, qualitative assay, use 84512)

84485 Trypsin; duodenal fluid

84488 feces, qualitative

84490 feces, quantitative, 24-hour collection

84510 Tyrosine

● New Code  ▲ Revised Code  + Add-On Code 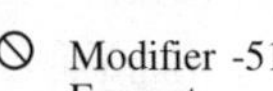 ⊘ Modifier -51 Exempt 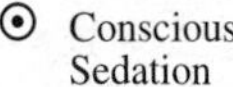 ⊙ Conscious Sedation

(Urate crystal identification, use 89060)

84512 Troponin, qualitative

(For Troponin, quantitative assay, use 84484)

84520 Urea nitrogen; quantitative

84525 semiquantitative (eg, reagent strip test)

84540 Urea nitrogen, urine

84545 Urea nitrogen, clearance

84550 Uric acid; blood

84560 other source

84577 Urobilinogen, feces, quantitative

84578 Urobilinogen, urine; qualitative

84580 quantitative, timed specimen

84583 semiquantitative

(Uroporphyrins, use 84120)

(Valproic acid (dipropylacetic acid), ues 80164)

84585 Vanillylmandelic acid (VMA), urine

84586 Vasoactive intestinal peptide (VIP)

84588 Vasopressin (antidiuretic hormone, ADH)

84590 Vitamin A

(Vitamin B-1, use 84425)

(Vitamin B-2, use 84252)

(Vitamin B-6, use 84207)

(Vitamin B-12, use 82607)

(Vitamin B-12, absorption (Schilling), see 78270, 78271)

Separate Procedure | Unlisted Procedure | CCI Comp. Code | Non-specific Procedure

(Vitamin C, use 82180)

(Vitamin D, see 82306, 82307, 82652)

(Vitamin E, use 84446)

84591 Vitamin, not otherwise specified

84597 Vitamin K

(VMA, use 84585)

84600 Volatiles (eg, acetic anhydride, carbon tetrachloride, dichloroethane, dichloromethane, diethylether, isopropyl alcohol, methanol)

(For acetaldehyde, use 82000)

(Volume, blood, RISA or Cr-51, see 78110, 78111)

84620 Xylose absorption test, blood and/or urine

(For administration, use 99070)

84630 Zinc

84681 C-peptide

84702 Gonadotropin, chorionic (hCG); quantitative

84703 qualitative

(For urine pregnancy test by visual color comparison, use 81025)

84830 Ovulation tests, by visual color comparison methods for human luteinizing hormone

84999 Unlisted chemistry procedure

HEMATOLOGY AND COAGULATION

(For blood banking procedures, see Transfusion Medicine)

(Agglutinins, see Immunology)

(Antiplasmin, use 85410)

(Antithrombin III, see 85300, 85301)

85002 Bleeding time

85004 Blood count; automated differential WBC count

85007 blood smear, microscopic examination with manual differential WBC count

85008 blood smear, microscopic examination without manual differential WBC count

(For other fluids (eg, CSF), see 89050, 89051)

85009 manual differential WBC count, buffy coat

(Eosinophils, nasal smear, use 89190)

85013 spun microhematocrit

85014 hematocrit (Hct)

85018 hemoglobin (Hgb)

(For other hemoglobin determination, see 83020-83069)

(For immunoassay, hemoglobin, fecal, use 86683)

85025 complete (CBC), automated (Hgb, Hct, RBC, WBC and platelet count) and automated differential WBC count

85027 complete (CBC), automated (Hgb, Hct, RBC, WBC and platelet count)

85032 manual cell count (erythrocyte, leukocyte, or platelet) each

85041 red blood cell (RBC), automated

(Do not report code 85041 in conjunction with 85025 or 85027)

85044 reticulocyte, manual

85045 reticulocyte, automated

85046 reticulocytes, automated, including one or more cellular parameters (eg, reticulocyte hemoglobin content (CHr), immature reticulocyte fraction (IRF), reticulocyte volume (mrv), RNA content), direct measurement

85048 leukocyte (WBC), automated

85049 platelet, automated

85055 Reticulated platelet assay

85060 Blood smear, peripheral, interpretation by physician with written report

85097 Bone marrow, smear interpretation

(For special stains, see 85540, 88312, 88313)

(For bone biopsy, see 20220, 20225, 20240, 20245, 20250, 20251)

85130 Chromogenic substrate assay

(Circulating anti-coagulant screen (mixing studies), see 85611, 85732)

85170 Clot retraction

85175 Clot lysis time, whole blood dilution

(Clotting factor I (fibrinogen), see 85384, 85385)

85210 Clotting; factor II, prothrombin, specific

(See also 85610-85613)

85220 factor V (AcG or proaccelerin), labile factor

85230 factor VII (proconvertin, stable factor)

85240 factor VIII (AHG), one stage

85244 factor VIII related antigen

85245 factor VIII, VW factor, ristocetin cofactor

85246 factor VIII, VW factor antigen

85247 factor VIII, von Willebrands factor, multimetric analysis

85250 factor IX (PTC or Christmas)

85260 factor X (Stuart-Prower)

85270 factor XI (PTA)

85280 factor XII (Hageman)

85290 factor XIII (fibrin stabilizing)

85291 factor XIII (fibrin stabilizing), screen solubility

85292 prekallikrein assay (Fletcher factor assay)

85293 high molecular weight kininogen assay (Fitzgerald factor assay)

85300 Clotting inhibitors or anticoagulants; antithrombin III, activity

85301 antithrombin III, antigen assay

85302 protein C, antigen

85303 protein C, activity

85305 protein S, total

85306 protein S, free

85307 Activated Protein C (APC) resistance assay

85335 Factor inhibitor test

85337 Thrombomodulin

(For mixing studies for inhibitors, use 85732)

85345 Coagulation time; Lee and White

85347 activated

85348 other methods

(Differential count, see 85007 et seq)

(Duke bleeding time, use 85002)

(Eosinophils, nasal smear, use 89190)

85360 Euglobulin lysis

(Fetal hemoglobin, see 83030, 83033, 85460)

85362 Fibrin(ogen) degradation (split) products (FDP)(FSP); agglutination slide, semiquantitative

(Immunoelectrophoresis, use 86320)

85366 paracoagulation

85370 quantitative

85378 Fibrin degradation products, D-dimer; qualitative or semiquantitative

85379 quantitative

(For ultrasensitive and standard sensitivity quantitative D-dimer, use 85379)

85380 ultrasensitive (eg., for evaluation for venous thromboembolism), qualitative or semiquantitative

85384 Fibrinogen; activity

85385 antigen

85390 Fibrinolysins or coagulopathy screen, interpretation and report

85396 Coagulation/fibrinolysis assay, whole blood (eg, viscoelastic clot assessment), including use of any pharmacologic additive(s), as indicated, including interpretation and written report, per day

85400 Fibrinolytic factors and inhibitors; plasmin

85410 alpha-2 antiplasmin

85415 plasminogen activator

85420 plasminogen, except antigenic assay

85421 plasminogen, antigenic assay

(Fragility, red blood cell, see 85547, 85555-85557)

85441 Heinz bodies; direct

85445 induced, acetyl phenylhydrazine

(Hematocrit (PCV), see 85014)

(Hemoglobin, see 83020-83068, 85018-85027)

85460 Hemoglobin or RBCs, fetal, for fetomaternal hemorrhage; differential lysis (Kleihauer-Betke)

(See also 83030, 83033)

(Hemolysins, see 86940, 86941)

85461 rosette

85475 Hemolysin, acid

(See also 86940, 86941)

85520 Heparin assay

85525 Heparin neutralization

85530 Heparin-protamine tolerance test

85536 Iron stain, peripheral blood

(For iron stains on bone marrow or other tissues with physician evaluation, use 88313)

85540 Leukocyte alkaline phosphatase with count

85547 Mechanical fragility, RBC

85549 Muramidase

(Nitroblue tetrazolium dye test, use 86384)

85555 Osmotic fragility, RBC; unincubated

85557 incubated

(Packed cell volume, use 85013)

(Partial thromboplastin time, see 85730, 85732)

(Parasites, blood (eg, malaria smears), use 87207)

(Plasmin, use 85400)

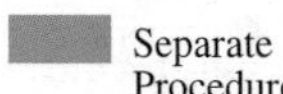 Separate Procedure | Unlisted Procedure | CCI Comp. Code | Non-specific Procedure

(Plasminogen, use 85420)

(Plasminogen activator, use 85415)

85576 Platelet; aggregation (in vitro), each agent

85597 Platelet neutralization

85610 Prothrombin time;

85611 substitution, plasma fractions, each

85612 Russell viper venom time (includes venom); undiluted

85613 diluted

(Red blood cell count, see 85025, 85027, 85041)

85635 Reptilase test

(Reticulocyte count, see 85044, 85045)

85651 Sedimentation rate, erythrocyte; non-automated

85652 automated

85660 Sickling of RBC, reduction

(Hemoglobin electrophoresis, use 83020)

(Smears (eg, for parasites, malaria), use 87207)

85670 Thrombin time; plasma

85675 titer

85705 Thromboplastin inhibition, tissue

(For individual clotting factors, see 85245-85247)

85730 Thromboplastin time, partial (PTT); plasma or whole blood

85732 substitution, plasma fractions, each

85810 Viscosity

(von Willebrand factor assay, see 85245-85247)

● New Code ▲ Revised Code + Add-On Code ⃠ Modifier -51 Exempt ⊙ Conscious Sedation

(WBC count, see 85025-85031, 85048, 89050)

85999 Unlisted hematology and coagulation procedure

IMMUNOLOGY

(Acetylcholine receptor antibody, see 83519, 86255, 86256)

(Actinomyces, antibodies to, use 86602)

(Adrenal cortex antibodies, see 86255, 86256)

86000 Agglutinins, febrile (eg, Brucella, Francisella, Murine typhus, Q fever, Rocky Mountain spotted fever, scrub typhus), each antigen

(For antibodies to infectious agents, see 86602-86804)

86001 Allergen specific IgG quantitative or semiquantitative, each allergen

(Agglutinins and autohemolysins, see 86940, 86941)

86003 Allergen specific IgE; quantitative or semiquantitative, each allergen

(For total quantitative IgE, use 82785)

86005 qualitative, multiallergen screen (dipstick, paddle or disk)

(For total qualitative IgE, use 83518)

(Alpha-1 antitrypsin, see 82103, 82104)

(Alpha-1 feto-protein, see 82105, 82106)

(Anti-AChR (acetylcholine receptor) antibody titer, see 86255, 86256)

(Anticardiolipin antibody, use 86147)

(Anti-DNA, use 86225)

(Anti-deoxyribonuclease titer, use 86215)

86021 Antibody identification; leukocyte antibodies

86022 platelet antibodies

86023 platelet associated immunoglobulin assay

86038 Antinuclear antibodies (ANA);

86039 titer

(Antistreptococcal antibody, ie, anti-DNAse, use 86215)

(Antistreptokinase titer, use 86590)

86060 Antistreptolysin 0; titer

(For antibodies to infectious agents, see 86602-86804)

86063 screen

(For antibodies to infectious agents, see 86602-86804)

(Blastomyces, antibodies to, use 86612)

(86064 deleted 2006 edition. For B cells, total count, use 86355)

86077 Blood bank physician services; difficult cross match and/or evaluation of irregular antibody(s), interpretation and written report

86078 investigation of transfusion reaction including suspicion of transmissible disease, interpretation and written report

86079 authorization for deviation from standard blood banking procedures (eg, use of outdated blood, transfusion of Rh incompatible units), with written report

(Brucella, antibodies to, use 86622)

(Candida, antibodies to, use 86628. For skin testing, use 86485)

86140 C-reactive protein;

(Candidiasis, use 86628)

86141 high sensitivity (hsCRP)

86146 Beta 2 Glycoprotein 1 antibody, each

86147 Cardiolipin (phospholipid) antibody, each lg class

86148 Anti-phosphatidylserine (phospholipid) antibody

(To report antiprothrombin (phospholipid cofactor) antibody, use Category III code 0030T)

86155 Chemotaxis assay, specify method

(Clostridium difficile toxin, use 87230)

(Coccidioides, antibodies, to, see 86635. For skin testing, use 86490)

86156 Cold agglutinin; screen

86157 titer

86160 Complement; antigen, each component

86161 functional activity, each component

86162 total hemolytic (CH50)

86171 Complement fixation tests, each antigen

(Coombs test, see 86880-86886)

86185 Counterimmunoelectrophoresis, each antigen

(Cryptococcus, antibodies to, use 86641)

86200 Cyclic citrullinated peptide (CCP), antibody

86215 Deoxyribonuclease, antibody

86225 Deoxyribonucleic acid (DNA) antibody; native or double stranded

(Echinococcus, antibodies to, see code for specific method)

(For HIV antibody tests, see 86701-86703)

86226 single stranded

(Anti D.S., DNA, IFA, eg, using C.Lucilae, see 86255 and 86256)

86235 Extractable nuclear antigen, antibody to, any method (eg, nRNP, SS-A, SS-B, Sm, RNP, Sc170, J01), each antibody

86243 Fc receptor

(Filaria, antibodies to, see code for specific method)

86255 Fluorescent noninfectious agent antibody; screen, each antibody

Separate Procedure | Unlisted Procedure | CCI Comp. Code | Non-specific Procedure

86256 titer, each antibody

(Fluorescent technique for antigen identification in tissue, use 88346; for indirect fluorescence, use 88347)

(FTA, see 86781)

(Gel (agar) diffusion tests, use 86331)

86277 Growth hormone, human (HGH), antibody

86280 Hemagglutination inhibition test (HAI)

(For rubella, use 86762)

(For antibodies to infectious agents, see 86602-86804)

86294 Immunoassay for tumor antigen, qualitative or semiquantitative (eg, bladder tumor antigen)

86300 Immunoassay for tumor antigen, quantitative; CA 15-3 (27.29)

86301 CA 19-9

86304 CA 125

(For measurement of serum HER-2/neu oncoprotein, see 83950)

(For hepatitis delta agent, antibody, use 86692)

86308 Heterophile antibodies; screening

(For antibodies to infectious agents, see 86602-86804)

86309 titer

(For antibodies to infectious agents, see 86602-86804)

86310 titers after absorption with beef cells and guinea pig kidney

(Histoplasma, antibodies to, use 86698. For skin testing, use 86510)

(For antibodies to infectious agents, see 86602-86804)

(Human growth hormone antibody, use 86277)

86316 Immunoassay for tumor antigen, other antigen, quantitative (eg, CA 50, 72-4, 549), each

● New Code ▲ Revised Code + Add-On Code ⊘ Modifier -51 Exempt ⊙ Conscious Sedation

86317 Immunoassay for infectious agent antibody, quantitative, not otherwise specified

(For immunoassay techniques for antigens, see 83516, 83518, 83519, 83520, 87301-87450, 87810-87899)

(For particle agglutination procedures, use 86403)

86318 Immunoassay for infectious agent antibody, qualitative or semiquantitative, single step method (eg, reagent strip)

86320 Immunoelectrophoresis; serum

86325 other fluids (eg, urine, cerebrospinal fluid) with concentration

86327 crossed (2-dimensional assay)

86329 Immunodiffusion; not elsewhere specified

86331 gel diffusion, qualitative (Ouchterlony), each antigen or antibody

86332 Immune complex assay

86334 Immunofixation electrophoresis; serum

86335 Immunofixation electrophoresis; other fluids with concentration (eg, urine, CSF)

86336 Inhibin A

86337 Insulin antibodies

86340 Intrinsic factor antibodies

(Leptospira, antibodies to, use 86720)

(Leukoagglutinins, use 86021)

86341 Islet cell antibody

86343 Leukocyte histamine release test (LHR)

86344 Leukocyte phagocytosis

Separate Procedure | Unlisted Procedure | CCI Comp. Code | Non-specific Procedure

86353 Lymphocyte transformation, mitogen (phytomitogen) or antigen induced blastogenesis

(Malaria antibodies, use 86750)

86355 B cells, total count

86357 Natural killer (NK) cells, total count

86359 T cells; total count

86360 absolute CD4 and CD8 count, including ratio

86361 absolute CD4 count

86367 Stem cells (ie, CD34), total count

(For flow cytometric immunophenotyping for the assessment of potential hematolymphoid neoplasia, see 88184-88189)

86376 Microsomal antibodies (eg, thyroid or liver-kidney), each

86378 Migration inhibitory factor test (MIF)

(Mitochondrial antibody, liver, see 86255, 86256)

(Mononucleosis, see 86308-86310)

(86379 deleted 2006 edition. For natural killer cells, total count, use 86357)

86382 Neutralization test, viral

86384 Nitroblue tetrazolium dye test (NTD)

(Ouchterlony diffusion, use 86331)

(Platelet antibodies, see 86022, 86023)

86403 Particle agglutination; screen, each antibody

86406 titer, each antibody

(Pregnancy test, see 84702, 84703)

(Rapid plasma reagin test (RPR), see 86592, 86593)

86430 Rheumatoid factor; qualitative

● New Code ▲ Revised Code + Add-On Code ⃠ Modifier -51 Exempt ⊙ Conscious Sedation

86431 quantitative

(Serologic test for syphilis, see 86592, 86593)

86480 Tuberculosis test, cell mediated immunity measurement of gamma interferon antigen response

86485 Skin test; candida

(For antibody, candida, use 86628)

86490 coccidioidomycosis

86510 histoplasmosis

(For histoplasma, antibody, use 86698)

86580 tuberculosis, intradermal

(For tuberculosis test, cell mediated immunity measurement of gamma interferon antigen response, use 86480)

(86585 deleted 2006 edition. To report tuberculosis testing by intradermal (Mantoux) text, use 86580)

(For skin tests for allergy, see 95010-95199)

(Smooth muscle antibody, see 86255, 86256)

(Sporothrix, antibodies to, see code for specific method)

86586 Unlisted antigen, each

(86587 deleted 2006 edition. For stem cells, total count, use 86367)

86590 Streptokinase, antibody

(For antibodies to infectious agents, see 86602-86804)

(Streptolysin O antibody, see antistreptolysin O, 86060, 86063)

86592 Syphilis test; qualitative (eg, VDRL, RPR, ART)

(For antibodies to infectious agents, see 86602-86804)

86593 quantitative

(For antibodies to infectious agents, see 86602-86804)

(Tetanus antibody, use 86774)

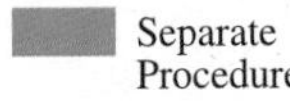 Separate Procedure 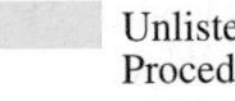 Unlisted Procedure 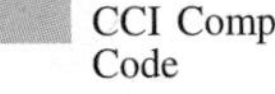 CCI Comp. Code 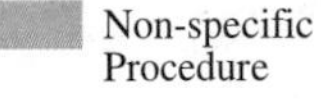 Non-specific Procedure

(Thyroglobulin antibody, use 86800)

(Thyroglobulin, use 84432)

(Thyroid microsomal antibody, use 86376)

(For toxoplasma antibody, see 86777-86778)

(For the detection of antibodies other than those to infectious agents, see specific antibody (eg, 86021, 86022, 86023, 86376, 86800, 86850-86870) or specific method (eg, 83516, 86255, 86256))

(For infectious agent/antigen detection, see 87260-87899)

86602 Antibody; actinomyces

86603 adenovirus

86606 Aspergillus

86609 bacterium, not elsewhere specified

86611 Bartonella

86612 Blastomyces

86615 Bordetella

86617 Borrelia burgdorferi (Lyme disease) confirmatory test (eg, Western blot or immunoblot)

86618 Borrelia burgdorferi (Lyme disease)

86619 Borrelia (relapsing fever)

86622 Brucella

86625 Campylobacter

86628 Candida

(For skin test, candida, use 86485)

86631 Chlamydia

86632 Chlamydia, IgM

(For chlamydia antigen, see 87270, 87320. For fluorescent antibody technique, see 86255, 86256)

86635 Coccidioides

86638 Coxiella Brunetii (Q fever)

86641 Cryptococcus

86644 cytomegalovirus (CMV)

86645 cytomegalovirus (CMV), IgM

86648 Diphtheria

86651 encephalitis, California (La Crosse)

86652 encephalitis, Eastern equine

86653 encephalitis, St. Louis

86654 encephalitis, Western equine

86658 enterovirus (eg, coxsackie, echo, polio)

(Trichinella, antibodies to, use 86784)

(Trypanosoma, antibodies to, see code for specific method)

(Tuberculosis, use 86580 for skin testing)

(Viral antibodies, see code for specific method)

86663 Epstein-Barr (EB) virus, early antigen (EA)

86664 Epstein-Barr (EB) virus, nuclear antigen (EBNA)

86665 Epstein-Barr (EB) virus, viral capsid (VCA)

86666 Ehrlichia

86668 Francisella Tularensis

86671 fungus, not elsewhere specified

86674 Giardia Lamblia

Separate Procedure | Unlisted Procedure | CCI Comp. Code | Non-specific Procedure

86677 Helicobacter Pylori

86682 helminth, not elsewhere specified

86684 Hemophilus influenza

86687 HTLV-I

86688 HTLV-II

86689 HTLV or HIV antibody, confirmatory test (eg, Western Blot)

86692 hepatitis, delta agent

(For hepatitis delta agent, antigen, use 87380)

86694 herpes simplex, non-specific type test

86695 herpes simplex, type 1

86696 herpes simplex, type 2

86698 histoplasma

86701 HIV-1

86702 HIV-2

86703 HIV-1 and HIV-2, single assay

(For HIV-1 antigen, use 87390)

(For HIV-2 antigen, use 87391)

(For confirmatory test for HIV antibody (eg, Western Blot), use 86689)

86704 Hepatitis B core antibody (HBcAb); total

86705 IgM antibody

86706 Hepatitis B surface antibody (HBsAb)

86707 Hepatitis Be antibody (HBeAb)

86708 Hepatitis A antibody (HAAb); total

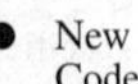 ● New Code 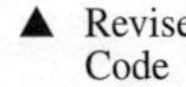 ▲ Revised Code + Add-On Code 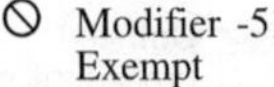 ⃠ Modifier -51 Exempt ⊙ Conscious Sedation

86709 IgM antibody

86710 Antibody; influenza virus

86713 Legionella

86717 Leishmania

86720 Leptospira

86723 Listeria monocytogenes

86727 lymphocytic choriomeningitis

86729 Lymphogranuloma Venereum

86732 mucormycosis

86735 mumps

86738 Mycoplasma

86741 Neisseria meningitidis

86744 Nocardia

86747 parvovirus

86750 Plasmodium (malaria)

86753 protozoa, not elsewhere specified

86756 respiratory syncytial virus

86757 Rickettsia

86759 rotavirus

86762 rubella

86765 rubeola

86768 Salmonella

86771 Shigella

86774 tetanus

86777 Toxoplasma

86778 Toxoplasma, IgM

86781 Treponema Pallidum, confirmatory test (eg, FTA-abs)

86784 trichinella

86787 varicella-zoster

● **86788** West Nile virus, IgM

● **86789** West Nile virus

86790 virus, not elsewhere specified

86793 Yersinia

86800 Thyroglobulin antibody

(For thyroglobulin, use 84432)

86803 Hepatitis C antibody;

86804 confirmatory test (eg, immunoblot)

TISSUE TYPING

(For pretransplant cross-match, see appropriate code or codes)

86805 Lymphocytotoxicity assay, visual crossmatch; with titration

86806 without titration

86807 Serum screening for cytotoxic percent reactive antibody (PRA); standard method

86808 quick method

86812 HLA typing; A, B, or C (eg, A10, B7, B27), single antigen

86813 A, B, or C, multiple antigens

86816 DR/DQ, single antigen

86817 DR/DQ, multiple antigens

86821 lymphocyte culture, mixed (MLC)

86822 lymphocyte culture, primed (PLC)

86849 Unlisted immunology procedure

TRANSFUSION MEDICINE

(For apheresis, see 36511-36512)

(For therapeutic phlebotomy, use 99195)

86850 Antibody screen, RBC, each serum technique

86860 Antibody elution (RBC), each elution

86870 Antibody identification, RBC antibodies, each panel for each serum technique

86880 Antihuman globulin test (Coombs test); direct, each antiserum

86885 indirect, qualitative, each antiserum

86886 indirect, titer, each antiserum

86890 Autologous blood or component, collection processing and storage; predeposited

86891 intra-or postoperative salvage

(For physician services to autologous donors, see 99201-99204)

86900 Blood typing; ABO

86901 Rh (D)

86903 antigen screening for compatible blood unit using reagent serum, per unit screened

86904 antigen screening for compatible unit using patient serum, per unit screened

86905 RBC antigens, other than ABO or Rh (D), each

86906 Rh phenotyping, complete

86910 Blood typing, for paternity testing, per individual; ABO, Rh and MN

86911 each additional antigen system

86920 Compatibility test each unit; immediate spin technique

86921 incubation technique

86922 antiglobulin technique

86923 electronic

(Do not use 86923 in conjunction with 86920-86922 for same unit crossmatch)

86927 Fresh frozen plasma, thawing, each unit

86930 Frozen blood, each unit; freezing (includes preparation)

86931 thawing

86932 freezing (includes preparation) and thawing

86940 Hemolysins and agglutinins; auto, screen, each

86941 incubated

86945 Irradiation of blood product, each unit

86950 Leukocyte transfusion

(For leukapheresis, see 36511-36512)

86960 Volume reduction of blood or blood product (eg, red blood cells or platelets), each unit

86965 Pooling of platelets or other blood products

86970 Pretreatment of RBCs for use in RBC antibody detection, identification, and/or compatibility testing; incubation with chemical agents or drugs, each

86971 incubation with enzymes, each

86972 by density gradient separation

86975 Pretreatment of serum for use in RBC antibody identification; incubation with drugs, each

86976 by dilution

86977 incubation with inhibitors, each

86978 by differential red cell absorption using patient RBCs or RBCs of known phenotype, each absorption

86985 Splitting of blood or blood products, each unit

86999 Unlisted transfusion medicine procedure

MICROBIOLOGY

87001 Animal inoculation, small animal; with observation

87003 with observation and dissection

87015 Concentration (any type), for infectious agents

(Do not report 87015 in conjunction with 87177)

87040 Culture, bacterial; blood, aerobic, with isolation and presumptive identification of isolates (includes anaerobic culture, if appropriate)

87045 stool, aerobic, with isolation and preliminary examination (eg, KIA, LIA), Salmonella and Shigella species

87046 stool, aerobic, additional pathogens, isolation and presumptive identification of isolates, each plate

87070 any other source except urine, blood or stool, aerobic, with isolation and presumptive identification of isolates

(For urine, use 87088)

87071 quantitative, aerobic with isolation and presumptive identification of isolates, any source except urine, blood or stool

(For urine, use 87088)

Separate Procedure

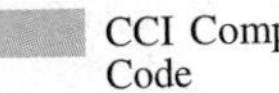

Unlisted Procedure

CCI Comp. Code

Non-specific Procedure

87073 quantitative, anaerobic with isolation and presumptive identification of isolates, any source except urine, blood or stool

(For definitive identification of isolates, use 87076 or 87077. for typing of isolates see 87140-87158)

87075 any source, except blood, anaerobic with isolation and presumptive identification of isolates

87076 anaerobic isolate, additional methods required for definitive identification, each isolate

(For gas liquid chromatography (GLC) or high pressure liquid chromatography (HPLC), use 87143)

87077 aerobic isolate, additional methods required for definitive identification, each isolate

(For gas liquid chromatography (GLC) or high pressure liquid chromatography (HPLC), use 87143)

87081 Culture, presumptive, pathogenic organisms, screening only;

87084 with colony estimation from density chart

87086 Culture, bacterial; quantitative colony count, urine

▲ **87088** with isolation and presumptive identification of each isolate, urine

87101 Culture, fungi (mold or yeast) isolation, with presumptive identification of isolates; skin, hair, or nail

87102 other source (except blood)

87103 blood

87106 Culture, fungi, definitive identification, each organism; yeast

(Use 87106 in addition to codes 87101, 87102 or 87103 when appropriate)

87107 mold

87109 Culture, mycoplasma, any source

87110 Culture, chlamydia, any source

(For immunofluorescence staining of shell vials, use 87140)

87116 Culture, tubercle or other acid-fast bacilli (eg, TB, AFB, mycobacteria) any source, with isolation and presumptive identification of isolates

87118 Culture, mycobacterial, definitive identification, each isolate

(For nucleic acid probe identification, use 87149)

(For GLC or HPLC identification, use 87143)

87140 Culture, typing; immunofluorescent method, each antiserum

87143 gas liquid chromatography (GLC) or high pressure liquid chromotography (HPLC) method

87147 immunologic method, other than immunofluorescence (eg, agglutination grouping), per antiserum

87149 identification by nucleic acid probe

87152 identification by pulse field gel typing

87158 other methods

87164 Dark field examination, any source (eg, penile, vaginal, oral, skin); includes specimen collection

87166 without collection

87168 Macroscopic examination; arthropod

87169 parasite

87172 Pinworm exam (eg, cellophane tape prep)

87176 Homogenization, tissue, for culture

87177 Ova and parasites, direct smears, concentration and identification

(Do not report 87177 in conjunction with 87015)

(For direct smears from a primary source, use 87207)

(For coccidia or microsporidia exam, use 87207)

(For complex special stain (trichrome, iron hematoxylin), use 87209)

(For nucleic acid probes in cytologic material, use 88365)

(For molecular diagnostics, see 83890-83898, 87470-87799)

87181 Susceptibility studies, antimicrobial agent; agar diffusion method, per agent (eg, antibiotic gradient strip)

87184 disk method, per plate (12 or fewer disks)

87185 enzyme detection (eg, beta lactamase), per enzyme

87186 microdilution or agar dilution (minimum inhibitory concentration (MIC) or breakpoint), each multi-antimicrobial, per plate

+ **87187** microdilution or agar dilution, minimum lethal concentration (MLC), each plate ((List separately in addition to code for primary procedure)

(Use 87187 in conjunction with 87186 or 87188)

87188 macrobroth dilution method, each agent

87190 mycobacteria, proportion method, each agent

(For other mycobacterial susceptibility studies, see 87181, 87184, 87186, or 87188)

87197 Serum bactericidal titer (Schlicter test)

87205 Smear, primary source with interpretation; Gram or Giemsa stain for bacteria, fungi, or cell types

87206 fluorescent and/or acid fast stain for bacteria, fungi, or cell types

87207 special stain for inclusion bodies or parasites (eg, malaria, coccidia, microsporidia, trypanosomes, herpes viruses)

(For direct smears with concentration and identification, use 87177)

(For thick smear preparation, use 87015)

(For fat, meat, fibers, nasal eosinophils, and starch, see miscellaneous section)

87209 complex special stain (eg, trichrome, iron hemotoxylin) for ova and parasites

87210 wet mount for infectious agents (eg, saline, India ink, KOH preps)

(For KOH examination of skin, hair or nails, see 87220)

87220 Tissue examination by KOH slide of samples from skin, hair, or nails for fungi or ectoparasite ova or mites (eg, scabies)

87230 Toxin or antitoxin assay, tissue culture (eg, Clostridium difficile toxin)

87250 Virus isolation; inoculation of embryonated eggs, or small animal, includes observation and dissection

87252 tissue culture inoculation, observation, and presumptive identification by cytopathic effect

87253 tissue culture, additional studies or definitive identification (eg, hemabsorption, neutralization, immunofluorescence stain) each isolate

(Electron microscopy, use 88348)

(Inclusion bodies in tissue sections, see 88304-88309; in smears, see 87207-87210; in fluids, use 88106)

87254 centrifuge enhanced (shell vial) technique, includes identification with immunofluorescence stain, each virus

(Report 87254 in addition to 87252 as appropriate)

87255 including identification by non-immunologic method, other than by cytopathic effect (eg., virus specific enzymatic activity)

87260 Infectious agent antigen detection by immunofluorescent technique; adenovirus

87265 Bordetella pertussis/parapertussis

87267 Enterovirus, direct fluorescent antibody (DFA)

87269 giardia

87270 Chlamydia trachomatis

Separate Procedure | Unlisted Procedure | CCI Comp. Code | Non-specific Procedure

87271 Cytomegalovirus, direct fluorescent antibody (DFA)

87272 cryptosporidium

87273 Herpes simplex virus type 2

87274 Herpes simplex virus 1

87275 Influenza B virus

87276 influenza A virus

87277 Legionella micdadei

87278 Legionella pneumophila

87279 Parainfluenza virus, each type

87280 respiratory syncytial virus

87281 Pneumocystis carinii

87283 Rubeola

87285 Treponema pallidum

87290 Varicella zoster virus

87299 not otherwise specified, each organism

87300 Infectious agent antigen detection by immunofluorescent technique, polyvalent for multiple organisms, each polyvalent antiserum

(For physican evaluation of infectious disease agents by immunofluorescence, use 88346)

87301 Infectious agent antigen detection by enzyme immunoassay technique, qualitative or semiquantitative, multiple step method; adenovirus enteric types 40/41

● **87305** Aspergillus

87320 Chlamydia trachomatis

87324 Clostridium difficile toxin(s)

87327 Cryptococcus neoformans

(For Cryptococcus latex agglutination, use 86403)

87328 cryptosporidium

87329 giardia

87332 cytomegalovirus

87335 Escherichia coli 0157

(For giardia antigen, use 87329)

87336 Entamoeba histolytica dispar group

87337 Entamoeba histolytica group

87338 Helicobacter pylori, stool

87339 Helicobacter pylori

(For H. pylori, stool, use 87338. For H. pylori, breath and blood by mass spectrometry, see 83013, 83014. For H. pylori, liquid scintillation counter, see 78267, 78268)

87340 hepatitis B surface antigen (HBsAg)

87341 hepatitis B surface antigen (HBsAg) neutralization

87350 hepatitis Be antigen (HBeAg)

87380 hepatitis, delta agent

87385 Histoplasma capsulatum

87390 HIV-1

87391 HIV-2

87400 Influenza, A or B, each

87420 respiratory syncytial virus

87425 rotavirus

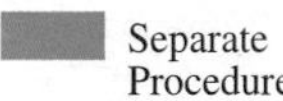
Separate Procedure
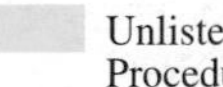
Unlisted Procedure
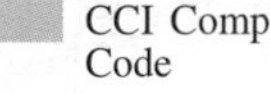
CCI Comp. Code
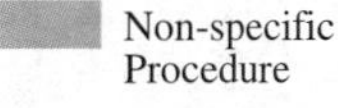
Non-specific Procedure

87427 Shiga-like toxin

87430 Streptococcus, group A

87449 Infectious agent antigen detection by enzyme immunoassay technique qualitative or semiquantitative; multiple step method, not otherwise specified, each organism

87450 single step method, not otherwise specified, each organism

87451 multiple step method, polyvalent for multiple organisms, each polyvalent antiserum

87470 Infectious agent detection by nucleic acid (DNA or RNA); Bartonella henselae and Bartonella quintana, direct probe technique

87471 Bartonella henselae and Bartonella quintana, amplified probe technique

87472 Bartonella henselae and Bartonella quintana, quantification

87475 Borrelia burgdorferi, direct probe technique

87476 Borrelia burgdorferi, amplified probe technique

87477 Borrelia burgdorferi, quantification

87480 Candida species, direct probe technique

87481 Candida species, amplified probe technique

87482 Candida species, quantification

87485 Chlamydia pneumoniae, direct probe technique

87486 Chlamydia pneumoniae, amplified probe technique

87487 Chlamydia pneumoniae, quantification

87490 Chlamydia trachomatis, direct probe technique

87491 Chlamydia trachomatis, amplified probe technique

87492 Chlamydia trachomatis, quantification

87495 cytomegalovirus, direct probe technique

87496 cytomegalovirus, amplified probe technique

87497 cytomegalovirus, quantification

● **87498** enterovirus, amplified probe technique

87510 Gardnerella vaginalis, direct probe technique

87511 Gardnerella vaginalis, amplified probe technique

87512 Gardnerella vaginalis, quantification

87515 hepatitis B virus, direct probe technique

87516 hepatitis B virus, amplified probe technique

87517 hepatitis B virus, quantification

87520 hepatitis C, direct probe technique

87521 hepatitis C, amplified probe technique

87522 hepatitis C, quantification

87525 hepatitis G, direct probe technique

87526 hepatitis G, amplified probe technique

87527 hepatitis G, quantification

87528 Herpes simplex virus, direct probe technique

87529 Herpes simplex virus, amplified probe technique

87530 Herpes simplex virus, quantification

87531 Herpes virus-6, direct probe technique

87532 Herpes virus-6, amplified probe technique

87533 Herpes virus-6, quantification

87534 HIV-1, direct probe technique

87535 HIV-1, amplified probe technique

87536 HIV-1, quantification

87537 HIV-2, direct probe technique

87538 HIV-2, amplified probe technique

87539 HIV-2, quantification

87540 Legionella pneumophila, direct probe technique

87541 Legionella pneumophila, amplified probe technique

87542 Legionella pneumophila, quantification

87550 Mycobacteria species, direct probe technique

87551 Mycobacteria species, amplified probe technique

87552 Mycobacteria species, quantification

87555 Mycobacteria tuberculosis, direct probe technique

87556 Mycobacteria tuberculosis, amplified probe technique

87557 Mycobacteria tuberculosis, quantification

87560 Mycobacteria avium-intracellulare, direct probe technique

87561 Mycobacteria avium-intracellulare, amplified probe technique

87562 Mycobacteria avium-intracellulare, quantification

87580 Mycoplasma pneumoniae, direct probe technique

87581 Mycoplasma pneumoniae, amplified probe technique

87582 Mycoplasma pneumoniae, quantification

87590 Neisseria gonorrhoeae, direct probe technique

87591 Neisseria gonorrhoeae, amplified probe technique

87592 Neisseria gonorrhoeae, quantification

87620 papillomavirus, human, direct probe technique

87621 papillomavirus, human, amplified probe technique

87622 papillomavirus, human, quantification

● **87640** Staphylococcus aureus, amplified probe technique

● **87641** Staphylococcus aureus, methicillin resistant, amplified probe technique

(For assays that detect methicillin resistance and identify Staphylococcus aureus using a single nucleic acid sequenc, use 87641)

87650 Streptococcus, group A, direct probe technique

87651 Streptococcus, group A, amplified probe technique

87652 Streptococcus, group A, quantification

● **87653** Streptococcus, group B, amplified probe technique

87660 Trichomonas vaginalis, direct probe technique

87797 Infectious agent detection by nucleic acid (DNA or RNA), not otherwise specified; direct probe technique, each organism

87798 amplified probe technique, each organism

87799 quantification, each organism

87800 Infectious agent detection by nucleic acid (DNA or RNA), multiple organisms; direct probe(s) technique

87801 amplified probe(s) technique

(For each specific organism nucleic acid detection from a primary source, see 87470-87660. For detection of specific infectious agents not otherwise specified, see 87797, 87798 or 87799 one time for each agent)

87802 Infectious agent antigen detection by immunoassay with direct optical observation; Streptococcus, group B

87803 Clostridium difficile toxin A

87804 Influenza

87807 respiratory syncytial virus

● **87808** Trichomonas vaginalis

87810 Infectious agent detection by immunoassay with direct optical observation; Chlamydia trachomatis

87850 Neisseria gonorrhoeae

87880 Streptococcus, group A

87899 not otherwise specified

87900 Infectious agent drug susceptibility phenotype prediction using regularly updated genotypic bioinformatics

87901 Infectious agent genotype analysis by nucleic acid (DNA or RNA) HIV 1, reverse transciptase and protease

(For infectious agent drug susceptibility phenotype prediction for HIV-1, use 87900)

87902 Hepatitis C virus

87903 Infectious agent phenotype analysis by nucleic acid (DNA or RNA) with drug resistance tissue culture analysis, HIV 1; first through 10 drugs tested

+ **87904** each additional drug tested (List separately in addition to code for primary procedure)

(Use 87904 in conjunction with code 87903)

87999 Unlisted microbiology procedure

ANATOMIC PATHOLOGY

POSTMORTEM EXAMINATION

88000 Necropsy (autopsy), gross examination only; without CNS

88005 with brain

88007 with brain and spinal cord

88012 infant with brain

88014 stillborn or newborn with brain

88016 macerated stillborn

88020 Necropsy (autopsy), gross and microscopic; without CNS

88025 with brain

88027 with brain and spinal cord

88028 infant with brain

88029 stillborn or newborn with brain

88036 Necropsy (autopsy), limited, gross and/or microscopic; regional

88037 single organ

88040 Necropsy (autopsy); forensic examination

88045 coroner's call

88099 Unlisted necropsy (autopsy) procedure

Separate Procedure | Unlisted Procedure | CCI Comp. Code | Non-specific Procedure

CYTOPATHOLOGY

When cytopathology codes are reported, the appropriate CPT code to bill is that which describes, to the highest level of specificity, what services were rendered. Accordingly, for a given specimen, only one code from a group of related codes describing a group of services that could be performed on a specimen with the same end result (e.g. 88104-88112, 88142- 88143, 88150-88154, 88164-88167, etc.) is to be reported.

If multiple services (i.e., separate specimens from different anatomic sites) are reported, modifier -59 should be used to indicate that different levels of service were provided for different specimens from different anatomic sites. This should be reflected in the cytopathologic reports. A cytopathology preparation from a fluid, washing, or brushing is to be reported using one code from the range of CPT codes 88104-88112. It is inappropriate to additionally use CPT codes 88160-88162 because the smears are included in the codes referable to fluids (or washings or brushings) and 88160-88162 references any other source which would exclude fluids, washings, or brushings.

(For cervicography, see Category III code 0003T)

(For collection of cytology specimens via mammary duct catheter lavage, report 0045T-0046T)

88104 Cytopathology, fluids, washings or brushings, except cervical or vaginal; smears with interpretation

▲ **88106** simple filter method with interpretation

▲ **88107** smears and simple filter preparation with interpretation

(For nongynecological selective cellular enhancement including filter transfer techniques, use 88112)

88108 Cytopathology, concentration technique, smears and interpretation (eg, Saccomanno technique)

(For cervical or vaginal smears, see 88150-88155)

(For gastric intubation with lavage, see 89130-89141, 91055)

(For x-ray localization, use 74340)

88112 Cytopathology, selective cellular enhancement technique with interpretation (eg, liquid based slide preparation method), except cervical or vaginal

(Do not report 88112 with 88108)

● New Code ▲ Revised Code + Add-On Code ⊘ Modifier -51 Exempt ⊙ Conscious Sedation

88125 Cytopathology, forensic (eg, sperm)

88130 Sex chromatin identification; Barr bodies

88140 peripheral blood smear, polymorphonuclear drumsticks

(For Guard stain, use 88313)

+ **88141** Cytopathology, cervical or vaginal (any reporting system), requiring interpretation by physician (List separately in addition to code for technical service)

(Use 88141 in conjunction with codes 88142-88154, 88164-88167, 88174-88175)

88142 Cytopathology, cervical or vaginal (any reporting system), collected in preservative fluid, automated thin layer preparation; manual screening under physician supervision

88143 with manual screening and rescreening under physician supervision

(For automated screening of automated thin layer preparation, see 88174, 88175)

88147 Cytopathology smears, cervical or vaginal; screening by automated system under physician supervision

88148 screening by automated system with manual rescreening under physician supervision

88150 Cytopathology, slides, cervical or vaginal; manual screening under physician supervision

88152 with manual screening and computer-assisted rescreening under physician supervision

88153 with manual screening and rescreening under physician supervision

88154 with manual screening and computer-assisted rescreening using cell selection and review under physician supervision

+ **88155** Cytopathology, slides, cervical or vaginal, definitive hormonal evaluation (eg, maturation index, karyopyknotic index, estrogenic index) (List separately in addition to code(s) for other technical and interpretation services)

Separate Procedure | Unlisted Procedure | CCI Comp. Code | Non-specific Procedure

(Use 88155 in conjunction with 88142-88154, 88164-88167, 88174-88175)

88160 Cytopathology, smears, any other source; screening and interpretation

88161 preparation, screening and interpretation

88162 extended study involving over 5 slides and/or multiple stains

(For aerosol collection of sputum, use 89350)

(For special stains, see 88312-88314)

88164 Cytopathology, slides, cervical or vaginal (the Bethesda System); manual screening under physician supervision

88165 with manual screening and rescreening under physician supervision

88166 with manual screening and computer-assisted rescreening under physician supervision

88167 with manual screening and computer-assisted rescreening using cell selection and review under physician supervision

(88170, 88171 have been deleted)

(To report collection of specimen via fine needle aspiration, see 10021, 10022)

88172 Cytopathology, evaluation of fine needle aspirate; immediate cytohistologic study to determine adequacy of specimen(s)

88173 interpretation and report

(For fine needle aspirate, see 10021, 10022)

(Do not report 88172, 88173 in conjunction with 88333 and 88334 for the same specimen)

88174 Cytopathology, cervical or vaginal (any reporting system), collected in preservative fluid, automated thin layer preparation; screening by automated system, under physician supervision

88175 with screening by automated system and manual rescreening or review, under physician supervision

(For manual screening, see 88142, 88143)

(88180 deleted 2005 edition. To report, use 88182, 88189)

88182 Flow cytometry; cell cycle or DNA analysis

(For DNA ploidy analysis by morphometric techniques, use 88358)

88184 Flow cytometry, cell surface, cytoplasmic, or nuclear marker, technical component only; first marker

\+ **88185** each additional marker (List separately in addition to code for first marker)

(Report 88185 in conjunction with 88184)

88187 Flow cytometry, interpretation; 2 to 8 markers

88188 9 to 15 markers

88189 16 or more markers

88199 Unlisted cytopathology procedure

(For electron microscopy, see 88348, 88349)

CYTOGENETIC STUDIES

When molecular diagnostic procedures are performed to test for oncologic or inherited disorder, use the appropriate modifier to specify probe type or condition tested.

(For acetylcholinesterase, use 82013)

(For alpha-fetoprotein, serum or amniotic fluid, see 82105, 82106)

(For laser microdissection of cells from tissue sample, see 88380)

88230 Tissue culture for non-neoplastic disorders; lymphocyte

88233 skin or other solid tissue biopsy

88235 amniotic fluid or chorionic villus cells

88237 Tissue culture for neoplastic disorders; bone marrow, blood cells

88239 solid tumor

88240 Cryopreservation, freezing and storage of cells, each cell line

(For therapeutic cryopreservation and storage, use 38207)

88241 Thawing and expansion of frozen cells, each aliquot

(For therapeutic thawing of previous harvest, use 38208)

88245 Chromosome analysis for breakage syndromes; baseline Sister Chromatid Exchange (SCE), 20-25 cells

88248 baseline breakage, score 50-100 cells, count 20 cells, 2 karyotypes (eg, for ataxia telangiectasia, Fanconi anemia, fragile X)

88249 score 100 cells, clastogen stress (eg, diepoxybutane, mitomycin C, ionizing radiation, UV radiation)

88261 Chromosome analysis; count 5 cells, 1 karyotype, with banding

88262 count 15-20 cells, 2 karyotypes, with banding

88263 count 45 cells for mosaicism, 2 karyotypes, with banding

88264 analyze 20-25 cells

88267 Chromosome analysis, amniotic fluid or chorionic villus, count 15 cells, 1 karyotype, with banding

88269 Chromosome analysis, in situ for amniotic fluid cells, count cells from 6-12 colonies, 1 karyotype, with banding

88271 Molecular cytogenetics; DNA probe, each (eg, FISH)

88272 chromosomal in situ hybridization, analyze 3-5 cells (eg, for derivatives and markers)

88273 chromosomal in situ hybridization, analyze 10-30 cells (eg, for microdeletions)

88274 interphase in situ hybridization, analyze 25-99 cells

88275 interphase in situ hybridization, analyze 100-300 cells

88280 Chromosome analysis; additional karyotypes, each study

88283 additional specialized banding technique (eg, NOR, C-banding)

88285 additional cells counted, each study

88289 additional high resolution study

88291 Cytogenetics and molecular cytogenetics, interpretation and report

88299 Unlisted cytogenetic study

SURGICAL PATHOLOGY

The CPT codes 88321-88325 are to be used to review slides, tissues, or other material obtained and prepared at a different location and referred to a pathologist for a second opinion. (These codes should not be reported by pathologists reporting a second opinion on slides, tissue, or material also examined and reported by another pathologist in the same provider group. Medicare generally does not pay twice for an interpretation of a given technical service (e.g., EKGs, radiographs, etc.).

CPT codes 88321- 88325 are reported with one unit of service regardless of the number of specimens, paraffin blocks, stained slides, etc. When reporting CPT codes 88321-88325, providers should not report other pathology CPT codes such as 88312, 88313, 88342, 88187, 88188, 88189, etc., for interpretation of stains, slides or material previously interpreted by another pathologist. CPT codes 88312, 88313 and 88342 may be reported with CPT code 88323 if provider performs and interprets these stains de novo.

CPT codes 88321-88325 are not to be used for a face-to-face evaluation of a patient. In the event that a physician provides an evaluation and management service to a patient and, in the course of this service, specimens obtained elsewhere are reviewed as well, this is part of the evaluation and management service and is not to be reported separately. Only the evaluation and management service would be reported.

Medicare does not pay for duplicate testing. CPT codes 88342 (immuno-cytochemistry, each antibody) and 88184, 88187, 88188, 88189 (flow cytometry) should not in general be reported for the same or similar specimens. The diagnosis should be established using one of these methods. The provider may report both CPT codes if both methods are required because the initial method is nondiagnostic or does not explain all the light microscopic findings. The provider can report both methods utilizing modifier -59 and document the need for both methods in the medical record.

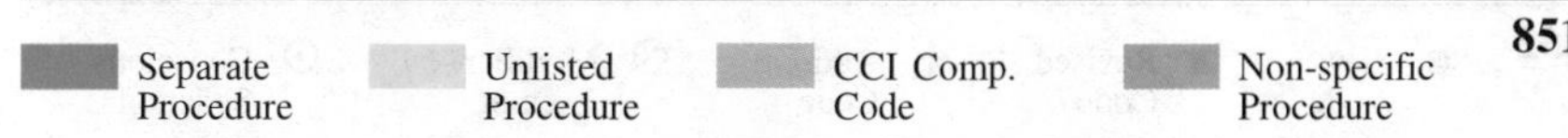

If the abnormal cells in two or more specimens are morphologically similar and testing on one specimen by one method (88342 or 88184, 88187, 88188, 88189) establishes the diagnosis, the same or other method should not be reported on the same or similar specimen. Similar specimens would include, but are not limited to: (1) blood and bone marrow; (2) bone marrow aspiration and bone marrow biopsy; (3) two separate lymph nodes; or (4) lymph node and other tissue with lymphoid infiltrate.

(Do not report 88302-88309 on the same specimen as part of Mohs surgery)

88300 Level I - Surgical pathology, gross examination only

88302 Level II - Surgical pathology, gross and microscopic examination

Appendix, Incidental
Fallopian Tube, Sterilization
Fingers/Toes, Amputation, Traumatic
Foreskin, Newborn
Hernia Sac, Any Location
Hydrocele Sac
Nerve
Skin, Plastic Repair
Sympathetic Ganglion
Testis, Castration
Vaginal Mucosa, Incidental
Vas Deferens, Sterilization

88304 Level III - Surgical pathology, gross and microscopic examination

Abortion, Induced
Abscess
Aneurysm - Arterial/Ventricular
Anus, Tag
Appendix, Other than Incidental
Artery, Atheromatous Plaque
Bartholin's Gland Cyst
Bone Fragment(s), Other than Pathologic Fracture
Bursa/Synovial Cyst
Carpal Tunnel Tissue
Cartilage, Shavings
Cholesteatoma
Colon, Colostomy Stoma
Conjunctiva - Biopsy/Pterygium
Cornea
Diverticulum - Esophagus/Small Intestine
Dupuytren's Contracture Tissue

● New Code ▲ Revised Code + Add-On Code ⊘ Modifier -51 Exempt ⊙ Conscious Sedation

Femoral Head, Other than Fracture
Fissue/Fistula
Foreskin, Other than Newborn
Gallbladder
Ganglion Cyst
Hematoma
Hemorrhoids
Hydatid of Morgagni
Intervertebral Disc
Joint, Loose Body
Meniscus
Mucocele, Salivary
Neuroma - Morton's/Traumatic
Pilonidal Cyst/Sinus
Polyps, Inflammatory - Nasal/Sinusoidal
Skin - Cyst/Tag/Debridement
Soft Tissue, Debridement
Soft Tissue, Lipoma
Spermatocele
Tendon/Tendon Sheath
Testicular Appendage
Thrombus or Embolus
Tonsil and/or Adenoids
Varicocele
Vas Deferens, Other than Sterilizaton
Vein, Varicosity

88305 Level IV - Surgical pathology, gross and microscopic examination

Abortion - Spontaneous/Missed
Artery, Biopsy
Bone Marrow, Biopsy
Bone Exostosis
Brain/Meninges, Other than for Tumor Resection
Breast Biopsy, Not Requiring Microscopic Evaluation of Surgical Margins
Breast, Reduction Mammoplasty
Bronchus, Biopsy
Cell Block, Any Source
Cervix, Biopsy
Colon, Biopsy
Duodenum, Biopsy
Endocervix, Curettings/Biopsy
Endometrium, Currettings/Biopsy
Esophagus, Biopsy
Extremity, Amputation, Traumatic
Fallopian Tube, Biopsy
Fallopian Tube, Ectopic Pregnancy
Femoral Head, Fracture

 Separate Procedure 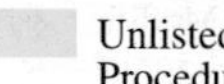 Unlisted Procedure CCI Comp. Code Non-specific Procedure

Fingers/Toes, Amputation, Non-Traumatic
Gingiva/Oral Mucosa, Biopsy
Heart Valve
Joint, Resection
Kidney, Biopsy
Larynx, Biopsy
Leiomyoma(s), Uterine Myomectomy - without Uterus
Lip, Biopsy/Wedge Resection
Lung, Transbronchial Biopsy
Lymph Node, Biopsy
Muscle, Biopsy
Nasal Mucosa, Biopsy
Nasopharynx/Oropharynx, Biopsy
Nerve, Biopsy
Odontogenic/Dental Cyst
Omentum, Biopsy
Ovary with or without Tube, Non-neoplastic
Ovary, Biopsy/Wedge Resection
Parathyroid Gland
Peritoneum, Biopsy
Pituitary Tumor
Placenta, Other than Third Trimester
Pleura/Pericardium - Biopsy/Tissue
Polyp, Cervical/Endometrial
Polyp, Colorectal
Polyp, Stomach/Small Intestine
Prostate, Needle Biopsy
Prostate, TUR
Salivary Gland, Biopsy
Sinus, Paranasal Biopsy
Skin, Other than Cyst/Tag/Debridement/Plastic Repair
Small Intestine, Biopsy
Soft Tissue, Other than Tumor/Mass/Lipoma/Debridement
Spleen
Stomach, Biopsy
Synovium
Testis, Other than Tumor/Biopsy/Castration
Thyroglossal Duct/Brachial Cleft Cyst
Tongue, Biopsy
Tonsil, Biopsy
Trachea, Biopsy
Ureter, Biopsy
Urethra, Biopsy
Urinary Bladder, Biopsy
Uterus, with or without Tubes and Ovaries, for Prolapse
Vagina, Biopsy
Vulva/Labia, Biopsy

88307 Level V - Surgical pathology, gross and microscopic examination

Adrenal, Resection
Bone - Biopsy/Curettings
Bone Fragment(s), Pathologic Fracture
Brain, Biopsy
Brain/Meninges, Tumor Resection
Breast, Excision of Lesion, Requiring Microscopic Evaluation of Surgical Margins
Breast, Mastectomy - Partial/Simple
Cervix, Conization
Colon, Segmental Resection, Other than for Tumor
Extremity, Amputation, Non-traumatic
Eye, Enucleation
Kidney, Partial/Total Nephrectomy
Larynx, Partial/Total Resection
Liver, Biopsy - Needle/Wedge
Lung, Wedge Biopsy
Lymph Nodes, Regional Resection
Mediastinum, Mass
Myocardium, Biopsy
Odontogenic Tumor
Ovary with or without Tube, Neoplastic
Pancreas, Biopsy
Placenta, Third Trimester
Prostate, Except Radical Resection
Salivary Gland
Sentinel Lymph Node
Small Intestine, Resection, Other Than for Tumor
Soft Tissue Mass (except Lipoma) - Biopsy/Simple Excision
Stomach - Subtotal/Total Resection, Other than for Tumor
Testis, Biopsy
Thymus, Biopsy
Thyroid, Total/Lobe
Ureter, Resection
Urinary Bladder, TUR
Uterus, with or without Tubes and Ovaries, Other than Neoplastic/Prolapse

88309 Level VI - Surgical pathology, gross and microscopic examination

Bone Resection
Breast, Mastectomy - with Regional Lymph Nodes
Colon, Segmental Resection for Tumor
Colon, Total Resection
Esophagus, Partial/Total Resection
Extremity, Disarticulation
Fetus, with Dissection

Larynx, Partial/Total Resection - with Regional Lymph Nodes
Lung - Total/Lobe/Segment Resection
Pancreas, Total/Subtotal Resection
Prostate, Radical Resection
Small Intestine, Resection for Tumor
Soft Tissue Tumor, Extensive Resection
Stomach - Subtotal/Total Resection for Tumor
Testis, Tumor
Tongue/Tonsil - Resection for Tumor
Urinary Bladder, Partial/Total Resection
Uterus, with or without Tubes and Ovaries, Neoplastic
Vulva, Total/Subtotal Resection

(For fine needle aspiration, see 10021, 10022)

(For evaluation of fine needle aspirate, see 88172-88173)

(Do not report 88302-88309 on the same specimen as part of Mohs surgery)

+ **88311** Decalcification procedure (List separately in addition to code for surgical pathology examination)

+ **88312** Special stains (List separately in addition to code for primary service); Group I for microorganisms (eg, Gridley, acid fast, methenamine silver), each

+ **88313** Group II, all other, (eg, iron, trichrome), except immunocytochemistry and immunoperoxidase stains, each

(For immunocytochemistry and immunoperoxidase tissue studies, use 88342)

+ **88314** histochemical staining with frozen section(s)

(Do not report 88314 with 17311-17315 for routine frozen section stain (eg., hematoxylin and eosin, toluidine blue), performed during Mohs surgery. When a nonroutine histochemical stain on frozen tissue is utilized, report 88314 with modifier -59)

88318 Determinative histochemistry to identify chemical components (eg, copper, zinc)

88319 Determinative histochemistry or cytochemistry to identify enzyme constituents, each

88321 Consultation and report on referred slides prepared elsewhere

88323 Consultation and report on referred material requiring preparation of slides

88325 Consultation, comprehensive, with review of records and specimens, with report on referred material

88329 Pathology consultation during surgery;

88331 first tissue block, with frozen section(s), single specimen

88332 each additional tissue block with frozen section(s)

88333 cytologic examination (eg, touch prep, squash prep), initial site

88334 cytologic examination (eg, touch prep, squash prep), each additional site

(For intraoperative consultation on a specimen requiring both frozen section and cytologic evaluation, use 88331 and 88334)

(For percutaneous needle biopsy requiring intraprocedural cytologic examination, use 88333)

(Do not report 88333 and 88334 for non-intraoperative cytologic examination, see 88160-88162)

(Do not report 88333 and 88334 for intraprocedural cytologic evaluation of fine needle aspirate, see 88172).

88342 Immunohistochemistry (including tissue immunoperoxidase), each antibody

(Do not report 88342 in conjunction with 88360 or 88361 for the same antibody)

(For quantitative or semiquantitative immunohistochemistry, see 88360, 88361)

88346 Immunofluorescent study, each antibody; direct method

88347 indirect method

88348 Electron microscopy; diagnostic

88349 scanning

88355 Morphometric analysis; skeletal muscle

88356 nerve

88358 tumor (eg, DNA ploidy)

(Do not report 88358 with 88313 unless each procedure is for a different special stain)

88360 Morphometric analysis, tumor immunohistochemistry (eg, Her-2/neu, estrogen receptor/progesterone receptor), quantitative or semiquantitative, each antibody; manual

88361 using computer-assisted technology

(Do not report 88360, 88361 with 88342 unless each procedure is for a different antibody)

(For morphometric analysis, in situ hybridization, see 88367, 88368)

(When semi-thin plastic-embedded sections are performed in conjunction with morphometric analysis, only the morphometric analysis should be coded; if performed as an independent procedure, see codes 88300-88309 for surgical pathology)

88362 Nerve teasing preparations

88365 In situ hybridization (eg, FISH), each probe

(Do not report 88365 in conjunction with 88367, 88368 for the same probe)

88367 Morphometric analysis, in situ hybridization, (quantitative or semi-quantitative) each probe; using computer-assisted technology

88368 manual

88371 Protein analysis of tissue by Western Blot, with interpretation and report;

88372 immunological probe for band identification, each

88380 Microdissection (eg, mechanical, laser capture)

88384 Array-based evaluation of multiple molecular probes; 11 through 50 probes

88385 51 through 250 probes

88386 251 through 500 probes

(For preparation of array-based evaluation, see 83890-83892, 83898-83901)

(For preparation and analyses of less than 11 probes, see 83890-83914)

88399 Unlisted surgical pathology procedure

TRANSCUTANEOUS PROCEDURES

88400 Bilirubin, total transcutaneous

OTHER PROCEDURES

89049 Caffeine halothane contracture test (CHCT) for malignant hyperthermia susceptibility, including interpretation and report

89050 Cell count, miscellaneous body fluids (eg, cerebrospinal fluid, joint fluid), except blood;

89051 with differential count

89055 Leukocyte assessment, fecal, qualitative or semiquantitative

▲ **89060** Crystal identification by light microscopy with or without polarizing lens analysis, tissue or any body fluid (except urine)

(Do not report 89060 for crystal identification on paraffin-embedded tissue)

89100 Duodenal intubation and aspiration; single specimen (eg, simple bile study or afferent loop culture) plus appropriate test procedure

89105 collection of multiple fractional specimens with pancreatic or gallbladder stimulation, single or double lumen tube

(For radiological localization, use 74340)

(For chemical analyses, see Chemistry, this section)

(Electrocardiogram, see 93000-93268)

(Esophagus acid perfusion test (Bernstein), see 91030)

89125 Fat stain, feces, urine, or respiratory secretions

Separate Procedure | Unlisted Procedure | CCI Comp. Code | Non-specific Procedure

89130 Gastric intubation and aspiration, diagnostic, each specimen, for chemical analyses or cytopathology;

89132 after stimulation

89135 Gastric intubation, aspiration, and fractional collections (eg, gastric secretory study); one hour

89136 two hours

89140 two hours including gastric stimulation (eg, histalog, pentagastrin)

89141 three hours, including gastric stimulation

(For gastric lavage, therapeutic, use 91105)

(For radiologic localization of gastric tube, use 74340)

(For chemical analyses, see 82926, 82928)

(Joint fluid chemistry, see Chemistry, this section)

89160 Meat fibers, feces

89190 Nasal smear for eosinophils

(Occult blood, feces, use 82270)

(Paternity tests, use 86910)

89220 Sputum, obtaining specimen, aerosol induced technique (separate procedure)

89225 Starch granules, feces

89230 Sweat collection by iontophoresis

89235 Water load test

89240 Unlisted miscellaneous pathology test

REPRODUCTIVE MEDICINE PROCEDURES

89250 Culture of oocyte(s)/embryo(s), less than 4 days;

89251 with co-culture of oocyte(s)/embryo(s)

(For extended culture of oocyte(s)/embryo(s), see 89272)

(89252 deleted 2004 edition. To report, use 89280-89281)

89253 Assisted embryo hatching, microtechniques (any method)

89254 Oocyte identification from follicular fluid

89255 Preparation of embryo for transfer (any method)

(89256 deleted 2004 edition. To report, use 89352)

89257 Sperm identification from aspiration (other than seminal fluid)

(For semen analysis, see 89300-89320)

(For sperm identification from testis tissue, use 89264)

89258 Cryopreservation; embryo(s)

89259 sperm

(For cryopreservation of reproductive tissue, testicular, use 89335)

(For cryopreservation of reproductive tissue, ovarian, use Category III code 0058T)

(For cryopreservation of oocyte(s), use Category III code 0059T)

89260 Sperm isolation; simple prep (eg, sperm wash and swim-up) for insemination or diagnosis with semen analysis

89261 complex prep (eg, Percoll gradient, albumin gradient) for insemination or diagnosis with semen analysis

(For semen analysis without sperm wash or swim-up, use 89320)

89264 Sperm identification from testis tissue, fresh or cryopreserved

(For biopsy of testis, see 54500, 54505)

Separate Procedure | Unlisted Procedure | CCI Comp. Code | Non-specific Procedure

(For sperm identification from aspiration, use 89257)

(For semen analysis, see 89300-89320)

89268 Insemination of oocytes

89272 Extended culture of oocyte(s)/embryo(s), 4-7 days

89280 Assisted oocyte fertiliation, microtechnique; less than or equal to 10 oocytes

89281 greater than 10 oocytes

89290 Biopsy, oocyte polar body or embryo blastomere, microtechnique (for pre-implantation genetic diagnosis); less than or equal to 5 embryos

89291 greater than 5 embryos

89300 Semen analysis; presence and/or motility of sperm including Huhner test (post coital)

89310 motility and count (not including Huhner test)

89320 complete (volume, count, motility, and differential)

(Skin tests, see 86485-86585 and 95010-95199)

89321 Semen analysis, presence and/or motility of sperm

(To report Hyaluronan binding assay (HBA), use Category III code 0087T)

89325 Sperm antibodies

(For medicolegal identification of sperm, use 88125)

89329 Sperm evaluation; hamster penetration test

89330 cervical mucus penetration test, with or without spinnbarkeit test

89335 Cryopreservation, reproductive tissue, testicular

(For cryopreservation of embryo(s), use 89258. For cryopreservation of sperm, use 89259)

● New Code ▲ Revised Code + Add-On Code ⊘ Modifier -51 Exempt ⊙ Conscious Sedation

(For cryopreservation of reproductive tissue, ovarian, use Category III code 0058T)

(For cryopreservation of oocyte, use Category III code 0059T)

89342 Storage, (per year); embryo(s)

89343 sperm/semen

89344 reproductive tissue, testicular/ovarian

89346 oocyte(s)

(89350 deleted 2004 edition. To report, use 89220)

89352 Thawing of cryopreserved; embryo(s)

89353 sperm/semen, each aliquot

89354 reproductive tissue, testicular/ovarian

(89355 deleted 2004 edition. To report, use 89225)

89356 oocytes, each aliquot

(89360 deleted 2004 edition. To report, use 89230)

(89365 deleted 2004 edition. To report, use 89235)

(89399 deleted 2004 edition. To report, use 89240)

This page intentionally left blank.

MEDICINE

MEDICINE SECTION OVERVIEW

The sixth section of the CPT coding system is the medicine section, which includes codes for immunizations, therapeutic or diagnostic injections, psychiatric services, dialysis, ophthalmology services, specialty specific diagnostic services, chemotherapy administration, physical medicine and rehabilitation services, osteopathic and chiropractic services. Within each subsection, the CPT codes are arranged by the type of service provided.

MEDICINE SUBSECTIONS

The MEDICINE section of CPT is divided into the following subsections:

Immune Globulins	90281-90399
Immunization Administration for Vaccines/Toxoids	90465-90474
Vaccines, Toxoids	90476-90749
Hydration, Therapeutic, Prophylactic, and Diagnostic Injections and Infusions	90760-90779
Psychiatry	90801-90899
Biofeedback	90901-90911
Dialysis	90918-90999
Gastroenterology	91000-91299
Ophthalmology	92002-92499
Special Otorhinolaryngologic Services	92502-92700
Cardiovascular	92950-93799
Non-Invasive Vascular Diagnostic Studies	93875-93990
Pulmonary	94002-94799
Allergy and Clinical Immunology	95004-95199
Endocrinology	95250-95251
Neurology and Neuromuscular Procedures	95805-96020
Medical Genetics and Genetic Counseling	96040
Central Nervous System Assessments/Tests	96101-96120
Health and Behavior Assessment/Intervention	96150-96155
Chemotherapy Administration	96401-96549
Photodynamic Therapy	96567-96571
Special Dermatological Procedures	96900-96999
Physical Medicine and Rehabilitation	97001-97799
Medical Nutrition Therapy	97802-97804
Acupuncture	97810-97814
Osteopathic Manipulative Treatment	98925-98929
Chiropractic Manipulative Tretment	98940-98943
Education/Training for Self-Management	98960-98962

continued

MED 90000

Separate Procedure | Unlisted Procedure | CCI Comp. Code | Non-specific Procedure

Special Services, Procedures and Reports	99000-99091
Qualifying Circumstances for Anesthesia	99100-99140
Moderate (Conscious) Sedation	99143-99150
Other Services and Procedures	99170-99199
Home Health Procedures/Services	99500-99602

Most of the subsections have special needs or instructions unique to that section which should be reviewed carefully before reporting.

MEDICINE SERVICES MODIFIERS

MEDICINE services and procedures may be modified under certain circumstances. When applicable, the modifying circumstance is identified by the addition of the appropriate modifier code. The following modifiers are frequently used with MEDICINE services.

-22 Unusual services

-26 Professional component

-51 Multiple procedures

This modifier may be used to report multiple medical procedures performed at the same session, as well as a combination of medical and surgical procedures.

-52 Reduced services

-76 Repeat procedure by same physician

-77 Repeat procedure by another physician

-90 Reference (outside) laboratory

-99 Multiple modifiers

MEDICINE CODES

IMMUNE GLOBULINS

Codes 90281-90399 identify the immune globulin product only and must be reported in addition to the administration codes 90765-90768, 90772, 90774, 90775 as appropriate. Immune globulin products listed here include broad-spectrum and anti-infective immune globulins, antitoxins, and various isoantibodies.

⊘ **90281** Immune globulin (Ig), human, for intramuscular use

⊘ **90283** Immune globulin (IgIV), human, for intravenous use

⊘ **90287** Botulinum antitoxin, equine, any route

⊘ **90288** Botulism immune globulin, human, for intravenous use

⊘ **90291** Cytomegalovirus immune globulin (CMV-IgIV), human, for intravenous use

⊘ **90296** Diphtheria antitoxin, equine, any route

⊘ **90371** Hepatitis B immune globulin (HBIg), human, for intramuscular use

⊘ **90375** Rabies immune globulin (RIg), human, for intramuscular and/or subcutaneous use

⊘ **90376** Rabies immune globulin, heat-treated (RIg-HT), human, for intramuscular and/or subcutaneous use

⊘ **90378** Respiratory syncytial virus immune globulin (RSV-IgIM), for intramuscular use, 50 mg, each SYNAGIS

⊘ **90379** Respiratory syncytial virus immune globulin (RSV-IgIV), human, for intravenous use

⊘ **90384** Rho(D) immune globulin (RhIg), human, full-dose, for intramuscular use

⊘ **90385** Rho(D) immune globulin (RhIg), human, mini-dose, for intramuscular use

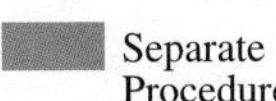
Separate Procedure
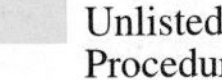
Unlisted Procedure
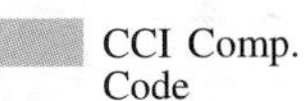
CCI Comp. Code
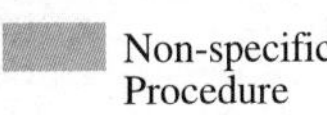
Non-specific Procedure

⊘ **90386** Rho(D) immune globulin (RhIgIV), human, for intravenous use

⊘ **90389** Tetanus immune globulin (TIg), human, for intramuscular use

⊘ **90393** Vaccinia immune globulin, human, for intramuscular use

⊘ **90396** Varicella-zoster immune globulin, human, for intramuscular use

⊘ **90399** Unlisted immune globulin

IMMUNIZATION ADMINISTRATION FOR VACCINES/TOXOIDS

Immunization is the administration of a vaccine or toxoid to stimulate the immune system to provide protection against disease. Immunizations are usually given in conjunction with an evaluation and management service. When an immunization is the only service performed, a minimal evaluation and management service code may be listed in addition to the injection code.

Coding Rules

1. *When an immunization is the only service provided, evaluation and management service code 99211, Minimal service, may be reported in addition to the immunization.*

2. *Immunization administration CPT codes must be reported in addition to the vaccine and toxoid CPT codes.*

3. *Supplies or equipment used to inject the vaccine or toxoid are not reported separately.*

IMMUNIZATION ADMINISTRATION

(For allergy testing, see 95004 et seq)

(For skin testing of bacterial, viral, fungal extracts, see 86485-86586)

(For therapeutic or diagnostic injections, see 90772-90779)

90465 Immunization administration under 8 years of age (includes percutaneous, intradermal, subcutaneous, or intramuscular injections) when the physician counsels the patient/family; first injection (single or combination vaccine/toxoid), per day

(Do not report 90465 in conjunction with 90467)

+ **90466** each additional injection (single or combination vaccine/toxoid), per day (List separately in addition to code for primary procedure)

(Use 90466 in conjunction with 90465 or 90467)

90467 Immunization administration under age 8 years (includes intranasal or oral routes of administration) when the physician counsels the patient/family; first administration (single or combination vaccine/toxoid), per day

(Do not report 90467 in conjunction with 90465)

+ **90468** each additional administration (single or combination vaccine/toxoid), per day (List separately in addition to code for primary procedure)

(Use 90468 in conjunction with 90465 or 90467)

90471 Immunization administration (includes percutaneous, intradermal, subcutaneous, or intramuscular injections); one vaccine (single or combination vaccine/toxoid)

(Do not report 90471 in conjunction with 90473)

+ **90472** each additional vaccine (single or combination vaccine/toxoid) (List separately in addition to code for primary procedure)

(Use 90472 in conjunction with code 90471 or 90473)

(For administration of immune globulins, see 90281-90399, 90760, 90761, 90765-90768, 90774)

(For intravesical administration of BCG vaccine, use 51720, and see 90586)

90473 Immunization administration by intranasal or oral route; one vaccine (single or combination vaccine/toxoid)

(Do not report 90473 in conjunction with 90471)

+ **90474** each additional vaccine (single or combination vaccine/toxoid) (List separately in addition to code for primary procedure)

(Use 90474 in conjunction with code 90471 or 90473)

VACCINES, TOXOIDS

Vaccines and toxoids are administered to provide protection from hepatitis, influenza, typhoid, measles, mumps, polio, and other diseases. Vaccine and toxoid CPT codes 90476-90749 identify the vaccine or toxoid only and must be reported in addition to immunization administration CPT codes.

(For immune globulins, see codes 90281-90399, and 90780-90784 for administration of immune globulins)

⊘ **90476** Adenovirus vaccine, type 4, live, for oral use

⊘ **90477** Adenovirus vaccine, type 7, live, for oral use

⊘ **90581** Anthrax vaccine, for subcutaneous use

⊘ **90585** Bacillus Calmette-Guerin vaccine (BCG) for tuberculosis, live, for percutaneous use

⊘ **90586** Bacillus Calmette-Guerin vaccine (BCG) for bladder cancer, live, for intravesical use

⊘ **90632** Hepatitis A vaccine, adult dosage, for intramuscular use

⊘ **90633** Hepatitis A vaccine, pediatric/adolescent dosage-2 dose schedule, for intramuscular use

⊘ **90634** Hepatitis A vaccine, pediatric/adolescent dosage-3 dose schedule, for intramuscular use

⊘ **90636** Hepatitis A and hepatitis B vaccine (HepA-HepB), adult dosage, for intramuscular use

⊘ **90645** Hemophilus influenza B vaccine (Hib), HbOC conjugate (4 dose schedule), for intramuscular use

⊘ **90646** Hemophilus influenza B vaccine (Hib), PRP-D conjugate, for booster use only, intramuscular use

⊘ **90647** Hemophilus influenza B vaccine (Hib), PRP-OMP conjugate (3 dose schedule), for intramuscular use

⊘ **90648** Hemophilus influenza B vaccine (Hib), PRP-T conjugate (4 dose schedule), for intramuscular use

⊘ **90649** Human papilloma virus (HPV) vaccine, types 6, 11, 16, 18 (quadrivalent), 3 dose schedule, for intramuscular use

● New Code ▲ Revised Code + Add-On Code ⊘ Modifier -51 Exempt ⊙ Conscious Sedation

⊘▲**90655** Influenza virus vaccine, split virus, preservative free, when administered to children 6-35 months of age, for intramuscular use

⊘▲**90656** Influenza virus vaccine, split virus, preservative free, when administered to individuals 3 years of age and older, for intramuscular use

⊘▲**90657** Influenza virus vaccine, split virus, when administered to children 6-35 months of age, for intramuscular use

⊘▲**90658** Influenza virus vaccine, split virus, when administered to individuals 3 years of age and older, for intramuscular use

(90659 deleted 2004 edition. To report influenza virus vaccine, split virus, see 90657 or 90658)

⊘ **90660** Influenza virus vaccine, live, for intranasal use

⊘ **90665** Lyme disease vaccine, adult dosage, for intramuscular use

⊘▲**90669** Pneumococcal conjugate vaccine, polyvalent, when administered to children younger than 5 years, for intramuscular use

⊘ **90675** Rabies vaccine, for intramuscular use

⊘ **90676** Rabies vaccine, for intradermal use

⊘ **90680** Rotavirus vaccine, pentavalent, 3 dose schedule, live, for oral use

⊘ **90690** Typhoid vaccine, live, oral

⊘ **90691** Typhoid vaccine, Vi capsular polysaccharide (ViCPs), for intramuscular use

⊘ **90692** Typhoid vaccine, heat- and phenol-inactivated (H-P), for subcutaneous or intradermal use

⊘ **90693** Typhoid vaccine, acetone-killed, dried (AKD), for subcutaneous use (U.S. military)

⊘ **90698** Diphtheria, tetanus toxoids, acellular pertussis vaccine, haemophilus influenza Type B, and poliovirus vaccine, inactivated (DTaP-Hib-IPV), for intramuscular use

(FDA approval pending)

⊘▲**90700** Diphtheria, tetanus toxoids, and acellular pertussis vaccine (DTaP), when administered to individuals younger than 7 years, for intramuscular use

⊘ **90701** Diphtheria, tetanus toxoids, and whole cell pertussis vaccine (DTP), for intramuscular use

⊘▲**90702** Diphtheria and tetanus toxoids (DT) adsorbed, when administered to individuals younger than 7 years, for intramuscular use

⊘ **90703** Tetanus toxoid adsorbed, for intramuscular use

⊘ **90704** Mumps virus vaccine, live, for subcutaneous use

⊘ **90705** Measles virus vaccine, live, for subcutaneous use

⊘ **90706** Rubella virus vaccine, live, for subcutaneous use

⊘ **90707** Measles, mumps and rubella virus vaccine (MMR), live, for subcutaneous use

⊘ **90708** Measles and rubella virus vaccine, live, for subcutaneous use

⊘ **90710** Measles, mumps, rubella, and varicella vaccine (MMRV), live, for subcutaneous use

⊘ **90712** Poliovirus vaccine, (any type(s)) (OPV), live, for oral use

⊘ **90713** Poliovirus vaccine, inactivated, (IPV), for subcutaneous or intramuscular use

⊘▲**90714** Tetanus and diphtheria toxoids (Td) adsorbed, preservative free, when administered to individuals 7 years or older, for intramuscular use

⊘▲**90715** Tetanus, diphtheria toxoids and acellular pertussis vaccine (Tdap), when administered to individuals 7 years or older, for intramuscular use

⊘ **90716** Varicella virus vaccine, live, for subcutaneous use

⊘ **90717** Yellow fever vaccine, live, for subcutaneous use

⊘▲**90718** Tetanus and diphtheria toxoids (Td) adsorbed, when administered to individuals 7 years or older, for intramuscular use

⊘ **90719** Diphtheria toxoid, for intramuscular use

⊘ **90720** Diphtheria, tetanus toxoids, and whole cell pertussis vaccine and Hemophilus influenza B vaccine (DTP-Hib), for intramuscular use

⊘ **90721** Diphtheria, tetanus toxoids, and acellular pertussis vaccine and Hemophilus influenza B vaccine (DtaP-Hib), for intramuscular use

⊘ **90723** Diphtheria, tetanus toxoids, acellular pertussis vaccine, Hepatitis B, and poliovirus vaccine, inactivated (DtaP-HepB-IPV), for intramuscular use

⊘ **90725** Cholera vaccine for injectable use

⊘ **90727** Plague vaccine, for intramuscular use

⊘▲**90732** Pneumococcal polysaccharide vaccine, 23-valent, adult or immunosuppressed patient dosage, when administered to individuals 2 years or older, for subcutaneous or intramuscular use

⊘ **90733** Meningococcal polysaccharide vaccine (any group(s)), for subcutaneous use

⊘ **90734** Meningococcal conjugate vaccine, serogroups A, C, Y and W-135 (tetravalent), for intramuscular use

⊘ **90735** Japanese encephalitis virus vaccine, for subcutaneous use

⊘ **90736** Zoster (shingles) vaccine, live, for subcutaneous injection

(FDA approval pending)

⊘ **90740** Hepatitis B vaccine, dialysis or immunosuppressed patient dosage (3 dose schedule), for intramuscular use

⊘ **90743** Hepatitis B vaccine, adolescent (2 dose schedule), for intramuscular use

⊘ **90744** Hepatitis B vaccine, pediatric/adolescent dosage (3 dose schedule), for intramuscular use

⊘ **90746** Hepatitis B vaccine, adult dosage, for intramuscular use

⊘ **90747** Hepatitis B vaccine, dialysis or immunosuppressed patient dosage (4 dose schedule), for intramuscular use

Separate Procedure | Unlisted Procedure | CCI Comp. Code | Non-specific Procedure

⊘ **90748** Hepatitis B and Hemophilus influenza B vaccine (HepB-Hib), for intramuscular use

⊘ **90749** Unlisted vaccine/toxoid

HYDRATION, THERAPEUTIC, PROPHYLACTIC, AND DIAGNOSTIC INJECTIONS AND INFUSIONS (EXCLUDES CHEMOTHERAPY)

CPT codes in this section are used to report hydration and infusions and injections for therapeutic, prophylactic and diagnostic purposes, other than chemotherapy

Coding Rules

1. *If a significant E/M service is performed, report the E/M service code with modifier -25 in addition to the infusion/injection codes.*
2. *Local anesthesia, IV initiation, access to indwelling IV, cath or port, flush after infusion, plus standard tubing, syringes and supplies are included if performed to facilitate the infusion.*
3. *For the administration of multiple drugs, report the service and material or drugs for each.*
4. *For the administration of multiple infusions or injections, only one initial service may be reported.*
5. *Include the actual time when reporting infusion codes that include time as a factor.*

HYDRATION

Hydration codes are used to report IV infusion of fluids and electrolytes such as normal saline, D5W, etc. These codes may not be used to report infusion of drugs or other substances. Direct physician supervision required for consent, safety and/or intraservice staff supervision

90760 Intravenous infusion, hydration; initial, up to 1 hour

(Do not report 90760 if performed as a concurrent infusion service)

▲+**90761** each additional hour (List separately in addition to code for primary procedure)

(Use 90761 in conjunction with 90760)

(Report 90761 for hydration infusion intervals of greater than 30 minutes beyond 1 hour increments)

(Report 90761 to identify hydration if provided as a secondary or subsequent service after a different initial service [90760, 90765, 90774, 96409, 96413] is provided)

THERAPEUTIC, PROPHYLACTIC, AND DIAGNOSTIC INJECTIONS AND INFUSIONS

CPT codes in this section are used to report a therapeutic, prophylactic or diagnostic intravenous (IV) infusion or injection for the administration of drugs and/or substances. Modes of infusion/injection include intravenous infusion, subcutaneous or intramuscular injection, intra-arterial or intravenous push.

Coding Rules

1. *Direct physician supervision is required.*
2. *The CPT codes in this section may not be used for chemotherapy infusions.*
3. *The substance or drug administered must be specified.*
4. *The fluid used to carry the drug(s) is incidental and may not be reported separately.*

(Do not report 90765-90779 with codes for which IV push or infusion is an inherent part of the procedure (eg, administration of contrast material for a diagnostic imaging study))

90765 Intravenous infusion, for therapy, prophylaxis, or diagnosis (specify substance or drug); initial, up to 1 hour

▲+90766 each additional hour (List separately in addition to code for primary procedure)

(Report 90766 in conjunction with 90765, 90767)

(Report 90766 for additional hour(s) of sequential infusion)

(Report 90766 for infusion intervals of greater than 30 minutes beyond 1 hour increments)

+ 90767 additional sequential infusion, up to 1 hour (List separately in addition to code for primary procedure)

(Report 90767 in conjunction with 90765, 90774, 96409, 96413 if provided as a secondary or subsequent service after a different initial service. Report 90767 only once per sequential infusion of same infusate mix)

+ 90768 concurrent infusion (List separately in addition to code for primary procedure)

(Report 90768 only once per encounter)

(Report 90768 in conjunction with 90765, 90766, 96413, 96415, 96416, 96422, 96423)

90772 Therapeutic, prophylactic or diagnostic injection (specify substance or drug); subcutaneous or intramuscular

(For administration of vaccines/toxoids, see 90465-90466, 90471-90472)

(Report 90772 for non-antineoplastic hormonal therapy injections)

(Report 96401 for anti-neoplastic nonhormonal injection therapy)

(Report 96402 for anti-neoplastic hormonal injection therapy)

(Do not report 90772 for injections given without direct physician supervision. To report, use 99211)

(90772 does not include injections for allergen immunotherapy. For allergen immunotherapy injections, see 95115-95117)

90773 intra-arterial

90774 intravenous push, single or initial substance/drug

+ 90775 each additional sequential intravenous push of a new substance/drug (List separately in addition to code for primary procedure)

(Use 90775 in conjunction with 90765, 90774, 96409, 96413)

(Report 90775 to identify intravenous push of a new substance/drug if provided as a secondary or subsequent service after a different initial service is provided)

90779 Unlisted therapeutic, prophylactic or diagnostic intravenous or intra-arterial injection or infusion

(For allergy immunizations, see 95004 et seq)

(90780 deleted 2006 edition. To report, see 90760, 90761, 90765-90768)

● New Code ▲ Revised Code + Add-On Code ⊘ Modifier -51 Exempt ⊙ Conscious Sedation

(90781 deleted 2006 edition. To report, see 90760, 90761, 90765-90768)

(90782 deleted 2006 edition. To report, use 90772)

(90783 deleted 2006 edition. To report, use 90773)

(90784 deleted 2006 edition. To report, use 90774)

(90788 deleted 2006 edition. To report, use 90772)

(90799 deleted 2006 edition. To report, use 90779)

PSYCHIATRY

(For repetitive transcranial magnetic stimulation for treatment of clinical depression, use Category III code 0018T)

Psychiatry is the study, treatment and prevention of mental disorders. Psychiatric services include diagnostic and therapeutic services in the hospital, office, or other outpatient setting. Psychiatric service CPT codes are used to report general psychiatry, clinical psychiatry, and psychiatric therapeutic services and procedures. Key coding issues include the type of psychotherapy, the place of service, the face-to-face time spent with the patient during psychotherapy, and whether evaluation and management services are furnished on the same date of service as psychotherapy.

Coding Rules

1. *Attending physicians reporting hospital care services in treating a psychiatric inpatient may use the full range of hospital evaluation and management service codes.*

2. *If the physician is active in the leadership or direction of a treatment team, a code may be selected based upon the services provided that day using Case Management CPT codes from evaluation and management services codes 99361-99362.*

3. *All procedures performed in addition to hospital care, such as electroconvulsive therapy or medical psychotherapy should be listed in addition to hospital care.*

4. *Psychiatric care may be reported without time dimensions, using CPT codes 90841 or 90845, or with time dimensions, using CPT codes 90843 or 90844, based upon practices customary in the local area.*

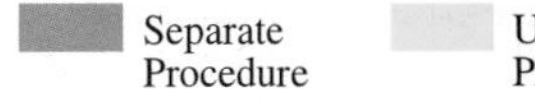

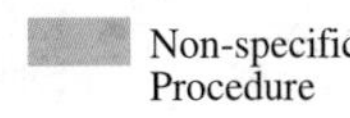

Non-specific Procedure

5. *The modifiers -52, reduced service, or -22, unusual service, may be used to report services that were less or more lengthy that the time-specified CPT codes define.*

PSYCHIATRIC CONSULTATIONS

Consultation services provided by psychiatrists are reported with evaluation and management consultation CPT codes. Psychiatric consultation services are limited to initial or follow-up evaluation and do not involve psychiatric treatment.

PSYCHIATRIC DIAGNOSTIC OR EVALUATIVE INTERVIEW PROCEDURES

90801 Psychiatric diagnostic interview examination

90802 Interactive psychiatric diagnostic interview examination using play equipment, physical devices, language interpreter, or other mechanisms of communication

PSYCHIATRIC THERAPEUTIC PROCEDURES

OFFICE OR OTHER OUTPATIENT FACILITY

Insight Oriented, Behavior Modifying and/or Supportive Psychotherapy

90804 Individual psychotherapy, insight oriented, behavior modifying and/or supportive, in an office or outpatient facility, approximately 20 to 30 minutes face-to-face with the patient;

90805 with medical evaluation and management services

90806 Individual psychotherapy, insight oriented, behavior modifying and/or supportive, in an office or outpatient facility, approximately 45 to 50 minutes face-to-face with the patient;

90807 with medical evaluation and management services

90808 Individual psychotherapy, insight oriented, behavior modifying and/or supportive, in an office or outpatient facility, approximately 75 to 80 minutes face-to-face with the patient;

90809 with medical evaluation and management services

Interactive Psychotherapy

90810 Individual psychotherapy, interactive, using play equipment, physical devices, language interpreter, or other mechanisms of non-verbal communication, in an office or outpatient facility, approximately 20 to 30 minutes face-to-face with the patient;

90811 with medical evaluation and management services

90812 Individual psychotherapy, interactive, using play equipment, physical devices, language interpreter, or other mechanisms of non-verbal communication, in an office or outpatient facility, approximately 45 to 50 minutes face-to-face with the patient;

90813 with medical evaluation and management services

90814 Individual psychotherapy, interactive, using play equipment, physical devices, language interpreter, or other mechanisms of non-verbal communication, in an office or outpatient facility, approximately 75 to 80 minutes face-to-face with the patient;

90815 with medical evaluation and management services

INPATIENT HOSPITAL, PARTIAL HOSPITAL OR RESIDENTIAL CARE FACILITY

Insight Oriented, Behavior Modifying and/or Supportive Psychotherapy

90816 Individual psychotherapy, insight oriented, behavior modifying and/or supportive, in an inpatient hospital, partial hospital or residential care setting, approximately 20 to 30 minutes face-to-face with the patient;

90817 with medical evaluation and management services

90818 Individual psychotherapy, insight oriented, behavior modifying and/or supportive, in an inpatient hospital, partial hospital or residential care setting, approximately 45 to 50 minutes face-to-face with the patient;

90819 with medical evaluation and management services

90821 Individual psychotherapy, insight oriented, behavior modifying and/or supportive, in an inpatient hospital, partial hospital or residential care setting, approximately 75 to 80 minutes face-to-face with the patient;

90822 with medical evaluation and management services

Interactive Psychotherapy

90823 Individual psychotherapy, interactive, using play equipment, physical devices, language interpreter, or other mechanisms of non-verbal communication, in an inpatient hospital, partial hospital or residential care setting, approximately 20 to 30 minutes face-to-face with the patient;

90824 with medical evaluation and management services

90826 Individual psychotherapy, interactive, using play equipment, physical devices, language interpreter, or other mechanisms of non-verbal communication, in an inpatient hospital, partial hospital or residential care setting, approximately 45 to 50 minutes face-to-face with the patient;

90827 with medical evaluation and management services

90828 Individual psychotherapy, interactive, using play equipment, physical devices, language interpreter, or other mechanisms of non-verbal communication, in an inpatient hospital, partial hospital or residential care setting, approximately 75 to 80 minutes face-to-face with the patient;

90829 with medical evaluation and management services

OTHER PSYCHOTHERAPY

90845 Psychoanalysis

90846 Family psychotherapy (without the patient present)

90847 Family psychotherapy (conjoint psychotherapy) (with patient present)

90849 Multiple-family group psychotherapy

90853 Group psychotherapy (other than of a multiple-family group)

90857 Interactive group psychotherapy

OTHER PSYCHIATRIC SERVICES OR PROCEDURES

(For repetitive transcranial magnetic stimulation for treatment of clinical depression, use Category III codes 0160T, 0161T)

90862 Pharmacologic management, including prescription, use, and review of medication with no more than minimal medical psychotherapy

90865 Narcosynthesis for psychiatric diagnostic and therapeutic purposes (eg, sodium amobarbital (Amytal) interview)

90870 Electroconvulsive therapy (includes necessary monitoring)

(90871 deleted 2006 edition.)

90875 Individual psychophysiological therapy incorporating biofeedback training by any modality (face-to-face with the patient), with psychotherapy (eg, insight oriented, behavior modifying or supportive psychotherapy); approximately 20-30 minutes

90876 approximately 45-50 minutes

90880 Hypnotherapy

90882 Environmental intervention for medical management purposes on a psychiatric patients behalf with agencies, employers, or institutions

90885 Psychiatric evaluation of hospital records, other psychiatric reports, psychometric and/or projective tests, and other accumulated data for medical diagnostic purposes

90887 Interpretation or explanation of results of psychiatric, other medical examinations and procedures, or other accumulated data to family or other responsible persons, or advising them how to assist patient

90889 Preparation of report of patient's psychiatric status, history, treatment, or progress (other than for legal or consultative purposes) for other physicians, agencies, or insurance carriers

90899 Unlisted psychiatric service or procedure

Separate Procedure 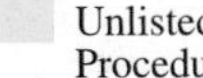 Unlisted Procedure 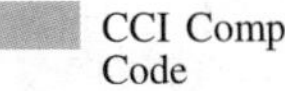 CCI Comp. Code 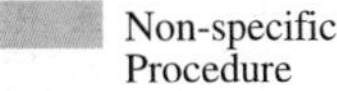 Non-specific Procedure

BIOFEEDBACK

Biofeedback is the process of detecting information about a patient's biological functions, eg. heart rate, breathing rate, skin temperature, and amount of muscle tension, picked up by surface electrodes (sensors) and electronically amplified to provide feedback, usually in the form of an audio-tone and/or visual read-out to the patient. Biofeedback training uses the information that has been monitored from the sensors attached to a muscle on the skin's surface, or to the skin only for thermal or other readings. With the help of a trained clinician, the patient can learn how to make voluntary changes in those biological functions and bring them under control.

Biofeedback services involve the use of electromyographic techniques to detect and record muscle activity. The CPT codes 95860- 95872 (EMG) should not be reported with biofeedback services based on the use of electromyography during a biofeedback session. If an EMG is performed as a separate medically necessary service for diagnosis or follow-up of organic muscle dysfunction, the appropriate EMG codes (e.g. CPT codes 95860-95872) may be reported.

Modifier -59 should be added to indicate that the service performed was a separately identifiable diagnostic service. Reporting only an objective electromyographic response to biofeedback is not sufficient to bill the codes referable to diagnostic EMG.

(For psychophysiological therapy incorporating biofeedback training, see 90875, 90876)

90901 Biofeedback training by any modality

90911 Biofeedback training, perineal muscles, anorectal or urethral sphincter, including EMG and/or manometry

(For incontinence treatment by pulsed magnetic neuromodulation, use Category III code 0029T)

(For testing of rectal sensation, tone and compliance, use 91120)

DIALYSIS

Dialysis is the process of passing body fluids through a membrane to remove harmful substances. Dialysis is used in the treatment of kidney failure. Key coding issues include the type of dialysis and the location of the service.

Coding Rules

1. *All evaluation and management services related to the patient's end stage renal disease that are rendered on a day when dialysis is performed and all other patient care services that are rendered during the dialysis procedure are included in the dialysis procedure CPT codes.*

2. *All evaluation and management services unrelated to the dialysis procedure that cannot be rendered during the dialysis session may be reported in addition to the dialysis procedure.*

3. *Supplies provided to dialysis patients not considered to be included with the dialysis service or procedure are reported using CPT code 99070 or HCPCS codes E1500-E1699 for DME, and A4650-A5149 for supplies for ESRD.*

END STAGE RENAL DISEASE SERVICES

90918 End stage renal disease (ESRD) related services per full month; for patients under two years of age to include monitoring for the adequacy of nutrition, assessment of growth and development, and counseling of parents

90919 for patients between two and eleven years of age to include monitoring for the adequacy of nutrition, assessment of growth and development, and counseling of parents

90920 for patients between twelve and nineteen years of age to include monitoring for the adequacy of nutrition, assessment of growth and development, and counseling of parents

90921 for patients twenty years of age and over

90922 End stage renal disease (ESRD) related services (less than full month), per day; for patients under two years of age

90923 for patients between two and eleven years of age

90924 for patients between twelve and nineteen years of age

90925 for patients twenty years of age and over

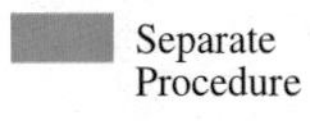

HEMODIALYSIS

(For home visit hemodialysis services performed by a non-physician health care professional, use 99512)

(For cannula declotting, see 36831, 36833, 36860, 36861)

(For declotting of implanted vascular access device or catheter by thrombolytic agent, use 36550)

(For collection of blood specimen from a partially or completely implantable venous access device, use 36540)

(For prolonged physician attendance, see 99354-99360)

90935 Hemodialysis procedure with single physician evaluation

90937 Hemodialysis procedure requiring repeated evaluation(s) with or without substantial revision of dialysis prescription

(90939 deleted 2006 edition. To report, use 90940)

90940 Hemodialysis access flow study to determine blood flow in grafts and arteriovenous fistulae by an indicator method

(For duplex scan of hemodialysis access, use 93990)

MISCELLANEOUS DIALYSIS PROCEDURES

(For insertion of intraperitoneal cannula or catheter, see 49420, 49421)

(For prolonged physician attendance, see 99354-99360)

90945 Dialysis procedure other than hemodialysis (eg, peritoneal, hemofiltration or other continuous replacement therapies), with single physician evaluation

(For home infusion of peritoneal dialysis, use 99559)

90947 Dialysis procedure other than hemodialysis (eg, peritoneal dialysis, hemofiltration, or other continuous renal replacement therapies) requiring repeated physician evaluations, with or without substantial revision of dialysis prescription

90989 Dialysis training, patient, including helper where applicable, any mode, completed course

90993 Dialysis training, patient, including helper where applicable, any mode, course not completed, per training session

90997 Hemoperfusion (eg, with activated charcoal or resin)

90999 Unlisted dialysis procedure, inpatient or outpatient

GASTROENTEROLOGY

Gastroenterology is the study and treatment of diseases of the stomach and digestive system. CPT codes listed in this subsection are used to report diagnostic services of the esophagus and/or stomach contents, and therapeutic services such as gastric intubation and lavage. Gastroenterology services are usually performed in conjunction with an evaluation and management service, such as a consultation or visit, and should be reported separately in addition to the evaluation and management service.

Gastroenterological tests included in CPT codes 91000-91299 are frequently complementary to endoscopic procedures. Esophageal and gastric washings for cytology are described as part of upper endoscopy (e.g. CPT code 43235); therefore, CPT codes 91000 (esophageal intubation) and 91055 (gastric intubation) are not separately reported when performed as part of an upper endoscopy.

Provocative testing (CPT code 91052) can be expedited during GI endoscopy (procurement of gastric specimens). When performed at the same time as GI endoscopy, CPT code 91052 is reported with modifier -52 indicating that a reduced level of service was performed.

(For duodenal intubation and aspiration, see 89100-89105)

(For gastrointestinal radiologic procedures, see 74210-74363)

(For esophagoscopy procedures, see 43200-43228; upper GI endoscopy 43234-43259; endoscopy, small intestine and stomal 44360-44393; proctosigmoidoscopy 45300-45321; sigmoidoscopy 45330-45339; colonscopy 45355-45385; anoscopy 46600-46615)

91000 Esophageal intubation and collection of washings for cytology, including preparation of specimens (separate procedure)

91010 Esophageal motility (manometric study of the esophagus and/or gastroesophageal junction) study;

91011 with mecholyl or similar stimulant

91012 with acid perfusion studies

Separate Procedure | Unlisted Procedure | CCI Comp. Code | Non-specific Procedure

91020 Gastric motility (manometric) studies

91022 Duodenal motility (manometric) study

(If gastrointestinal endoscopy is performed, use 43235)

(If fluoroscopy is performed, use 76000)

(If gastric motility study is performed, use 91020)

91030 Esophagus, acid perfusion (Bernstein) test for esophagitis

(91032 deleted 2005 edition. To report, see 91034, 91035)

(91033 deleted 2005 edition. To report, see 91034, 91035)

91034 Esophagus, gastroesophageal reflux test; with nasal catheter pH electrode(s) placement, recording, analysis and interpretation

91035 with mucosal attached telemetry pH electrode placement, recording, analysis and interpretation

91037 Esophageal function test, gastroesophageal reflux test with nasal catheter intraluminal impedance electrode(s) placement, recording, analysis and interpretation;

91038 prolonged (greater than 1 hour, up to 24 hours)

91040 Esophageal balloon distension provocation study

(For balloon dilatation with endoscopy, see 43220, 43249, 43456, or 43458)

91052 Gastric analysis test with injection of stimulant of gastric secretion (eg, histamine, insulin, pentagastrin, calcium and secretin)

(For gastric biopsy by capsule, peroral, via tube, one or more specimens, use 43600)

(For gastric laboratory procedures, see also 89130-89141)

91055 Gastric intubation, washings, and preparing slides for cytology (separate procedure)

(For gastric lavage, therapeutic, use 91105)

(91060 deleted 2007 edition)

● New Code ▲ Revised Code + Add-On Code ⦸ Modifier -51 Exempt ⊙ Conscious Sedation

(For biopsy by capsule, small intestine, per oral, via tube (one or more specimens), use 44100)

91065 Breath hydrogen test (eg, for detection of lactase deficiency), fructose intolerance, bacterial overgrowth, or oro-cecal gastrointestinal transit)

(For H. pylori breath test analysis, use 83013 for non-radioactive (C-13) isotope or 78268 for radioactive (C-14) isotope)

91100 Intestinal bleeding tube, passage, positioning and monitoring

91105 Gastric intubation, and aspiration or lavage for treatment (eg, for ingested poisons)

(For cholangiography, see 47500, 74320)

(For abdominal paracentesis, see 49080, 49081; with instillation of medication, see 96440, 96445)

(For peritoneoscopy, use 49320; with biopsy, use 49321)

(For peritoneoscopy and guided transhepatic cholangiography, use 47560; with biopsy, use 47561)

(For splenoportography, see 38200, 75810)

91110 Gastrointestinal tract imaging, intraluminal (eg, capsule endoscopy), esophagus through ileum, with physician interpretation and report

(Visualization of the colon is not reported separately)

(Append modifier -52 if the ileum is not visualized)

● **91111** Gastrointestinal tract imaging, intraluminal (eg, capsule endoscopy), esophagus with physician interpretation and report

(Do not report 91111 in conjunction with 91110)

91120 Rectal sensation, tone, and compliance test (ie, response to graded balloon distention)

(For biofeedback training, use 90911)

(For anorectal manometry, use 91122)

91122 Anorectal manometry

91123 Pulsed irrigation of fecal impaction

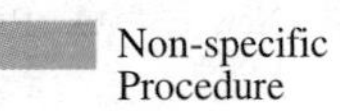

GASTRIC PHYSIOLOGY

91132 Electrogastrography, diagnostic, transcutaneous;

91133 with provocative testing

OTHER PROCEDURES

91299 Unlisted diagnostic gastroenterology procedure

OPHTHALMOLOGY

(For surgical procedures, see Surgery, Eye and Ocular Adnexa, 65091 et seq)

Ophthalmology is the study and treatment of diseases of the eye. Ophthalmological diagnostic and treatment services are reported using CPT Medicine codes 92002-92499.

Coding Rules

1. *Minimal, brief and limited office services, and hospital, home, extended care, emergency department and consultations are reported using appropriate evaluation and management service codes.*

2. *Surgical procedures on the eye(s) are reported using CPT codes from the Eye and Ocular Adnexa subsection of the SURGERY section of CPT.*

3. *To report intermediate ophthalmological services, the following must be performed and documented: a) evaluation of new or existing condition, b) complications of new diagnostic or management problems (not necessarily related to the primary diagnosis), c) history, d) general medical observation e) external ocular and adnexal examination, f) other diagnostic procedures as indicated, and g) may include the use of mydriasis. Intermediate ophthalmological services do not usually include determination of refractive state but may in an established patient under continuing active treatment.*

4. *To report comprehensive ophthalmological services the following must be performed and documented: a) reported as a single service but may be performed at more than one session, b) history, c) general medical observation, d) external and ophthalmoscopic examination, e) gross visual fields, f) basic sensorimotor examination, g. may include, as indicated; biomicroscopy, examination with cycloplegia or mydriasis and tonometry, h) always includes initiation of diagnostic and treatment programs.*

5. *For both intermediate and comprehensive ophthalmological services, service components, such as slip lamp examination, keratomy,*

● New Code ▲ Revised Code + Add-On Code ⃠ Modifier -51 Exempt ⊙ Conscious Sedation

ophthalmoscopy, retinoscopy, tonometry and motor evaluation are not reported separately.

For procedures requiring intravenous injection of dye or other diagnostic agent, insertion of an intravenous catheter and dye injection are necessary to accomplish the procedure and are included in the procedure. Accordingly, HCPCS/CPT codes 36000 (introduction of a needle or catheter), 36410 (venipuncture), G0345-G0350 (90760-90768 in 2006)(IV infusion), and G0353-G0354 (90774-90775 in 2006)(IV injection)as well as selective vascular catheterization codes are not to be separately reported with services requiring intravenous injection (e.g. CPT codes 92230, 92235, 92240, 92287, for angioscopy and angiography).

Fundus photography (CPT code 92250) and scanning ophthalmic computerized diagnostic imaging (CPT code 92135) are generally mutually exclusive of one another in that a provider would use one technique or the other to evaluate fundal disease. However, there are a limited number of clinical conditions where both techniques are medically reasonable and necessary on the ipsilateral eye. In these situations, both CPT codes may be reported appending modifier -59 to CPT code 92250.

GENERAL OPHTHALMOLOGICAL SERVICES

General ophthalmological services (e.g. CPT codes 92002-92014) describe components of the ophthalmologic examination. When evaluation and management codes are reported, these general ophthalmological service codes (e.g. CPT codes 92002-92014) are not to be reported; the same services would be represented by both series of codes.

NEW PATIENT

92002 Ophthalmological services: medical examination and evaluation with initiation of diagnostic and treatment program; intermediate, new patient

92004 comprehensive, new patient, one or more visits

ESTABLISHED PATIENT

92012 Ophthalmological services: medical examination and evaluation, with initiation or continuation of diagnostic and treatment program; intermediate, established patient

92014 comprehensive, established patient, one or more visits

(For surgical procedures, see Surgery, Eye and Ocular Adnexa, 65091 et seq)

SPECIAL OPHTHALMOLOGICAL SERVICES

Special ophthalmological services are defined as a level of service in which a special evaluation of part of the visual system is made which goes beyond the services usually included under general ophthalmological services, or in which special treatment is given. Fluorescein angioscopy, quantitative visual field examination, or extended color vision examination should be specifically reported as special ophthalmological services.

Special ophthalmologic services represent specific services not described as part of a general or routine ophthalmological examination. Special ophthalmological services are recognized as significant, separately identifiable services.

92015 Determination of refractive state

92018 Ophthalmological examination and evaluation, under general anesthesia, with or without manipulation of globe for passive range of motion or other manipulation to facilitate diagnostic examination; complete

92019 limited

92020 Gonioscopy (separate procedure)

(For gonioscopy under general anesthesia, use 92018)

● **92025** Computerized corneal topography, unilateral or bilateral, with interpretation and report

(Do not report 92025 in conjunction with 65710-65755)

(92025 is not used for manual keratoscopy, which is part of a single system of E/M or ophthalmological service)

92060 Sensorimotor examination with multiple measurements of ocular deviation (eg, restrictive or paretic muscle with diplopia) with interpretation and report (separate procedure)

92065 Orthoptic and/or pleoptic training, with continuing medical direction and evaluation

92070 Fitting of contact lens for treatment of disease, including supply of lens

92081 Visual field examination, unilateral or bilateral, with interpretation and report; limited examination (eg, tangent screen, Autoplot, arc perimeter, or single stimulus level automated test, such as Octopus 3 or 7 equivalent)

92082 intermediate examination (eg, at least 2 isopters on Goldmann perimeter, or semiquantitative, automated suprathreshold screening program, Humphrey suprathreshold automatic diagnostic test, Octopus program 33)

92083 extended examination (eg, Goldmann visual fields with at least 3 isopters plotted and static determination within the central 30 degrees, or quantitative, automated threshold perimetry, Octopus programs G-1, 32 or 42, Humphrey visual field analyzer full threshold programs 30-2, 24-2, or 30/60-2)

(Gross visual field testing (eg, confrontation testing) is a part of general ophthalmological services and is not reported separately)

92100 Serial tonometry (separate procedure) with multiple measurements of intraocular pressure over an extended time period with interpretation and report, same day (eg, diurnal curve or medical treatment of acute elevation of intraocular pressure)

92120 Tonography with interpretation and report, recording indentation tonometer method or perilimbal suction method

92130 Tonography with water provocation

92135 Scanning computerized ophthalmic diagnostic imaging (eg, scanning laser) with interpretation and report, unilateral

92136 Ophthalmic biometry by partial coherence interferometry with intraocular lens power calculation

92140 Provocative tests for glaucoma, with interpretation and report, without tonography

OPHTHALMOSCOPY

92225 Ophthalmoscopy, extended, with retinal drawing (eg, for retinal detachment, melanoma), with interpretation and report; initial

92226 subsequent

92230 Fluorescein angioscopy with interpretation and report

92235 Fluorescein angiography (includes multiframe imaging) with interpretation and report

92240 Indocyanine-green angiography (includes multiframe imaging) with interpretation and report

92250 Fundus photography with interpretation and report

92260 Ophthalmodynamometry

(For opthalmoscopy under general anesthesia, use 92018)

OTHER SPECIALIZED SERVICES

92265 Needle oculoelectromyography, one or more extraocular muscles, one or both eyes, with interpretation and report

92270 Electro-oculography with interpretation and report

92275 Electroretinography with interpretation and report

(For electronystagmography for vestibular function studies, see 92541 et seq)

(For ophthalmic echography (diagnostic ultrasound), see 76511-76529)

92283 Color vision examination, extended, eg, anomaloscope or equivalent

(Color vision testing with pseudoisochromatic plates (such as HRR or Ishihara) is not reported separately. It is included in the appropriate general or ophthalmological service, or 99172)

92284 Dark adaptation examination with interpretation and report

92285 External ocular photography with interpretation and report for documentation of medical progress (eg, close-up photography, slit lamp photography, goniophotography, stereo-photography)

92286 Special anterior segment photography with interpretation and report; with specular endothelial microscopy and cell count

92287 with fluorescein angiography

CONTACT LENS SERVICES

(For therapeutic or surgical use of contact lens, see 68340, 92070)

92310 Prescription of optical and physical characteristics of and fitting of contact lens, with medical supervision of adaptation; corneal lens, both eyes, except for aphakia

(For prescription and fitting of one eye, add modifier -52)

92311 corneal lens for aphakia, one eye

92312 corneal lens for aphakia, both eyes

92313 corneoscleral lens

92314 Prescription of optical and physical characteristics of contact lens, with medical supervision of adaptation and direction of fitting by independent technician; corneal lens, both eyes except for aphakia

(For prescription and fitting of one eye, add modifier -52)

92315 corneal lens for aphakia, one eye

92316 corneal lens for aphakia, both eyes

92317 corneoscleral lens

92325 Modification of contact lens (separate procedure), with medical supervision of adaptation

92326 Replacement of contact lens

(For prescription, fitting, and/or medical supervision of ocular prosthetic adaptation by a physician, see Evaluation and Management services or General Ophthalmological service codes 92002-92014)

(92330 deleted 2006 edition.)

(92335 deleted 2006 edition.)

Separate Procedure | Unlisted Procedure | CCI Comp. Code | Non-specific Procedure

SPECTACLE SERVICES (INCLUDING PROSTHESIS FOR APHAKIA)

92340 Fitting of spectacles, except for aphakia; monofocal

92341 bifocal

92342 multifocal, other than bifocal

92352 Fitting of spectacle prosthesis for aphakia; monofocal

92353 multifocal

92354 Fitting of spectacle mounted low vision aid; single element system

92355 telescopic or other compound lens system

92358 Prosthesis service for aphakia, temporary (disposable or loan, including materials)

92370 Repair and refitting spectacles; except for aphakia

92371 spectacle prosthesis for aphakia

(92390 deleted 2006 edition. For supply of spectacles or contact lenses, use the appropriate supply codes)

(92391 deleted 2006 edition. For supply of spectacles or contact lenses, use the appropriate supply codes)

(92392 deleted 2006 edition. For supply of spectacles or contact lenses, use the appropriate supply codes)

(92393 deleted 2006 edition. For supply of spectacles or contact lenses, use the appropriate supply codes)

(92395 deleted 2006 edition. For supply of spectacles or contact lenses, use the appropriate supply codes)

(92396 deleted 2006 edition. For supply of spectacles or contact lenses, use the appropriate supply codes)

OTHER PROCEDURES

92499 Unlisted ophthalmological service or procedure

SPECIAL OTORHINOLARYNGOLOGIC SERVICES

Otorhinolaryngology is the study and treatment of diseases of the head and neck, including the ears, nose and throat. Diagnostic or treatment procedures usually included in a comprehensive otorhinolaryngologic evaluation or office visit, are reported as an integrated medical service, using CPT evaluation and management service codes.

Code 92506 is used to report evaluation of speech production, receptive language, and expressive language abilities. Tests may examine speech sound production, articulatory movements of oral musculature, the patient's ability to understand the meaning and intent of written and verbal expressions, and the appropriate formulation and utterance of expressive thought. In contrast, 92626 and 92627 are reported for an evaluation of auditory rehabilitation status determining the patient's ability to use residual hearing in order to identify the acoustic characteristics of sounds associated with speech communication.

CPT coding for otorhinolaryngologic services involves a number of tests that can be performed qualitatively by confrontation during physical examination or quantitatively with electrical recording equipment. The CPT definition specifies which is the case for each code. CPT codes 92552-92557, and 92561- 92588 can be performed qualitatively or quantitatively but according to CPT definition these can be reported only if calibrated electronic equipment is used. Confrontational estimation of these tests by the physician is part of the evaluation and management service.

Speech language pathologists may perform services coded as CPT codes 92507, 92508, or 92526. They do not perform services coded as CPT codes 97110, 97112, 97150, 97530, or 97532 which are generally performed by physical or occupational therapists. Speech language pathologists should not report CPT codes 97110, 97112, 97150, 97530, or 97532 as unbundled services included in the services coded as 92507, 92508, or 92526.

Coding Rules

1. *Component procedures, such as otoscopy, rhinoscopy, tuning fork test, which may be provided as part of a comprehensive service are not reported separately.*

2. *Special otorhinolaryngologic diagnostic or treatment services not usually included in a comprehensive otorhinolaryngologic evaluation or office visit are reported separately.*

3. *All otorhinolaryngologic services include medical diagnostic evaluation. Technical procedures, which may or may not be performed by the physician personally, are often part of the service, but should not be mistaken to constitute the service itself.*

(For laryngoscopy with stroboscopy, use 31579)

92502 Otolaryngologic examination under general anesthesia

92504 Binocular microscopy (separate diagnostic procedure)

92506 Evaluation of speech, language, voice, communication, and/or auditory processing

92507 Treatment of speech, language, voice, communication, and/or auditory processing disorder; individual

92508 group, two or more individuals

(92510 deleted 2006 edition.)

(For auditory rehabilitation, prelingual hearing loss, use 92630)

(For auditory rehabilitation, postlingual hearing loss, use 92633)

(For cochlear implant programming, see 92601-92604)

92511 Nasopharyngoscopy with endoscope (separate procedure)

92512 Nasal function studies (eg, rhinomanometry)

92516 Facial nerve function studies (eg, electroneuronography)

92520 Laryngeal function studies (ie, aerodynamic testing and acoustic testing)

(For performance of a single test, use modifier 52)

(To report flexible fiberoptic laryngeal evaluation of swallowing and laryngeal sensory testing, see 92611-92617)

(To report other testing of laryngeal function (eg, electroglottography), use 92700)

92526 Treatment of swallowing dysfunction and/or oral function for feeding

VESTIBULAR FUNCTION TESTS, WITH OBSERVATION AND EVALUATION BY PHYSICIAN, WITHOUT ELECTRICAL RECORDING

92531 Spontaneous nystagmus, including gaze

92532 Positional nystagmus test

92533 Caloric vestibular test, each irrigation (binaural, bithermal stimulation constitutes four tests)

92534 Optokinetic nystagmus test

VESTIBULAR FUNCTION TESTS, WITH RECORDING (eg, ENG, PENG), AND MEDICAL DIAGNOSTIC EVALUATION

92541 Spontaneous nystagmus test, including gaze and fixation nystagmus, with recording

92542 Positional nystagmus test, minimum of 4 positions, with recording

92543 Caloric vestibular test, each irrigation (binaural, bithermal stimulation constitutes four tests), with recording

92544 Optokinetic nystagmus test, bidirectional, foveal or peripheral stimulation, with recording

92545 Oscillating tracking test, with recording

92546 Sinusoidal vertical axis rotational testing

\+ **92547** Use of vertical electrodes (List separately in addition to code for primary procedure)

(Use 92547 in conjunction with codes 92541-92546)

(For unlisted vestibular tests, use 92700)

92548 Computerized dynamic posturography

Separate Procedure
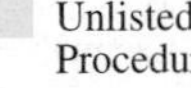
Unlisted Procedure
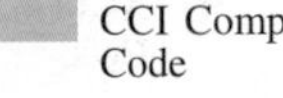
CCI Comp. Code
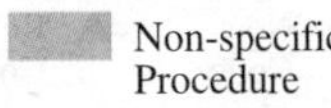
Non-specific Procedure

AUDIOLOGIC FUNCTION TESTS WITH MEDICAL DIAGNOSTIC EVALUATION

(For evaluation of speech, language and/or hearing problems through observation and assessment of performance, use 92506)

92551 Screening test, pure tone, air only

92552 Pure tone audiometry (threshold); air only

92553 air and bone

92555 Speech audiometry threshold;

92556 with speech recognition

92557 Comprehensive audiometry threshold evaluation and speech recognition (92553 and 92556 combined)

(For hearing aid evaluation and selection, see 92590-92595)

92559 Audiometric testing of groups

92560 Bekesy audiometry; screening

92561 diagnostic

92562 Loudness balance test, alternate binaural or monaural

92563 Tone decay test

92564 Short increment sensitivity index (SISI)

92565 Stenger test, pure tone

92567 Tympanometry (impedance testing)

92568 Acoustic reflex testing; threshold

92569 decay

92571 Filtered speech test

92572 Staggered spondaic word test

(92573 deleted 2007 edition. To report the Lombard test, see 92700)

● New Code ▲ Revised Code + Add-On Code ⦸ Modifier -51 Exempt ⊙ Conscious Sedation

92575 Sensorineural acuity level test

92576 Synthetic sentence identification test

92577 Stenger test, speech

92579 Visual reinforcement audiometry (VRA)

92582 Conditioning play audiometry

92583 Select picture audiometry

92584 Electrocochleography

92585 Auditory evoked potentials for evoked response audiometry and/or testing of the central nervous system; comprehensive

92586 limited

92587 Evoked otoacoustic emissions; limited (single stimulus level, either transient or distortion products)

92588 comprehensive or diagnostic evaluation (comparison of transient and/or distortion product otoacoustic emissions at multiple levels and frequencies)

(92589 deleted 2005 edition)

(For central auditory function evaluation, see 92620, 92621)

92590 Hearing aid examination and selection; monaural

92591 binaural

92592 Hearing aid check; monaural

92593 binaural

92594 Electroacoustic evaluation for hearing aid; monaural

92595 binaural

92596 Ear protector attenuation measurements

92597 Evaluation for use and/or fitting of voice prosthetic device to supplement oral speech

Separate Procedure | Unlisted Procedure | CCI Comp. Code | Non-specific Procedure

(To report augmentative and alternative communication device services, see 92605, 92607, 92608)

EVALUATIVE AND THERAPEUTIC SERVICES

(For placement of cochlear implant, use 69930)

92601 Diagnostic analysis of cochlear implant, patient under 7 years of age; with programming

92602 subsequent reprogramming

(Do not report 92602 in addition to 92601)

(For aural rehabilitation services following cochlear implant, including evaluation of rehabilitation status, see 92626-92627, 92630-92633)

92603 Diagnostic analysis of cochlear implant, age 7 years or older; with programming

92604 subsequent reprogramming

(Do not report 92604 in addition to 92603)

92605 Evaluation for prescription of non-speech-generating augmentative and alternative communication device

92606 Therapeutic service(s) for the use of non-speech-generating device, including programming and modification

92607 Evaluation for prescription for speech-generating augmentative and alternative communication device, face-to-face with the patient; first hour

(For evaluation for prescription of a non-speech-generating device, use 92605)

+ **92608** each additional 30 minutes (List separately in addition to code for primary procedure)

(Use 92608 in conjunction with 92607)

92609 Therapeutic services for the use of speech-generating device, including programming and modification

(For therapeutic service(s) for the use of a non-speech-generating device, use 92606)

92610 Evaluation of oral and pharyngeal swallowing function

(For motion fluoroscopic evaluation of swallowing function, use 92611)

(For flexible endoscopic examination, use 92612-92617)

92611 Motion fluoroscopic evaluation of swallowing function by cine or video recording

(For radiological supervision and interpretation, use 74230)

(For evaluation of oral and pharyngeal swallowing function, use 92610)

(For flexible fiberoptic diagnostic laryngoscopy, use 31575. Do not report 31575 in conjunction with 92612-92617)

92612 Flexible fiberoptic endoscopic evaluation of swallowing by cine or video recording;

(If flexible fiberoptic or endoscopic evaluation of swallowing is performed without cine or video recording, use 92700)

92613 physician interpretation and report only

(To report an evaluation of oral and pharyngeal swallowing function, use 92610)

(To report motion fluoroscopic evaluation of swallowing function, use 92611)

92614 Flexible fiberoptic endoscopic evaluation, laryngeal sensory testing by cine or video recording;

(If flexible fiberoptic or endoscopic evaluation of swallowing is performed without cine or video recording, use 92700)

92615 physician interpretation and report only

92616 Flexible fiberoptic endoscopic evaluation of swallowing and laryngeal sensory testing by cine or video recording;

(If flexible fiberoptic or endoscopic evaluation of swallowing is performed without cine or video recording, use 92700)

92617 physician interpretation and report only

92620 Evaluation of central auditory function, with report; initial 60 minutes

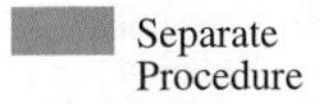 Separate Procedure  Unlisted Procedure 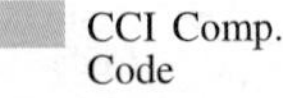 CCI Comp. Code 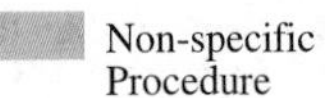 Non-specific Procedure

92621 each additional 15 minutes

(Do not report 92620, 92621 in conjunction with 92506)

92625 Assessment of tinnitus (includes pitch, loudness matching, and masking)

(Do not report 92625 in conjunction with 92562)

(For unilateral assessment, use modifier 52)

92626 Evaluation of auditory rehabilitation status; first hour

+ **92627** each additional 15 minutes (List separately in addition to code for primary procedure)

(Use 92627 in conjunction with 92626)

(When reporting 92626, 92627, use the face-to-face time with the patient or family)

92630 Auditory rehabilitation; pre-lingual hearing loss

92633 post-lingual hearing loss

SPECIAL DIAGNOSTIC PROCEDURES

● **92640** Diagnostic analysis with programming of auditory brainstem implant, per hour

(Report nonprogramming services separately [eg., cardiac monitoring])

OTHER PROCEDURES

92700 Unlisted otorhinolaryngological service or procedure

CARDIOVASCULAR

Cardiovascular services refers to the study and treatment of diseases of the heart and vascular (arteries and veins) system. Cardiovascular services CPT codes are used to report therapeutic services such as cardiopulmonary resuscitation (CPR), cardioversion and percutaneous transluminal coronary angioplasty (PTCA) and diagnostic procedures such as electrocardiography, echocardiography and cardiac catheterization.

Cardiovascular medicine services include non-invasive and invasive diagnostic testing (including intracardiac testing) as well as therapeutic services (e.g. electrophysiological procedures).

When cardiopulmonary resuscitation is performed without other evaluation and management services (e.g. a physician responds to a "code blue" and directs cardiopulmonary resuscitation with the patient's attending physician then resuming the care of the patient after the patient has been revived), only the CPT code 92950 for CPR should be reported. Levels of critical care services and prolonged management services are determined by time; when CPT code 92950 is reported, the time required to perform CPR is not included in critical care or other timed evaluation and management services.

In keeping with the policies outlined previously, procedures routinely performed as part of a comprehensive service are included in the comprehensive service and not separately reported. A number of therapeutic and diagnostic cardiovascular procedures (e.g. CPT codes 92950-92998, 93501-93545, 93600-93624, 93640-93652) routinely utilize intravenous or intra-arterial vascular access, routinely require electrocardiographic monitoring, and frequently require agents administered by injection or infusion techniques; accordingly, separate codes for routine access, monitoring, injection or infusion services are not to be reported.

Fluoroscopic guidance procedures are integral to invasive intravascular procedures and are included in those services. In unique circumstances, where these services are performed, not as an integral part of the procedure, the appropriate code can be separately reported with modifier -59. When supervision and interpretation codes are identified in the CPT code book for a given procedure, these can be separately reported.

Cardiac output measurement (e.g. CPT codes 93561-93562) is routinely performed during cardiac catheterization procedures per CPT definition and, therefore, CPT codes 93561-93562 are not to be reported with cardiac catheterization codes.

THERAPEUTIC SERVICES AND PROCEDURES

(For non-surgical septal reduction therapy (eg, alcohol ablation), use Category III code 0024T)

92950 Cardiopulmonary resuscitation (eg, in cardiac arrest)

(See also critical care services, 99291, 99292)

⊙ **92953** Temporary transcutaneous pacing

(For physician direction of ambulance or rescue personnel outside the hospital, use 99288)

Separate Procedure | Unlisted Procedure | CCI Comp. Code | Non-specific Procedure

⊙ **92960** Cardioversion, elective, electrical conversion of arrhythmia; external

⊙ **92961** internal (separate procedure)

(Do not report 92961 in addition to codes 93662, 93618-93624, 93631, 93640-93642, 93650-93652, 93741-93744)

92970 Cardioassist-method of circulatory assist; internal

92971 external

(For balloon atrial-septostomy, use 92992)

(For placement of catheters for use in circulatory assist devices such as intra-aortic balloon pump, use 33970)

⊙+**92973** Percutaneous transluminal coronary thrombectomy (List separately in addition to code for primary procedure)

(Use 92973 in conjunction with codes 92980, 92982)

⊙+**92974** Transcatheter placement of radiation delivery device for subsequent coronary intravascular brachytherapy (List separately in addition to code for primary procedure)

(Use 92974 in conjunction with codes 92980, 92982, 92995, 93508)

(For intravascular radioelement application, see 77781-77784)

⊙ **92975** Thrombolysis, coronary; by intracoronary infusion, including selective coronary angiography

92977 by intravenous infusion

(For thrombolysis of vessels other than coronary, see 37201, 75896)

(For cerebral thrombolysis, use 37195)

⊙+**92978** Intravascular ultrasound (coronary vessel or graft) during diagnostic evaluation and/or therapeutic intervention including imaging supervision, interpretation and report; initial vessel (List separately in addition to code for primary procedure)

⊙+**92979** each additional vessel (List separately in addition to code for primary procedure)

(Use 92979 in conjunction with code 92978)

● New Code ▲ Revised Code + Add-On Code ⊘ Modifier -51 Exempt ⊙ Conscious Sedation

(Intravascular ultrasound services include all transducer manipulations and repositioning within the specific vessel being examined, both before and after therapeutic intervention (eg, stent placement)

⊙ **92980** Transcatheter placement of an intracoronary stent(s), percutaneous, with or without other therapeutic intervention, any method; single vessel

⊙+**92981** each additional vessel (List separately in addition to code for primary procedure)

(Use 92981 in conjunction with code 92980)

(Codes 92980, 92981 are used to report coronary artery stenting. Coronary angioplasty (92982, 92984) or atherectomy (92995, 92996), in the same artery, is considered part of the stenting procedure and is not reported separately. Codes 92973 (percutaneous transluminal coronary thrombectomy), 92974 (coronary brachytherapy) and 92978, 92979 (intravascular ultrasound) are add-on codes for reporting procedures performed in addition to coronary stenting, atherectomy, and angioplasty and are not included in the "therapeutic interventions" in 92980)

(To report additional vessels treated by angioplasty or atherectomy only during the same session, see 92984, 92996)

(To report transcatheter placement of radiation delivery device for coronary intravascular brachytherapy, use 92974)

(For intravascular radioelement application, see 77781-77784)

⊙ **92982** Percutaneous transluminal coronary balloon angioplasty; single vessel

⊙+**92984** each additional vessel (List separately in addition to code for primary procedure)

(Use 92984 in conjunction with codes 92980, 92982, 92995)

(For stent placement following completion of angioplasty or atherectomy, see 92980, 92981)

(To report transcatheter placement of radiation delivery device for coronary intravascular brachytherapy, use 92974)

(For intravascular radioelement application, see 77781-77784)

⊙ **92986** Percutaneous balloon valvuloplasty; aortic valve

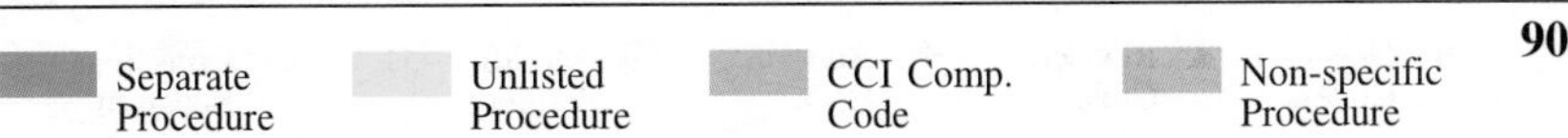

⊙ **92987** mitral valve

92990 pulmonary valve

92992 Atrial septectomy or septostomy; transvenous method, balloon (eg, Rashkind type) (includes cardiac catheterization)

92993 blade method (Park septostomy) (includes cardiac catheterization)

⊙ **92995** Percutaneous transluminal coronary atherectomy, by mechanical or other method, with or without balloon angioplasty; single vessel

⊙+**92996** each additional vessel (List separately in addition to code for primary procedure)

(Use 92996 in conjunction with code(s) 92980, 92982, 92995)

(For stent placement following completion of angioplasty or atherectomy, see 92980, 92981)

(To report additional vessels treated by angioplasty only during the same session, use 92984)

92997 Percutaneous transluminal pulmonary artery balloon angioplasty; single vessel

+ **92998** each additional vessel (List separately in addition to code for primary procedure)

(Use 92998 in conjunction with code 92997)

CARDIOGRAPHY

Routine monitoring of EKG rhythm and review of daily hemodynamics, including cardiac outputs, is a part of critical care evaluation and management. Separate billing for review of EKG rhythm strips and cardiac output measurements (e.g. CPT codes 93040-93042, 93561, 93562) and critical care services is inappropriate.

An exception to this may include a sudden change in patient status associated with a change in cardiac rhythm requiring a return to the ICU or telephonic transmission to review a rhythm strip. If reported separately, time included for this service is not included in the critical care time calculated for the critical care service.

(For echocardiography, see 93303-93350)

93000 Electrocardiogram, routine ECG with at least 12 leads; with interpretation and report

93005 tracing only, without interpretation and report

93010 interpretation and report only

(For ECG monitoring, see 99354-99360)

93012 Telephonic transmission of post-symptom electrocardiogram rhythm strip(s), 24-hour attended monitoring, per 30 day period of time; tracing only

93014 physician review with interpretation and report only

93015 Cardiovascular stress test using maximal or submaximal treadmill or bicycle exercise, continuous electrocardiographic monitoring, and/or pharmacological stress; with physician supervision, with interpretation and report

93016 physician supervision only, without interpretation and report

93017 tracing only, without interpretation and report

93018 interpretation and report only

(For inert gas rebreathing measurement, see Category III codes 0104T, 0105T)

93024 Ergonovine provocation test

93025 Microvolt T-wave alternans for assessment of ventricular arrhythmias

93040 Rhythm ECG, one to three leads; with interpretation and report

93041 tracing only without interpretation and report

93042 interpretation and report only

93224 Electrocardiographic monitoring for 24 hours by continuous original ECG waveform recording and storage, with visual superimposition scanning; includes recording, scanning analysis with report, physician review and interpretation

Separate Procedure | Unlisted Procedure | CCI Comp. Code | Non-specific Procedure

93225 recording (includes hook-up, recording, and disconnection)

93226 scanning analysis with report

93227 physician review and interpretation

93230 Electrocardiographic monitoring for 24 hours by continuous original ECG waveform recording and storage without superimposition scanning utilizing a device capable of producing a full miniaturized printout; includes recording, microprocessor-based analysis with report, physician review and interpretation

93231 recording (includes hook-up, recording, and disconnection)

93232 microprocessor-based analysis with report

93233 physician review and interpretation

93235 Electrocardiographic monitoring for 24 hours by continuous computerized monitoring and non-continuous recording, and real-time data analysis utilizing a device capable of producing intermittent full-sized waveform tracings, possibly patient activated; includes monitoring and real-time data analysis with report, physician review and interpretation

93236 monitoring and real-time data analysis with report

93237 physician review and interpretation

93268 Patient demand single or multiple event recording with presymptom memory loop, 24-hour attended monitoring, per 30 day period of time; includes transmission, physician review and interpretation

93270 recording (includes hook-up, recording, and disconnection)

93271 monitoring, receipt of transmissions, and analysis

93272 physician review and interpretation only

(For postsymptom recording, see 93012, 93014)

(For implanted patient activated cardiac event recording, see 33282, 93727)

93278 Signal-averaged electrocardiography (SAECG), with or without ECG

● New Code ▲ Revised Code + Add-On Code ⊘ Modifier -51 Exempt ⊙ Conscious Sedation

(For interpretation and report only, use 93278 with modifier -26)

(For unlisted cardiographic procedure, use 93799)

ECHOCARDIOGRAPHY

An echocardiogram is an ultrasound of the heart. Using standard ultrasound techniques, two-dimensional slices of the heart can be imaged. The latest ultrasound systems employ 3D real-time imaging. The standard echocardiogram is also known as a transthoracic echocardiogram, or TTE. In this case, the echocardiography transducer (or probe) is placed on the chest wall (or thorax) of the subject, and images are taken through the chest wall. This is a non-invasive, highly accurate and quick assessment of the overall health of the heart.

Another method to perform an echocardiogram is to insert a specialized scope containing an echocardiography transducer (TOE probe) into the patient's esophagus and record pictures from there. This is known as a transesophageal echocardiogram, or TEE. The advantages of TEE over TTE are clearer images, since the transducer is closer to the heart. Some structures are better imaged with the TEE. These structures include the aorta, the pulmonary artery, the valves of the heart, and the left and right atria. While TTE can be performed easily and without pain for the patient, TEE may require light sedation and a local anesthetic lubricant for the esophagus. Unlike the TTE, the TEE is considered an invasive procedure.

In addition to creating two-dimensional pictures of the cardiovascular system, the echocardiogram can also produce accurate assessment of the direction of blood flow and the velocity of blood and cardiac tissue at any arbitrary point using Doppler ultrasound. This allows assessment of cardiac valve areas and function, any abnormal communications between the left and right side of the heart, any leaking of blood through the valves (valvular regurgitation), and calculation of the cardiac output as well as the ejection fraction.

(For fetal echocardiography, see 76825-76828)

93303 Transthoracic echocardiography for congenital cardiac anomalies; complete

93304 follow-up or limited study

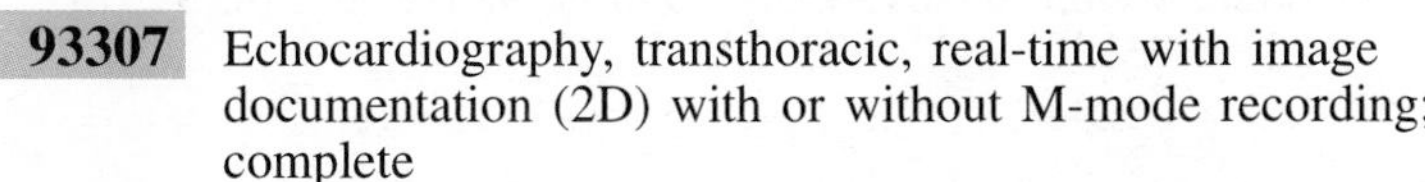

93307 Echocardiography, transthoracic, real-time with image documentation (2D) with or without M-mode recording; complete

93308 follow-up or limited study

⊙ **93312** Echocardiography, transesophageal, real time with image documentation (2D) (with or without M-mode recording); including probe placement, image acquisition, interpretation and report

⊙ **93313** placement of transesophageal probe only

⊙ **93314** image acquisition, interpretation and report only

⊙ **93315** Transesophageal echocardiography for congenital cardiac anomalies; including probe placement, image acquisition, interpretation and report

⊙ **93316** placement of transesophageal probe only

⊙ **93317** image acquisition, interpretation and report only

⊙ **93318** Echocardiography, transesophageal (TEE) for monitoring purposes, including probe placement, real time 2-dimensional image acquisition and interpretation leading to ongoing (continuous) assessment of (dynamically changing) cardiac pumping function and to therapeutic measures on an immediate time basis

+ **93320** Doppler echocardiography, pulsed wave and/or continuous wave with spectral display (List separately in addition to codes for echocardiographic imaging); complete

(Use 93320 in conjunction with codes 93303, 93304, 93307, 93308, 93312, 93314, 93315, 93317, 93350)

+ **93321** follow-up or limited study (List separately in addition to codes for echocardiographic imaging)

(Use 93321 in conjunction with codes 93303, 93304, 93307, 93308, 93312, 93314, 93315, 93317, 93350)

+ **93325** Doppler echocardiography color flow velocity mapping (List separately in addition to codes for echocardiography)

(Use 93325 in conjunction with codes 76825, 76826, 76827, 76828, 93303, 93304, 93307, 93308, 93312, 93314, 93315, 93317, 93320, 93321, 93350)

93350 Echocardiography, transthoracic, real-time with image documentation (2D), with or without M-mode recording, during rest and cardiovascular stress test using treadmill, bicycle exercise and/or pharmacologically induced stress, with interpretation and report

(The appropriate stress testing code from the 93015-93018 series should be reported in addition to 93350 to capture the exercise stress portion of the study)

CARDIAC CATHETERIZATION

A coronary catheterization is a minimally invasive procedure to access the coronary circulation and blood filled chambers of the heart using a catheter. It is performed for both diagnostic and interventional (treatment) purposes.

Specifically, coronary catheterization is a visually interpreted test performed to recognize occlusion, stenosis, restenosis, thrombosis or aneurysmal enlargement of the coronary artery lumens, heart chamber size, heart muscle contraction performance and some aspects of heart valve function. Important internal heart and lung blood pressures, not measurable from outside the body, can be accurately measured during the test. The relevant problems that the test deals with most commonly occur as a result of advanced atherosclerosis, atheroma activity within the wall of the coronary arteries. Less frequently, other issues, valvular, heart muscle or arrhythmia issues are the primary focus of the test.

Coronary artery luminal narrowing reduces the flow reserve for oxygenated blood to the heart, typically producing intermittent angina if very advanced; luminal occlusion usually produces a heart attack. However, it has been increasingly recognized, since the late 1980s, that coronary catheterization does not allow the recognition of the presence or absence of coronary atherosclerosis itself, only significant luminal changes which have occurred as a result of end stage complications of the atherosclerotic process. See IVUS and atheroma for a better understanding of this issue.

Coronary catheterization is performed in a cardiac catheterization lab, usually located within a hospital.

Catheterization to treat luminal disease

By changing the diagnostic catheter to a guiding catheter, physicians can also pass a variety of instruments through the catheter and into the artery to a lesion site. The most commonly used are guide wires and the balloon dilation catheters.

By injecting radiocontrast agent through a tiny passage extending down the balloon catheter and into the balloon, the balloon is progressively expanded. The hydraulic pressures are chosen and applied by the physician, according to how the balloon within the stenosis responds. The radiocontrast filled balloon is watched under fluoroscopy (it typically assumes a "dog bone" shape imposed on the outside of the balloon by the stenosis as the balloon is expanded), as it opens. As much hydraulic brute force is applied as judged needed and visualized to be effective to make the stenosis of the artery lumen visibly enlarge.

Additionally, several other devices can be advanced into the artery via a guiding catheter. These include laser catheters, stent catheters, IVUS catheters, Doppler catheter, pressure or temperature measurement catheter and various clot and grinding or removal devices. Most of these devices have turned out to be niche devices, only useful in a small percentage of situations or for research.

Stents, specially manufactured expandable stainless steel mesh tubes, mounted on a balloon catheter, are the most commonly used device beyond the balloon catheter. When the stent/balloon device is positioned within the stenosis, the balloon is inflated which, in turn, expands the stent and the artery. The balloon is removed and the stent remains in place, supporting the inner artery walls in the more open, dilated position.

⊘⊙93501 Right heart catheterization

(For bundle of His recording, use 93600)

⊘ 93503 Insertion and placement of flow directed catheter (eg, Swan-Ganz) for monitoring purposes

(For subsequent monitoring, see 99356-99357)

⊘⊙93505 Endomyocardial biopsy

⊘⊙93508 Catheter placement in coronary artery(s), arterial coronary conduit(s), and/or venous coronary bypass graft(s) for coronary angiography without concomitant left heart catheterization

(93508 is to be used only when left heart catheterization 93510, 93511, 93524, 93526 is not performed)

(93508 is to be used only once per procedure)

(To report transcatheter placement of radiation delivery device for coronary intravascular brachytherapy, use 92974)

(For intravascular radioelement application, see 77781-77784)

⊘⊙93510 Left heart catheterization, retrograde, from the brachial artery, axillary artery or femoral artery; percutaneous

⊘⊙93511 by cutdown

⊘⊙93514 Left heart catheterization by left ventricular puncture

⊘⊙93524 Combined transseptal and retrograde left heart catheterization

⊘⊙**93526** Combined right heart catheterization and retrograde left heart catheterization

⊘⊙**93527** Combined right heart catheterization and transseptal left heart catheterization through intact septum (with or without retrograde left heart catheterization)

⊘⊙**93528** Combined right heart catheterization with left ventricular puncture (with or without retrograde left heart catheterization)

⊘⊙**93529** Combined right heart catheterization and left heart catheterization through existing septal opening (with or without retrograde left heart catheterization)

⊘⊙**93530** Right heart catheterization, for congenital cardiac anomalies

⊘ **93531** Combined right heart catheterization and retrograde left heart catheterization, for congenital cardiac anomalies

⊘ **93532** Combined right heart catheterization and transseptal left heart catheterization through intact septum with or without retrograde left heart catheterization, for congenital cardiac anomalies

⊘ **93533** Combined right heart catheterization and transseptal left heart catheterization through existing septal opening, with or without retrograde left heart catheterization, for congenital cardiac anomalies

(When injection procedures are performed in conjunction with cardiac catheterization, these services do not include introduction of catheters but do include repositioning of catheters when necessary and use of automatic power injectors. Injection procedures 93539-93545 represent separate identifiable services and may be coded in conjunction with one another when appropriate. The technical details of angiography, supervision of filming and processing, interpretation and report are not included. To report imaging supervision, interpretation and report, use 93555 and/or 93556. Modifier -51 should not be appended to 93539-93556)

⊘⊙**93539** Injection procedure during cardiac catheterization; for selective opacification of arterial conduits (eg, internal mammary), whether native or used for bypass

⊘⊙**93540** for selective opacification of aortocoronary venous bypass grafts, one or more coronary arteries

⊘⊙**93541** for pulmonary angiography

Separate Procedure | Unlisted Procedure | CCI Comp. Code | Non-specific Procedure

⊘⊙93542 for selective right ventricular or right atrial angiography

⊘⊙93543 for selective left ventricular or left atrial angiography

⊘⊙93544 for aortography

⊘⊙93545 for selective coronary angiography (injection of radiopaque material may be by hand)

(To report imaging supervision and interpretation, use 93555)

⊘⊙93555 Imaging supervision, interpretation and report for injection procedure(s) during cardiac catheterization; ventricular and/or atrial angiography

⊘⊙93556 pulmonary angiography, aortography, and/or selective coronary angiography including venous bypass grafts and arterial conduits (whether native or used in bypass)

(Codes 93561 and 93562 are not to be used with cardiac catheterization codes)

⊙ 93561 Indicator dilution studies such as dye or thermal dilution, including arterial and/or venous catheterization; with cardiac output measurement (separate procedure)

⊙ 93562 subsequent measurement of cardiac output

(For radioisotope method of cardiac output, see 78472, 78473 or 78481)

⊙+93571 Intravascular Doppler velocity and/or pressure derived coronary flow reserve measurement (coronary vessel or graft) during coronary angiography including pharmacologically induced stress; initial vessel (List separately in addition to code for primary procedure)

⊙+93572 each additional vessel (List separately in addition to code for primary procedure)

(Intravascular distal coronary blood flow velocity measurements include all Doppler transducer manipulations and repositioning within the specific vessel being examined, during coronary angiography or therapeutic intervention (eg, angioplasty))

(For unlisted cardiac catheterization procedure, use 93799)

REPAIR OF SEPTAL DEFECT

93580 Percutaneous transcatheter closure of congenital interatrial communication (i.e., fontan fenestration, atrial septal defect) with implant

(Percutaneous transcatheter closure of atrial septal defect includes a right hear catheterization procedure. Code 93580 includes injection of contrast for atrial and ventricular angiograms. Codes 93501, 93529-93533, 93539, 93543, 93555 should not be reported separately in addition to code 93580)

93581 Percutaneous transcatheter closure of a congenital ventricular septal defect with implant

(Percutaneous transcatheter closure of ventricular septal defect (i.e., fontan fenestration) includes a right heart catheterization procedure. Code 93581 includes injection of contrast for atrial and ventricular angiograms. Codes 93501, 93529-93533, 93539, 93543, 93555 should not be reported separately in addition to 93581)

(For ventricular septal defect closure via transmyocardial implant delivery, see 0166T, 0167T)

(For echocardiographic services performed in addition to 93580, 93581, see 93303-93317 as appropriate)

INTRACARDIAC ELECTROPHYSIOLOGICAL PROCEDURES/STUDIES

Intracardiac electrophysiology study (EPS) involves placing wire electrodes within the heart to determine the characteristics of heart arrhythmias. Before performing EPS, which is invasive, the cardiologist will try to identify a suspected arrhythmia using other, less invasive tests like ambulatory cardiac monitoring. If the abnormal rhythm is not detected by these other methods and symptoms suggest an arrhythmia, EPS may be recommended. Additional reasons that EPS may be considered include:

- *To find the location of a known arrhythmia and determine the best therapy*
- *To assess the severity of the arrhythmia and determine if the patient is at risk for future cardiac events, especially sudden cardiac death*
- *To evaluate the effectiveness of medication in controlling an arrhythmia*
- *To determine if the focus (the place where the arrhythmia is coming from) should be ablated*

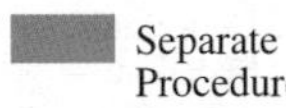 Separate Procedure 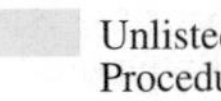 Unlisted Procedure 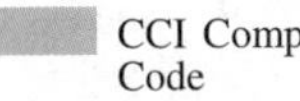 CCI Comp. Code 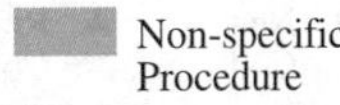 Non-specific Procedure

- *To evaluate the need for a permanent pacemaker or an implantable cardioverter-defibrillator (ICD)*

During EPS, the cardiologist inserts a catheter through a small incision in a groin vein after cleansing the site and numbing it with a local anesthetic. This catheter is equipped with an electrode connected to electrocardiographic monitors. The catheter is then carefully threaded into the heart using an x-ray imaging technique called fluoroscopy to guide the insertion. Electrodes are placed in the heart to measure electrical activity along the heart's conduction system and within heart muscle cells themselves.

Normal electrical activity is signaled from the heart's natural pacemaker known as the sinoatrial (SA) node. It then travels through the atria, the atrioventricular (AV) node, and the ventricles. Abnormal electrical activity can occur anywhere along this conduction system, including in the muscle cells of either the atria or ventricles. The electrodes inserted during EPS will map the type of arrhythmia the patient has and where the problem arises in the heart.

If ablation is thought to be the appropriate therapy, it is performed at the time of EPS.

⃠ **93600** Bundle of His recording

⃠ **93602** Intra-atrial recording

⃠ **93603** Right ventricular recording

(93604, 93606 have been deleted. To report, see 93603, 93609 and 93622 as appropriate)

⊙+**93609** Intraventricular and/or intra-atrial mapping of tachycardia site(s) with catheter manipulation to record from multiple sites to identify origin of tachycardia (List separately in addition to code for primary procedure)

(Use 93609 in conjunction with codes 93620, 93651, 93652)

(Do not report 93609 in addition to 93613)

⃠ **93610** Intra-atrial pacing

⃠ **93612** Intraventricular pacing

(Do not report 93612 in conjunction with codes 93620-93622)

⊙+**93613** Intracardiac electrophysiologic 3-dimensional mapping (List separately in addition to code for primary procedure)

(Use 93613 in conjunction with codes 93620, 93651, 93652)

● New Code ▲ Revised Code + Add-On Code ⃠ Modifier -51 Exempt ⊙ Conscious Sedation

(Do not report 93613 in addition to 93609)

⊘⊙**93615** Esophageal recording of atrial electrogram with or without ventricular electrogram(s);

⊘⊙**93616** with pacing

⊘⊙**93618** Induction of arrhythmia by electrical pacing

(For intracardiac phonocardiogram, use 93799)

⊘⊙**93619** Comprehensive electrophysiologic evaluation with right atrial pacing and recording, right ventricular pacing and recording, His bundle recording, including insertion and repositioning of multiple electrode catheters without induction or attempted induction of arrhythmia

(Do not report 93619 in conjunction with codes 93600, 93602, 93610, 93612, 93618 or 93620-93622)

⊘⊙**93620** Comprehensive electrophysiologic evaluation including insertion and repositioning of multiple electrode catheters with induction or attempted induction of arrhythmia; with right atrial pacing and recording, right ventricular pacing and recording, His bundle recording

(Do not report 93620 in conjunction with codes 93600, 93602, 93610, 93612, 93618 or 93619)

⊙+**93621** with left atrial pacing and recording from coronary sinus or left atrium (List separately in addition to code for primary procedure)

(Use 93621 in conjunction with code 93620)

⊙+**93622** with left ventricular pacing and recording (List separately in addition to code for primary procedure)

(Use 93622 in conjunction with code 93620)

+ **93623** Programmed stimulation and pacing after intravenous drug infusion (List separately in addition to code for primary procedure)

(Use 93623 in conjunction with codes 93619, 93620)

⊘⊙**93624** Electrophysiologic follow-up study with pacing and recording to test effectiveness of therapy, including induction or attempted induction of arrhythmia

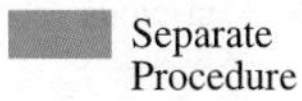 Separate Procedure 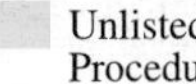 Unlisted Procedure 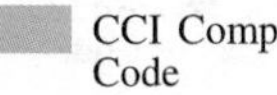 CCI Comp. Code 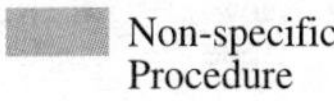 Non-specific Procedure

⊘ **93631** Intra-operative epicardial and endocardial pacing and mapping to localize the site of tachycardia or zone of slow conduction for surgical correction

⊘⊙**93640** Electrophysiologic evaluation of single or dual chamber pacing cardioverter-defibrillator leads including defibrillation threshold evaluation (induction of arrhythmia, evaluation of sensing and pacing for arrhythmia termination) at time of initial implantation or replacement;

⊘⊙**93641** with testing of single or dual chamber pacing cardioverter-defibrillator pulse generator

(For subsequent or periodic electronic analysis and/or reprogramming of single or dual chamber pacing cardioverter-defibrillators, see 93642, 93741-93744)

⊘⊙**93642** Electrophysiologic evaluation of single or dual chamber pacing cardioverter-defibrillator (includes defibrillation threshold evaluation, induction of arrhythmia, evaluation of sensing and pacing for arrhythmia termination, and programming or reprogramming of sensing or therapeutic parameters)

⊘⊙**93650** Intracardiac catheter ablation of atrioventricular node function, atrioventricular conduction for creation of complete heart block, with or without temporary pacemaker placement

⊘⊙**93651** Intracardiac catheter ablation of arrhythmogenic focus; for treatment of supraventricular tachycardia by ablation of fast or slow atrioventricular pathways, accessory atrioventricular connections or other atrial foci, singly or in combination

⊘⊙**93652** for treatment of ventricular tachycardia

⊘ **93660** Evaluation of cardiovascular function with tilt table evaluation, with continuous ECG monitoring and intermittent blood pressure monitoring, with or without pharmacological intervention

(For testing of autonomic nervous system function, see 95921-95923)

\+ **93662** Intracardiac echocardiography during therapeutic/diagnostic intervention, including imaging supervision and interpretation (List separately in addition to code for primary procedure)

(Use 93662 in conjunction with 92987, 93527, 93532, 93580, 93581, 93621, 93622, 93651, or 93652, as appropriate)

(Do not report 92961 in addition to 93662)

● New Code ▲ Revised Code + Add-On Code ⊘ Modifier -51 Exempt ⊙ Conscious Sedation

PERIPHERAL ARTERIAL DISEASE REHABILITATION

Peripheral Arterial Disease (PAD) rehabilitation is an outpatient service for patients diagnosed with peripheral artery disease—a disorder of the vessels of the legs or arms resulting in pain. Rehabilitation consists of a series of sessions involving physical exercise, using a motorized treadmill and various other pieces of exercise equipment to permit each patient to achieve symptom-limited claudication. Claudication is taken from the Latin word 'to limp' and refers to the pain that occurs in PAD patients when they exercise. A medically supervised walking program can improve the symptoms of claudication and lead to an enhanced quality of life.

Each rehabilitation session lasts about 45 to 60 minutes and is supervised by an exercise physiologist or nurse. A patient's claudication threshold and other cardiovascular limitations are monitored and adjustments are made to the workload during the exercises.

PAD rehabilitation requires a physician's referral. The referring physician receives progress notes about his or her patient's progress in the program.

93668 Peripheral arterial disease (PAD) rehabilitation, per session

NONINVASIVE PHYSIOLOGIC STUDIES AND PROCEDURES

(For arterial cannulization and recording of direct arterial pressure, use 36620)

(For radiographic injection procedures, see 36000-36299)

(For vascular cannulization for hemodialysis, see 36800-36821)

(For chemotherapy for malignant disease, see 96409-96549)

(For penile plethysmography, use 54240)

93701 Bioimpedance, thoracic, electrical

93720 Plethysmography, total body; with interpretation and report

93721 tracing only, without interpretation and report

93722 interpretation and report only

(For regional plethysmography, see 93875-93931)

93724 Electronic analysis of antitachycardia pacemaker system (includes electrocardiographic recording, programming of device, induction and termination of tachycardia via implanted pacemaker, and interpretation of recordings)

93727 Electronic analysis of implantable loop recorder (ILR) system (includes retrieval of recorded and stored ECG data, physician review and interpretation of retrieved ECG data and reprogramming)

93731 Electronic analysis of dual-chamber pacemaker system (includes evaluation of programmable parameters at rest and during activity where applicable, using electrocardiographic recording and interpretation of recordings at rest and during exercise, analysis of event markers and device response); without reprogramming

93732 with reprogramming

93733 Electronic analysis of dual chamber internal pacemaker system (may include rate, pulse amplitude and duration, configuration of wave form, and/or testing of sensory function of pacemaker), telephonic analysis

93734 Electronic analysis of single chamber pacemaker system (includes evaluation of programmable parameters at rest and during activity where applicable, using electrocardiographic recording and interpretation of recordings at rest and during exercise, analysis of event markers and device response); without reprogramming

93735 with reprogramming

93736 Electronic analysis of single chamber internal pacemaker system (may include rate, pulse amplitude and duration, configuration of wave form, and/or testing of sensory function of pacemaker), telephonic analysis

93740 Temperature gradient studies

93741 Electronic analysis of pacing cardioverter-defibrillator (includes interrogation, evaluation of pulse generator status, evaluation of programmable parameters at rest and during activity where applicable, using electrocardiographic recording and interpretation of recordings at rest and during exercise, analysis of event markers and device response); single chamber or wearable cardioverter-defibrillator system, without reprogramming

(Do not report 93741 in conjunction with 93745)

93742 single chamber or wearable cardioverter-defibrillator system, with reprogramming

(Do not report 93742 in conjunction with 93745)

93743 dual chamber, without reprogramming

93744 dual chamber, with reprogramming

93745 Initial set-up and programming by a physician of wearable cardioverter-defibrillator includes initial programming of system, establishing baseline electronic ECG, transmission of data to data repository, patient instruction in wearing system and patient reporting of problems or events

(Do not report 93745 in conjunction with 93741, 93742)

93760 Thermogram; cephalic

93762 peripheral

93770 Determination of venous pressure

(For central venous cannulization see 36555-36556, 36500)

93784 Ambulatory blood pressure monitoring, utilizing a system such as magnetic tape and/or computer disk, for 24 hours or longer; including recording, scanning analysis, interpretation and report

93786 recording only

93788 scanning analysis with report

93790 physician review with interpretation and report

OTHER PROCEDURES

93797 Physician services for outpatient cardiac rehabilitation; without continuous ECG monitoring (per session)

93798 with continuous ECG monitoring (per session)

93799 Unlisted cardiovascular service or procedure

Separate Procedure | Unlisted Procedure | CCI Comp. Code | Non-specific Procedure

NON-INVASIVE VASCULAR DIAGNOSTIC STUDIES

Vascular studies refers to diagnostic procedures performed to determine blood flow and/or the condition of arteries and/or veins. Vascular studies include patient care required to perform the studies, supervision of the studies and interpretation of the study results with copies for patient records of hard copy output with analysis of all data, including bi-directional vascular flow or imaging when provided.

The use of a simple hand-held or other Doppler device that does not produce hard copy output, or that produces a record that does not permit analysis of bi-directional vascular flow, is considered to be part of the physical examination of the vascular system and is not reported separately. To report unilateral non-invasive diagnostic studies, add modifier -52 to the basic code.

A Duplex Scan is defined as "An ultrasonic scanning procedure with display of both two-dimensional structure and motion with time and Doppler ultrasonic signal documentation with spectral analysis and/or color flow velocity mapping or imaging.

Coding Rules

1. *Non-invasive vascular studies are usually performed in addition to evaluation and management service, such as a consultation or visit, and should be reported separately in addition to the evaluation and management service.*

2. *All of the non-invasive vascular services fall under the Medicare Purchased Diagnostic Services guidelines; therefore, reporting should be as instructed by your local Medicare carrier.*

CEREBROVASCULAR ARTERIAL STUDIES

A complete transcranial Doppler (TCD) study (93886) includes ultrasound evaluation of the right and left anterior circulation territories and the posterior circulation territory (to include vertebral arteries and basilar artery). In a limited TCD study (93888) there is ultrasound evaluation of two or fewer of these territories. For TCD, ultrasound evaluation is a reasonable and concerted attempt to identify arterial signals through an acoustic window.

93875 Non-invasive physiologic studies of extracranial arteries, complete bilateral study (eg, periorbital flow direction with arterial compression, ocular pneumoplethysmography, Doppler ultrasound spectral analysis)

93880 Duplex scan of extracranial arteries; complete bilateral study

93882 unilateral or limited study

(To report common carotid intima-media thickness (IMT) study for evaluation of atherosclerotic burden or coronary heart disease risk factor assessment, use Category III code 0126T)

93886 Transcranial Doppler study of the intracranial arteries; complete study

93888 limited study

93890 vasoreactivity study

93892 emboli detection without intravenous microbubble injection

93893 emboli detection with intravenous microbubble injection

(Do not report 93890-93893 in conjunction with 93888)

EXTREMITY ARTERIAL STUDIES (INCLUDING DIGITS)

93922 Non-invasive physiologic studies of upper or lower extremity arteries, single level, bilateral (eg, ankle/brachial indices, Doppler waveform analysis, volume plethysmography, transcutaneous oxygen tension measurement)

93923 Non-invasive physiologic studies of upper or lower extremity arteries, multiple levels or with provocative functional maneuvers, complete bilateral study (eg, segmental blood pressure measurements, segmental Doppler waveform analysis, segmental volume plethysmography, segmental transcutaneous oxygen tension measurements, measurements with postural provocative tests, measurements with reactive hyperemia)

93924 Non-invasive physiologic studies of lower extremity arteries, at rest and following treadmill stress testing, complete bilateral study

93925 Duplex scan of lower extremity arteries or arterial bypass grafts; complete bilateral study

93926 unilateral or limited study

93930 Duplex scan of upper extremity arteries or arterial bypass grafts; complete bilateral study

93931 unilateral or limited study

EXTREMITY VENOUS STUDIES (INCLUDING DIGITS)

93965 Non-invasive physiologic studies of extremity veins, complete bilateral study (eg, Doppler waveform analysis with responses to compression and other maneuvers, phleborheography, impedance plethysmography)

93970 Duplex scan of extremity veins including responses to compression and other maneuvers; complete bilateral study

93971 unilateral or limited study

VISCERAL AND PENILE VASCULAR STUDIES

93975 Duplex scan of arterial inflow and venous outflow of abdominal, pelvic, scrotal contents and/or retroperitoneal organs; complete study

93976 limited study

93978 Duplex scan of aorta, inferior vena cava, iliac vasculature, or bypass grafts; complete study

93979 unilateral or limited study

93980 Duplex scan of arterial inflow and venous outflow of penile vessels; complete study

93981 follow-up or limited study

EXTREMITY ARTERIAL-VENOUS STUDIES

93990 Duplex scan of hemodialysis access (including arterial inflow, body of access and venous outflow)

(For measurement of hemodialysis access flow using indicator dilution methods, use 90940)

PULMONARY

Pulmonary disease is concerned with diseases of the lungs and airways. The Pulmonologist diagnoses and treats pneumonia, cancer, pleurisy, asthma, occupational diseases, bronchitis, sleep disorders, emphysema, and other complex disorders of the lungs. Pulmonologists test lung functions in many ways, endoscope the bronchial airways and prescribe and monitor mechanical assistance to ventilation. Many pulmonary disease physicians are also expert in critical care.

Pulmonary services refer to diagnostic procedures performed to determine air flow, blood gases, and the condition of the lungs and respiratory system. Pulmonary services include the laboratory procedure(s), interpretation, and physician's services (except surgical and anesthesia services) unless otherwise stated. It is common for pulmonologists to provide interpretation services only, under contract to medical facilities.

CPT coding for pulmonary function tests includes both comprehensive and component codes to accommodate variation among pulmonary function laboratories. As a result of these code combinations, several issues are addressed in this policy section.

Alternate methods of reporting data obtained during a spirometry or other pulmonary function session cannot be separately reported. Specifically, the flow volume loop is an alternative method of calculating a standard spirometric parameter. The CPT code 94375 is included in standard spirometry (rest and exercise) studies.

When a physician who is in attendance for a pulmonary function study, obtains a limited history, and performs a limited examination referable specifically to the pulmonary function testing, separately coding for an evaluation and management service is not appropriate. If a significant, separately identifiable service is performed unrelated to the technical performance of the pulmonary function test, an evaluation and management service may be reported.

When multiple spirometric determinations are necessary (e.g. CPT code 94070) to complete the service described in the CPT code, only one unit of service is reported.

Complex pulmonary stress testing (e.g. CPT code 94621) is a comprehensive stress test with a number of component tests separately defined in the CPT code book. It is inappropriate to separately code venous access, EKG monitoring, spirometric parameters performed before, during and after exercise, oximetry, O2 consumption, CO2 production, rebreathing cardiac output calculations, etc., when performed as part of a complex pulmonary stress test. It is also inappropriate to bill for a cardiac stress test and the component codes used to perform a simple pulmonary stress test (CPT code 94620), when a complex pulmonary stress test is performed. If using a standard exercise protocol, serial electrocardiograms are obtained, and a separate report describing a cardiac stress test (professional component) is included in the medical record, the professional components for both a cardiac and pulmonary stress test may be reported. Modifier -59 should be reported with the secondary procedure. Both tests must satisfy the requirement for medical necessity. (Since a complex pulmonary stress test includes electrocardiographic recordings, the technical components for both the cardiac stress test and the pulmonary stress test should not be reported separately.)

VENTILATOR MANAGEMENT

● **94002** Ventilation assist and management, initiation of pressure or volume preset ventilators for assisted or controlled breathing; hospital inpatient/observation, initial day

● **94003** hospital inpatient/observation, each subsequent day

● **94004** nursing facility, per day

(Do not report 94002-94004 in conjunction with E/M services 99201-99499)

● **94005** Home ventilator management care plan oversight of a patient (patient not present) in home, domiciliary or rest home (eg, assisted living) requiring review of status, review of laboratories and other studies and revision of orders and respiratory care plan (as appropriate),within a calendar month, 30 min. or more

(Do not report 94005 in conjunction with 99339-99340, 99374-99378)

(Ventilator management care plan oversight is reported separately from home or domiciliary, rest home [eg., assisted living] services. A physician may report 94005, when performed, including when a different physician reports 99339-99340, 99374-99378 for the same 30 days)

OTHER PROCEDURES

94010 Spirometry, including graphic record, total and timed vital capacity, expiratory flow rate measurement(s), with or without maximal voluntary ventilation

94014 Patient-initiated spirometric recording per 30-day period of time; includes reinforced education, transmission of spirometric tracing, data capture, analysis of transmitted data, periodic recalibration and physician review and interpretation

94015 recording (includes hook-up, reinforced education, data transmission, data capture, trend analysis, and periodic recalibration)

94016 physician review and interpretation only

94060 Bronchodilation responsiveness, spirometry as in 94010, pre- and post-bronchodilator administration

(Report bronchodilator supply separately with 99070 or appropriate supply code)

(For prolonged exercise test for bronchospasm with pre- and post-spirometry, use 94620)

94070 Bronchospasm provocation evaluation, multiple spirometric determinations as in 94010, with administered agents (eg, antigen(s), cold air, methacholine)

(Report antigen(s) administration separately with 99070 or appropriate supply code)

94150 Vital capacity, total (separate procedure)

94200 Maximum breathing capacity, maximal voluntary ventilation

94240 Functional residual capacity or residual volume: helium method, nitrogen open circuit method, or other method

94250 Expired gas collection, quantitative, single procedure (separate procedure)

94260 Thoracic gas volume

(For plethysmography, see 93720-93722)

94350 Determination of maldistribution of inspired gas: multiple breath nitrogen washout curve including alveolar nitrogen or helium equilibration time

94360 Determination of resistance to airflow, oscillatory or plethysmographic methods

94370 Determination of airway closing volume, single breath tests

94375 Respiratory flow volume loop

94400 Breathing response to CO2 (CO2 response curve)

Separate Procedure | Unlisted Procedure | CCI Comp. Code | Non-specific Procedure

94450 Breathing response to hypoxia (hypoxia response curve)

(For high altitude simulation test (HAST), see 94452, 94453)

94452 High altitude simulation test (HAST), with physician interpretation and report;

(For obtaining arterial blood gases, use 36600)

(Do not report 94452 in conjunction with 94453, 94760, 94761)

94453 with supplemental oxygen titration

(For obtaining arterial blood gases, use 36600)

(Do not report 94453 in conjunction with 94452, 94760, 94761)

⊘●**94610** Intrapulmonary surfactant administration by a physician through endotracheal tube

(Do not report 94610 in conjunction with 99293-99296)

(For endotracheal intubation, use 31500)

(Report 94610 once per dosing episode)

▲ **94620** Pulmonary stress testing; simple (eg, 6-minute walk, prolonged exercise test for bronchospasm with pre- and post-spirometry and oximetry)

94621 complex (including measurements of CO2 production, O2 uptake, and electrocardiographic recordings)

94640 Pressurized or nonpressurized inhalation treatment for acute airway obstruction or for sputum induction for diagnostic purposes (eg., with an aerosol generator, nebulizer, metered dose inhaler or intermittent positive pressure breathing (IPPB) device)

(For more than one inhalation treatment performed on the same date, append modifier -76)

(For continuous inhalation treatment of 1 hour or more, see 94644, 94645)

94642 Aerosol inhalation of pentamidine for pneumocystis carinii pneumonia treatment or prophylaxis

● **94644** Continuous inhalation treatment with aerosol medication for acute airway obstruction; first hour

(For services of less than 1 hour, use 94640)

●+94645 each additional hour (List separately in addition to code primary procedure)

(Use 94645 in conjunction with 94644)

(94656 deleted 2007 edition, see 94002, 94004)

(94657 deleted 2007 edition, see 94003, 94004)

94660 Continuous positive airway pressure ventilation (CPAP), initiation and management

94662 Continuous negative pressure ventilation (CNP), initiation and management

94664 Demonstration and/or evaluation of patient utilization of an aerosol generator, nebulizer, metered dose inhaler or IPPB device

(94664 can be reported one time only per day of service)

94667 Manipulation chest wall, such as cupping, percussing, and vibration to facilitate lung function; initial demonstration and/or evaluation

94668 subsequent

94680 Oxygen uptake, expired gas analysis; rest and exercise, direct, simple

94681 including CO2 output, percentage oxygen extracted

94690 rest, indirect (separate procedure)

(For single arterial puncture, use 36600)

94720 Carbon monoxide diffusing capacity (eg, single breath, steady state)

94725 Membrane diffusion capacity

94750 Pulmonary compliance study (eg, plethysmography, volume and pressure measurements)

Separate Procedure 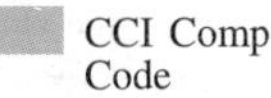 Unlisted Procedure CCI Comp. Code 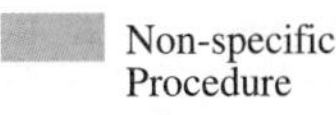 Non-specific Procedure

94760 Noninvasive ear or pulse oximetry for oxygen saturation; single determination

(For blood gases, see 82803-82810)

94761 multiple determinations (eg, during exercise)

94762 by continuous overnight monitoring (separate procedure)

94770 Carbon dioxide, expired gas determination by infrared analyzer

(For bronchoscopy, see 31622-31656)

(For placement of flow directed catheter, use 93503)

(For venipuncture, use 36410)

(For central venous catheter placement, see 36488-36491)

(For arterial puncture, use 36600)

(For arterial catheterization, use 36620)

(For thoracentesis, use 32000)

(For phlebotomy, therapeutic, use 99195)

(For lung biopsy, needle, use 32405)

(For intubation, orotracheal or nasotracheal, use 31500)

94772 Circadian respiratory pattern recording (pediatric pneumogram), 12 to 24 hour continuous recording, infant

(Separate procedure codes for electromyograms, EEG, ECG, and recordings of respiration are excluded when 94772 is reported)

● **94774** Pediatric home apnea monitoring event recording including respiratory rate, pattern and heart rate per 30-day period of time; includes monitor attachment, download of data, physician review, interpretation, and preparation of a report

(Do not report 94774 in conjunction with 94775-94777 during the same reporting period)

● **94775** monitor attachment only (includes hook-up, initiation of recording and disconnection)

● **94776** monitoring, download of information, receipt of transmission(s) and analyses by computer only

● New Code ▲ Revised Code + Add-On Code ⃠ Modifier -51 Exempt ⊙ Conscious Sedation

● **94777** physician review, interpretation and preparation of report only

(When oxygen saturation monitoring is used in addition to heart rate and respiratory monitoring, it is not reported separately)

(Do not report 94774-94777 in conjunction with 93224-93272)

(Do not report apnea recording device separately)

(For sleep study, see 95805-95811)

94799 Unlisted pulmonary service or procedure

ALLERGY AND CLINICAL IMMUNOLOGY

Allergy and Immunology refers to diagnostic services performed to determine a patient's sensitivity to specific substances, the treatment of patients with allergens by the administration or allergenic extracts, and/or medical conference services.

The CPT coding system divides allergy and clinical immunology into testing and immunotherapy. Immunotherapy is divided into codes that include preparation of the antigen when it is administered at the same session and when it is prepared but delivered for immunotherapy by a different physician. Several specific issues are identified regarding allergy testing and immunotherapy.

If percutaneous or intracutaneous (intradermal)single test (CPT codes 95004 or 95024) and "sequential and incremental" tests (CPT codes 95010, 95015, or 95027) are performed on the same date of service, both the "sequential and incremental" test and single test codes may be reported if the tests are for different allergens or different dilutions of the same allergen. The unit of service to report is the number of separate tests. Do not report both a single test and a sequential and incremental test for the same dilution of an allergen. For example, if the single test for an antigen is positive and the provider proceeds to sequential and incremental tests with three additional different dilutions of the same antigen, the provider may report one unit of service for the single test code and three units of service for the sequential and incremental test code.

When photo patch tests (e.g. CPT code 95052) are performed (same antigen/same session) with patch or application tests, only the photo patch testing should be reported. Additionally, if photo testing is performed including application or patch testing, the code for photo patch testing (CPT code 95052) is to be reported, not CPT code 95044 (patch or application tests) and CPT code 95056 (photo tests).

Evaluation and management codes reported with allergy testing or allergy immunotherapy are appropriate only if a significant, separately identifiable service is administered. Obtaining informed consent, is included in the immunotherapy. If

E & M services are reported, medical documentation of the separately identifiable service should be in the medical record.

Allergy testing is not performed on the same day as allergy immunotherapy in standard medical practice. These codes should, therefore, not be reported together. Additionally, the testing becomes an integral part to rapid desensitization kits (CPT code 95180) and would therefore not be reported separately.

ALLERGY TESTING

(For allergy laboratory tests, see 86000-86999)

(For therapy for severe or intractable allergic disease, see 90765-90768, 90772, 90774, 90775)

95004 Percutaneous tests (scratch, puncture, prick) with allergenic extracts, immediate type reaction, specify number of tests

95010 Percutaneous tests (scratch, puncture, prick) sequential and incremental, with drugs, biologicals or venoms, immediate type reaction, specify number of tests

● **95012** Nitric oxide expired gas determination

(For nitric oxide determination by spectroscopy, use Category III code 0064T)

95015 Intracutaneous (intradermal) tests, sequential and incremental, with drugs, biologicals, or venoms, immediate type reaction, specify number of tests

95024 Intracutaneous (intradermal) tests with allergenic extracts, immediate type reaction, specify number of tests

95027 Intracutaneous (intradermal) tests, sequential and incremental, with allergenic extracts for airborne allergens, immediate type reaction, specify number of tests

95028 Intracutaneous (intradermal) tests with allergenic extracts, delayed type reaction, including reading, specify number of tests

95044 Patch or application test(s) (specify number of tests)

95052 Photo patch test(s) (specify number of tests)

95056 Photo tests

95060 Ophthalmic mucous membrane tests

95065 Direct nasal mucous membrane test

95070 Inhalation bronchial challenge testing (not including necessary pulmonary function tests); with histamine, methacholine, or similar compounds

95071 with antigens or gases, specify

(For pulmonary function tests, see 94060, 94070)

95075 Ingestion challenge test (sequential and incremental ingestion of test items, eg, food, drug or other substance such as metabisulfite)

(95078 deleted 2007 edition)

ALLERGEN IMMUNOTHERAPY

Allergen immunotherapy CPT codes include the professional services necessary for allergen immunotherapy. Evaluation and management service codes may be reported in addition to allergen immunotherapy if other identifiable services are provided at the same time.

95115 Professional services for allergen immunotherapy not including provision of allergenic extracts; single injection

95117 two or more injections

95120 Professional services for allergen immunotherapy in prescribing physicians office or institution, including provision of allergenic extract; single injection

95125 two or more injections

95130 single stinging insect venom

95131 two stinging insect venoms

95132 three stinging insect venoms

95133 four stinging insect venoms

95134 five stinging insect venoms

Separate Procedure
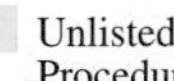
Unlisted Procedure
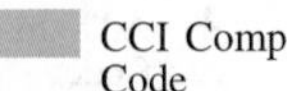
CCI Comp. Code
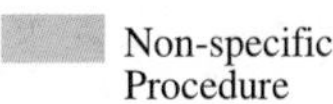
Non-specific Procedure

95144 Professional services for the supervision of preparation and provision of antigens for allergen immunotherapy; single dose vials(s) (specify number of vials)

(A single dose vial contains a single dose of antigen administered in one injection)

95145 Professional services for the supervision of preparation and provision of antigens for allergen immunotherapy (specify number of doses); single stinging insect venom

95146 two single stinging insect venoms

95147 three single stinging insect venoms

95148 four single stinging insect venoms

95149 five single stinging insect venoms

95165 Professional services for the supervision of preparation and provision of antigens for allergen immunotherapy; single or multiple antigens (specify number of doses)

95170 whole body extract of biting insect or other arthropod (specify number of doses)

(For allergy immunotherapy reporting, a dose is the amount of antigen(s) administered in a single injection from a multiple dose vial)

95180 Rapid desensitization procedure, each hour (eg, insulin, penicillin, equine serum)

95199 Unlisted allergy/clinical immunologic service or procedure

(For skin testing of bacterial, viral, fungal extracts, see 95028, 86485-86586)

(For special reports on allergy patients, use 99080)

(For testing procedures such as radioallergosorbent testing (RAST), rat mast cell technique (RMCT), mast cell degranulation test (MCDT), lymphocytic transformation test (LTT), leukocyte histamine release (LHR), migration inhibitory factor test (MIF), transfer factor test (TFT), nitroblue tetrazolium dye test (NTD), see Immunology section in Pathology or use 95199)

ENDOCRINOLOGY

95250 Ambulatory continuous glucose monitoring of interstitial tissue fluid via a subcutaneous sensor for up to 72 hours; sensor placement, hook-up, calibration of monitor, patient training, removal of sensor, and printout of recording

(Do not report 95250 in conjunction with 99091)

95251 physician interpretation and report

(Do not report 95250, 95251 in conjunction with 99091)

NEUROLOGY AND NEUROMUSCULAR PROCEDURES

Neurology refers to the study and treatment of the nervous system. Neurology services are usually performed in conjunction with a medical consultation. The consultation should be reported separately using the appropriate evaluation and management consultation code.

Neurologic services are typically consultative, and any of the levels of consultation (99241-99255) may be appropriate.

The EEG, autonomic function, evoked potential, reflex tests, EMG, NCV, and MEG services (95812-95829 and 95860-95967) include recording, interpretation by a physician, and report. For interpretation only, use modifier 26. For EMG guidance, see 95873, 95874.

The CPT coding system defines codes for neuromuscular diagnostic or therapeutic services not requiring surgical procedures. Sleep testing, nerve and muscle testing and electroencephalographic procedures are included. The CPT code book guidelines regarding sleep testing are very precise and should be reviewed carefully before billing for these services.

Sleep testing differs from polysomnography in that the latter requires the presence of sleep staging. Sleep staging includes a qualitative and quantitative assessment of sleep as determined by standard sleep scoring techniques. Accordingly, at the same session, a "sleep study" and "polysomnography" are not reported together.

Polysomnography requires at least one central and usually several other EEG electrodes. EEG procurement for polysomnography (sleep staging) differs greatly from that required for diagnostic EEG testing (i.e. speed of paper, number of channels, etc.). Accordingly, EEG testing is not to be reported with polysomnography unless performed separately; the EEG tests, if rendered with a separate report, are to be reported with modifier -59, indicating that this represents a different session from the sleep study.

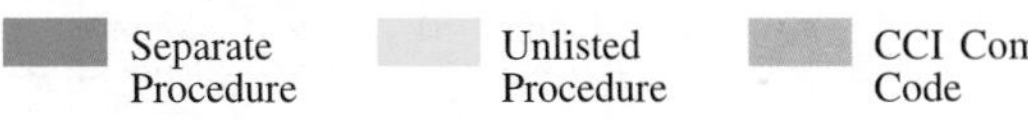

Continuous electroencephalographic monitoring services (CPT codes 95950-95962) represent different services than those provided during sleep testing; accordingly these codes are only to be reported when a separately identifiable service is performed and documented. Additionally, billing standard EEG services would only be appropriate if a significant, separately identifiable service is provided. These codes are to be reported with modifier -59 to indicate that a different service is clearly documented.

When nerve testing (EMG, nerve conduction velocity, etc.) is performed to assess the level of paralysis during anesthesia or during mechanical ventilation, the series of CPT codes 95851-95937 are not to be separately reported; these codes reflect significant, separately identifiable diagnostic services requiring a formal report in the medical record. Additionally, electrical stimulation used to identify or locate nerves as part of a procedure involving treatment of a cranial or peripheral nerve (e.g. nerve block, nerve destruction, neuroplasty, transection, excision, repair, etc.) is part of the primary procedure.

Intraoperative neurophysiology testing (CPT code 95920) should not be reported by the physician performing an operative procedure since it is included in the global package. However, when performed by a different physician during the procedure, it is separately reportable by the second physician. The physician performing an operative procedure should not bill other 90000 neurophysiology testing codes for intraoperative neurophysiology testing since they are also included in the global package.

The NCCI edit with column one CPT code 95903 (Motor nerve conduction studies with F-wave study, each nerve) and column two CPT code 95900 (Motor nerve conduction studies without F-wave study, each nerve) is often bypassed by utilizing modifier -59. Use of modifier -59 with the column two CPT code 95900 of this NCCI edit is only appropriate if the two procedures are performed on different nerves or in separate patient encounters.

(For repetitive transcranial magnetic stimulation for treatment of clinical depression, see Category III codes 0160T, 0161T)

(Do not report codes 95860-95875 in addition to 96000-96004)

SLEEP TESTING

Polysomnography includes sleep staging that is refined to include a 1-4 lead electroencephalogram (EEG), an electro-oculogram (EOG), and a submental electromyogram (EMG). For a study to be reported as polysomnography, sleep must be recorded and staged. Additional parameters of sleep include:

Electrocardiogram (ECG)

airflow

ventilation and respiratory effort

gas exchange by oximetry, transcutaneous monitoring, or end tidal gas analysis

extremity muscle activity, motor activity-movement

extended EEG monitoring

penile tumescence

gastroesophageal reflux

continuous blood pressure monitoring

snoring

body positions, etc.

For a study to be reported as a polysomnogram:

studies must be performed for 6 hours

sleep must be recorded and staged

an attendant must be present throughout the course of the study

Diagnostic testing is covered when a patient has the symptoms or complaints of one of the following conditions:

Narcolepsy - Narcolepsy is a neurologic disorder of unknown etiology characterized predominantly by abnormalities of REM, some abnormalities of NREM sleep and the presence of excessive daytime sleepiness often with involuntary daytime sleep episodes (e.g., while driving, in the middle of a meal, amnesiac episodes).

Sleep Apnea - Sleep Apnea is defined as a cessation of airflow for at least 10 seconds. These cessations of breathing may be due to either an occlusion of the airway (obstructive sleep apnea), absence of respiratory effort (central sleep apnea), or a combination of these factors (mixed sleep apnea).

Parasomnias - Parasomnias are a group of behavioral disorders during sleep that are associated with brief or partial arousals but not with marked sleep disruption or impaired daytime alertness. The presenting complaint is usually related to the behavior itself.

(Report with a -52 modifier if less than 6 hours of recording or in other cases of reduced services as appropriate)

(For unattended sleep study, use 95806)

95805 Multiple sleep latency or maintenance of wakefulness testing, recording, analysis and interpretation of physiological measurements of sleep during multiple trials to assess sleepiness

95806 Sleep study, simultaneous recording of ventilation, respiratory effort, ECG or heart rate, and oxygen saturation, unattended by a technologist

95807 Sleep study, simultaneous recording of ventilation, respiratory effort, ECG or heart rate, and oxygen saturation, attended by a technologist

95808 Polysomnography; sleep staging with 1-3 additional parameters of sleep, attended by a technologist

95810 sleep staging with 4 or more additional parameters of sleep, attended by a technologist

95811 sleep staging with 4 or more additional parameters of sleep, with initiation of continuous positive airway pressure therapy or bilevel ventilation, attended by a technologist

ROUTINE ELECTROENCEPHALOGRAPHY (EEG)

95812 Electroencephalogram (EEG) extended monitoring; 41-60 minutes

95813 greater than one hour

95816 Electroencephalogram (EEG) including recording awake and drowsy

95819 including recording awake and asleep

95822 recording in coma or sleep only

95824 cerebral death evaluation only

95827 all night recording

(For 24-hour EEG monitoring, see 95950-95953 or 95956)

(For EEG during nonintracranial surgery, use 95955)

(For Wada test, use 95958)

(For digital analysis of EEG, use 95957)

95829 Electrocorticogram at surgery (separate procedure)

95830 Insertion by physician of sphenoidal electrodes for electroencephalographic (EEG) recording

MUSCLE AND RANGE OF MOTION TESTING

95831 Muscle testing, manual (separate procedure) with report; extremity (excluding hand) or trunk

95832 hand, with or without comparison with normal side

95833 total evaluation of body, excluding hands

95834 total evaluation of body, including hands

95851 Range of motion measurements and report (separate procedure); each extremity (excluding hand) or each trunk section (spine)

95852 hand, with or without comparison with normal side

95857 Tensilon test for myasthenia gravis;

(95858 deleted 2006 edition.)

ELECTROMYOGRAPHY AND NERVE CONDUCTION TESTS

95860 Needle electromyography; one extremity with or without related paraspinal areas

95861 two extremities with or without related paraspinal areas

(For dynamic electromyography performed during motion analysis studies, see 96002-96003)

95863 three extremities with or without related paraspinal areas

95864 four extremities with or without related paraspinal areas

95865 larynx

(Do not report modifier 50 in conjunction with 95865)

Separate Procedure | Unlisted Procedure | CCI Comp. Code | Non-specific Procedure

(For unilateral procedure, report modifier 52 in conjunction with 95865)

95866 hemidiaphragm

95867 cranial nerve supplied muscle(s), unilateral

95868 cranial nerve supplied muscles, bilateral

95869 thoracic paraspinal muscles (excluding T1 or T12

95870 limited study of muscles in one extremity or non-limb (axial) muscles (unilateral or bilateral), other than thoracic paraspinal, cranial nerve supplied muscles, or sphincters

(To report a complete study of the extremities, see 95860-95864)

(For anal or urethral sphincter, detrusor, urethra, perineum musculature, see 51785-51792)

(For eye muscles, use 92265)

95872 Needle electromyography using single fiber electrode, with quantitative measurement of jitter, blocking and/or fiber density, any/all sites of each muscle studied

+ **95873** Electrical stimulation for guidance in conjunction with chemodenervation (List separately in addition to code for primary procedure)

+ **95874** Needle electromyography for guidance in conjunction with chemodenervation (List separately in addition to code for primary procedure)

(Use 95873, 95874 in conjunction with 64612-64614)

(Do not report 95874 in conjunction with 95873)

(Do not report 95873, 95874 in conjunction with 95860-95870)

95875 Ischemic limb exercise test with serial specimen(s) acquisition for muscle(s) metabolite(s)

⦸ **95900** Nerve conduction, amplitude and latency/velocity study, each nerve; motor, without F-wave study

⦸ **95903** motor, with F-wave study

⊘ **95904** sensory

(Report 95900, 95903, and/or 95904 only once when multiple sites on the same nerve are stimulated or recorded)

INTRAOPERATIVE NEUROPHYSIOLOGY

\+ **95920** Intraoperative neurophysiology testing, per hour (List separately in addition to code for primary procedure)

(Use code 95920 in conjunction with the study performed, 92585, 95822, 95860, 95861, 95867, 95868, 95870, 95900, 95904, 95925-95937)

(Code 95920 describes ongoing electrophysiologic testing and monitoring performed during surgical procedures. Code 95920 is reported per hour of service, and includes only the ongoing electrophysiologic monitoring time distinct from performance of specific type(s) of baseline electrophysiologic study(ies) (95860, 95861, 95867, 95868, 95870, 95900, 95904, 95928, 95929, 95933-95937) or interpretation of specific type(s) of baseline electrophysiologic study(ies) (92585, 95822, 95870, 95925-95928, 95929, 95930). The time spent performing or interpreting the baseline electrophysiologic study(ies) should not be counted as intraoperative monitoring, but represents separately reportable procedures. Code 95920 should be used once per hour even if multiple electrophysiologic studies are performed. The baseline electrophysiologic study(ies) should be used once per operative session.)

(For electrocorticography, use 95829)

(For intraoperative EEG during nonintracranial surgery, use 95955)

(For intraoperative functional cortical or subcortical mapping, see 95961-95962)

(For intraoperative neurostimulator programming and analysis, see 95970-95975)

AUTONOMIC FUNCTION TESTS

95921 Testing of autonomic nervous system function; cardiovagal innervation (parasympathetic function), including two or more of the following: heart rate response to deep breathing with recorded R-R interval, Valsalva ratio, and 30:15 ratio

95922 vasomotor adrenergic innervation (sympathetic adrenergic function), including beat-to-beat blood pressure and R-R interval changes during Valsalva maneuver and at least five minutes of passive tilt

95923 sudomotor, including one or more of the following: quantitative sudomotor axon reflex test (QSART), silastic sweat imprint, thermoregulatory sweat test, and changes in sympathetic skin potential

EVOKED POTENTIALS AND REFLEX TESTS

95925 Short-latency somatosensory evoked potential study, stimulation of any/all peripheral nerves or skin sites, recording from the central nervous system; in upper limbs

95926 in lower limbs

95927 in the trunk or head

(To report a unilateral study, use modifier -52)

(For auditory evoked potentials, use 92585)

95928 Central motor evoked potential study (transcranial motor stimulation); upper limbs

95929 lower limbs

95930 Visual evoked potential (VEP) testing central nervous system, checkerboard or flash

95933 Orbicularis oculi (blink) reflex, by electrodiagnostic testing

95934 H-reflex, amplitude and latency study; record gastrocnemius/soleus muscle

95936 record muscle other than gastrocnemius/soleus muscle

(To report a bilateral study, use modifier -50)

95937 Neuromuscular junction testing (repetitive stimulation, paired stimuli), each nerve, any one method

SPECIAL EEG TESTS

95950 Monitoring for identification and lateralization of cerebral seizure focus, electroencephalographic (eg, 8 channel EEG) recording and interpretation, each 24 hours

95951 Monitoring for localization of cerebral seizure focus by cable or radio, 16 or more channel telemetry, combined electroencephalographic (EEG) and video recording and interpretation (eg, for presurgical localization), each 24 hours

95953 Monitoring for localization of cerebral seizure focus by computerized portable 16 or more channel EEG, electroencephalographic (EEG) recording and interpretation, each 24 hours

95954 Pharmacological or physical activation requiring physician attendance during EEG recording of activation phase (eg, thiopental activation test)

95955 Electroencephalogram (EEG) during nonintracranial surgery (eg, carotid surgery)

95956 Monitoring for localization of cerebral seizure focus by cable or radio,16 or more channel telemetry, electroencephalographic (EEG) recording and interpretation, each 24 hours

95957 Digital analysis of electroencephalogram (EEG) (eg, for epileptic spike analysis)

95958 Wada activation test for hemispheric function, including electroencephalographic (EEG) monitoring

95961 Functional cortical and subcortical mapping by stimulation and/or recording of electrodes on brain surface, or of depth electrodes, to provoke seizures or identify vital brain structures; initial hour of physician attendance

+ **95962** each additional hour of physician attendance (List separately in addition to code for primary procedure)

(Use 95962 in conjunction with code 95961)

95965 Magnetoencephalography (MEG), recording and analysis; for spontaneous brain magnetic activity (eg, epileptic cerebral cortex localization)

95966 for evoked magnetic fields, single modality (eg, sensory, motor, language, or visual cortex localization)

+ **95967** for evoked magnetic fields, each additional modality (eg, sensory, motor, language, or visual cortex localization) (List separately in addition to code for primary procedure)

Separate Procedure | Unlisted Procedure | CCI Comp. Code | Non-specific Procedure

(Use 95967 in conjunction with code 95966)

(For electroencephalography performed in addition to magnetoencephalography, see 95812-95827)

(For somatosensory evoked potentials, auditory evoked potentials, and visual evoked potentials performed in addition to magnetic evoked field responses, see 92585, 95925, 95926, and/or 95930)

(For computerized tomography performed in addition to magnetoencephalography, see 70450-70470, 70496)

(For magnetic resonance imaging performed in addition to magnetoencephalography, see 70551-70553)

NEUROSTIMULATORS, ANALYSIS-PROGRAMMING

(For insertion of neurostimulator pulse generator, see 61885, 63685, 64590)

(For revision or removal of neurostimulator pulse generator or receiver, see 61888, 63688, 64595)

(For implantation of neurostimulator electrodes, see 43647, 43881, 61850-61875, 63650-63655, 64553-64580, 0155T, 0157T. For revision or removal of neurostimulator electrodes, see 43648, 43882, 61880, 63660, 64585, 0156T, 0158T)

95970 Electronic analysis of implanted neurostimulator pulse generator system (eg, rate, pulse amplitude and duration, configuration of wave form, battery status, electrode selectability, output modulation, cycling, impedance and patient compliance measurements); simple or complex brain, spinal cord, or peripheral (ie, cranial nerve, peripheral nerve, autonomic nerve, neuromuscular) neurostimulator pulse generator/transmitter, without reprogramming

95971 simple spinal cord, or peripheral (ie, peripheral nerve, autonomic nerve, neuromuscular) neurostimulator pulse generator/transmitter, with intraoperative or subsequent programming

95972 complex spinal cord, or peripheral (except cranial nerve) neurostimulator pulse generator/transmitter, with intraoperative or subsequent programming, first hour

+ 95973 complex spinal cord, or peripheral (except cranial nerve) neurostimulator pulse generator/transmitter, with intraoperative or subsequent programming, each additional

30 minutes after first hour (List separately in addition to code for primary procedure)

(Use 95973 in conjunction with code 95972)

95974 complex cranial nerve neurostimulator pulse generator/transmitter, with intraoperative or subsequent programming, with or without nerve interface testing, first hour

+ **95975** complex cranial nerve neurostimulator pulse generator/transmitter, with intraoperative or subsequent programming, each additional 30 minutes after first hour (List separately in addition to code for primary procedure)

(Use 95975 in conjunction with code 95974)

(For electronic analysis, programming, and reprogramming of gastric neurostimulator pulse generator, lesser curvature [morbid obesity], use Category III code 0162T)

+ **95978** Electronic analysis of implanted neurostimulator pulse generator system (eg, rate, pulse amplitude and duration, battery status, electrode selectability and polarity, impedance and patient compliance measurements), complex deep brain neurostimulator pulse generator/transmitter, with initial or subsequent programming; first hour

+ **95979** each additional 30 minutes after first hour (List separately in addition to code for primary procedure)

(Use 95979 in conjunction with 95978)

OTHER PROCEDURES

95990 Refilling and maintenance of implantable pump or reservoir for drug delivery, spinal (intrathecal, epidural) or brain (intraventricular);

(For analysis and/or reprogramming of implantable infusion pump, see 62367-62368)

(For refill and maintenance of implanted infusion pump or reservoir for systemic drug therapy (eg., chemotherapy or insulin) use 96522)

95991 administered by physician

95999 Unlisted neurological or neuromuscular diagnostic procedure

Separate Procedure | Unlisted Procedure | CCI Comp. Code | Non-specific Procedure

MOTION ANALYSIS

(For performance of needle electromyography procedures, see 95860-95875)

(For gait training, use 97116)

96000 Comprehensive computer-based motion analysis by video-taping and 3-D kinematics;

96001 with dynamic plantar pressure measurements during walking

96002 Dynamic surface electromyography, during walking or other functional activities, 1-12 muscles

96003 Dynamic fine wire electromyography, during walking or other functional activities, 1 muscle

(Do not report codes 96002, 96003 in conjunction with 95860-95864, 95869-95872)

96004 Physician review and interpretation of comprehensive computer based motion analysis, dynamic plantar pressure measurements, dynamic surface electromyography during walking or other functional activities, and dynamic fine wire electromyography, with written report

FUNCTIONAL BRAIN MAPPING

Code 96020 includes selection and administration of testing of language, memory, cognition, movement, sensation, and other neurological functions when conducted in association with functional neuroimaging, monitoring of performance of this testing, and determination of validity of neurofunctional testing relative to separately interpreted functional magnetic resonance images.

● **96020** Neurofunctional testing selection and administration during noninvasive imaging functional brain mapping, with test administered entirely by a physician or psychologist, with review of test results and report

(For functional magnetic resonance imaging [fMRI], brain, use 70555)

(Do not report 96020 in conjunction with 96101-96103, 96116-96120)

(Do not report 96020 in conjunction with 70554)

(Evaluation and Management services codes should not be reported on the same day as 96020)

MEDICAL GENETICS AND GENETIC COUNSELING SERVICES

These sevices are provided by trained genetic counselors and may include obtaining a structured family genetic history, pedigree construction, analysis for genetic risk assessment, and counseling of the patient and family. These activities may be provided during one or more sessions and may include review of medical data and family information, face-to-face interviews, and counseling services.

● **96040** Medical genetics and genetic counseling services, each 30 minutes face-to-face with patient/family

(For genetic counseling and education provided by a physician to an individual, see the appropriate E/M codes)

(For genetic counseling and education provided by a physician to a group, use 99078)

(For education regarding genetic risks by a nonphysician to a group, see 98961, 98962)

(For genetic counseling and/or risk factor reduction intervention provided by a physician to patient(s) without symptoms or established disease, see 99401-99412)

CENTRAL NERVOUS SYSTEM ASSESSMENTS/TESTS (eg, NEURO-COGNITIVE, MENTAL STATUS, SPEECH TESTING)

Neurobehavioral status exam (CPT code 96115) should not be reported when a mini-mental status examination is performed. CPT code 96115 may never be reported with psychiatric diagnostic examinations (CPT codes 90801 or 90802). CPT code 96115 may be reported with other psychiatric services or evaluation and management services only if a complete neurobehavioral status exam is performed. If a mini-mental status examination is performed by a physician, it is included in the evaluation and management service.

(For development of cognitive skills, see 97532, 97533)

(96100 deleted 2006 edition. To report, see 96101, 96102, 96103)

(For mini-mental status examination performed by a physician, see E/M services codes)

96101 Psychological testing (includes psychodiagnostic assessment of emotionality, intellectual abilities, personality and psychopathology, eg, MMPI, Rorshach, WAIS), per hour of the psychologist's or physician's time, both face-to-face time with the patient and time interpreting test results and preparing the report

96102 Psychological testing (includes psychodiagnostic assessment of emotionality, intellectual abilities, personality and psychopathology, eg, MMPI and WAIS), with qualified health care professional interpretation and report, administered by technician, per hour of technician time, face-to-face

96103 Psychological testing (includes psychodiagnostic assessment of emotionality, intellectual abilities, personality and psychopathology, eg, MMPI), administered by a computer, with qualified health care professional interpretation and report

96105 Assessment of aphasia (includes assessment of expressive and receptive speech and language function, language comprehension, speech production ability, reading, spelling, writing, eg, by Boston Diagnostic Aphasia Examination) with interpretation and report, per hour

96110 Developmental testing; limited (eg, Developmental Screening Test II, Early Language Milestone Screen), with interpretation and report

96111 extended (includes assessment of motor, language, social, adaptive and/or cognitive functioning by standardized developmental instruments) with interpretation and report

(96115 deleted 2006 edition. To report, use 96116)

96116 Neurobehavioral status exam (clinical assessment of thinking, reasoning and judgment, eg, acquired knowledge, attention, language, memory, planning and problem solving, and visual spatial abilities), per hour of the psychologist's or physician's time, both face-to-face time with the patient and time interpreting test results and preparing the report

(96117 deleted 2006 edition. To report, see 96118, 96119, 96120)

96118 Neuropsychological testing (eg, Halstead-Reitan Neuropsychological Battery, Wechsler Memory Scales and Wisconsin Card Sorting Test), per hour of the psychologist's or physician's time, both face-to-face time with the patient and time interpreting test results and preparing the report

● New Code ▲ Revised Code + Add-On Code ⊘ Modifier -51 Exempt ⊙ Conscious Sedation

96119 Neuropsychological testing (eg, Halstead-Reitan Neuropsychological Battery, Wechsler Memory Scales and Wisconsin Card Sorting Test), with qualified health care professional interpretation and report, administered by technician, per hour of technician time, face-to-face

96120 Neuropsychological testing (eg, Wisconsin Card Sorting Test), administered by a computer, with qualified health care professional interpretation and report

HEALTH AND BEHAVIOR ASSESSMENT/INTERVENTION

(For health and behavior assessment and/or intervention performed by a physician, see Evaluation and Management or Preventive Medicine services codes)

96150 Health and behavior assessment (eg, health-focused clinical interview, behavioral observations, psychophysicological monitoring, health-oriented questionnaires), each 15 minutes face-to-face with the patient; intial assessment

96151 re-assessment

96152 Health and behavior intervention, each 15 minutes, face-to-face; individual

96153 group (2 or more patients)

96154 family (with the patient present)

96155 family (without the patient present),

CHEMOTHERAPY ADMINISTRATION

Chemotherapy is the process of treating cancer with chemicals formulated to harm or destroy the cancer cells. Chemotherapy agents are administered via intravenous or infusion methods. Chemotherapy administration may be coded when administered by a physician or a qualified assistant under the supervision of a physician, excluding chemotherapy administered by hospital or home health agency personnel.

Chemotherapy administration codes include codes for the administration of chemotherapeutic agents by multiple routes, the most common being the intravenous route. Separate payment is allowed for chemotherapy administration by push and by infusion technique on the same day. For a given date of service

Separate Procedure | Unlisted Procedure | CCI Comp. Code | Non-specific Procedure

only one initial service code may be reported unless it is medically reasonable and necessary that the drug or substance administrations occur at separate vascular access sites. To report two different initial service codes use NCCI associated modifiers.

Although CPT code 99211 is not reportable with chemotherapy and no chemotherapy drug or substance administration HCPCS/CPT codes, other office/outpatient evaluation and management CPT codes (99201-99205, 99212-99215) are separately reportable with modifier -25 if the physician provides a significant and separately identifiable E & M service.

Drug administration services performed in hospital facilities including emergency departments are not separately reportable by physicians. Drug administration services performed in an Ambulatory Surgical Center (ASC) related to a Medicare approved ASC payable procedure are not separately reportable by physicians. Hospital outpatient facilities may bill separately for drug administration services when appropriate.

Flushing or irrigation of an implanted vascular access port or device prior to or subsequent to the administration of chemotherapeutic or non-chemotherapeutic drugs is integral to the chemotherapy drug administration service and is not separately reportable.

CPT code 96522 describes the refilling and maintenance of an implantable pump or reservoir for systemic drug delivery. The pump or reservoir must be capable of programmed release of a drug at a prescribed rate. CPT code 96522 should not be reported for accessing a nonprogrammable implantable intravenous device for the provision of infusion(s) or chemotherapy administration. These codes should not be reported for accessing or flushing an indwelling peripherally-placed intravenous catheter port (external to skin), subcutaneous port, or non-programmable subcutaneous pump. Accessing and flushing these devices is an inherent service facilitating these infusion(s) and is not reported separately.

CPT code 96522 and CPT code 96521 (refilling and maintenance of portable pump) should not be reported with CPT code 96416 (initiation of prolonged intravenous chemotherapy infusion (more than eight hours), requiring use of a portable or implantable pump) or CPT code 96425 (chemotherapy administration, intra-arterial; infusion technique, initiation of prolonged infusion (more than eight hours) requiring the use of a portable or implantable pump).

CPT codes 96416 and 96425 include the initial filling and maintenance of a portable or implantable pump. CPT codes 96522 and 96521 are used to report subsequent refilling of the pump.

Chemotherapy Drugs

Chemotherapy administration CPT codes do not include provision of the chemotherapy agent. CPT code 96545 is used to report provision of the

● New Code ▲ Revised Code + Add-On Code ⊘ Modifier -51 Exempt ⊙ Conscious Sedation

chemotherapy agent for non-Medicare patients. For Medicare patients, choose HCPCS codes from the series J9000-J9999 to report chemotherapy drugs.

Preparation of chemotherapy agent(s) is included in the service for administration of the agent. Report separate CPT codes for each parenteral method of administration employed when chemotherapy is administered by different techniques.

(For declotting a catheter or port, use 36550)

(For home infusion services, see 99601-99602)

INJECTION AND INTRAVENOUS INFUSION CHEMOTHERAPY

(96400 deleted 2006 edition. To report, see 96401, 96402)

96401 Chemotherapy administration, subcutaneous or intramuscular; non-hormonal anti-neoplastic

96402 hormonal anti-neoplastic

96405 Chemotherapy administration; intralesional, up to and including 7 lesions

96406 intralesional, more than 7 lesions

(96408 deleted 2006 edition. To report, use 96409)

96409 intravenous, push technique, single or initial substance/drug

(96410 deleted 2006 edition. To report, use 96413)

+ **96411** intravenous, push technique, each additional substance/drug (List separately in addition to code for primary procedure)

(Use 96411 in conjunction with 96409, 96413)

(96412 deleted 2006 edition. To report, use 96415)

96413 Chemotherapy administration, intravenous infusion technique; up to 1 hour, single or initial substance/drug

(96414 deleted 2006 edition. To report, use 96416)

▲**+96415** each additional hour (List separately in addition to code for primary procedure)

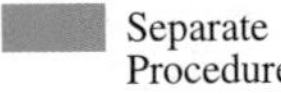
Separate Procedure
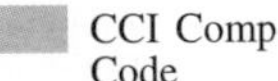
Unlisted Procedure
CCI Comp. Code
Non-specific Procedure

(Use 96415 in conjunction with 96413)

(Report 96415 for infusion intervals of greater than 30 minutes beyond 1-hour increments)

(Report 90761 to identify hydration, or 90766, 90767, 90775 to identify therapeutic, prophylactic, or diagnostic drug infusion or injection, if provided as a secondary or subsequent service in association with 96413)

96416 initiation of prolonged chemotherapy infusion (more than 8 hours), requiring use of a portable or implantable pump

(For refilling and maintenance of a portable pump or an implantable infusion pump or reservoir for drug delivery, see 96521-96523)

+ **96417** each additional sequential infusion (different substance/drug), up to 1 hour (List separately in addition to code for primary procedure)

(Use 96417 in conjunction with 96413)

(Report only once per sequential infusion. Report 96415 for additional hour(s) of sequential infusion)

INTRA-ARTERIAL CHEMOTHERAPY

96420 Chemotherapy administration, intra-arterial; push technique

96422 infusion technique, up to one hour

▲+**96423** infusion technique, each additional hour (List separately in addition to code for primary procedure)

(Use 96423 in conjunction with code 96422)

(Report 96423 for infusion intervals of greater than 30 minutes beyond 1-hour increments)

(For regional chemotherapy perfusion via membrane oxygenator perfusion pump to an extremity, use 36823)

96425 infusion technique, initiation of prolonged infusion (more than 8 hours), requiring the use of a portable or implantable pump

(For refilling and maintenance of a portable pump or an implantable infusion pump or reservoir for drug delivery, see 96521-96523)

OTHER CHEMOTHERAPY

(For collection of blood specimen from a completely implantable venous access device, use 36540)

96440 Chemotherapy administration into pleural cavity, requiring and including thoracentesis

96445 Chemotherapy administration into peritoneal cavity, requiring and including peritoneocentesis

96450 Chemotherapy administration, into CNS (eg, intrathecal), requiring and including spinal puncture

(For intravesical (bladder) chemotherapy administration, use 51720)

(For insertion of subarachnoid catheter and reservoir for infusion of drug, see 62350, 62351, 62360, 62361, 62362; for insertion of intraventricular catherter and reservoir, see 61210, 61215)

(96520 deleted 2006 edition. To report, use 96521)

96521 Refilling and maintenance of portable pump

96522 Refilling and maintenance of implantable pump or reservoir for drug delivery, systemic (eg, intravenous, intra-arterial)

(For refilling and maintenance of an implantable infusion pump for spinal or brain drug infusion, use 95990-95991)

96523 Irrigation of implanted venous access device for drug delivery systems

(Do not report 96523 if an injection or infusion is provided on the same day)

(96530 deleted 2006 edition. To report, use 96522)

96542 Chemotherapy injection, subarachnoid or intraventricular via subcutaneous reservoir, single or multiple agents

(96545 deleted 2006 edition.)

(For radioactive isotope therapy, use 79005)

96549 Unlisted chemotherapy procedure

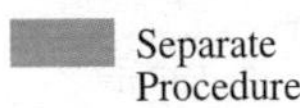
Separate Procedure

Unlisted Procedure

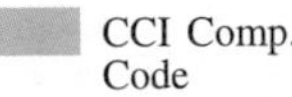
CCI Comp. Code

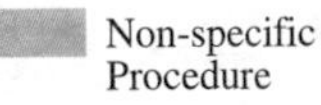
Non-specific Procedure

PHOTODYNAMIC THERAPY

Photodynamic therapy (PDT) is a two-part treatment for esophageal cancer, gastric cancer, and lung cancer using a photosensitizing drug activated by red, non-thermal laser light.

(To report ocular photodynamic therapy, use 67221)

96567 Photodynamic therapy by external application of light to destroy premalignant and/or malignant lesions of the skin and adjacent mucosa (eg, lip) by activation of photosensitive drug(s), each phototherapy exposure session

+ **96570** Photodynamic therapy by endoscopic application of light to ablate abnormal tissue via activation of photosensitive drug(s); first 30 minutes (List separately in addition to code for endoscopy or bronchoscopy procedures of lung and esophagus)

+ **96571** each additional 15 minutes (List separately in addition to code for endoscopy or bronchoscopy procedures of lung and esophagus)

(96570, 96571 are to be used in addition to bronchoscopy, endoscopy codes)

(Use 96570, 96571 in conjunction with codes 31641, 43228 as appropriate)

SPECIAL DERMATOLOGICAL PROCEDURES

(For whole body photography, use 96904)

(For intralesional injections, see 11900, 11901)

(For Tzanck smear, see 88160-88161)

96900 Actinotherapy (ultraviolet light)

96902 Microscopic examination of hairs plucked or clipped by the examiner (excluding hair collected by the patient) to determine telogen and anagen counts, or structural hair shaft abnormality

● **96904** Whole body integumentary photography, for monitoring of high risk patients with dysplastic nevus syndrome or a history of dysplastic nevi, or patients with a personal or familial history of melanoma

96910 Photochemotherapy; tar and ultraviolet B (Goeckerman treatment) or petrolatum and ultraviolet B

96912 psoralens and ultraviolet A (PUVA)

96913 Photochemotherapy (Goeckerman and/or PUVA) for severe photoresponsive dermatoses requiring at least four to eight hours of care under direct supervision of the physician (includes application of medication and dressings)

96920 Laser treatment for inflammatory skin disease (psoriasis); total area less than 250 sq cm

96921 250 sq cm to 500 sq cm

96922 over 500 sq cm

96999 Unlisted special dermatological service or procedure

PHYSICAL MEDICINE AND REHABILITATION

Physical medicine is the diagnosis, treatment, and prevention of disease with the aid of physical agents such as light, heat, cold, water, electricity or with mechanical devices. Physical medicine services may be provided by physicians or physical therapists. Physical medicine and rehabilitation CPT codes are divided into three sections: Modalities, Procedures and Tests and Measurements. Other services performed by medical professionals specializing in physical medicine and/or physical therapy include: muscle testing, range of joint motion, electromyography, biofeedback training by EMG, and transcutaneous nerve stimulation (TNS).

With one exception providers should not report more than one physical medicine and rehabilitation therapy service for the same fifteen minute time period. The only exception involves a supervised modality defined by CPT codes 97010-97028 which may be reported for the same fifteen minute time period as other therapy services. Some CPT codes for physical medicine and rehabilitation services include an amount of time in their code descriptors.

Coding Rules

1. *The physician or therapist is required to be in constant attendance when reporting CPT codes for modalities and procedures.*

2. *The physical medicine procedure CPT codes specify treatment to one area, initial 30 minutes, and provide CPT codes to report each additional 15 minutes of treatment.*

SPECIAL PHYSICAL MEDICINE CODING ISSUES

Many worker's compensation and casualty insurance companies use pre-CPT coding systems, such as CRVS, and do not use any form of diagnostic coding, relying instead on special reports to justify the procedures performed and services provided. As the majority of physical medicine services are performed for accidents and injuries, many work related, the medical professional performing these services must be informed of the specific reporting requirements in the area that they practice.

PHYSICAL MEDICINE AND REHABILITATION SERVICES

(For muscle testing, range of joint motion, electromyography, see 95831 et seq)

(For biofeedback training by EMG, use 90901)

(For transcutaneous nerve stimulation (TNS), use 64550)

97001 Physical therapy evaluation

97002 Physical therapy re-evaluation

97003 Occupational therapy evaluation

97004 Occupational therapy re-evaluation

97005 Athletic training evaluation

97006 Athletic training re-evaluation

MODALITIES

SUPERVISED

97010 Application of a modality to one or more areas; hot or cold packs

97012 traction, mechanical

97014 electrical stimulation (unattended)

(For acupuncture with electrical stimulation, see 97813, 97814)

97016 vasopneumatic devices

97018 paraffin bath

(97020 deleted 2006 edition. To report, use 97024)

97022 whirlpool

97024 diathermy (eg, microwave)

97026 infrared

97028 ultraviolet

CONSTANT ATTENDANCE

97032 Application of a modality to one or more areas; electrical stimulation (manual), each 15 minutes

97033 iontophoresis, each 15 minutes

97034 contrast baths, each 15 minutes

97035 ultrasound, each 15 minutes

97036 Hubbard tank, each 15 minutes

97039 Unlisted modality (specify type and time if constant attendance)

THERAPEUTIC PROCEDURES

97110 Therapeutic procedure, one or more areas, each 15 minutes; therapeutic exercises to develop strength and endurance, range of motion and flexibility

97112 neuromuscular reeducation of movement, balance, coordination, kinesthetic sense, posture, and/or proprioception for sitting and/or standing activities

97113 aquatic therapy with therapeutic exercises

97116 gait training (includes stair climbing)

(Use 96000-96003 to report comprehensive gait and motion analysis procedures)

97124 massage, including effleurage, petrissage and/or tapotement (stroking, compression, percussion)

Separate Procedure | Unlisted Procedure | CCI Comp. Code | Non-specific Procedure

(For myofascial release, use 97140)

97139 Unlisted therapeutic procedure (specify)

97140 Manual therapy techniques (eg, mobilization/ manipulation, manual lymphatic drainage, manual traction), one or more regions, each 15 minutes

97150 Therapeutic procedure(s), group (2 or more individuals)

(Report 97150 for each member of group)

(Group therapy procedures involve constant attendance of the physician or therapist, but by definition do not require one-on-one patient contact by the physician or therapist)

(For manipulation under general anesthesia, see appropriate anatomic section in Musculoskeletal System)

(For osteopathic manipulative treatment (OMT), see 98925-98929)

(97504 deleted 2006 edition. To report, use 97760)

(97520 deleted 2006 edition. To report, use 97761)

97530 Therapeutic activities, direct (one-on-one) patient contact by the provider (use of dynamic activities to improve functional performance), each 15 minutes

97532 Development of cognitive skills to improve attention, memory, problem solving, (includes compensatory training), direct (one-on-one) patient contact by the provider, each 15 minutes

97533 Sensory integrative techniques to enhance sensory processing and promote adaptive responses to environmental demands, direct (one-on-one) patient contact by the provider, each 15 minutes

97535 Self-care/home management training (eg, activities of daily living (ADL) and compensatory training, meal preparation, safety procedures, and instructions in use of assistive technology devices/adaptive equipment) direct one-on-one contact by provider, each 15 minutes

97537 Community/work reintegration training (eg, shopping, transportation, money management, avocational activities and/or work environment/modification analysis, work task analysis, use

● New Code ▲ Revised Code + Add-On Code ⊘ Modifier -51 Exempt ⊙ Conscious Sedation

of assistive technology device/adaptive equipment), direct one-on-one contact by provider, each 15 minutes

(For wheelchair management/propulsion training, use 97542)

97542 Wheelchair management (eg, assessment, fitting, training), each 15 minutes

97545 Work hardening/conditioning; initial 2 hours

+ 97546 each additional hour (List separately in addition to code for primary procedure)

(Use 97546 in conjunction with code 97545)

ACTIVE WOUND CARE MANAGEMENT

(Do not report 97597-97602 in conjunction with 11040-11044)

97597 Removal of devitalized tissue from wound(s), selective debridement, without anesthesia (eg, high pressure waterjet with/without suction, sharp selective debridement with scissors, scalpel and forceps), with or without topical application(s), wound assessment, and instruction(s) for ongoing care, may include use of a whirlpool, per session; total wound(s) surface area less than or equal to 20 square centimeters

97598 total wound(s) surface area greater than 20 square centimeters

(97601 deleted 2005 edition. To report, use 97597, 97598)

97602 Removal of devitalized tissue from wound(s), non-selective debridement, without anesthesia (eg, wet-to-moist dressings, enzymatic, abrasion), including topical application(s), wound assessment, and instruction(s) for ongoing care, per session

97605 Negative pressure wound therapy (eg, vacuum assisted drainage collection), including topical application(s), wound assessment, and instruction(s) for ongoing care, per session; total wound(s) surface area less than or equal to 50 square centimeters

97606 total wound(s) surface area greater than 50 square centimeters

Separate Procedure 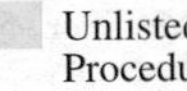 Unlisted Procedure 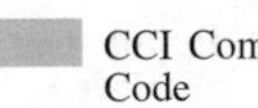 CCI Comp. Code 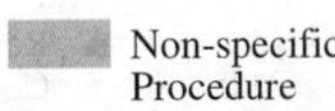 Non-specific Procedure

TESTS AND MEASUREMENTS

(For muscle testing, manual or electrical, joint range of motion, electromyography or nerve velocity determination, see 95831-95904)

(97703 deleted 2006 edition. To report, use 97762)

97750 Physical performance test or measurement (eg, musculo-skeletal, functional capacity), with written report, each 15 minutes

97755 Assistive technology assessment (eg, to restore, augment or compensate for existing function, optimize functional tasks and/or maximize environmental accessibility), direct one-on-one contact by provider, with written report, each 15 minutes

(To report augmentative and alternative communication devices, use 92605 or 92607)

ORTHOTIC MANAGEMENT AND PROSTHETIC MANAGEMENT

97760 Orthotic(s) management and training (including assessment and fitting when not otherwise reported), upper extremity(s), lower extremity(s) and/or trunk, each 15 minutes

(Code 97760 should not be reported with 97116 for the same extremity)

97761 Prosthetic training, upper and/or lower extremity(s), each 15 minutes

97762 Checkout for orthotic/prosthetic use, established patient, each 15 minutes

OTHER PROCEDURES

(For extracorporeal shock wave musculoskeletal therapy, see Category III codes 0019T, 0101T, 0102T)

(97780 deleted 2005 edition. To report, see 97810, 97811)

(97781 deleted 2005 edition. To report, see 97813, 97814)

97799 Unlisted physical medicine/rehabilitation service or procedure

MEDICAL NUTRITION THERAPY

Medical nutrition therapy (MNT) is the assessment of nutritional status followed by nutritional therapy. The nutrition assessment includes review and analysis of 1) medical, nutrition and medication histories, 2) physical examination, 3) anthropometric measurements, and 4) laboratory test values. Nutrition therapy may include 1) diet modification, 2) counseling and education, 3) disease self-management skills training, and 4) administration of specialized therapies such as medical foods, intravenous or tube feedings.

97802 Medical nutrition therapy; initial assessment and intervention, individual, face-to-face with the patient, each 15 minutes

97803 re-assessment and intervention, individual, face-to-face with the patient, each 15 minutes

97804 group (2 or more individual(s)), each 30 minutes

(For medical nutrition therapy assessment and/or intervention performed by a physician, see Evaluation and Management or Preventive Medicine service codes)

ACUPUNCTURE

97810 Acupuncture, one or more needles; without electrical stimulation, initial 15 minutes of personal one-on-one contact with the patient

(Do not report 97810 in conjunction with 97813)

+ **97811** without electrical stimulation, each additional 15 minutes of personal one-on-one contact with the patient, with re-insertion of needle(s) (List separately in addition to code for primary procedure)

(Use 97811 in conjunction with 97810, 97813)

97813 with electrical stimulation, initial 15 minutes of personal one-on-one contact with the patient

(Do not report 97813 in conjunction with 97810)

+ **97814** with electrical stimulation, each additional 15 minutes of personal one-on-one contact with the patient, with re-insertion of needle(s) (List separately in addition to code for primary procedure)

(Use 97814 in conjunction with 97810, 97813)

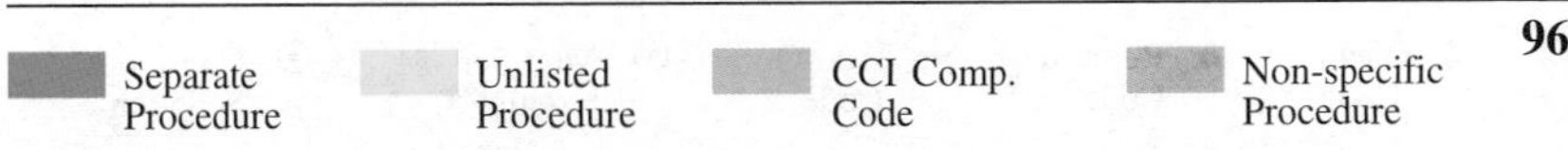

OSTEOPATHIC MANIPULATIVE TREATMENT

Osteopathic medicine is a system of therapy based on the theory that the body is capable of making its own remedies against disease and other toxic conditions when it is in normal structural relationship and has favorable environmental conditions and adequate nutrition. Osteopathic manipulative treatment (OMT) is a form of manual treatment applied by a physician to eliminate or alleviate somatic dysfunction and related disorders. This treatment may be accomplished by a variety of techniques.

Osteopathic Manipulative Treatment (OMT) is subject to Global Surgery Rules. Per Medicare Anesthesia Rules a provider performing OMT cannot separately report anesthesia services such as nerve blocks or epidural injections for OMT. In addition, per Medicare Global Surgery Rules, postoperative pain management after OMT (e.g., nerve block, epidural injection) is not separately reportable. Epidural or nerve block injections performed on the same date of service as OMT and unrelated to the MT may be reported with OMT using modifier -59.

Coding Rules

1. *Evaluation and management services may be reported separately, if, and only if the patient's condition requires a significant separately identifiable evaluation and management service, above and beyond the usual pre-service and post service work associated with the osteopathic manipulation.*

2. *CPT codes in this section are used to report OMT services provided in any location.*

OSTEOPATHIC MANIPULATIVE TREATMENT CODES

98925 Osteopathic manipulative treatment (OMT); one to two body regions involved

98926 three to four body regions involved

98927 five to six body regions involved

98928 seven to eight body regions involved

98929 nine to ten body regions involved

CHIROPRACTIC MANIPULATIVE TREATMENT

Chiropractic medicine is a system of diagnosis and treatment based on the theory that irritation of the nervous system by mechanical, chemical or psychic factors is the cause of disease. Chiropractic services may include office visits, diagnostic tests, physical therapy, and/or chiropractic manipulation. Chiropractic manipulation treatment (CMT) is a form of manual treatment applied by a chiropractic physician to eliminate or alleviate somatic dysfunction and related disorders.

Coding Rules

1. *Chiropractic manipulation treatment includes a pre-manipulation patient assessment.*

2. *Evaluation and management services provided in conjunction with CMT may be reported separately with the addition of CPT modifier -25, along with any diagnostic tests or other therapy provided.*

REPORTING CHIROPRACTIC MANIPULATION TO MEDICARE

Medicare restricts the number of times the CMT code may be reported, provides a maximum reimbursement amount per year, and requires extensive supporting documentation as described below:

Documentation of Treatment Phase

Proper documentation of the treatment phase is extremely important when submitting claims for chiropractic services to Medicare. The treatment phase consists of the date the course of treatment was initiated and the number of treatments rendered to date. Proper documentation enables Medicare to process your claims quickly and accurately. For payment of chiropractic claims, the following information must be on the CMS1500 claim form:

1. *The service must be manual manipulation of the spine. This service is reported by CPT codes 98940-98943.*

2. *The primary diagnosis must be subluxation of the spine, either so stated or identified by a term descriptive of the subluxation. The following diagnoses are acceptable because they would always involve a subluxation:*

Intervertebral disc disorders	*722.0-722.9*
Curvatures of the spine	*737.0-737.9*
Spondylolisthesis	*738.4,756.12*
Nonallopathic lesions	*739.1-739.4*
Spondylolysis	*756.11*

3. *The level of subluxation must be stated.*

4. *The symptoms related to the level of subluxation must be given.*

5. *The date of the confirming x-ray must be on the claim. Note that the x-ray must have been taken within 12 months prior to or 3 months after the course of treatment was initiated.*

6. *The date this course of treatment was initiated and the number of treatments rendered since the start of this course must be on the claim.*

Special Situations

If a patient returns with a new condition or injury, this represents a new treatment phase. The treatment phase information should reflect when you first saw the patient for this condition. Do not use the date you first saw the patient for an earlier course of treatment. Note on your CMS1500 claim form that this is a new condition. Remember that a new documenting x-ray may be required.

In the case of chronic conditions, an x-ray older than 12 months may be acceptable. For coverage of chronic conditions such as scoliosis, spondylolysis, and spondylolisthesis, there must be a reasonable expectation that there is a restorative potential. Remember that maintenance care is not covered by Medicare.

Chiropractic Manipulative Treatment Medicare covers chiropractic manipulative treatment (CMT) of five spinal regions. Physical therapy services described by CPT codes 97112, 97124 and 97140 are not separately reportable when performed in a spinal region undergoing CMT. If these physical therapy services are performed in a different region than CMT and the provider is eligible to report physical therapy codes under the Medicare program, the provider may report CMT and the above physical therapy codes using modifier -59.

CHIROPRACTIC MANIPULATIVE TREATMENT CODES

98940 Chiropractic manipulative treatment (CMT); spinal, one to two regions

98941 spinal, three to four regions

98942 spinal, five regions

98943 extraspinal, one or more regions

● New Code ▲ Revised Code + Add-On Code ⊘ Modifier -51 Exempt ⊙ Conscious Sedation

EDUCATION AND TRAINING FOR PATIENT SELF-MANAGEMENT

The CPT codes in this section are used to report physician prescribed educational and training services provided by a non-physician healthcare professional. To qualify for reporting under this section a standardized curriculum must be followed. These services are provided in 30 minute intervals and may be provided to individuals and/or groups.

(For counseling and education provided by a physician to an individual, see the appropriate Evaluation and Management codes)

(For counseling and education provided by a physician to a group, use 99078)

(For counseling and/or risk factor reduction intervention provided by a physician to patient(s) without symptoms or established disease, see 99401-99412)

(For medical nutrition therapy, see 97802-97804)

(For health and behavior assessment/intervention that is not part of a standardized curriculum, see 96150-96155)

(For education provided as genetic counseling services, use 96040. For education to a group regarding genetic risks, see 98961, 98962)

98960 Education and training for patient self-management by a qualified, nonphysician health care professional using a standardized curriculum, face-to-face with the patient (could include caregiver/family) each 30 minutes; individual patient

98961 2-4 patients

98962 5-8 patients

SPECIAL SERVICES, PROCEDURES AND REPORTS

The MEDICINE section of CPT includes a subsection Special Services and Reports, with CPT codes 99000-99090 which provides the reporting physician with a means of identifying the completion of special reports and services that are an adjunct to the basic services rendered. The specific special services code reported indicates the special circumstances under which a basic procedure is performed.

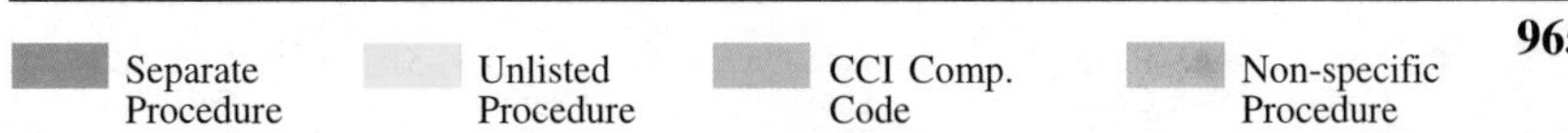

The proper use of Special Services CPT codes can result in a significant increase in reimbursement. Most codes in this section are "add on" codes which means that they are used in addition to whatever other CPT codes describe the procedures or services performed.

MISCELLANEOUS SERVICES

99000 Handling and/or conveyance of specimen for transfer from the physician's office to a laboratory

99001 Handling and/or conveyance of specimen for transfer from the patient in other than a physician's office to a laboratory (distance may be indicated)

99002 Handling, conveyance, and/or any other service in connection with the implementation of an order involving devices (eg, designing, fitting, packaging, handling, delivery or mailing) when devices such as orthotics, protectives, prosthetics are fabricated by an outside laboratory or shop but which items have been designed, and are to be fitted and adjusted by the attending physician

(For routine collection of venous blood, use 36415)

99024 Postoperative follow-up visit, normally included in the surgical package, to indicate that an evaluation and management service was performed during a postoperative period for a reason(s) related to the origianl procedure

(As a component of a surgical "package," see Surgery guidelines)

(99025 deleted 2004 edition.)

99026 Hospital mandated on call service; in-hospital, each hour

99027 out-of-hospital, each hour

(For physician standby services requiring prolonged physician attendance, use 99360, as appropriate. Time spent performing separately reportable procedure(s) or service(s) should not be included in the time reported as mandated on call service)

99050 Services provided in the office at times other than regularly scheduled office hours, or days when the office is normally closed (eg, holidays, Saturday or Sunday), in addition to basic service

● New Code ▲ Revised Code + Add-On Code ⊘ Modifier -51 Exempt ⊙ Conscious Sedation

99051 Service(s) provided in the office during regularly scheduled evening, weekend, or holiday office hours, in addition to basic service

(99052 deleted 2006 edition.)

99053 Service(s) provided between 10:00 PM and 8:00 AM at 24-hour facility, in addition to basic service

(99054 deleted 2006 edition.)

99056 Service(s) typically provided in the office, provided out of the office at request of patient, in addition to basic service

99058 Service(s) provided on an emergency basis in the office, which disrupts other scheduled office services, in addition to basic service

99060 Service(s) provided on an emergency basis, out of the office, which disrupts other scheduled office services, in addition to basic service

99070 Supplies and materials (except spectacles), provided by the physician over and above those usually included with the office visit or other services rendered (list drugs, trays, supplies, or materials provided)

(For supply of spectacles, use the appropriate supply codes)

99071 Educational supplies, such as books, tapes, and pamphlets, provided by the physician for the patient's education at cost to physician

99075 Medical testimony

99078 Physician educational services rendered to patients in a group setting (eg, prenatal, obesity, or diabetic instructions)

99080 Special reports such as insurance forms, more than the information conveyed in the usual medical communications or standard reporting form

(Do not report 99080 in conjunction with 99455, 99456 for the completion of Workmen's Compensation forms)

99082 Unusual travel (eg, transportation and escort of patient)

Separate Procedure | Unlisted Procedure | CCI Comp. Code | Non-specific Procedure

99090 Analysis of clinical data stored in computers (eg, ECGs, blood pressures, hematologic data)

(For physician/health care professional collection and interpretation of physiologic data stored/transmitted by patient/caregiver, see 99091)

(Do not report 99090 if other more specific CPT codes exist, eg, 93014, 93227, 93233, 93272 for cardiographic services; 95250 for continuous glucose monitoring, 97750 for musculoskeletal function testing)

99091 Collection and interpretation of physiologic data (eg, ECG, blood pressure, glucose monitoring) digitally stored and/or transmitted by the patient and/or caregiver to the physician or other qualified health care professional, requiring a minimum of 30 minutes of time

QUALIFYING CIRCUMSTANCES FOR ANESTHESIA

(For explanation of these services, see Anesthesia guidelines)

+ **99100** Anesthesia for patient of extreme age, under 1 year and over 70 (List separately in addition to code for primary anesthesia procedure)

(For procedure performed on infants less than 1 year of age at time of surgery, see 00326, 00834, 00836)

+ **99116** Anesthesia complicated by utilization of total body hypothermia (List separately in addition to code for primary anesthesia procedure)

+ **99135** Anesthesia complicated by utilization of controlled hypotension (List separately in addition to code for primary anesthesia procedure)

+ **99140** Anesthesia complicated by emergency conditions (specify) (List separately in addition to code for primary anesthesia procedure)

(An emergency is defined as existing when delay in treatment of the patient would lead to a significant increase in the threat to life or body part)

● New Code ▲ Revised Code + Add-On Code ⃠ Modifier -51 Exempt ⊙ Conscious Sedation

MODERATE (CONSCIOUS) SEDATION

(99141 deleted 2006 edition. To report, see 99143-99145)

(99142 deleted 2006 edition. To report, see 99143-99145)

⊘ **99143** Moderate sedation services (other than those services described by codes 00100-01999) provided by the same physician performing the diagnostic or therapeutic service that the sedation supports, requiring the presence of an independent trained observer to assist in the monitoring of the patient's level of consciousness and physiological status; under 5 years of age, first 30 minutes intra-service time

⊘ **99144** age 5 years or older, first 30 minutes intra-service time

+ **99145** each additional 15 minutes intra-service time (List separately in addition to code for primary service)

(Use 99145 in conjunction with 99143, 99144)

⊘ **99148** Moderate sedation services (other than those services described by codes 00100-01999), provided by a physician other than the health care professional performing the diagnostic or therapeutic service that the sedation supports; under 5 years of age, first 30 minutes intra-service time

⊘ **99149** age 5 years or older, first 30 minutes intra-service time

+ **99150** each additional 15 minutes intra-service time (List separately in addition to code for primary service)

(Use 99150 in conjunction with 99148, 99149)

OTHER SERVICES AND PROCEDURES

99170 Anogenital examination with colposcopic magnification in childhood for suspected trauma

(For conscious sedation, use 99143-99150)

99172 Visual function screening, automated or semi-automated bilateral quantitative determination of visual acuity, ocular alignment, color vision by pseudoisochromatic plates, and field of vision (may include all or some screening of the determination(s) for contrast sensitivity, vision under glare)

(This service must employ graduated visual acuity stimuli that allow a quantitative determination of visual acuity (eg, Snellen chart). This service may not be used in addition to a gernal ophthalmological service or an E/M service)

(Do not report 99172 in conjunction with code 99173)

99173 Screening test of visual acuity, quantitative, bilateral

(The screening test used must employ graduated visual acuity stimuli that allow a quantitative estimate of visual acuity (eg, Snellen chart). Other identifiable services unrelated to this screening test provided at the same time may be reported separately (eg, preventive medicine services). When acuity is measured as part of a general ophthalmological service or of an E/M service of the eye, it is a diagnostic examination and not a screening test.)

(Do not report 99173 in conjunction with code 99172)

99175 Ipecac or similar administration for individual emesis and continued observation until stomach adequately emptied of poison

(For diagnostic intubation, see 82926-82928, 89130-89141)

(For gastric lavage for diagnostic purposes, see 91055)

99183 Physician attendance and supervision of hyperbaric oxygen therapy, per session

(Evaluation and Management services and/or procedures (eg, wound debridement) provided in a hyperbaric oxygen treatment facility in conjunction with a hyperbaric oxygen therapy session should be reported separately)

99185 Hypothermia; regional

99186 total body

99190 Assembly and operation of pump with oxygenator or heat exchanger (with or without ECG and/or pressure monitoring); each hour

99191 45 minutes

99192 30 minutes

99195 Phlebotomy, therapeutic (separate procedure)

● New Code ▲ Revised Code + Add-On Code ⊘ Modifier -51 Exempt ⊙ Conscious Sedation

99199 Unlisted special service, procedure or report

HOME HEALTH PROCEDURES/SERVICES

Home health procedures/services codes are used by non-physician health care professionals to report services provided in the patient's residence. Physicians should use home visit codes 99341-99350.

99500 Home visit for prenatal monitoring and assessment to include fetal heart rate, non-stress test, uterine monitoring, and gestational diabetes monitoring

99501 Home visit for postnatal assessment and follow-up care

99502 Home visit for newborn care and assessment

99503 Home visit for respiratory therapy care (eg, bronchodilator, oxygen therapy, respiratory assessment, apnea evaluation)

99504 Home visit for mechanical ventilation care

99505 Home visit for stoma care and maintenance including colostomy and cystostomy

99506 Home visit for intramuscular injections

99507 Home visit for care and maintenance of catheter(s) (eg, urinary, drainage, and enteral)

99509 Home visit for assistance with activities of daily living and personal care

(To report self-care/home management training, see 97535)

(To report home medical nutrition assessment and intervention services, see 97802-97804)

(To report home speech therapy services, see 92507-92508)

99510 Home visit for individual, family, or marriage counseling

99511 Home visit for fecal impaction management and enema administration

99512 Home visit for hemodialysis

(For home infusion of peritoneal dialysis, use 99601, 99602)

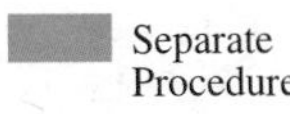 Separate Procedure 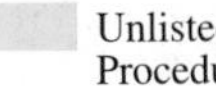 Unlisted Procedure 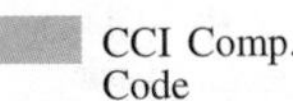 CCI Comp. Code 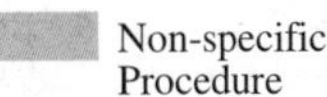 Non-specific Procedure

99600 Unlisted home visit service or procedure

HOME INFUSION PROCEDURES/SERVICES

Home infusion procedures codes are used to report per diem home visits for the purpose of administering infusions. With the exception of the infusion drug; all materials, equipments and supplies are included in the basic code. Drugs used for the infusion are coded separately.

99601 Home infusion/specialty drug administration, per visit (up to 2 hours)

+ 99602 each additional hour (List separately in addition to code for primary procedure)

(Use 99602 in conjunction with 99601)

CATEGORY II CODES

This section of the CPT coding system is the Category II Performance Measurement section. The primary purpose of this section is to provide classification codes which will allow the collection of data for performance measurement.

The assignment of a Category II code to a given service or procedure does not mean that the particular service or procedure is endorsed, approved, safe or has applicability to clinical practice. The Category II code simply provides a mechanism to identify and review performance measurements.

The most current codes and their implementation dates can be found on the Web at http://www.ama-assn.org/go/cpt.

(For blood pressure measured, use 2000F)

(0002F deleted 2005 edition. To report use 1000F)

(0003F deleted 2005 edition. To report see 1034F-1036F)

(0004F deleted 2005 edition. To report use 4000F)

(For tobacco use cessation intervention, pharmacologic therapy, use 4001F)

(0006F deleted 2005 edition. To report use 4002F)

(0007F deleted 2005 edition. To report use 4006F)

(0008F deleted 2005 edition. To report use 4009F)

(0009F deleted 2005 edition. To report use 1002F)

(0010F deleted 2005 edition)

(0011F deleted 2005 edition. To report use 4011F)

MODIFIERS

The following performance measurement modifiers may be used for Category II codes to indicate that a service specified in the associate measure(s) was considered but, due to either medical, patient or system circumstance(s) documented in the medical record, the service was not provided. These modifiers serve as denominator exclusions from the performance measure.

Category II modifiers should only be reported with Category II codes; they should not be reported with Category I or Category III codes. In addition, the modifiers in the Category II section should only be used where specified in the guidelines, reporting instructions, parenthetic notes, or code descriptor language listed in the Cateogry II section..

1P Performance Measure Exclusion Modifier due to Medical Reasons:

Includes:

- Not indicated (absence of organ/limb, already received/performed, other)
- Contraindicated (patient allergic history, potential adverse drug interaction, other)

2P Performance Measure Exclusion Modifier due to Patient Reason:

Includes:

- Patient declined
- Economic, social or religious reasons
- Other patient reasons

3P Performance Measure Exclusion Modifier due to System Reason:

Includes:

- Resources to perform the services not available
- Insurance coverage/payor-related limitations
- Other reasons attributable to health care delivery system

COMPOSITE CODES

Composite codes combine several measures grouped within a single code descriptor to facilitate reporting for a clinical condition when all components are met. If only some of the components are met, or if services are provided in addition to those included in the composite code, they may be reported individually using the corresponding CPT Category II codes for those services.

▲ **0001F** Heart failure assessed (includes assessment of all the following components):

Blood pressure measured (2000F)[1]

Level of activity assessed (1003F)[1]

Clinical symptoms of volume overload (excess) assessed (1004F)[1]

Weight, recorded (2001F)[1]

Clinical signs of volume overload (excess) assessed (2002F)[1]

(To report blood pressure measured, use 2000F)

0005F Osteoarthritis assessed

Includes assessment of all the following components:

Osteoarthritis symptoms and functional status assessed (1006F)[1]

Use of anti-inflammatory or over-the-counter (OTC) analgesic medications assessed (1007F)[1]

Initial examination of the involved joint(s) (includes visual inspection, palpation, range of motion) (2004F)[1]

(To report tobacco use cessation intervention, use 4001F)

● **0012F** Community-acquired bacterial pneumonia assessment (includes all of the following components) (CAP)[1]:

Co-morbid conditions assessed (1026F)[1]

Vital signs recorded (2010F)[1]

Mental status assessed (2014F)[1]

Hydration status assessed (2018F)[1]

PATIENT MANAGEMENT

Patient management codes describe utilization measures or measures of patient care provided for specific clinical purposes (eg, prenatal care, pre- and post-surgical care).

0500F Initial prenatal care visit (report at first prenatal encounter with health care professional providing obstetrical care. Report also date of visit and, in a separate field, the date of the last menstrual period-LMP)[2]

Footnotes

[1]Physician Consortium for Performance Improvement, www.ama-assn.org/go/quality

[2]National Committee on Quality Assurance (NCQA), Health Employer Data Information Set (HEDIS®), www.ncqa.org

0501F Prenatal flow sheet documented in medical record by first prenatal visit (documentation includes at minimum blood pressure, weight, urine protein, uterine size, fetal heart tones, and estimated date of delivery). Report also: date of visit and, in a separate field, the date of the last menstrual period-LMP (note: if reporting 0501F prenatal flow sheet, it is not necessary to report 0500F initial prenatal care visit)[1]

0502F Subsequent prenatal care visit

[Excludes: patients who are seen for a condition unrelated to pregnancy or prenatal care (eg, an upper respiratory infection; patients seen for consultation only, not for continuing care)]

0503F Postpartum care visit[2]

PATIENT HISTORY

Patient history codes describe measures for select aspects of patient history or review of systems.

▲ **1000F** Tobacco use assessed (CAD, CAP, COPD, PV)[1] (DM)[4]

(1001F deleted 2007 edition. To report smoking use, tobacco use, or non-use of tobacco products, see 1034F-1036F)

1002F Anginal symptoms and level of activity, assessed[1]

1003F Level of activity assessed

1004F Clinical symptoms of volume overload (excess) assessed

1005F Asthma symptoms evaluated (includes physician documentation of numeric frequency of symptoms or patient completion of an asthma assessment tool/survey/questionnaire)

1006F Osteoarthritis symptoms and functional status assessed (may include the use of a standardized scale or the completion of an assessment questionnaire, such as the SF-36, AAOS Hip & Knee Questionnaire)

[Instructions: report when osteoarthritis is addressed during the patient encounter]

1007F Use of anti-inflammatory or analgesic over-the-counter (OTC) medications for symptom relief assessed

1008F Gastrointestinal and renal risk factors assessed for patients on prescribed or OTC non-steroidal anti-inflammatory drug (NSAID)

● **1015F** Chronic obstructive pulmonary disease (COPD) symptoms assessed (Includes assessment of at least one of the following: dyspnea, cough/sputum, wheezing), or respiratory symptom assessment tool completed (COPD)[1]

● **1018F** Dyspnea assessed, not present (COPD)[1]

● **1019F** Dyspnea assessed, present (COPD)[1]

● **1022F** Pneumococcus immunization status assessed (CAP, COPD)[1]

● **1026F** Co-morbid conditions assessed (eg, includes assessment for presence or absence of: malignancy, liver disease, congestive heart failure, cerebrovascular disease, renal disease, chronic obstructive pulmonary disease, asthma, diabetes, other co-morbid conditions) (CAP)[1]

● **1030F** Influenza immunization status assessed (CAP)[1]

● **1034F** Current tobacco smoker (CAD, CAP, COPD, PV)[1] (DM)[4]

● **1035F** Current smokeless tobacco user (eg, chew, snuff) (PV)[1]

● **1036F** Current tobacco non-user (CAD, CAP, COPD, PV)[1] (DM)[4]

● **1038F** Persistent asthma (mild, moderate or severe) (Asthma)[1]

● **1039F** Intermittent asthma (Asthma)[1]

PHYSICAL EXAMINATION

Physical examination codes describe aspects of physical examination or clinical assessment.

2000F Blood pressure, measured[1]

2001F Weight recorded

2002F Clinical signs of volume overload (excess) assessed

(2003F deleted 2007 edition)

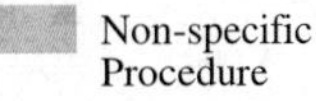

Separate Procedure | Unlisted Procedure | CCI Comp. Code | Non-specific Procedure

2004F Initial examination of the involved joint(s) (includes visual inspection, palpation, range of motion)

[Instructions: report only for initial osteoarthritis visit or for visits for new joint involvement]

● **2010F** Vital signs recorded (includes at minimum: temperature, pulse, respiration, and blood pressure)(CAP)[1]

● **2014F** Mental status assessed (normal/mildly impaired/severely impaired) (CAP)[1]

● **2018F** Hydration status assessed (normal/mildly dehydrated/severely dehydrated) (CAP)[1]

● **2022F** Dilated retinal eye exam with interpretation by an ophthalmologist or optometrist documented and reviewed (DM)[4]

● **2024F** Seven standard field stereoscopic photos with interpretation by an ophthalmologist or optometrist documented and reviewed (DM)[4]

● **2026F** Eye imaging validated to match diagnosis from seven standard field stereoscopic photos results documented and reviewed (DM)[4]

● **2028F** Foot examination performed (includes examination through visual inspection, sensory exam with monofilament, and pulse exam - report when any of the three components are completed) (DM)[4]

DIAGNOSTIC/SCREENING PROCESSES OR RESULTS

Diagnostic/screening processes or results codes describe results of tests ordered (clinical laboratory tests, radiological or other procedural examinations).

(3000F deleted 2007 edition. To report blood pressure, use the corresponding systolic codes (3076F and 3077F) and diastolic codes (3078F, 3079F, 3080F))

(3002F deleted 2007 edition. To report blood presure, use the corresponding systolic codes (3076F and 3077F)) and diastolic codes (3078F, 3079F, 3080F))

● **3006F** Chest X-ray results documented and reviewed (CAP)[1]

● New Code ▲ Revised Code + Add-On Code ⊘ Modifier -51 Exempt ⊙ Conscious Sedation

● **3011F** Lipid panel results documented and reviewed (must include total cholesterol, HDL-C, triglycerides and calculated LDL-C) (CAD)[1]

● **3014F** Screening mammography results documented and reviewed (PV)[1]

● **3017F** Colorectal cancer screening results documented and reviewed (PV)[1]

(Includes: fecal occult blood testing annually, flexible sigmoidoscopy every 5 years, annual fecal occult blood testing plus flexible sigmoidoscopy every 5 years, double-contrast barium enema every 5 years, or colonoscopy every 10 years)

● **3020F** Left ventricular function (LVF) assessment (eg, echocardiography, nuclear test, or ventriculography) documented in the medical record (Includes quantitative or qualitative assessment results)(CHF)[1]

● **3021F** Left ventricular ejection fraction (LVEF) 40% or documentation of moderately or severely depressed left ventricular systolic function (CAD, HF)[1]

● **3022F** Left ventricular ejection fraction (LVEF) 40% or documentation as normal or mildly depressed left ventricular systolic function (CAD, HF)[1]

● **3023F** Spirometry results documented and reviewed (COPD)[1]

● **3025F** Spirometry test results demonstrate FEV1/FVC70% with COPD symptoms (eg, dyspnea, cough/sputum, wheezing) (CAP, COPD)[1]

● **3027F** Spirometry test results demonstrate FEV1/FVC70% or patient does not have COPD symptoms (COPD)[1]

● **3028F** Oxygen saturation results documented and reviewed (Includes assessment through pulse oximetry or arterial blood gas measurement) (CAP, COPD)[1]

● **3035F** Oxygen saturation 88 % or a Pa02 55 mm Hg (COPD)[1]

● **3037F** Oxygen saturation 88% or PaO2 55 mmHg (COPD)[1]

● **3040F** Functional expiratory volume (FEV1) 40% of predicted value (COPD)[1]

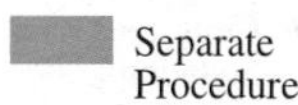 Separate Procedure 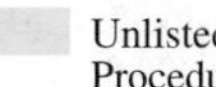 Unlisted Procedure 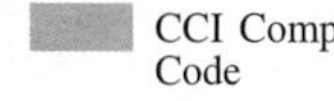 CCI Comp. Code 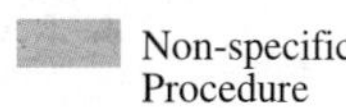 Non-specific Procedure

● **3042F** Functional expiratory volume (FEV1) 40% of predicted value (COPD)[1]

● **3046F** Most recent hemoglobin A1c level > 9.0% (DM)[4]

● **3047F** Most recent hemoglobin A1c level 9.0% (DM)[4]

● **3048F** Most recent LDL-C 100 mg/dL (DM)[4]

● **3049F** Most recent LDL-C 100-129 mg/dL (DM)[4]

● **3050F** Most recent LDL-C 130 mg/dL (DM)[4]

● **3060F** Positive microalbuminuria test result documented and reviewed (DM)[4]

● **3061F** Negative microalbuminuria test result documented and reviewed (DM)[4]

● **3062F** Positive macroalbuminuria test result documented and reviewed (DM)[4]

● **3066F** Documentation of treatment for nephropathy (eg, patient receiving dialysis, patient being treated for ESRD, CRF, ARF, or renal insufficiency, any visit to a nephrologist) (DM)[4]

● **3072F** Low risk for retinopathy (no evidence of retinopathy in the prior year) (DM)[4]

● **3076F** Most recent systolic blood pressure 140 mm Hg (HTN)[1] (DM)[4]

● **3077F** Most recent systolic blood pressure 140 mm Hg (HTN)[1] (DM)[4]

● **3078F** Most recent diastolic blood pressure 80 mm Hg (HTN)[1] (DM)[4]

● **3079F** Most recent diastolic blood pressure 80-89 mm Hg (HTN)[1] (DM)[4]

● **3080F** Most recent diastolic blood pressure 90 mm Hg (HTN)[1] (DM)[4]

THERAPEUTIC, PREVENTIVE OR OTHER INTERVENTIONS

Therapeutic, preventive or other interventions codes describe pharmacologic, procedural, or behavioral therapies, including preventive services such as patient education and counseling.

4000F Tobacco use cessation intervention, counseling[1]

4001F Tobacco use cessation intervention, pharmacologic therapy[1]

4002F Statin therapy, prescribed[1]

4003F Patient education, written/oral, appropriate for patients with heart failure performed

4006F Beta-blocker therapy, prescribed[1]

▲ **4009F** Angiotensin converting enzyme (ACE) inhibitor or angiotensin receptor blocker (ARB) therapy, prescribed[1]

4011F Oral antiplatelet therapy, prescribed (eg, aspirin, clopidogrel/ Plavix, or combination of aspirin and dipyridamole/Aggrenox)[1]

4012F Warfarin therapy prescribed

4014F Written discharge instructions provided to heart failure patients discharged home. (Instructions include all of the following components: activity level, diet, discharge medications, follow-up appointment, weight monitoring, what to do if symptoms worsen)

[Excludes patients < 18 years of age]

▲ **4015F** Persistent asthma, preferred long term control medication or an acceptable alternative treatment, prescribed (Asthma[1])

[Note: There are no medical exclusion criteria]

(Do not report modifier 1P with 4015F)

(To report patient reasons for not prescribing, use modifier 2P)

4016F Anti-inflammatory/analgesic agent prescribed

[Use for prescribed or continued medication(s), including over-the-counter medication(s)]

4017F Gastrointestinal prophylaxis for NSAID use prescribed

4018F Therapeutic exercise for the involved joint(s) instructed or physical or occupational therapy prescribed

● **4025F** Inhaled bronchodilator prescribed (COPD)[1]

● **4030F** Long term oxygen therapy prescribed (more than fifteen hours per day) (COPD)[1]

● **4033F** Pulmonary rehabilitation exercise training recommended (COPD)[1]

(Report 4033F with 1019F)

● **4035F** Influenza immunization recommended (COPD)[1]

● **4037F** Influenza immunization ordered or administered (COPD, PV)[1]

● **4040F** Pneumococcal immunization ordered or administered (COPD)[1]

● **4045F** Appropriate empiric antibiotic prescribed (See measure developer's Web site for definition of appropriate antibiotic) (CAP)[1]

● **4050F** Hypertension plan of care documented as appropriate (HTN)[1]

FOLLOW-UP OR OTHER OUTCOMES

Follow-up or other outcomes codes describe review and communication of test results to patients, patient satisfaction or experience with care, patient functional status, and patient morbidity and mortality.

(No codes at this time.)

PATIENT SAFETY

Patient safety codes that describe patient safety practices.

● **6005F** Rationale (eg, severity of illness and safety) for level of care (eg, home, hospital) documented (CAP)[1]

● New Code ▲ Revised Code + Add-On Code ⊘ Modifier -51 Exempt ⊙ Conscious Sedation

CATEGORY III CODES

CATEGORY III SECTION OVERVIEW

The eighth section of the CPT coding system is the Category III Emerging Technology section. The primary purpose of this section is to provide classification codes which will allow the collection of data on emerging technology services and procedures.

The assignment of a Category III code to a given service or procedure does not mean that the particular service or procedure is endorsed, approved, safe or has applicability to clinical practice. The Category III code simply provides a mechanism to identify and review emerging services and procedures.

Category III codes consist of four numbers followed by the letter "T." There is no particular organization to the codes listed in this section.

CATEGORY III CODES

(0001T deleted 2005 edition. To report, use 34803)

(0003T deleted 2007 edition)

(0005T deleted 2005 edition. To report, see 0075T, 0076T)

(0006T deleted 2005 edition. To report, see 0075T, 0076T)

(0007T deleted 2005 edition. To report, see 0075T, 0076T)

(0008T deleted 2007 edition)

(0009T deleted 2005 edition. To report, use 58356)

(0010T deleted 2006 edition. To report, use 86480)

(0012T deleted 2005 edition. To report, use 29866)

(0013T deleted 2005 edition. To report, use 29867, 27415)

(0014T deleted 2005 edition. To report, use 29868)

0016T Destruction of localized lesion of choroid (eg, choroidal neovascularization), transpupillary thermotherapy

0017T Destruction of macular drusen, photocoagulation

(0018T deleted 2007 edition, see 0160T, 0161T)

0019T Extracorporeal shock wave involving musculoskeletal system, not otherwise specified, low energy

(For application of high energy extracorporeal shock wave involving musculoskeletal system not otherwise specified, use 0101T)

(For application of high energy extracorporeal shock wave involving lateral humeral epicondyle, use 0102T)

(0020T deleted 2006 edition. To report, use 28890)

(0021T deleted 2007 edition)

(0023T deleted 2006 edition. To report, use 87900)

0024T Non-surgical septal reduction therapy (eg, alcohol ablation), for hypertrophic obstructive cardiomyopathy, with coronary arteriograms, with or without temporary pacemaker

(0025T deleted 2004 edition. To report, use 76514)

0026T Lipoprotein, direct measurement, intermediate density lipoproteins (IDL) (remnant lipoproteins)

0027T Endoscopic lysis of epidural adhesions with direct visualization using mechanical means (eg., spinal endoscopic catheter system) or solution injection (eg., normal saline) including radiologic localization and epidurography

(For diagnostic epidurography, use 64999)

0028T Dual energy x-ray absorptiometry (DEXA) body composition study, one or more sites

0029T Treatment(s) for incontinence, pulsed magnetic neuromodulation, per day

0030T Antiprothrombin (phospholipid cofactor) antibody, each Ig class

0031T Speculoscopy;

0032T with directed sampling

(0033T deleted 2006 edition. For endovascular repair of descending thoracic aorta, involving coverage of left subclavian artery origin, use 33880)

(0034T deleted 2006 edition. For endovascular repair of descending thoracic aorta, not involving coverage of left subclavian artery origin, use 33881)

(0035T deleted 2006 edition. For proximal extension during endovascular repair of descending thoracic aorta, use 33883. Distal extensions are included in 33880, 33881. Distal extensions performed after endovascular repair of descending thoracic aorta are reported with 33886)

(0036T deleted 2006 edition. For additional proximal extensions use 33884. Additional distal extensions during endovascular repair of descending thoracic aorta are included in 33880, 33881. Additional distal extensions placed after endovascular repair of thoracic aorta are included in 33886)

(0037T deleted 2006 edition. For open subclavian to carotid artery transposition performed in conjunction with endovascular thoracic aortic repair by neck incision, use 33889)

(0038T deleted 2006 edition. For endovascular repair of descending thoracic aorta, involving coverage of left subclavian artery origin, radiological supervision and interpretation, use 75956)

(0039T deleted 2006 edition. For endovascular repair of descending thoracic aorta, not involving coverage of left subclavian artery origin, radiological supervision and interpretation, use 75957)

(0040T deleted 2006 edition. For placement of proximal extension prosthesis for endovascular repair of descending thoracic aorta, radiological supervision and interpretation, use 75958. For placement of distal extension prosthesis after thoracic endovascular repair of descending thoracic aorta, radiological supervision and interpretation, use 75959)

0041T Urinalysis infectious agent detection, semi-quantitative analysis of volatile compounds

0042T Cerebral perfusion analysis using computed tomography with contrast administration, including post-processing of parametric

Separate Procedure | Unlisted Procedure | CCI Comp. Code | Non-specific Procedure

maps with determination of cerebral blood flow, cerebral blood volume, and mean transit time

0043T Carbon monoxide, expired gas analsysis (eg., ETCOc/hemolysis breath test)

(0044T deleted 2007 edition, see 96904)

(0045T deleted 2007 edition, see 96904)

0046T Catheter lavage of a mammary duct(s) for collection of cytology specimen(s), in high risk individuals (GAIL risk scoring or prior personal history of breast cancer), each breast; single duct

0047T each additional duct

0048T Implantation of a ventricular assist device, extracorporeal, percutaneous transseptal access, single or dual cannulation

+ **0049T** Prolonged extracorporeal percutaneous transseptal ventricular assist device, greater than 24 hours, each subsequent 24 hour period (List separately in addition to code for primary procedure)

(Use 0049T in conjunction with 0048T)

0050T Removal of a ventricular assist device, extracorporeal, percutaneous transseptal access, single or dual cannulation

0051T Implantation of a total replacement heart system (artificial heart) with recipient cardiectomy

(For implantation of heart assist or ventricular assist device, see 33975, 33976)

0052T Replacement or repair of thoracic unit of a total replacement heart system (artificial heart)

(For replacement or repair of other implantable components in a total replacement heart system (artificial heart), use 0053T)

0053T Replacement or repair of implantable component or components of total replacement heart system (artificial heart), excluding thoracic unit

(For replacement or repair of a thoracic unit of a total replacement heart system (artificial heart), use 0052T)

● New Code ▲ Revised Code + Add-On Code ⊘ Modifier -51 Exempt ⊙ Conscious Sedation

+ **0054T** Computer-assisted musculoskeletal surgical navigational orthopedic procedure, with image-guidance based on fluoroscopic images (List separately in addition to code for primary procedure)

+ **0055T** Computer-assisted musculoskeletal surgical navigational orthopedic procedure, with image-guidance based on CT/MRI images (List separately in addition to code for primary procedure)

(When CT and MRI are both performed, report 0055T only once)

+ **0056T** Computer assisted musculoskeletal surgical navigational orthopedic procedure, image-less (List separately in addition to code for primary procedure)

(0057T deleted 2005 edition. To report, use 43257)

0058T Cryopreservation; reproductive tissue, ovarian

0059T oocyte(s)

(For cryopreservation of embryo(s), sperm and testicular reproductive tissue, see 89258, 89259, 89335)

0060T Electrical impedance scan of the breast, bilateral (risk assessment device for breast cancer)

0061T Destruction/reduction of malignant breast tumor including breast carcinoma cells in the margins, microwave phased array thermotherapy, disposable catheter with combined temperature monitoring probe and microwave sensor, externally applied microwave energy, including interstitial placement of sensor

(For imaging guidance performed in conjunction with 0061T, see 76942, 76998)

▲ **0062T** Percutaneous intradiscal annuloplasty, any method except electrothermal, unilateral or bilateral including fluoroscopic guidance; single level

+ **0063T** one or more additional levels (List separately in addition to 0062T for primary procedure)

(For CT or MRI guidance and localization for needle placement and annuloplasty in conjunction with 0062T, 0063T, see 77012, 77021)

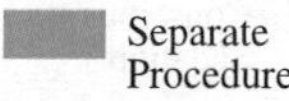

Separate Procedure | Unlisted Procedure | CCI Comp. Code | Non-specific Procedure

(For intradiscal electrothermal annuloplasty, see 22526-22527)

0064T Spectroscopy, expired gas analysis (eg, nitric oxide/carbon dioxide test)

0065T Ocular photoscreening, with interpretation and report, bilateral

(Do not report 0065T in conjunction with 99172 or 99173)

0066T Computed tomographic (CT) colonography (ie, virtual colonoscopy); screening

0067T diagnostic

(Do not report 0066T or 0067T in conjunction with 72192-72194, 74150-74170)

+ **0068T** Acoustic heart sound recording and computer analysis; with interpretation and report (List separately in addition to codes for electrocardiography)

(Use 0068T in conjunction with 93000)

+ **0069T** acoustic heart sound recording and computer analysis only (List separately in addition to codes for electrocardiography)

(Use 0069T in conjunction with 93005)

+ **0070T** interpretation and report only (List separately in addition to codes for electrocardiography)

(Use 0070T in conjunction with 93010)

0071T Focused ultrasound ablation of uterine leiomyomata, including MR guidance; total leiomyomata volume less than 200 cc of tissue

0072T total leiomyomata volume greater or equal to 200 cc of tissue

(Do not report 0071T, 0072T in conjunction with 51702 or 77022)

0073T Compensator-based beam modulation treatment delivery of inverse planned treatment using three or more high resolution (milled or cast) compensator convergent beam modulated fields, per treatment session

(For treatment planning, use 77301)

(Do not report 0073T in conjunction with 77401-77416, 77418)

ONLINE MEDICAL EVALUATION

0074T Online evaluation and management service, per encounter, provided by a physician, using the Internet or similar electronic communications network, in response to a patient's request, established patient

0075T Transcatheter placement of extracranial vertebral or intrathoracic carotid artery stent(s), including radiologic supervision and interpretation, percutaneous; initial vessel

\+ **0076T** each additional vessel (List separately in addition to code for primary procedure)

(Use 0076T in conjunction with 0075T)

(When the ipsilateral extracranial vertebral or intrathoracic carotid arteriogram (including imaging and selective catheterization) confirms the need for stenting, then 0075T and 0076T include all ipsilateral extracranial vertebral or intrathoracic selective carotid catheterization, all diagnostic imaging for ipsilateral extracranial vertebral or intrathoracic carotid artery stenting, and all related radiologic supervision and interpretation. If stenting is not indicated, then the appropriate codes for selective catheterization and imaging should be reported in lieu of code 0075T or 0076T.)

0077T Implanting and securing cerebral thermal perfusion probe, including twist drill or burr hole, to measure absolute cerebral tissue perfusion

(0078T-0081T should be reported in accordance with the Endovascular Abdominal Aneurysm Repair guidelines established for 34800-34826)

0078T Endovascular repair using prosthesis of abdominal aortic aneurysm, pseudoaneurysm or dissection, abdominal aorta involving visceral branches (superior mesenteric, celiac and/or renal artery(s))

(Do not report 0078T in conjunction with 34800-34805, 35081, 35102, 35452, 35454, 35472, 37205-37208)

(Report 0078T in conjunction with 35454, 37205-37208 when these procedures are performed outside the target zone of the endoprosthesis)

+ 0079T Placement of visceral extension prosthesis for endovascular repair of abdominal aortic aneurysm involving visceral vessels, each visceral branch (List separately in addition to code for primary procedure)

(Use 0079T in conjunction with 0078T)

(Do not report 0079T in conjunction with 34800-34805, 35081, 35102, 35452, 35454, 35472, 37205-37208)

(Report 0079T in conjunction with 35454, 37205-37208 when these procedures are performed outside the target zone of the endoprosthesis)

0080T Endovascular repair of abdominal aortic aneurysm, pseudoaneurysm or dissection, abdominal aorta involving visceral vessels (superior mesenteric, celiac or renal), using fenestrated modular bifurcated prosthesis (two docking limbs), radiological supervision and interpretation

(Do not report 0080T in conjunction with 34800-34805, 35081, 35102, 35452, 35454, 35472, 37205-37208)

(Report 0080T in conjunction with 35454, 37205-37208 when these procedures are performed outside the target zone of the endoprosthesis)

+ 0081T Placement of visceral extension prosthesis for endovascular repair of abdominal aortic aneurysm involving visceral vessels, each visceral branch, radiological supervision and interpretation (List separately in addition to code for primary procedure)

(Use 0081T in conjunction with 0080T)

(Do not report 0081T in conjunction with 34800-34805, 35081, 35102, 35452, 35454, 35472, 37205-37208)

(Report 0081T in conjunction with 35454, 37205-37208 when these procedures are performed outside the target zone of the endoprosthesis)

(0082T deleted 2007 edition, see 77371, 77373)

(0083T deleted 2007 edition, see 77371, 77373)

0084T Insertion of a temporary prostatic urethral stent

0085T Breath test for heart transplant rejection

0086T Left ventricular filling pressure indirect measurement by computerized calibration of the arterial waveform response to Valsalva maneuver

0087T Sperm evaluation, hyaluronan binding assay

0088T Submucosal radiofrequency tissue volume reduction of tongue base, one or more sites, per session (ie, for treatment of obstructive sleep apnea syndrome)

0089T Actigraphy testing, recording, analysis and interpretation (minimum of three-day recording)

▲ **0090T** Total disc arthroplasty (artificial disc), anterior approach, including diskectomy to prepare interspace (other than for decompression) cervical; single interspace

(0091T deleted 2007 edition. To report total disc lumbar arthroplasty, use 22857)

\+ **0092T** each additional interspace (List separately in addition to code for primary procedure)

(Use 0092T in conjunction with 0090T)

(For total disc lumbar arthroplasty of additional interspaces, use 0163T)

(Do not report 0092T in conjunction with 22857)

▲ **0093T** Removal of total disc arthroplasty, anterior approach, cervical; single interspace

(0094T deleted 2007 edition. To report removal of total disc lumbar arthroplasty, use 22865)

\+ **0095T** each additional interspace (List separately in addition to code for primary procedure)

(Use 0095T in conjunction with 0093T)

(For removal of total disc lumbar arthroplasty additional interspaces, use 0164T)

(Do not report 0095T in conjunction with 22865)

▲ **0096T** Revision of total disc arthroplasty, anterior approach, cervical; single interspace

(Do not report 0096T in conjunction with 0093T)

Separate Procedure | Unlisted Procedure | CCI Comp. Code | Non-specific Procedure

(0097T deleted 2007 edition. To report revision of total disc lumbar arthroplasty, use 22862)

+ 0098T each additional interspace (List separately in addition to code for primary procedure)

(Use 0098T in conjunction with 0096T)

(0090T-0098T include fluoroscopy when performed)

(Do not report 0090T-0098T in conjunction with 22851, 49010, when performed at the same level)

(Do not report 0098T in conjunction with 22862, 0095T)

(For revision of total disc lumbar arthroplasty additional interspaces, use 0165T)

(For decompression, see 63001-63048)

0099T Implantation of intrastromal corneal ring segments

0100T Placement of a subconjunctival retinal prosthesis receiver and pulse generator, and implantation of intra-ocular retinal electrode array, with vitrectomy

0101T Extracorporeal shock wave involving musculoskeletal system, not otherwise specified, high energy

(For application of low energy musculoskeletal system extracorporeal shock wave, use 0019T)

0102T Extracorporeal shock wave, high energy, performed by a physician, requiring anesthesia other than local, involving lateral humeral epicondyle

(For application of low energy musculoskeletal system extracorporeal shock wave, use 0019T)

0103T Holotranscobalamin, quantitative

0104T Inert gas rebreathing for cardiac output measurement; during rest

0105T during exercise

0106T Quantitative sensory testing (QST), testing and interpretation per extremity; using touch pressure stimuli to assess large diameter sensation

● New Code ▲ Revised Code + Add-On Code ⦸ Modifier -51 Exempt ⊙ Conscious Sedation

0107T using vibration stimuli to assess large diameter fiber sensation

0108T using cooling stimuli to assess small nerve fiber sensation and hyperalgesia

0109T using heat-pain stimuli to assess small nerve fiber sensation and hyperalgesia

0110T using other stimuli to assess sensation

0111T Long-chain (C20-22) omega-3 fatty acids in red blood cell (RBC) membranes

(For very long chain fatty acids, use 82726)

MEDICATION THERAPY MANAGEMENT

0115T Medication therapy management service(s) provided by a pharmacist, individual, face-to-face with patient, initial 15 minutes, with assessment, and intervention if provided; initial encounter

0116T subsequent encounter

+ **0117T** each additional 15 minutes (List separately in addition to code for primary service)

(Use 0117T in conjunction with 0115T, 0116T)

(0120T deleted 2007 edition, see 19105)

0123T Fistulization of sclera for glaucoma, through ciliary body

0124T Conjunctival incision with posterior juxtascleral placement of pharmacological agent (does not include supply of medication)

0126T Common carotid intima-media thickness (IMT) study for evaluation of atherosclerotic burden or coronary heart disease risk factor assessment

0130T Validated, statistically reliable, randomized, controlled, single-patient clinical investigation of FDA approved chronic care drugs, provided by a pharmacist, interpretation and report to the prescribing health care professional

0133T Upper gastrointestinal endoscopy, including esophagus, stomach, and either the duodenum and/or jejunum as appropriate, with injection of implant material into and along the muscle of the lower esophageal sphincter (eg, for treatment of gastroesophageal reflux disease)

0135T Ablation, renal tumor(s), unilateral, percutaneous, cryotherapy

0137T Biopsy, prostate, needle, saturation sampling for prostate mapping

(Do not report 0137T in conjunction with 76942)

0140T Exhaled breath condensate pH

● **0141T** Pancreatic islet cell transplantation through portal vein, percutaneous

(For open approach, use 0142T)

(For laparoscopic approach, use 0143T)

(For percutaneous portal vein catheterization, use 36481)

(For radiological supervision and interpretation, use 75887)

● **0142T** Pancreatic islet cell transplantation through portal vein, open

(For percutaneous approach, use 0141T)

(For laparoscopic approach, use 0143T)

(Do not report 0142T in conjunction with 49000, 49002)

● **0143T** Laparoscopy, surgical, pancreatic islet cell transplantation through portal vein

(For percutaneous approach, use 0141T)

(For open approach, use 0142T)

(Do not report 0143T in conjunction with 49320)

● **0144T** Computed tomography, heart, without contrast material, including image post processing and quantitative evaluation of coronary calcium

(Do not report 0144T in conjunction with 0145T-0151T)

● New Code ▲ Revised Code + Add-On Code ⃠ Modifier -51 Exempt ⊙ Conscious Sedation

● **0145T** Computed tomography, heart, without contrast material followed by contrast material(s) and further sections, including cardiac gating and 3D image post processing; cardiac structure and morphology

(For cardiac structure and morphology in congenital heart disease, use 0150T)

● **0146T** computed tomographic angiography of coronary arteries (including native and anomalous coronary arteries, coronary bypass grafts), without quantitative evaluation of coronary calcium

● **0147T** computed tomographic angiography of coronary arteries (including native and anomalous coronary arteries, coronary bypass grafts), with quantitative evaluation of coronary calcium

(Do not report 0147T in conjunction with 0144T)

● **0148T** cardiac structure and morphology and computed tomographic angiography of coronary arteries (including native and anomalous coronary arteries, coronary bypass grafts), without quantitative evaluation of coronary calcium

● **0149T** cardiac structure and morphology and computed tomographic angiography of coronary arteries (including native and anomalous coronary arteries, coronary bypass grafts), with quantitative evaluation of coronary calcium

(Do not report 0149T in conjunction with 0144T)

● **0150T** cardiac structure and morphology in congenital heart disease

●+**0151T** Computed tomography, heart, without contrast material followed by contrast material(s) and further sections, including cardiac gating and 3D image post processing, function evaluation (left and right ventricular function, ejection-fraction and segmental wall motion) (List separately in addition to code for primary procedure)

(Use 0151T in conjunction with 0145T-0150T)

●+**0153T** Transcatheter placement of wireless physiologic sensor in aneurysmal sac during endovascular repair, including radiological supervision and interpretation and instrument calibration (List separately in addition to code for primary procedure)

(Use 0153T in conjunction with 34800, 34802, 34803, 34804, 34805, 34900)

(0153T includes deployment of the sensor, repositioning if required, and intraoperative calibration)

● **0154T** Non-invasive physiologic study of implanted wireless pressure sensor in aneurysmal sac following endovascular repair, complete study including recording, analysis of pressure and waveform tracings, interpretation and report

(Do not report 0154T in conjunction with 0153T)

● **0155T** Laparoscopy, surgical; implantation or replacement of gastric stimulation electrodes, lesser curvature (ie, morbid obesity)

● **0156T** Laparoscopy, surgical; revision or removal of gastric stimulation electrodes, lesser curvature (ie, morbid obesity)

(For open approach, see 0157T, 0158T)

(For insertion of gastric neurostimulator pulse generator, use 64590)

(For revision or removal of gastric neurostimulator pulse generator, use 64595)

(For electronic analysis andprogramming of gastric neurostimulator pulse generator, see 95999)

● **0157T** Laparotomy, implantation or replacement of gastric stimulation electrodes, lesser curvature (ie, morbid obesity)

● **0158T** Laparotomy, revision or removal of gastric stimulation electrodes, lesser curvature (ie, morbid obesity)

(For laparoscopic approach, see 0155T, 0156T)

(For insertion of gastric neurostimulator pulse generator, use 64590)

(For revision or removal of gastric neurostimulator pulse generator, use 64595)

(For electronic analysis and programming of gastric neurostimulator pulse generator, see 95999)

(For electronic analysis, programming and reprogramming of gastric neurostimulator, use 0162T)

●+0159T Computer-aided detection, including computer algorithm analysis of MRI image data for lesion detection/characterization, pharmacokinetic analysis, with further physician review for interpretation, breast MRI (List separately in addition to code for primary procedure)

(Use 0159T in conjunction with 77058, 77059)

● 0160T Therapeutic repetitive transcranial magnetic stimulation treatment planning

(Pre-treatment determination of optimal magnetic field strength via titration, treatment location determination and stimulation parameter and protocol programming in the therapeutic use of high power, focal magnetic pulses for the direct, noninvasive modulation of cortical neurons)

● 0161T Therapeutic repetitive transcranial magnetic stimulation treatment delivery and management, per session

(Treatment session using high power, focal magnetic pulses for the direct, noninvasive modulation of cortical neurons. Clinical evaluation, safety monitoring and treatment parameter review in the therapeutic use of high power, focal magnetic pulses for the direct, noninvasive modulation of cortical neurons)

● 0162T Electronic analysis and programming, reprogramming of gastric neurostimulator (ie, morbid obesity)

●+0163T Total disc arthroplasty (artificial disc), anterior approach, including discectomy to prepare interspace (other than for decompression), lumbar, each additional interspace

(Use 0163T in conjunction with 22857)

●+0164T Removal of total disc arthroplasty, anterior approach, lumbar, each additional interspace

(Use 0164T in conjunction with 22865)

●+0165T Revision of total disc arthroplasty, anterior approach, lumbar, each additional interspace

(Use 0165T in conjunction with 22862)

(0163T-0165T include fluoroscopy when performed)

(Do not report 0163T-0165T in conjunction with 22851, 49010, when performed at the same level)

(For cervical total disc arthroplasty procedures, see 0090T-0098T)

(For decompression, see 63001-63048)

● **0166T** Transmyocardial transcatheter closure of ventricular septal defect, with implant; without cardiopulmonary bypass

● **0167T** Transmyocardial transcatheter closure of ventricular septal defect, with implant; with cardiopulmonary bypass

(Do not report 0166T, 0167T in conjunction with 32020, 33210, 33211)

(For ventricular septal defect closure via percutaneous transcatheter implant delivery, use 93581)

● **0168T** Rhinophototherapy, intranasal application of ultraviolet and visible light, bilateral

● **0169T** Stereotactic placement of infusion catheter(s) in the brain for delivery of therapeutic agent(s), including computerized stereotactic planning and burr hole(s)

(Do not report code 0169T in conjunction with 20660, 61107, 61795)

● **0170T** Repair of anorectal fistula with plug (eg, porcine small intestine submucosa [SIS])

(For repair of anal fistula using fibrin glue, use 46706)

(Do not report 0170T in conjunction with 15430, 15431)

ALPHABETICAL INDEX

The alphabetical index includes listings by procedure, CPT® headings and sub-headings and anatomic site. Procedures and services commonly known by their acronyms, eponyms, homonyms or other designations are also included. The alphabetical index of CPT® PLUS is unique in that both indexes to specific page numbers and indexes to CPT code numbers are included.

HOW TO USE THE ALPHABETICAL INDEX

When using the alphabetical index to locate CPT codes, use the following search sequence:

- *Look for the CPT HEADING for the general category of surgical procedure(s) or medical service(s) or TOPIC for instructional and/or explanatory information.*
- *Look for the CPT Sub-heading for the organ system(s) involved or service(s) performed or the TOPIC sub-heading for the instructional or explanatory issue. Scan the index listings to determine if the specific procedure or service or topic is listed.*
- *For CPT codes, use the thumb-tab indexes to locate the appropriate CPT code section. If the specific procedure or service was listed in the index, locate the procedure or service in the CPT code section and verify the full description of the CPT code before using. If the specific procedure or service was not listed in the index, first locate the organ system and/or medical service sub-heading and then review the CPT code section until you locate the specific procedure and/or service.*
- *For instructional and/or explanatory topics, turn to the page number specified in the alphabetical index.*
- *Alternately, look for SYNONYMS, HOMONYMS, EPONYMS or ACRONYMS.*

This page intentionally left blank.

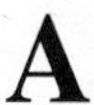

Abbe-Estlander procedure ~ 40527, 40761
Abdomen
- abdominal wall
  - removal
    - mesh ~ 11008
    - prosthesis ~ 11008
  - repair hernia ~ 49491-49496, 49501, 49507, 49521, 49590
  - tumor excision ~ 22900
  - unlisted services and procedures ~ 22999
- abscess
  - incision and drainage ~ 49020, 49040
    - open ~ 49040
    - percutaneous ~ 49021
- angiography ~ 74175, 75635
- artery ligation ~ 37617
- biopsy ~ 49000
- bypass graft ~ 35907
- cannula/catheter removal ~ 49422
- celiotomy for staging ~ 49220
- CT scan ~ 74150-74175, 75635
- cyst destruction/excision ~ 49200-49201
- drainage fluid ~ 49080-49081
- ectopic pregnancy ~ 59130
- endometrioma destruction/excision ~ 49200-49201
- exploration ~ 49000-49002
  - blood vessel ~ 35840
  - staging ~ 58960
- incision ~ 49000
  - staging ~ 58960
- incision and drainage pancreatitis ~ 48000
- infraumbilical panniculectomy ~ 15830
- injection
  - air ~ 49400
  - contrast material ~ 49400
- insertion
  - catheter ~ 49419-49421
  - venous shunt ~ 49425
- intraperitoneal
  - catheter removal ~ 49422
  - shunt
    - ligation ~ 49428
    - removal ~ 49429
- laparotomy, staging ~ 49220
- magnetic resonance imaging (MRI) ~ 74181-74183
- needle biopsy mass ~ 49180
- peritoneocentesis ~ 49080-49081
- radical resection ~ 51597
- repair
  - blood vessel ~ 35221
    - with other graft ~ 35281
    - with vein graft ~ 35251
  - hernia ~ 49491-49525, 49560-49587
  - suture ~ 49900
- revision venous shunt ~ 49426

Abdomen ~ *continued*
- suture ~ 49900
- tumor destruction/excision ~ 49200-49201
- ultrasound ~ 76700-76705
- unlisted services and procedures ~ 49999
- wound exploration penetrating ~ 20102
- X-ray ~ 74000-74022

Abdominal aorta ~ *see* aorta, abdominal
Abdominal aortic aneurysm ~ 0078T-0081T, 34800-34805, 34825-34832, 35081-35103, 75952, 75953
Abdominal deliveries ~ *see* cesarean delivery
Abdominal hysterectomy ~ *see* hysterectomy, abdominal
Abdominal lymphangiogram ~ 75805, 75807
Abdominal paracentesis ~ *see* abdomen, drainage
Abdominal radiographies ~ 74000-74022
Abdominal wall
- debridement, infected ~ 11005-11006
- reconstruction ~ 49905
- removal
  - mesh ~ 11008
  - prosthesis ~ 11008
- surgery ~ 22999
- tumor excision ~ 22900

Abdominohysterectomy ~ *see* hysterectomy, abdominal
Abdominopelvic amputation ~ 27290
Abdominoplasty
- excision ~ 15847

Ablation
- anal
  - polyp ~ 46615
  - tumor ~ 46615
- bone tumor ~ 20982
- colon tumor ~ 45339
- CT scan guidance ~ 77013
- endometrial ~ 58353-58356, 58563
- endometrium ultrasound guidance ~ 58356
- heart arrthymogenic focus ~ 93650-93652
- liver tumor
  - laparoscopic ~ 47370-47371
  - open ~ 47380-47382
- lung
  - tumor
    - radiofrequency ~ 32998
- pulmonary tumor ~ 32998
- radiofrequency ~ 32998
- magnetic resonance guidance ~ 77022
- parenchymal tissue
  - CT scan guidance ~ 77013
- prostate ~ 55873
- renal cyst ~ 50541
- renal mass ~ 50542
- turbinate mucosa ~ 30801-30802
- ultrasound
  - guidance ~ 76940
  - uterine tumor ~ 0071T-0072T
- uterine tumor, ultrasound, focused ~ 0071T-0072T
- vein, endovenous ~ 36475-36479

Abortion
incomplete ~ 59812
induced by
dilation and curettage ~ 59840
dilation and evacuation ~ 59841
saline ~ 59850-59851
vaginal suppositories ~ 59855-59856
missed
first trimester ~ 59820
second trimester ~ 59821
septic ~ 59830
spontaneous ~ 59812
therapeutic
by saline ~ 59850
with dilation and curettage ~ 59851
with hysterectomy ~ 59852
with hysterectomy ~ 59100, 59852, 59857
Abrasion
skin
chemical peel ~ 15788-15793
dermabrasion ~ 15780-15783
lesion ~ 15786-15787
salabrasion ~ 15810-15811
Abscess
abdomen ~ 49040-49041
incision and drainage
open ~ 49040
percutaneous ~ 49021
anal, incision and drainage ~ 46045-46050
ankle ~ 27603
appendix, incision and drainage ~ 44900
open ~ 44900
percutaneous ~ 44901
arm, lower ~ 25028
excision ~ 25145
incision and drainage ~ 25035
arm, upper, incision and drainage ~ 23930-23935
auditory canal, external ~ 69020
Bartholin's gland, incision and drainage ~ 56420
bladder, incision and drainage ~ 51080
brain
drainage ~ 61150-61151
excision ~ 61514, 61522
incision and drainage ~ 61320-61321
breast, incision and drainage ~ 19020
carpals, incision, deep ~ 25035
clavicle sequestrectomy ~ 23170
drainage, with X-ray ~ 75989
ear, external
complicated ~ 69005
simple ~ 69000
elbow, incision and drainage ~ 23930-23935
epididymis, incision and drainage ~ 54700
excision
olecranon process ~ 24138
radius ~ 24136
ulna ~ 24138
eyelid, incision and drainage ~ 67700
facial bones, excision ~ 21026
finger ~ 26010-26011

Abscess ~ *continued*
incision and drainage ~ 26034
foot, incision ~ 28005
gums, incision and drainage ~ 41800
hand, incision and drainage ~ 26034
hematoma, incision and drainage ~ 27603
hip, incision and drainage ~ 26990-26992
humeral head ~ 23174
humerus
excision ~ 24134
incision and drainage ~ 23935
kidney incision and drainage ~ 50020
open ~ 50020
percutaneous ~ 50021
leg, lower,incision and drainage ~ 27603
liver ~ 47010
drainage, open ~ 47010
injection ~ 47015
repair ~ 47300
localization, nuclear medicine ~ 78806-78807
lung, percutaneous drainage ~ 32200-32201
lymph node, incision and drainage ~ 38300-38305
lymphocele drainage ~ 49062
mandible, excision ~ 21025
mouth, incision and drainage ~ 40800-40801, 41005-41009, 41015-41018
nasal septum, incision and drainage ~ 30020
neck, incision and drainage ~ 21501-21502
ovarian incision and drainage ~ 58820-58822
abdominal approach ~ 58822
vaginal approach ~ 58820
ovary, drainage, percutaneous ~ 58823
palate, incision and drainage ~ 42000
paraurethral gland, incision and drainage ~ 53060
parotid gland drainage ~ 42300-42305
pelvic, drainage, percutaneous ~ 58823
pelvis, incision and drainage ~ 26990-26992, 45000
pericolic, drainage, percutaneous ~ 58823
perineum, incision and drainage ~ 56405
perirenal or renal
drainage ~ 50020-50021
percutaneous ~ 50021
peritoneum
incision and drainage
open ~ 49020
percutaneous ~ 49021
prostate
incision and drainage ~ 55720-55725
transurethral drainage ~ 52700
radius, incision, deep ~ 25035
rectum, incision and drainage ~ 45005-45020, 46040, 46060
retroperitoneal ~ 49060-49061
drainage
open ~ 49060
percutaneous ~ 49061
salivary gland, drainage ~ 42300-42320
scapula, sequestrectomy ~ 23172

Abscess ~ *continued*
scrotum, incision and drainage ~ 54700, 55100
shoulder, drainage ~ 23030
Skene's gland, incision and drainage ~ 53060
skin
incision and drainage ~ 10060-10061
puncture aspiration ~ 10160
soft tissue, incision ~ 20000-20005
subdiaphragmatic ~ 49040-49041
sublingual gland, drainage ~ 42310-42320
submaxillary gland, drainage ~ 42310-42320
subphrenic ~ 49040-49041
testis, incision and drainage ~ 54700
thoracostomy ~ 32020
thorax, incision and drainage ~ 21501-21502
throat, incision and drainage ~ 42700-42725
tongue, incision and drainage ~ 41000-41006
tonsil, incision and drainage ~ 42700
ulna, incision, deep ~ 25035
urethra, incision and drainage ~ 53040
uvula, incision and drainage ~ 42000
vagina, incision and drainage ~ 57010
vulva, incision and drainage ~ 56405
wrist
excision ~ 25145
incision and drainage ~ 25028, 25035
X-ray ~ 76080
Absorptiometry
dual energy
body composition ~ 0028T
bone
appendicular ~ 77081
axial skeleton ~ 77080
vertebral ~ 77082
dual photon, bone ~ 78351
radiographic, photodensity ~ 77083
single photon, bone ~ 78350
Absorption spectrophotometry, atomic ~ 82190
Accessory nerve, spinal ~ 63191
Accessory, toes ~ 28344
ACE (angiotensin converting enzyme) ~ 82164
Acetabuloplasty ~ 27120-27122
Acetabulum
fracture
closed treatment ~ 27220-27222
open treatment ~ 27226-27228
with manipulation ~ 27222
without manipulation ~ 27220
reconstruction ~ 27120
with resection, femoral head ~ 27122
tumor, excision ~ 27076
Acetaldehyde, blood ~ 82000
Acetaminophen, urine ~ 82003
Acetic anhydrides ~ 84600
Acetone, blood or urine ~ 82009-82010
Acetone body ~ 82009-82010
Acetylcholinesterase, blood or urine ~ 82013
AcG ~ 85220
Achilles tendon
incision ~ 27605-27606
lengthening ~ 27612
repair ~ 27650-27654
Achillotomy ~ 27605-27606
Acid(s)
adenylic ~ 82030
amino ~ 82127-82139
aminolevulinic ~ see aminolevulinic acid (ALA)
ascorbic ~ 82180
bile ~ 82239
deoxyribonucleic ~ 86225-86226
fatty ~ see fatty acid
folic ~ 82747
gastric ~ 82926-82928
glycocholic ~ 82240
guanylic ~ 83008
lactic ~ 83605
n-acetylneuraminic ~ 84275
n-acetylneuraminic ~ 84275
phenylethylbarbituric ~ 82205
uric ~ see uric acid
Acidity/alkalinity ~ *see* pH
Acid diethylamide, lysergic ~ 80102-80103, 80299
Acid fast bacilli (AFB), culture ~ 87116
Acid fast stain ~ 88312
Acid perfusion test, esophagus ~ 91012, 91030
Acid phosphatase ~ 84060-84066
Acid probes, nucleic ~ *see* nucleic acid probes
Acid reflux test, esophagus ~ 91034-91038
Acne surgery
incision and drainage
abscess ~ 10060-10061
comedones ~ 10040
cyst ~ 10040
milia, multiple ~ 10040
pustules ~ 10040
Acne treatment
abrasion ~ 15786-15787
chemical peel ~ 15788-15793
cryotherapy ~ 17340
dermabrasion ~ 15780-15783
exfoliation
chemical ~ 17360
salabrasion ~ 15810-15811
Acoustic evoked brain stem potential ~ 92585-92586
Acoustic neuroma (*see also* brainstem, skull base surgery) ~ 61510, 61518, 61520-61521, 61526-61530, 61545, 62164
Acoustic recording, heart sounds, with computer analysis ~ 0068T-0070T
Acromioclavicular joint, arthrocentesis ~ 20605
arthrotomy ~ 23044
with biopsy ~ 23101
dislocation ~ 23540-23552
open treatment ~ 23550-23552
X-ray ~ 73050
Acromion,excision, shoulder ~ 23130

Acromionectomy, partial ~ 23130
Acromioplasty ~ 23415-23420
partial ~ 23130
ACTH releasing factor ~ 80412
Actinomyces, antibody ~ 86602
Actinomycosis ~ 86000
Actinomycotic infection ~ 86000
Actinotherapy ~ see dermatology ~ 96900
Activated factor X ~ 85260
Activated partial thomboplastin time ~ 85730-85732
Activation, lymphocyte ~ 86353
Activities of daily living ~ *see* physical medicine/therapy/occupational therapy
Activity, glomerular procoagulant ~ *see* thromboplastin
Acupuncture
with electrical stimulation ~ 97813-97814
without electrical stimulation ~ 97810-97811
Acute poliomyelitis ~ *see* polio
Acylcarnitines ~ 82016-82017
Adamantinoma, pituitary ~ *see* craniopharyngioma
Addam operation ~ 26040-26045
Adductor tenotomy of hip ~ 27000-27003
Adenoidectomy ~ 42820-42821, 42830-42836
Adenoids
excision ~ 42830-42836
with tonsils ~ 42820-42821
unlisted services and procedures ~ 42999
Adenoma
pancreas, excision ~ 48120
thyroid gland excision ~ 60200
Adenosine 3'5' monophosphate ~ 82030
Adenosine diphosphate, blood ~ 82030
Adenosine monophosphate (AMP), blood ~ 82030
Adenovirus
antibody ~ 86603
antigen detection
enzyme immunoassay ~ 87301
immunofluorescense ~ 87260
Adenovirus vaccine ~ *see* vaccines
Adenylic acid ~ *see* adenosine monophosphate (AMP)
ADH (antidiuretic hormone) ~ 84588
Adhesions
epidural ~ 0027T, 62263-62264
eye
corneovitreal ~ 65880
incision
anterior segment ~ 65860-65870
posterior segment ~ 65875
intermarginal, construction ~ 67880
transposition of tarsal plate ~ 67882
intestinal, enterolysis ~ 44005
laparoscopic ~ 44200
intracranial, lysis ~ 62161
intrauterine, lysis ~ 58559
labial, lysis ~ 56441
lungs, lysis ~ 32124
pelvic, lysis ~ 58660, 58662, 58740
Adhesions ~ *continued*
penile, lysis, post-circumcision ~ 54162
preputial, lysis ~ 54450
urethral, lysis ~ 53500
Adipectomy ~ *see* lipectomy
ADL ~ *see* activities of daily living
Administration immunization
each additional vaccine/toxoid ~ 90472, 90474
with counseling ~ 90466, 90468
one vaccine/toxoid ~ 90471, 90473
with counseling ~ 90465, 90467
ADP ~ *see* adenosine diphosphate
ADP phosphocreatine phosphotransferase ~ *see* CPK
Adrenal cortex hormone ~ *see* corticosteroids
Adrenal gland
biopsy ~ 60540-60545
excision
laparoscopy ~ 60650
retroperitoneal tumor ~ 60545
exploration ~ 60540-60545
nuclear medicine, imaging ~ 78075
Adrenal medulla ~ *see* medulla
Adrenalectomy ~ 60540
anesthesia ~ 00866
laparoscopic ~ 50545
Adrenalin ~ 80424, 82382-82384
blood ~ 82383
urine ~ 82384
Adrenaline-noradrenaline
testing ~ 82382-82384
Adrenocorticotropic hormone (ACTH) ~ 80400-80406, 80412, 80418, 82024
blood or urine ~ 82024
stimulation panel ~ 80400-80406
Adrenogenital syndrome ~ 56805, 57335
Adult T cell leukemia lymphoma virus I ~ *see* HTLV I
Advanced life support ~ 99281-99288
physician direction ~ 99288
Advancement
genioglossus ~ 21199
tendon foot ~ 28238
Advancement flap ~ 14000-14350
Aerosol inhalation ~ *see* pulmonology, therapeutic
pentamidine ~ 94642
AFB ~ *see* acid fast bacilli
Afferent nerve ~ *see* sensory nerve
AFP ~ *see* alpha-fetoprotein
After hours medical services ~ 99050-99054
Agents, anticoagulant ~ 85300-85305, 85307
Agglutinin
cold ~ 86156-86157
febrile ~ 86000
Aggregation, platelet ~ 85576
AHG ~ 85210-85293
AICD (pacing cardioverter-defibrillator) ~ *see* defibrillator, heart; pacemaker, heart
Aid, hearing ~ *see* hearing aid
AIDS antibodies ~ 86689, 86701-86703

AIDS virus ~ *see* HIV-1
Akin operation ~ 28296-28299
ALA ~ *see* aminolevulinic acid
Alanine 2 oxoglutarate aminotransferase ~ 84460
Alanine amino (ALT) ~ 84460
Alanine transaminase ~ 84460
Albarran test ~ 89235
Albumin
ischemia modified ~ 82045
serum ~ 82040
urine ~ 82042-82044
Alcohol
breath ~ 82075
ethyl
blood ~ 82055
urine ~ 82055
ethylene glycol ~ 82693
dehydrogenase ~ 84588
isopropyl ~ 84600
methyl ~ 84600
Aldolase, blood ~ 82085
Aldosterone
blood ~ 82088
suppression evaluation ~ 80408
urine ~ 82088
Alimentary canal ~ *see* gastrointestinal tract
Alkaline phosphatase ~ 84075-84080
leukocyte ~ 85540
WBC ~ 85540
Alkaloids ~ *see* specific drug
urine ~ 82101
Allergen bronchial provocation tests ~ 95070-95071
Allergen challenge, endobronchial ~ 95070-95071
Allergen immunotherapy
allergen
prescription/ supply/injection ~ 95120-95125
with extract supply ~ 95144
injection ~ 95115-95117
antigens ~ 95144
IgE ~ 86003-86005
IgG ~ 86001
insect venom
prescription/supply ~ 95145-95149
prescription/supply/injection ~ 95130-95134
prescription/supply ~ 95165
insect, whole body ~ 95170
rapid desensitization ~ 95180
Allergy services/procedures ~ 95004-95199
education and counseling ~ 99201-99215
unlisted services and procedures ~ 95199
Allergy tests
challenge test
bronchial ~ 95070-95071
ingestion ~ 95075
eye allergy ~ 95060
food allergy ~ 95075
intradermal
allergen extract ~ 95024-95028
biologicals ~ 95015
Allergy tests ~ *continued*
drugs ~ 95015
incremental ~ 95027
venoms ~ 95015
nasal mucous membrane test ~ 95065
nose allergy ~ 95065
patch
application tests ~ 95044
photo patch ~ 95052
photosensitivity ~ 95056
skin tests
allergen extract ~ 95004
biologicals ~ 95010
drugs ~ 95010
venoms ~ 95010
Allogeneic donor, lymphocyte infusion ~ 38242
Allogeneic transplantation ~ *see* homograft
Allograft
aortic valve ~ 33406, 33413
bone, structural ~ 20931
cartilage, knee ~ 27415
lung transplant ~ 32850
skin ~ 15350-15351
spine surgery
morselized ~ 20930
structural ~ 20931
Allograft preparation
heart ~ 33933, 33944
intestines ~ 44715-44721
kidney ~ 50323-50329
liver ~ 47143-47147
lung ~ 32855-32856, 33933
pancrease ~ 48551-48552
renal ~ 50323-50329
Allotransplantation
intestines ~ 44135-44136
renal ~ 50360-50365
removal ~ 50370
Almen test ~ 82270
Alpha-1 antitrypsin ~ 82103-82104, 99565
Alpha-2 antiplasmin ~ 85410
Alpha-fetoprotein
amniotic fluid ~ 82106
serum ~ 82105, 82107
Alphatocopherol ~ 84446
ALT ~ 84460
Altemeier procedure ~ (*see* anus) 45130-45135
Aluminum, blood ~ 82108
Alveolafracture
closed treatment ~ 21421
open treatment ~ 21422-21423
Alveolar cleft
ungrafted bilateral ~ 21147
ungrafted unilateral ~ 21146
Alveolar nerve
avulsion ~ 64738
incision ~ 64738
transection ~ 64738

Alveolar ridge fracture
closed treatment ~ 21440
open treatment ~ 21445
Alveolectomy ~ 41830
Alveoloplasty ~ 41874
Alveolus, excision ~ 41830
Amide, procaine ~ *see* procainamide
Amikacin, assay ~ 80150
Amine, vaginal fluid ~ 82120
Amino acids ~ 82127-82139
Aminolevulinic acid (ALA), blood or urine ~ 82135
Aminotransferase ~ *see* transaminase
Aminotransferase, alanine ~ 84460
Aminotransferase, aspartate ~ 84450
Amitriptyline, assay ~ 80152
Ammonia
blood ~ 82140
urine ~ 82140
Amniocenteses ~ 59000
with amniotic fluid reduction ~ 59001
induced abortion ~ 59850
with dilation and curettage ~ 59851
with dilation and evacuation ~ 59851
with hysterectomy ~ 59852
Amnioinfusion, transabdominal ~ 59070
Amnion ~ 59001
amniocentesis ~ 59000
with amniotic fluid reduction ~ 59001
amnioinfusion, transabdominal ~ 59070
Amniotic fluid
alpha-fetoprotein ~ 82106
scan ~ 82143
testing ~ 83661, 83663-83664
Amniotic membrane ~ 59001
Amobarbital ~ 82205
AMP ~ 82030
AMP, cyclic ~ 82030
Amphetamine, blood or urine ~ 82145
Amputation ~ *see* radical resection; replantation
ankle ~ 27888
arm, lower ~ 25900-25905, 25915
revision ~ 25907-25909
arm, upper ~ 24900-24920
and shoulder ~ 23900-23921
revision ~ 24925-24930
with implant ~ 24931-24935
cervix, total ~ 57530
ear
partial ~ 69110
total ~ 69120
finger ~ 26910-26952
foot ~ 28800-28805
hand at metacarpal ~ 25927
at wrist ~ 25920
revision ~ 25922
revision ~ 25924, 25929-25931
interpelviabdominal ~ 27290
interthoracoscapular ~ 23900
leg, lower ~ 27598, 27880-27882
revision ~ 27884-27886

Amputation ~ *continued*
leg, upper ~ 27590-27592
at hip ~ 27290-27295
revision ~ 27594-27596
metacarpal ~ 26910
metatarsal ~ 28810
nose ~ *see* resection, nose
penis
partial ~ 54120
radical ~ 54130-54135
total ~ 54125
thumb ~ 26910-26952
toe ~ 28810-28825
tuft of distal phalanx ~ 11752
upper extremity ~ 24940
cineplasty ~ 24940
Amylase
blood ~ 82150
urine ~ 82150
ANA ~ 86038-86039
Anabolic steroid ~ *see* androstenedione
Anal abscess ~ *see* abscess, anal
Anal bleeding ~ *see* anus, hemorrhage
Anal fistula ~ *see* fistula, anal
Anal fistulectomy ~ 46288, 46706
Anal fistulotomy ~ 46270, 46280
Anal sphincter
dilation ~ 45905
incision ~ 46080
Anal ulceration ~ *see* anus, fissure
Analgesia ~ *see* anesthesia; sedation 99141-99142
Analgesic cutaneous electrostimulation ~ 64550
Analysis
computer data ~ 99090
electroencephalogram, digital ~ 95957
electronic
drug infusion pump ~ 62367-62368
pacing cardioverter-defibrillator ~ see pacemaker, heart ~ 93741-93744
pulse generator ~ 95970-95971
physiologic data, remote ~ 99091
protein, tissue western blot ~ 88372
semen, sperm isolation ~ 89260-89261
spectrum ~ *see* spectrophotometry
Anaspadias ~ *see* epispadias
Anastomosis
aorta-pulmonary artery ~ 33606
arteriovenous fistula
direct ~ 36821
with bypass graft ~ 35686
with graft ~ 36825-36830, 36832
artery
to aorta ~ 33606
to artery, cranial ~ 61711
bile duct
to bile duct ~ 47800
to intestines ~ 47760, 47780
bile duct to gastrointestinal ~ 47785
bladder, to intestine ~ 51960

Anastomosis ~ *continued*
broncho-bronchial ~ 32486
caval to mesenteric ~ 37160
colorectal ~ 44620
epididymis
to vas deferens
bilateral ~ 54901
unilateral ~ 54900
excision trachea ~ 31780-31781
fallopian tube ~ 58750
gallbladder to intestines ~ 47720-47740
hepatic duct ~ see hepatic duct, anastomosis
hepatic duct to intestines ~ 47765, 47802
ileo-anal ~ 45113
intestines
colo-anal ~ 45119
cystectomy ~ 51590
enterocystoplasty ~ 51960
resection, laparoscopic ~ 44202-44205
intestine to intestine ~ 44130
intrahepatic portosystemic ~ 37182-37183
jejunum ~ 43825
lacrimal sac to conjunctival sac ~ see conjunctivorhinostomy
microvascular, free transfer, jejunum ~ 43496
nerve
facial to hypoglossal ~ 64868
facial to phrenic ~ 64870
oviduct ~ 58750
pancreas ~ see pancreas, anastomosis
pancreas to intestines ~ 48520-48540, 48548
portocaval ~ 37140
pulmonary ~ 33606
renoportal ~ 37145
splenorenal ~ 37180-37181
stomach ~ 43825
to duodenum ~ 43810, 43855
revision ~ 43850
to jejunum ~ 43820, 43860-43865
tubotubal ~ 58750
ureter
to bladder ~ 50780-50785
to colon ~ 50810-50815
removal ~ 50830
to intestine ~ 50800, 50820-50825
removal ~ 50830
to kidney ~ 50727-50750
to ureter ~ 50727, 50760-50770
vein, saphenopopliteal ~ 34530
vein to vein ~ 37140-37160, 37182-37183
Anatomic pathology services ~ 88000-88099
Anderson tibial lengthening ~ *see* ankle 27715
Androstanediol glucuronide ~ 82154
Androstanolone ~ 82651
Androstenedione, blood or urine ~ 82157
Androstenolone ~ 82626
Androsterone, blood or urine ~ 82160

Anesthesia ~ 00100-01999
Abbe-Estlander procedure ~ 00102
abdomen
abdominal wall ~ 00700, 00730, 00800-00802, 00820, 00836
Halsted repair ~ 00750-00756
blood vessels ~ 00770, 00880-00882
endoscopy ~ 00740, 00810
extraperitoneal ~ 00860-00862, 00866-00870
hernia repair ~ 00830-00836
Halsted repair ~ 00750-00756
intraperitoneal ~ 00790-00797, 00840-00842
abdominoperineal resection ~ 00844
abortion, induced ~ 01964
Achilles tendon repair ~ 01472
acromioclavicular joint ~ 01620
adrenalectomy ~ 00866
amniocentesis ~ 00842
aneurysm
axillary-brachial ~ 01652
knee ~ 01444
popliteal artery ~ 01444
angiography ~ 01920
ankle ~ 00400, 01462-01522
anorectal procedure ~ 00902
anus ~ 00902
arm
lower ~ 00400, 01810-01820, 01830-01860
upper ~ 00400, 01710-01782
arrhythmias ~ 00410
arteriography ~ 01916
arteriovenous fistula ~ 01432, 01784
arthroplasty
hip ~ 01214-01215
knee ~ 01402
arthroscopic procedures
ankle ~ 01464
elbow ~ 01732-01740
foot ~ 01464
hip ~ 01202
knee ~ 01382, 01400
shoulder ~ 01622-01630
wrist ~ 01829-01830
auditory canal, external, removal foreign body ~ 69205
axilla ~ 00400, 01610-01682
back skin ~ 00300
Batch-Spittler-McFaddin operation ~ 01404
biopsy ~ 00100
liver ~ 00702
bladder ~ 00870, 00912
brain ~ 00210-00218, 00220-00222
breast ~ 00402-00406
bronchi ~ 00542
intrathoracic repair of trauma ~ 00548
reconstruction ~ 00539
bronchoscopy ~ 00520
burns
debridement and/or excision ~ 01951-01953
dressings and/or debridement ~ 16010-16015
burr hole ~ 00214

Anesthesia ~ *continued*
bypass graft
leg, lower ~ 01500
leg, upper ~ 01270
shoulder, axillary ~ 01654-01656
cardiac catheterization ~ 01920
cast, knee ~ 01420
cast application
forearm, wrist and hand ~ 01860
leg ~ 01490
pelvis ~ 01130
shoulder ~ 01680-01682
central venous circulation ~ 00532
cervical cerclage ~ 00948
cervix ~ 00948
cesarean delivery ~ 01961, 01963
chemonucleolysis ~ 00634
chest ~ 00400-00406, 00410, 00470-00474, 00522, 00530-00539, 00542, 00546-00550
chest skin ~ 00400
childbirth
cesarean delivery ~ 01961, 01963, 01968-01969
external cephalic version ~ 01958
vaginal delivery ~ 01960, 01967
clavicle ~ 00450-00454
cleft lip repair ~ 00102
cleft palate repair ~ 00172
colpectomy ~ 00942
colporrhaphy ~ 00942
colpotomy ~ 00942
corneal transplant ~ 00144
cranioplasty ~ 00215
culdoscopy ~ 00950
cystectomy ~ 00864
cystolithotomy ~ 00870
cystourethroscopy
local ~ 52265
spinal ~ 52260
decortication ~ 00542
defibrillator ~ 00534, 00560
diaphragm ~ 00540-00541
disarticulation
hip ~ 01212
knee ~ 01404
shoulder ~ 01634
diskography ~ 01905
dressing change ~ 15852
drug administration, epidural or subarachnoid ~ 01996
ear ~ 00120-00126
elbow ~ 00400, 01710-01782
electrocoagulation, intracranial nerve ~ 00222
electroconvulsive therapy ~ 00104
embolectomy
arm, upper ~ 01772
femoral ~ 01274
femoral artery ~ 01274
forearm, wrist and hand ~ 01842
leg, lower ~ 01502

Anesthesia ~ *continued*
endoscopy
arm, lower ~ 01830
gastrointestinal ~ 00740
intestines ~ 00810
uterus ~ 00952
vagina ~ 00950
esophagus ~ 00320, 00500
external cephalic version ~ 01958
external fixation system
adjustment/revision ~ 20693
removal ~ 20694
eye ~ 00140-00148
cornea ~ 00144
iridectomy ~ 00147
iris ~ 00147
eyelid ~ 00103
facial bones ~ 00190-00192
fallopian tube, ligation ~ 00851
femoral artery, ligation ~ 01272
femur ~ 01220-01234, 01340-01360
fibula ~ 01390-01392
foot ~ 00400, 01462-01522
forearm ~ 00400, 01810-01820, 01830-01860
Fowler-Stephens orchiopexy ~ 00930
gastrocnemius recession ~ 01474
gastrointestinal endoscopy ~ 00740
genitalia
female ~ 00940-00952, 01958-01969
male ~ 00920-00938
great vessels of chest ~ 00560-00563
hand ~ 00400, 01810-01820, 01830-01860
Harrington rod technique ~ 00670
head ~ 00222, 00300
muscles ~ 00300
nerves ~ 00300
heart ~ 00560-00566, 00580
coronary artery bypass grafting ~ 00566
electrophysiology/ablation ~ 00537
transplant ~ 00580
hepatectomy, partial ~ 00792
hernia repair, abdomen
lower ~ 00830-00836
upper ~ 00750-00752, 00756
hip ~ 01200-01215
humerus ~ 01620, 01730, 01742-01744, 01758
hysterectomy ~ 01962
cesarean ~ 01963, 01969
radical ~ 00846
vaginal ~ 00944
hysterosalpingography ~ 00952
hysteroscopy ~ 00952
induced abortion ~ 01964
inferior vena cava ligation ~ 00882
injections, nerve ~ 01991-01992
integumentary system
anterior trunk ~ 00400
arm, upper ~ 00400
axilla ~ 00400
elbow ~ 00400
extremity ~ 00400

Anesthesia ~ *continued*
forearm ~ 00400
hand ~ 00400
head ~ 00300
knee ~ 00400
leg, lower ~ 00400
leg, upper ~ 00400
neck ~ 00300
perineum ~ 00400
popliteal area ~ 00400
posterior pelvis ~ 00300
posterior trunk ~ 00300
shoulder ~ 00400
wrist ~ 00400
intestines, endoscopy ~ 00810
intracranial procedures ~ 00210-00218, 00220-00222
intraoral procedures ~ 00170-00176
intrathoracic procedures
bronchi ~ 00539, 00548
trachea ~ 00539, 00548
intrathoracic system ~ 00500, 00520-00529, 00530-00539, 00540-00548, 00550, 00560-00566, 00580
iridectomy ~ 00147
Keen operation ~ 00604
kidney ~ 00862, 00868, 00872-00873
knee ~ 00400, 01320-01444
knee skin ~ 00400
laminectomy ~ 00604
laparoscopy ~ 00790-00792, 00840
larynx ~ 00320, 00326
leg
lower ~ 00400, 01462-01522
upper ~ 01200-01274
lens ~ 00142
Leriche operation ~ 00622
life support for organ donor ~ 01990
ligation, fallopian tube ~ 00851
lithotripsy ~ 00872-00873
liver ~ 00702, 00796
transplant ~ 00796
liver hemorrhage ~ 00792
lumbar puncture ~ 00635
lungs ~ 00522, 00539, 00540-00548
transplant ~ 00580
lymphadenectomy ~ 00934-00936
lymphatic system ~ 00320
mammoplasty ~ 00402
marcellation operation ~ 00944
mediastinoscopy ~ 00528-00529
mediastinum ~ 00528-00529, 00540-00541
mouth ~ 00170-00172
myelography ~ 01905
myringotomy ~ 69421
neck ~ 00300, 00320-00322, 00350-00352
nephrectomy ~ 00862
neuraxial
cesarean delivery ~ 01968-01969
labor ~ 01967-01969
vaginal delivery ~ 01967
neurectomy ~ 01180-01190

Anesthesia ~ *continued*
nose ~ 00160-00164
removal, foreign body ~ 30310
omphalocele ~ 00754
ophthalmoscopy ~ 00148
orchiectomy ~ 00926-00928
orchiopexy ~ 00930
Torek procedure ~ 00930
organ harvesting, brain dead patient ~ 01990
osteoplasty, tibia/fibula ~ 01484
osteotomy
humerus ~ 01742
tibia/fibula ~ 01484
other procedures ~ 01990, 01996-01999
otoscopy ~ 00124
pacemaker insertion ~ 00530
pacing cardioverter/defibrillator ~ 00534
pancreas ~ 00794
pancreatectomy ~ 00794
panniculectomy ~ 00802
patella ~ 01390-01392
pectus excavatum ~ 00474
pelvic exenteration ~ 00848
pelvis ~ 00400, 00865, 01112-01190
amputation ~ 01140
bone ~ 01120
bone marrow ~ 01112
examination ~ 57400
extraperitoneal ~ 00864
intraperitoneal ~ 00844-00848
repair ~ 01173
skin ~ 00300, 00400
penis ~ 00932-00938
pericardial sac ~ 00560-00563
perineum ~ 00904-00908
pharynx ~ 00174-00176
phleborrhaphy
arm, upper ~ 01782
forearm, wrist, and hand ~ 01852
pleura ~ 00540-00541
needle biopsy ~ 00522
pneumocentesis ~ 00524
popliteal area ~ 00400, 01320, 01430-01444
prognathism ~ 00192
prostate ~ 00865, 00908, 00914
prostatectomy
perineal ~ 00908
radical ~ 00865
Walsh modified radical ~ 00865
radiologic procedures ~ 01905-01922
arterial, therapeutic ~ 01924-01926
venous/lymphatic, therapeutic ~ 01930-01933
renal procedures ~ 00862
repair of skull ~ 00215
replacement
ankle ~ 01486
elbow ~ 01760
hip ~ 01212-01215
knee ~ 01402
shoulder ~ 01638
wrist ~ 01832

Anesthesia ~ *continued*
restriction, gastric
for obesity ~ 00797
retropharyngeal tumor excision ~ 00174
rib resection ~ 00470-00474
sacroiliac joint ~ 01160-01170, 27096
salivary glands ~ 00100
Scheie procedure ~ 00147
sedation, analgesia ~ 99141-99142
seminal vesicles ~ 00922
shoulder ~ 00400, 00450-00454, 01610-01682
dislocation, closed treatment ~ 23655
shunt, spinal fluid ~ 00220
sinuses, accessory ~ 00160-00164
skull ~ 00190
skull fracture, elevation ~ 00215
special circumstances
emergency ~ 99140
extreme age ~ 99100
hypotension ~ 99135
hypothermia ~ 99116
spinal instrumentation ~ 00670
spinal manipulation ~ 00640
spine and spinal cord ~ 00600-00604, 00620-00670
cervical ~ 00600-00604, 00640-00670
injection ~ 62310-62319
lumbar ~ 00630-00635, 00640, 00670
thoracic ~ 00620-00626, 00640, 00670
vascular ~ 00670
sternoclavicular joint ~ 01620
sternum ~ 00550
stomach, restriction, for obesity ~ 00797
Strayer procedure ~ 01474
subdural taps ~ 00212
suture removal ~ 15850-15851
sympathectomy
lumbar ~ 00632
thoracolumbar ~ 00622
symphysis pubis ~ 01160-01170
tenodesis ~ 01716
tenoplasty ~ 01714
tenotomy ~ 01712
testis ~ 00924-00930
thoracoplasty ~ 00472
thoracoscopy ~ 00528-00529, 00540-00541
thoracotomy ~ 00540-00541
thorax ~ 00400-00406, 00410, 00450-00454, 00470-00474
thromboendarterectomy ~ 01442
thyroid ~ 00320-00322
tibia ~ 01390-01392, 01484
trachea ~ 00320, 00326, 00542
reconstruction ~ 00539
transplantation
cornea ~ 00144
heart ~ 00580
kidney ~ 00868
liver ~ 00796, 01990
lungs ~ 00580
organ harvesting ~ 01990

Anesthesia ~ *continued*
transurethral procedures ~ 00910-00918
tubal ligation ~ 00851
tuffier vaginal hysterectomy ~ 00944
TURP ~ 00914
tympanostomy ~ 00120
tympanotomy ~ 00126
unlisted services and procedures ~ 01999
urethra ~ 00910, 00918-00920, 00942
urethrocystoscopy ~ 00910
urinary bladder ~ 00864, 00870, 00912
urinary tract ~ 00860
uterus ~ 00952
vagina ~ 00940-00942, 00950
dilation ~ 57400
removal, foreign body ~ 57415
vaginal delivery ~ 01960
vas deferens, excision ~ 00921
vascular access ~ 00532
vascular shunt ~ 01844
vascular surgery
abdomen, lower ~ 00880-00882
abdomen, upper ~ 00770
arm, lower ~ 01840-01852
arm, upper ~ 01770-01782
brain ~ 00216
elbow ~ 01770-01782
hand ~ 01840-01852
knee ~ 01430-01444
leg, lower ~ 01500-01522
leg, upper ~ 01260-01274
neck ~ 00350-00352
shoulder ~ 01650-01670
wrist ~ 01840-01852
vasectomy ~ 00921
venography ~ 01916
ventriculography ~ 00214, 01920
vertebral process, fracture/dislocation, closed treatment ~ 22315
vertebroplasty ~ 01905
vitrectomy ~ 00145
vitreoretinal surgery ~ 00145
vitreous body ~ 00145
vulva ~ 00906
vulvectomy ~ 00906
Wertheim operation ~ 00846
wrist ~ 00400, 01810-01860

Aneurysm repair
abdominal aorta ~ 0078T-0081T, 34800-34805, 34825-34832, 35081-35103, 75952-75953
axillary artery ~ 35011-35013
basilar artery ~ 61698, 61702
brachial artery ~ 35011-35013
carotid artery ~ 35001-35002, 61613, 61697, 61700, 61703
celiac artery ~ 35121-35122
femoral artery ~ 35141-35142
hepatic artery ~ 35121-35122
iliac artery ~ 34900, 35131-35132, 75953-75954
innominate artery ~ 35021-35022

Aneurysm repair ~ *continued*
intracranial artery ~ 61705-61708
mesenteric artery ~ 35121-35122
popliteal artery ~ 35151-35152
radial artery ~ 35045
renal artery ~ 35121-35122
splenic artery ~ 35111-35112
subclavian artery ~ 35001-35002, 35021-35022
thoracic aorta ~ 0033T-0040T
thoracoabdominal aorta ~ 33877
ulnar artery ~ 35045
vascular malformation or carotid-cavernous fistula ~ 61710
vertebral artery ~ 61698, 61702
Angel dust ~ 83992
Angina assessment ~ *see* performance measure
Angiocardiographies ~ *see* heart, angiography
Angiography ~ 75600-75605, 75630, 93544
abdomen ~ 74175, 74185, 75635, 75726
abdominal aorta ~ 0080T-0081T, 75635, 75952-75953
adrenal ~ 75731-75733
aorta, injection ~ 93544
arm artery ~ 73206, 75710-75716
arteriovenous shunt ~ 75790
brachial artery ~ 75658
brain ~ 70496
carotid artery ~ 75660-75671
cervical
bilateral ~ 75680
unilateral ~ 75676
chest ~ 71275, 71555
coronary artery ~ 93556
flow velocity measurement during angiography ~ 93571-93572
coronary bypass ~ 93556
endovascular repair ~ 0080T-0081T, 75952-75953
extremity, lower ~ 73725
extremity, upper ~ 73225
fluorescein ~ 92235
head ~ 70496, 70544-70546
artery ~ 75650
heart vessels, injection ~ 93545
indocyanine-green ~ 92240
left heart, injection ~ 93543
leg artery ~ 73706, 75635, 75710-75716
lung, injection ~ 93539-93545
mammary artery ~ 75600-75605, 75630, 75756, 93544
neck ~ 70498, 70547-70549
artery ~ 75650
nuclear medicine ~ 78445
other artery ~ 75774
pelvic artery ~ 72198, 75736
pelvis ~ 72191
pulmonary ~ 75741-75746
renal artery ~ 75722-75724
right heart, injection ~ 93542
spinal artery ~ 75705
spinal canal ~ 72159

Angiography ~ *continued*
thorax ~ 71275
transcatheter therapy
embolization ~ 75894, 75898
infusion ~ 75894, 75898
vertebral ~ 75685
Angioma ~ see lesion, skin
Angioplasties, coronary balloon ~ see percutaneous transluminal angioplasty
Angioplasty
aorta
intraoperative ~ 35452
percutaneous ~ 35472
axillary artery, intraoperative ~ 35458
brachiocephalic artery
intraoperative ~ 35458
percutaneous ~ 35475
coronary artery, percutaneous transluminal ~ 92982-92984
femoral artery
intraoperative ~ 35456
percutaneous ~ 35474
iliac artery
intraoperative ~ 35454
percutaneous ~ 35473
percutaneous transluminal angioplasty ~ 92982-92984
popliteal artery
intraoperative ~ 35456
percutaneous ~ 35474
pulmonary artery, percutaneous transluminal ~ 92997-92998
renal artery
intraoperative ~ 35450
percutaneous ~ 35471
subclavian artery, intraoperative ~ 35458
tibioperoneal artery
intraoperative ~ 35459
percutaneous ~ 35470
transluminal
arterial ~ 75962-75968
venous ~ 75978
venous
intraoperative ~ 35460
percutaneous ~ 35476
visceral artery
intraoperative ~ 35450
percutaneous ~ 35471
Angioscopy, non-coronary vessels ~ 35400
Angiotensin converting enzyme (ACE) ~ 82164
Angiotensin forming enzyme ~ 80408, 80416, 84244
Angiotensin I ~ 84244
riboflavin ~ 84252
Angiotensin II, blood or urine ~ 82163
Angle deformity, reconstruction toe ~ 28313
Anhydride, carbonic ~ 82374
Anhydrides, acetic ~ 84600
Animal inoculation ~ 87001-87003, 87250

Ankle
(see also fibula; leg, lower; tibia; tibiofibular joint)
abscess, incision and drainage ~ 27603
amputation ~ 27888
arthrocentesis ~ 20605
arthrodesis ~ 27870
arthrography ~ 73615
arthroplasty ~ 27700-27703
arthroscopy, surgical ~ 29891-29899
arthrotomy ~ 27610-27612, 27620-27626
biopsy ~ 27613-27614, 27620
bursa, incision and drainage ~ 27604
disarticulation ~ 27889
dislocation
closed treatment ~ 27840-27842
open treatment ~ 27846-27848
exploration ~ 27610, 27620
fracture
lateral ~ 27786-27814
medial ~ 27760-27766, 27808-27814
trimalleolar ~ 27816-27823
fusion ~ 27870
hematoma, incision and drainage ~ 27603
incision ~ 27607
injection, radiologic ~ 27648
lesion excision ~ 27630
magnetic resonance imaging (MRI) ~ 73721-73723
manipulation ~ 27860
removal
foreign body ~ 27610, 27620
implant ~ 27704
loose body ~ 27620
repair
Achilles tendon ~ 27650-27654
ligament ~ 27695-27698
tendon ~ 27612, 27680-27687
strapping ~ 29540
synovium, excision ~ 27625-27626
tenotomy ~ 27605-27606
tumor, excision ~ 27615-27619
unlisted services and procedures ~ 27899
X-ray ~ 73600-73610
with contrast ~ 73615
Ankylosis (surgical) ~ see arthrodesis
Annuloplasty, percutaneous, intradiscal ~ 0062T-0063T, 22526-22527
Anogenital region ~ see perineum
Anoplasty, stricture ~ 46700-46705
Anorectal myectomy ~ 45108
Anorectal procedure, biofeedback ~ 90911
Anorectovaginoplasty ~ 46744-46746
Anoscopy
ablation, polyp/tumor ~ 46615
biopsy ~ 46606
dilation ~ 46604
exploration ~ 46600
hemorrhage ~ 46614
removal
foreign body ~ 46608
polyp/tumor ~ 46610-46612
Antebrachium ~ 20805
Antecedent, plasma thromboplastin ~ 85270
Antepartum care
vaginal delivery ~ 59400, 59425-59426
with cesarean delivery ~ 59510
previous ~ 59610, 59618
Anterior ramus of thoracic nerve ~ see intercostal nerve
Anthrax vaccine ~ 90476-90749
Anthrogon ~ 80418, 80426, 83001
Anti Australia antigens ~ see antibody, hepatitis B
Anti D immunoglobulin ~ 90384-90386
Anti-human globulin consumption test ~ 86880
Anti-phospholipid antibody ~ 86147
Antiactivator, plasmin ~ 85410
Antibiotic administration, injection ~ 90788
Antibiotic sensitivity ~ 87181-87184, 87188
enzyme detection ~ 87185
minimum bactericidal concentration ~ 87187
minimum inhibitory concentration ~ 87186
Antibody ~ (*see also* antibody identification) 86376
actinomyces ~ 86602
adenovirus ~ 86603
antinuclear ~ 86038-86039
antiphosphatidylserine (phospholipid) ~ 86148
antiprothrombin ~ 0030T
antistreptolysin O ~ 86060-86063
aspergillus ~ 86606
bacterium ~ 86609
bartonella ~ 86611
beta 2 glycoprotein 1 ~ 86146
blastomyces ~ 86612
blood crossmatch ~ 86920-86922
bordetella ~ 86615
borrelia ~ 86618-86619
brucella ~ 86622
campylobacter ~ 86625
candida ~ 86628
cardiolipin ~ 86147
chlamydia ~ 86631-86632
coccidioides ~ 86635
coxiella burnetii ~ 86638
cryptococcus ~ 86641
cytomegalovirus ~ 86644-86645
cytotoxic screen ~ 86807-86808
deoxyribonuclease ~ 86215
deoxyribonucleic acid (DNA) ~ 86225-86226
diphtheria ~ 86648
ehrlichia ~ 86666
encephalitis ~ 86651-86654
enterovirus ~ 86658
Epstein-Barr virus ~ 86663-86665
fluorescent ~ 86255-86256
francisella tularensis ~ 86668
fungus ~ 86671
giardia lamblia ~ 86674
growth hormone ~ 86277
helicobacter pylori ~ 86677
helminth ~ 86682
hemophilus influenza ~ 86684

Antibody ~ *continued*
hepatitis, delta agent ~ 86692
hepatitis A ~ 86708-86709
hepatitis B
core ~ 86704
IgM ~ 86705
surface ~ 86706
hepatitis Be ~ 86707
hepatitis C ~ 86803-86804
herpes simplex ~ 86694-86696
heterophile ~ 86308-86310
histoplasma ~ 86698
HIV ~ 86689, 86701-86703
HIV 1 ~ 86701, 86703
HIV 2 ~ 86702-86703
HTLV I ~ 86687, 86689
HTLV II ~ 86688
influenza virus ~ 86710
insulin ~ 86337
intrinsic factor ~ 86340
islet cell ~ 86341
legionella ~ 86713
leptospira ~ 86720
listeria monocytogenes ~ 86723
Lyme disease ~ 86617
lymphocytic choriomeningitis ~ 86727
lymphogranuloma venereum ~ 86729
microsomal ~ 86376
mucormycosis ~ 86732
mumps ~ 86735
mycoplasma ~ 86738
neisseria meningitidis ~ 86741
nocardia ~ 86744
nuclear antigen ~ 86235
other virus ~ 86790
parvovirus ~ 86747
phospholipid ~ 86147
phospholipid cofactor ~ 0030T
plasmodium ~ 86750
platelet ~ 86022-86023
protozoa ~ 86753
red blood cell ~ 86850-86870
respiratory syncytial virus (RSV) ~ 86756
rickettsia ~ 86757
rotavirus ~ 86759
rubella ~ 86762
rubeola ~ 86765
salmonella ~ 86768
shigella ~ 86771
sperm ~ 89325
streptokinase ~ 86590
tetanus ~ 86774
thyroid-stimulating ~ 84445
thyroglobulin ~ 86800
toxoplasma ~ 86777-86778
treponema pallidum ~ 86781
trichinella ~ 86784
varicella-zoster ~ 86787
viral ~ 86280
West Nile virus ~ 86788-86789
white blood cell ~ 86021
yersinia ~ 86793

Antibody identification
leukocyte antibodies ~ 86021
platelet ~ 86022-86023
red blood cell, pretreatment ~ 86970-86972
serum, pretreatment ~ 86975-86978
Antibody neutralization test ~ 86382
Antibody receptor ~ 86243
Anticoagulant ~ 85300-85305, 85307
Antidiabetic hormone ~ 82943
Antidiuretic hormone measurement~ 84588
AntiDNA autoantibody ~ 86038-86039
Antigen(s)
allergen immunotherapy ~ 95144
Australia ~ 87340-87341
bronchial provocation tests ~ see bronchial challenge test
carcinoembryonic ~ 82378
CD4 ~ 86360
CD8 ~ 86360
CD142 ~ see thromboplastin
CD143 ~ 82164
E ~ 87350
hepatitis ~ see hepatitis antigen
hepatitis B ~ 87515-87517
prostate specific ~ 84152-84153
Antigen detection
direct fluorescence ~ 87265-87272, 87276, 87278, 87280, 87285-87290
bordetella ~ 87265
chlamydia trachomatis ~ 87270
cryptosporidium ~ 87272
cytomegalovirus ~ 87271
enterovirus ~ 87267
giardia ~ 87269
influenza A ~ 87276
legionella pneumophila ~ 87278
not otherwise specified ~ 87299
respiratory syncytial virus ~ 87280
treponema pallidum ~ 87285
varicella-zoster ~ 87290
enzyme immunoassay ~ 87301-87451
adenovirus ~ 87301
aspergillus ~ 87305
chlamydia trachomatis ~ 87320
clostridium difficile ~ 87324
cryptococcus neoformans ~ 87327
cryptosporidium ~ 87328
cytomegalovirus ~ 87332
entomoeba histolytica dispar group ~ 87336
entomoeba histolytica group ~ 87337
escherichia coli 0157 ~ 87335
giardia ~ 87329
helicobacter pylori ~ 87338-87339
hepatitis Be antigen (HBeAg) ~ 87350
hepatitis B surface antigen (HBsAg) ~ 87340
hepatitis B surface antigen (HBsAg) neutralization ~ 87341
hepatitis delta agent ~ 87380
histoplasma capsulatum ~ 87385
HIV 1 ~ 87390
HIV 2 ~ 87391
influenza A ~ 87400

Antigen detection ~ *continued*
influenza B ~ 87400
multiple step method ~ 87301-87449
polyvalent ~ 87451
not otherwise specified ~ 87449, 87451
respiratory syncytial virus ~ 87420
rotavirus ~ 87425
shigella-like toxin ~ 87427
single step method ~ 87450
streptococcus, group A ~ 87430
immunofluorescence ~ 87260-87300
adenovirus ~ 87260
herpes simplex ~ 87273-87274
influenza B ~ 87275
legionella micdadei ~ 87277
not otherwise specified ~ 87299
parainfluenza virus ~ 87279
pneumocystis carinii ~ 87281
polyvalent ~ 87300
rubeola ~ 87283
Antihemophilic factor B ~ 85250
Antihemophilic factor C ~ 85270
Antihemophilic globulin (AHG) ~ 85240
Antihuman globulin ~ 86880-86886
Antimony ~ 83015
Antinuclear antibodies (ANA) ~ 86038-86039
Antiplasmin, alpha 2 ~ Antigen detection
Antiplatelet therapy ~ see performance measures
Antiprotease, alpha 1 ~ 82103-82104, 99565
Antiprothrombin antibody ~ 0030T
Antistreptococcal antibody ~ 86215
Antistreptokinase titer ~ 86590
Antistreptolysin O ~ 86060-86063
Antithrombin III ~ 85300-85301
Antithrombin VI (six) ~ 85362-85380
Antitoxin assay ~ 87230
Antiviral antibody ~ 86280
Antrostomy, sinus, maxillary ~ 31256-31267
Antrotomy, sinus
maxillary ~ 31020-31032
transmastoid ~ 69501
Antrum of highmore ~ see sinuses, maxillary
Antrum puncture
sinus
maxillary ~ 31000
sphenoid ~ 31002
Anus ~ see also hemorrhoids; rectum
ablation ~ 46615
abscess, incision and drainage ~ 46045-46050
biofeedback ~ 90911
biopsy, endoscopy ~ 46606
crypt, excision ~ 46210-46211
dilation, endoscopy ~ 46604
endoscopy
biopsy ~ 46606
dilation ~ 46604
exploration ~ 46600
hemorrhage ~ 46614
removal
foreign body ~ 46608

Anus ~ *continued*
polyp ~ 46610, 46612
tumor ~ 46610, 46612
excision, tag ~ 46220, 46230
exploration, endoscopy ~ 46600
fissure
destruction ~ 46940-46942
excision ~ 46200
fistula
excision ~ 46270-46285
repair ~ 46706
hemorrhage, endoscopic control ~ 46614
hemorrhoids
clot excision ~ 46320
destruction ~ 46934-46936
excision ~ 46250-46262
injection ~ 46500
ligation ~ 46221, 46945-46946
stapling ~ 46947
suture ~ 46945-46946
imperforated, repair ~ 46715-46742
incision, septum ~ 46070
lesion
destruction ~ 46900-46917, 46924
excision ~ 45108, 46922
manometry ~ 91122
placement, seton ~ 46020
reconstruction ~ 46742
congenital absence ~ 46730-46740
sphincter ~ 46750-46751, 46760-46762
with graft ~ 46753
with implant ~ 46762
removal
foreign body ~ 46608
seton ~ 46030
suture ~ 46754
wire ~ 46754
repair
anovaginal fistula ~ 46715-46716
cloacal anomaly ~ 46748
fistula ~ 46706
stricture ~ 46700-46705
sphincter
electromyography ~ 51784-51785
needle ~ 51785
unlisted services and procedures ~ 46999
Aorta
abdominal
aneurysm ~ 0078T-0081T, 34800-34805, 34825-34832, 35081-35103, 75952-75953
thromboendarterectomy ~ 35331
anastomosis, to pulmonary artery ~ 33606
angiogram, radiologic injection ~ 93539-93545
angioplasty ~ 35452
aortography ~ 75600-75630
balloon ~ 33967, 33970
catheterization
catheter ~ 36200
intracatheter/needle ~ 36160
circulation assist ~ 33967, 33970

Aorta ~ *continued*
conduit to heart ~ 33404
excision, coarctation ~ 33840-33851
insertion
balloon device ~ 33967
graft ~ 33330-33335
intracatheter/needle ~ 36160
-pulmonary art transposition ~ 33770-33781
removal, balloon assist device ~ 33968, 33971
repair ~ 33320-33322, 33802-33803
coarctation ~ 33840-33851
graft ~ 33860-33877
hypoplastic or interrupted aortic arch
with cardiopulmonary bypass ~ 33853
without cardiopulmonary bypass ~ 33852
sinus of Valsalva ~ 33702-33720
suspension ~ 33800
suture ~ 33320-33322
thoracic, aneurysm ~ 0033T-0040T
valve
incision ~ 33415
repair ~ 33400-33403
left ventricle ~ 33414
supravalvular stenosis ~ 33417
replacement ~ 33405-33413
X-ray with contrast ~ 75600-75630
Aortic sinus ~ 33702-33720
Aortic stenosis
repair ~ 33415
supravalvular ~ 33417
Aortic valve ~ see heart, aortic valve
Aortic valve replacement ~ 33405-33413
Aortocoronary bypass ~ 33503-33505, 33510-33516
Aortography ~ (see angiography) 75600-75605, 75630, 93544
serial ~ 75625
with iliofemoral artery ~ 75630
Aortoiliac
embolectomy ~ 34151-34201
thrombectomy ~ 34151-34201
Aortopexy ~ 33800
Aortoplasty, supravalvular stenosis ~ 33417
AP ~ see voiding pressure studies
Apert-Gallais syndrome ~ see adrenogenital syndrome
Aphasia testing ~ (see neurology, diagnostic) 96105
Apheresis, therapeutic ~ 36511-36516
Apical-aortic conduit ~ 33404
Apicectomy
with mastoidectomy ~ 69605
petrous ~ 69530
Apoaminotransferase, aspartate ~ see transaminase, glutamic oxaloacetic
Apolipoprotein, blood or urine ~ 82172
Appendectomy ~ 44950-44960
laparoscopic ~ 44970
Appendiceal abscess ~ see abscess, appendix
Appendico-vesicostomy, cutaneous ~ 50845
Appendix
abscess
incision and drainage
open ~ 44900
percutaneous ~ 44901
excision ~ 44950-44960
Application
allergy tests ~ 95044
bone fixation device
multiplane ~ 20692
uniplane ~ 20690
caliper ~ 20660
cranial tongs ~ 20660
fixation device, shoulder ~ 23700
halo
cranial ~ 20661
thin skull osteology ~ 20664
femoral ~ 20663
maxillofacial fixation ~ 21100
pelvic ~ 20662
interdental fixation device ~ 21110
neurostimulation ~ 64550
radioelement ~ 77761-77778
surface ~ 77789
with ultrasound ~ 76965
stereotactic frame ~ 20660
Application of external fixation device ~ see fixation device, application, external
APPT ~ see thromboplastin, partial, time
Aquatic therapy ~ 97113
Aqueous shunt
to extraocular reservoir ~ 66180
revision ~ 66185
Arch, zygomatic ~ see zygomatic arch
Arm
see also radius; ulna; wrist
lower
abscess ~ 25028
excision ~ 25145
incision and drainage, bone ~ 25035
amputation ~ 24900-24920, 25900-25905, 25915
cineplasty ~ 24940
revision ~ 25907-25909
angiography ~ 73206
artery ligation ~ 37618
biopsy ~ 25065-25066
bursa, incision and drainage ~ 25031
bypass graft ~ 35903
cast ~ 29075
CT scan ~ 73200-73206
decompression ~ 25020-25025
exploration, blood vessel ~ 35860
fasciotomy ~ 24495, 25020-25025
hematoma ~ 25028
lesion, tendon sheath, excision ~ 25110
magnetic resonance imaging (MRI) ~ 73218-73220, 73223
reconstruction, ulna ~ 25337
removal, foreign body ~ 25248

Arm ~ *continued*
repair
blood vessel with other graft ~ 35266
blood vessel with vein graft ~ 35236
decompression ~ 24495
muscle ~ 25260-25263, 25270
secondary muscle or tendon ~ 25272-25274
tendon ~ 25260-25263, 25270, 25280-25295, 25310-25316
secondary ~ 25265
tendon sheath ~ 25275
replantation ~ 20805
splint ~ 29125-29126
tenotomy ~ 25290
tumor, excision ~ 25075-25077
ultrasound ~ 76880
unlisted services and procedures ~ 25999
X-ray ~ 73090
with upper arm ~ 73092
removal, foreign body, forearm or wrist ~ 25248
repair
muscle ~ 24341
tendon ~ 24341
upper
abscess, incision and drainage ~ see elbow; humerus ~ 23930
amputation ~ 23900-23921, 24900-24920
cineplasty ~ 24940
revision ~ 24925-24930
with implant ~ 24931-24935
anesthesia ~ 00400, 01710-01782
angiography ~ 73206
artery, ligation ~ 37618
biopsy ~ 24065-24066
bypass graft ~ 35903
cast ~ 29065
CT scan ~ 73200-73206
exploration, blood vessel ~ 35860
hematoma, incision and drainage ~ 23930
magnetic resonance imaging (MRI) ~ 73218-73220, 73223
muscle revision ~ 24330-24331
removal
cast ~ 29705
foreign body ~ 24200-24201
repair
blood vessel with other graft ~ 35266
blood vessel with vein graft ~ 35236
muscle transfer ~ 24301, 24320
tendon ~ 24332
tendon lengthening ~ 24305
tendon revision ~ 24320
tendon transfer ~ 24301
tenotomy ~ 24310
replantation ~ 20802
splint ~ 29105
tumor, excision ~ 24075-24077
ultrasound ~ 76880
unlisted services and procedures ~ 24999

Arm ~ *continued*
wound exploration, penetrating ~ 20103
X-ray, with lower arm, infant ~ 73092
Arnold-Chiari malformation repair ~ 61343
Arrest, epiphyseal ~ see epiphyseal arrest
Arrhythmogenic focus
heart
catheter ablation ~ 93650-93652
destruction ~ 33250-33251, 33261
Arsenic ~ 83015
blood or urine ~ 82175
ART (syphilis test) ~ 86592, 86593
Arterial
catheterization ~ see cannulation, arterial
dilation, transluminal ~ see angioplasty, transluminal
grafting for coronary artery bypass ~ see bypass graft, coronary artery, arterial
pressure ~ see blood pressure
puncture ~ 36600
Arteriography, aorta ~ see aortography
Arteriosus, ductus ~ see ductus arteriosus
Arteriosus, truncus ~ see truncus arteriosus
Arteriotomy ~ see incision, artery; transection, artery
Arteriovenous anastomosis ~ 36818-36820
Arteriovenous fistula
cannulization vein ~ 36815
repair
abdomen ~ 35182
acquired or traumatic ~ 35189
head ~ 35180
acquired or traumatic ~ 35188
lower extremity ~ 35184
acquired or traumatic ~ 35190
neck ~ 35180
acquired or traumatic ~ 35188
thorax ~ 35182
acquired or traumatic ~ 35189
upper extremity ~ 35184
acquired or traumatic ~ 35190
revision, hemodialysis graft or fistula
without thrombectomy ~ 36832
with thrombectomy ~ 36833
thrombectomy
dialysis graft, without revision ~ 36831
graft ~ 36870
Arteriovenous malformation
cranial, repair ~ 61680-61692, 61705-61708
spinal
excision ~ 63250-63252
injection ~ 62294
repair ~ 63250-63252
Arteriovenous shunt
angiography ~ 75790
catheterization ~ 36145
Artery
abdomen
angiography ~ 75726
catheterization ~ 36245-36248
ligation ~ 37617

Artery ~ *continued*
adrenal, angiography ~ 75731-75733
anastomosis, cranial ~ 61711
angioplasty ~ 75962-75968
aorta
angioplasty ~ 35452
atherectomy ~ 35481, 35491
aortoiliac
embolectomy ~ 34151-34201
thrombectomy ~ 34151-34201
aortoiliofemoral ~ 35363
arm
angiography ~ 75710-75716
harvest of artery for coronary artery bypass graft ~ 35600
atherectomy
open ~ 35480-35485
percutaneous ~ 35490-35495
axillary
aneurysm ~ 35011-35013
angioplasty ~ 35458
bypass graft ~ 35516-35522, 35533, 35616-35623, 35650, 35654
embolectomy ~ 34101
thrombectomy ~ 34101
thromboendarterectomy ~ 35321
basilar, aneurysm ~ 61698, 61702
biopsy, transcatheter ~ 75970
brachial
aneurysm ~ 35011-35013
angiography ~ 75658
bypass graft ~ 35510, 35512, 35522-35525
catheterization ~ 36120
embolectomy ~ 34101
exploration ~ 24495
exposure ~ 34834
thrombectomy ~ 34101
thromboendarterectomy ~ 35321
brachiocephalic
angioplasty ~ 35458
atherectomy ~ 35484, 35494
catheterization ~ 36215-36218
bypass graft, with composite graft ~ 35681-35683
cannulization
for extra corporeal circulation ~ 36823
to vein ~ 36810-36815
carotid
aneurysm ~ 35001-35002, 61697-61705
vascular malformation or carotid-cavernous fistula ~ 61710
angiography ~ 75660-75680
bypass graft ~ 35501-35510, 35526, 35601-35606, 35626, 35642
catheterization ~ 36100
decompression ~ 61590-61591, 61595-61596
embolectomy ~ 34001
exploration ~ 35701
ligation ~ 37600-37606, 61611-61612
thrombectomy ~ 34001
thromboendarterectomy ~ 35301, 35390
transection ~ 61611-61612

Artery ~ *continued*
celiac
aneurysm ~ 35121-35122
bypass graft ~ 35531, 35631
embolectomy ~ 34151
thrombectomy ~ 34151
thromboendarterectomy ~ 35341
chest, ligation ~ 37616
coronary
angiography ~ 93556
atherectomy ~ 92995-92996
bypass ~ 33517-33519
arterial ~ 33533-33536
bypass venous graft ~ 33510-33516
graft ~ 33503-33505
ligation ~ 33502
repair ~ 33500-33506
thrombectomy, percutaneous ~ 92973
digital, sympathectomy ~ 64820
ethmoidal, ligation ~ 30915
extracranial, vascular studies, non-invasive, physiologic ~ 93875
extra corporeal circulation, for regional chemotherapy of extremity ~ 36823
extremities, vascular studies ~ 93922-93923
extremity
bypass graft revision ~ 35879-35881
catheterization ~ 36140
ligation ~ 37618
femoral
aneurysm ~ 35141-35142
angioplasty ~ 35456
atherectomy ~ 35483, 35493
bypass graft ~ 35521, 35533, 35551-35558, 35566, 35621, 35646-35647, 35651-35661, 35666, 35700
bypass in-situ ~ 35583-35585
embolectomy ~ 34201
exploration ~ 35721
exposure ~ 34812-34813
thrombectomy ~ 34201
thromboendarterectomy ~ 35371-35372
great vessel, repair ~ 33770-33781
head, angiography ~ 75650
hepatic, aneurysm ~ 35121-35122
iliac
aneurysm ~ 35131-35132, 75954
angioplasty ~ 35454
atherectomy ~ 35482, 35492
bypass graft ~ 35563, 35663
embolectomy ~ 34151-34201
exposure ~ 34820, 34833
graft ~ 34900
occlusion device ~ 34808
thrombectomy ~ 34151-34201
thromboendarterectomy ~ 35351, 35361-35363
iliofemoral
bypass graft ~ 35548-35549, 35565, 35665
thromboendarterectomy ~ 35355, 35363
X-ray with contrast ~ 75630

Artery ~ *continued*
innominate
aneurysm ~ 35021-35022
embolectomy ~ 34001-34101
thrombectomy ~ 34001-34101
thromboendarterectomy ~ 35311
leg
angiography ~ 75710-75716
catheterization ~ 36245-36248
mammary, angiography ~ 75756
maxillary, ligation ~ 30920
mesenteric
aneurysm ~ 35121-35122
bypass graft ~ 35531, 35631
embolectomy ~ 34151
thrombectomy ~ 34151
thromboendarterectomy ~ 35341
middle cerebral artery, fetal, vascular studies ~ 76821
neck
angiography ~ 75650
ligation ~ 37615
nose, incision ~ 30915-30920
other angiography ~ 75774
other artery, exploration ~ 35761
pelvic
angiography ~ 75736
catheterization ~ 36245-36248
peripheral arterial rehabilitation ~ 93668
peroneal
bypass graft ~ 35566-35571, 35666-35671
bypass in-situ ~ 35585-35587
embolectomy ~ 34203
thrombectomy ~ 34203
thromboendarterectomy ~ 35305-35306
popliteal
aneurysm ~ 35151-35152
angioplasty ~ 35456
atherectomy ~ 35483, 35493
bypass graft ~ 35551-35556, 35571, 35623, 35651, 35656, 35671, 35700
bypass in-situ ~ 35583, 35587
embolectomy ~ 34203
exploration ~ 35741
thrombectomy ~ 34203
thromboendarterectomy ~ 35303
pulmonary
anastomosis ~ 33606
angiography ~ 75741-75746
repair ~ 33690
radial, aneurysm ~ 35045
embolectomy ~ 34111
sympathectomy ~ 64821
thrombectomy ~ 34111
rehabilitation ~ 93668
reimplantation
carotid ~ 35691, 35694-35695
subclavian ~ 35693-35695
vertebral ~ 35691-35693
visceral ~ 35697

Artery ~ *continued*
renal
aneurysm ~ 35121-35122
angiography ~ 75722-75724
angioplasty ~ 35450
atherectomy ~ 35480, 35490
bypass graft ~ 35536, 35560, 35631-35636
embolectomy ~ 34151
thrombectomy ~ 34151
thromboendarterectomy ~ 35341
repair
aneurysm ~ 36834, 61697-61708
angioplasty ~ 75962-75968
revision
hemodialysis graft or fistula
without thrombectomy ~ 36832
with thrombectomy ~ 36833
spine, angiography ~ 75705
splenic
aneurysm ~ 35111-35112
bypass graft ~ 35536, 35636
subclavian
aneurysm ~ 35001-35002, 35021-35022
angioplasty ~ 35458
bypass graft ~ 35506, 35511-35516, 35526, 35606-35616, 35626, 35645
embolectomy ~ 34001-34101
thrombectomy ~ 34001-34101
thromboendarterectomy ~ 35301-35311
unlisted services and procedures ~ 37799
superficial palmar arch, sympathectomy ~ 64823
temporal
biopsy ~ 37609
ligation ~ 37609
thoracic, catheterization ~ 36215-36218
thrombectomy
hemodialysis graft or fistula ~ 36831
other than hemodialysis graft or fistula ~ 35875, 36870
tibial
bypass graft ~ 35566-35571, 35623, 35666-35671
bypass in-situ ~ 35585-35587
embolectomy ~ 34203
thrombectomy ~ 34203
thromboendarterectomy ~ 35305-35306
tibioperoneal
angioplasty ~ 35459, 35470
atherectomy ~ 35485, 35495
transcatheter therapy, with angiography ~ 75894-75898
transposition
carotid ~ 0037T, 35691, 35694-35695
subclavian ~ 0037T, 35693-35695
vertebral ~ 35691-35693
ulnar
aneurysm ~ 35045
embolectomy ~ 34111
sympathectomy ~ 64822
thrombectomy ~ 34111
unlisted services and procedures ~ 37799

Artery ~ *continued*
vertebral
aneurysm ~ 35005, 61698, 61702
angiography ~ 75685
bypass graft ~ 35508, 35515, 35642-35645
catheterization ~ 36100
decompression ~ 61597
thromboendarterectomy ~ 35301
visceral
angioplasty ~ 35450
atherectomy ~ 35480, 35490
reimplantation ~ 35697
Artery catheterization, pulmonary ~ see catheterization, pulmonary artery
Arthrectomy, elbow ~ 24155
Arthrocentesis
intermediate joint ~ 20605
large joint ~ 20610
small joint ~ 20600
Arthrodesis
ankle ~ 27870
tibiotalar and fibulotalar joints ~ 29899
carpometacarpal joint
hand ~ 26843-26844
thumb ~ 26841-26842
cervical anterior, with discectomy ~ 22554
elbow ~ 24800-24802
finger joint ~ 26852
interphalangeal ~ 26860-26863
metacarpophalangeal ~ 26850
foot joint ~ 28730-28735, 28740
pantalar ~ 28705
subtalar ~ 28725
triple ~ 28715
with advancement ~ 28737
with lengthening ~ 28737
hand joint ~ 26843-26844
hip joint ~ 27284-27286
intercarpal joint ~ 25820
with autograft ~ 25825
interphalangeal joint ~ 26860-26863
great toe ~ 28755
with tendon transfer ~ 28760
intervertebral disc
removal ~ 0093T, 0095T, 0164T, 22865
revision ~ 0096T-0098T, 0165T, 22862
total replacement ~ 0090T, 0092T, 0163T, 22857
knee ~ 27580
metacarpophalangeal joint ~ 26850-26852
metatarsophalangeal joint, great toe ~ 28750
pubic symphysis ~ 27282
radioulnar joint, with resection of ulna ~ 25830
sacroiliac joint ~ 27280
shoulder ~ see shoulder, arthrodesis
shoulder joint ~ 23800
with autogenous graft ~ 23802
talus
pantalar ~ 28705
subtalar ~ 28725
triple ~ 28715

Arthrodesis ~ *continued*
tarsal joint ~ 28730-28735, 28740
with advancement ~ 28737
with lengthening ~ 28737
tarsometatarsal joint ~ 28730-28735, 28740
thumb joint ~ 26841-26842
tibiofibular joint ~ 27871
vertebra
additional interspace
anterior/anterolateral approach ~ 22585
lateral extracavitary ~ 22534
posterior ~ 22632
cervical
anterior/anterolateral approach ~ 22548
posterior/posterolateral and/or lateral traverse process ~ 22590-22600
lumbar
anterior/anterolateral approach ~ 22558
lateral extracavitary ~ 22533
posterior/interbody ~ 22630
posterior/posterolateral and/or lateral transverse process ~ 22612
spinal deformity
anterior approach ~ 22808-22812
posterior approach ~ 22800-22804
spinal fusion, exploration ~ 22830
thoracic
anterior/anterolateral approach ~ 22556
lateral extracavitary ~ 22532
posterior/posterolateral and/or lateral traverse process ~ 22610
vertebrae, posterior ~ 22614
wrist ~ 25800
with graft ~ 25810
with sliding graft ~ 25805
Arthrography
ankle ~ 73615
injection ~ 27648
elbow ~ 73085
injection ~ 24220
hip ~ 73525
injection ~ 27093-27095
knee ~ 73580
injection ~ 27370
sacroiliac joint ~ 73542
injection ~ 27096
shoulder ~ 73040
injection ~ 23350
temporomandibular joint (TMJ) ~ 70328-70332
injection ~ 21116
wrist ~ 73115
injection ~ 25426
Arthroplasties, knee replacement ~ 27438, 27445
Arthroplasty
ankle ~ 27700-27703
elbow ~ 24360
total replacement ~ 24363
with implant ~ 24361-24362
hip ~ 27132
partial replacement ~ 27125

Arthroplasty ~ *continued*
revision ~ 27134-27138
total replacement ~ 27130
interphalangeal joint ~ 26535-26536
knee ~ 27437-27443, 27446-27447
revision ~ 27486-27487
with prosthesis ~ 27438, 27445
metacarpophalangeal joint ~ 26530-26531
radius ~ 24365
with implant ~ 24366
reconstruction, prosthesis, hip ~ 27125
shoulder joint with implant ~ 23470-23472
temporomandibular joint ~ 21240-21243
wrist ~ 25447
carpal ~ 25443
lunate ~ 25444
navicular ~ 25443
radius ~ 25441
revision ~ 25449
total replacement ~ 25446
trapezium ~ 25445
ulna ~ 25442
with implant ~ 25441-25445
wrist (pseudarthrosis type) ~ 25332
Arthropods, examination ~ 87168
Arthroscopy
diagnostic
elbow ~ 29830
hip ~ 29860
knee ~ 29870
metacarpophalangeal joint ~ 29900
shoulder ~ 29805
temporomandibular joint ~ 29800
wrist ~ 29840
surgical
ankle ~ 29891-29899
elbow ~ 29834-29838
hip ~ 29861-29863
knee ~ 29871-29889
cartilage allograft ~ 29867
cartilage autograft ~ 29866
meniscal transplantation ~ 29868
metacarpophalangeal joint ~ 29901-29902
shoulder ~ 29806-29827
temporomandibular joint ~ 29804
wrist ~ 29843-29848
unlisted services and procedures ~ 29999
Arthrotomy
acromioclavicular joint ~ 23044
ankle ~ 27610-27612, 27620
ankle joint ~ 27625-27626
carpometacarpal joint ~ 26070
with biopsy, synovium
with synovial biopsy ~ 26100
elbow ~ 24000
capsular release ~ 24006
with joint exploration ~ 24101
with synovectomy ~ 24102
with synovial biopsy ~ 24100
finger joint ~ 26075
interphalangeal
with synovial biopsy ~ 26110

Arthrotomy ~ *continued*
metacarpophalangeal
with biopsy, synovium ~ 26105
glenohumeral joint ~ 23040
hip ~ 27033
for infection
with drainage ~ 27030
with synovectomy ~ 27054
interphalangeal joint ~ 26080, 26110
toe ~ 28024, 28054
intertarsal joint ~ 28020, 28050
knee ~ 27310, 27330-27335, 27403, 29868
metacarpophalangeal joint ~ 26075, 26105
metatarsophalangeal joint ~ 28022, 28052
shoulder ~ 23044, 23105-23107
shoulder joint ~ 23100-23101
exploration and/or removal of loose or foreign body ~ 23107
sternoclavicular joint ~ 23044
tarsometatarsal joint ~ 28020, 28050
temporomandibular joint ~ 21010
with biopsy
acromioclavicular joint ~ 23101
glenohumeral joint ~ 23100
hip joint ~ 27052
knee joint ~ 27330
sacroiliac joint
hip joint ~ 27050
sternoclavicular joint ~ 23101
with synovectomy
glenohumeral joint ~ 23105
sternoclavicular joint ~ 23106
wrist ~ 25040, 25100-25107
Articular ligament ~ see ligament
Artificial abortion ~ see abortion
Artificial cardiac pacemaker ~ see heart, pacemaker
Artificial eye ~ see prosthesis
Artificial genitourinary sphincter ~ see prosthesis, urethral sphincter
Artificial insemination ~ 58976
intra-cervical ~ 58321
intra-uterine ~ 58322
sperm washing ~ 58323
Artificial knee joints ~ 27438, 27445
Artificial penis ~ see penile prosthesis
Artificial pneumothorax ~ 32960
Arytenoid, excision, endoscopic ~ 31560-31561
Arytenoid cartilage
excision ~ 31400
repair ~ 31400
Arytenoidectomy ~ 31400
endoscopic ~ 31560
Arytenoidopexy ~ 31400
Ascorbic acid, blood ~ 82180
Aspartate aminotransferase ~ 84450
Aspergillus
antibody ~ 86606
antigen detection
enzyme immunoassay ~ 87305

Aspiration ~ see puncture aspiration
amniotic fluid
diagnostic ~ 59000
therapeutic ~ 59001
bladder ~ 51000-51010
bone marrow ~ 38220
brain lesion, stereotactic ~ 61750-61751
bronchi, endoscopy ~ 31645-31646
bursa ~ 20600-20610
catheter
nasotracheal ~ 31720
tracheobronchial ~ 31725
chest ~ 32000-32002
cyst
bone ~ 20615
kidney ~ 50390
pelvis ~ 50390
spinal cord ~ 62268
thyroid ~ 60001
duodenal ~ 89100-89105
fetal fluid ~ 59074
ganglion cyst ~ 20612
hydrocele, tunica vaginalis ~ 55000
joint ~ 20600-20610
laryngoscopy
direct ~ 31515
lens material ~ 66840
liver ~ 47015
lung ~ 32420
lung puncture ~ 32420
nail ~ 11740
nucleus of disk, lumbar ~ 62287
orbital contents ~ 67415
pelvis, endoscopy ~ 49322
pericardium ~ 33010-33011
pleural cavity ~ 32000-32002
puncture, cyst, breast ~ 19000-19001
spinal cord, stereotaxis ~ 63615
spinal puncture ~ see spinal tap
syrinx, spinal cord ~ 62268
thyroid ~ 60001
trachea
nasotracheal ~ 31720
puncture ~ 31612
tunica vaginalis, hydrocele ~ 55000
vitreous ~ 67015
Aspiration lipectomies ~ 15876-15879
Aspiration of bone marrow from donor for transplant ~ 38230
Assay, very long chain fatty acids ~ 82726
Assay tobramycin ~ 80200
Assisted circulation ~ see circulation assist
AST ~ 84450
Astragalectomy ~ 28130
Astragalus ~ see talus
Asymmetry, face ~ 21247
Ataxia telangiectasia, chromosome analysis ~ 88248
Ataxy, telangiectasia ~ 88248
Atherectomy ~ 75992-75996
open
aorta ~ 35481
brachiocephalic ~ 35484
femoral ~ 35483
iliac ~ 35482
popliteal ~ 35483
renal ~ 35480
tibioperoneal ~ 35485
visceral ~ 35480
percutaneous
aorta ~ 35491
brachiocephalic ~ 35494
coronary ~ see artery, coronary ~ 92995-92996
femoral ~ 35493
iliac ~ 35492
popliteal ~ 35493
renal ~ 35490
tibioperoneal ~ 35495
visceral ~ 35490
X-ray
peripheral artery ~ 75992-75993
renal artery ~ 75994
visceral artery ~ 75995-75996
ATLV ~ see HTLV I
ATLV antibodies ~ 86688
Atomic absorption spectroscopy ~ 0064T, 82190
ATP creatine phosphotranferase ~ 82550-82552
Atresia
choanal ~ 30540-30545
congenital, auditory canal, external, reconstruction ~ 69320
Atria, reconstruction ~ 33254-33256, 33265-33266
Atrial electrogram ~ see cardiology, diagnostic
esophageal recording ~ 93615-93616
Atrial fibrillation ~ see fibrillation, atrial
Atrioseptopexy ~ see heart, repair, atrial septum
Atrioseptoplasty ~ see heart, repair, atrial septum
Attachment ~ see fixation
Atticotomy ~ 69631, 69635
Audiologic function tests ~ 92590-92595
acoustic reflex ~ 92568
acoustic reflex decay ~ 92569
audiometry
Bekesy ~ 92560-92561
comprehensive ~ 92557
conditioning play ~ 92582
groups ~ 92559
pure tone ~ 92552-92553
select picture ~ 92583
speech ~ 92555-92556
visual reinforcement ~ 92579
central auditory function ~ 92620-92621
diagnostic analysis
auditory brainstem implant ~ 92640
electrocochleography ~ 92584

Audiologic function tests ~ *continued*
evoked otoacoustic emission ~ 92587-92588
filtered speech ~ 92571
loudness balance ~ 92562
screening ~ 92551
sensorineural acuity ~ 92575
short increment sensitivity index ~ 92564
staggered spondaic word test ~ 92572
Stenger test ~ 92565, 92577
synthetic sentence test ~ 92576
tinnitus assessment ~ 92625
tone decay ~ 92563
Audiometry, Bekesy ~ 92560-92561
brainstem evoked response ~ 92585-92586
comprehensive ~ 92557
conditioning play ~ 92582
groups ~ see ear, nose and throat ~ 92559
pure tone ~ 92552-92553
select picture ~ 92583
speech ~ 92555-92556
tympanometry ~ 92567
Auditory brain stem evoked response ~ 92585-92586
Auditory canal
decompression ~ 61591
external
abscess, incision and drainage ~ 69020
biopsy ~ 69105
lesion, excision ~ 69140-69155
reconstruction
for congenital atresia ~ 69320
for stenosis ~ 69310
removal
cerumen ~ 69210
ear wax ~ 69210
foreign body ~ 69200-69205
internal, decompression ~ 69960
Auditory atresia, external ~ 69320
Auditory evoked otoacoustic emission ~ 92587-92588
Auditory evoked potentials ~ 92585-92586, 92590-92595
Auditory labyrinth ~ see ear, inner
Auditory meatus, X-ray ~ 70134
Auditory system surgical procedures ~ 69000-69990
Auditory tube ~ see eustachian tube
Augmentation
chin ~ 21120, 21123
malar ~ 21270
mammoplasty ~ 19324-19325
mandibular body
with bone graft ~ 21127
with prosthesis ~ 21125
osteoplasty, facial bones ~ 21208
Augmented histamine test ~ 91052
Aural rehabilitation ~ 92510
Auricle (heart) ~ see atria
Auricular fibrillation ~ fibrillation, atria
Auricular prosthesis ~ 21086
Australia antigen ~ 87340-87341
Autograft
bone
local ~ 20936
morselized ~ 20937
structural ~ 20938
chondrocytes, knee ~ 27412
for spine surgery
local ~ 20936
morselized ~ 20937
structural ~ 20938
Autologous blood transfusion ~ 86890-86891
Autologous transplantation ~ see autograft
Automated data, nuclear medicine ~ 78890-78891
Autonomic nervous system function ~ see neurology, diagnostic; neurophysiologic testing
Autoprothrombin
C ~ 85260
I ~ 85230
II ~ 85250
III ~ 85260
Autopsy
coroner's exam ~ 88045
forensic exam ~ 88040
gross and micro exam ~ 88020-88029
gross exam ~ 88000-88016
organ ~ 88037
regional ~ 88036
unlisted services and procedures ~ 88099
Autotransfusion, blood ~ 86890-86891
Autotransplant ~ see autograft
Autotransplantation, renal ~ 50380
Avulsion
nails ~ 11730-11732
nerve ~ 64732-64772
AV fistula ~ see arteriovenous fistula
AV shunt ~ see arteriovenous shunt
Axillary arteries ~ see artery, axillary
Axillary nerve, injection, anesthetic ~ 64417
Axis, dens ~ 22548

B

B antibodies, hepatitis ~ see antibody, hepatitis B
B antigens, hepatitis ~ 87515-87517
B complex vitamins, B12 absorption ~ 78270-78272
B-DNA ~ 86225-86226
B-hexosaminidase ~ 83080
B1 vitamin ~ see 84425
B6 vitamin ~ 84207
B12 vitamin ~ 82607-82608
Babcock operation ~ 37700-37735, 37780
Bacillus Calmette Guerin vaccine ~ see BCG vaccine

Back/ flank
biopsy ~ 21920-21925
repair, hernia ~ 49540
strapping ~ 29220
tumor
excision ~ 21930
radical resection ~ 21935
wound exploration
penetrating ~ 20102
Backbone ~ see spine
Bacteria culture
additional methods ~ 87077
aerobic ~ 87040-87071
anaerobic ~ 87073-87076
blood ~ 87040
other source ~ 87070-87075
screening ~ 87081
stool ~ 87045-87046
urine ~ 87086-87088
Bacterial endotoxins ~ 87176
Bacterial overgrowth breath test ~ 91065
Bactericidal titer, serum ~ 87197
Bacterium, antibody ~ 86609
Baer ~ 92585-92586
Baker's cyst ~ 27345
Baker tube, intestine decompression ~ 44021
Balanoplasty ~ see penis, repair
Baldy-Webster operation ~ 58400
Balkan grippe ~ 86000, 86638
Balloon
angioplasties, coronary ~ see percutaneous transluminal angioplasty
angioplasty ~ see angioplasty
assisted device, aorta ~ 33967-33974, 93727
Band, pulmonary artery ~ 33690
Banding, artery
fistula ~ 37607
pulmonary ~ 33690
Bank, blood ~ see blood banking
Bankart procedure ~ 23450-23462
Barany caloric test ~ 92533
Barbiturates, blood or urine ~ 82205
Bardenheurer operation ~ 37616
Bariatric surgery ~ 43644-43645, 43842-43848
Barium ~ 83015
Barium enema ~ 74270-74280
Barker operation ~ 28120, 28130
Barr bodies ~ 88130
Barr procedure ~ 27690-27692
Bartholin's gland
abscess, incision and drainage ~ 56420
cyst, repair ~ 56440
excision ~ 56740
marsupialization ~ 56440
Bartonella
antibody ~ 86611
detection ~ 87470-87472
Basic life services ~ 99450
Basic proteins, myelin ~ 83873
Basilar arteries ~ 61698, 61702
Batch-Spittler-McFaddin operation ~ 27598
BCG vaccine ~ 90585, 90586
Be antigens, hepatitis ~ 87350
Bed sores ~ see debridement; skin graft and flap; 15920-15999
Bekesy audiometry ~ 92560-92561
Belsey IV procedure ~ see fundoplasty
Bender-Gestalt test ~ 96100
Benedict test for urea ~ 81005
Benign cystic mucinous tumour ~ see ganglion
Benign neoplasm of cranial nerves ~ see cranial nerve
Bennett fracture ~ see phalanx, finger; 26720-26727
Bennett procedure ~ see revision; 27385-27386, 27400, 27430
Benzidine test ~ 82270, 82272
Benzodiazepine, assay ~ 80154
Benzoyl cholinesterase ~ 82480-82482
Bernstein test ~ 91012, 91030
Beryllium ~ 83015
Beta-2 -microglobulin
blood ~ 82232
urine ~ 82232
Beta-hydroxydehydrogenase ~ 80406
Beta 2 glycoprotein 1 antibody ~ 86146
Beta blocker therapy ~ see performance measures
Beta glucosidase ~ 82963
Beta hypophamine ~ 84588
Beta lipoproteins ~ 83700-83704, 83721
Beta test ~ see psychiatric diagnosis ~ 96100
Bethesda system ~ 88164-88167
Bicarbonate ~ 82374
Biceps tendon, insertion ~ 24342
Bichloride, methylene ~ 84600
Bicuspid valve ~ see mitral valve
Bifrontal craniotomy ~ 61557
Bilaminate skin substitute/ neodermis ~ see tissue
repair ~ see tissue, culture; 15100-15101, 15120-15121
Bile acids ~ 82239
blood ~ 82240
Bile duct ~ see gallbladder
anastomosis, cyst ~ 47719
with intestines ~ 47760, 47780-47785
biopsy, endoscopy ~ 47553
catheterization ~ 75982
change catheter tube ~ 75984
cyst
excision ~ 47715
repair ~ 47719
destruction, calculi (stone) ~ 43265
dilation, endoscopy ~ 43271, 47555-47556
drainage, transhepatic ~ 75980
endoscopy
biopsy ~ 47553
destruction
calculi (stone) ~ 43265
tumor ~ 43272
dilation ~ 43271, 47555-47556
exploration ~ 47552

Bile duct ~ *continued*
intraoperative ~ 47550
removal
calculi (stone) ~ 43264, 47554
foreign body ~ 43269
stent ~ 43269
specimen collection ~ 43260
sphincterotomy ~ 43262
sphincter pressure ~ 43263
tube placement ~ 43267-43268
exploration
atresia ~ 47700
endoscopy ~ 47552
incision, sphincter ~ 43262, 47460
incision and drainage ~ 47420-47425
insertion
catheter ~ 47510, 47525, 75982
revision ~ 47530
stent ~ 47511, 47801
nuclear medicine, imaging ~ 78223
reconstruction, anastomosis ~ 47800
removal
calculi (stone) ~ 43264, 47420-47425
percutaneous ~ 47630
foreign body ~ 43269
stent ~ 43269
repair ~ 47701
cyst ~ 47719
gastrointestinal tract ~ 47785
with intestines ~ 47760, 47780
tube placement
nasobiliary ~ 43267
stent ~ 43268
tumor
destruction ~ 43271
excision ~ 47711-47712
unlisted services and procedures ~ 47999
X-ray
guide dilation ~ 74360
with contrast ~ 74300-74320
calculus removal ~ 74327
guide catheter ~ 74328, 74330
Bile duct, common, cystic dilatation ~ see cyst, choledochal
Bilirubin
blood ~ 82247-82248
feces ~ 82252
total
direct ~ 82247-82248
transcutaneous ~ 88400
Billroth I or II ~ 43631-43635, 43845
Bilobectomy ~ 32482
Bimone ~ 84402
Binding globulin, testosterone-estradiol ~ 84270
Binet-Simon test ~ 96100
Binet test ~ 96100
Binet-Simon test, binocular microscopy ~ 92504
Biofeedback ~ 90901-90911
anorectal ~ 90911
psychiatric treatment ~ 90875-90876
Biofeedback training ~ 90901-90911
Bioimpedance
breast ~ 0060T
thorax ~ 93701
Biological skin grafts ~ 15300-15336
Biometry, eye ~ 76516-76519, 92136
Biopsies, needle ~ see needle biopsy
Biopsy ~ see brush biopsy; needle biopsy
abdomen ~ 49000
adrenal gland ~ 60540-60545
anal, endoscopy ~ 46606
ankle ~ 27613-27614, 27620
arm, lower ~ 25065-25066
arm, upper ~ 24065-24066
artery, temporal ~ 37609
auditory canal, external ~ 69105
back/flank ~ 21920-21925
bile duct, endoscopy ~ 47553
bladder ~ 52354
cystourethroscope ~ 52204
cystourethroscopy ~ 52224, 52250
blood vessel, transcatheter ~ 75970
bone ~ 20220-20245
bone marrow ~ 38221
brain ~ 61140
stereotactic ~ 61750-61751
brainstem ~ 61575-61576
breast ~ 19100-19103
stereotactic localization ~ 77031
bronchi
catheterization ~ 31717
endoscopic ~ 31625-31629, 31632-31633
brush
bronchi ~ 31717
renal pelvis ~ 52007
ureter ~ 52007
with cystourethroscopy ~ 52204
carpometacarpal joint, synovium ~ 26100
cervix ~ 57454-57455, 57460, 57500, 57520
chorionic villus ~ 59015
colon ~ 44025, 44100
endoscopy ~ 44389, 45380, 45391, 45392
multiple, with colostomy, cecostomy ~ 44322
colon-sigmoid, endoscopy ~ 45305, 45331
conjunctiva ~ 68100
cornea ~ 65410
duodenum ~ 44010
ear, external ~ 69100
elbow ~ 24065-24066, 24101
synovium ~ 24100
embryo blastomere ~ 89290-89291
endometrium ~ 58100, 58558
epididymis ~ 54800-54865
esophagus, endoscopy ~ 43202
eye muscle ~ 67346
eyelid ~ 67810
forearm, soft tissue ~ 25065-25066
gallbladder, endoscopy ~ 43261
gastrointestinal, upper, endoscopy ~ 43239
hand joint, synovium ~ 26100
heart ~ 93505

Biopsy ~ *continued*
hip ~ 27040-27041
joint ~ 27052
hypopharynx ~ 42802
ileum, endoscopy ~ 44382
interphalangeal joint
finger ~ 26110
toe ~ 28054
intertarsal joint, toe ~ 28050
intestines, small ~ 44020, 44100
endoscopy ~ 44361, 44377
kidney ~ 50200-50205
endoscopic ~ 50555-50557, 50574-50576, 52354
knee ~ 27323-27324
synovium ~ 27330
knee joint, synovium ~ 27330
lacrimal gland ~ 68510
lacrimal sac ~ 68525
larynx, endoscopy ~ 31510, 31576
leg
lower ~ 27613-27614
upper ~ 27323-27324
lip ~ 40490
liver ~ 47000-47001, 47100
lung
needle ~ 32405
thoracotomy ~ 32095-32100
lymph nodes ~ 38500-38530
injection procedure, for identification of sentinel node ~ 38792
laparoscopic ~ 38570-38572
needle ~ 38505
open ~ 38500, 38510-38530
superficial ~ 38500
mediastinum ~ 39400
needle ~ 32405
metacarpophalangeal joint ~ 26105
metatarsophalangeal joint ~ 28052
mouth ~ 40808, 41108
muscle ~ 20200-20206
nail ~ 11755
nasopharynx ~ 42804-42806
neck ~ 21550
nerve ~ 64795
nose
endoscopic ~ 31237
intranasal ~ 30100
oocyte polar body ~ 89290-89291
orbit ~ 61332
exploration ~ 67400, 67450
fine needle aspiration ~ 67415
oropharynx ~ 42800
ovary ~ 58900
palate ~ 42100
pancreas ~ 48100
pelvis ~ 27040-27041
penis ~ 54100
deep structures ~ 54105
percutaneous needle, spinal cord ~ 62269
perineum ~ 56605-56606
peritoneum, endoscopic ~ 47561

Biopsy ~ *continued*
pharynx ~ 42800-42806
pleura
needle ~ 32400-32402
thoracotomy ~ 32095-32100
pleural, open ~ 32402
prostate ~ 55700-55705
rectum ~ 45100
retroperitoneal area ~ 49010
sacroiliac joint ~ 27050
salivary gland ~ 42405
shoulder
deep ~ 23066
soft tissue ~ 23065
shoulder joint ~ 23100-23101
sinus, sphenoid ~ 31050-31051
skin ~ see skin, biopsy
skin lesion ~ 11100-11101
spinal cord ~ 63275-63290
percutaneous ~ 62269
stereotaxis ~ 63615
stomach ~ 43600-43605
tarsometatarsal joint, synovial ~ 28050
testis ~ 54500-54505
thorax ~ 21550
throat ~ 42800-42806
tongue ~ 41100-41105
transcatheter ~ 37200
ureter ~ 52354
endoscopic ~ 50955-50957, 50974-50976
urethra ~ 52204, 52354, 53200
uterus
endometrial ~ 58100
endoscopic ~ 58558
uvula ~ 42100
vagina ~ 57100-57105, 57421
vein ~ 75970
vertebral body ~ 20250-20251
vulva ~ 56605-56606, 56821
with arthrotomy
acromioclavicular joint ~ 23101
glenohumeral joint ~ 23100
sternoclavicular joint ~ 23101
with cystourethroscopy ~ 52354
wrist ~ 25065-25066, 25100-25101
Biostatistics ~ 76516-76519, 92136
Biosterol ~ 84590
Biotinidase ~ 82261
Birthing room, newborn care ~ 99431
Bischof procedure ~ 63170-63172
Bismuth ~ 83015
Bizzozero's corpuscle/cell ~ see blood, platelet
Bladder
abscess, incision and drainage ~ 51080
anastomosis ~ 51960
aspiration ~ 51000-51010
biopsy ~ 52204
catheterization ~ 51045, 51701-51703
change tube ~ 51705-51710
creation, stoma ~ 51980
cyst, urachal, excision ~ 51500
destruction, endoscopic ~ 52214-52224, 52354

Bladder ~ *continued*
dilation, ureter ~ 52260-52265, 52341-52342, 52344-52345
diverticulum
excision ~ 51525
incision ~ 52305
resection ~ 52305
endoscopy ~ 52000
biopsy ~ 52204, 52354
catheterization ~ 52005, 52010
destruction ~ 52214-52224, 52400
dilation ~ 52260-52265
diverticulum ~ 52305
evacuation, clot ~ 52001
excision, tumor ~ 52234-52240, 52355
exploration ~ 52351
injection ~ 52283
lithotripsy ~ 52353
radiotracer ~ 52250
removal
calculus ~ 52310-52315, 52352
foreign body ~ 52310-52315
sphincter surgery ~ 52277
tumor, excision ~ 52355
ureter surgery ~ 52290-52300
urethral syndrome ~ 52285
with urethrotomy ~ 52270-52276
excision
partial ~ 51550-51565
total ~ 51570, 51580, 51590-51597
with nodes ~ 51575, 51585, 51595
transurethral ~ 52640
tumor ~ 52234-52240
incision
catheter ~ 51045
with destruction ~ 51020-51030
with radiotracer ~ 51020
incision and drainage ~ 51040
injection, radiologic ~ 51600-51610
insertion, stent ~ 51045, 52334
instillation, drugs ~ 51720
irrigation ~ 51700
lesion, destruction ~ 51030
neck, endoscopy, injection of implant material ~ 51715
excision ~ 51520
nuclear medicine, residual study ~ 78730
radiotracer ~ 52250
reconstruction, and urethra ~ 51800-51820
with intestines ~ 51960
removal
calculus ~ 51050, 52310-52315
foreign body ~ 52310-52315
urethral stent ~ 52310-52315
repair
diverticulum ~ 52305
exstrophy ~ 51940
fistula ~ 44660-44661, 45800-45805, 51880-51925
neck ~ 51845
wound ~ 51860-51865

Bladder ~ *continued*
resection ~ 52500
sphincter surgery ~ 52277
suspension ~ 51990
suture
fistula ~ 44660-44661, 45800-45805, 51880-51925
wound ~ 51860-51865
tumor, excision ~ 51530
unlisted services and procedures ~ 53899
urethrocystography ~ 74450-74455
urethrotomy ~ 52270-52276
urinary incontinence procedures, laparoscopy ~ 51990-51992
pulsed magnetic neuromodulation ~ 0029T
X-ray ~ 74430
with contrast ~ 74450-74455
Bladder voiding pressure studies ~ 51795
Blalock-Hanlon procedure ~ 33735-33737
Blalock-Taussig procedure ~ see shunt, great vessel
Blastocyst implantation ~ see implantation
Blastocyst transfer ~ see embryo transfer
Blastogenesis ~ 86353
Blastomyces, antibody ~ 86612
Blastomycosis, european ~ see cryptococcus
Blast cells ~ see stem cell
Blast transformation ~ 86353
Bleeding ~ see also hemorrhage
anal ~ 46614
disorder ~ 85390
time ~ 85002
tube, passage and placement ~ 91100
uterine ~ 59160
vaginal ~ 57180
Blepharoplasty ~ 15820-15823, 67950
anesthesia ~ 00103
Blepharoptosis
repair ~ 67901-67909
frontalis muscle technique ~ 67901
with fascial sling ~ 67902
superior rectus technique with fascial sling ~ 67906
tarso levator resection/advancement
external approach ~ 67904
internal approach ~ 67903
Blepharorrhaphy ~ 67875
Blepharospasm, chemodenervation ~ 64612
Blepharotomy ~ 67700
Blister ~ see bulla
Blom-Singer prosthesis ~ 31611
Blood ~ 85025-85027
bleeding time ~ 85002
collection, for autotransfusion
intraoperative ~ 86891
preoperative ~ 86890
feces ~ 82270
by hemoglobin immunoassay ~ 82274
gastric contents ~ 82273
hemoglobin concentration ~ 85046
nuclear medicine
flow imaging ~ 78445

Blood ~ *continued*
plasma iron ~ 78160
red cell ~ 78140
red cell survival ~ 78130-78135
osmolality ~ 83930
other source ~ 82273
plasma, exchange ~ 36514-36516
platelet
aggregation ~ 85576
automated count ~ 85049
count ~ 85008
manual count ~ 85032
stem cell
count ~ 86587
donor search ~ 38204
harvesting ~ 38205-38206
transplantation ~ 38240-38242
cell concentration ~ 38215
cryopreservation ~ 38207, 88240
plasma depletion ~ 38214
platelet depletion ~ 38213
red blood cell depletion ~ 38212
T-cell depletion ~ 38210
thawing ~ 38208-38209, 88241
tumor cell depletion ~ 38211
washing ~ 38209
transfusion ~ 36430
exchange ~ 36455
newborn ~ 36450
fetal ~ 36460
push, infant ~ 36440
unlisted services and procedures ~ 85999
urine ~ 83491
viscosity ~ 85810
Blood, occult ~ 82270-82272
Blood banking
frozen blood preparation ~ 86930-86932
frozen plasma preparation ~ 86927
physician services ~ 86077-86079
Blood cell
CD4 and CD8, including ratio ~ 86360
enzyme activity ~ 82657
exchange ~ 36511-36513
red ~ see red blood cell (RBC)
sedimentation rate
automated ~ 85652
manual ~ 85651
white ~ see leukocyte
Blood cell count
automated ~ 85049
B-cells ~ 86064
blood smear ~ 85007-85008
differential WBC count ~ 85004-85007, 85009
hematocrit ~ 85014
hemoglobin ~ 85018
hemogram
added indices ~ 85025-85027
automated ~ 85025-85027
manual ~ 85032
microhematocrit ~ 85013
natural killer (NK) cells ~ 86379
Blood cell count ~ *continued*
red ~ 85032-85041
red blood cells ~ 85032-85041
reticulocyte ~ 85044-85046
stem cells ~ 86587
T-cells ~ 86359-86361
white ~ 85032, 85048, 89055
white blood cells ~ 85032, 85048, 89055
Blood clot
assay ~ 85396
clotting factor ~ 85250-85293
clotting factor test ~ 85210-85244
clotting inhibitors ~ 85300-85302, 85305, 85307
clot lysis time ~ 85175
clot retraction ~ 85170
coagulation time ~ 85345-85348
Blood coagulation
defect ~ 85390
disorders ~ 34401-34490, 35875-35876, 50230
factor ~ 85210-85293
factor I ~ 85384-85385
factor II ~ 85210
factor III ~ see thromboplastin
factor IV ~ see calcium
factor VII ~ 85230
factor VIII ~ 85210-85293
factor IX ~ 85250
factor X ~ 85260
factor X, activated ~ 85260
factor XI ~ 85270
factor XIII ~ 85290-85291
test ~ 85999
Blood component removal ~ 36511-36516
Blood count, complete ~ 85025-85027
Blood flow check, graft ~ 15860, 90939-90940
Blood gases
CO2 ~ 82803
HCO3 ~ 82803
O2 saturation ~ 82805-82810
pCO2 ~ 82803
pH ~ 82800-82803
pO2 ~ 82803
Blood letting ~ 99195
Blood lipoprotein ~ see lipoprotein
Blood pool imaging ~ 78472-78473, 78481-78483, 78494-78496
Blood pressure ~ see performance measures
left ventricular filling ~ 0086T
monitoring, 24 hour ~ 93784-93790
venous ~ 93770
Blood products
irradiation ~ 86945
pooling ~ 86965
splitting ~ 86985
Blood sample, fetal ~ 59030
Blood serum ~ see serum
Blood smear ~ 85060
Blood syndrome, chromosome analysis ~ 88245-88248

Blood tests
nuclear medicine
iron, chelatable ~ 78172
iron absorption ~ 78162
iron utilization ~ 78170
plasma volume ~ 78110-78111
platelet survival ~ 78190-78191
red cell volume ~ 78120-78121
whole blood volume ~ 78122
panels
electrolyte ~ 80051
general health panel ~ 80050
hepatic function ~ 80076
hepatitis, acute ~ 80074
lipid panel ~ 80061
metabolic
basic ~ 80048
comprehensive ~ 80053
obstetric panel ~ 80055
renal function ~ 80069
volume determination ~ 78122
Blood transfusion, autologous ~ 86890-86891
Blood typing, ABO only ~ 86900
antigen screen ~ 86903-86904
crossmatch ~ 86920-86922
other RBC antigens ~ 86905
paternity testing ~ 86910-86911
Rh (D) ~ 86901
Rh phenotype ~ 86906
Blood urea nitrogen ~ 84520-84525
Blood vessels ~ see also artery; vein
angioscopy, non-coronary ~ 35400
endoscopy, surgical ~ 37500
excision, arteriovenous malformation ~ 63250-63252
exploration
abdomen ~ 35840
chest ~ 35820
extremity ~ 35860
neck ~ 35800
great, suture ~ 33320-33322
harvest
endoscopic ~ 33508
lower extremity vein ~ 35572
upper extremity artery ~ 35600
upper extremity vein ~ 35500
kidney, repair ~ 50100
repair
abdomen ~ see aneurysm repair; fistula, repair
with composite graft ~ 35681-35683
with other graft ~ 35281
with vein graft ~ 35251
aneurysm ~ 61705-61708
arteriovenous malformation ~ 61680-61692, 61705-61710, 63250-63252
chest
with composite graft ~ 35681-35683
with other graft ~ 35271-35276
with vein graft ~ 35241-35246
direct ~ 35201-35226
finger ~ 35207
Blood vessels ~ *continued*
graft defect ~ 35870
hand ~ 35207
lower extremity ~ 35226
with composite graft ~ 35681-35683
with other graft ~ 35281
with vein graft ~ 35251
neck
with composite graft ~ 35681-35683
with other graft ~ 35261
with vein graft ~ 35231
upper extremity ~ 35206
with composite graft ~ 35681-35683
with other graft ~ 35266
with vein graft ~ 35236
shunt creation, direct ~ 36818, 36821
thomas shunt ~ 36835
with bypass graft ~ 35686
with graft ~ 36825-36830
shunt revision, with graft ~ 36832
Blood, occult ~ see occult blood
Bloom syndrome, chromosome analysis ~ 88245
Blotting, western ~ see western blot
Blot test, ink ~ 96100
Blow-out fracture, orbital floor ~ 21385-21395
Blue, dome cyst ~ 19000-19001
BMT ~ 38240-38242
Boarding home care ~ 99321-99333
Bodies
acetone ~ 82009-82010
Barr ~ 88130
carotid ~ see carotid body
ciliary ~ see ciliary body
Heinz ~ 85441-85445
inclusion ~ see inclusion bodies
ketone ~ 82009-82010
Body cast
halo ~ 29000
removal ~ 29700, 29710-29715
repair ~ 29720
Risser jacket ~ 29010-29015
turnbuckle jacket ~ 29020-29025
upper body and head ~ 29040
upper body and legs ~ 29046
upper body and one leg ~ 29044
upper body only ~ 29035
Body composition, dual energy X-ray absorptiometry ~ 0028T
Body fluid, crystal identification ~ 89060
Body of vertebra ~ see vertebral, body
Body section
X-ray ~ 76100
motion ~ 76101-76102
Body system, neurologic ~ ***78699***
Boil ~ 10060-10061
Boil, vulva ~ 56405
Bone ~ see also specific bone***
ablation, tumor ~ 20982
biopsy ~ 20220-20245
carpal ~ see carpal bone

Bone ~ *continued*
cheek ~ see cheekbone
CT scan, density study ~ 77078-77079
cyst
drainage ~ 20615
injection ~ 20615
dual energy X-ray absorptiometry ~ 77080-77081
excision
epiphyseal bar ~ 20150
facial bones ~ 21026
mandible ~ 21025
facial ~ see facial bone
fixation
caliper ~ 20660
cranial tong ~ 20660
halo ~ 20661-20663, 21100
interdental ~ 21110
multiplane ~ 20692
pin/wire ~ 20650
skeletal, humeral epicondyle, percutaneous ~ 24566
stereotactic frame ~ 20660
uniplane ~ 20690
hyoid ~ 21495
insertion
needle ~ 36680
osseointegrated implant, for external speech processor/cochlear stimulator ~ 69714-69718
metatarsal ~ see metatarsal
nasal ~ see nasal bone
navicular ~ see navicular
nuclear medicine
density study ~ 78350-78351
imaging ~ 78300-78320
spect ~ 78320
unlisted services and procedures ~ 78399
protein ~ 83937
removal, fixation device ~ 20670-20680
replacement, osseointegrated implant, for external speech processor/cochlear stimulator ~ 69717-69718
scan ~ see bone, nuclear medicine; nuclear medicine
semilunar ~ see lunate
sesamoid ~ see sesamoid bone
tarsal ~ see ankle
temporal ~ see temporal bone
X-ray
age study ~ 77072
dual energy absorptiometry ~ 77080-77081
length study ~ 77073
osseous survey ~ 77074-77077
Bone 4-carboxyglutamic protein ~ 83937
Bone conduction hearing device, electromagnetic
implantation/replacement ~ 69710
removal/repair ~ 69711
Bone density study
appendicular skeleton ~ 77079, 77081
axial skeleton ~ 77078, 77080
Bone density study ~ *continued*
ultrasound ~ 76977
vertebral fracture assessment ~ 77082
Bone graft
augmentation mandibular body ~ 21127
femur ~ 27170
fracture orbit ~ 21408
harvesting ~ 20900-20902
malar area ~ 21210
mandible ~ 21215
mandibular ramus ~ 21194
maxilla ~ 21210
microvascular anastomosis
fibula ~ 20955
other ~ 20962
nasal area ~ 21210
nasomaxillary complex fracture ~ 21348
open treatment, craniofacial separation ~ 21436
osteocutaneous flap ~ 20969-20973
reconstruction
mandibular rami ~ 21194
midface ~ 21145-21160
skull ~ 61316
excision ~ 62148
spine surgery
allograft
morselized ~ 20930
structural ~ 20931
autograft
local ~ 20936
morselized ~ 20937
structural ~ 20938
vascular pedicle ~ 25430
Bone healing
electrical stimulation
invasive ~ 20975
noninvasive ~ 20974
ultrasound stimulation ~ 20979
Bone infection ~ 20000-20005
Bone marrow
aspiration ~ 38220
harvesting ~ 38230
magnetic resonance imaging (MRI) ~ 77084
needle biopsy ~ 38221
nuclear medicine, imaging ~ 78102-78104
smear ~ 85097
T-cell transplantation ~ 38240-38242
trocar biopsy ~ 38221
Bone plate, mandible ~ 21244
Bone scan ~ see bone, nuclear medicine; nuclear medicine
Bone spur ~ 69140
Bone wedge reversal, osteotomy ~ 21122
Bordetella
antibody ~ 86615
antigen detection
direct fluorescence ~ 87265
Borrelia, antibody ~ 86618-86619
Borrelia burgdorferi ab ~ 86617
Borreliosis, Lyme ~ 86617-86618
Borthen operation ~ 66165

Bost fusion ~ 25800
Bosworth operation ~ see arthrodesis, vertebrae; fasciotomy; 23540-23552
Bottle type procedure ~ 55060
Botulinum toxin ~ see chemodenervation
Boutonniere deformity ~ 26426-26428
Bowel ~ see intestine
Bowleg repair ~ 27455-27457
Boyce operation ~ 50040-50045
Boyd hip disarticulation ~ see radical resection; replantation; 27590-27592
Brace ~ see cast for leg cast ~ 29358
Brachial arteries ~ see artery, brachial
Brachial plexus
decompression ~ 64713
injection anesthetic ~ 64415-64416
neuroplasty ~ 64713
release ~ 64713
repair/suture ~ 64861
Brachiocephalic artery ~ see artery, brachiocephalic
Brachycephaly ~ 21175
Brachytherapy ~ 77761-77778, 77789
dose plan ~ 77326-77328
remote afterloading
1 to 4 positions ~ 77781
5 to 8 positions ~ 77782
9 to 12 positions ~ 77783
over 12 positions ~ 77784
over 4 positions ~ 77781-77784
unlisted services and procedures ~ 77799
Bradykinin, blood or urine ~ 82286
Brain ~ see also brainstem; skull base surgery; 61480
abscess
drainage ~ 61150-61151
excision ~ 61514, 61522
incision and drainage ~ 61320-61321
adhesions, lysis ~ 62161
anesthesia ~ 00210-00218, 00220-00222
angiography ~ 70496
biopsy ~ 61140
stereotactic ~ 61750-61751
catheter
irrigation ~ 62194, 62225
replacement ~ 62160, 62194, 62225
cisternography ~ 70015
computer assisted, surgery ~ 61795
cortex, magnetic stimulation ~ 0160T-0161T
craniopharyngioma, excision ~ 61545
CT scan ~ 0042T, 70450-70470, 70496
cyst
drainage ~ 61150-61151, 62161-62162
excision ~ 61516, 61524, 62162
Doppler, transcranial ~ 93886-93893
epileptogenic focus, excision ~ 61534, 61536
excision
amygdala ~ 61566
choroid plexus ~ 61544
hemisphere ~ 61542-61543
hippocampus ~ 61566
other lobe ~ 61323, 61539-61540

Brain ~ *continued*
temporal lobe ~ 61537-61538
exploration
infratentorial ~ 61305
supratentorial ~ 61304
hematoma
drainage ~ 61154
incision and drainage ~ 61312-61315
implantation
chemotherapy agent ~ 61517
electrode ~ 61850-61875
pulse generator ~ 61885-61886
receiver ~ 61885-61886
thermal profusion probe ~ 0077T
incision
corpus callosum ~ 61541
frontal lobe ~ 61490
mesencephalic tract ~ 61480
subpial ~ 61567
insertion, catheter ~ 61210
electrode ~ 61531-61533, 61850-61875
pulse generator ~ 61885-61886
receiver ~ 61885-61886
reservoir ~ 61210-61215
lesion
aspiration stereotactic ~ 61750-61751
excision ~ 61534, 61536, 61600-61608, 61615-61616
magnetic resonance imaging (MRI) ~ 70551-77055
intraoperative ~ 70557-70559
meningioma, excision ~ 61512, 61519
myelography ~ 70010
nuclear medicine
blood flow ~ 78610-78615
cerebrospinal fluid ~ 78630-78650
imaging ~ 78600-78607
vascular flow ~ 78610
positron emission tomography ~ 78608-78609
removal
electrode ~ 61535, 61880
foreign body ~ 61570, 62163
pulse generator ~ 61888
receiver ~ 61888
shunt ~ 62256-62258
repair
dura ~ 61618
wound ~ 61571
shunt
creation ~ 62180-62192, 62200-62223
removal ~ 62256-62258
replacement ~ 62160, 62194, 62225-62230, 62256-62258
reprogramming ~ 62252
skull
transcochlear approach ~ 61596
transcondylar approach ~ 61597
transpetrosal approach ~ 61598
transtemporal approach ~ 61595
skull base
craniofacial approach ~ 61580-61585
infratemporal approach ~ 61590-61591

Brain ~ *continued*
orbitocranial-zygomatic approach ~ 61592
stereotactic, aspiration ~ 61750-61751
biopsy ~ 61750-61751
create lesion ~ 61720-61735, 61790-61791
localization for placement of therapy fields ~ 61770
radiation treatment ~ 77432
radiosurgery ~ 61793
surgery ~ 61795
trigeminal tract ~ 61791
transection, subpial ~ 61567
tumor, excision ~ 61510, 61518, 61520-61521, 61526-61530, 61545, 62164
X-ray, with contrast ~ 70010-70015
Brainstem ~ see also brain
auditory evoked potential ~ 92585-92586
biopsy ~ 61575-61576
decompression ~ 61575-61576
evoked potentials ~ 92585-92586
lesion, excision ~ 61575-61576
Brain coverings ~ 61512, 61519
Brain death, determination ~ 95824
Brain surface electrode, stimulation ~ 95961-95962
Brain tumor
acoustic neuroma ~ 61510, 61518, 61520-61521, 61526-61530, 61545, 62164
craniopharyngioma ~ 61545
meningioma ~ 61512, 61519
Brain ventriculography ~ see ventriculography
Branchial cleft cyst excision ~ 42810-42815
Branchioma ~ 42810-42815
Breast
ablation
cryosurgery ~ 19105
abscess
incision and drainage ~ 19020
augmentation ~ 19324-19325
bioimpedance ~ 0060T
biopsy ~ 19100-19103
catheter placement, for interstitial radioelement application ~ 19296-19298
cyst, puncture aspiration ~ 19000-19001
excision
biopsy ~ 19100-19103
capsules ~ 19371
chest wall tumor ~ 19260-19272
cyst ~ 19120
lactiferous duct fistula ~ 19112
lesion ~ 19120-19126, 19301
by needle localization ~ 19125-19126
mastectomy ~ 19300-19307
nipple exploration ~ 19110
exploration ~ 19020
implants
insertion ~ 19340-19342
preparation of moulage ~ 19396
removal ~ 19328-19330
supply ~ 19396
incision, capsules ~ 19370
injection, radiologic ~ 19030
Breast ~ *continued*
magnetic resonance imaging (MRI) ~ 77058-77059
mammoplasty
augmentation ~ 19324-19325
reduction ~ 19318
mastopexy ~ 19316
metallic localization clip placement ~ 19295
needle biopsy ~ 19100
needle wire placement ~ 19290-19291
periprosthetic capsulectomy ~ 19371
periprosthetic capsulotomy ~ 19370
reconstruction ~ 19357-19369
augmentation ~ 19324-19325
mammoplasty ~ 19318-19325
nipple ~ 19350-19355
areola ~ 19350
revision ~ 19380
with free flap ~ 19364
with latissimus dorsi flap ~ 19361
with other techniques ~ 19366
with tissue expander ~ 19357
with transverse rectus abdominis myocutaneous flap ~ 19367-19369
reduction ~ 19318
removal
capsules ~ 19371
modified radical ~ 19307
partial ~ 19300-19302
radical ~ 19305-19306
simple, complete ~ 19303
subcutaneous ~ 19304
repair, suspension ~ 19316
stereotactic localization ~ 77031
ultrasound ~ 76645
unlisted services and procedures ~ 19499
X-ray ~ 77055-77057
localization nodule ~ 77032
with computer-aide detection ~ 77051-77052
Breathing, inspiratory positive-pressure ~ see intermittent positive pressure breathing (IPPB)
Breath odor alcohol ~ 82075
Breath test
alcohol, ethyl ~ 82075
heart transplant rejection detection ~ 0085T
helicobacter pylori ~ 78267-78268, 83013-83014
hydrogen ~ 91065
Bricker procedure, intestines anastomosis ~ 50820
Bristow procedure ~ 23450-23462
Brock operation ~ 33470-33474
Broken, nose ~ see fracture, nasal bone
Bronchi
aspiration, endoscopic ~ 31645-31646
biopsy, endoscopic ~ 31625-31629, 31632-31633
catheterization
with bronchial brush biopsy ~ 31717
endoscopy
aspiration ~ 31645-31646

Bronchi ~ *continued*
biopsy ~ 31625-31629, 31632-31633
destruction, tumor ~ 31641
dilation ~ 31630-31631, 31636-31638
excision, lesion ~ 31640
exploration ~ 31622
foreign body removal ~ 31635
fracture ~ 31630
injection ~ 31656
lesion ~ 31640-31641
stenosis ~ 31641
tumor ~ 31640-31641
ultrasound ~ 31620
exploration, endoscopic ~ 31622
fracture, endoscopy ~ 31630
injection, X-ray ~ 31656, 31715
needle biopsy ~ 31629, 31633
reconstruction ~ 31770
graft repair ~ 31770
stenosis ~ 31775
removal, foreign body ~ 31635
repair, fistula ~ 32815
stenosis, endoscopic treatment ~ 31641
stent
placement ~ 31636-31637
revision ~ 31638
tumor, excision ~ 31640
ultrasound ~ 31620
unlisted services and procedures ~ 31899
X-ray, with contrast ~ 71040-71060
Bronchial
alveolar lavage ~ 31624
brushings/protected brushing ~ 31623
brush biopsy, with catheterization ~ 31717
challenge test ~ 95070-95071, 95075
with antigens, gases ~ 95070
with chemicals ~ 95071
lavage ~ 31624
Broncho-bronchial anastomosis ~ 32486
Bronchoalveolar lavage ~ 31624
Bronchography ~ 71040-71060
injection, transtracheal ~ 31715
segmental, injection ~ 31656
Bronchoplasty ~ 32501
excision stenosis and anastomosis ~ 31775
graft repair ~ 31770
Bronchopneumonia, hiberno-vernal ~ 86000, 86638
Bronchopulmonary lavage ~ 31624
Bronchoscopy
alveolar lavage ~ 31624
aspiration ~ 31645-31646
biopsy ~ 31625-31629, 31632-31633
brushing/protected brushing ~ 31623
catheter placement, intracavitary radioelement ~ 31643
dilation ~ 31630-31631, 31636-31638
exploration ~ 31622
fracture ~ 31630
injection ~ 31656
needle biopsy ~ 31629, 31633
Bronchoscopy ~ *continued*
removal
foreign body ~ 31635
tumor ~ 31640-31641
stenosis ~ 31641
stent placement ~ 31631, 31636-31637
stent revision ~ 31638
ultrasound ~ 31620
X-ray contrast ~ 31656
Bronchospasm evaluation ~ 94010-94070
Bronkodyl ~ 80198
Brow ptosis, repair ~ 67900
Brucella ~ 86000
antibody ~ 86622
Bruise ~ see hematoma
Brunschwig operation ~ see hip ~ 45126, 58240
Brush biopsy ~ see biopsy; needle biopsy
bronchi ~ 31717
Brush border ab ~ 86308-86310
Bucca ~ see cheek
Buccal mucosa ~ 40818
Bulbourethral gland, excision ~ 53250
Bulla
incision and drainage
puncture aspiration ~ 10160
lung
excision-plication ~ 32141
endoscopic ~ 32655
Bun ~ see urea nitrogen ~ 84520-84525
Bunion repair ~ 28296-28299
Chevron procedure ~ 28296
concentric procedure ~ 28296
Joplin procedure ~ 28294
Keller procedure ~ 28292
Lapidus procedure ~ 28297
Mayo procedure ~ 28292
McBride procedure ~ 28292
Mitchell procedure ~ 28296
Silver procedure ~ 28290
with implant ~ 28293
Burgess amputation ~ 27889
Burhenne procedure ~ see gallbladder ~ 43264, 47420-47425
Burkitt herpesvirus ~ 86663-86665
Burns
allograft ~ 15350-15351
debridement ~ 01951-01953, 15002-15005, 16010-16030
dressings ~ 16010-16030
escharotomy ~ 16035-16036
excision ~ 01951-01953
initial treatment ~ 16000
tissue culture skin grafts ~ 15100-15121, 15342-15343
xenograft ~ 15400-15401
Burrow's operation ~ 14000-14350
Burr hole
anesthesia ~ 00214
skull
biopsy brain ~ 61140
catheterization ~ 61210

Burr hole ~ *continued*
drainage
abscess ~ 61150-61151
cyst ~ 61150-61151
hematoma ~ 61154-61156
exploration
infratentorial ~ 61253
supratentorial ~ 61250
for implant of neurostimulator array ~ 61863-61868
injection, contrast media ~ 61120
insertion, catheter ~ 61210
reservoir ~ 61210
Bursa
ankle ~ 27604
arm, lower ~ 25031
elbow
excision ~ 24105
incision and drainage ~ 23931
femur, excision ~ 27062
foot, incision and drainage ~ 28001
hip, incision and drainage ~ 26991
injection ~ 20600-20610
ischial, excision ~ 27060
joint
aspiration ~ 20600-20610
drainage ~ 20600-20610
injection ~ 20600-20610
knee, excision ~ 27340
leg, lower ~ 27604
palm, incision and drainage ~ 26025-26030
pelvis, incision and drainage ~ 26991
shoulder, drainage ~ 23031
wrist ~ 25031
excision ~ 25115-25116
Bursectomy ~ see excision, bursa
Bursitis, radiohumeral ~ 24350-24356
Bursocentesis ~ 20600-20610
Button, nasal septal prosthesis, insertion ~ 30220
Butyrylcholine esterase ~ 82480-82482
Bypass, cardiopulmonary ~ 33926
Bypass graft
aortobi-iliac ~ 35538, 35638
aortobifemoral ~ 35540
aortofemoral ~ 35539
axillary artery ~ 35516-35522, 35533, 35616-35623, 35650, 35654
brachial artery ~ 35510, 35512, 35522-35525
carotid artery ~ 35501-35510, 35526, 35601-35606, 35626, 35642
celiac artery ~ 35531, 35631
coronary artery
angiography ~ 93556
arterial ~ 33533-33536
venous graft ~ 33510-33516
excision
abdomen ~ 35907
extremity ~ 35903
neck ~ 35901
thorax ~ 35905
Bypass graft ~ *continued*
femoral artery ~ 35521, 35533, 35551-35558, 35566, 35621, 35646-35647, 35651-35661, 35666, 35700
harvest
endoscopic ~ 33508
upper extremity vein ~ 35500
iliac artery ~ 35563, 35663
iliofemoral artery ~ 35548-35549, 35565, 35665
mesenteric artery ~ 35531, 35631
peroneal artery ~ 35566-35571, 35666-35671
placement, vein patch ~ 35685
popliteal artery ~ 35551-35558, 35571, 35623, 35651, 35656, 35671, 35700
renal artery ~ 35536, 35560, 35631-35636
reoperation ~ 35700
repair
abdomen ~ 35907
extremity ~ 35903
lower extremity, with composite graft ~ 35681-35683
neck ~ 35901
thorax ~ 35905
revascularization
extremity ~ 35903
neck ~ 35901
thorax ~ 35905
revision
lower extremity
femoral artery ~ 35883-35884
with angioplasty ~ 35879
with vein interposition ~ 35881
secondary repair ~ 35870
splenic artery ~ 35536, 35636
subclavian artery ~ 35506, 35511-35516, 35526, 35606-35616, 35626, 35645
thrombectomy, other than hemodialysis graft or fistula ~ 35875-35876
tibial artery ~ 35566-35571, 35623, 35666-35671
vertebral artery ~ 35508, 35515, 35642-35645
with composite graft ~ 35681
Bypass in-situ
femoral artery ~ 35582-35585
peroneal artery ~ 35585-35587
popliteal artery ~ 35583, 35587
tibial artery ~ 35585-35587

C

C vitamin ~ 82180
C-13
urea breath test ~ 83013-83014
urease activity ~ 83013-83014
C-14
urea breath test ~ 78267-78268
urease activity ~ 83013-83014
C-peptide ~ 80432, 84681

C-reactive protein ~ 86140-86141
C-section ~ see cesarean delivery
CABG ~ see coronary artery bypass graft (CABG) ~ 33503-33505, 33510-33516
Cadmium, urine ~ 82300
Calcaneal spur ~ 28119
Calcaneus
craterization ~ 28120
cyst, excision ~ 28100-28103
diaphysectomy ~ 28120
excision ~ 28118-28120
fracture
open treatment ~ 28415-28420
percutaneous fixation ~ 28406
without manipulation ~ 28400
with manipulation ~ 28405-28406
repair, osteotomy ~ 28300
saucerization ~ 28120
tumor, excision ~ 27647, 28100-28103
X-ray ~ 73650
Calcareous deposits, subdeltoid, removal ~ 23000
Calcifediol, blood or urine ~ 82306
Calcifediol assay ~ 82307
Calciferol, blood or urine ~ 82307
Calcification ~ see calcium, deposits
Calciol ~ 82306
Calcitonin
blood or urine ~ 82308
stimulation panel ~ 80410
Calcium, blood, infusion test ~ 82331
deposits ~ see removal, calculi (stone) ~ 65205-65265
ionized ~ 82330
total ~ 82310
urine ~ 82340
Calcium-binding protein, vitamin K-dependent ~ 83937
Calcium-pentagastrin stimulation ~ 80410
Calculus
analysis ~ 82355-82370
destruction
bile duct ~ 43265
pancreatic duct ~ 43265
removal
bile duct ~ 43264, 47554, 74327
bladder ~ 51050, 52310-52318, 52352
kidney ~ 50060-50081, 50130, 50561, 50580, 52352
pancreatic duct ~ 43264
ureter ~ 50610-50630, 50961, 50980, 51060-51065, 52320-52325, 52352
urethra ~ 52310-52315, 52352
Calculus of kidney ~ 50060-50081, 50130, 50561, 50580, 52352
Caldwell-Luc procedure ~ 21385
sinusotomy ~ 31030-31032
Caliper, application/removal ~ 20660
Callander knee disarticulation ~ 27598
Callosum, corpus ~ 61541
Calmette Guerin Bacillus vaccine ~ see BCG vaccine
Caloric vestibular test ~ 92533
Calycoplasty ~ 50405
Camey enterocystoplasty ~ 50825
CAMP ~ 82030
Campbell procedure ~ 27422
Campylobacter, antibody ~ 86625
Campylobacter pylori ~ see helicobacter pylori
Canal, ear ~ see auditory canal
Canal, semicircular ~ 69820, 69840
Canaloplasty ~ 69631, 69635
Candida
antibody ~ 86628
skin test ~ 86485
Cannulation ~ 36821
arterial ~ 36620-36625
sinus
maxillary ~ 31000
sphenoid ~ 31002
thoracic duct ~ 38794
Cannulation, renoportal ~ 37145
Cannulization ~ see catheterization
arteriovenous ~ 36145, 36810-36815
declotting ~ 36550, 36860-36861
ecmo ~ 36822
external, declotting ~ 36860-36861
vas deferens ~ 55200
vein to vein ~ 36800
Canthocystostomy ~ 68745, 68750
Canthopexy
lateral ~ 21282
medial ~ 21280
Canthoplasty ~ 67950
Canthorrhaphy ~ 67880-67882
Canthotomy ~ 67715
Canthus, reconstruction ~ 67950
Cap, cervical ~ 57170
Capsule ~ 26516-26518
elbow
arthrotomy ~ 24006
excision ~ 24006
foot ~ 28264
interphalangeal joint
excision ~ 26525
incision ~ 26525
knee ~ 27435
metacarpophalangeal joint
excision ~ 26520
incision ~ 26520
metatarsophalangeal joint, release ~ 28289
shoulder, incision ~ 23020
wrist, excision ~ 25320
Capsulectomy, breast, periprosthetic ~ 19371
Capsulodesis, metacarpophalangeal joint ~ 26516-26518
Capsulorrhaphy
anterior ~ 23450-23462
multi-directional instability ~ 23466
posterior ~ 23465
wrist ~ 25320

Capsulotomy, breast, periprosthetic ~ 19370
foot ~ 28260-28262
hip, with release, flexor muscles ~ 27036
interphalangeal joint ~ 28272
knee ~ 27435
metacarpophalangeal joint ~ 26520
metatarsophalangeal joint ~ 28270
toe ~ 28270-28272
wrist ~ 25085
Captopril ~ 80416-80417
Carbamazepine, assay ~ 80156-80157
Carbazepin ~ 80156-80157
Carbinol ~ 84600
Carbohydrate deficient transferrin ~ 82373
Carbon dioxide, blood or urine ~ 82374
Carbon monoxide, blood ~ 82375-82376
Carbon tetrachloride ~ 84600
Carboxycathepsin ~ 82164
Carboxyhemoglobin ~ 82375-82376
Carbuncle, incision and drainage ~ 10060-10061
Carcinoembryonal antigen ~ 82378
Carcinoembryonic antigen ~ 82378
Cardiac ~ see coronary
Cardiac arrhythmia, tachycardia ~ 93609
Cardiac atria ~ see atria
Cardiac catheterization
combined left and right heart ~ 93526-93529
combined right and retrograde left
congenital cardiac anomalies ~ 93531
combined right and transseptal left
congenital cardiac anomalies ~ 93532-93533
for biopsy ~ 93505
for dilution studies ~ 93561-93562
imaging ~ 93555-93556
injection ~ see catheterization, cardiac ~ 93539-93545
left heart ~ 93510-93524
pacemaker ~ 33210
right, congenital cardiac anomalies ~ 93530
right heart ~ 93501-93503
Cardiac electroversion ~ 92960-92961
Cardiac event recorder
implantation ~ 33282
removal ~ 33284
Cardiac magnetic resonance imaging (CMRI)
complete study ~ 75554
limited study ~ 75555
morphology ~ 75553
velocity flow mapping ~ 75556
Cardiac massage, thoracotomy ~ 32160
Cardiac muscle ~ see myocardium
Cardiac neoplasm ~ 33120-33130
Cardiac output, indicator dilution ~ 93561-93562
Cardiac pacemaker ~ see heart, pacemaker
Cardiac rehabilitation ~ 93797-93798
Cardiac septal defect ~ 33813-33814
Cardiac transplantation ~ 33935, 33945
Cardiectomy, donor ~ 33930, 33940
Cardioassist ~ 0049T, 92970-92971
Cardiolipin antibody ~ 86147
Cardiology ~ see electrocardiography
diagnostic
acoustic recording with computer analysis
heart sounds ~ 0068T-0070T
atrial electrogram
esophageal recording ~ 93615-93616
cardio-defibrillator
evaluation and testing ~ 93640-93642, 93741-93744
echocardiography
Doppler ~ 93303-93321, 93662
intracardiac ~ 93662
transesophageal ~ 93318
transthoracic ~ 93303-93317, 93350
electrocardiogram
evaluation ~ 93000, 93010, 93014
microvolt t-wave alternans ~ 93025
monitoring ~ 93224-93237
patient-demand ~ 93268-93272
rhythm ~ 93040-93042
tracing ~ 93005
transmission ~ 93012
ergonovine provocation test ~ 93024
hemodynamic monitoring non-invasive ~ 0086T
implantable loop recorder system ~ 93727
intracardiac pacing and mapping ~ 93631
3-D mapping ~ 93613
follow-up study ~ 93624
stimulation and pacing ~ 93623
intracardiac pacing and recording
arrhythmia induction ~ 93618-93620
bundle of His ~ 93600
comprehensive ~ 93619-93622
intra-atrial ~ 93602, 93610
right ventricle ~ 93603
tachycardia sites ~ 93609
ventricular ~ 93612
intravascular ultrasound ~ 92978-92979
left ventricle pressure measurement ~ 0086T
pacemaker testing ~ 93642
antitachycardia system ~ 93724
dual chamber ~ 93731-93733
leads ~ 93641
single chamber ~ 93734-93736
perfusion imaging ~ see nuclear medicine ~ 78460-78461
stress tests
cardiovascular ~ 93015-93018
drug induced ~ 93024
multiple gated acquisition (MUGA) ~ 78473
tilt table evaluation ~ 93660
therapeutic
cardio-defibrillator
initial set-up and programming ~ 93745
cardioassist ~ 92970-92971
cardioversion ~ 92960-92961
intravascular ultrasound ~ 92978-92979
pacing
transcutaneous, temporary ~ 92953
thrombolysis ~ 92975-92977

Cardiology ~ *continued*
thrombolysis, coronary ~ 92977
valvuloplasty, percutaneous ~ 92986-92990
Cardiomyotomy ~ 32665, 43330-43331
Cardioplasty ~ 43320
Cardiopulmonary bypass ~ 32852, 32854, 32851-32854, 33935
Cardiopulmonary resuscitation ~ 92950
Cardiotomy ~ 33310-33315
Cardiovascular stress test ~ 93015-93018
Cardiovascular system
medical services ~ 92950-93799
surgical procedures ~ 33000-39599
Cardioversion ~ 92960-92961
Care, custodial ~ see nursing facility services
Care, intensive ~ 99298-99300
Care, neonatal intensive ~ see intensive care, neonatal
Care, self ~ see self care
Care plan oversight services ~ 99339-99340, 99374-99380
Carneous mole ~ see abortion
Carnitine ~ 82379
Carotene ~ 82380
Caroticum, glomus ~ 60605, 60600
Carotid artery
aneurysm repair
vascular malformation or carotid-cavernous fistula ~ 61710
excision ~ 60605
ligation ~ 37600-37606
stent, transcatheter placement ~ 0075T-0076T
transection, with skull base surgery ~ 61609
Carotid body
lesion
carotid artery ~ 60605
excision ~ 60600
Carpals, incision and drainage ~ 25035
Carpal bone ~ see wrist
arthroplasty, with implant ~ 25443
cyst, excision ~ 25130-25136
dislocation
closed treatment ~ 25690
open treatment ~ 25695
excision ~ 25210-25215
partial ~ 25145
fracture
closed treatment ~ 25622, 25630
open treatment ~ 25628, 25645
without manipulation ~ 25630
with manipulation ~ 25624, 25635
incision and drainage ~ 26034
insertion, vascular pedicle ~ 25430
osteoplasty ~ 25394
repair ~ 25431-25440
sequestrectomy ~ 25145
tumor, excision ~ 25130-25136
Carpal tunnel, injection, therapeutic ~ 20526
Carpal tunnel syndrome, decompression ~ 64721
Carpectomy ~ 25210-25215
Carpometacarpal joint
arthrodesis
hand ~ 26843-26844
thumb ~ 26841-26842
arthrotomy ~ 26070
biopsy, synovium ~ 26100
dislocation
closed treatment ~ 26670
with manipulation ~ 26675-26676
open treatment ~ 26685-26686
exploration ~ 26070
fusion
hand ~ 26843-26844
thumb ~ 26841-26842
removal, foreign body ~ 26070
repair ~ 25447
synovectomy ~ 26130
Cartilage, arytenoid ~ 31560-31561
Cartilage, ear ~ 21235
Cartilage graft
ear to face ~ 21235
harvesting ~ 20910-20912
rib to face ~ 21230
Cartilaginous exostoses ~ 69140
Case management services
anticoagulant management ~ 99363-99364
team conferences ~ 99361-99373
telephone calls ~ 99361-99373
Cast ~ see also splint ~ 29358
body, Risser jacket ~ 29010-29015
body cast
halo ~ 29000
turnbuckle jacket ~ 29020-29025
upper body and head ~ 29040
upper body and legs ~ 29046
upper body and one leg ~ 29044
upper body only ~ 29035
clubfoot ~ 29450
cylinder ~ 29365
finger ~ 29086
hand ~ 29085
hip ~ 29305-29325
leg, rigid total contact ~ 29445
long arm ~ 29065
long leg ~ 29345-29355, 29365, 29450
long leg brace ~ 29358
patellar tendon bearing (PTB) ~ 29435
removal ~ 29700-29715
repair ~ 29720
short arm ~ 29075
short leg ~ 29405-29435, 29450
shoulder ~ 29049-29058
walking ~ 29355, 29425
revision ~ 29440
wedging ~ 29740-29750
windowing ~ 29730
wrist ~ 29085
Casting, unlisted services and procedures ~ 29799
Castration ~ see orchiectomy

Castration, female ~ 58262-58263, 58291-58292, 58552, 58554, 58661, 58940-58943
Cat scan ~ see CT scan
Cataract
excision ~ 66830
incision ~ 66820-66821
laser ~ 66821
stab incision ~ 66820
removal/extraction
extracapsular ~ 66982, 66984
intracapsular ~ 66983
Catecholamines ~ 80424, 82382-82384
blood ~ 82383
urine ~ 82382
Cathepsin-D ~ 82387
Catheter ~ see cannulization; venipuncture
aspiration
nasotracheal ~ 31720
tracheobronchial ~ 31725
bladder ~ 51701-51703
irrigation ~ 51700
breast cytology ~ 0046T-0047T
declotting ~ 36550
exchange
arterial ~ 37209, 75900
peritoneal ~ 49423
intracatheter, irrigation ~ 99507
obstruction clearance ~ 36596
pericatheter obstruction
clearance ~ 36595
placement
breast
for intracavitary radioelement application ~ 19296-19298
bronchus
for intracavitary radioelement application ~ 31643
removal
central venous ~ 36589
peritoneum ~ 49422
spinal cord ~ 62355
repair, central venous ~ 36575
replacement, central venous ~ 36580-36581, 36584
repositioning ~ 36597
Catheterization ~ see also catheter
abdomen ~ 49420-49421
abdominal artery ~ 36245-36248
aorta ~ 36160-36215
arterial
cutdown ~ 36625
intracatheter/needle ~ 36100-36140
percutaneous ~ 36620
arteriovenous shunt ~ 36145
bile duct ~ 47530
change ~ 47525
percutaneous ~ 47510
bladder ~ 51010, 51045
brachiocephalic artery ~ 36215-36218
Catheterization ~ ***continued***
brain ~ 61210
replacement ~ 62160, 62194, 62225
cardiac
combined left and right heart ~ 93526-93529
combined right and retrograde left
for congenital cardiac anomalies ~ 93531
combined right and transseptal left
for congenital cardiac anomalies ~ 93532-93533
flow directed ~ 93503
for biopsy ~ 93505
for dilution studies ~ 93561-93562
imaging ~ 93555-93556
injection ~ 93539-93545
left heart ~ 93510-93524
pacemaker ~ 33210
right heart ~ 36013, 93501
for congenital cardiac anomalies ~ 93530
central ~ 36555-36566
cerebral artery ~ 36215
cystourethroscopy, ejaculatory duct ~ 52010
ureteral ~ 52005
ear, middle ~ 69405
eustachian tube ~ 69405
fallopian tube ~ 58345, 74742
intracardiac, ablation ~ 93650-93652
jejunum, for enteral ~ 44015
kidney
drainage ~ 50392
with ureter ~ 50393
legs ~ 36245-36248
nasotracheal ~ 31720
newborn, umbilical vein ~ 36510
pelvic artery ~ 36245-36248
peripheral ~ 36568-36571
placement, arterial coronary conduit, without concomitant left heart catheterization ~ 93508
coronary artery, without concomitant left heart catheterization ~ 93508
venous coronary bypass graft
without concomitant left heart catheterization ~ 93508
pleural cavity ~ 32019
portal vein ~ 36481
pulmonary artery ~ 36013-36015
radioelement application ~ 55875
removal
fractured catheter ~ 75961
obstructive material
intracatheter ~ 36596
pericatheter ~ 36595
salivary duct ~ 42660
skull ~ 61107
spinal cord ~ 62350-62351
thoracic artery ~ 36215-36218
tracheobronchi ~ 31725
umbilical artery ~ 36660
umbilical vein ~ 36510

Catheterization ~ *continued*
ureter
endoscopic ~ 50553, 50572, 50953, 50972, 52005
injection ~ 50394, 50684
manometric studies ~ 50396, 50686
uterus
radiology ~ 58340
vena cava ~ 36010
venous
central line ~ 36555-36556, 36568-36569, 36580, 36584
first order ~ 36011
intracatheter/needle ~ 36000
organ blood ~ 36500
second order ~ 36012
umbilical vein ~ 36510
ventricular ~ 61020-61026, 61210-61215
Cauda equina ~ see spinal cord
decompression ~ 63005-63011, 63017, 63047-63048, 63055-63057, 63087-63091
exploration ~ 63005-63011, 63017
Cauterization
anal fissure ~ 46940-46942
cervix ~ 57522
cryocautery ~ 57511
electro or thermal ~ 57510
laser ablation ~ 57513
chemical, granulation tissue ~ 17250
everted punctum ~ 68705
lower esophageal sphincter, thermal, via endoscopy ~ 0057T
nasopharyngeal hemorrhage ~ 42970
nose, hemorrhage ~ 30901-30906
skin lesion ~ 11055-11057, 17000-17004
skin tags ~ 11200-11201
turbinate mucosa ~ 30801-30802
Cavernitides, fibrous ~ see Peyronie disease
Cavernosography, corpora ~ 54230
Cavernosometry ~ 54231
Cavities, pleural ~ see pleural cavity
Cavus foot correction ~ 28309
CBC ~ see blood cell count ~ 85025-85027
CCL4 ~ 84600
CCU visit ~ 99289-99292
CD142 antigens ~ see thromboplastin
CD143 antigens ~ 82164
CD4 ~ 86360
CD8 ~ 86360
CEA ~ 82378
Cecil repair ~ 46744-46746
Cecostomy ~ 44300
Celiac plexus
destruction ~ 64680
injection
anesthetic ~ 64530
neurolytic ~ 64680
Celiac trunk artery ~ see artery, celiac
Celioscopy ~ see endoscopy, peritoneum
Celiotomy ~ 49000
abdomen, for staging ~ 49220
Cell count, body fluid ~ 89050-89051
Cell, blood ~ see blood cell
Cell, islet ~ 86341
Cell, mother ~ see stem cell
Cell-stimulating hormone, interstitial ~ 80418, 80426, 83002
Cellobiase ~ 82963
Cellular inclusion ~ see inclusion bodies
Central shunt ~ 33764
Central nervous system assessments or tests ~ 96101-96120
Central venous catheter placement
insertion
central ~ 36555-36558
peripheral ~ 36568-36569
repair ~ 36575
replacement ~ 36580-36585
repositioning ~ 36597
Central venous catheter removal ~ 36589
Cephalic version, of fetus, external ~ 59412
Cephalocele ~ 62120-62121
Cephalogram, orthodontic ~ 70350
Cerclage, cervix ~ 57700
abdominal ~ 59325
removal under anesthesia ~ 59871
vaginal ~ 59320
Cerebellopontine angle tumor ~ see brainstem; skull base surgery ~ 61480, 61510, 61518, 61520-61521, 61526-61530, 61545, 62164
Cerebral cortex decortication ~ see decortication
Cerebral death ~ 95824
Cerebral hernia ~ 62120-62121
Cerebral perfusion analysis ~ 0042T
Cerebral thermography ~ 93760
Cerebral ventriculographies ~ see ventriculography
Cerebral vessels, occlusion ~ 61623
Cerebrose ~ 82760
Cerebrospinal fluid ~ 86325
nuclear imaging ~ 78630-78650
Cerebrospinal fluid leak ~ 63744
brain, repair ~ 61618-61619, 62100
nasal/sinus endoscopy, repair ~ 31290-31291
spinal cord, repair ~ 63707-63709
Cerebrospinal fluid shunt ~ 63740, 63746
creation ~ 62180-62192, 62200-62223
irrigation ~ 62194
removal ~ 62256-62258
replacement ~ 62160, 62194, 62225-62230
reprogramming ~ 62252
Ceruloplasmin ~ 82390
Cerumen, removal ~ 69210
Cervical cap ~ 57170
Cervical lymphadenectomy ~ 38720-38724
Cervical mucus penetration test ~ 89330
Cervical plexus, injection, anesthetic ~ 64413
Cervical pregnancy ~ 59140
Cervical puncture ~ 61050-61055
Cervical smears ~ 88141, 88155, 88164-88167, 88174-88175
Cervical spine ~ see vertebra, cervical

Cervical sympathectomy ~ 64802
Cervicectomy ~ 57530
Cervicography ~ 0003T
Cervicoplasty ~ 15819
Cervicothoracic ganglia ~ 64510
Cervix ~ see cytopathology
amputation, total ~ 57530
biopsy ~ 57500, 57520
colposcopy ~ 57454-57455, 57460
cauterization ~ 57522
cryocautery ~ 57511
electro or thermal ~ 57510
laser ablation ~ 57513
cerclage ~ 57700
abdominal ~ 59325
removal under anesthesia ~ 59871
vaginal ~ 59320
cervicography ~ 0003T
colposcopy ~ 57452-57461
conization ~ 57461, 57520-57522
curettage, endocervical ~ 57454, 57456, 57505
dilation
canal ~ 57800
stump ~ 57558
dilation and curettage ~ 57558
ectopic pregnancy ~ 59140
excision
radical ~ 57531
stump
abdominal approach ~ 57540-57545
vaginal approach ~ 57550-57556
total ~ 57530
exploration, endoscopy ~ 57452
insertion
dilation ~ 59200
laminaria ~ 59200
prostaglandin ~ 59200
sensor, fetal oximetry ~ 0021T
repair, cerclage ~ 57700
abdominal ~ 59325
suture ~ 57720
vaginal ~ 59320
unlisted services and procedures ~ 58999
Cesarean delivery
antepartum care ~ 59610, 59618
delivery
after attempted vaginal delivery ~ 59618
delivery only ~ 59620
postpartum care ~ 59622
routine care ~ 59610, 59618
delivery only ~ 59514
postpartum care ~ 59515
routine care ~ 59510
tubal ligation at time of ~ 58611
with hysterectomy ~ 59525
CGMP ~ 83008
Chalazion, excision ~ 67805
multiple
different lids ~ 67805
same lid ~ 67801
single ~ 67800
under anesthesia ~ 67808
Challenge tests, bronchial ingestion ~ 95070-95075
Chambers procedure ~ 28300
Change
catheter
bile duct ~ 75984
fetal position
by manipulation ~ 59412
tube or stent
endoscopic
bile or pancreatic duct ~ 43269
Change, gastrostomy tube ~ 43760
Change of, dressing ~ 15852
Cheek
bone
excision ~ 21030, 21034
fracture
closed treatment with manipulation ~ 21355
open treatment ~ 21360-21366
reconstruction ~ 21270
fascia graft ~ 15840
muscle graft ~ 15841-15845
muscle transfer ~ 15845
Cheilectomy, metatarsophalangeal joint release ~ 28289
Cheiloplasty ~ 40650-40654
Cheiloschisis ~ 30460-30462, 40700-40761
Cheilotomy ~ 40806
Chemical cauterization, granulation tissue ~ 17250
Chemical exfoliation ~ 17360
Chemical peel ~ 15788-15793
Chemiluminescent assay ~ 82397
Chemistry tests ~ 82000-84999
Chemocauterization
corneal epithelium ~ 65435
with chelating agent ~ 65436
Chemodenervation
cervical spinal muscle ~ 64613
extraocular muscle ~ 67345
extremity muscle ~ 64614
facial muscle ~ 64612
trunk muscle ~ 64614
Chemonucleolysis ~ 62292
Chemosurgery
Mohs technique ~ 17311-17315
skin lesion ~ 17004, 17110, 17270, 17280
Chemotaxis assay ~ 86155
Chemotherapy
administration ~ 96401-96549
arterial catheterization ~ 36640
bladder instillation ~ 51720
CNS ~ 61517, 96450
extracorporeal circulation, extremity ~ 36823
home infusion procedures ~ 99601-99602
intra-arterial ~ 96420-96425
intralesional ~ 96405-96406
intramuscular ~ 96400
intravenous ~ 96408-96414
kidney instillation ~ 50391
peritoneal cavity ~ 96445

Chemotherapy ~ *continued*
pleural cavity ~ 96440
pump services
implantable ~ 96530
maintenance ~ 95990-95991
portable ~ 96520
reservoir filling ~ 96542
subcutaneous ~ 96400
supply of agent ~ 96545
unlisted services and procedures ~ 96549
ureteral instillation ~ 50391
Chest ~ see mediastinum; thorax
angiography ~ 71275
artery, ligation ~ 37616
CT scan ~ 71250-71275
exploration, blood vessel ~ 35820
magnetic resonance imaging (MRI) ~ 71550-71552
repair, blood vessel ~ 35211-35216
with other graft ~ 35271-35276
with vein graft ~ 35241-35246
ultrasound ~ 76604
wound exploration, penetrating ~ 20101
X-ray ~ 71010-71035
complete (four views), with fluoroscopy ~ 71034
insertion pacemaker ~ 71090
partial (two views)
with fluoroscopy ~ 71023
stereo ~ 71015
with fluoroscopy ~ 71090
Chest, funnel ~ 21740, 21742-21743
Chest cavity, bypass graft ~ 35905
endoscopy
exploration ~ 32601-32606
surgical ~ 32650-32665
Chest wall ~ 94667-94668
manipulation ~ 94667-94668
reconstruction ~ 49904
trauma ~ 32820
repair ~ 32905
closure ~ 32810
fistula ~ 32906
tumor, excision ~ 19260-19272
unlisted services and procedures ~ 32999
Chest wall fistula ~ 32906
Chevron procedure ~ 28296
Chiari osteotomy of the pelvis ~ 27158
Chicken pox vaccine ~ 90716
Child procedure ~ 48140-48146, 48150, 48153-48154, 48160
Chin
repair
augmentation ~ 21120
osteotomy ~ 21121-21123
Chinidin ~ 80194
Chiropractic manipulation (CMT) ~ 98940-98943
Chiropractic treatment
spinal
extraspinal ~ 98940-98943
Chlamydia
antibody ~ 86631-86632
antigen detection
direct fluorescence ~ 87270
enzyme immunoassay ~ 87320
culture ~ 87110
Chloramphenicol ~ 82415
Chloride
blood ~ 82435
other source ~ 82438
spinal fluid ~ 82438
urine ~ 82436
Chloride, methylene ~ 84600
Chlorinated hydrocarbons ~ 82441
Chlorohydrocarbon ~ 82441
Chlorpromazine ~ 84022
Choanal atresia, repair ~ 30540-30545
Cholangiography
injection ~ 47500-47505
intraoperative ~ 74300-74301
percutaneous ~ 74320
with laparoscopy ~ 47560-47561
postoperative ~ 74305
repair
with bile duct exploration ~ 47700
with cholecystectomy ~ 47563, 47605, 47620
Cholangiopancreatography ~ see bile duct; pancreatic duct ~ 43260
repair ~ see bile duct; pancreatic duct
with biopsy ~ 43261
with surgery ~ 43262-43267, 43269
Cholangiostomy ~ 47400
Cholangiotomy ~ 47400
Cholecalciferol ~ 82306
Cholecystectomy ~ 47562-47564, 47600-47620
any method ~ 47562-47564
with cholangiography ~ 47563, 47605, 47620
with exploration common duct ~ 47564, 47610
Cholecystenterostomy ~ 47570, 47720-47741
Cholecystography ~ 74290-74291
Cholecystotomy ~ 47480, 48001
percutaneous ~ 47490
Choledochoplasty ~ 47701
Choledochoscopy ~ 47550
Choledochostomy ~ 47420-47425
Choledochotomy ~ 47420-47425
Choledochus, cyst ~ see cyst, choledochal
Cholera vaccine, injectable ~ 90725
Cholesterol
measurement ~ 83721
serum ~ 82465
testing ~ 83718-83719
Cholinesterase, blood ~ 82480-82482
Choline esterase I ~ 82013
Choline esterase II ~ 82480-82482
Cholylglycine, blood ~ 82240
Chondroitin sulfate ~ 82485
Chondromalacia patella, repair ~ 27418
Chondropathia patellae ~ 27418

Chondrosteoma ~ 69140
Chopart procedure ~ see radical resection; replantation ~ 28800-28805
Chordotomies ~ 63194-63199
Chorioangioma ~ see lesion, skin
Choriogonadotropin ~ 80414-80415, 84702-84703
Choriomeningitides, lymphocytic ~ 86727
Chorionic gonadotropin ~ 80414, 84702-84703
stimulation ~ 80414-80415
Chorionic growth hormone ~ 83632
Chorionic tumor ~ 59100, 59870
Chorionic villi ~ 59015
Chorionic villus, biopsy ~ 59015
Choroid, destruction, lesion ~ 0016T, 67220-67225
Choroid plexus, excision ~ 61544
Christmas factor ~ 85250
Chromaffinoma, medullary ~ 80424
Chromatin, sex ~ 88130
Chromatography
column/mass spectrometry ~ 82541-82544
gas-liquid or HPLC ~ 82486, 82491-82492
paper ~ 82487-82488
thin-layer ~ 82489
Chromium ~ 82495
Chromogenic substrate assay ~ 85130
Chromosome analysis ~ 59000
added study ~ 88280-88289
amniotic fluid ~ 88267-88269
culture ~ 88235
biopsy culture, tissue ~ 88233
bone marrow culture ~ 88237
chorionic villus ~ 88267
5 cells ~ 88261
15-20 cells ~ 88262
20-25 cells ~ 88264
45 cells ~ 88263
culture ~ 88235
for breakage syndromes ~ 88245-88249
fragile-X ~ 88248
lymphocyte culture ~ 88230
pregnancy associated plasma protein-A ~ 84163
skin culture, tissue ~ 88233
tissue culture ~ 88239
unlisted services and procedures ~ 88299
Chromotubation ~ 58350
oviduct ~ 58350
Chronic erection ~ see priapism
Chronic interstitial cystitides ~ 52260-52265
Ciliary body
cyst
destruction
cryotherapy ~ 66720
cyclodialysis ~ 66740
cyclophotocoagulation ~ 66710, 66711
diathermy ~ 66700
nonexcisional ~ 66770
destruction ~ 66770
cyclophotocoagulation ~ 66710, 66711
endoscopic ~ 66711
Ciliary body ~ ***continued***
lesion, destruction ~ 66770
repair ~ 66680
Cimino type procedure ~ 36821
Cinefluorographies ~ see cineradiography
Cineplasty, arm, lower or upper ~ 24940
Cineradiography
esophagus ~ 74230
pharynx ~ 70371, 74230
speech evaluation ~ 70371
swallowing evaluation ~ 74230
unlisted services and procedures ~ 76120-76125
Circulation, extracorporeal ~ 33960-33961
Circulation assist
aortic ~ 33967, 33970
balloon ~ 33967, 33970
external ~ 33960-33961
Circulatory assist ~ see circulation assist
Circumcision
repair ~ 54163
surgical excision ~ 54161
newborn ~ 54160
with clamp or other device ~ 54150
newborn ~ 54150
Cisternal puncture ~ 61050-61055
Cisternography ~ 70015
nuclear ~ 78630
Citrate, blood or urine ~ 82507
Clagett procedure ~ 32810
Clavicle
craterization ~ 23180
cyst
excision ~ 23140
with allograft ~ 23146
with autograft ~ 23145
diaphysectomy ~ 23180
dislocation
acromioclavicular joint
closed treatment ~ 23540-23545
open treatment ~ 23550-23552
sternoclavicular joint
closed treatment ~ 23520-23525
open treatment ~ 23530-23532
without manipulation ~ 23540
excision ~ 23170
partial ~ 23120, 23180
total ~ 23125
fracture
closed treatment
without manipulation ~ 23500
with manipulation ~ 23505
open treatment ~ 23515
pinning, wiring ~ 23490
prophylactic treatment ~ 23490
repair osteotomy ~ 23480-23485
saucerization ~ 23180
sequestrectomy ~ 23170
tumor, excision ~ 23140, 23146, 23200
with autograft ~ 23145
radical resection ~ 23200
X-ray ~ 73000

Clavicula ~ see clavicle
Claviculectomy
partial ~ 23120
total ~ 23125
Claw finger repair ~ 26499
Cleft, branchial ~ see branchial cleft
Cleft cyst, branchial ~ 42810-42815
Cleft foot, reconstruction ~ 28360
Cleft hand, repair ~ 26580
Cleft lip
repair ~ 40700-40761
rhinoplasty ~ 30460-30462
Cleft palate
repair ~ 42200-42225
rhinoplasty ~ 30460-30462
Clinical act of insertion ~ see insertion
Clinical chemistry test ~ 84999
Clinical pathology ~ 80500-80502
Clitoroplasty, intersex state ~ 56805
Closed [transurethral] biopsy of bladder ~ 52224, 52250
Clostridial tetanus ~ 86280
Clostridium botulinum toxin ~ see chemodenervation
Clostridium difficile
antigen detection
enzyme immunoassay ~ 87324
by immunoassay
with direct optical observation ~ 87803
Clostridium tetani AB ~ 86774
Closure
anal fistula ~ 46288
atrioventricular valve ~ 33600
cranial sutures, premature ~ see craniosynostosis
cystostomy ~ 51880
enterostomy ~ 44625-44626
esophagostomy ~ 43420-43425
fistula, vesicouterine ~ 51920-51925
gastrostomy ~ 43870
lacrimal fistula ~ 68770
lacrimal punctum
plug ~ 68761
thermocauterization, ligation or laser surgery ~ 68760
meningocele spinal ~ 63700-63702
rectovaginal fistula ~ 57300-57308
semilunar valve ~ 33602
septal defect ~ 33615
ventricular ~ 33675-33677, 0166T-0167T, 93581
sternotomy ~ 21750
vagina ~ 57120
ventricular tunnel ~ 33722
Clot ~ 34401-34490, 35875-35876, 50230
Clotting disorder ~ 85390
Clotting factor ~ 85210-85293
Clotting inhibitors ~ 85300-85305, 85307
Clotting operation ~ 11765
Clotting test
protein C ~ 85303, 85307
protein S ~ 85306
Clotting time ~ 85345-85348
Clot lysis time ~ 85175
Clot retraction ~ 85170
Clubfoot cast ~ 29450
wedging ~ 29750
CMG ~ 51725-51726
CMRI ~ see cardiac magnetic resonance imaging
CMV ~ see cytomegalovirus
CNPB (continuous negative pressure breathing) ~ 94662
Co-factor I , heparin ~ 85300-85301
CO2 ~ 82374
Coagulation
blood ~ see blood clot
defect ~ 85390
factor ~ 85210-85293
factor I (fibrinogen) ~ 85384, 85385
factor II (prothrombin) ~ 85210
factor III (thromboplastin) ~ 85730, 85732
factor IV (calcium) ~ 82310
factor V (AcG or proaccelerin) ~ 85220
factor VII (proconvertin) ~ 85230
factor VIII (AHG) ~ 85240-85247
factor IX (Christmas factor) ~ 85250
factor X (thrombokinase) (Stuart-Prower factor) ~ 85260
factor XI (plasma thromboplastin antecedent, PTA) ~ 85270
factor XII (Hageman factor) ~ 85280
factor XIII (fibrin stabilizing factor) ~ 85290, 85291
light ~ see photocoagulation
time ~ 85345-85348
unlisted services and procedures ~ 85999
Coagulin ~ see thromboplastin
Coagulopathy ~ 85390
assay ~ 85130
Cocaine
blood or urine ~ 82520
screen ~ 82486
Coccidioides, antibody ~ 86635
Coccidioidin test ~ 86590
Coccidioidomycosis, skin test ~ 86490
Coccygeal spine fracture ~ 27200, 27202
Coccygectomy ~ 15920-15922, 27080
Coccyx
excision ~ 27080
fracture
closed treatment ~ 27200
open treatment ~ 27202
tumor, excision ~ 49215
X-ray ~ 72220
Cochlear device
insertion ~ 69930
programming ~ 92601-92604
Codeine, alkaloid screening ~ 82101
Codeine screen ~ 82486
Cofactor protein S ~ 85305, 85306
Coffey operation ~ 58400
Cognitive function tests ~ see neurology, diagnostic ~ 96116

Cognitive skills development ~ 97532
Cold agglutinin ~ 86156-86157
Cold pack treatment ~ 97010
Cold preservation ~ see cryopreservation
Cold therapies ~ see cryotherapy
Colectomy
partial ~ 44140
with anastomosis ~ 44140
laparoscopic ~ 44204, 44207-44208
with coloproctostomy ~ 44145-44146
with colostomy ~ 44141-44144
laparoscopic ~ 44206, 44208
with ileocolostomy, laparoscopic ~ 44205
with ileostomy ~ 44144
with ileum removal ~ 44160
with transcanal approach ~ 44147
total
laparoscopic ~ 44210-44212
with protectomy and ileostomy ~ 44210-44212
without protectomy ~ 44210
open
with complete proctectomy ~ 45121
with ileostomy ~ 44150-44151
with protectomy ~ 44155-44158
Collagen cross links ~ 82523
Collagen injection ~ 11950-11954
Collar bone ~ see clavicle
Collateral ligament
ankle repair ~ 27695-27698
interphalangeal joint ~ 26545
knee
joint repair ~ 27409
repair ~ 27405
metacarpophalangeal joint ~ 26540-26542
Collection and processing
allogenic blood harvesting of stem cells ~ 38205
autologous blood
harvesting of stem cells ~ 38206
intraoperative ~ 86891
preoperative ~ 86890
specimen
capillary blood ~ 36416
venous blood ~ 36415, 36540
washings
esophagus ~ 91000
stomach ~ 91055
Colles fracture ~ 25600-25605
Colles fracture reversed ~ see Smith fracture
Collins syndrome, Treacher ~ 21150-21151
Collis procedure ~ 43326, 43842-43843
Colon ~ see also colon-sigmoid
biopsy ~ 44025, 44100, 44322
endoscopic ~ 44389, 45380, 45391, 45392
colostomy, revision ~ 44340-44346
colotomy ~ 44322
colostomy ~ 44320
CT scan
virtual colonoscopy ~ 0066T-0067T
colonography ~ 0066T-0067T

Colon ~ *continued*
destruction
lesion ~ 44393, 45383
tumor ~ 44393, 45383
endoscopy
biopsy ~ 44389, 45380, 45391, 45392
destruction
lesion ~ 44393
tumor ~ 44393, 45383
dilation ~ 45386
exploration ~ 44388, 45378, 45381, 45386
hemorrhage ~ 44391, 45382
injection, submucosal ~ 45381
placement, stent ~ 45387
removal
foreign body ~ 44390, 45379
polyp ~ 44392, 45384-45385
tumor ~ 45384-45385
specimen collection ~ 45380
via colotomy ~ 45355
via stoma ~ 44388-44397
virtual ~ 0066T-0067T
excision
partial ~ 44140-44147, 44160
laparoscopic ~ 44204-44208
total ~ 44150-44156
laparoscopic ~ 44210-44212
exploration ~ 44025
endoscopy ~ 44388, 45378, 45381, 45386
hemorrhage, endoscopic control ~ 44391, 45382
hernia ~ 44050
incision
creation, stoma ~ 44320-44322
exploration ~ 44025
revision, stoma ~ 44340-44346
lavage, intraoperative ~ 44701
lesion
destruction ~ 45383
excision ~ 44110-44111
lysis, adhesions ~ 44005
obstruction ~ 44025-44050
reconstruction, bladder from ~ 50810
removal
foreign body ~ 44025, 44390, 45379
polyp ~ 44392
repair
diverticula ~ 44605
fistula ~ 44650-44661
hernia ~ 44050
malrotation ~ 44055
obstruction ~ 44050
ulcer ~ 44605
volvulus ~ 44050
wound ~ 44605
stoma closure ~ 44620-44625
suture
diverticula ~ 44605
fistula ~ 44650-44661
plication ~ 44680
stoma ~ 44620-44625
ulcer ~ 44605

Colon ~ *continued*
wound ~ 44605
tumor, destruction ~ 45383
ultrasound, endoscopic ~ 45391-45392
X-ray with contrast, barium enema ~ 74270-74280
Colon-sigmoid ~ see also colon
biopsy, endoscopy ~ 45331
dilation, endoscopy ~ 45340
endoscopy
ablation
polyp ~ 45339
tumor ~ 45339
biopsy ~ 45331
dilation ~ 45340
exploration ~ 45330, 45335
hemorrhage ~ 45334
needle biopsy ~ 45342
placement, stent ~ 45327, 45345
removal
foreign body ~ 45332
polyp ~ 45333, 45338
tumor ~ 45333, 45338
ultrasound ~ 45341-45342
volvulus ~ 45337
exploration, endoscopy ~ 45330, 45335
hemorrhage, endoscopy ~ 45334
needle biopsy, endoscopy ~ 45342
removal, foreign body ~ 45332
repair, volvulus, endoscopy ~ 45337
ultrasound, endoscopy ~ 45341-45342
Colonna procedure ~ 27120
Colonography, CT scan ~ 0066T-0067T
Colonoscopy
biopsy ~ 45380, 45392
collection specimen ~ 45380
via colotomy ~ 45355
destruction
lesion ~ 45383
tumor ~ 45383
dilation ~ 45386
hemorrhage control ~ 45382
injection, submucosal ~ 45381
placement, stent ~ 45387
removal
foreign body ~ 45379
polyp ~ 45384-45385
tumor ~ 45384-45385
ultrasound ~ 45391-45392
via stoma ~ 44388-44390
biopsy ~ 44389
destruction
of lesion ~ 44393
of tumor ~ 44393
exploration ~ 44388
hemorrhage ~ 44391
placement, stent ~ 44397
removal
foreign body ~ 44390
polyp ~ 44392, 44394
tumor ~ 44392, 44394
virtual ~ 0066T-0067T
Colorrhaphy ~ 44604
Color vision examination ~ 92283
Colostomy ~ 44320, 45563
abdominal, establishment ~ 50810
home visit ~ 99505
intestine, large, with suture ~ 44605
perineal, establishment ~ 50810
revision ~ 44340
paracolostomy hernia ~ 44345-44346
Colotomy ~ 44025
Colpectomy
partial ~ 57106
total ~ 57110
with hysterectomy ~ 58275-58280
with repair of enterocele ~ 58280
Colpo-urethrocystopexy ~ 58152, 58267, 58293
Marshall-Marchetti-Krantz procedure ~ 58152, 58267, 58293
Pereyra procedure ~ 58267, 58293
Colpoceliocentesis ~ 57020
Colpocentesis ~ 57020
Colpocleisis ~ 57120
Colpohysterectomies ~ 58260, 58290-58294, 58550, 58553
Colpoperineorrhaphy ~ 57210
Colpopexy
extra-peritoneal ~ 57282
intra-peritoneal ~ 57283
laparoscopic ~ 57425
open ~ 57280
Colpoplasty ~ see repair, vagina
Colporrhaphy
anterior ~ 57240, 57289
with insertion of mesh ~ 57267
with insertion of prosthesis ~ 57267
anteroposterior ~ 57260-57265
with enterocele repair ~ 57265
with insertion of mesh ~ 57267
with insertion of prosthesis ~ 57267
nonobstetrical ~ 57200
posterior ~ 57250
with insertion of mesh ~ 57267
with insertion of prosthesis ~ 57267
Colposcopy
biopsy ~ 56821, 57421, 57454-57455, 57460
cervix ~ 57421, 57452-57461
exploration ~ 57452
loop electrode excision ~ 57460
loop electrode conization ~ 57461
perineum ~ 99170
vagina ~ 57420-57421
vulva ~ 56820
biopsy ~ 56821
Colpotomy
drainage, abscess ~ 57010
exploration ~ 57000
Colprosterone ~ 84144
Columna vertebralis ~ see spine
Column chromatography/mass spectrometry ~ 82541-82544
Combined heart-lung transplantation ~ 33935

Combined right and left heart cardiac catheterization ~ 93526-93529
Comedones, removal ~ 10040
Commissurotomy, right ventricle ~ 33476-33478
Common sensory nerve, repair/suture ~ 64834
Common truncus ~ 33786
Communication device
non-speech-generating ~ 92605-92606
speech-generating ~ 92606-92609
Community/work reintegration training ~ 97537
Compatibility test, blood ~ 86920
Complement
antigen ~ 86160
fixation test ~ 86171
functional activity ~ 86161
hemolytic, total ~ 86162
total ~ 86162
Complete blood count (CBC) ~ see also blood cell count ~ 85025-85027
Complete colectomy ~ see colectomy, total
Complete pneumonectomy ~ 32488
Complete transposition of great vessels ~ 33770-33781
Complex, factor IX ~ 85250
Complex, vitamin B ~ 78270-78272
Component removal, blood ~ 36511-36516
Composite graft ~ 15760-15770, 35681-35683
Compound B ~ 82528
Compound F ~ 80400-80406, 80418-80420, 80436, 82530
Compression, nerve, median ~ 64721
Computed tomographic scintigraphy ~ 78607
Computed tomography (CT) ~ see CT scan; specific anatomic site
Computer assisted navigation, orthopedic surgery ~ 0054T-0056T
Computer analysis, acoustic recording, heart sounds ~ 0068T-0070T
Computer data analysis ~ 99090
Computer-aided detection, mammography ~ 77051-77052
Computerized emission tomography ~ 78607
Concentration, hydrogen ion ~ see pH
Concentration, minimum inhibitory ~ 87186
Concentration of specimen ~ 87015
Concentric procedure ~ 28296
Conchae nasale ~ 30930
Concha Bullosa resection
with nasal/sinus endoscopy ~ 31240
Conduction, nerve ~ see nerve conduction
Conduit, ileal ~ 50690
Condyle
humerus
fracture
closed treatment ~ 24576-24577
open treatment ~ 24579
percutaneous ~ 24582
metatarsal, excision ~ 28288
phalanges, toe, excision ~ 28126
Condyle, mandibular ~ 21247, 21465
Condylectomy
temporomandibular joint ~ 21050
with skull base surgery ~ 61596-61597
Condyloma, destruction ~ 54050-54065
Conference, medical, with interdisciplinary team ~ 99361-99373
Confirmation, drug ~ 80102
Confirmatory consultations ~ see consultation
new or established patient ~ 99271-99275
Congenital arteriovenous malformation ~ see arteriovenous malformation
Congenital elevation of scapula ~ 23400
Congenital heart septum defect ~ 33813-33814
Congenital kidney abnormality
nephrolithotomy ~ 50070
pyeloplasty ~ 50405
pyelotomy ~ 50135
Congenital laryngocele ~ 31300
Congenital vascular anomaly ~ see vascular malformation
Conisation ~ 57461, 57520-57522
Conization, cervix ~ 57461, 57520-57522
Conjoint psychotherapy ~ 90846-90849, 99510
Conjunctiva
biopsy ~ 68100
cyst, incision and drainage ~ 68020
fistulize for drainage, with tube ~ 68750
without tube ~ 68745
graft ~ 65782
harvesting ~ 68371
harvesting ~ 68371
insertion stent ~ 68750
lesion
destruction ~ 68135
excision ~ 68110-68130
over 1 cm ~ 68115
with adjacent sclera ~ 68130
reconstruction ~ 68320-68335
symblepharon, with graft ~ 68335
with flap
bridge or partial ~ 68360
total ~ 68362
repair
symblepharon
division ~ 68340
with graft ~ 68335
without graft ~ 68330
wound
direct closure ~ 65270
mobilization and rearrangement ~ 65272-65273
unlisted services and procedures ~ 68399
Conjunctivo-tarso-Muller resection ~ 67908
Conjunctivocystorhinostomy ~ 68745-68750
Conjunctivodacryocystostomy ~ 68745-68750
Conjunctivoplasty ~ 68320-68330
reconstruction cul de sac, with extensive rearrangement ~ 68326
with graft ~ 68326
buccal mucous membrane ~ 68328

Conjunctivoplasty ~ *continued*
with extensive rearrangement ~ 68320
with graft ~ 68320
buccal mucous membrane ~ 68325
Conjunctivorhinostomy
with tube ~ 68750
without tube ~ 68745
Conscious sedation ~ 99143-99150
Construction
finger
toe to hand transfer ~ 26551-26556
neobladder ~ 51596
vagina
with graft ~ 57292
without graft ~ 57291
Consultation(s) ~ 99241-99255
clinical pathology ~ 80500-80502
confirmatory ~ 99271-99275
new or established patient ~ 99271-99275
follow-up inpatient, established patient ~ 99261-99263
initial inpatient ~ 99251-99255
new or established patient ~ 99251-99255
office and/or other outpatient ~ 99241-99245
new or established patient ~ 99241-99245
psychiatric, with family ~ 90887
radiation therapy, radiation physics ~ 77336-77370
surgical pathology ~ 88321-88325
intraoperation ~ 88329-88332
X-ray ~ 76140
Consumption test, antiglobulin ~ 86880
Contact lens services
fittings and prescription ~ 92070, 92310-92313
modification ~ 92325
prescription ~ 92314-92317
replacement ~ 92326
supply ~ 92391, 92396
Continuous negative pressure breathing (CNPD) ~ 94662
Continuous positive airway pressure (CPAP) ~ 94660
Contouring
silicone injections ~ 11950-11954
tumor, facial bone ~ 21029
Contraception
cervical cap
fitting ~ 57170
diaphragm
fitting ~ 57170
intrauterine device (IUD)
insertion ~ 58300
removal ~ 58301
Contraceptive capsules, implantable
insertion ~ 11975
removal ~ 11976
with reinsertion ~ 11977
Contraceptive device, intrauterine ~ 58300-58301
Contracture
elbow, release
with radical resection of capsule ~ 24149
palm, release ~ 26121-26125
thumb, release ~ 26508
Contracture of palmar fascia ~ 26040-26045
Contralateral ligament repair, knee ~ 27405
Contrast aortogram ~ 75600-75605, 75630, 93544
Contrast bath therapy ~ see also physical medicine/therapy/occupational therapy ~ 97034
Contrast material
injection via peritoneal catheter ~ 49424
Contrast phlebogram ~ see venography
Contusion ~ see hematoma
Converting enzyme, angiotensin ~ 82164
Coombs test ~ 86880
Copper ~ 82525
Coprobilinogen, feces ~ 84577
Coproporphyrin ~ 84120
Coracoacromial ligament release ~ 23415
Coracoid process transfer ~ 23462
Cord
spermatic ~ see spermatic cord
spinal ~ see spinal cord
vocal ~ see vocal cords
Cordectomy ~ 31300
Cordocentesis ~ 59012
Cordotomy ~ 63194-63199
Corectomy ~ see excision, iris
Coreoplasty ~ 66762
Cornea
biopsy ~ 65410
curettage ~ 65435-65436
with chelating agent ~ 65436
epithelium, excision ~ 65435-65436
with chelating agent ~ 65436
lesion
destruction ~ 65450
excision ~ 65400
with graft ~ 65426
without graft ~ 65420
pachymetry ~ 76514
prosthesis ~ 65770
pterygium, excision ~ 65420
puncture ~ 65600
relaxing incisions ~ 65772-65775
repair
astigmatism ~ 65772-65775
wedge resection ~ 65775
with glue ~ 65286
wound
nonperforating ~ 65275
perforating ~ 65280-65285
tissue glue ~ 65286
reshape
epikeratoplasty ~ 65765
keratomileusis ~ 65760
keratoprosthesis ~ 65767

Cornea ~ *continued*
scraping, smear ~ 65430
tattoo ~ 65600
thickness measurement ~ 76514
transplantation
autograft or homograft
lamellar ~ 65710
penetrating ~ 65730-65755
for aphakia ~ 65750
Coronary
atherectomy, percutaneous ~ 92995-92996
thrombectomy, percutaneous ~ 92973
Coronary angioplasty, transluminal balloon ~ see percutaneous transluminal angioplasty
Coronary artery
insertion, stent ~ 92980-92981
ligation ~ 33502
placement, radiation delivery device ~ 92974
repair ~ 33500-33506
Coronary artery bypass graft (CABG) ~ 33503-33505, 33510-33516
arterial ~ 33533-33536
arterial-venous ~ 33517-33523
harvest, upper extremity artery ~ 35600
reoperation ~ 33530
venous ~ 33510-33516
Coronary endarterectomy ~ 33572
Coroner's exam ~ 88045
Coronoidectomy, temporomandibular joint ~ 21070
Corpectomy ~ 63101-63103
Corpora cavernosa
corpus spongiosum shunt ~ 54430
glans penis fistulization ~ 54435
injection ~ 54235
irrigation, priapism ~ 54220
saphenous vein shunt ~ 54420
X-ray with contrast ~ 74445
Corpora cavernosa, plastic induration ~ see Peyronie disease
Corpora cavernosography ~ 74445
Corpus callosum, transection ~ 61541
Corpus vertebrae (vertebrale) ~ see vertebral body
Correction (of)
cleft palate ~ 42200-42225
lid retraction ~ 67911
malrotation of duodenum ~ 44055
syndactyly ~ 26560-26562
ureteropelvic junction ~ 50400-50405, 50544
Cortex decortication, cerebral ~ see decortication
Cortical mapping
transection, by electric stimulation ~ 95961-95962
Corticoids ~ 83491
Corticoliberin ~ 80412
Corticosteroids
blood ~ 83491
urine ~ 83491
Corticosteroid binding globulin ~ 84449
Corticosteroid binding protein ~ 84449
Corticosterone, blood or urine ~ 82528
Corticotropic releasing hormone (CRH) ~ 80412
Cortisol ~ 80400-80406, 80418-80420, 80436, 82530
stimulation ~ 80412
total ~ 82533
Cortisol binding globulin ~ 84449
Costectomy ~ 19260-19272, 32900
Costen syndrome ~ see temporomandibular joint (TMJ)
Costotransversectomy ~ 21610
Cothromboplastin ~ 85230
Cotte operation ~ see revision ~ 58400-58410
Cotton procedure, Bohler procedure ~ 28405
Counseling ~ 99381-99397
Counseling and/or risk factor reduction intervention - preventive medicine, individual counseling ~ 99401-99404
Count
blood cell ~ see blood cell count
blood platelet ~ 85008
cell ~ 89050-89051
complete blood ~ 85025-85027
erythrocyte ~ 85032-85041
leukocyte ~ 85032, 85048, 89055
reticulocyte ~ 85044-85045
Counterimmunoelectrophoresis ~ 86185
Counters, cell ~ 89050-89051
Countershock, electric ~ 92960-92961
Coventry tibial wedge osteotomy ~ 27455-27457, 27705, 27709-27712
Cowper's gland, excision ~ 53250
Coxa ~ see hip
Coxiella burnetii, antibody ~ 86638
Coxsackie, antibody ~ 86658
CPAP ~ 94660
CPK, blood ~ 82550-82552
CPR (cardiopulmonary resuscitation) ~ 92950
Cranial bone
halo, thin skull osteology ~ 20664
reconstruction, extracranial ~ 21181-21184
tumor, excision ~ 61563-61564
Cranial halo ~ 20661
Cranial nerve ~ see specific nerve
avulsion ~ 64732-64760, 64771
decompression ~ 61458, 64716
implantation, electrode ~ 64553, 64573
incision ~ 64732-64752, 64760, 65771
injection
anesthetic ~ 64400-64408, 64412
neurolytic ~ 64600-64610
insertion, electrode ~ 64553, 64573
neuroplasty ~ 64716
release ~ 64716
repair, suture, with or without graft ~ 64864-64865
section ~ 61460
transection ~ 64732-64760, 64771
transposition ~ 64716
Cranial nerve II ~ see optic nerve
Cranial nerve V (five) ~ see trigeminal nerve

Cranial nerve VII (seven) ~ see facial nerve
Cranial nerve X (ten) ~ see vagus nerve
Cranial nerve XI (eleven) ~ see accessory nerve
Cranial nerve XII (twelve) ~ 64868
Cranial tongs
application/removal ~ 20660
removal ~ 20665
Craniectomy ~ see also craniotomy ~ 61501
decompression ~ 61322-61323, 61340-61343
exploratory ~ 61304-61305
extensive, for multiple suture craniosynostosis ~ 61558-61559
for electrode ~ 61860-61875
release stenosis ~ 61550-61552
surgical ~ 61312-61315, 61320-61323, 61440-61480, 61500-61516, 61518-61522
Craniofacial procedures, unlisted services and procedures ~ 21299
Craniofacial separation
closed treatment ~ 21431
open treatment ~ 21432-21436
wire fixation ~ 21431
Craniomegalic skull, reduction ~ 62115-62117
Craniopharyngioma, excision ~ 61545
Cranioplasty ~ 62120
encephalocele repair ~ 62120
for defect ~ 62140-62141, 62145
with autograft ~ 62146-62147
with bone graft ~ 61316, 62146-62147
Craniostenosis ~ see craniosynostosis
Craniosynostosis
bifrontal craniotomy ~ 61557
extensive craniectomy ~ 61558-61559
Craniotomy ~ see burr hole; drill hole; puncture ~ 61501
bifrontal ~ 61557
decompression ~ 61322-61323
exploratory ~ 61304-61305
for craniosynostosis ~ 61556-61557
for encephalocele ~ 62121
for implant of neurostimulators ~ 61850-61875
frontal ~ 61556
parietal ~ 61556
surgery ~ 61312-61315, 61320-61323, 61440, 61490, 61546, 61570-61571, 61582-61583, 61590, 61592, 61760, 62120
with bone flap ~ 61510-61516, 61526-61530, 61533-61545, 61566-61567
Cranium ~ see skull
Craterization
calcaneus ~ 28120
clavicle ~ 23180
femur ~ 27070-27071, 27360
fibula ~ 27360, 27641
hip ~ 27070
humerus ~ 23184, 24140
ileum ~ 27070
metacarpal ~ 26230
metatarsal ~ 28122
olecranon process ~ 24147

Craterization ~ ***continued***
phalanges
finger ~ 26235-26236
toe ~ 28124
pubis ~ 27070
radius ~ 24145, 25151
scapula ~ 23182
talus ~ 28120
tarsal ~ 28122
tibia ~ 27360, 27640
ulna ~ 24147, 25150
Creatine ~ 82553-82554
blood or urine ~ 82540
Creatine kinase, total ~ 82550
Creatine phosphokinase
blood ~ 82552
total ~ 82550
Creatinine
blood ~ 82565
clearance ~ 82575
other source ~ 82570
urine ~ 82570-82575
Creation
arteriovenous
fistula/autogenous graft ~ 36825
colonic reservoir ~ 45119
complete heart block ~ 93650
defect ~ 40720
ileal reservoir ~ 44158, 45113
lesion ~ 61790, 63600
mucofistula ~ 44144
pericardial window ~ 32659
recipient site ~ 15002-15005
shunt
cerebrospinal fluid ~ 62200
subarachnoid, lumbar-peritoneal ~ 63740
subarachnoid-subdural ~ 62190
ventriculo ~ 62200
sigmoid bladder ~ 50810
speech prosthesis ~ 31611
stoma
bladder ~ 51980
kidney ~ 50395
renal pelvis ~ 50395
tympanic membrane ~ 69433-69436
ureter ~ 50860
ventral hernia ~ 39503
CRF ~ 80412
CRH ~ see corticotropic releasing hormone (CRH)
Cricoid cartilage split, larynx ~ 31587
Cricothyroid membrane, incision ~ 31605
Cristobalite ~ 84285
Critical care services ~ 99289-99292
evaluation and management ~ 99291-99292
gastric intubation ~ 91105
interfacility transport ~ 99289-99290
ipecac administration for poison ~ 99175
neonatal
initial ~ 99295
low birth weight infant ~ 99298-99299
subsequent ~ 99296

Critical care services ~ *continued*
pediatric
initial ~ 99293
interfacility transport ~ 99289-99290
subsequent ~ 99294, 99299
Cross finger flap ~ 15574
Crossmatch ~ 86920-86922
Crossmatching, tissue ~ 86812-86817, 86821-86822
Cruciate ligament
arthroscopic repair ~ 29888-29889
repair ~ 27407-27409
knee
with collateral ligament ~ 27409
Cryoablation ~ 17000-17286, 47371, 47381
Cryofibrinogen ~ 82585
Cryofixation ~ see cryopreservation
Cryoglobulin ~ 82595
Cryopreservation
cells ~ 38207-38209, 88240-88241
embryo ~ 89258
for transplantation ~ 32850, 33930, 33940, 44132, 47133, 47140, 48550, 50300-50320, 50547
freezing and storage ~ 38207, 88240
oocyte ~ 0059T
ovarian tissue ~ 0058T
sperm ~ 89259
testes ~ 89335
thawing
embryo ~ 89352
oocytes ~ 89353
reproductive tissue ~ 89354
sperm ~ 89356
Cryosurgery ~ see destruction ~ 17000-17286, 47371, 47381
fibroadenoma
breast ~ 19105
labyrinthotomy ~ 69801
lesion
mouth ~ 40820
penis ~ 54056, 54065
vagina ~ 57061-57065
vulva ~ 56501-56515
Cryotherapy
acne ~ 17340
destruction, ciliary body ~ 66720
lesion
cornea ~ 65450
retina ~ 67208, 67227
retinal detachment
prophylaxis ~ 67141
repair ~ 67101
trichiasis, correction ~ 67825
Cryptectomy ~ 46210-46211
Cryptococcus
antibody ~ 86641
antigen detection, enzyme immunoassay ~ 87327
Cryptococcus neoformans, antigen detection, enzyme immunoassay ~ 87327
Cryptorchism ~ 54550-54560
Cryptosporidium
antigen detection
direct fluorescence ~ 87272
enzyme immunoassay ~ 87328
Crystal identification, any body fluid ~ 89060
CSF ~ see cerebrospinal fluid leak
CT scan
bone, density study ~ 77078-77079
drainage ~ 75989
follow-up study ~ 76380
guidance
localization ~ 77011
needle placement ~ 77012
parenchymal tissue ablation ~ 77013
radiation therapy ~ 77014
vertebroplasty ~ 72292
other planes ~ 76375
unlisted services and procedures ~ 76497
with contrast ~ 70460
abdomen ~ 74160
arm ~ 73201
brain ~ 0042T, 70460
cerebral blood flow/volume ~ 0042T
ear ~ 70481
face ~ 70487
head ~ 70460
leg ~ 73701
maxilla ~ 70487
neck ~ 70491
orbit ~ 70481
pelvis ~ 72193
sella tucica ~ 70481
spine
cervical ~ 72126
lumbar ~ 72132
thoracic ~ 72129
thorax ~ 71260
without and with contrast
abdomen ~ 74170-74175, 75635
arm ~ 73202-73206
brain ~ 70470, 70496
chest ~ 71275
ear ~ 70482
face ~ 70488
head ~ 70470, 70496
leg ~ 73702-73706, 75635
maxilla ~ 70488
neck ~ 70492, 70498
orbit ~ 70482
pelvis ~ 72191, 72194
sella turcica ~ 70482
spine, cervical ~ 72127
lumbar ~ 72133
thoracic ~ 72130
thorax ~ 71270-71275
without contrast ~ 70450
abdomen ~ 74150
arm ~ 73200
brain ~ 70450
colon
colonography ~ 0066T-0067T
virtual colonoscopy ~ 0066T-0067T

CT scan ~ *continued*
ear ~ 70480
face ~ 70486
head ~ 70450
leg ~ 73700
maxilla ~ 70486
neck ~ 70490
orbit ~ 70480
pelvis ~ 72192
sella turcica ~ 70480
spine
cervical ~ 72125
lumbar ~ 72131
thoracic ~ 72128
thorax ~ 71250
CT scan, radionuclide ~ 78607
Cuff, rotator ~ 23410-23420
Culdocentesis ~ 57020
Culture
acid fast bacilli ~ 87116
amniotic fluid
chromosome analysis ~ 88235
bacteria, additional methods ~ 87077
aerobic ~ 87040-87070
anaerobic ~ 87073-87076
blood ~ 87040
other ~ 87070-87073
screening ~ 87081
stool ~ 87045-87046
urine ~ 87086-87088
bone marrow, chromosome analysis ~ 88237
chlamydia ~ 87110
chorionic villus, chromosome analysis ~ 88235
fertilized oocyte
for in vitro fertilization ~ 89250
co-culture of embryo ~ 89251
fungus
blood ~ 87103
hair ~ 87101
identification ~ 87106
nail ~ 87101
other ~ 87102
skin ~ 87101
lymphocyte, chromosome analysis ~ 88230
mold ~ 87107
mycobacteria ~ 87116-87118
mycoplasma ~ 87109
oocyte/embryo ~ 89250
co-culture of oocyte/embryo ~ 89251
extended culture ~ 89272
pathogen, by kit ~ 87084
skin, chromosome analysis ~ 88233
tissue
toxin/antitoxin ~ 87230
virus ~ 87252-87253
tubercle bacilli ~ 87116
typing ~ 87140-87158
unlisted services and procedures ~ 87999
yeast ~ 87106

Curettage ~ 59840
cervix, endocervical ~ 57454, 57456, 57505
cornea ~ 65435-65436
chelating agent ~ 65436
hydatidiform mole ~ 59870
postpartum ~ 59160
uterus ~ 58356
Curettage and dilatation ~ 59840
Curettement, skin lesion ~ 11055-11057, 17004, 17110, 17270, 17280
Curietherapy ~ 77761-77778, 77789
Custodial care ~ see domiciliary services; nursing facility services
Cutaneolipectomy ~ *see* lipectomy
Cutaneous-vesicostomy ~ 51980
Cutaneous electrostimulation, analgesic ~ 64550
Cutaneous tag ~ 11200-11201
Cutaneous tissue ~ see integumentary system
CVS ~ 59015
Cyanacobalamin ~ 82607-82608
Cyanide
blood ~ 82600
tissue ~ 82600
Cyanocobalamin ~ 82607-82608
Cyclic AMP ~ 82030
Cyclic GMP ~ 83008
Cyclic somatostatin ~ 84307
Cyclocryotherapy ~ 66720
Cyclodialysis, destruction ciliary body ~ 66740
Cyclophotocoagulation, destruction ciliary body ~ 66710
Cyclosporine, assay ~ 80158
Cyst
abdomen, destruction/excision ~ 49200-49201
ankle
capsule ~ 27630
tendon sheath ~ 27630
Bartholin's gland excision ~ 56440, 56740
repair ~ 56440
bile duct ~ 47715
bladder, excision ~ 51500
bone
drainage ~ 20615
injection ~ 20615
brain
drainage ~ 61150-61151, 61156, 62161-62162
excision ~ 61516, 61524, 62162
branchial cleft, excision ~ 42810-42815
breast
incision and drainage ~ 19020
puncture aspiration ~ 19000-19001
calcaneus ~ 28100-28103
carpal ~ 25130-25136
choledochal ~ 47715, 47719
ciliary body, destruction ~ 66770
clavicle, excision ~ 23140-23146
conjunctiva ~ 68020
dermoid, nose, excision ~ 30124-30125

Cyst ~ *continued*
drainage
contrast injection ~ 49424
with X-ray ~ 76080
excision
cheekbone ~ 21030
clavicle ~ 23140
with allograft ~ 23146
with autograft ~ 23145
femur ~ 27355-27358
ganglion ~ see ganglion
humerus
with allograft ~ 23156
with autograft ~ 23155
hydatid ~ 86171, 86280
lymphatic ~ 49062, 49323
maxilla ~ 21030
mediastinum ~ 32662
olecranon process
with allograft ~ 24126
with autograft ~ 24125
pericardial ~ 32661
pilonidal ~ 11770-11772
radius
with allograft ~ 24126
with autograft ~ 24125
scapula ~ 23140
with allograft ~ 23146
with autograft ~ 23145
ulna
with allograft ~ 24126
with autograft ~ 24125
zygoma ~ 21030
facial bones
excision ~ 21030
femur ~ 27065-27067
fibula ~ 27635-27638
ganglion, aspiration/injection ~ 20612
gums, incision and drainage ~ 41800
hip ~ 27065-27067
humerus
excision ~ 23150-23156, 24110
with allograft ~ 24116
with autograft ~ 24115
ileum ~ 27065-27067
incision and drainage ~ 10060-10061
pilonidal ~ 10080-10081
iris, destruction ~ 66770
kidney
ablation ~ 50541
aspiration ~ 50390
excision ~ 50280-50290
injection ~ 50390
X-ray ~ 74470
knee
Baker's ~ 27345
excision ~ 27347
leg, lower
capsule ~ 27630
tendon sheath ~ 27630

Cyst ~ *continued*
liver ~ 47010
drainage ~ 47010
open ~ 47010
repair ~ 47300
lung
incision and drainage ~ 32200
removal ~ 32140
lymph node
axillary/cervical
excision ~ 38550-38555
mandible, excision ~ 21040, 21046-21047
maxilla, excision ~ 21030, 21048-21049
mediastinal, excision ~ 39200
metacarpal ~ 26200-26205
metatarsal ~ 28104-28107
mouth ~ 41005-41009, 41015-41018
incision and drainage ~ 40800-40801
mullerian duct, excision ~ 55680
nose, excision ~ 30124-30125
olecranon ~ 24120
ovarian
excision ~ 58925
incision and drainage ~ 58800-58805
pancreas ~ 48500
anastomosis ~ 48520-48540
excision ~ 48120
pelvis
aspiration ~ 50390
injection ~ 50390
pericardial, excision ~ 33050
phalanges
finger ~ 26210-26215
toe ~ 28108
pilonidal
excision ~ 11770-11772
incision and drainage ~ 10080-10081
pubis ~ 27065-27067
radius ~ 24120, 25120-25126
Rathke's pouch ~ 61545
removal, skin ~ 10040
retroperitoneal, destruction/excision ~ 49200-49201
salivary gland creation
destruction/excision, fistula ~ 42325-42326
drainage ~ 42409
excision ~ 42408
scapula, excision ~ 23140-23146
seminal vesicle, excision ~ 55680
skin, puncture aspiration ~ 10160
spinal cord
aspiration ~ 62268
incision and drainage ~ 63172-63173
sublingual gland drainage ~ 42409
excision ~ 42408
talus ~ 28100-28103
tarsal ~ 28104-28107
thyroglossal duct
excision ~ 60280-60281
incision and drainage ~ 60000

Cyst ~ *continued*
thyroid gland aspiration ~ 60001
excision ~ 60200
injection ~ 60001
tibia ~ 27635-27638
tongue ~ 41000-41006, 41015
ulna ~ 24120, 25120-25126
urachal, bladder, excision ~ 51500
vaginal, excision ~ 57135
wrist ~ 25130-25136
excision ~ 25111-25112
zygoma
excision ~ 21030
Cyst ovary ~ see ovary, cyst
Cystatins, kininogen ~ 85293
Cystectomy
complete ~ 51570
with bilateral pelvic lymphadenectomy ~ 51575, 51585, 51595
with continent diversion ~ 51596
with ureteroileal conduit ~ 51590
with ureterosigmoidostomy ~ 51580
ovarian ~ 58925
laparoscopic ~ 58661
partial
complicated ~ 51555
reimplantation of ureters ~ 51565
simple ~ 51550
Cystic hygroma ~ 38550-38555
Cystine, urine ~ 82615
Cystitis, interstitial ~ 52260-52265
Cystography ~ 74430
injection ~ 52281
radiologic ~ 51600
Cystolithotomy ~ 51050
Cystometrogram ~ 51725-51726
Cystoplasty ~ 51800
Cystorrhaphy ~ 51860-51865
Cystoscopy ~ 52000
Cystoscopy, with biopsy ~ 52224, 52250
Cystostomy
change tube ~ 51705-51710
closure ~ 51880
home visit ~ 99505
with fulguration ~ 51020
with insertion radioactive material ~ 51020
with urethrectomy
female ~ 53210
male ~ 53215
Cystotomy
excision
bladder diverticulum ~ 51525
bladder tumor ~ 51530
repair of ureterocele ~ 51535
vesical neck ~ 51520
repair of ureterocele ~ 51535
with calculus basket extraction ~ 51065
with destruction intravesical lesion ~ 51030
with drainage ~ 51040
with fulguration ~ 51020

Cystotomy ~ *continued*
with insertion
radioactive material ~ 51020
ureteral catheter ~ 51045
with removal calculus ~ 51050, 51065
Cystourethrogram, retrograde ~ 51610
Cystourethropexy ~ 51840-51841
Cystourethroplasty ~ 51800-51820
Cystourethroscopy ~ 52000, 52351, 52601, 52647-52648, 53500
biopsy ~ 52204, 52354
brush ~ 52007
calibration and/or dilation urethral stricture or stenosis ~ 52281
catheterization
ejaculatory duct ~ 52010
ureteral ~ 52005
destruction, lesion ~ 52400
dilation
bladder ~ 52260-52265
intra-renal stricture ~ 52343, 52346
ureter ~ 52341-52342, 52344-52345
urethra ~ 52281
evacuation, clot ~ 52001
female urethral syndrome ~ 52285
incision, ejaculatory duct ~ 52402
injection of implant material ~ 52327
insertion
indwelling ureteral stent ~ 50947, 52332
radioactive substance ~ 52250
ureteral guide wire ~ 52334
urethral stent ~ 52282
lithotripsy ~ 52353
manipulation of ureteral calculus ~ 52330
meatotomy, ureteral ~ 52290-52305
removal
calculus ~ 52310-52315, 52320-52325, 52352
foreign body ~ 52310-52315
urethral stent ~ 52310-52315
resection
ejaculatory duct ~ 52402
external sphincter ~ 52277
tumor ~ 52355
urethral syndrome ~ 52285
vasectomy, transurethral ~ 52402
vasotomy
transurethral ~ 52402
with direct vision internal urethromtomy ~ 52276
with ejaculatory duct catheterization ~ 52010
with fulguration ~ 52214, 52354
lesion ~ 52224
tumor ~ 52234-52240
with internal urethrotomy
female ~ 52270
male ~ 52275
with steroid injection ~ 52283
with ureteral catheterization ~ 52005
with ureteral meatotomy ~ 52290-52305
Cytochrome reductase, lactic ~ 83615-83625

Cytogenetic studies ~ 88271-88275, 88291, 88299
molecular, DNA probe ~ 88271-88275, 88291, 88365
unlisted services and procedures ~ 88299
Cytomegalovirus
antibody ~ 86644-86645
antigen detection
direct fluorescence ~ 87271
enzyme immunoassay ~ 87332
nucleic acid ~ 87495-87497
Cytometries, flow ~ 88184-88189
Cytopathology ~ 99104-88199
cervical or vaginal
requiring interpretation by physician ~ 88141
thin layer prep ~ 88142-88143, 88174-88175
concentration technique ~ 88108
evaluation ~ 88172
fluids, washings, brushings ~ 88104-88108
forensic ~ 88125
other source ~ 88160-88162
selective cellular enhancement technique ~ 88112
smears, cervical or vaginal ~ 88141-88167, 88174-88175
unlisted services and procedures ~ 88199
Cytoscopy ~ 52000
Cytosol aminopeptidase ~ 83670
Cytotoxic screen
lymphocyte ~ 86805-86806
percent reactive antibody (PRA) ~ 86807-86808
serum antibodies ~ 86807-86808

D

D and C ~ 59840
D and E ~ 59841
D-xylose absorption test ~ 84620
Dacryoadenectomy
partial ~ 68505
total ~ 68500
Dacryocystectomy ~ 68520
Dacryocystogram ~ 68850, 70170
Dacryocystography ~ 68850, 70170
nuclear imaging ~ 78660
Dacryocystorhinostomy ~ 68720
total, with nasal/sinus endoscopy ~ 31239
Dacryocystostomies ~ 68420
Dacryocystotomy ~ 68420
Daily living activities ~ 97535, 99509
Damus-Kaye-Stansel procedure ~ 33606
Dana operation ~ 63185-63190
Dandy operation ~ 62180, 62200-62201
Dark adaptation examination ~ 92284
Dark field examination ~ 87164-87166
Darkroom test ~ 92140
Darrach procedure ~ 25150-25151, 25240
Day test ~ 82270, 82272
De Quervain's disease treatment ~ 25000
Death, brain ~ 95824
Debridement
brain ~ 62010
burns ~ 01951-01953, 16010-16030
mastoid cavity
complex ~ 69222
simple ~ 69220
metatarsophalangeal joint ~ 28289
muscle
infected ~ 11004-11006
nails ~ 11720-11721
nose
endoscopic ~ 31237
pancreatic tissue ~ 48105
skin
eczematous ~ 11000-11001
full thickness ~ 11041
infected ~ 11000-11006
with open fracture and/or dislocation ~ 11010-11012
partial thickness ~ 11040
subcutaneous tissue ~ 11042-11044
infected ~ 11004-11006
sternum ~ 21627
wound
non-selective ~ 97602
selective ~ 97597-97598
Debulking procedure
ovary/pelvis ~ 58952-58954
Decompression ~ see section
arm, lower ~ 24495, 25020-25025
auditory canal, internal ~ 69960
brainstem ~ 61575-61576
cauda equina ~ 63011, 63017, 63047-63048, 63056-63057, 63087-63091
cranial nerve ~ 61458
esophagogastric varices ~ 37181
facial nerve ~ 61590
intratemporal
lateral to geniculate ganglion ~ 69720, 69740
medial to geniculate ganglion ~ 69725, 69745
total ~ 69955
finger ~ 26035
gasserian ganglion
sensory root ~ 61450
hand ~ 26035-26037
intestines
small ~ 44021
jejunostomy
laparoscopic ~ 44201
leg, fasciotomy ~ 27600-27602
nerve ~ 64702-64727
root ~ 63020-63048, 63055-63103
nucleus of disk
lumbar ~ 62287
optic nerve ~ 67570
orbit ~ 61330
removal of bone ~ 67414, 67445

Decompression ~ *continued*
skull ~ 61322-61323, 61340-61345
spinal cord ~ 63001-63017, 63045-63103,
cauda equina ~ 63005
tarsal tunnel release ~ 28035
volvulus ~ 45321, 45337
with nasal/sinus endoscopy
optic nerve ~ 31294
orbit wall ~ 31292-31293
wrist ~ 25020-25025
Decortication
lung
endoscopic ~ 32651-32652
with parietal pleurectomy ~ 32320
partial ~ 32225
total ~ 32220
Decubiti ~ see pressure ulcer (decubitus)
Decubitus ulcers ~ see debridement; pressure ulcer (decubitus); skin graft and flap
Deetjeen's body ~ see blood, platelet
Defect, coagulation ~ 85390
Defect, heart septal ~ 33813-33814
Defect, septal closure, atrial ~ see heart, repair, atrial septum
Deferens, ductus ~ see vas deferens
Defibrillation ~ 92960-92961
Defibrillator, heart ~ see pacemaker, heart
evaluation and testing ~ 93640-93642, 93741-93744
insertion single/dual chamber
electrodes ~ 33216-33217, 33224-33225, 33249
pulse generator ~ 33240
removal single/dual chamber
electrodes ~ 33243-33244
pulse generator ~ 33241
repair ~ 33218-33220
repositioning single/dual chamber
electrodes ~ 33215, 33226
revise pocket chest ~ 33223
wearable device ~ 93741-93742, 93745
Deformity, boutonniere ~ 26426-26428
Deformity, Sprengel's ~ 23400
Degenerative, articular cartilage, patella ~ 27418
Degradation products, fibrin ~ 85362-85380
Dehydroepiandrosterone ~ 82626
Dehydroepiandrosterone sulfate ~ 82627
Dehydrogenase, 6-phosphogluconate ~ 84085
Dehydrogenase, alcohol ~ 84588
Dehydrogenase, glucose-6-phosphate ~ 82955-82960
Dehydrogenase, glutamate ~ 82965
Dehydrogenase, isocitrate ~ 83570
Dehydrogenase, lactate ~ 83615-83625
Dehydrogenase, malate ~ 83775
Dehydroisoandrosterone sulfate ~ 82626
Delay of flap, skin graft ~ 15600-15630
Deligation, ureter ~ 50940
Deliveries, abdominal ~ see cesarean delivery
Delivery ~ see cesarean delivery; vaginal delivery
Delorme operation ~ see pericardiectomy
Denervation
hip
femoral ~ 27035
obturator ~ 27035
sciatic ~ 27035
Denervation, sympathetic ~ 64802-64818
Denis-Browne splint ~ 29590
Dens axis ~ 22548
Denver developmental screening test ~ 96100
Denver shuntpatency test ~ 78291
Denver Krupic procedure ~ 66180
Denver-Krupin procedure ~ 66180
Deoxycorticosterone ~ 82633
Deoxycortisol ~ 80436, 82634
Deoxyephedrine ~ 82145
Deoxyribonuclease antibody ~ 86215
Deoxyribonuclease I ~ 86215
Deoxyribonucleic acid antibody ~ 86225-86226
Depilation ~ see removal, hair
Depletion
plasma ~ 38214
platelet ~ 38213
T-cell ~ 38210
tumor cell ~ 38211
Deposit calcium ~ 82310, 82330, 82340
Depth electrode
insertion ~ 61760
Derma-fat-fascia graft ~ 15770
Dermabrasion ~ 15780-15783
Dermatology medical procedures ~ 96900-96999
actinotherapy ~ 96900
examination of hair, microscopic ~ 96902
ultraviolet A treatment ~ 96912
ultraviolet B treatment ~ 96910-96913
ultraviolet light treatment ~ 96900-96913
unlisted services and procedures ~ 96999
Dermatoplasty, septal ~ 30620
Dermoid ~ 30124-30125
Derrick-Burnet disease ~ 86000, 86638
Descending abdominal aorta ~ see aorta, abdominal
Desipramine, assay ~ 80160
Desmotomy ~ 23415, 29848
Desoxycorticosterone ~ 82633
Desoxycortone ~ 82633
Desoxyephedrine ~ 82145
Desoxynorephedrin ~ 82145
Desoxyphenobarbital ~ 80188
Desquamation ~ 17360
Destruction
acne ~ 17340-17360
cryotherapy ~ 17340
arrhythmogenic focus, heart ~ 33250-33251, 33261
bladder ~ 51020, 52214-52224, 52354
calculus
bile duct ~ 43265
kidney ~ 50590
pancreatic duct ~ 43265

Destruction ~ *continued*
chemical cauterization, granulation tissue ~ 17250
ciliary body
cryotherapy ~ 66720
cyclodialysis ~ 66740
cyclophotocoagulation ~ 66710-66711
diathermy ~ 66700
endoscopic ~ 66711
cyst
abdomen ~ 49200-49201
ciliary body ~ 66770
iris ~ 66770
retroperitoneal ~ 49200-49201
endometrial ablation ~ 58356
endometriomas
abdomen ~ 49200-49201
retroperitoneal ~ 49200-49201
fissure, anal ~ 46940-46942
hemorrhoids ~ 46934-46936
kidney ~ 52354
endoscopic ~ 50557, 50576
lesion
anal ~ 46900-46917, 46924
bladder ~ 51030
breast ~ 0061T
choroid ~ 0016T, 67220-67225
ciliary body ~ 66770
colon ~ 45383
conjunctiva ~ 68135
cornea ~ 65450
eyelid ~ 67850
facial ~ 17000-17004, 17280-17286
gastrointestinal, upper ~ 43258
gums ~ 41850
intestines
large ~ 44393
small ~ 44369
iris ~ 66770
mouth ~ 40820
nose, intranasal ~ 30117-30118
palate ~ 42160
penis
cryosurgery ~ 54056
electrodesiccation ~ 54055
extensive ~ 54065
laser surgery ~ 54057
simple ~ 54050-54060
surgical excision ~ 54060
pharynx ~ 42808
prostrate ~ 45320
thermotherapy ~ 53850-53853
microwave ~ 53850
radio frequency ~ 53852
rectum ~ 45320
retina
cryotherapy, diathermy ~ 67208, 67227
photocoagulation ~ 0017T, 67210, 67228
radiation by implantation of source ~ 67218

Destruction ~ *continued*
skin
benign ~ 17000-17250
malignant ~ 17260-17286, 96567
premalignant ~ 96567
spinal cord ~ 62280-62282
ureter ~ 52341-52342, 52344-52345
urethra ~ 52400, 53265
uvula ~ 42160
vagina
extensive ~ 57065
simple ~ 57061
vascular, cutaneous ~ 17106-17108
vulva
extensive ~ 56515
simple ~ 56501
molluscum contagiosum ~ 17110
muscle endplate
cervical spinal ~ 64613
extraocular ~ 67345
extremity ~ 64614
facial ~ 64612
trunk ~ 64614
nerve ~ 64600-64681
laryngeal, recurrent ~ 31595
polyp
aural ~ 69540
nose ~ 30110-30115
urethra ~ 53260
prostate ~ 55873
prostate tissue, transurethral thermotherapy ~ 53850-53853
sinus, frontal ~ 31080-31085
Skene's gland ~ 53270
skin lesion
benign ~ 17000-17004
fifteen or more lesions ~ 17004
two - fourteen lesions ~ 17003
malignant ~ 17260-17286
by photodynamic therapy ~ 96567
premalignant ~ 17000-17004
fifteen or more lesions ~ 17004
by photodynamic therapy ~ 96567
two - fourteen lesions ~ 17003
tonsil, lingual ~ 42870
tumor
abdomen ~ 49200-49201
bile duct ~ 43272
breast ~ 0061T
chemosurgery ~ 17311-17315
colon ~ 45383
intestines
large ~ 44393
small ~ 44369
pancreatic duct ~ 43272
rectum ~ 45190, 46937-46938
retroperitoneal ~ 49200-49201
urethra ~ 53220
tumor or polyp, rectum ~ 45320
turbinate mucosa ~ 30801-30802

Destruction ~ *continued*
ureter ~ 52354
endoscopic ~ 50957, 50976
urethra ~ 52214-52224, 52354
prolapse ~ 53275
warts, flat ~ 17110-17111
with cystourethroscopy ~ 52354
Determination, blood pressure ~ see blood pressure
Developmental testing ~ 96110-96111
Device
iliac artery occlusion device insertion ~ 34808
venous access
collection of blood specimen ~ 36540
fluoroscopic guidance ~ 36598, 77001
insertion
central ~ 36560-36566
peripheral ~ 36570-36571
obstruction clearance ~ 36595-36596
imaging ~ 75901-75902
removal ~ 36590
repair ~ 36576
replacement ~ 36582-36583, 36585
catheter ~ 36578
ventricular assist, extracorporeal removal ~ 0050T
Device, intrauterine ~ 58300-58301
Device, orthotic ~ 97760, 97762
Device handling ~ 99002
Dexamethasone suppression test ~ 80420
DHA sulfate ~ 82627
Dhea ~ 82626
Dhea sulfate ~ 82627
DHT ~ 82651
Diagnosis, psychiatric ~ see psychiatric diagnosis
Diagnostic amniocentesis ~ 59000
Diagnostic aspiration of anterior chamber of eye ~ 65800
Diagnostic radiology ~ 70010-76499
Diagnostic skin and sensitization tests ~ see allergy tests
Diagnostic ultrasound ~ 76506-76999
Diagnostic ultrasound of heart ~ see echocardiography
Dialyses, peritoneal ~ 90945-90947
Dialysis
arteriovenous fistula revision without thrombectomy ~ 36832
arteriovenous shunt ~ 36145
revision with thrombectomy ~ 36833
thrombectomy ~ 36831
end stage renal disease ~ 90918-90925
hemodialysis ~ 90935-90937
blood flow study ~ 90939-90940
hemoperfusion ~ 90997
patient training
completed course ~ 90989
per session ~ 90993
peritoneal ~ 90945-90947
unlisted services and procedures ~ 90999
Dialysis, extracorporeal ~ 90935-90937
Dialysis services ~ 90918-90999
Diaphragm
repair
for eventration ~ 39545
hernia ~ 39502-39541
laceration ~ 39501
resection ~ 39560-39561
unlisted procedures ~ 39599
vagina
fitting ~ 57170
Diaphragm contraception ~ 57170
Diaphysectomy
calcaneus ~ 28120
clavicle ~ 23180
femur ~ 27360
fibula ~ 27360, 27641
humerus ~ 23184, 24140
metacarpal ~ 26230
metatarsal ~ 28122
olecranon process ~ 24147
phalanges
finger ~ 26235-26236
toe ~ 28124
radius ~ 24145, 25151
scapula ~ 23182
talus ~ 28120
tarsal ~ 28122
tibia ~ 27360, 27640
ulna ~ 24147, 25150
Diastase ~ 82150
Diastasis ~ see separation
Diathermy ~ 97024
destruction ciliary body ~ 66700
lesion retina ~ 67208, 67227
retinal detachment
prophylaxis ~ 67141
repair ~ 67101
surgical ~ 17000-17286
Dibucaine number ~ 82638
Dichloride, methylene ~ 84600
Dichlorides, ethylene ~ 84600
Dichloroethane ~ 84600
Dichloromethane ~ 84600
Diethylamide, lysergic acid ~ 80102-80103, 80299
Diethylether ~ 84600
Differential count ~ 85032, 85048, 89055
Differentiation reversal factor ~ 85210
Diffusion test, gel ~ 86329-86331
Digestive system, surgical procedures ~ 40490-49999
Digestive tract ~ see gastrointestinal tract
Digit replantation ~ 20816-20822
Digital artery sympathectomy ~ 64820
Digital slit-beam radiograph ~ see scanogram
Digits pinch graft ~ 15050
Digoxin assay ~ 80162
Dihydrocodeinone ~ 82646
Dihydrocodeinone screen ~ 82486
Dihydroepitestosterone ~ 82651
Dihydrohydroxycodeinone ~ 80102-80103, 83925

Dihydromorphinone ~ 82486, 82649
Dihydrotestosterone ~ 82651
Dihydroxyethanes ~ 82693
Dihydroxyvitamin D ~ 82652
Dilatation, transluminal arterial ~ 75962-75968
Dilation ~ 59840
anal
endoscopy ~ 46604
sphincter ~ 45905
bile duct
endoscopy ~ 43271, 47555-47556
stricture ~ 74363
bladdercystourethroscopy ~ 52260-52265
bronchiendoscopy ~ 31630, 31636-31638
cervix
canal ~ 57800
stump ~ 57558
colon endoscopy ~ 45386
colon-sigmoid endoscopy ~ 45340
esophagus ~ 43450-43458
balloon ~ 43220, 43249
endoscopy ~ 43220, 43226, 43249
surgical ~ 43510
intestines, small endoscopy ~ 44370
kidney ~ 50395
intra-renal stricture ~ 52343, 52346
lacrimal punctum ~ 68801
larynx
endoscopy ~ 31528-31529
pancreatic duct
endoscopy ~ 43271
rectum
endoscopy ~ 45303
sphincter ~ 45910
salivary duct ~ 42650-42660
trachea
endoscopy ~ 31630-31631, 31636-31638
ureter ~ 50395, 52341-52342, 52344-52345
endoscopy ~ 50553, 50572, 50953, 50972
urethra ~ 52260-52265
general ~ 53665
suppository and/or instillation ~ 53660-53661
urethral
stenosis ~ 52281
stricture ~ 52281, 53600-53621
vagina ~ 57400
Dilation and curettage ~ 59840
cervix ~ 57558, 57800
corpus uteri ~ 58120
hysteroscopy ~ 58558
postpartum ~ 59160
with amniotic injections ~ 59851
with vaginal suppositories ~ 59856
Dilation and evacuation ~ 59841
with amniotic injections ~ 59851
Dimethadione ~ 82654
Dioxide, carbon ~ 82374
Dioxide, silicon ~ 84285
Dipeptidyl peptidase A ~ 82164
Diphenylhydantoin ~ 80185-80186
Diphosphate, adenosine ~ 82030
Diphtheria ~ 86648
Dipropylacetic acid assay ~ 80164
Direct pedicle flap formation ~ 15570-15576
Disability evaluation services
basic life and/or disability evaluation ~ 99450
work-related or medical disability evaluation ~ 99455-99456
Disarticulation
ankle ~ 27889
hip ~ 27295
knee ~ 27598
shoulder ~ 23920-23921
wrist ~ 25920, 25924
revision ~ 25922
Disc, intervertebral ~ see intervertebral disk
Discectomies ~ 63075-63078
percutaneous ~ 62287
Discharge, body substance ~ see drainage
Discharge services
hospital ~ 99238-99239
nursing facility ~ 99315-99316
observation care ~ 99234-99236
Discission
cataract
laser surgery ~ 66821
stab incision ~ 66820
vitreous strands ~ 67030
Discography ~ see diskography
Discolysis ~ 62292
Disease
Durand-Nicolas-Favre ~ 86729
Erb-Goldflam ~ 95857
Heine-Medin ~ see polio
hydatid ~ see echinococcosis
Lyme ~ see Lyme disease
Ormond ~ see retroperitoneal fibrosis
Peyronie ~ see Peyronie disease
Posada-Wernicke ~ 86490
Disease/organ panel ~ see organ or disease oriented panel
Diskectomy ~ 63075-63078
additional segment ~ 22226
arthrodesis
additional interspace ~ 22534, 22585
cervical ~ 22554
lumbar ~ 22533, 22558, 22630
thoracic ~ 22532, 22556
cervical ~ 22220
lumbar ~ 22224, 22630
percutaneous ~ 62287
thoracic ~ 22222
Diskography
cervical disk ~ 72285
injection ~ 62290-62291
lumbar disk ~ 72295
thoracic ~ 72285
Disk chemolyses, intervertebral ~ 62292
Dislocated joint ~ see dislocation

Dislocation
acromioclavicular joint, open treatment ~ 23550-23552
ankle
closed treatment ~ 27840-27842
open treatment ~ 27846-27848
carpal
closed treatment ~ 25690
open treatment ~ 25695
carpometacarpal joint ~ 26670
closed treatment
with manipulation ~ 26675-26676
open treatment ~ 26685-26686
percutaneous fixation ~ 26676
clavicle
closed treatment ~ 23540-23545
open treatment ~ 23550-23552
without manipulation ~ 23540
with manipulation ~ 23545
closed treatment
carpometacarpal joint ~ 26670-26675
metacarpophalangeal ~ 26700-26706
thumb ~ 26641
elbow
closed treatment ~ 24600-24605, 24640
open treatment ~ 24615
hip joint
closed treatment ~ 27250-27252, 27265-27266
congenital ~ 27256-27259
open treatment ~ 27253-27254, 27258-27259
without trauma ~ 27265-27266
interphalangeal joint
closed treatment ~ 26770-26775
open treatment ~ 26785
percutaneous fixation ~ 26776
toe
closed treatment ~ 28660-28665
open treatment ~ 28675
percutaneous fixation ~ 26770-26776, 28666
with manipulation ~ 26770
knee ~ 27560-27562
closed treatment ~ 27550-27552, 27560-27562
open treatment ~ 27556-27558, 27566, 27730
recurrent ~ 27420-27424
lunate
closed treatment ~ 25690
open treatment ~ 25695
with manipulation ~ 25690, 26670-26676, 26700-26706
metacarpophalangeal joint
closed treatment ~ 26700-26706
open treatment ~ 26715
metatarsophalangeal joint
closed treatment ~ 28630-28635
open treatment ~ 28645
percutaneous fixation ~ 28636

Dislocation ~ *continued*
open treatment ~ 26685-26686
patella
closed treatment ~ 27560-27562
open treatment ~ 27566
recurrent ~ 27420-27424
pelvic ring
closed treatment ~ 27193-27194
open treatment ~ 27217-27218
percutaneous fixation ~ 27216
without manipulation ~ 27193-27194
percutaneous fixation
metacarpophalangeal ~ 26705
peroneal tendons ~ 27675-27676
radiocarpal joint ~ 25660
radio-ulnar joint ~ 25520-25526
radius
closed treatment ~ 24640
with fracture
closed treatment ~ 24620
open treatment ~ 24635
shoulder
closed treatment with manipulation ~ 23650-23655
open treatment ~ 23660
with greater tuberosity fracture
closed treatment ~ 23665
open treatment ~ 23670
with surgical or anatomical neck fracture
closed treatment ~ 23675
open treatment ~ 23680
skin debridement ~ 11010-11012
sternoclavicular joint
closed treatment
without manipulation ~ 23520
with manipulation ~ 23525
open treatment ~ 23530-23532
talotarsal joint
closed treatment ~ 28570-28575
open treatment ~ 28546
percutaneous fixation ~ 28576
tarsal
closed treatment ~ 28540-28545
open treatment ~ 28555
percutaneous fixation ~ 28546
tarsometatarsal joint
closed treatment ~ 28600-28605
open treatment ~ 28615
percutaneous fixation ~ 28606
temporomandibular joint
closed treatment ~ 21480-21485
open treatment ~ 21490
thumb
closed treatment ~ 26641-26645
open treatment ~ 26665
percutaneous fixation ~ 26650
with fracture ~ 26645
open treatment ~ 26665
percutaneous fixation ~ 26650-26665
with manipulation ~ 26641-26650

Dislocation ~ *continued*
tibiofibular joint
closed treatment ~ 27830-27831
open treatment ~ 27832
vertebra
additional segment, open treatment ~ 22328
cervical
open treatment ~ 22326
closed treatment ~ 22305
without manipulation ~ 22310
with manipulation, casting and/or bracing ~ 22315
lumbar, open treatment ~ 22325
thoracic, open treatment ~ 22327
wrist
closed treatment ~ 25660, 25675, 25680
intercarpal ~ 25660
open treatment ~ 25670
open treatment ~ 25670, 25685
percutaneous fixation ~ 25671
radiocarpal ~ 25660
open treatment ~ 25670
radioulnar
closed treatment ~ 25675
open treatment ~ 25676
percutaneous fixation ~ 25671
with fracture
closed treatment ~ 25680
open treatment ~ 25685
with manipulation ~ 25660, 25675, 25680
Disorder
blood coagulation ~ 85390
penis ~ see penis
retinal ~ see retina
Displacement therapy
nose ~ 30210
Dissection
hygroma, cystic
axillary/cervical ~ 38550-38555
lymph nodes ~ 38542
neck, radical ~ see radical neck dissection
Distention ~ see dilation
Diverticula, Meckel's ~ 44800
Diverticulectomy ~ 44800
esophagus ~ 43130-43135
Meckel's ~ 44800
Diverticulum
bladder ~ see bladder, diverticulum
Meckel's, excision ~ 44800
repair, urethra ~ 53400-53405
Division
isthmus, horseshoe kidney ~ 50540
muscle, foot ~ 28250
plantar fascia, foot ~ 28250
Division, scalenus anticus muscle ~ 21700-21705
Di-amphetamine ~ 82145
DMO ~ 82654
DNA antibody ~ 86225-86226
endonuclease ~ 86215
probe ~ see cytogenetics studies ~ 83896
DNAse antibody ~ 86215
Domiciliary services ~ 99324-99340
discharge services ~ 99315-99316
established patient ~ 99331-99333
new patient ~ 99321-99323
Donor procedures
conjunctival graft ~ 68371
heart/lung excision ~ 33930
heart excision ~ 33940
liver segment ~ 47140-47142
stem cells
donor search ~ 38204
Dopamine ~ 80424, 82382-82384
blood ~ 82383-82384
urine ~ 82382, 82384
Doppler echocardiography ~ 76827-76828, 93307-93308, 93320-93350
extracranial ~ 93875
intracardiac ~ 93662
transesophageal ~ 93318
transthoracic ~ 93303-93317
Doppler scan
arterial studies ~ 93922-93924
extremities ~ 93922-93924
fetal
middle cerebral artery ~ 76821
umbilical artery ~ 76820
extremities ~ 93965
intracranial arteries ~ 93886-93888
Dorsal vertebra ~ 22101, 22112
Dose plan ~ see dosimetry
Dosimetry
radiation therapy ~ 77300, 77331
brachytherapy ~ 77326-77328
intensity modulation ~ 77301
teletherapy ~ 77305-77321
Double-stranded DNA ~ 86225-86226
Doxepin
assay ~ 80166
DPH ~ 80185-80186
Drainage ~ see also excision; incision; incision and drainage
abdomen
abdomen fluid ~ 49080-49081
abscess
appendix ~ 44900-.44901
percutaneous ~ 44901
brain ~ 61150-61151
eyelid ~ 67700
liver ~ 47010-47011
ovary, percutaneous ~ 58823
pelvic, percutaneous ~ 58823
pericolic, percutaneous ~ 58823
perirenal or renal ~ 50020-50021
percutaneous ~ 50021
prostate ~ 52700
retroperitoneal ~ 49060-49061
percutaneous ~ 49061
subdiaphragmatic or subphrenic ~ 49040-49041
percutaneous ~ 49040-49041
with X-ray ~ 75989

Drainage ~ *continued*
amniotic fluid
diagnostic aspiration ~ 59000
therapeutic aspiration ~ 59001
bile duct, transhepatic ~ 75980
brain fluid ~ 61070
bursa ~ 20600-20610
cerebrospinal fluid ~ 61000-61020, 61050, 61070, 62272
cervical fluid ~ 61050
cisternal fluid ~ 61050
cyst
bone ~ 20615
brain ~ 61150-61151, 62161-62162
breast ~ 19000-19001
ganglion ~ 20612
liver ~ 47010-47011
percutaneous ~ 47011
salivary gland ~ 42409
sublingual gland ~ 42409
with fistula ~ 42325-42326
extraperitoneal lymphocele
laparoscopic ~ 49323
open ~ 49062
eye
anterior chamber paracentesis
with diagnostic aspiration of aqueous ~ 65800
with therapeutic release of aqueous ~ 65805
removal blood ~ 65815
removal of vitreous and/or discission anterior hyaloid membrane ~ 65810
fetal fluid ~ 59074
ganglion cyst ~ 20612
hematoma
brain ~ 61154-61156
vagina ~ 57022-57023
hematoma, subungual ~ 11740
joint ~ 20600-20610
liver
abscess or cyst ~ 47010-47011
percutaneous ~ 47011
lymphocele, endoscopic ~ 49323
onychia ~ 10060-10061
orbit ~ 67405, 67440
pancreas
pseudocyst ~ 48510-48511
percutaneous ~ 48511
paronychia ~ 10060-10061
pericardial sac ~ 32659
pericardium ~ 33010-33011
pseudocyst
gastrointestinal, upper
transmural endoscopic ~ 43240
pancreas ~ 48510
open ~ 48510
percutaneous ~ 48511
puncture
chest ~ 32000-32002
skin ~ 10040-10180

Drainage ~ *continued*
spinal cord
cerebrospinal fluid ~ 62272
subdural fluid ~ 61000-61001
urethra
extravasation ~ 53080-53085
ventricular fluid ~ 61020
Drainage implant, glaucoma ~ 66180, 66185
Dressings
burns ~ 16010-16030
change
anesthesia ~ 15852
Drez procedure ~ see incision, spinal cord ~ 63200
Dril ~ 36838
Drill hole, skull
catheter ~ 61107
drain hematoma ~ 61108
exploration ~ 61105
implant electrode ~ 61850, 61863-61868
Drinking test for glaucoma ~ 92140
Drug ~ see drug assay; specific drug
analysis
tissue preparation ~ 80103
confirmation ~ 80102
infusion ~ 62360-62362
Drugs, anticoagulant ~ 85300-85305, 85307
Drug assay
amikacin ~ 80150
amitriptyline ~ 80152
benzodiazepine ~ 80154
carbamazepine ~ 80156-80157
cyclosporine ~ 80158
desipramine ~ 80160
digoxin ~ 80162
dipropylacetic acid ~ 80164
doxepin ~ 80166
ethosuximide ~ 80168
gentamicin ~ 80170
gold ~ 80172
haloperidol ~ 80173
imipramine ~ 80174
lidocaine ~ 80176
lithium ~ 80178
nortriptyline ~ 80182
phenobarbital ~ 80184
phenytoin ~ 80185-80186
primidone ~ 80188
procainamide ~ 80190-80192
quantitative, other ~ 80299
quinidine ~ 80194
salicylate ~ 80196
tacrolimus ~ 80197
theophylline ~ 80198
Tobramycin ~ 80200
topiramate ~ 80201
vancomycin ~ 80202
Drug delivery implant
insertion ~ 11981
maintenance and refill
brain ~ 95990
epidural ~ 95990-95991

Drug delivery implant ~ *continued*
intra-arterial ~ 96530
intrathecal ~ 95990-95991
intravenous ~ 96530
intraventricular ~ 95990-95991
removal ~ 11982-11983
with reinsertion ~ 11983
Drug instillation ~ see instillation, drugs
Drug management
psychiatric ~ 90862
Drug screen ~ 80100-80101, 82486
Drug testing ~ 80100-80103
DST ~ 80420
DTaP-HepB-IPV immunization ~ 90723
DTaP immunization ~ 90721
DTP immunization ~ 90701, 90720
DT shots ~ 90702
Dual X-ray absorptiometry (DXA)
appendicular ~ 77081
axial skeleton ~ 77080
body composition ~ 0028T
vertebral fracture ~ 77082
Dual photon absorptiomety ~ 78351
Duct
bile ~ see bile duct
hepatic ~ see hepatic duct
mammary, lavage ~ 0046T-0047T
nasolacrimal ~ see nasolacrimal duct
omphalomesenteric ~ 44800
pancreatic ~ see pancreatic duct
salivary ~ see salivary duct
Stensen's ~ see parotid duct
thoracic ~ see thoracic duct
Ductogram, mammary ~ galactogram
Ductus arteriosus repair ~ 33820-33824
Ductus deferens ~ see vas deferens
Duhamel procedure ~ 45110, 45112, 45119-45120
Dunn operation ~ 28730-28735, 28740
Duodenotomy ~ 44010
Duodenum
biopsy ~ 44010
exclusion ~ 48547
exploration ~ 44010
incision ~ 44010
removal
foreign body ~ 44010
X-ray ~ 74260
Duplex scan ~ see vascular studies
arterial studies
aorta ~ 93978-93979
extracranial ~ 93880-93882
lower extremity ~ 93925-93926
penile ~ 93980-93981
upper extremity ~ 93930-93931
visceral ~ 93975-93979
hemodialysis access ~ 93990
venous studies
extremity ~ 93970-93971
penile ~ 93980-93981
Dupuy-Dutemp operation ~ see reconstruction, eyelid; revision
Dupuytren's contracture ~ 26040-26045
Durand-Nicolas-Favre disease ~ 86729
Dust, Angel ~ 83992
Duvries operation ~ 01714
Dwyer procedure ~ 28300
DXA ~ see dual X-ray absorptiometry (DXA)
Dynamometry ~ 28300
venous studies ~ 28300
with ophthalmoscopy ~ 92260
D & C yellow no. 7 (seven) ~ see fluorescein
D 2, vitamin ~ 82307
D galactose ~ 82760
D glucose ~ 80422-80424, 80430-80435, 95250-95251
D vitamin ~ 82307, 82652

E

E1 ~ 82679
E2 ~ 82670
E3 ~ 82677
Ear
collection of blood ~ 36415-36416
drum ~ see tympanic membrane ~ 69420-69421, 69433-69436, 69450, 69610-69620
external
abscess incision and drainage
complicated ~ 69005
simple ~ 69000
biopsy ~ 69100
excision
partial ~ 69110
total ~ 69120
hematoma
incision and drainage ~ 69000-69005
reconstruction ~ 69300
unlisted services and procedures ~ 69399
inner
CAT scan ~ 70480-70482
excision labyrinth ~ 69905-69910
exploration endolymphatic sac ~ 69805-69806
incision ~ 69820
labyrinth ~ 69801-69802
semicircular canal ~ 69840
insertion cochlear device ~ 69930
semicircular canal ~ 69820
unlisted services and procedures ~ 69949
middle
CAT scan ~ 70480-70482
catheterization ~ 69405
exploration ~ 69440
inflation
with catheterization ~ 69400
without catheterization ~ 69401

Ear ~ *continued*
insertion
baffle ~ 69410
catheter ~ 69405
lesion excision ~ 69540
reconstruction
tympanoplasty with antrotomy or mastoidectomy ~ 69635-69637
tympanoplasty with mastoidectomy ~ 69641-69646
tympanoplasty without mastoidectomy ~ 69631-69633
removal ventilating tube ~ 69424
repair
oval window ~ 69666
round window ~ 69667
revision, stapes ~ 69662
tumor excision ~ 69550-69554
unlisted services and procedures ~ 69799
outer, CAT scan ~ 70480-70482
Ear canal ~ see auditory canal
Ear cartilage graft to face ~ 21235
Ear lobes, pierce ~ 69090
Ear, nose, and throat ~ see also hearing aid services ~ 92700
audiologic function tests
acoustic reflex ~ 92568
acoustic reflex decay ~ 92569
audiometry
Bekesy ~ 92560-92561
comprehensive ~ 92557
conditioning play ~ 92582
evoked response ~ 92585-92586
groups ~ 92559
pure tone ~ 92552-92553
select picture ~ 92583
speech ~ 92555-92556
brainstem evoked response ~ 92585-92586
central auditory function ~ 92620-92621
ear protector evaluation ~ 92596
electrocochleography ~ 92584
filtered speech ~ 92571
hearing aid evaluation ~ 92590-92595
Lombard test ~ 92700
loudness balance ~ 92562
screening test ~ 92551
sensorineural acuity ~ 92575
short increment sensitivity index (SISI) ~ 92564
staggered spondaic word test ~ 92572
Stenger test ~ 92565, 92577
synthetic sentence test ~ 92576
tone decay ~ 92563
tympanometry ~ 92567
audiometry
evoked otoacoustic emissions ~ 92587-92588
visual reinforcement ~ 92579
binocular microscopy ~ 92504
facial nerve function study ~ 92516
hearing, language, and speech evaluation ~ 92506

Ear, nose and throat ~ *continued*
laryngeal function study ~ 92520
nasal function study ~ 92512
nasopharyngoscopy ~ 92511
vestibular function tests
additional electrodes ~ 92547
caloric tests ~ 92533, 92543
nystagmus
optokinetic ~ 92534, 92544
positional ~ 92532, 92542
spontaneous ~ 92531, 92541
posturography ~ 92548
torsion swing test ~ 92546
tracking tests ~ 92545
Ear protector attenuation ~ see also hearing aid services ~ 92596
Ear wax ~ 69210
Ebstein anomaly repair ~ 33468
ECG ~ see electrocardiography
Echinococcosis ~ 86171, 86280
Echocardiography
cardiac ~ 93320-93350
intracardiac ~ 93662
transesophageal ~ 93318
transthoracic ~ 93303-93317
Doppler ~ 93303-93317, 93320-93321, 93662
fetal heart ~ 76825-76826
Doppler
complete ~ 76827
follow-up or repeat study ~ 76828
for congenital anomalies
transesophageal ~ 93315-93317
transthoracic ~ 93303-93304
intracardiac ~ 93662
transesophageal ~ 93318
for congenital anomalies ~ 93315-93317
transthoracic ~ 93303-93318, 93350
for congenital anomalies ~ 93303-93304
Echoencephalography ~ 76506
Echography
abdomen ~ 76700-76705
arm ~ 76880
breast ~ 76645
cardiac ~ 93303-93317, 93320-93321, 93350, 93662
guidance ~ 76932
chest ~ 76604
extracranial arteries ~ 93880-93882
eyes ~ 76511-76529
follow-up ~ 76970
head ~ 76536
heart imaging guidance ~ 76932
hip infant ~ 76885-76886
intracranial arteries ~ 93886-93893
intraoperative ~ 76998
kidney transplant ~ 76776
leg ~ 76880
neck ~ 76536
pelvis ~ 76856-76857
placement therapy fields ~ 76950
pregnant uterus ~ 76801-76828

Echography ~ *continued*
prostate ~ 76872-76873
retroperitoneal ~ 76770-76775
scrotum ~ 76870
spine ~ 76800
transvaginal ~ 76817, 76830
unlisted services and procedures ~ 76999
vagina ~ 76817, 76830
Echotomography ~ see echography
ECMO ~ see extracorporeal membrane oxygenation
ECS ~ see emission computerized tomography
ECSF (erythrocyte colony stimulating factor) ~ 82668
ECT ~ see emission computerized tomography
Ectasia ~ see dilation
Ectopic pregnancy ~ see obstetrical care
abdominal ~ 59130
cervix ~ 59140
interstitial
partial resection uterus ~ 59136
total hysterectomy ~ 59135
laparoscopy ~ 59150
with salpingectomy and/or oophorectomy ~ 59151
tubal ~ 59121
with salpingectomy and/or oophorectomy ~ 59120
Ectropion, repair
excision tarsal wedge ~ 67916
extensive ~ 67917
suture ~ 67914
thermocauterization ~ 67915
Education services, group ~ 99078
Education supplies ~ 99071
EEG ~ see electroencephalography (EEG)
Egg (ova) ~ 87177
Ehrlichia antibody ~ 86666
EKG ~ see electrocardiogram
Elastase ~ 82656
Elbow ~ see also humerus; radius; ulna
abscess, incision and drainage ~ 23930, 23935
anesthesia ~ 00400, 01710-01782
arthrectomy ~ 24155
arthrocentesis ~ 20605
arthrodesis ~ 24800-24802
arthroplasty ~ 24360
with implant ~ 24361-24362
total replacement ~ 24363
arthroscopy
diagnostic ~ 29830
surgical ~ 29834-29838
arthrotomy ~ 24000
capsular release ~ 24006
with joint exploration ~ 24101
with synovectomy ~ 24102
with synovial biopsy ~ 24101
biopsy ~ 24065-24066, 24101
bursa, incision and drainage ~ 23931
Elbow ~ *continued*
dislocation
closed treatment ~ 24600-24605, 24640
open treatment ~ 24615
subluxate ~ 24640
excision ~ 24155
bursa ~ 24105
synovium ~ 24102
exploration ~ 24000, 24101
fracture
Monteggia ~ 24620-24635
open treatment ~ 24586-24587
hematoma, incision and drainage ~ 23930
implant, removal ~ 24164
incision and drainage ~ 24000
injection, arthrography, radiologic ~ 24220
magnetic resonance imaging (MRI) ~ 73221
manipulation ~ 24300
radical resection, capsule, soft tissue and bone with contracture release ~ 24149
removal
foreign body ~ 24000, 24101, 24200-24201
implant ~ 24160
loose body ~ 24101
repair
epicondylitis ~ 24350
fasciotomy ~ 24350-24356
flexorplasty ~ 24330
hemiepiphyseal arrest ~ 24470
ligament ~ 24343-24346
muscle ~ 24341
muscle transfer ~ 24301
tendon ~ 24340-24342
lengthening ~ 24305
transfer ~ 24301
tennis elbow ~ 24350-24356
Steindler advancement ~ 24330
strapping ~ 29260
tumor excision ~ 24075-24077
unlisted services and procedures ~ 24999
X-ray ~ 73070-73080
with contrast ~ 73085
Elbow, golfer ~ 24350-24356
Elbows, tennis ~ 24350-24356
Electrical stimulation
bone healing
invasive ~ 20975
noninvasive ~ 20974
brain surface ~ 95961-95962
physical therapy
attended, manual ~ 97032
unattended ~ 97014
Electric countershock ~ 92960-92961
Electric stimulation ~ see electrical stimulation
Electric stimulation, transcutaneous ~ 64550
Electro-hydraulic procedure ~ 52325
Electro-oculography ~ 92270
Electroanalgesia ~ 64550

Electrocardiography
twenty-four hour monitoring ~ 93224-93237
evaluation ~ 93000, 93010, 93014
monitoring ~ 93271
patient-demand recording transmission and evaluation ~ 93270
patient-demand transmission and evaluation interpretation ~ 93272
rhythm
evaluation ~ 93042
microvolt T-wave alternans ~ 93025
tracing ~ 93041
tracing and evaluation ~ 93040
signal averaged ~ 93278
transmission ~ 93012
Electrocautery ~ see also destruction ~ 17000-17286
Electrochemistry ~ 17380
Electroconvulsive therapy ~ 90870-90871
Electrocortiogram, intraoperative ~ 95829
Electrode, depth ~ 61760
Electrodesiccation ~ 17000-17286
lesion, penis ~ 54055
Electroejaculation ~ 55870
Electroencephalography (EEG) ~ 95816
brain death ~ 95824
coma ~ 95822
digital analysis ~ 95957
electrode placement ~ 95830
intraoperative ~ 95955
monitoring ~ 95812-95813, 95950-95953, 95956
with drug activation ~ 95954
with physical activation ~ 95954
with wada activation ~ 95958
sleep ~ 95822, 95827
standard ~ 95819
Electrogastrography ~ 91132-91133
Electrogram, atrial esophageal recording ~ 93615-93616
Electrolysis ~ 17380
Electromyographs ~ see electromyography, needle
Electromyography
anorectal with biofeedback ~ 90911
fine wire dynamic ~ 96004
needle
extremities ~ 95861-95864
extremity ~ 95860
face and neck muscles ~ 95867-95868
ocular ~ 92265
other than thoracic paraspinal ~ 95870
single fiber electrode ~ 95872
thoracic paraspinal muscles ~ 95869
sphincter muscles
anus ~ 51784-51785
needle ~ 51785
urethra ~ 51784-51785
needle ~ 51785
surface dynamic ~ 96002-96004
Electron microscopy ~ 88348-88349
Electronic analysis
drug infusion pump ~ 62367-62368
implantable loop recorder system ~ 93727
neurostimulator pulse generator ~ 95970-95979
pacing cardioverter-defibrillator ~ 93741-93744
Electrophoresis
counterimmuno- ~ 86185
immuno- ~ 86320-86327
immunofixation ~ 86334-86335
protein ~ 84165-84166
unlisted services and procedures ~ 82664
Electrophysiology procedure ~ 93600-93660
Electroretinogram ~ 92275
Electroretinography ~ 92275
Electrostimulation, analgesic cutaneous ~ 64550
Electrosurgery, trichiasis correction ~ 67825
Electroversion, cardiac ~ 92960-92961
Elevation, scapula, congenital ~ 23400
Elliot operation ~ 66130
Eloesser procedure ~ 32035-32036
Eloesser thoracoplasty ~ 32905
Embolectomy
aortoiliac artery ~ 34151-34201
axillary artery ~ 34101
brachial artery ~ 34101
carotid artery ~ 34001
celiac artery ~ 34151
femoral ~ 34201
iliac ~ 34151-34201
innominate artery ~ 34001-34101
mesentery artery ~ 34151
peroneal artery ~ 34203
popliteal artery ~ 34203
pulmonary artery ~ 33910-33916
radial artery ~ 34111
renal artery ~ 34151
subclavian artery ~ 34001-34101
tibial artery ~ 34203
ulnar artery ~ 34111
Embolization
leiomyomata ~ 37210
Embryo
biopsy ~ 89290-89291
cryopreservation ~ 89258
cryopreserved preparation thawing ~ 89352
culture ~ 89250
with co-culture oocyte ~ 89251
hatching assisted microtechnique ~ 89253
preparation for transfer ~ 89255
storage ~ 89342
Embryonated eggs inoculation ~ 87250
Embryo/fetus monitoring ~ 59050-59051, 99500
Embryo implantation ~ see implantation
Embryo transfer
in vitro fertilization ~ 58974-58976
intrafallopian transfer ~ 58976
intrauterine transfer ~ 58974

Emergency department services ~ 99281-99288
anesthesia ~ 99140
physician direction of advanced life support ~ 99288
Emesis induction ~ 99175
EMG ~ see electromyography, needle
Emission-computed tomography, single-photon ~ 78607
Emission computerized tomography ~ 78607
EMI scan ~ see CAT scan
Emmet operation ~ 59300
Empyema
closure, chest wall ~ 32810
lung ~ 21501-21502
thoracostomy ~ 32020-32036
Empyemectomy ~ 32540
Encephalitis
antibody ~ 86651-86654
Encephalitis virus vaccine ~ 90735
Encephalocele
repair ~ 62120
craniotomy ~ 62121
Encephalon ~ see brain
End stage renal disease services ~ 90918-90925
End-expiratory pressure, positive ~ 94660
Endarterectomy
coronary artery ~ 33572
pulmonary ~ 33916
Endemic flea-borne typhus ~ 86000
Endobronchial challenge tests ~ 95070-95071
Endocavitary fulguration ~ 17000-17286
Endocrine, pancreas ~ 86341
Endocrine system surgical procedures 60000-60699
Endolymphatic sac
exploration
with shunt ~ 69806
without shunt ~ 69805
Endometrial ablation ~ 0009T, 58353
exploration via hysteroscopy ~ 58563
Endometrioma
abdomen
destruction/excision ~ 49200-49201
retroperitoneal
destruction/excision ~ 49200-49201
Endometriosis, adhesive ~ 58559
Endometrium
ablation ~ 58356
biopsy ~ 58100, 58558
Endonuclease, DNA ~ 86215
Endoscopic retrograde cannulation of pancreatic duct (ERCP) ~ 43260
Endoscopies, pleural ~ see thoracoscopy
Endoscopy ~ see arthroscopy; thoracoscopy
adrenal gland
biopsy ~ 60650
excision ~ 60650
anus
biopsy ~ 46606
dilation ~ 46604

Endoscopy ~ *continued*
exploration ~ 46600
hemorrhage ~ 46614
removal
foreign body ~ 46608
polyp ~ 46610, 46612
tumor ~ 46610, 46612
atria ~ 33265-33266
bile duct
biopsy ~ 47553
destruction
calculi (stone) ~ 43265
tumor ~ 43272
dilation ~ 43271, 47555-47556
exploration ~ 47552
intraoperative ~ 47550
percutaneous ~ 47552-47555
removal
calculi (stone) ~ 43264, 47554
foreign body ~ 43269
stent ~ 43269
specimen collection ~ 43260
sphincter pressure ~ 43263
sphincterotomy ~ 43262
tube placement ~ 43267-43268
bladder ~ 52000
biopsy ~ 52204, 52354
catheterization ~ 52005, 52010
destruction ~ 52354
lesion ~ 52400
evacuation clot ~ 52001
excision tumor ~ 52355
exploration ~ 52351
lithotripsy ~ 52353
removal calculus ~ 52352
urethral stent ~ 52282
bladder neck
injection of implant material ~ 51715
brain shunt creation ~ 62201
bronchi
aspiration ~ 31645-31646
biopsy ~ 31625-31629, 31632-31633
destruction
lesion ~ 31641
tumor ~ 31641
dilation ~ 31630-31631, 31636-31638
exploration ~ 31622
injection ~ 31656
lesion destruction ~ 31641
needle biopsy ~ 31629, 31633
placement stent ~ 31631, 31636-31637
revision stent ~ 31638
specimen collection ~ 31623-61324
stenosis ~ 31641
tumor destruction ~ 31641
ultrasound ~ 31620
cervix
biopsy ~ 57454-57455, 57460
curettage ~ 57454, 57456
exploration ~ 57452
loop electrode biopsy ~ 57460
loop electrode conization ~ 57461

Endoscopy ~ *continued*
chest cavity
exploration ~ 32601-32606
surgical ~ 32650-32665
colon
biopsy ~ 44389, 45380, 45392
destruction
lesion ~ 44393, 45383
tumor ~ 44393, 45383
exploration ~ 45378
hemorrhage ~ 44391, 45382
injection ~ 45381
placement stent ~ 45387
removal
foreign body ~ 44390, 45379
polyp ~ 44392, 45384-45385
tumor ~ 44392, 45384-45385
specimen collection ~ 45380
ultrasound ~ 45391-45392
via colotomy ~ 45355
via stoma ~ 44388-44393, 44397
virtual ~ 0066T-0067T
colon-sigmoid
ablation
polyp ~ 45339
tumor ~ 45339
biopsy ~ 45331
dilation ~ 45340
exploration ~ 45330, 45335
hemorrhage ~ 45334
needle biopsy ~ 45342
placement stent ~ 45327, 45345
removal
foreign body ~ 45332
polyp ~ 45333, 45338
tumor ~ 45333, 45338
specimen collection ~ 45331
ultrasound ~ 45341-45342
volvulus ~ 45337
esophagus
biopsy ~ 43202
dilation ~ 43220-43226
exploration ~ 43200
hemorrhage ~ 43227
injection ~ 43201, 43204
insertion stent ~ 43219
needle biopsy ~ 43232
removal
foreign body ~ 43215
polyp ~ 43216-43217, 43228
tumor ~ 43216, 43228
ultrasound ~ 43231-43232
vein ligation ~ 43205
eye ~ 66990
foot, plantar fasciotomy ~ 29893
gastrointestinal, upper
biopsy ~ 43239
catheterization ~ 43241
destruction of lesion ~ 43258
dilation ~ 43245, 43248-43249
drainage of pseudocyst ~ 43240
exploration ~ 43234-43235

Endoscopy ~ *continued*
foreign body ~ 43247
gastric bypass ~ 43644-43645
gastroenterostomy ~ 43644-43645
hemorrhage ~ 43255
inject varices ~ 43243
injection ~ 43236
needle biopsy ~ 43238, 43242
removal ~ 43247, 43250-43251
roux-en-y ~ 43644
stent placement ~ 43256
suturing ~ 0008T
thermal radiation ~ 43257
tube placement ~ 43246
ultrasound ~ 43237-43242, 43259, 76975
vein ligation ~ 43244
ileum via stoma ~ 44383
intestines, small
biopsy ~ 44361, 44377
destruction
lesion ~ 44369
tumor ~ 44369
diagnostic ~ 44376
exploration ~ 44360
hemorrhage ~ 44366, 44378
insertion
stent ~ 44370, 44379
tube ~ 44379
pelvic pouch ~ 44385-44386
removal
foreign body ~ 44363
lesion ~ 44365
polyp ~ 44364-44365
tube placement ~ 44372
tube revision ~ 44373
via stoma ~ 44380-44383
tumor ~ 44364-44365
intracranial ~ 62160-62165
kidney
biopsy ~ 50555, 50574-50576, 52354
catheterization ~ 50553, 50572
destruction ~ 50557, 50576, 52354
dilation of ureter ~ 50553
excision tumor ~ 52355
exploration ~ 52351
lithotripsy ~ 52353
removal
calculus ~ 50561, 50580, 52352
foreign body ~ 50561, 50580
via incision ~ 50562-50580
via stoma ~ 50551-50561
larynx
biopsy ~ 31510, 31535-31536
direct ~ 31515-31571
exploration ~ 31505, 31520-31526, 31575
fiberoptic ~ 31575-31579
indirect ~ 31505-31513
operative ~ 31530-31561
removal
foreign body ~ 31530-31531
lesion ~ see endoscopic ~ 31511, 31545-31546

Endoscopy ~ *continued*
lysis device ~ 0027T
mediastinoscopy
biopsy ~ 39400
exploration ~ 39400
nose
diagnostic ~ 31231-31235
surgical ~ 31237-31294
unlisted services and procedures ~ 31299
pancreatic duct
destruction
calculi (stone) ~ 43265
tumor ~ 43272
dilation ~ 43271
removal
calculi (stone) ~ 43264
foreign body ~ 43269
stent ~ 43269
specimen collection ~ 43260
sphincter pressure ~ 43263
sphincterotomy ~ 43262
tube placement ~ 43267-43268
pelvis
aspiration ~ 49322
destruction of lesion ~ 58662
lysis of adhesions ~ 58660
oviduct surgery ~ 58670-58671
removal of adnexal structures ~ 58661
peritoneum
biopsy ~ 47561
drainage lymphocele ~ 49323, 54690
radiologic ~ 47560
rectum
biopsy ~ 45305
destruction tumor ~ 45320
dilation ~ 45303
exploration ~ 45300
hemorrhage ~ 45317
removal
foreign body ~ 45307
polyp ~ 45308-45315
tumor ~ 45308-45315
volvulus ~ 45321
spleen, removal ~ 38120
testis, removal ~ 54690
trachea
dilation ~ 31630-31631, 31636-31638
via tracheostomy ~ 31615
ureter
biopsy ~ 50955-50957, 50974-50976, 52354
catheterize ~ 50953, 50972
destruction ~ 50957, 50976, 52354
excision tumor ~ 52355
exploration ~ 52351
injection of implant material ~ 52327
lithotripsy ~ 52353
manipulation of ureteral calculus ~ 52330
placement stent ~ 50947
removal
calculus ~ 50961, 50980, 52352
foreign body ~ 50961, 50980

Endoscopy ~ *continued*
resection ~ 52355
via incision ~ 50970-50980
via stoma ~ 50951-50961
ureteral
biopsy ~ 52007
catheterization ~ 52005
urethra ~ 52000
biopsy ~ 52204, 52354
catheterization ~ 52010
destruction ~ 52354
lesion ~ 52400
evacuation clot ~ 52001
excision tumor ~ 52355
exploration ~ 52351
incision ejaculatory duct ~ 52402
injection of implant material ~ 51715
lithotripsy ~ 52353
removal calculus ~ 52352
resection ejaculatory duct ~ 52402
vasectomy ~ 52402
vasotomy ~ 52402
uterus
anesthesia ~ 00952
hysteroscopy
diagnostic ~ 58555
with division/resection intrauterine septum ~ 58560
with lysis of intrauterine adhesions ~ 58559
placement fallopian tube ~ 58565
removal
endometrial ~ 58563
impacted foreign body ~ 58562
leiomyomata ~ 58561
surgical with biopsy ~ 58558
vagina
anesthesia ~ 00950
biopsy ~ 57454
exploration ~ 57452
vascularsurgical ~ 33508, 37500-37501
virtual colon ~ 0066T-0067T
Endosteal implant
reconstruction
mandible ~ 21248-21249
maxilla ~ 21248-21249
Endothelioma, dural ~ 61512, 61519
Endotracheal intubation ~ 31500
Endotracheal tube
intubation ~ 31500
Endovascular repair ~ 0033T-0040T, 0078T-0081T, 34800-34805, 34812-34826, 34833-34900
angiography ~ 75952-75954
imaging neck ~ 0037T
Endovascular therapy
ablation, vein ~ 36475-36479
occlusion ~ 61623
Enema
home visit for fecal impaction ~ 99511
intussusception ~ 74283
therapeutic, for intussusception ~ 74283

Energies, electromagnetic ~ 86945
ENT ~ see ear nose and throat ~ 92700
Entamoeba histolytica
antigen detection
enzyme immunoassay ~ 87336-87337
Enterectomy ~ 44120-44121, 44126-44128, 44137, 44202
donor ~ 44132-44133
with enterostomy ~ 44125
Enterocele
repair ~ 57556
hysterectomy
with colpectomy ~ 58280
Enterocystoplasty ~ 51960
Camey ~ 50825
Enteroenterostomy ~ see anastomosis, intestines
Enterolysis ~ 44005
laparoscopic ~ 44200
Enteropancreatostomy ~ see anastomosis, pancreas to intestines
Enterorrhaphy ~ 44602-44603, 44615
Enterostomy ~ 44300
closure ~ 44625-44626
with enterectomy
intestine, small ~ 44125
Enterotomy ~ 44615
Enterovirus
antibody ~ 86658
Entropion
repair ~ 67921-67924
excision tarsal wedge ~ 67923
suture ~ 67921
thermocauterization ~ 67922
Enucleation
eye
with implant ~ 65103
muscles attached ~ 65105
without implant ~ 65101
pleural ~ 32540
Enucleation, cyst, ovarian ~ 58925
Environmental intervention
for psychiatric patients ~ 90882
Enzyme
angiotensin converting ~ 82164
angiotensin-forming ~ 80408, 80416, 84244
Enzyme activity ~ 82657
radioactive substrate ~ 82658
EOG ~ 92270
Eosinocyte ~ 89190
Eosinophils
nasal smear ~ 89190
Epiandrosterone ~ 82666
Epicondylitides, lateral humeral ~ 24350-24356
Epicondylitis, radiohumeral ~ 24350-24356
Epidemic parotitis ~ see mumps
Epididymectomy
bilateral ~ 54861
unilateral ~ 54860
Epididymis
abscess, incision and drainage ~ 54700
anastomosis
to vas deferens
bilateral ~ 54901
unilateral ~ 54900
biopsy ~ 54800, 54865
epididymography ~ 74440
excision
bilateral ~ 54861
unilateral ~ 54860
exploration biopsy ~ 54865
hematoma, incision and drainage ~ 54700
lesion
excision
local ~ 54830
spermatocele ~ 54840
needle biopsy ~ 54800
spermatocele excision ~ 54840
unlisted services and procedures ~ 55899
X-ray with contrast ~ 74440
Epididymograms ~ 55300
Epididymography ~ 74440
Epididymoplasty ~ 54900-54901
Epididymovasostomy
bilateral ~ 54901
unilateral ~ 54900
Epidural
electrode
insertion ~ 61531
removal ~ 61535
injection ~ 62281-62282 62310-62319, 64479-64484
lysis ~ 0027T, 62263-62264
Epidural anesthesia ~ see anesthesia; epidural
Epidurography ~ 72275
Epigastric hernia repair ~ 49572
Epiglottidectomy ~ 31420
Epiglottis excision ~ 31420
Epikeratoplasty ~ 65767
Epilation ~ 17380
Epinephrine ~ 80424, 82382-82384
blood ~ 82383-82384
urine ~ 82384
Epiphysis ~ see bone; specific bone
Epiphyseal arrest
femur ~ 20150, 27185, 27475, 27479-27485, 27742
fibula ~ 20150, 27477-27485, 27730-27742
radius ~ 20150, 25450-25455
tibia ~ 20150, 27477-27485, 27730, 27734-27742
ulna ~ 20150, 25450-25455
Epiphyseal separation
radius
closed treatment ~ 25600
open treatment ~ 25607-25609
Epiphysiodesis ~ see epiphyseal arrest
Epiploectomy ~ 49255
Episiotomy ~ 59300

Epispadias
penis reconstruction ~ 54385
repair ~ 54380-54390
with extrophy of bladder ~ 54390
with incontinence ~ 54380-54390
Epistaxis ~ 30901-30906
with nasal/sinus endoscopy ~ 31238
EPO ~ see erythropoietin
Epstein-Barr virus
antibody ~ 86663-86665
Equina, cauda ~ see cauda equina
ERCP ~ see bile duct; pancreatic duct ~ 43260
ERG ~ 92275
Ergocalciferol ~ 82307
Ergocalciferols ~ 82307
Ergonovine provocation test ~ 93024
Erythrocyte ~ see red blood cell (RBC)
Erythrocyte AB ~ see antibody, red blood cell
Erythrocyte count ~ 85032-85041
Erythropoietin ~ 82668
Escharotomy, burns ~ 16035-16036
Escherichia coli 0157
antigen detection, enzyme immunoassay ~ 87335
ESD ~ see endoscopy, gastrointestinal, upper
Esophageal
acid infusion test ~ 91012, 91030
polyp ~ 43228
tumor ~ 43228
varices
ligation ~ 43205, 43400
transection/repair ~ 43401
Esophagectomy
partial ~ 43116-43124
total ~ 43107-43113, 43124
Esophagoenterostomy with total gastrectomy ~ 43620
Esophagogastroduodenoscopies ~ see endoscopy, gastrointestinal, upper
Esophagogastromyotomy ~ 32665, 43330-43331
Esophagogastrostomy ~ 43320
Esophagojejunostomy ~ 43340-43341
Esophagomyotomy ~ 32665, 43330-43331
Esophagorrhaphy ~ 43405
Esophagoscopies ~ see endoscopy, esophagus
Esophagostomy ~ 43350-43352
closure ~ 43420-43425
Esophagotomy ~ 43020, 43045
Esophagotracheal fistula ~ see fistula, tracheoesophageal
Esophagus
acid perfusion test ~ 91030
acid reflux tests ~ 91034-91038
balloon distention provocation study ~ 91040
biopsy endoscopy ~ 43202
cineradiography ~ 74230
dilation
endoscopic ~ 43220-43226, 43248-43249
surgical ~ 43510

Esophagus ~ *continued*
endoscopy
biopsy ~ 43202
dilation ~ 43220-43226
exploration ~ 43200
hemorrhage ~ 43227
injection ~ 43201, 43204
insertion stent ~ 43219
needle biopsy ~ 43232
removal
foreign body ~ 43215
polyp ~ 43216-43217, 43228
tumor ~ 43216, 43228
ultrasound ~ 43231-43232
vein ligation ~ 43205
excision
diverticula ~ 43130-43135
partial ~ 43116-43124
total ~ 43107-43113, 43124
exploration endoscopy ~ 43200
hemorrhage ~ 43227
incision ~ 43020, 43045
muscle ~ 43030
injection
sclerosing agent ~ 43204
submucosal ~ 43201
insertion
stent ~ 43219
tamponade ~ 43460
tube ~ 43510
intubation with specimen collection ~ 91000
lesion excision ~ 43100-43101
ligation ~ 43405
motility study ~ 78258, 91010-92012
needle biopsy endoscopy ~ 43232
nuclear medicine
imaging (motility) ~ 78258
reflux study ~ 78262
reconstruction ~ 43300, 43310, 43313
creation stoma ~ 43350-43352
esophagostomy ~ 43350
fistula ~ 43305, 43312, 43314
gastrointestinal ~ 43360-43361
removal
foreign bodies ~ 43020, 43045, 43215, 74235
lesion ~ 43216
polyp ~ 43216-43217, 43228
repair ~ 43300, 43310, 43313
esophagogastric fundoplasty ~ 43324-43325
laparoscopic ~ 43280
esophagogastrostomy ~ 43320
esophagojejunostomy ~ 43340-43341
fistula ~ 43305, 43312, 43314, 43420-43425
muscle ~ 43330-43331
pre-existing perforation ~ 43405
varices ~ 43401
wound ~ 43410-43415
suture ~ 43405
wound ~ 43410-43415
ultrasoundendoscopy ~ 43231-43232

Esophagus ~ *continued*
unlisted services and procedures ~ 43289, 43499
vein ligation ~ 43205, 43400
video ~ 74230
X-ray ~ 74220
Esophagus, varix ~ 43205, 43400-43401
Esophagus neoplasm ~ 43228
Established patient
confirmatory consultations ~ 99271-99275
domiciliary or rest home visit ~ 99331-99333
emergency department services ~ 99281-99285
home services ~ 99347-99350
hospital inpatient services ~ 99221-99239
hospital observation services ~ 99217-99220
initial inpatient consultations ~ 99251-99255
office and/or other outpatient consultations ~ 99241-99245
office visit ~ 99211-99215
online evaluation and management services ~ 0074T
outpatient visit ~ 99211-99215
Establishment
colostomy
abdominal ~ 50810
perineal ~ 50810
Estes operation ~ 58825
Estlander procedure ~ 40525
Estradiol ~ 82670
response ~ 80414
Estriol
blood or urine ~ 82677
Estrogen
blood or urine ~ 82671-82672
receptor ~ 84233
Estrone blood or urine ~ 82679
Ethanediols ~ 82693
Ethanol
blood ~ 82055
breath ~ 82075
urine ~ 82055
Ethchlorovynol ~ 82690
Ethchlorvinol ~ 82690
Ethchlorvynol
blood ~ 82690
urine ~ 82690
Ethmoid fracture with fixation ~ 21340
Ethmoid, sinus ~ see sinus, ethmoid
Ethmoidectomy ~ 31200-31205
endoscopic ~ 31254-31255
skull base surgery ~ 61580-61581
with nasal/sinus endoscopy ~ 31254-31255
Ethosuccimid ~ 80168
Ethosuximide ~ 80168
assay ~ 80168
Ethylene dichlorides ~ 84600
Ethyl alcohol ~ 82055, 82075
Ethylene glycol ~ 82693
Ethylmethylsuccimide ~ 80168
Etiocholanolone ~ 82696
Etiocholanolone measurement ~ 82696
ETOH ~ 82055
Euglobulin lysis ~ 85360
European blastomycosis ~ see cryptococcus
Eustachian tube
catheterization ~ 69405
inflation
myringotomy ~ 69420
anesthesia ~ 69421
with catheterization ~ 69400
without catheterization ~ 69401
insertion, catheter ~ 69405
Eutelegenesis ~ 58976
Evacuation
cervical pregnancy ~ 59140
hematoma
brain ~ 61312-61315
subungual ~ 11740
hydatidiform mole ~ 59870
Evaluation and management services codes ~ 99200-99499
assistive technology, assessment ~ 97755
athletic training
evaluation ~ 97005
re-evaluation ~ 97006
basic life and/or disability evaluation services ~ 99450
care plan oversight services ~ 99374-99380
home health agency care ~ 99374
hospice ~ 99377-99378
nursing facility ~ 99379-99380
case management services ~ 99361-99373
consultation ~ 99241-99275
critical care ~ 99291-99292
interfacility pediatric transport ~ 99289-99290
domiciliary or rest home ~ 99321-99333
emergency department ~ 99281-99288
health behavior
assessment ~ 96150
family intervention ~ 96154-96155
group intervention ~ 96153
individual intervention ~ 96152
re-assessment ~ 96151
home services ~ 99341-99350
hospital ~ 99221-99233
discharge ~ 99238-99239
hospital services, observation care ~ 99217-99220
insurance exam ~ 99455-99456
internet communication ~ 0074T
low birthweight infant ~ 99298-99299
medical
with individual psychotherapy
hospital or residential care ~ 90817, 90819, 90822, 90824, 90827, 90829
office or outpatient ~ 90805, 90807, 90809
with individual psychotherapy, interactive
office or outpatient ~ 90811, 90813, 90815
neonatal intensive care ~ 99295-99296
newborn care ~ 99431-99440
nursing facility ~ see nursing facility services ~ 99301-99313

Evaluation and management services codes ~ *continued*
occupation therapy evaluation ~ 97003
re-evaluation ~ 97004
office and other outpatient ~ 99201-99215
online ~ 0074T
pediatric critical care ~ 99293-99294
pediatric interfacility transport ~ 99289-99290
physical therapy evaluation ~ 97001
re-evaluation ~ 97002
physician standby services ~ 99360
preventive services ~ 99381-99429
prolonged services ~ 99356-99357
psychiatric records or reports ~ 90885
psychiatric residential treatment facility care ~ 99301-99313
unlisted services and procedures ~ 99499
work-related and/or medical disability evaluation ~ 99450
Evaluation studies, drug, pre-clinical ~ 80100-80101, 82486
Evisceration
ocular contents
with implant ~ 65093
without implant ~ 65091
pelvic ~ 45126, 58240
Evocative/suppression testing ~ 80400-80440
stimulation panel ~ 80410
Evoked potential ~ see audiologic function tests
auditory brainstem ~ 92585-92586
central motor
transcranial motor stimulation ~ 95928-95929
somatosensory testing ~ 95925-95927
visual, CNS ~ 95930
Ewart procedure ~ 42226-42227
Excavatum, pectus ~ 21740-21743
Exchange
arterial catheter ~ 37209, 75900
drainage catheter
under radiologic guidance ~ 49423
intraocular lens ~ 66986
transfusion ~ 36455
Excision ~ see debridement; destruction
abscess
brain ~ 61514, 61522
olecranon process ~ 24138
radius ~ 24136
ulna ~ 24138
acromion
shoulder ~ 23130
adenoids ~ 42830-42836
adenoma thyroid gland ~ 60200
adrenal gland ~ 60540
with excision retroperitoneal tumor ~ 60545
laparoscopic ~ 60650
alveolus ~ 41830
anal crypt ~ 46210-46211
anal fissure ~ 46200
anal tag ~ 46220, 46230

Excision ~ *continued*
aorta coarctation ~ 33840-33851
appendix ~ 44950-44960
arteriovenous malformation
spinal ~ 63250-63252
arytenoid cartilage ~ 31400
endoscopic ~ 31560-31561
atrial septum ~ 33735-33737
Bartholin's gland ~ 56740
bladder
diverticulum ~ 51525
neck ~ 51520
partial ~ 51550-51565
total ~ 51570, 51580, 51590-51597
with nodes ~ 51575, 51585, 51595
transurethral ~ 52640
tumor ~ 51530
bladder neck contracture, postoperative ~ 52640
bone
facial ~ 21026
mandible ~ 21025
postoperative
femur ~ 20150
fibula ~ 20150
radius ~ 20150
tibia ~ 20150
ulna ~ 20150
bone abscess
facial ~ 21026
mandible ~ 21025
brain
amygdala ~ 61566
epileptogenic focus ~ 61536
hemisphere ~ 61542-61543
hippocampus ~ 61566
other lobe ~ 61323, 61539-61540
temporal lobe ~ 61537-61538
brain lobe ~ 61323, 61537-61540
breast
biopsy ~ 19100-19103
chest wall tumor ~ 19260-19272
cyst ~ 19120-19126
lactiferous duct fistula ~ 19112
lesion ~ 19120-19126
by needle localization ~ 19125-19126
mastectomy ~ 19300-19307
nipple exploration ~ 19110
bulbourethral gland ~ 53250
bullae
lung ~ 32141
endoscopic ~ 32655
burns ~ 01951-01953, 15002-15005
bursa
elbow ~ 24105
femur ~ 27062
ischial ~ 27060
knee ~ 27340
wrist ~ 25115-25116
bypass graft ~ 35901-35907
calcaneus ~ 28118-28120

Excision ~ *continued*
calculi (stone)
parotid gland ~ 42330, 42340
salivary gland ~ 42330-42340
sublingual gland ~ 42330
submandibular gland ~ 42330-42335
carotid artery ~ 60605
carpal ~ 25145, 25210-25215
cartilage
knee joint ~ 27332-27333
shoulder joint ~ 23101
temporomandibular joint ~ 21060
wrist ~ 25107
caruncle
urethra ~ 53265
cataract
secondary ~ 66830
cervix
radical ~ 57531
stump
abdominal approach ~ 57540-57545
vaginal approach ~ 57550-57556
total ~ 57530
chalazion
multiple
different lids ~ 67805
same lid ~ 67801
single ~ 67800
with anesthesia ~ 67808
chest wall tumor ~ 19260-19272
choroid plexus ~ 61544
clavicle
partial ~ 23120, 23180
sequestrectomy ~ 23170
total ~ 23125
tumor
radical resection ~ 23200
coccyx ~ 27080
colon
excision
partial ~ 44140-44147, 44160
with anastomosis ~ 44140
total ~ 44150-44158
laparoscopic
with anastomosis ~ 44204, 44207-44208
with colostomy ~ 44206, 44208
with ileocolostomy ~ 44205
condyle, temporomandibular joint ~ 21050
constricting ring
finger ~ 26596
cornea
epithelium ~ 65435
with chelating agent ~ 65436
scraping ~ 65430
coronoidectomy ~ 21070
Cowper's gland ~ 53250
cranial bone tumor ~ 61563-61564
cyst ~ see also ganglion cyst
bile duct ~ 47715
bladder ~ 51500
brain ~ 61516, 61524, 62162
branchial ~ 42810-42815

Excision ~ *continued*
calcaneus ~ 28100-28103
carpal ~ 25130-25136
cheekbone ~ 21030
clavicle ~ 23140
with allograft ~ 23146
with autograft ~ 23145
facial bone ~ 21030
femur ~ 27065-27067, 27355-27358
fibula ~ 27635-27638
finger ~ 26160
foot ~ 28090
hand ~ 26160
hip ~ 27065-27067
humerus ~ 23150, 24110
with allograft ~ 23156, 24116
with autograft ~ 23155, 24115
ileum ~ 27065-27067
kidney ~ 50280-50290
knee ~ 27345-27347
lung ~ 32140
mandible ~ 21040, 21046-21047
maxilla ~ 21030, 21048-21049
mediastinal ~ 39200
mediastinum ~ 32662
metacarpal ~ 26200-26205
metatarsal ~ 28104-28107
mullerian duct ~ 55680
nose ~ 30124-30125
olecranon ~ 24120
olecranon process
with allograft ~ 24126
with autograft ~ 24125
ovarian ~ 58925
pericardial ~ 33050
endoscopic ~ 32661
phalanges ~ 26210-26215
toe ~ 28108
pilonidal ~ 11770-11772
pubis ~ 27066-27067
radius ~ 24120, 25120-25126
with allograft ~ 24126
with autograft ~ 24125
salivary gland ~ 42408
scapula ~ 23140
with allograft ~ 23146
with autograft ~ 23145
seminal vesicle ~ 55680
sublingual gland ~ 42408
talus ~ 28100-28103
tarsal ~ 28104-28107
thyroglossal duct ~ 60280-60281
thyroid gland ~ 60200
tibia ~ 27635-27638
toe ~ 28092
ulna ~ 24120, 25120-25126
with allograft ~ 24126
with autograft ~ 24125
urachalbladder ~ 51500
vaginal ~ 57135

Excision ~ *continued*
destruction of the vestibule of the mouth ~ 40808-40820
diverticulum, Meckel's ~ 44800
ear, external
partial ~ 69110
total ~ 69120
elbow joint ~ 24155
electrode ~ 57522
embolectomy/thrombectomy
aortoiliac artery ~ 34151-34201
axillary artery ~ 34101
brachial artery ~ 34101
carotid artery ~ 34001
celiac artery ~ 34151
femoral artery ~ 34201
heart ~ 33310-33315
iliac artery ~ 34151-34201
innominate artery ~ 34001-34101
mesentery artery ~ 34151
peroneal artery ~ 34203
popliteal artery ~ 34203
radial artery ~ 34111
renal artery ~ 34151
subclavian artery ~ 34001-34101
tibial artery ~ 34203
ulnar artery ~ 34111
embolism, pulmonary artery ~ 33910-33916
empyema
lung ~ 32540
pleural ~ 32540
epididymis
bilateral ~ 54861
unilateral ~ 54860
epiglottis ~ 31420
esophagus
diverticula ~ 43130-43135
partial ~ 43116-43124
total ~ 43107-43113, 43124
eye ~ 65101, 65103, 65109
fallopian tube
salpingectomy ~ 58700
salpingo-oophorectomy ~ 58720
fascia ~ see fasciectomy
femur ~ 27360
partial ~ 27070-27071
fibula ~ 27360, 27455-27457, 27641
fistula
anal ~ 46270-46285
foot
fasciectomy ~ 28060
radical ~ 28060-28062
gallbladder ~ 47600-47620
cholecystectomy ~ 47562-47564
with cholangiography ~ 47563
with exploration common duct ~ 47564
ganglion cyst
knee ~ 27347
wrist ~ 25111-25112
gingiva ~ 41820

Excision ~ *continued*
gums ~ 41820
alveolus ~ 41830
operculum ~ 41821
heart
donor ~ 33940
heart/lung
donor ~ 33930
hemangioma ~ 11400-11446
hemorrhoids ~ 46221, 46250
clot ~ 46320
complex ~ 46260-46262
with fissurectomy ~ 46257-46258
simple ~ 46255
hip, partial ~ 27070-27071
hippocampus ~ 61566
humeral head
resection ~ 23195
sequestrectomy ~ 23174
humerus ~ 23184, 23220-23222, 24134, 24140, 24150-24151
hydrocele
spermatic cord ~ 55500
tunica vaginalis ~ 55040-55041
bilateral ~ 55041
unilateral ~ 55040
hygroma, cystic, axillary/cervical ~ 38550-38555
hymenotomy ~ 56700
ileum
ileoanal reservoir ~ 45136
partial ~ 27070-27071
inner ear ~ 69905-69910
interphalangeal joint
toe ~ 28160
intervertebral disk
decompression ~ 63075-63078
hemilaminectomy ~ 63040, 63043-63044
herniated ~ 63020-63044, 63055-63066
intestine
laparoscopic
with anastomosis ~ 44202-44203
intestines
donor ~ 44132-44133
intestines, small ~ 44120-44128
transplantation ~ 44137
iris
iridectomy
with corneoscleral or corneal section ~ 66600
with cyclectomy ~ 66605
optical ~ 66635
peripheral ~ 66625
sector ~ 66630
kidney
donor ~ 50300-50320, 50547
partial ~ 50240
recipient ~ 50340
transplantation ~ 50370
with ureters ~ 50220-50236
kneecap ~ 27350

Excision ~ *continued*
labyrinth
with mastoidectomy ~ 69910
transcanal ~ 69905
lacrimal gland
partial ~ 68505
total ~ 68500
lacrimal sac ~ 68520
larynx
partial ~ 31367-31382
with pharynx ~ 31390-31395
total ~ 31360-31365
lesion
anal ~ 45108, 46922
ankle ~ 27630
arthroscopic ~ 29891
auditory canal, external
exostosis ~ 69140
radical with neck dissection ~ 69155
radical without neck dissection ~ 69150
soft tissue ~ 69145
bladder ~ 52224
brain ~ 61534, 61536-61540
brainstem ~ 61575-61576
carotid body ~ 60600-60605
colon ~ 44110-44111
conjunctiva ~ 68110-68130
over 1cm ~ 68115
with adjacent sclera ~ 68130
cornea ~ 65400
without graft ~ 65420
ear, middle ~ 69540
epididymis
local ~ 54830
spermatocele ~ 54840
esophagus ~ 43100-43101
eye ~ 65900
eyelid
multiple, different lids ~ 67805
multiple, same lid ~ 67801
single ~ 67800
under anesthesia ~ 67808
without closure ~ 67840
femur ~ 27062
finger ~ 26160
foot ~ 28080, 28090
gums ~ 41822-41828
hand ~ 26160
intestines ~ 44110
small ~ 43250, 44111
intraspinal ~ 63265-63273
knee ~ 27347
larynx, endoscopic ~ 31545-31546
leg, lower ~ 27630
meniscus ~ 27347
mesentery ~ 44820
mouth ~ 40810-40816, 41116
nerve ~ 64774-64792
neuroma ~ 64778
nose, intranasal ~ 30117-30118
orbit ~ 61333
lateral approach ~ 67420

Excision ~ *continued*
palate ~ 42104-42120
pancreas ~ 48120
penis ~ 54060
surgical excision penile plaque ~ 54110-54112
pharynx ~ 42808
rectum ~ 45108
sclera ~ 66130
skin
benign ~ 11400-11471
malignant ~ 11600-11646
skull ~ 61500, 61615-61616
spermatic cord ~ 55520
spinal cord ~ 63300-63308
stomach ~ 43611
talus, arthroscopic ~ 29891
testis ~ 54512
tibia, arthroscopic ~ 29891
toe ~ 28092
tongue ~ 41110-41114
urethra ~ 52224, 53265
uterus ~ 59100
leiomyomata ~ 58140, 58545-58546, 58561
uvula ~ 42104-42107
wrist tendon ~ 25110
lesion, arthroscopic
ankle ~ 29891
talus ~ 29891
tibia ~ 29891
lesion, tendon sheath
arm, lower ~ 25110
lip ~ 40500-40530
frenum ~ 40819
liver
extensive ~ 47122
lobectomy ~ 47125-47130
partial ~ 47120, 47125-47130, 47140-47142
total ~ 47133
lung
bronchus resection ~ 32486
bullae, endoscopic ~ 32655
chest resection ~ 32520-32525
completion ~ 32488
emphysematous ~ 32491
lobe ~ 32480-32482
segment ~ 32484
total ~ 32440-32445
wedge resection ~ 32500
endoscopic ~ 32657
lung/heart donor ~ 33930
lymph nodes ~ 38500, 38510-38530
abdominal ~ 38747
inguinofemoral ~ 38760-38765
limited, for staging
para-aortic ~ 38562
pelvic ~ 38562
retroperitoneal ~ 38564
pelvic ~ 38770

Excision ~ *continued*
radical
axillary ~ 38740-38745
cervical ~ 38720-38724
suprahyoid ~ 38700
retroperitoneal transabdominal ~ 38780
thoracic ~ 38746
mandibular exostosis ~ 21031
mastoid
complete ~ 69502
radical ~ 69511
modified ~ 69505
petrous apicectomy ~ 69530
simple ~ 69501
maxilla exotosis ~ 21032
maxillary torus palatinus ~ 21032
meningioma, brain ~ 61512, 61519
meniscectomy, temporomandibular joint ~ 21060
metacarpal ~ 26230
metatarsal ~ 28110-28114, 28122, 28140
condyle ~ 28288
mouth, frenum ~ 40819
mucosa
gums ~ 41828
mouth ~ 40818
nail fold ~ 11765
nails ~ 11750-11752
nerve
foot ~ 28055
leg, upper ~ 27325
sympathetic ~ 64802-64818
neurofibroma ~ 64788-64790
neurolemmoma ~ 64788-64792
neuroma ~ 64774-64786
nose
dermoid cyst
complex ~ 30125
simple ~ 30124
polyp ~ 30110-30115
rhinectomy ~ 30150-30160
skin ~ 30120
submucous resection
nasal septum ~ 30520
turbinate ~ 30140
turbinate ~ 30130-30140
odontoid process ~ 22548
olecranon process ~ 24147
omentum ~ 49255
ovary ~ 58720
partial
oophorectomy ~ 58940
ovarian malignancy ~ 58943
peritoneal malignancy ~ 58943
tubal malignancy ~ 58943
wedge resection ~ 58920
total ~ 58940-58943
oviduct ~ 58720
palate ~ 42120, 42145

Excision ~ *continued*
pancreas
ampulla of Vater ~ 48148
duct ~ 48148
partial ~ 48140-48146, 48150, 48153-48154, 48160
peripancreatic tissue ~ 48105
total ~ 48155-48160
parathyroid gland ~ 60500-60502
parotid gland ~ 42340
partial ~ 42410-42415
total ~ 42420-42426
patella ~ 27350, 27424
penile adhesions, post-circumcision ~ 54162
penis
frenulum ~ 54164
partial ~ 54120
prepuce ~ 54150-54161, 54163
radical ~ 54130-54135
total ~ 54125
pericardium ~ 33030-33031
endoscopic ~ 32659
petrous temporal
apex ~ 69530
phalanges
fingers ~ 26235-26236
toe ~ 28124-28126, 28150-28160
pharynx ~ 42145
with larynx ~ 31390-31395
partial ~ 42890
resection ~ 42892-42894
pituitary gland ~ 61546-61548
pleura ~ 32310-32320
endoscopic ~ 32656
polyp
intestines ~ 43250
nose
extensive ~ 30115
simple ~ 30110
sinus ~ 31032
urethra ~ 53260
pressure ulcers ~ see also skin graft and flap ~ 15920-15999
prostate
abdominoperineal ~ 45119
partial ~ 55801, 55821-55831
perineal ~ 55801-55815
radical ~ 55810-55815, 55840-55845
regrowth ~ 52630
residual obstructive tissue ~ 52620
retropubic ~ 55831-55845
suprapubic ~ 55821
transurethral ~ 52601, 52612-52614
pterygium, with graft ~ 65426
pubis, partial ~ 27070-27071
radical synovium wrist ~ 25115-25116
radius ~ 24130, 24136, 24145, 24152-24153, 25145
styloid process ~ 25230

Excision ~ *continued*
rectum
with colon ~ 45121
partial ~ 45111, 45113-45116, 45123
prolapse ~ 45130-45135
stricture ~ 45150
total ~ 45119-45120
redundant skin of eyelid ~ 15820-15823
ribs ~ 21600-21616, 32900
scapula
ostectomy ~ 23190
partial ~ 23182
sequestrectomy ~ 23172
tumor
radical resection ~ 23210
sclera ~ 66160
scrotum ~ 55150
semilunar cartilage of knee ~ 27332-27333
seminal vesicle ~ 55650
sesamoid bone
foot ~ 28315
sinus
ethmoid ~ 31200-31205
maxillary ~ 31225-31230
Skene's gland ~ 53270
skin
excess ~ 15830-15839, 15847
lesion
benign ~ 11400-11471
malignant ~ 11600-11646
nose ~ 30120
skin graft, preparation of site ~ 15000
skull ~ 61501
spermatic veins ~ 55530-55540
abdominal approach ~ 55535
hernia repair ~ 55540
spleen ~ 38100-38102
laparoscopic ~ 38120
stapes
with footplate drill out ~ 69661
without foreign material ~ 69660
sternum ~ 21620, 21630-21632
stomach
partial ~ 43631-43639, 43845
total ~ 43620-43622
sublingual gland ~ 42450
submandibular gland ~ 42440, 42508
sweat glands
axillary ~ 11450-11451
inguinal ~ 11462-11463
perianal ~ 11470-11471
perineal ~ 11470-11471
umbilical ~ 11470-11471
synovium
ankle ~ 27625-27626
carpometacarpal joint ~ 26130
elbow ~ 24102
hip joint ~ 27054
interphalangeal joint ~ 26140
intertarsal joint ~ 28070
knee joint ~ 27334-27335

Excision ~ *continued*
metacarpophalangeal joint ~ 26135
metatarsophalangeal joint ~ 28072
shoulder ~ 23105-23106
tarsometatarsal joint ~ 28070
wrist ~ 25105, 25118-25119
talus ~ 28120, 28130
tarsal ~ 28116, 28122
temporal bone ~ 69535
temporal, petrous apex ~ 69530
tendon
arm
lower ~ 25109
finger ~ 26180, 26390, 26415
hand ~ 26390, 26415
palm ~ 26170
tendon sheath
finger ~ 26145
foot ~ 28086-28088
palm ~ 26145
wrist ~ 25115-25116
testis
laparoscopic ~ 54690
partial ~ 54522
radical ~ 54530-54535
simple ~ 54520
tumor ~ 54530-54535
thrombectomy
axillary vein ~ 34490
bypass graft ~ 35875-35876
femoropopliteal vein ~ 34401-34451
iliac vein ~ 34401-34451
subclavian vein ~ 34471-34490
vena cava ~ 34401-34451
thromboendarterectomy
aorta, abdominal ~ 35331
aortoiliofemoral ~ 35363
axillary artery ~ 35321
brachial artery ~ 35321
carotid artery ~ 35301, 35390
celiac artery ~ 35341
femoral artery ~ 35371-35372
iliac ~ 35361-35363
iliac artery ~ 35351
iliofemoral artery ~ 35355, 35363
innominate artery ~ 35311
mesenteric artery ~ 35341
peroneal artery ~ 35305-35306
popliteal artery ~ 35303
renal artery ~ 35341
subclavian artery ~ 35301-35311
tibial artery ~ 35305-35306
vertebral artery ~ 35301
thymus gland ~ 60521
thyroid gland for malignancy
partial ~ 60210-60225
removal all thyroid tissue ~ 60260
secondary ~ 60260

Excision ~ *continued*
total ~ 60240
cervical approach ~ 60271
sternal split/transthoracic approach ~ 60270
limited neck dissection ~ 60252
radical neck dissection ~ 60254
tibia ~ 27360, 27640
tongue
complete ~ 41140-41155
frenum ~ 41115
with mouth resection ~ 41150-41153
partial ~ 41120-41135
with radical neck ~ 41135, 41145-41155
tonsils ~ 42825-42826
lingual ~ 42870
radical ~ 42842-42845
tag ~ 42860
with adenoids ~ 42820-42821
torus mandibularis ~ 21031
trachea stenosis ~ 31780-31781
transcervical approach ~ 60520
tricuspid valve ~ 33460
tumor
abdominal wall ~ 22900
acetabulum ~ 27076
ankle ~ 27615-27619
arm, lower ~ 25075-25077
arm, upper ~ 24075-24077
back/flank ~ 21930
bile duct ~ 47711-47712
bladder ~ 51530, 52234-52240, 52355
brain ~ 61510, 61518, 61520-61521, 61526-61530, 61545, 62164
bronchi ~ 31640
calcaneus ~ 27647, 28100-28103
carpal ~ 25130-25136
cheekbone ~ 21030, 21034, 21048-21049
clavicle ~ 23140
with allograft ~ 23146
with autograft ~ 23145
ear, middle
extended ~ 69554
transcanal ~ 69550
transmastoid ~ 69552
elbow ~ 24075-24077
esophagus endoscopic ablation ~ 43228
facial bones ~ 21029-21030, 21034-21040, 21046-21049
facial tissue ~ 21015
femur ~ 27065-27067, 27355-27358, 27365
fibula ~ 27635-27638, 27646
finger ~ 26115-26117
foot ~ 28043-28046
gums ~ 41825-41827
hand ~ 26115-26117
heart ~ 33120-33130
hip ~ 27047-27049, 27065-27067
radical ~ 27075-27076

Excision ~ *continued*
humerus ~ 23150, 23220-23222, 24110-24115
with allograft ~ 23156, 24116
with autograft ~ 23155, 24116
ileum ~ 27065-27067
innominate ~ 27077
intestines, small ~ 43250
ischial ~ 27078-27079
kidney ~ 52355
knee ~ 27327-27329, 27365
lacrimal gland
frontal approach ~ 68540
involving osteotomy ~ 68550
larynx ~ 31300
endoscopic ~ 31540-31541, 31578
leg, lower ~ 27615-27619
leg, upper ~ 27327-27329
mandible ~ 21040-21047
maxilla ~ 21030, 21034, 21048-21049
mediastinal ~ 39220
mediastinum ~ 32662
metacarpal ~ 26200-26205
radical ~ 26250-26255
metatarsal ~ 28104-28107, 28173
neck ~ 21555-21557
olecranon process ~ 24120
with allograft ~ 24126
with autograft ~ 24125
parotid gland ~ 42410-42426
pelvis ~ 27047-27049
pericardial ~ 33050
pericardium ~ 32661
phalanges ~ 26210-26215, 26260-26262
toe ~ 26215, 28108, 28175
pituitary gland ~ 61546-61548, 62165
presacral ~ 49215
pubis ~ 27065-27067
radius ~ 24120-24125, 25120-25126, 25170
rectum ~ 45160-45170
sacrococcygeal ~ 49215
scapula ~ 23140
with allograft ~ 23146
with autograft ~ 23145
shoulder ~ 23075-23077
skull ~ 61500
spermatocele ~ 54840
spinal cord ~ 63275-63290
spleen, total ~ 38100
sternum ~ 21630
stomach ~ 43610
talus ~ 27647, 28100-28103
tarsal ~ 28104-28107, 28171
thorax ~ 21555-21557
thyroid ~ 60200
tibia ~ 27635-27638, 27645-27646
trachea
cervical ~ 31785
thoracic ~ 31786
ulna ~ 24120-24125, 25120-25126, 25170
ureter ~ 52355

Excision ~ *continued*
urethra ~ 52234-52240, 52355, 53220
uterus
abdominal approach ~ 58140, 58146
vaginal approach ~ 58145
vagina ~ 57135
vertebra, lumbar ~ 22102
vertebra, thoracic ~ 22101
wrist ~ 25075-25077
zygoma ~ 21030, 21034
turbinate ~ 30130-30140
tympanic nerve ~ 69676
ulcer
stomach ~ 43610
ulna ~ 24147, 25145
complete ~ 25240
partial ~ 25150-25151, 25240
umbilicus ~ 49250
ureter ~ 50650-50660
ureterocele ~ 51535
urethra
diverticulum ~ 53230-53235
prolapse ~ 53275
total
female ~ 53210
male ~ 53215
uterus
laparoscopic ~ 58550
leiomyomata ~ 58546
partial ~ 58180
radical ~ 58210, 58285
removal tubes and/ or ovaries ~ 58262-58263, 58291, 58552, 58554
total ~ 58150-58152, 58200
vaginal ~ 58260, 58290-58294, 58550, 58553
with colpectomy ~ 58275-58280
with colpo-urethrocystopexy ~ 58267, 58293
with repair of enterocele ~ 58270, 58292, 58294
uvula ~ 42140-42145
vagina
closure ~ 57120
complete
with removal of paravaginal tissue ~ 57111
with removal of vaginal wall ~ 57110
with removal of paravaginal tissue with lymphadenectomy ~ 57112
partial
with removal of paravaginal tissue with lymphadenectomy ~ 57109
with removal of paravaginal tissue ~ 57107
with removal of vaginal wall ~ 57106
repair of enterocele ~ 58280
septum ~ 57130
total ~ 57110
with hysterectomy ~ 58275-58280

Excision ~ *continued*
varicocele
spermatic cord ~ 55530-55540
abdominal approach ~ 55535
hernia repair ~ 55540
vas deferens ~ 55250
vascular malformation
finger ~ 26115
hand ~ 26115
vein, varicose ~ 37765-37766
vertebra
additional segment ~ 22103, 22116
cervical ~ 22110
for tumor ~ 22100, 22110
lumbar ~ 22102
for tumor ~ 22114
thoracic ~ 22112
for tumor ~ 22101
vertebral body
decompression ~ 63081-63103
lesion ~ 63300-63308
vitreous ~ 67039
with retinal surgery ~ 67038
total
pars plana approach ~ 67036
with epiretinal membrane stripping ~ 67038
vulva
radical
complete ~ 56633-56640
partial ~ 56630-56632
simple
complete ~ 56625
partial ~ 56620
Exclusion
duodenum ~ 48547
small intestine ~ 44700
Exenteration
eye
removal orbital contents ~ 65110
therapeutic removal of bone ~ 65112
with muscle or myocutaneous flap ~ 65114
pelvis ~ 45126, 58240
Exercise stress tests ~ 93015-93018
Exercise test ~ see also electromyography, needle
ischemic limb ~ 95875
Exercise therapy ~ 97110-97113
Exfoliation, chemical ~ 17360
Exocrine, pancreas ~ see pancreas
Exomphalos ~ 49600-49611
Exostectomy ~ 28288, 28290
Exostoses ~ 69140
Exostoses, cartilaginous ~ 69140
Exostosis excision ~ 69140
Expander, skin, inflatable ~ see tissue, expander
Expired gas analysis ~ 0043T, 0064T, 94250, 94680-94690, 94770
carbon monoxide breath test ~ 0043T

Exploration
abdomen ~ 49000-49002
penetrating wound ~ 20102
staging ~ 58960
adrenal gland ~ 60540-60545
anal endoscopy ~ 46600
ankle ~ 27610, 27620
arm, lower ~ 25248
artery
brachial ~ 24495
carotid ~ 35701
femoral ~ 35721
other ~ 35761
popliteal ~ 35741
back, penetrating wound ~ 20102
bile duct
atresia ~ 47700
endoscopy ~ 47552-47553
blood vessel
abdomen ~ 35840
chest ~ 35820
extremity ~ 35860
neck ~ 35800
brain
via burr hole
infratentorial ~ 61253
supratentorial ~ 61250
infratentorial ~ 61305
supratentorial ~ 61304
breast ~ 19020
bronchi endoscopy ~ 31622
bronchoscopy ~ 31622
cauda equina ~ 63005-63011, 63017
chest penetrating wound ~ 20101
colon endoscopic ~ 44388, 45378
colon-sigmoid endoscopic ~ 45330, 45335
common bile duct with cholecystectomy ~ 47610
duodenum ~ 44010
ear, inner
endolymphatic sac
with shunt ~ 69806
without shunt ~ 69805
ear, middle ~ 69440
elbow ~ 24000, 24101
epididymis ~ 54865
esophagus endoscopy ~ 43200
extremity penetrating wound ~ 20103
finger joint ~ 26075-26080
flank penetrating wound ~ 20102
gallbladder ~ 47480
gastrointestinal tract, upper endoscopy ~ 43234-43236
hand joint ~ 26070
heart ~ 33310-33315
hepatic duct ~ 47400
hip ~ 27033
interphalangeal joint toe ~ 28024
intertarsal joint ~ 28020
intestines, small
endoscopy ~ 44360
enterotomy ~ 44020

Exploration ~ *continued*
kidney ~ 50010, 50045, 50120
knee ~ 27310, 27331
lacrimal duct ~ 68810
canaliculi ~ 68840
with anesthesia ~ 68811
with insertion tube or stent ~ 68815
larynx ~ 31320
endoscopy ~ 31505, 31520-31526, 31575
liver wound ~ 47361-47362
mediastinum ~ 39000-39010
metatarsophalangeal joint ~ 28022
nasolacrimal duct ~ 68810
with anesthesia ~ 68811
with insertion tube or stent ~ 68815
neck
lymph nodes ~ 38542
penetrating wound ~ 20100
nipple ~ 19110
nose endoscopy ~ 31231-31235
orbit ~ 61332-61334
with/without biopsy ~ 67450
without bone flap ~ 67400
parathyroid gland ~ 60500-60505
pelvis ~ 49320
prostate ~ 55860
with nodes ~ 55862-55865
rectum
endoscopic ~ 45300
injury ~ 45562-45563
retroperitoneal area ~ 49010
scrotum ~ 55110
shoulder joint ~ 23040-23044, 23107
sinus
frontal ~ 31070-31075
maxillary ~ 31020-31030
skull ~ 61105
spinal cord ~ 63001-63011, 63015-63017, 63040-63044
spine fusion ~ 22830
stomach ~ 43500
tarsometatarsal joint ~ 28020
testis, undescended ~ 54550-54560
toe joint ~ 28024
ureter ~ 50600
vagina ~ 57000
endocervical ~ 57452
wrist ~ 25101, 25248
joint ~ 25040
Exploration, larynx by incision ~ 31320
Exploratory laparotomy ~ 49000-49002
Expression lesion, conjunctiva ~ 68040
Exteriorization, small intestine ~ 44300
External auditory canal ~ see auditory canal
External cephalic version ~ 59412
External ear ~ see ear, external
External extoses ~ 69140
External fixation
adjustment/revision ~ 20693
application ~ 20690-20692
mandibular fracture
open treatment ~ 21454

External fixation ~ *continued*
percutaneous treatment ~ 21452
removal ~ 20694
Extirpation, lacrimal sac ~ 68520
Extracorporeal circulation ~ 33960-33961
for regional chemotherapy
extremity ~ 36823
Extracorporeal dialyses ~ 90935-90937
Extracorporeal membrane oxygenation cannulization ~ 36822
Extracorporeal photochemotherapies ~ 36522
Extracorporeal shock wave therapy ~ see lithotripsy
musculoskeletal ~ 0019T
plantar fascia ~ 0020T
Extracranial intracranial ~ 61623
Extraction lens
extracapsular ~ 66940
intracapsular ~ 66920
for dislocated lens ~ 66930
Extraction, cataract ~ 66830
Extradural anesthesia ~ see anesthesia; epidural
Extradural injection ~ 62281-62282, 62310-62319, 64479-64484
Extraocular muscle ~ 67340
Extrauterine pregnancy ~ see ectopic pregnancy
Extravasation blood ~ see hemorrhage
Extremity
lower
harvest of vein for bypass graft ~ 35500
harvest of vein for vascular reconstruction ~ 35572
revision ~ 35879-35881
upper
harvest of artery for coronary artery bypass graft ~ 35600
harvest of vein for bypass graft ~ 35500
repair blood vessel ~ 35206
wound exploration penetrating wound ~ 20103
Eye
biometry ~ 76516-76519, 92136
drainage anterior chamber
discission of anterior hyaloid membrane ~ 65810
with diagnostic aspiration of aqueous ~ 65800
with removal of blood ~ 65815
with removal of vitreous and/or with therapeutic release of aqueous ~ 65805
endoscopy ~ 66990
goniotomy ~ 65820
incision
adhesions
anterior synechiae ~ 65860, 65870
corneovitreal adhesions ~ 65880
goniosynechiae ~ 65865
posterior synechiae ~ 65875
anterior chamber ~ 65820
trabeculae ~ 65850

Eye ~ *continued*
injection
air ~ 66020
medication ~ 66030
insertion, implantation
drug delivery system ~ 67027
foreign material for reinforcement ~ 65155
muscles attached ~ 65140
muscles, not attached ~ 65135
reinsertion ~ 65150
scleral shell ~ 65130
interferometry biometry ~ 92136
lesion excision ~ 65900
nerve destruction ~ 67345
paracentesis anterior chamber
with diagnostic aspiration of aqueous ~ 65800
removal of blood ~ 65815
removal of vitreous and/or discission anterior hyaloid membrane ~ 65810
with therapeutic release of aqueous ~ 65805
radial keratotomy ~ 65771
reconstruction
graft
conjunctiva ~ 65782
stem cell ~ 65781
transplantation
amniotic membrane ~ 65780
removal
blood clot ~ 65930
bone ~ 65112
foreign body
conjunctival embedded ~ 65210
conjunctival superficial ~ 65205
corneal with slit lamp ~ 65222
corneal without slit lamp ~ 65220
intraocular ~ 65235-65265
implant ~ 65175
anterior segment ~ 65920
muscles, not attached ~ 65103
posterior segment ~ 67120-67121
repair
conjunctiva
by mobilization and rearrangement without hospitalization ~ 65272
by mobilization and rearrangement with hospitalization ~ 65273
direct closure ~ 65270
cornea
nonperforating ~ 65275
perforating ~ 65280-65285
muscles ~ 65290
sclera
anterior segment ~ 66250
with graft ~ 66225
without graft ~ 66220
with tissue glue ~ 65286
trabeculae ~ 65855
wound
by mobilization and rearrangement ~ 65272-65273
direct closure ~ 65270

Eye ~ *continued*
shunt, aqueous to extraocular reservoir ~ 66180
ultrasound ~ 76510-76514
biometry ~ 76516-76519
foreign body ~ 76529
unlisted services and procedures
anterior segment ~ 66999
posterior segment ~ 67299
with muscle or myocutaneous flap ~ 65114
muscles attached ~ 65105
ocular contents
without implant ~ 65091
with implant ~ 65093
orbital contents ~ 65110
without implant ~ 65101
X-ray ~ 70030
Eye and ocular adnexa, surgical procedures 65091-68899
Eyebrow repair
ptosis ~ 67900
Eyeglasses ~ 92340-92342
Eyelashes
repair trichiasis
epilation
by forceps only ~ 67820
by other than forceps ~ 67825
incision of lid margin ~ 67830
with free mucous membrane graft ~ 67835
Eyelid
abscess, incision and drainage ~ 67700
biopsy ~ 67810
blepharoplasty ~ 15820-15823
chalazion
excision ~ 67805
with anesthesia ~ 67808
multiple ~ 67801-67805
single ~ 67800
closure by suture ~ 67875
incision
canthus ~ 67715
sutures ~ 67710
injection, subconjunctival ~ 68200
lesion
destruction ~ 67850
excision
with anesthesia ~ 67808
without closure ~ 67840
multiple ~ 67801-67805
single ~ 67800
reconstruction
canthus ~ 67950
total ~ 67973-67975
total eyelid
lower ~ 67973-67975
second stage ~ 67975
upper ~ 67974
transfer of tarsoconjunctival flap from opposing eyelid ~ 67971
removal foreign body ~ 67938

Eyelid ~ *continued*
repair ~ 21280-21282
blepharoptosis
conjunctivo-tarso-muller's muscle-levator resection ~ 67908
frontalis muscle technique ~ 67901-67094
reduction overcorrection of ptosis ~ 67909
superior rectus technique with fascial sling ~ 67906
ectropion
blepharoplasty ~ 67914
suture ~ 67914
entropion
excision tarsal wedge ~ 67923
extensive ~ 67924
suture ~ 67921
thermocauterization ~ 67922
excisional ~ 67961
over one-fourth of lid margin ~ 67966
lagophthalmos ~ 67912
lashes
epilation, by forceps only ~ 67820
epilation, by other than forceps ~ 67825
lid margin ~ 67830-67835
wound
full thickness ~ 67935
partial thickness ~ 67930
repair with graft retraction ~ 67911
skin graft
full thickness ~ 67961
split ~ 67961
suture ~ 67880
with transposition of tarsal plate ~ 67882
tissue transfer, adjacent ~ 67961
unlisted services and procedures ~ 67999
Eyelid ptoses ~ see blepharoptosis
Eye allergy test ~ 95060
Eye evisceration ~ 65091, 65093
Eye exam
established patient ~ 92012-92014
new patient ~ 92002-92004
with anesthesia ~ 92018-92019
Eye exercises, training ~ 92065
Eye muscles
biopsy ~ 67346
repair
strabismus
adjustable sutures ~ 67335
exploration and/or repair detached extraocular muscle ~ 67340
one vertical muscle ~ 67314
on patient with previous surgery ~ 67331
posterior fixation suture ~ 67334
recession or resection ~ 67311-67312
release of scar tissue without detaching extraocular muscle ~ 67343
two or more vertical muscles ~ 67316
with scarring extraocular muscles ~ 67332
with superior oblique muscle ~ 67318
transposition ~ 67320
unlisted services and procedures ~ 67399
Eye prosthesis ~ see prosthesis

Eye socket ~ see orbit ~ 21385-21395, 21260-21263, 21267-21268, 67415
E antigens ~ 87350
E B virus ~ 86663-86665
E vitamin ~ 84446

F

Face
CT scan ~ 70486-70488
lesion
destruction ~ 17000-17004, 17280-17286
lift ~ 15824-15828
magnetic resonance imaging (MRI) ~ 70540-70543
tumor resection ~ 21015
Facial asymmetries ~ 21247
Facial bones ~ see also mandible; maxilla
abscess excision ~ 21026
reconstruction
secondary ~ 21275
repair ~ 21208-21209
tumor
excision ~ 21029-21034
resection
radical ~ 21015
X-ray ~ 70140-70150
Facial nerve
anastomosis
to hypoglossal ~ 64868
to phrenic nerve ~ 64870
to spinal accessory ~ 64866
avulsion ~ 64742
decompression ~ 61590, 61596
intratemporal
lateral to geniculate ganglion ~ 69720, 69740
medial to geniculate ganglion ~ 69725, 69745
total ~ 69955
function study ~ 92516
incision ~ 64742
injection
anesthetic ~ 64402
mobilization ~ 61590
repair
lateral to geniculate ganglion ~ 69740
medial to geniculate ganglion ~ 69745
repair/suture
with or without graft ~ 64864-64865
suture
lateral to geniculate ganglion ~ 69740
medial to geniculate ganglion ~ 69745
transection ~ 64742
Facial nerve paralysis
graft ~ 15840-15845
repair ~ 15840-15845
Facial prosthesis impression ~ 21088
Facial rhytidectomy ~ 15824-15828
Factor
ACTH-releasing ~ 80412
antinuclear ~ 86038-86039
blood coagulation ~ 85210-85293
Factor I ~ 85384-85385
Factor II ~ 85210
Factor III ~ see thromboplastin
Factor inhibitor test ~ 85335
Factor IV ~ see calcium
Factor IXix ~ 85250
Factor rheumatoid ~ 86430-86431
Factor VII ~ 85230
Factor VIII ~ 85210-85293
Factor X ~ 85260
Factor X, activated ~ 85260
Factor XA inhibitor ~ 85300-85301
Factor XI ~ 85270
Factor XII ~ 85280
Factor XIII ~ 85290-85291
Fitzgerald ~ 85293
Fletcher ~ 85293
hyperglycemic-glycogenolytic ~ 82943
intrinsic ~ 83528
sulfation ~ 84305
Fallopian tube
anastomosis ~ 58750
catheterization ~ 58345, 74742
destruction endoscopy ~ 58670
ectopic pregnancy ~ 59121
with salpingectomy and/or oophorectomy ~ 59120
excision ~ 58700-58720
ligation ~ 58600-58611
lysis adhesions ~ 58740
occlusion ~ 58615
endoscopy ~ 58671
placement, implant for occlusion ~ 58568
pregnancy ~ 59121
repair ~ 58752
anastomosis ~ 58750
create stoma ~ 58770
tumor resection ~ 58950, 58952-58956
unlisted services and procedures ~ 58999
X-ray ~ 74742
Fallot, tetralogy of ~ 33692-33697, 33924
Family psychotherapy ~ 90846-90849, 99510
Fanconi anemia chromosome analysis ~ 88248
Farnsworth-Munsell color test ~ 92283
Farr test ~ 82784-82787
Fasanella-Servat procedure ~ 67908
Fascia graft ~ 15840
Fascia lata graft harvesting ~ 20920-20922
Fascial defect repair ~ 50728
Fascial graft
free microvascular anastomosis ~ 15758
open treatment, sternoclavicular dislocation ~ 23532

Fasciectomy
foot ~ 28060
radical ~ 28060-28062
palm ~ 26121-26125
Fasciocutaneous flaps ~ 15732-15738
Fasciotomy
arm, lower ~ 24495, 25020-25025
elbow ~ 24350-24356
foot ~ 28008
hand decompression ~ 26037
hip ~ 27025
knee ~ 27305, 27496-27499
leg, lower ~ 27600-27602, 27892-27894
leg, upper ~ 27305, 27496-27499, 27892-27894
palm ~ 26040-26045
plantar endoscopic ~ 29893
thigh ~ 27025
toe ~ 28008
wrist ~ 25020-25023
FAST ~ see allergen immunotherapy
Fat
feces ~ 82705-82715
removal, lipectomy ~ 15876-15879
Fatty acid
blood ~ 82725
very long chain ~ 82726
Fat stain
feces ~ 89125
respiratory secretions ~ 89125
sputum ~ 89125
urine ~ 89125
Favre-durand disease ~ 86729
FC receptor ~ 86243
FDP ~ 85362-85380
Fe (iron) ~ 83540
Feedback, psychophysiologic (see biofeedback) ~ 90901-90911
Female castration ~ 58262-58263, 58291-58292, 58552, 58554, 58661, 58940-58943
Female genital system, surgical procedures ~ 56405-58999
Female gonad ~ see ovary
Femoral arteries ~ see artery, femoral
Femoral nerve
injection, anesthetic ~ 64447-64448
Femoral stem prosthesis ~ 27132
Femoral vein ~ 34501
Femur ~ see hip; knee; leg, upper
abscess, incision ~ 27303
bursa, excision ~ 27062
craterization ~ 27070, 27360
cyst, excision ~ 27065-27067, 27355-27358
diaphysectomy ~ 27360
drainage ~ 27303
excision ~ 27070, 27360
epiphyseal bar ~ 20150
fracture ~ 27244
closed treatment ~ 27501-27503
distal ~ 27508, 27510, 27514
distal, medial or lateral condyle ~ 27509
Femur ~ *continued*
epiphysis ~ 27516-27519
intertrochanteric ~ 27244
intertrochanteric
closed treatment ~ 27238
treatment with implant ~ 27244
with implant ~ 27245
with manipulation ~ 27240
neck
closed treatment ~ 27230-27232
open treatment ~ 27236
percutaneous fixation ~ 27235
open treatment ~ 27245, 27506-27507, 27511-27513
percutaneous fixation ~ 27509
pertrochanteric ~ 27244
pertrochanteric
closed treatment ~ 27238
treatment with implant ~ 27244
with implant ~ 27245
with manipulation ~ 27240
shaft ~ 27500, 27502, 27506-27507
subtrochanteric ~ 27244
subtrochanteric
closed treatment ~ 27238
treatment with implant ~ 27244
with implant ~ 27245
with manipulation ~ 27240
supracondylar ~ 27501-27503, 27509, 27511-27513
transcondylar ~ 27501-27503, 27509, 27511-27513
trochanteric
closed treatment ~ 27246
open treatment ~ 27248
without manipulation ~ 27501
with manipulation ~ 27503
halo ~ 20663
lesion excision ~ 27062
osteoplasty
lengthening ~ 27466-27468
shortening ~ 27465, 27468
osteotomywithout fixation ~ 27448
prophylactic treatment ~ 27187, 27495
realignment ~ 27454
reconstruction ~ 27468
at knee ~ 27442-27443, 27446
lengthening ~ 27466-27468
shortening ~ 27465, 27468
repair ~ 27470-27472
epiphysis ~ 27181, 27475, 27742
arrest ~ 27185
muscle transfer ~ 27110
osteotomy ~ 27140, 27151-27156, 27161-27165, 27450-27454
with graft ~ 27170
saucerization ~ 27070, 27360
tumor excision ~ 27065-27067, 27355-27358, 27365
X-ray ~ 73550
Fenestration, pericardium ~ 33015

Fenestration procedure
semicircular canal ~ 69820
revision ~ 69840
tracheostomy ~ 31610
Fern test ~ 87210
Ferric chloride, urine ~ 81005
Ferrihemoglobin ~ 83045-83050
Ferritin, blood or urine ~ 82728
Ferroxidase ~ (ceruloplasmin) 82390
Fertility control ~ see contraception
Fertility test
semen analysis ~ 89300-89321
sperm analysis
cervical mucus penetration test ~ 89330
hamster penetration ~ 89329
Fertilization, assisted
oocyte ~ 89250, 89251
microtechnique ~ 89280-89281
with co-culture ~ 89251
Fertilization in vitro ~ 58321-58322
Fetal biophysical profile ~ 76818-76819
Fetal contraction stress test ~ 59020
Fetal hemoglobin ~ 85461
Fetal lung maturity assessment; lecithin sphingomyelin ratio ~ 83661
Fetal monitoring ~ 59050-59051, 99500
Fetal non-stress test ~ 59025
ultrasound ~ 76818
Fetal procedure
amnioinfusion ~ 59070
cord occlusion ~ 59072
fluid drainage ~ 59074
shunt placement ~ 59076
unlisted ~ 59897
Fetal testing
amniotic fluid lung maturity ~ 83661, 83663-83664
heart ~ 76825-76826
Doppler
complete ~ 76827
follow-up or repeat study ~ 76828
hemoglobin ~ 83030-83033, 85460
ultrasound ~ 76801-76828
heart ~ 76825
middle cerebral artery ~ 76821
umbilical artery ~ 76820
Fetuin ~ 82105-82106
Fever, Australian Q ~ 86000, 86638
Fever, Japanese river ~ 86000
Fibrillation, atrial ~ 33254-33256, 33265-33266
Fibrillation, heart ~ see heart, fibrillation
Fibrin
degradation products ~ 85362-85380
deposit removal ~ 32150
stabilizing factor ~ 85290-85291
Fibrinase ~ 85400
Fibrinogen ~ 85384-85385
Fibrinolysin ~ 85400
Fibrinolysins ~ 85390
Fibrinolysis
alpha-2 antiplasmin ~ 85410
assay ~ 85396
plasmin ~ 85400
plasminogen ~ 85420-85421
plasminogen activator ~ 85415
Fibroadenoma, excision ~ 19120-19126
ablation
cryosurgical ~ 19105
Fibroblastoma, arachnoidal ~ 61512, 61519
Fibrocutaneous tags ~ 11200-11201
Fibromatosis, Dupuytren's ~ 26040-26045
Fibromatosis, penile ~ see Peyronie disease
Fibromyoma ~ 58140, 58545-58546, 58561
Fibronectin, fetal ~ 82731
Fibrosis, penile ~ see Peyronie disease
Fibrosis, retroperitoneal ~ 50715
Fibrous cavernitides ~ see Peyronie disease
Fibrous dysplasia ~ 21029, 21181-21184
Fibula ~ see ankle; knee; tibia
bone graft with microvascular anastomosis ~ 20955
craterization ~ 27360, 27641
cyst excision ~ 27635-27638
diaphysectomy ~ 27360, 27641
excision ~ 27360, 27641
epiphyseal bar ~ 20150
fracture
malleolus ~ 27786-27814
shaft ~ 27780-27784
incision ~ 27607
osteoplasty lengthening ~ 27715
repair
epiphysis ~ 27477-27485, 27730-27742
osteotomy ~ 27707-27712
saucerization ~ 27360, 27641
tumor excision ~ 27635-27638, 27646
X-ray ~ 73590
Figure of eight cast ~ 29049
Filariasis ~ 86280
Filtering operation ~ see incision, sclera, fistulization
Filtration implant, glaucoma ~ 66180, 66185
Fimbrioplasty ~ 58760
laparoscopic ~ 58672
Fine needle aspiration ~ 10021-10022
evaluation ~ 88172-88173
Finger ~ see phalanx, finger
abscess
bone, incision and drainage ~ 26034
incision and drainage ~ 26010-26011
amputation ~ 26951-26952
with exploration or removal ~ 26910
arthrocentesis ~ 20600
arthrodesis
interphalangeal joint ~ 26860-26863
metacarpophalangeal joint ~ 26850-26852
bone, incision and drainage ~ 26034
cast ~ 29086
collection of blood ~ 36415-36416
decompression ~ 26035

Finger ~ *continued*
excision
constricting ring ~ 26596
tendon ~ 26180, 26390, 26415
insertion, tendon graft ~ 26392
magnetic resonance imaging (MRI) ~ 73221
reconstruction
extra digit ~ 26587
toe to hand transfer ~ 26551-26556
removal
implantation ~ 26320
tube ~ 26392, 26416
repair
blood vessel ~ 35207
claw finger ~ 26499
extra digit ~ 26587
macrodactylia ~ 26590
tendon
extensor ~ 26415-26434, 26445-26449, 26460
flexor ~ 26356-26358, 26440-26442, 26455
volar plate ~ 26548
web finger ~ 26560-26562
replantation ~ 20816-20822
reposition ~ 26555
sesamoidectomy ~ 26185
splint ~ 29130-29131
strapping ~ 29280
tendon sheath
excision ~ 26145
incision ~ 26055
incision and drainage ~ 26020
tenotomy ~ 26060, 26460
flexor ~ 26455
tumor excision ~ 26115-26117
unlisted services and procedures ~ 26989
X-ray ~ 73140
Finger flap, tissue transfer ~ 14350
Finger joint ~ see intercarpal joint
Finney operation ~ 43810, 43850-43855
FISH ~ 88365
Fishberg concentration test ~ 89235
Fissurectomy, anal ~ 46200
Fissure in ano ~ 46200, 46949-46942
Fistula
anal, repair ~ 46288, 46706
autogenous graft ~ 36825
bronchi, repair ~ 32815
carotid-cavernous, repair ~ 61710
chest wall, repair ~ 32906
conjunctiva
without tube ~ 68745
with tube or stent ~ 68750
enterovesical
closure ~ 44660-44661
kidney ~ 50520-50526
lacrimal gland closure ~ 68770
dacryocystorhinostomy ~ 68720
nose repair ~ 30580-30600
oval window ~ 69666
postauricular ~ 69700

Fistula ~ *continued*
rectovaginal
abdominal approach ~ 57305
transperineal approach ~ 57308
with concomitant colostomy ~ 57307
round window ~ 69667
sclera
iridencleisis or iridotasis ~ 66165
sclerectomy with punch or scissors with iridectomy ~ 66160
thermocauterization with iridectomy ~ 66155
trabeculectomy ab externo in absence previous surgery ~ 66170
trabeculectomy ab externo with scarring ~ 66172
trephination with iridectomy ~ 66150
suture
kidney ~ 50520-50526
ureter ~ 50920-50930
trachea ~ 31755
tracheoesophageal
repair ~ 43305, 43312, 43314
speech prothesis ~ 31611
ureter ~ 50920-50930
urethra ~ 53400-53405
urethrovaginal ~ 57310
with bulbocavernosus transplant ~ 57311
vesicouterine closure ~ 51920-51925
vesicovaginal
closure ~ 51900
transvesical and vaginal approach ~ 57330
vaginal approach ~ 57320
X-ray ~ 76080
Fistulectomy, anal ~ 46060, 46270-46285
Fistulization
conjunction to nasal cavity ~ 68745
esophagus ~ 43350-43352
intestines ~ 44300-44346
lacrimal sac to nasal cavity ~ 68720
penis ~ 54435
pharynx ~ 42955
repair salivary cyst, sublingual ~ 42325-42326
tracheopharyngeal ~ 31755
Fistulization, interatrial ~ 33735-33737
Fistulotomy, anal ~ 46270, 46280
Fitting
cervical cap ~ 57170
contact lens ~ 92070, 92310-92313
diaphragm ~ 57170
low vision aid ~ 92354-92355
ocular prosthesis ~ 92330
spectacles ~ 92340-92342
spectacle prosthesis ~ 92352-92353
Fitzgerald factor ~ 85293
Fixation, interdental without fracture ~ 21497
Fixation, external ~ see external fixation
Fixation, kidney ~ see nephropexy
Fixation, rectum ~ see proctopexy
Fixation, tongue ~ see tongue, fixation

Fixation (device) ~ see application; bone, fixation; spinal instrumentation
application, external ~ 20690-20692
pelvic, insertion ~ 22848
removal
external ~ 20694
internal ~ 20670-20680
sacrospinous ligament, vaginal prolapse ~ 57282
shoulder ~ 23700
skeletal, humeral epycondyle, percutaneous ~ 24566
spinal
insertion ~ 22841-22847
prosthetic ~ 22851
reinsertion ~ 22849
Fixation test, complement ~ 86171
Flank ~ see back/flank
Flap ~ see skin graft and flap
free, breast reconstruction ~ 19364
grafts ~ 15570-15738, 15842
latissimus dorsi breast reconstruction ~ 19361
omentum ~ 49905
omentum, free, with microvascular anastomosis ~ 49906
transverse rectus abdominis myocutaneous breast reconstruction ~ 19367-19369
Flatfoot correction ~ 28735
Flea typhus ~ 86000
Fletcher factor ~ 85292
Flow cytometry ~ 88182-88189
Flow-volume loop, pulmonary ~ 94375
Fluid
amniotic ~ see amniotic fluid
body ~ 89060
cerebrospinal ~ 86325
collection, incision and drainage, skin ~ 10140
Fluorescein
angiography, ocular ~ 92287
intravenous injection
vascular flow check, graft ~ 15860
Fluorescein angiography ~ 92235
Fluorescent in situ hybridization ~ 88365
Fluoride
blood ~ 82735
urine ~ 82735
Fluoroscopy
bile duct
calculus removal ~ 74327
guide catheter ~ 74328, 74330
chest ~ 31628
bronchoscopy ~ 31622-31640
complete (four views) ~ 71034
partial (two views) ~ 71023
drain abscess ~ 75989
GI tract
guide intubation ~ 74340
hourly ~ 76000-76001
introduction GI tube ~ 74340
larynx ~ 70370
nasogastric ~ 43752
needle biopsy ~ 77002
Fluoroscopy ~ ***continued***
orogastric ~ 43752
pancreatic duct, guide catheter ~ 74329-74330
pharynx ~ 70370
renal guide catheter ~ 74475
spine/paraspinous, guide catheter/needle ~ 77003
unlisted services and procedures ~ 76496
ureter guide catheter ~ 74480
venous access device ~ 36598, 77001
Flurazepam, blood or urine ~ 82742
Flush aortogram ~ 75722-75724
FNA ~ see fine needle aspiration
Foam stability test ~ 83662
Fold, vocal ~ see vocal cords
Foley operation pyeloplasty ~ 50400-50405, 50544
Foley Y-pyeloplasty ~ 50400-50405
Folic acid ~ 82747
blood ~ 82746
Follicle stimulating hormone (FSH) ~ 80418, 80426, 83001
Folliculin ~ 82679
Follitropin ~ 80418, 80426, 83001
Follow-up inpatient consultations ~ 99251-99255
Follow-up services
inpatient consultations ~ 99261-99263
post-op ~ 99024
Fontan procedure ~ 33600-33617
Food allergy test ~ 95075
Foot ~ see metatarsal ~ 28456
amputation ~ 28800-28805
bursa incision and drainage ~ 28001
capsulotomy ~ 28260-28264
cast ~ 29450
fasciectomy ~ 28060
radical ~ 28060-28062
fasciotomy ~ 28008
endoscopic ~ 29893
incision ~ 28002-28005
joint ~ see tarsometatarsal joint ~ 28570-28576, 28585
magnetic resonance imaging (MRI) ~ 73721-73723
lesion excision ~ 28080, 28090
magnetic resonance imaging (MRI) ~ 73718-73720
nerve
excision ~ 28055
incision ~ 28035
neuroma excision ~ 28080
reconstruction cleft foot ~ 28360
removal foreign body ~ 28190-28193
repair
muscle ~ 28250
tendon ~ 28200-28230, 28234-28238
replantation ~ 20838
sesamoid excision ~ 28315
splint ~ 29590
strapping ~ 29540, 29590

Foot ~ *continued*
suture tendon ~ 28200-28210
tendon sheath excision ~ 28086-28088
tenotomy ~ 28230, 28234
tumor excision ~ 28043-28046
unlisted services and procedures ~ 28899
X-ray ~ 73620-73630
Foot abscess ~ 28005
Forearm ~ see arm, lower ~ 20805
Forehead
reconstruction ~ 21179-21180, 21182-21184
midface ~ 21159-21160
reduction ~ 21137-21139
Forehead and orbital rim
reconstruction ~ 21172-21180
Foreign body removal
anal ~ 46608
arm
lower ~ 25248
upper ~ 24200, 24201
auditory canal, external ~ 69200
with anesthesia ~ 69205
bronchi ~ 31635
colon ~ 44025, 44390, 45332, 45379
conjunctival, embedded ~ 65210
cornea ~ 65220, 65222
duodenum ~ 44010
external eye ~ 65205
eyelid ~ 67938
finger ~ 26075, 26080
foot ~ 28190, 28193
gum ~ 41805
hand ~ 26070
hip ~ 27033, 27086, 27087
intraocular ~ 65235
knee joint ~ 27310, 27331, 27372
lacrimal duct/gland ~ 68530
larynx ~ 31511, 31530, 31531, 31577
leg, upper ~ 27372
lung ~ 32151
mandible ~ 41806
maxillary sinus ~ 31299
mediastinum ~ 39000, 39010
mouth ~ 40804, 40805
nose ~ 30300
with anesthesia ~ 30310
lateral rhinotomy ~ 30320
orbit ~ 61334, 67413, 67430
pancreatic duct ~ 43269
pelvis ~ 27086, 27087
penis ~ 54115
pericardium ~ 33020
endoscopic ~ 32658
pharynx ~ 42809
pleura ~ 32150, 32151
endoscopic ~ 32653
rectum ~ 45307, 45915
scrotum ~ 55120
shoulder ~ 23040, 23044
complicated ~ 23332
deep ~ 23331

Foreign body removal ~ *continued*
subcutaneous 23330
skin with debridement ~ 11010-11012
subcutaneous ~ 10120, 10121
with debridement ~ 11010-11012
ureter ~ 50961, 50980
urethra ~ 52310, 52315
uterus ~ 58562
vagina ~ 57415
Forensic exam ~ 88040
cytopathology ~ 88125
phosphatase, acid ~ 84061
Foreskin of penis ~ 54450
Formycin diphosphate ~ 85362-85380
Fournier's gangrene ~ 11004-11006
Fowler-Stephens orchiopexy ~ 54640, 54650, 54692
Fowler-Stephens procedure ~ 54650
Fox operation ~ 67921-67924
Fraction, factor IX (nine) ~ 85250
Fracture
acetabulum
closed treatment ~ 27220-27222
with manipulation ~ 27222
without manipulation ~ 27220
open treatment ~ 27226-27228
alveola
closed treatment ~ 21421
open treatment ~ 21422-21423
alveolar ridge
closed treatment ~ 21440
open treatment ~ 21445
ankle
closed treatment ~ 27816-27818
lateral ~ 27786-27814
with manipulation ~ 27818
without manipulation ~ 27816
medial ~ 27760-27766, 27808-27814
open treatment ~ 27822-27823
trimalleolar ~ 27816-27823
ankle bone
medial ~ 27760-27762
Bennett's thumb fracture
with dislocation ~ 26645, 26650
open treatment ~ 26665
bronchi endoscopy ~ 31630
calcaneus
closed treatment ~ 28400-28405
with manipulation ~ 28405-28406
without manipulation ~ 28400
open treatment ~ 28415-28420
percutaneous fixation ~ 28436
carpal
closed treatment
with manipulation ~ 25624, 25635
without manipulation ~ 25622, 25630
open treatment ~ 25628, 25645
carpal scaphoid, closed treatment ~ 25622
cheekbone
with manipulation ~ 21355
open treatment ~ 21360-21366

Fracture ~ *continued*
clavicle
closed treatment
with manipulation ~ 23505
without manipulation ~ 23500
open treatment ~ 23515
closed treatment ~ 27520
coccyx
closed treatment ~ 27200
open treatment ~ 27202
Colles ~ see Colles fracture
Colles-reversed ~ see Smith fracture
elbow
Monteggia
closed treatment ~ 24620
open treatment ~ 24635
open treatment ~ 24586-24587
femur ~ 27244
closed treatment ~ 27230, 27238-27240, 27246, 27500-27503, 27508, 27510, 27516-27517
with manipulation ~ 27232
distal ~ 27508, 27510, 27514
epiphysis ~ 27516-27519
intertrochanteric ~ 27244
closed treatment ~ 27238
intramedullary implant ~ 27245
open treatment ~ 27244
with implant ~ 27245
with manipulation ~ 27240
neck
closed treatment ~ 27230
with manipulation ~ 27232
open treatment ~ 27236
percutaneous fixation ~ 27235
open treatment ~ 27245, 27248, 27506-27507, 27511-27514, 27519
percutaneous fixation ~ 27235, 27509
pertrochanteric
closed treatment ~ 27238
with manipulation ~ 27240
intramedullary implant shaft ~ 27245, 27500, 27502, 27506-27507
open treatment ~ 27245, 27245
subtrochanteric
closed treatment ~ 27238
with manipulation ~ 27240
intramedullary implant ~ 27245
open treatment ~ 27245
supracondylar ~ 27501-27503, 27509, 27511-27513
transcondylar ~ 27501-27503, 27509, 27511-27513
trochanteric
closed treatment ~ 27246
open treatment ~ 27248
with manipulation ~ 27232, 27502-27503, 27510
without manipulation ~ 27230, 27238, 27246, 27500-27501, 27508, 27516-27517, 27520

Fracture ~ *continued*
fibula
closed treatment ~ 27780-27781, 27786-27788, 27808-27810
malleolus ~ 27786-27814
open treatment ~ 27784, 27792, 27814
shaft ~ 27780-27786, 27808
with manipulation ~ 27788, 27810
without manipulation ~ 27780-27781
frontal sinus, open treatment ~ 21343-21344
great toe
closed treatment ~ 28490
without manipulation ~ 28490
heel
closed treatment
with manipulation ~ 28405-28406
without manipulation ~ 28400
open treatment ~ 28415-28420
humerus
closed treatment ~ 24500-24505
with manipulation ~ 23605
without manipulation ~ 23600
condyle
closed treatment ~ 24576-24577
open treatment ~ 24579
percutaneous ~ 24582
epicondyle
closed treatment ~ 24560-24565
open treatment ~ 24575
skeletal fixation, percutaneous ~ 24566
greater tuberosity fracture
closed treatment with manipulation ~ 23625
closed treatment without manipulation ~ 23620
open treatment ~ 23630
open treatment ~ 23615-23616
shaft ~ 24500-24505, 24516
open treatment ~ 24515
supracondylar
closed treatment ~ 24530-24535
open treatment ~ 24545-24546
percutaneous fixation ~ 24538
transcondylar
closed treatment ~ 24530-24535
open treatment ~ 24545-24546
percutaneous fixation ~ 24538
with dislocation
closed treatment ~ 23665
open treatment ~ 23670
with shoulder dislocation
closed treatment ~ 23675
open treatment ~ 23680
hyoid bone
closed treatment
manipulation ~ 21494
without manipulation ~ 21493
open treatment ~ 21495
ilium
open treatment ~ 27215, 27218
percutaneous fixation ~ 27216

Fracture ~ *continued*
knee ~ 27520
arthroscopic treatment ~ 29850-29851
open treatment ~ 27524
larynx
closed treatment
with manipulation ~ 31586
without manipulation ~ 31585
open treatment ~ 31584
malar area
open treatment ~ 21360-21366
with bone graft ~ 21366
with manipulation ~ 21355
mandible
closed treatment
interdental fixation ~ 21453
with manipulation ~ 21451
without manipulation ~ 21450
open treatment ~ 21454-21470
external fixation ~ 21454
with interdental fixation ~ 21462
without interdental fixation ~ 21461
percutaneous treatment ~ 21452
maxilla
closed treatment ~ 21421
open treatment ~ 21422-21423
metacarpal
closed treatment ~ 26600-26605
with fixation ~ 26607
with manipulation ~ 26605-26607
without manipulation ~ 26600
open treatment ~ 26615
percutaneous fixation ~ 26608
metatarsal
closed treatment ~ 28470-28475
with manipulation ~ 28475-28476
without manipulation ~ 28450, 28470
open treatment ~ 28485
percutaneous fixation ~ 28476
Monteggia ~ see fracture, ulna ~ 24620-24635
nasal bone
closed treatment ~ 21310-21320
with manipulation ~ 21315-21320
without manipulation ~ 21310
open treatment ~ 21325-21335
nasal septum
closed treatment ~ 21337
open treatment ~ 21336
nasal turbinate therapeutic ~ 30930
nasoethmoid
open treatment ~ 21338-21339
percutaneous treatment ~ 21340
with fixation ~ 21340
nasomaxillary
closed treatment ~ 21345
open treatment ~ 21346-21348
with bone grafting ~ 21348
with fixation ~ 21345-21347
navicular
closed treatment ~ 25622
open treatment ~ 25628
with manipulation ~ 25624

Fracture ~ *continued*
odontoid
open treatment
with graft ~ 22319
without graft ~ 22318
orbit
closed treatment
with manipulation ~ 21401
without manipulation ~ 21400
open treatment ~ 21406-21408
blowout fracture ~ 21385-21395
orbital floor
blow out ~ 21385-21395
palate
closed treatment ~ 21421
open treatment ~ 21422-21423
patella
closed treatment, without manipulation ~ 27520
open treatment ~ 27524
pelvic ring
closed treatment ~ 27193-27194
without manipulation ~ 27193-27194
open treatment
anterior ~ 27217
posterior ~ 27218
percutaneous fixation ~ 27216
phalanges
articular
closed treatment ~ 26740
open treatment ~ 26746
with manipulation ~ 26742
closed treatment ~ 26742, 28510
articular ~ 26740
distal ~ 26750
with manipulation ~ 26755
distal ~ 26755-26756
closed treatment ~ 26750
open treatment ~ 26765
percutaneous fixation ~ 26756
finger/thumb
closed treatment ~ 26720-26725
with manipulation ~ 26725-26727
shaft ~ 26720, 26727
great toe ~ 28490
closed treatment ~ 28495
with manipulation ~ 28495-28496
open treatment ~ 28505
percutaneous fixation ~ 28496
open treatment ~ 26735, 26746
distal ~ 26765
shaft
closed treatment ~ 26725
open treatment ~ 26735
percutaneous fixation ~ 26727
toe
closed treatment ~ 28515
with manipulation ~ 28515
without manipulation ~ 28510
open treatment ~ 28525
with manipulation ~ 26742, 26755
without manipulation ~ 26740, 26750

Fracture ~ *continued*
radius
closed treatment ~ 25560-25565
Colles ~ 25600-25605
distal ~ 25600-25606
open treatment ~ 25607-25609
Smith ~ 25600-25605
head/neck
closed treatment ~ 24650-24655
open treatment ~ 24665-24666
open treatment ~ 25515, 25607-25609
percutaneous fixation ~ 25606
shaft ~ 25500, 25525-25526
closed treatment ~ 25500-25505, 25520
open treatment ~ 25515, 25525-25526, 25574
with manipulation ~ 25565, 25605
without manipulation ~ 25560, 25600
with ulna ~ 25560-25565
open treatment ~ 25575
rib
closed treatment ~ 21800
external fixation ~ 21810
open treatment ~ 21805
scaphoid
closed treatment ~ 25622
open treatment ~ 25628
with dislocation
closed treatment ~ 25680
open treatment ~ 25685
with manipulation ~ 25624
scapula
closed treatment
with manipulation ~ 23575
without manipulation ~ 23570
open treatment ~ 23585
sesamoid
closed treatment ~ 28530
foot ~ 28530-28531
open treatment ~ 28531
skin debridement ~ 11010-11012
skull ~ 62000-62010
sternum
closed treatment ~ 21820
open treatment ~ 21825
talus
closed treatment ~ 28430-28435
open treatment ~ 28445
with manipulation ~ 28435-28436
without manipulation ~ 28430
tarsal
open treatment ~ 28465
percutaneous fixation ~ 28456
with manipulation ~ 28455-28456
thumb
open treatment ~ 26665
with dislocation ~ 26645-26650
tibia ~ 27759
arthroscopic treatment ~ 29855-29856

Fracture ~ *continued*
closed treatment ~ 27530-27532, 27538, 27750-27752, 27760-27762, 27808-27810, 27824-27825
distal ~ 27824-27828
intercondylar ~ 27538-27540
malleolus ~ 27760-27766, 27808-27814
open treatment ~ 27535-27536, 27540, 27758, 27766, 27814, 27826-27828
percutaneous fixation ~ 27756
plateau ~ 27530-27536, 29855-29856
shaft ~ 27750-27759
with manipulation ~ 27752, 27760-27762, 27810
without manipulation ~ 27530, 27750, 27760-27762, 27808, 27825
trachea, endoscopy ~ 31630
ulna
closed treatment ~ 25560-25565
olecranon
closed treatment ~ 24670-24675
open treatment ~ 24685
open treatment ~ 25574-25575
shaft
closed treatment ~ 25530-25535
open treatment ~ 25545, 25574
styloid process
closed treatment ~ 25650
open treatment ~ 25652
percutaneous fixation ~ 25651
with dislocation ~ 24620, 24635
closed treatment ~ 24620
Monteggia ~ 24620-24635
open treatment ~ 24635
with manipulation ~ 25535, 25565
with radius ~ 25560-25565
open treatment ~ 25575
without manipulation ~ 25530, 25560
vertebra
additional segment, open treatment ~ 22328
cervical, open treatment ~ 22326
closed treatment
with manipulation, casting and/or bracing ~ 22315
without manipulation ~ 22310
lumbar, open treatment ~ 22325
posterior, open treatment ~ 22325-22327
thoracic, open treatment ~ 22327
with shoulder dislocation
closed treatment ~ 23675
open treatment ~ 23680
vertebral process, closed treatment ~ 22305
wrist, with dislocation
closed treatment ~ 25680
open treatment ~ 25685
zygomatic arch
open treatment ~ 21356-21366
with manipulation ~ 21355

Fragile-X chromosome analysis ~ 88248

Fragility
red blood cell
mechanical ~ 85547
osmotic ~ 85555-85557
Frames, stereotactic ~ 20660
Francisella ~ 86000
antibody ~ 86668
Fredet-Ramstedt procedure ~ 43520
Free E3 ~ 82677
Free skin graft ~ 15050-15321, 15340-15366, 15420-15431, 15757
Free T4 (four) ~ 84439
Frei disease ~ 86729
Frenectomy ~ 40819, 41115
Frenectomy, lingual ~ 41115
Frenotomy ~ 40806, 41010
Frenulectomy ~ 40819
Frenuloplasty ~ 41520
Frenum lip, incision ~ 40806
Frenumectomy ~ 40819
Frickman operation ~ see proctopexy
Frontal craniotomy ~ 61556
Frontal sinus ~ see sinus, frontal
Frontal sinusotomy ~ 31070-31075
Frost suture ~ 67875
Frozen blood preparation ~ 86930-86932
Fructose ~ 84375
semen ~ 82757
Fructose intolerance breath test ~ 91065
Fruit sugar ~ 84375
FSF ~ 85290-85291
FSH ~ 80418, 80426, 83001
FT-4 ~ 84439
Fulguration ~ see destruction
bladder ~ 51020
cystourethroscopy with ~ 52214
lesion ~ 52224
tumor ~ 52234-52240
ureter ~ 50957-50959, 50976-50978
ureterocele
ectopic ~ 52301
orthotopic ~ 52300
Fulguration, endocavitary ~ 17000-17286
Full thickness graft ~ 15200-15261
Function, study, nasal ~ 92512
Function test, lung ~ see pulmonology, diagnostic
Function test, vestibular ~ see vestibular function tests
Fundoplasty
esophagogastric ~ 43324-43325
laparoscopic ~ 43280
with gastroplasty ~ 43326
Fundoplication ~ 43324-43325
Fungus
antibody ~ 86671
culture
blood ~ 87103
hair ~ 87101
identification ~ 87106
nail ~ 87101
other ~ 87102
Fungus ~ *continued*
skin ~ 87101
tissue exam ~ 87220
Funnel chest ~ 21740-21743
Furuncle
incision and drainage ~ 10060-10061
vulva ~ 56405
Fusion ~ see arthrodesis
pleural cavity ~ 32005
thumb in opposition ~ 26820
Fusion, epiphyseal-diaphyseal ~ see epiphyseal arrest
Fusion, joint ~ see arthrodesis
Fusion, joint, ankle ~ 27870
Fusion, joint, interphalangeal, finger ~ 26860-26863

G

Gago procedure ~ 33463-33465
Gait training ~ 97116
Galactogram ~ 77053-77054
injection ~ 19030
Galactokinase, blood ~ 82759
Galactose
blood ~ 82760
urine ~ 82760
Galactose-1-phosphate
uridyl transferase ~ 82775-82776
Gallbladder ~ see also bile duct
anastomosis with intestines ~ 47720-47741
excision ~ 47562-47564, 47600-47620
exploration ~ 47480
incision ~ 47490
incision and drainage ~ 47480
nuclear medicine, imaging ~ 78223
removal, calculi (stone) ~ 47480
repair
with gastroenterostomy ~ 47741
with intestines ~ 47720-47740
unlisted services and procedures ~ 47999
X-ray with contrast ~ 74290-74291
Galvanocautery ~ 17000-17286
Galvanoionization ~ 97033
Gamete intrafallopian transfer ~ see GIFT
Gamete transfer, in vitro fertilization ~ 58976
Gamma camera imaging ~ see nuclear medicine
Gamma glutamyl transferase ~ 82977
Gamma seminoprotein ~ 84152-84153
Gammacorten ~ 80420
Gammaglobulin, blood ~ 82784-82787
Gamulin Rh ~ 90384-90386
Ganglia, trigeminal ~ 61450, 61790
Ganglion cyst ~ 61450, 61790
aspiration/injection ~ 20612
drainage ~ 20612
injection, anesthetic ~ 64505, 64510
wrist excision ~ 25111-25112

Ganglion, Gasser's ~ 61450, 61790
Ganglion cervicothoracicum ~ 64510
Ganglion pterygopalatinum ~ 64505
Gardner operation ~ 63700-63702
Gardnerella vaginalis detection ~ 87510-87512
Gasserian ganglion
sensory root
decompression ~ 61450
section ~ 61450
stereotactic ~ 61790
Gasser ganglion ~ 61450, 61790
Gastrectomy
partial ~ 43631-43639, 43845
with gastrojejunostomy ~ 43632
total ~ 43621-43622
with esophagoenterostomy ~ 43620
with gastroduodenostomy ~ 43631
Gastric
acid ~ 82926-82928
analysis test ~ 91052
electrodes
implantation
laparoscopic
neurostimulator ~ 43647
stimulation ~ 0155T
open
neurostimulator ~ 43881
stimulation ~ 0157T
removal
laparoscopic
neurostimulator ~ 43648
stimulation ~ 0156T
open
neurostimulator ~ 43882
stimulation ~ 0156T
replacement
laparoscopic
neurostimulator ~ 43647
stimulation ~ 0156T
open
neurostimulator ~ 43881
stimulation ~ 0157T
revision
laparoscopic
neurostimulator ~ 43648
stimulation ~ 0156T
open
neurostimulator ~ 43882
stimulation ~ 0158T
intubation ~ 89130-89141, 91105
lavage, therapeutic ~ 91105
tests, manometry ~ 91020
ulcer disease ~ 43610
Gastrin ~ 82938-82941
Gastrocnemius recession, leg, lower ~ 27687
Gastroduodenostomy ~ 43810, 43850-43855
Gastroenterology, diagnostic services ~ 91000-91299
breath hydrogen test ~ 91065
esophagus tests
acid perfusion ~ 91030
acid reflux ~ 91032-91033
Gastroenterology, d/x services ~ ***continued***
balloon distension provocation study ~ 91040
intubation with specimen collection ~ 91000
motility study ~ 91010-91012
gastroesophageal reflux test ~ 91034-91038
gastric tests, manometry ~ 91020
intestine bleeding tube ~ 91100
manometry ~ 91020
rectum sensation, tone, and compliance test ~ 91120
rectum/anus manometry ~ 91122
stomach
intubation with specimen prep ~ 91055
stimulation of secretion ~ 91052
unlisted services and procedures ~ 91299
Gastroenterostomy
for obesity ~ 43644-43645, 43842-43848
Gastroesophageal reflux test ~ 91034-91038
Gastrointestinal exam
nuclear medicine
blood loss study ~ 78278
protein loss study ~ 78282
shunt testing ~ 78291
unlisted services and procedures ~ 78299
Gastrointestinal tract
imaging intraluminal ~ 91110-91111
reconstruction ~ 43360-43361
upper dilation ~ 43249
X-ray ~ 74240-74245
with contrast ~ 74246-74249
guide dilator ~ 74360
guide intubation ~ 74340-74350
Gastrointestinal, upper
biopsy, endoscopy ~ 43239
dilation
endoscopy ~ 43245
esophagus ~ 43248
endoscopy
catheterization ~ 43241
destruction lesion ~ 43258
dilation ~ 43245
drainage pseudocyst ~ 43240
exploration ~ 43234-43235
hemorrhage ~ 43255
inject varices ~ 43243
injection ~ 43236
needle biopsy ~ 43242, 43238
removal
foreign body ~ 43247
lesion ~ 43251
polyp ~ 43251
tumor ~ 43251
stent placement ~ 43256
suturing esophagogastric junction ~ 0008T
thermal radiation ~ 43257
tube placement ~ 43246
ultrasound ~ 43237-43238, 43242, 43259, 76975
exploration endoscopy ~ 43234-43235
hemorrhage endoscopic control ~ 43255

Gastrointestinal, upper ~ *continued*
injection
submucosal ~ 43236
varices ~ 43243
lesion destruction ~ 43258
ligation of vein ~ 43244
needle biopsy, endoscopy ~ 43238, 43242
removal
foreign body ~ 43247
lesion ~ 43250
polyp ~ 43250-43251
tumor ~ 43250
tube placement, endoscopy ~ 43246
ultrasound endoscopy ~ 43237-43238, 43242, 43259, 76975
Gastrojejunostomy ~ 43860-43865
with duodenal exclusion ~ 48547
with partial gastrectomy ~ 43632
with vagotomy ~ 43825
without vagotomy ~ 43820
Gastroplasty evision for obesity ~ 43644-43645, 43842-43848
Gastroplasty with esophagogastric fundoplasty ~ 43326, 43842-43843
Gastrorrhaphy ~ 43840
Gastroschises ~ 49605
Gastrostomy
closure ~ 43870
laparoscopic, temporary ~ 43653
temporary ~ 43830
laparoscopic ~ 43653
neonatal ~ 43831
with pancreatic drain ~ 48001
with pyloroplasty ~ 43640
with vagotomy ~ 43640
Gastrostomy tube
change of ~ 43760
directed placement, endoscopic ~ 43246
insertion, percutaneous ~ 43750
percutaneous ~ 43750
repositioning ~ 43761
Gastrotomy ~ 43500-43501, 43510
GDH ~ 82965
Gel diffusion ~ 86331
Gel diffusion test ~ 86329-86331
Gene product ~ see protein
Genioplasty ~ 21120-21123
augmentation ~ 21120, 21123
osteotomy ~ 21121-21123
Genitourinary sphincter, artificial ~ 53444-53449
Genotype analysis
by nucleic acid
infectious agent
HIV-1 protease/reverse transcriptase ~ 87901
hepatitis C virus ~ 87902
Gentamicin ~ 80170
assay ~ 80170
Gentamycin level ~ 80170
Gentiobiase ~ 82963
GERD ~ 91034-91038
German measles ~ 86762, 90706
Gestational trophoblastic tumor ~ 59100, 59870
GGT ~ 82977
GI tract ~ see gastrointestinal tract
Giardia
antigen detection
immunofluorescence ~ 87269
enzyme immunoassay ~ 87329
Giardia lamblia
antibody ~ 86674
Gibbons stent ~ 52332
GIF ~ 84307
GIFT (gamete intrafallopian transfer) ~ 58976
Gillies approach
fracture, zygomatic arch ~ 21356
Gill operation ~ 63012
Gingiva ~ see gums
Gingiva, abscess ~ see abscess
fracture ~ see 41800 ~ gums
zygomatic arch ~ 41800
Gingivectomy ~ 41820
Gingivoplasty ~ 41872
Girdlestone laminectomy ~ see laminectomy
Girdlestone procedure ~ 27120
G1A protein (bone) ~ 83937
Gland ~ see specific gland
Glasses ~ see spectacle services
Glaucoma
cryotherapy ~ 66720
cyclophotocoagulation ~ 66710, 66711
diathermy ~ 66700
fistulization of sclera ~ 66150
provocative test ~ 92140
Glaucoma drainage implant ~ 66180, 66185
GLC ~ 82486
Glenn procedure ~ 33766-33767
Glenohumeral joint
arthrotomy ~ 23040
with biopsy ~ 23100
with synovectomy ~ 23105
exploration ~ 23107
removalforeign or loose body ~ 23107
Glenoid Fossa reconstruction ~ 21255
GLN ~ 82975
Globulin
antihuman ~ 86880-86886
corticosteroid-binding ~ 84449
immune ~ 90281-90399
Rh immune ~ 90384-90386
sex hormone binding ~ 84270
thyroxine-binding ~ 84442
Glomerular procoagulant activity ~ see thromboplastin
Glomus caroticum ~ 60600, 60605
Glossectomies ~ see excision, tongue
Glossopexy ~ 41500
Glossorrhaphy ~ 41510
Glucagon ~ 82943
tolerance panel ~ 80422-80424
tolerance test ~ 82946

Glucose ~ 80422-80424, 80430-80435, 95250
blood test ~ 82947-82950, 82962
body fluid ~ 82945
interstitial fluid continuous monitoring ~ 95250
tolerance test ~ 82951-82952
with tolbutamide ~ 82953
Glucose-6-phosphate dehydrogenase ~ 82955-82960
Glucose phosphate isomerase ~ 84087
Glucosidase ~ 82963
Glucuronide androstanediol ~ 82154
Glue
cornea wound ~ 65286
sclera wound ~ 65286
Glukagon ~ see glucagon
Glutamate dehydrogenase, blood ~ 82965
Glutamate pyruvate transaminase ~ 84460
Glutamic
alanine transaminase ~ 84460
aspartic transaminase ~ 84450
dehydrogenase ~ 82965
Glutamine ~ 82975
Glutamyltransferase, gamma ~ 82977
Glutathione ~ 82978
Glutathione reductase ~ 82979
Glutethimide ~ 82980
Glycanhydrolase, N-acetylmuramide ~ 85549
Glycated hemoglobins ~ 83036
Glycated protein ~ 82985
Glycerol, phosphatidyl ~ 84081
Glycerol, phosphoglycerides ~ 84081
Glycerophosphatase ~ 84075-84080
Glycinate, theophylline sodium ~ 80198
Glycocholic acid ~ 82240
Glycohemoglobin ~ 83036
Glycol, ethylene ~ 82693
Glycosaminoglycan ~ 83864-83866
GMP (guanosine monophosphate), cyclic ~ 83008
Goeckerman treatment ~ 96910-96913
Gol-Vernet operation
pyelotomy, exploration 50120
Gold assay ~ 80172
Goldwaite procedure ~ 27422
Golfer's elbow ~ 24350-24356
Gonadectomy, female ~ 58262-58263, 58291-58292, 58552, 58554, 58661, 58940-58943
Gonadectomy, male ~ 54520, 54522, 54530-54535, 54690
Gonadotropin
chorionic ~ 84702-84703
FSH ~ 83001
ICSH ~ 83002
LH ~ 83002
panel ~ 80426
Gonioscopy ~ 92020
Goniotomy ~ 65820
Gonococcus ~ 87590-87592, 87850
Goodenough Harris drawing test ~ 96100
GOTT ~ 84450
GPUT ~ 82775-82776
Graft ~ see bone graft; bypass graft
anal ~ 46753
aorta ~ 33840-33851, 33860-33877
artery
coronary ~ 33503-33505
bone ~ 38240-38242
harvesting ~ 20900-20902
microvascular anastomosis ~ 20955-20962
osteocutaneous flap with microvascular anastomosis ~ 20969-20973
vascular pedicle ~ 25430
bone and skin ~ 20969-20973
cartilage
ear to face ~ 21235
harvesting ~ 20910-20912
rib to face ~ 21230
conjunctiva ~ 65782
harvesting ~ 68371
cornea, with lesion excision ~ 65426
cornea transplant
in aphakia ~ 65750
lamellar ~ 65710
penetrating ~ 65730
in pseudophakia ~ 65755
dura, spinal cord ~ 63710
endovascular ~ 34900
eye
amniotic membrane ~ 65780
conjunctiva ~ 65782
stem cell ~ 65781
facial nerve paralysis ~ 15840-15845
fascia, cheek ~ 15840
fascia lata, harvesting ~ 20920-20922
gum mucosa ~ 41870
heart ~ 33935, 33945
heart lung ~ 33935
kidney ~ see kidney, transplantation
liver ~ 47135-47136
lung ~ 32851-32854, 33935
muscle, cheek ~ 15841-15845
nail bed reconstruction ~ 11762
nerve ~ 64885-64907
oral mucosa ~ 40818
organ ~ see transplantation
pancreas ~ 48160, 48550, 48554-48556
skin
biological ~ 15300-15336
blood flow check, graft ~ 15860
vascular flow check, graft ~ 15860
tendon
finger ~ 26392
hand ~ 26392
harvesting ~ 20924
tissue harvesting ~ 20926
vein cross-over ~ 34520
Grain alcohol ~ see alcohol, ethyl
Granulation tissue cauterization, chemical ~ 17250
Great toe
free osteocutaneous flap with microvascular anastomosis ~ 20973

Great vessels
shunt
aorta to pulmonary artery
ascending ~ 33755
descending ~ 33762
central ~ 33764
subclavian to pulmonary artery ~ 33750
vena cava to pulmonary artery ~ 33766-33767
unlisted services and procedures ~ 33999
Great vessels transposition ~ 33770-33781
Greater tuberosity fracture
with shoulder dislocation
closed treatment ~ 23665
open treatment ~ 23670
Greater vestibular gland ~ see Bartholin's gland
Green operation ~ (scapulopexy) 23400
Gridley stain ~ 88312
Grippe, Balkan ~ 86000, 86638
Gritti operation ~ 27590-27592
Groin repair, hernia ~ 49550-49557
Group health education ~ 99078
Grouping, blood ~ see blood typing
Growth factors, insulin-like ~ 84305
Growth hormone ~ 83003
human ~ 80418, 80428-80430, 86277
Growth hormone release inhibiting factor ~ 84307
GTT (hydatidiform mole) ~ 82951, 82952
Guaiac test, blood in feces ~ 82270
Guanosine monophosphate (GMP) ~ 83008
Guanosine monophosphate, cyclic ~ 83008
Guanylic acids ~ 83008
Guard stain ~ 88313
Gullett ~ see esophagus
Gums
abscess, incision and drainage ~ 41800
alveolus, excision ~ 41830
cyst, incision and drainage ~ 41800
excision
gingiva ~ 41820
operculum ~ 41821
graft, mucosa ~ 41870
hematoma, incision and drainage ~ 41800
lesion
destruction ~ 41850
excision ~ 41822-41828
mucosa, excision ~ 41828
reconstruction
alveolus ~ 41874
gingiva ~ 41872
removal, foreign body ~ 41805
tumor, excision ~ 41825-41827
unlisted services and procedures ~ 41899
Gunning-Lieben test ~ 82009-82010
Guthrie test ~ 84030

H

H flu ~ see Hemophilus influenza
H-reflex study ~ 95934-95936
HAAb (antibody, hepatitis) ~ 86708, 86709
HAA (hepatitis associated antigen) ~ 87340-87380, 87515-87527
Haemoglobin F ~ see fetal hemoglobin
Haemorrhage ~ see hemorrhage
Haemorrhage rectum ~ see hemorrhage, rectum
Hageman factor ~ 85280
Hair
electrolysis ~ 17380
KOH examination ~ 87220
microscopic evaluation ~ 96902
removal ~ see removal, hair
transplant
punch graft ~ 15775-15776
strip graft ~ 15220-15221
HAI test ~ see hemagglutination inhibition test
Hallux ~ see great toe
Halo
body cast ~ 29000
cranial ~ 20661
for thin skull osteology ~ 20664
femur ~ 20663
maxillofacial ~ 21100
pelvic ~ 20662
removal ~ 20665
Haloperidol assay ~ 80173
Halsted mastectomy ~ see mastectomy, radical
Halsted hernia repair ~ 49495
Ham test ~ 85475
Hammertoe repair ~ 28285-28286
Hamster penetration test ~ 89329
Hand ~ see also carpometacarpal joint; intercarpal joint
amputation
at metacarpal ~ 25927
revision ~ 25924, 25929-25931
at wrist ~ 25920
revision ~ 25922
arthrodesis
carpometacarpal joint ~ 26843-26844
intercarpal joint ~ 25820-25825
bone, incision and drainage ~ 26034
cast ~ 29085
decompression ~ 26035-26037
fracture metacarpal ~ 26600
insertion tendon graft ~ 26392
magnetic resonance imaging (MRI) ~ 73218-73223
reconstruction tendon pulley ~ 26500-26502
removal
implantation ~ 26320
tube/rod ~ 26390-26392, 26416
repair
blood vessel ~ 35207

Hand ~ *continued*
cleft hand ~ 26580
muscle ~ 26591-26593
tendon
extensor ~ 26410-26416, 26426-26428, 26433-26437
flexor ~ 26350-26358, 26440
profundus ~ 26370-26373
replantation ~ 20808
strapping ~ 29280
tendon excision ~ 26390
extensor ~ 26415
tenotomy ~ 26450, 26460
tumor excision ~ 26115-26117
unlisted services and procedures ~ 26989
X-ray ~ 73120-73130
Handling
device ~ 99002
radioelement ~ 77790
specimen ~ 99000-99001
Hand abscess ~ see abscess, hand
Hand phalange ~ see finger, bone
Hanganutziu Deicher antibodies ~ see antibody, heterophile
Haptoglobin ~ 83010-83012
Hard palate ~ see palate
Harelip operation ~ see cleft lip, repair
Harii procedure ~ 25430
Harrington rod
insertion ~ 22840
removal ~ 22850
Hartmann procedure
open ~ 44143
laparoscopic ~ 44206
Harvesting
bone graft ~ 20900-20902
bone marrow ~ 38230
cartilage graft ~ 20910-20912
conjunctival graft ~ 68371
eggs, in vitro fertilization ~ 58970
endoscopic, vein for bypass graft ~ 33508
fascia lata graft ~ 20920-20922
intestines ~ 44132-44133
kidney ~ 50300-50320, 50547
liver ~ 47133, 47140-47142
lower extremity vein for vascular reconstruction ~ 35572
stem cell ~ 38205-38206
tendon graft ~ 20924
tissue grafts ~ 20926
upper extremity
artery for coronary artery bypass graft ~ 35600
vein for bypass graft ~ 35500
Hauser procedure ~ 27420
Hayem's elementary corpuscle ~ see blood, platelet
Haygroves procedure ~ 27120, 27122
HBcAb ~ 86704, 86705
HBeAb ~ 86707
HBeAg ~ 87350
HBsAb ~ 86706
HBsAg (hepatitis B surface antigen) ~ 87340
HCG ~ 84702, 84703
HCO3 ~ see bicarbonate
Hct (hematocrit) ~ 85014
HCV antibodies ~ see antibody, hepatitis C
HDL (high density lipoprotein) ~ 83718
Head
angiography ~ 70496, 70544-70546
CT scan ~ 70450-70470, 70496
excision ~ 21015-21070
fracture and/or dislocation ~ 21310-21497
incision ~ 21010, 61316, 62148
introduction or removal ~ 21076-21116
lipectomy, suction assisted ~ 15876
magnetic resonance angiography (MRA) ~ 70544-70546
nerve graft ~ 64885-64886
other procedures ~ 21299, 21499
repair/revision and/or reconstruction ~ 21120-21296
ultrasound exam ~ 76506, 76536
unlisted services and procedures ~ 21499
X-ray ~ 70350
Head rings, stereotactic ~ see stereotactic frame
Headbrace
application ~ 21100
application/removal ~ 20661
Heaf TB test ~ 86580
Health and behavior assessment ~ 96150-96155
Health risk assessment instrument ~ 99420
Hearing aid
bone conduction
implantation ~ 69710
removal ~ 69711
repair ~ 69711
replacement ~ 69710
check ~ 92592-92593
services
electroacoustic test ~ 92594-92595
examination ~ 92590-92591
Hearing evaluation ~ 92510
Hearing tests ~ see audiologic function tests; hearing evaluation
Hearing therapy ~ 92507-92510, 92601-92604
Heart
ablation, ventricular septum, non-surgical ~ 0024T
allograft preparation ~ 33933-33934
angiography, injection ~ 93542-93543
aortic arch
with cardiopulmonary bypass ~ 33853
without cardiopulmonary bypass ~ 33852
aortic valve
repair, left ventricle ~ 33414
replacement ~ 33405-33413
arrhythmogenic focus
catheter ablation ~ 93650-93652
destruction ~ 33250-33251, 33261
atria ~ see atria

Heart ~ *continued*
biopsy ~ 93505
ultrasound imaging guidance ~ 76932
blood vessel repair ~ 33320-33322
cardiac output measurements ~ 93561-93562
cardiac rehabilitation ~ 93797-93798
cardioassist ~ 92970-92971
ventricular assist device, extracorporeal ~ 0049T
cardiopulmonary bypass with lung transplant ~ 32852, 32854
catheterization ~ 93501, 93510-93533
combined right and retrograde left for congenital cardiac anomalies ~ 93531
combined right and transseptal left for congenital cardiac anomalies ~ 93532-93533
flow-directed ~ 93503
right, for congenital cardiac anomalies ~ 93530
closure
septal defect ~ 33615
valve, atrioventricular ~ 33600
semilunar ~ 33602
commissurotomy right ventricle ~ 33476-33478
destruction arrhythmogenic focus ~ 33250, 33261
electrical recording
acoustic heart sound ~ 0068T-0070T
3-D mapping ~ 93613
atria ~ 93602
atrial electrogram, esophageal (or trans-esophageal) ~ 93615-93616
bundle of His ~ 93600
comprehensive ~ 93619-93622
right ventricle ~ 93603
tachycardia sites ~ 93609
electroconversion ~ 92960-92961
electrophysiologic follow-up study ~ 93624
excision
donor ~ 33930, 33940
tricuspid valve ~ 33460
exploration ~ 33310-33315
fibrillation, atrial ~ 33254-33256, 33265-33266
great vessels ~ see great vessels
heart-lung bypass ~ see cardiopulmonary bypass
heart-lung transplantation ~ see transplantation, heart-lung
hemodynamic monitoring, non-invasive ~ 0086T
implantation
artificial heart, intracorporeal ~ 0051T
total replacement heart system, intracorporeal ~ 0051T
ventricular assist device ~ 33976
extracorporeal ~ 0048T
intracorporeal ~ 33979
incision
atrial ~ 33254-33256
exploration ~ 33310-33315

Heart ~ *continued*
injection, radiologic ~ 93542-93543
insertion
balloon device ~ 33973
electrode ~ 33210-33211, 33216-33217, 33224-33225
pacemaker ~ 33206-33208
catheter ~ 33210
pulse generator ~ 33212-33213
ventricular assist device ~ 33975
intraoperative pacing and mapping ~ 93631
ligation, fistula ~ 37607
magnetic resonance imaging (MRI) ~ 75552-75553
mitral valve ~ see mitral valve
muscle ~ see myocardial
myocardium
imaging ~ 78466-78469
perfusion study ~ 78460-78465
nuclear medicine
blood flow study ~ 78414
blood pool imaging ~ 78472-78473, 78481-78483, 78494-78496
myocardial imaging ~ 78466-78469
myocardial perfusion ~ 78460-78465
shunt detection ~ 78428
unlisted services and procedures ~ 78499
open chest massage ~ 32160
output ~ see cardiac output
pacemaker
conversion ~ 33214
insertion ~ 33206-33208
pulse generator ~ 33212-33213
removal ~ 33233-33237
replacement ~ 33206-33208
catheter ~ 33210
upgrade ~ 33214
pacing
arrhythmia induction ~ 93618
atria ~ 93610
transcutaneous, temporary ~ 92953
ventricular ~ 93612
pacing cardioverter-defibrillator
evaluation and testing ~ 93640-93642, 93740-93744
insertion single/dual chamber electrodes ~ 33216-33217, 33224-33225, 33249
pulse generator ~ 33240
repositioning single/dual chamber electrodes ~ 33215, 33226
wearable device ~ 93741-93742, 93745
positron emission tomography (PET)~ 78459
perfusion study ~ 78491-78492
pulmonary valve ~ see pulmonary valve
rate increase ~ see tachycardia
reconstruction
atrial septum ~ 33735-33737
vena cava ~ 34502
recording acoustic ~ 0068T

Heart ~ *continued*
reduction, ventricular septum, non-surgical ~ 0024T
removal
balloon device ~ 33974
electrode ~ 33238
ventricular assist device ~ 33977-33978
extracorporeal ~ 0050T
intracorporeal ~ 33980
removal single/dual chamber
electrodes ~ 33243-33244
pulse generator ~ 33241
repair ~ 33218-33220
repair
anomaly ~ 33615-33617
aortic sinus ~ 33702-33722
artificial heart, intracorporeal ~ 0052T, 0053T
atrial septum ~ 33641, 33647
atrioventricular canal ~ 33660-33665
complete ~ 33670
prosthetic valve ~ 33670
atrioventricular valve ~ 33660-33665
cor triatriatum ~ 33732
electrode ~ 33218
fenestration ~ 93580
infundibular ~ 33476-33478
mitral valve ~ 33420-33430
myocardium ~ 33542
outflow tract ~ 33476-33478
postinfarction ~ 33542-33545
prosthetic valve dysfunction ~ 33496
septal defect ~ 33608-33610, 33660, 33813-33814, 93581
sinus of valsalva ~ 33702-33722
sinus venosus ~ 33645
tetralogy of Fallot ~ 33692-33697, 33924
total replacement heart system
intracorporeal ~ 0052T, 0053T
tricuspid valve ~ 33463-33468
ventricle ~ 33611-33612
obstruction ~ 33619
ventricular septum ~ 33545, 33647, 33681-33688, 33692-33697, 93581
ventricular tunnel ~ 33722
wound ~ 33300-33305
replacement
artificial heart, intracorporeal ~ 0052T, 0053T
electrode ~ 33210-33211, 33217
mitral valve ~ 33430
total replacement heart system, intracorporeal ~ 0052T, 0053T
tricuspid valve ~ 33465
repositioning
electrode ~ 33215, 33217, 33226
tricuspid valve ~ 33468
resuscitation ~ 92950
septal defect ~ see septal defect
stimulation and pacing ~ 93623
thrombectomy ~ 33310-33315
transplantation ~ 33935, 33945

Heart ~ *continued*
allograft preparation ~ 33933, 33944
tricuspid valve ~ see tricuspid valve
tumor excision ~ 33120-33130
unlisted services and procedures ~ 33999
ventriculography ~ see ventriculography
ventriculomyectomy ~ 33416
wound repair ~ 33300-33305
Heart sounds, acoustic recording, with computer analysis ~ 0068T-0070T
Heart vessels
angioplasty, percutaneous ~ 92982-92984
insertion graft ~ 33330-33335
thrombolysis ~ 92975-92977
valvuloplasty, percutaneous ~ 92986-92990
Heat unstable haemoglobin ~ see hemoglobin, thermolabile
Heavy lipoproteins ~ see lipoprotein
Heavy metal ~ 83015-83018
Heel ~ 36415-36416
X-ray ~ 73650
Heel bone ~ see calcaneus
Heel fracture ~ see calcaneus, fracture
Heel spur excision ~ 28119
Heine-Medin disease ~ see polio
Heine operation ~ see cyclodialysis
Heinz bodies ~ 85441-85445
Helicobacter pylori
antibody ~ 86677
antigen detection enzyme immunoassay ~ 87338-87339
blood test ~ 83009
breath test ~ 78267-78268, 83013-83014
stool ~ 87338
urease activity ~ 83009, 83013-83014
Heller procedure ~ 32665, 43330-43331
Helminth antibody ~ 86682
Hemagglutination inhibition test ~ 86280
Hemangioma ~ 17106-17108
Hemapheresis ~ 36511-36516
Hematochezia ~ 82270, 82274
Hematologic test ~ see blood tests
Hematology and coagulation ~ 85002-85999
Hematoma
ankle ~ 27603
arm, lower ~ 25028
arm, upper, incision and drainage ~ 23930
brain
drainage ~ 61154-61156
evacuation ~ 61312-61315
incision and drainage ~ 61312-61315
drain ~ 61108
ear, external
complicated ~ 69005
simple ~ 69000
elbow, incision and drainage ~ 23930
epididymis, incision and drainage ~ 54700
gums, incision and drainage ~ 41800
hip ~ 26990
incision and drainage
neck ~ 21501-21502
skin ~ 10140

Hematoma ~ *continued*
thorax ~ 21501-21502
knee ~ 27301
leg, lower ~ 27603
leg, upper ~ 27301
mouth ~ 41005-41009, 41015-41018
incision and drainage ~ 40800-40801
nasal septum, incision and drainage ~ 30020
nose, incision and drainage ~ 30000-30020
pelvis ~ 26990
scrotum, incision and drainage ~ 54700
shoulder, drainage ~ 23030
skin
incision and drainage ~ 10140
puncture aspiration ~ 10160
subdural ~ 61108
subungual, evacuation ~ 11740
testis, incision and drainage ~ 54700
tongue ~ 41000-41006, 41015
vagina, incision and drainage ~ 57022-57023
wrist ~ 25028
Hematopoietic stem cell transplantation ~ see stem cell, transplantation
Hematopoietin ~ see erythropoietin
Hematuria ~ see blood, urine
Hemic and lymphatic systems, surgical procedures ~ 38100-38999
Hemiepiphyseal arrest, elbow ~ 24470
Hemifacial microsomia, reconstruction, mandibular condyle ~ 21247
Hemilaminectomy ~ 63020-63044
Hemilaryngectomy ~ 31370-31382
Hemipelvectomies ~ see amputation, interpelviabdominal
Hemiphalangectomy, toe ~ 28160
Hemispherectomy
partial ~ 61543
total ~ 61542
Hemocytoblast ~ see stem cell
Hemodialysis ~ 90935-90937
blood flow study ~ 90939-90940
duplex scan of access ~ 93990
Hemodynamic monitoring, non-invasive left ventricular ~ 0086T
Hemofiltration ~ 90945-90947
Hemoglobin ~ 83036
analysis, O2 affinity ~ 82820
carboxyhemoglobin ~ 82375-82376
chromatography ~ 83021
concentration ~ 85046
electrophoresis ~ 83020
fetal ~ 83030-83033, 85460-85461
fractionation and quantitation ~ 83020
glycated ~ 83036
methemoglobin ~ 83045-83050
non-automated ~ 83026
plasma ~ 83051
sulfhemoglobin ~ 83055-83060
thermolabile ~ 83065-83068
urine ~ 83069
Hemoglobin, glycosylated ~ see glycohemoglobin
Hemoglobin F (fetal)
chemical ~ 83030
qualitative ~ 83033
Hemogram
added indices ~ 85025-85027
automated ~ 85025-85027
manual ~ 85014-85018, 85032
Hemolysins ~ 85475
with agglutinins ~ 86940-86941
Hemolytic complement ~ see complement, hemolytic
Hemolytic complement, total ~ see complement, hemolytic, total
Hemoperfusion ~ 90997
Hemophil ~ see clotting factor
Hemophilus influenza
antibody ~ 86684
B vaccine ~ 90645-90648, 90720-90721, 90748
Hemorrhage
abdomen ~ 49002
anal, endoscopic control ~ 46614
bladder, postoperative ~ 52606
chest cavity, endoscopic control ~ 32654
colon, endoscopic control ~ 44391, 45382
colon-sigmoid, endoscopic control ~ 45334
esophagus, endoscopic control ~ 43227
gastrointestinal, upper, endoscopic control ~ 43255
intestines, small, endoscopic control ~ 44366, 44378
liver, control ~ 47350
lung ~ 32110
nasal
cauterization ~ 30901-30906
endoscopic control ~ 31238
nasopharynx ~ 42970-42972
oropharynx ~ 42960-42962
rectum, endoscopic control ~ 45317
throat ~ 42960-42962
uterus, postpartum ~ 59160
vagina ~ 57180
Hemorrhoidectomy
complex ~ 46260
with fissurectomy ~ 46261-46262
external complete ~ 46250
ligature ~ 46221
simple ~ 46255
with fissurectomy ~ 46257-46258
Hemorrhoidopexy ~ 46947
Hemorrhoids
destruction ~ 46934-46936
incision, external ~ 46083
injection, sclerosing solution ~ 46500
ligation ~ 46945-46946
stapling ~ 46947
suture ~ 46945-46946
Hemosiderin ~ 83070-83071
Hemothorax, thoracostomy ~ 32020
Heparin ~ see clotting inhibitors ~ 85520
neutralization ~ 85525
protamine tolerance test ~ 85530

Heparin cofactor I ~ see antithrombin III
Hepatectomy
extensive ~ 47122
left lobe ~ 47125
partial
donor ~ 47140-47142
lobe ~ 47120
right lobe ~ 47130
total
donor ~ 47133
Hepaticodochotomy ~ see hepaticostomy
Hepaticoenterostomy ~ 47802
Hepaticostomy ~ 47400
Hepaticotomy ~ 47400
Hepatic abscess ~ see abscess, liver
Hepatic arteries ~ see artery, hepatic
Hepatic artery aneurysm ~ see artery, hepatic, aneurysm
Hepatic duct
anastomosis, with intestines ~ 47765, 47802
exploration ~ 47400
incision and drainage ~ 47400
nuclear medicine imaging ~ 78223
removalcalculi (stone) ~ 47400
repair, with intestines ~ 47765, 47802
unlisted services and procedures ~ 47999
Hepatic haemorrhage ~ see hemorrhage, liver
Hepatic portal vein ~ see vein, hepatic portal
Hepatic portoenterostomies ~ see hepaticoenterostomy
Hepatic transplantation ~ see liver, transplantation
Hepatitis A and hepatitis B ~ 90636
Hepatitis antibody
A ~ 86708-86709
B
B core ~ 86704-86705
B surface ~ 86706
Be ~ 86707
C ~ 86803-86804
delta agent ~ 86692
IgG ~ 86704, 86708
IgM ~ 86704-86705, 86708-86709
Hepatitis antigen
B ~ 87515-87517
B surface ~ 87340-87341
Be ~ 87350
C ~ 87520-87522
delta agent ~ 87380
G ~ 87525-87527
Hepatitis A vaccine
adolescent/pediatric
2 dose schedule ~ 90633
3 dose schedule ~ 90634
adult dosage ~ 90632
Hepatitis B and Hib ~ 90748
Hepatitis B vaccine dosage
adolescent ~ 90743
adult ~ 90746
immunosuppressed ~ 90740, 90747
pediatric/adolescent ~ 90744
Hepatitis B virus e antibody ~ see antibody, hepatitis
Hepatitis B virus surface ab ~ see antibody, hepatitis B, surface
Hepatorrhaphy ~ see liver, repair
Hepatotomy
abscess ~ 47010-47011
percutaneous ~ 47011
cyst ~ 47010-47011
percutaneous ~ 47011
Hernia repair
abdominal ~ 49590
incisional ~ 49560
recurrent ~ 49565
diaphragmatic ~ 39502-39541
epigastric ~ 49570
incarcerated ~ 49572
femoral ~ 49550
incarcerated ~ 49553
recurrent ~ 49555
recurrent incarcerated ~ 49557
incisional, incarcerated ~ 49561
inguinal ~ 49491, 49495-49500, 49505
incarcerated ~ 49492, 49496, 49501, 49507, 49521
laparoscopic ~ 49650-49651
recurrent ~ 49520
sliding ~ 49525
strangulated ~ 49492
lumbar ~ 49540
lung ~ 32800
orchiopexy ~ 54640
recurrent incisional
incarcerated ~ 49566
reducible ~ 49565
with spermatic cord ~ 55540
spigelian ~ 49590
umbilicus
incarcerated ~ 49582, 49587
reducible ~ 49580, 49585
Hernia, cerebral ~ see encephalocele
Hernia, rectovaginal ~ see rectocele
Hernia, umbilical ~ see omphalocele
Heroin, alkaloid screening ~ 82101
Heroin screen ~ 82486
Herpes simplex
antibody ~ 86696
antigen detection
immunofluorescence ~ 87273-87274
nucleic acid ~ 87528-87530
identification smear and stain ~ 87207
Herpes smear and stain ~ 87207
Herpes virus-4 (gamma), human ~ see Epstein-Barr virus
Herpes virus-6 (six) detection ~ 87531-87533
Herpetic vesicle destruction ~ 54050-54065
Heteroantibodies ~ see antibody, heterophile
Heterograft, skin ~ 15400
Heterologous transplant ~ see xenograft
Heterologous transplantation ~ see heterograft
Heterophile antibody ~ 86308-86310

Heterotropia ~ see strabismus
Hex b ~ see b-hexosaminidase
Hexadecadrol ~ see dexamethasone
Hexosephosphate isomerase ~ see phosphohexose isomerase
Heyman procedure ~ 27179, 28264
Hgb (hemoglobin) ~ 85018
HGH (human growth hormone) ~ 80418, 80428, 80430, 83003, 86277
Hg factor ~ see glucagon
HHV-4 ~ see Epstein-Barr virus
HIAA (hydroxyindolacetic acid, urine) 83497
Hibb operation ~ 22841
Hib vaccine
4 dose schedule
HbOC ~ 90645
PRP-T ~ 90648
PRP-D
booster ~ 90646
PRP-OMP
3 dose schedule ~ 90647
Hickmann catheterization ~ see cannulization; catheterization, venous, central line; venipuncture
Hidradenitis (see also sweat gland)
excision ~ 11450-11471
suppurative, incision and drainage ~ 10060-10061
Highly selective vagotomy ~ see vagotomy, highly selective
Highmore antrum ~ see sinuses, maxillary
High altitude simulation test ~ 94452-94453
High density lipoprotein ~ 83718
High molecular weight kininogen ~ 85293
Hill procedure ~ 43324
laparoscopic ~ 43280
Hinton positive ~ 86592, 86593
Hip joint
arthroplasty ~ 27132
revision ~ 27134-27138
arthrotomy ~ 27052
biopsy ~ 27052
capsulotomy, with release, flexor muscles ~ 27036
dislocation ~ 27250-27252
congenital ~ 27256-27259
open treatment ~ 27253-27254
without trauma ~ 27265-27266
manipulation ~ 27275
reconstruction, revision ~ 27134-27138
synovium
excision ~ 27054
arthroscopic ~ 29863
total replacement ~ 27132
Hip ~ see also femur; pelvis
abscess, incision and drainage ~ 26990
arthrocentesis ~ 20610
arthrodesis ~ 27284-27286
arthrography ~ 73525
arthroplasty ~ 27130-27132
arthroscopy ~ 29860-29863
arthrotomy ~ 27030-27033
Hip ~ ***continued***
biopsy ~ 27040-27041
bone, drainage ~ 26992
bursa, incision and drainage ~ 26991
capsulectomy with release, flexor muscles ~ 27036
cast ~ 29305-29325
craterization ~ 27070
cyst, excision ~ 27065-27067
denervation ~ 27035
echography, infant ~ 76885-76886
endoprosthesis ~ see prosthesis, hip
excision ~ 27070
exploration ~ 27033
fasciotomy ~ 27025
fusion ~ 27284-27286
hematoma, incision and drainage ~ 26990
injectio, radiologic ~ 27093-27096
reconstruction, total replacement ~ 27130
removal
cast ~ 29710
foreign body ~ 27033, 27086-27087
arthroscopic ~ 29861
loose body
arthroscopic ~ 29861
prosthesis ~ 27090-27091
repair
muscle transfer ~ 27100-27105, 27111
osteotomy ~ 27146-27156
tendon ~ 27097
saucerization ~ 27070
stem prosthesis ~ see arthroplasty, hip
strapping ~ 29520
tenotomy
abductor tendon ~ 27006
adductor tendon ~ 27000-27003
iliopsoas ~ 27005
total replacement ~ 27130-27132
tumor
excision ~ 27047-27049, 27065-27067
radical ~ 27075-27076
ultrasound, infant ~ 76885-76886
X-ray ~ 73500-73520, 73540
with contrast ~ 73525
intraoperative ~ 73530
Hip stem prostheses ~ see arthroplasty, hip
Hippocampus excision ~ 61566
Histamine ~ 83088
Histamine release test ~ 86343
Histochemistry ~ 88318-88319
Histocompatibility testing ~ see tissue typing
Histoplasma
antibody ~ 86698
antigen ~ 87385
Histoplasma capsulatum, antigen detection, enzyme immunoassay ~ 87385
Histoplasmin test ~ see histoplasmosis, skin test
Histoplasmoses ~ see histoplasmosis
Histoplasmosis skin test ~ 86510
History and physical ~ 57410

HIV
antibody ~ 86701-86703
confirmation test ~ 86689
HIV-1
antigen detection
enzyme immunoassay ~ 87390
HIV-2
antigen detection
enzyme immunoassay ~ 87391
HK3 kallikrein ~ see prostate specific antigen
HLA typing ~ 86812-86817
HMRK ~ see Fitzgerald factor
HMW kininogen ~ see Fitzgerald factor
Hoffman apparatus ~ 20690
Hofmeister operation (gastrectomy, total) ~ 43632
Holographic imaging ~ 76375
Holten test ~ 82575
Home health services ~ 99500-99600
activities of daily living ~ 99509
apnea care ~ 94774-94777
catheter care ~ 99507
enema administration ~ 99511
established patient ~ 99347-99350
hemodialysis ~ 99512
home infusion procedures ~ 99601-99602
individual or family counseling ~ 99510
intramuscular injections ~ 99506
mechanical ventilation ~ 99504
newborn care ~ 99502
new patient ~ 99341-99345
postnatal assessment ~ 99501
prenatal monitoring ~ 99500
respiratory therapy ~ 99503
sleep studies ~ 95805-95811
stoma care ~ 99505
unlisted services and procedures ~ 99600
Home visits ~ 99341-99350
Homocystine ~ 83090
urine ~ 82615
Homogenization, tissue ~ 87176
Homograft, skin ~ 15350
Homologous grafts ~ see graft
Homologous transplantation ~ see homograft
Homovanillic acid, urine ~ 83150
Hormone adrenocorticotrophic (ACTH) ~ 80400-80406, 80412, 80418, 82024
corticotropic-releasing ~ 80412
growth ~ see human growth hormone
human growth ~ 80418, 80428, 80430, 86277, 83003
interstitial cell-stimulating ~ see luteinizing hormone (LH)
luteinizing hormone (LH) ~ 80418, 80426, 83002
parathyroid ~ 83970
pituitary lactogenic (prolactin) ~ 80418, 80440, 84146
placental lactogen ~ 83632
somatotropin release-inhibiting (somatostatin) ~ 84307
Hormone adrenocorticotrophic (ACTH) ~ ***continued***
thyroid-stimulating (TSH) ~ 80418, 80438-80440, 80443
Hormone-binding globulin, sex ~ see globulin, sex hormone binding
Hormones, adrenal cortex ~ see corticosteroids
Hormones, antidiuretic ~ see antidiuretic hormone
Hormone assay
ACTH ~ 82024
aldosterone, blood or urine ~ 82088
androstenedione, blood or urine ~ 82157
androsterone, blood or urine ~ 82160
angiotensin II ~ 82163
corticosterone ~ 82528
cortisol, total ~ 82533
dehydroepiandrosterone ~ 82626
dihydroelestosterone ~ 82651
dihydrotestosterone ~ 82651
epiandrosterone ~ 82666
estradiol ~ 82670
estriol ~ 82677
estrogen ~ 82671-82672
estrone ~ 82679
follicle stimulating hormone (FSH) ~ 83001
growth hormone, human ~ 83003
hydroxyprogesterone ~ 83498-83499
luteinizing hormone ~ 83002
somatotropin ~ 83003
testosterone ~ 84403
vasopressin ~ 84588
Hormone pellet implantation ~ 11980
Hospital discharge services ~ 99238-99239
Hospital services ~ 99217-99239
inpatient services ~ 99238-99239
discharge services ~ 99238-99239
initial care, new or established patient ~ 99221-99223
initial hospital care ~ 99221-99223
newborn ~ 99431-99433
prolonged services ~ 99356-99357
subsequent hospital care ~ 99231-99233
observation
discharge services ~ 99234-99236
initial care ~ 99218-99220
new or established patient ~ 99218-99220
same day admission, discharges services ~ 99234-99236
subsequent newborn care ~ 99433
Hot pack treatment ~ 97010
House calls ~ 99341-99350
Howard test ~ 52005
HPL ~ (lactogen, human placental) 83632
HTLV I antibody
confirmatory test ~ 86689
detection ~ 86687
HTLV II antibody ~ 86688
HTLV III ~ see HIV
HTLV III antibodies ~ see antibody, HIV
HTLV IV ~ see HIV-2
Hubbard tank therapy ~ 97036, 97113

Hue test ~ 92283
Huggin operation ~ 54520
Huhner test ~ 89300, 89320
Human chorionic gonadotropin ~ see chorionic gonadotropin
Human chorionic somatomammotropin ~ see lactogen, human placental
Human cytomegalovirus group ~ see cytomegalovirus
Human growth hormone(HGH) ~ 80418, 80428-80430
Human herpes virus 4 ~ see Epstein-Barr virus
Human immunodeficiency virus ~ see HIV
Human immunodeficiency virus 1 ~ see HIV-1
Human immunodeficiency virus 2 ~ see HIV-2
Human papillomavirus detection ~ 87620-87622
Human placental lactogen ~ 83632
Human T cell leukemia virus I ~ see HTLV I
Human T cell leukemia virus II ~ see HTLV II
Human T cell leukemia virus I antibodies ~ see antibody, HTLV IHuman T cell leukemia virus II antibodies ~ see antibody, HTLV II
Humeral epicondylitides, lateral (tennis elbow) ~ 24350-24356
Humeral fracture ~ see fracture, humerus
Humerus ~ see arm, upper; shoulder
abscess
incision and drainage ~ 23935
craterization ~ 23184, 24140
cyst
excision ~ 23150, 24110
with allograft ~ 23156, 24116
with autograft ~ 23155, 24115
diaphysectomy ~ 23184, 24140
excision ~ 23174, 23184, 23195, 24134, 24140, 24150-24151
fracture
closed treatment ~ 24500-24505
with manipulation ~ 23605
without manipulation ~ 23600
condyle
closed treatment ~ 24576-24577
open treatment ~ 24579
percutaneous fixation ~ 24582
epicondyle
closed treatment ~ 24560-24565
open treatment ~ 24575
skeletal fixation, percutaneous ~ 24566
greater tuberosity fracture
closed treatment with manipulation ~ 23625
closed treatment without manipulation ~ 23620
open treatment ~ 23630
open treatment ~ 23615-23616
shaft ~ 24500-24505, 24516
Humerus ~ *continued*
open treatment ~ 24515
supracondylar
closed treatment ~ 24530-24535
open treatment ~ 24545-24546
percutaneous fixation ~ 24538
transcondylar
closed treatment ~ 24530-24535
open treatment ~ 24545-24546
percutaneous fixation ~ 24538
with dislocation ~ 23665-23670
osteomyelitis ~ 24134
pinning, wiring ~ 23491, 24498
prophylactic treatment ~ 23491, 24498
radical resection ~ 23220-23222
repair ~ 24430
with graft ~ 24435
nonunion, malunion ~ 24430-24435
osteoplasty ~ 24420
osteotomy ~ 24400-24410
resection head ~ 23195
saucerization ~ 23184, 24140
sequestrectomy ~ 23174, 24134
tumor
excision ~ 23150, 23220-23222, 24110
with allograft ~ 23156, 24116
with autograft ~ 23155, 24115
X-ray ~ 73060
Hummelshein operation ~ see strabismus, repair
Humor shunt, aqueous ~ 66180, 66185
HVA (homovanillic acid) ~ 83150
Hyaluron binding assay ~ 0087T
Hybridization probes, DNA ~ see nucleic acid probe
Hydatid disease ~ see echinococcosis
Hydatidiform mole
evacuation and curettage ~ 59870
excision ~ 59100
Hydration ~ 90760-90761
Hydrocarbons, chlorinated ~ 82441
Hydrocele
aspiration ~ 55000
excision
bilateral, tunica vaginalis ~ 55041
unilateral
spermatic cord ~ 55500
tunica vaginalis ~ 55040
repair ~ 55060
Hydrochloric acid, gastric ~ see acid, gastric
Hydrochloride, vancomycin ~ see vancomycin
Hydrocodon ~ see dihydrocodeinone
Hydrogen ion concentration ~ see pH
Hydrolase, acetylcholine ~ see acetylcholinesterase
Hydrolase, triacylglycerol ~ see lipase
Hydrolases, phosphoric monoester ~ see phosphatase
Hydrotherapy (Hubbard tank) ~ 97036, 97113
Hydrotubation ~ 58350
Hydroxyacetanilide ~ see acetaminophen

Hydroxycorticosteroid ~ 83491
Hydroxyindolacetic acid ~ 83497
urine ~ 83497
Hydroxypregnenolone ~ 80406, 84143
Hydroxyprogesterone ~ 80402-80406, 83498-83499
Hydroxyproline ~ 83500-83505
Hydroxytyramine ~ see dopamine
Hygroma, cystic, axillary/cervical, excision ~ 38550-38555
Hymen
excision ~ 56700
incision ~ 56442
Hymenal ring
revision ~ 56700
Hymenectomy ~ 56700
Hymenotomy ~ 56442
Hyoid
bone, fracture
closed treatment
with manipulation ~ 21494
without manipulation ~ 21493
open treatment ~ 21495
muscle, incision and suspension ~ 21685
Hyperbaric oxygen pressurization ~ 99183
Hypercycloidal X-ray ~ 76101-76102
Hyperdactylies ~ see supernumerary digit
Hyperglycemic glycogenolytic factor ~ see glucagon
Hypertelorism of orbit ~ see orbital hypertelorism
Hyperthermia therapy ~ see thermotherapy
Hyperthermia treatment ~ 77600-77620
Hypnotherapy ~ 90880
Hypodermis ~ see subcutaneous tissue
Hypogastric plexus
destruction ~ 64681
injection
anesthetic ~ 64517
neurolytic ~ 64681
Hypoglossal-facial anastomosis ~ see anastomosis, nerve, facial to hypoglossal
Hypoglossal nerve
anastomosis, to facial nerve ~ 64868
Hypopharynges ~ see hypopharynx
Hypopharynx, biopsy ~ 42802
Hypophysectomy ~ 61546-61548, 62165
Hypophysis ~ see pituitary gland
Hypopyrexia ~ see hypothermia
Hypospadias repair ~ 54300, 54352
complications ~ 54340-54348
first stage ~ 54304
proximal penile or penoscrotal ~ 54332
one stage
meatal advancement ~ 54322
perineal ~ 54336
urethroplasty
local skin flaps ~ 54324
local skin flaps and mobilization of urethra ~ 54326
local skin flaps, skin graft patch and/or island flap ~ 54328
Hypospadias repair ~ *continued*
urethroplasty for second stage ~ 54308-54316
free skin graft ~ 54316
urethroplasty for third stage ~ 54318
Hypothermia ~ 99185-99186
Hypoxia
breathing response ~ 94450
high altitude simulation test ~ 94452-94453
Hysterectomy
abdominal
radical ~ 58210
resection of ovarian malignancy ~ 58951, 58953-58956
supracervical ~ 58180
total ~ 58150, 58200, 58956
with colpo-urethrocystopexy ~ 58152
with partial vaginectomy ~ 58200
with omentectomy ~ 58956
cesarean
after cesarean delivery ~ 59525
with closure of vesicouterine fistula ~ 51925
laparoscopic ~ 58541-58544
radical ~ 58548
removal lesion ~ 59100
supracervical
laparoscopic ~ 58541-58544
vaginal ~ 58260-58270, 58290-58294, 58550-58554
with colpectomy ~ 58275-58280
with colpo-urethrocystopexy ~ 58267, 58293
laparoscopic ~ 58550
radical ~ 58285
removal tubes/ovaries ~ 58262-58263, 58291-58292, 58552, 58554
repair of enterocele ~ 58263, 58292, 58294
Hysterolysis ~ 58559
Hysteroplasty ~ 58540
Hysterorrhaphy ~ 58520, 59350
Hysterosalpingography ~ 74740
catheterization ~ 58345
injection procedure ~ 58340
Hysterosalpingostomy ~ see implantation, tubouterine
Hysteroscopy
ablation, endometrial ~ 58563
diagnostic ~ 58555
lysis adhesions ~ 58559
placement fallopian tube implants ~ 58565
removal
impacted foreign body ~ 58562
leiomyomata ~ 58561
resection of intrauterine septum ~ 58560
surgical with biopsy ~ 58558
unlisted services and procedures ~ 58579
Hysterosonography ~ 76831
Hysterotomy ~ 59100
induced abortion
with amniotic injections ~ 59852
with vaginal suppositories ~ 59857
Hysterotrachelectomy ~ 57530

I

I, angiotensin ~ see angiotensin I
1 antibodies, HTLV ~ see antibody, HTLV-1
I, coagulation factor ~ see fibrinogenI, heparin cofactor ~ see antithrombin
IIIICCE ~ see extraction, lens, intracapsular
Ichthyosis, sex linked ~ see syphilis test
ICSH ~ see luteinizing hormone (LH)
Identification
  oocyte, from follicular fluid ~ 89254
  sperm
    from aspiration ~ 89257
    from tissue ~ 89264
IDH (isocitric dehydrogenase, blood) ~ 83570
Ig ~ see immune globulins
IgE ~ 86003-86005
IgG ~ 86001
II, coagulation factor ~ see prothrombin
II, cranial nerve ~ see optic nerve
Ileal conduit visualization ~ 50690
Ileoscopy via stoma ~ 44383
Ileostomy ~ 44310, 45136
  continent (Kock procedure) ~ 44316
  revision ~ 44312-44314
Iliac arteries ~ see artery, iliac
Iliac crest (free osteocutaneous flap with microvascular anastomosis) ~ 20970
Iliohypogastric nerve, injection anesthetic ~ 64425
Ilioinguinal nerve, injection anesthetic ~ 64425
Ilium
  craterization ~ 27070
  cyst excision ~ 27065-27067
  excision ~ 27070
  fracture, open treatment ~ 27215, 27218
  saucerization ~ 27070
  tumor excision ~ 27065-27067
Ilizarov procedure, Monticelli type ~ (see also application, bone fixation device) 20692
Imaging ~ see vascular studies
Imaging, gamma camera ~ see nuclear medicine
Imaging, magnetic resonance ~ see magnetic resonance imaging (MRI)
Imaging, ultrasonic ~ see echography
Imbrication, diaphragm ~ 39545
Imidobenzyle ~ 80174
Imipramine assay ~ 80174
Immune complex assay ~ 86332
Immune globulins ~ 90281-90399
  antitoxin
    botulinum ~ 90287
    diphtheria ~ 90296
  botulism ~ 90288
  cytomegalovirus ~ 90291
  hepatitis B ~ 90371
  human ~ 90281-90283
Immune globulins ~ *continued*
  rabies ~ 90375-90376
  respiratory syncytial virus ~ 90378-90379
  Rho (D) ~ 90384-90386
  tetanus ~ 90389
  unlisted immune globulin ~ 90399
  vaccinia ~ 90393
  varicella-zoster ~ 90396
Immune globulin administration ~ 90780-90784
Immune globulin E ~ 86003-86005
Immunization administration ~ 90465-90474
  one vaccine/toxoid ~ 90471, 90473
    with counseling ~ 90465, 90467
  each additional vaccine/toxoid ~ 90472, 90474
    with counseling ~ 90466, 90468
Immunizations
  active
    acellular pertussis ~ 90700, 90721-90723
    BCG ~ 90585, 90586
    cholera ~ 90725
    diphtheria ~ 90700-90702, 90718-90723
    diphtheria, tetanus, pertussis (DTP) ~ 90701, 90720
    diphtheria, tetanus, acellular influenza B and poliovirus inactivated ~ 90698
    hemophilus influenza B ~ 90645-90648, 90720-90721, 90748
    hepatitis A ~ 90632-90636
    hepatitis B ~ 90740-90748
    influenza ~ 90655-90660
    influenza B ~ 90645-90648
    Japanese encephalitis ~ 90735
    Lyme disease ~ 90665
    measles ~ 90705
    measles, mumps, rubella (MMR) ~ 90707
    measles, mumps, rubella, varicella ~ 90710
    measles, rubella ~ 90708
    meingococcal ~ 90733, 90734
    mumps ~ 90704
    plague ~ 90727
    pneumococcal ~ 90732
    poliomyelitis ~ 90713
    poliovirus ~ 90712
    rabies ~ 90675, 90676
    rotavirus vaccine ~ 90680
    rubella ~ 90706
    tetanus ~ 90700-90703, 90715, 90718, 90720-90723
    typhoid ~ 90690-90693
    varicella (chicken pox) ~ 90716
    yellow fever ~ 90717
  passive
    hyperimmune serum globulin ~ 90287-90399
    immune serum globulin ~ 90281, 90283
  unlisted services and procedures ~ 90749
Immunoassay
  analyte ~ 83519-83520
  infectious agent ~ 86317-86318, 87449-87451
  nonantibody ~ 83516-83519
  tumor antigen ~ 86294, 86316
    CA 125 ~ 86304

Immunoassay ~ *continued*
CA 15-3 ~ 86300
CA 19-9 ~ 86301
Immunoblotting, Western ~ see Western Blot
Immunochemical, lysozyme (muramidase) ~ see lysozyme
Immunocytochemistry ~ 88342
Immunodeficiency virus, human ~ see HIV
Immunodeficiency virus type 1 , human ~ see HIV 1
Immunodeficiency virus type 2 , human ~ see HIV 2
Immunodiffusion ~ 86329-86331
Immunoelectrophoresis ~ 86320-86327, 86334-86335
Immunofixation electrophoresis ~ 86334-86335
Immunofluorescent study ~ 88346-88347
Immunogen ~ see antigen
Immunoglobulin ~ 82787
platelet associated ~ 86023
thyroid stimulating ~ 84445
Immunoglobulin E ~ 86003-86005
Immunoglobulin receptor assay ~ 86243
Immunologic skin test ~ see skin, tests
Immunology ~ 86000-86849
Immunotherapies, allergen ~ see allergen immunotherapy
Impedance testing ~ (see also audiologic function tests) 92567
Imperfectly descended testis ~ 54550, 54560
Implantation
artificial heart, intracorporeal ~ 0051T
bone, for external speech processor/cochlear stimulator ~ 69714-69718
brain
chemotherapy ~ 61517
thermal perfusion probe ~ 0077T
cardiac event recorder ~ 33282
contraceptive capsules ~ 11975, 11977
drug delivery device ~ 11981, 11983, 61517
electrode
brain ~ 61850-61875
gastric implantation
laparoscopic
neurostimulator ~ 43647
stimulator ~ 0155T
open
neurostimulator ~ 43881
stimulator ~ 0157T
nerve ~ 64553-64581
spinal cord ~ 63650-63655
eye
anterior segment ~ 65920
aqueous shunt to extraocular placement or replacement of pegs ~ 65125
posterior segment
extraocular ~ 67120
intraocular ~ 67121
reservoir ~ 66180
vitreous, drug delivery system ~ 67027
fallopian tube ~ 58565

Implantation ~ *continued*
hearing aid hormone pellet(s)
bone conduction ~ 69710
hip prosthesis ~ see arthroplasty, hip
hormone pellet ~ 11980
intraocular lens ~ see insertion, intraocular lens
joint ~ see arthroplasty
mesh
hernia repair ~ 49568
vaginal repair ~ 57267
nerve
into bone ~ 64787
into muscle ~ 64787
neurostimulators
gastric
implantation
laparoscopic
neurostimulator ~ 43647
stimulation ~ 0155T
oprn
neurostimulator ~ 43881
stimulator ~ 0157T
pulse generator ~ 61885
receiver ~ 61886
ovum ~ 58976
pulse generator
brain ~ 61885-61886
spinal cord electrode array ~ 63685
receiver
brain ~ 61885-61886
nerve ~ 64590
spinal cord ~ 63685
removal ~ 20670-20680
elbow ~ 24164
radius ~ 24164
reservoir vascular access device
declotting ~ 36550
total replacement heart system
intracorporeal ~ 0051T
tubouterine ~ 58752
ventricular assist device ~ 33976
extracorporeal ~ 0048T
intracorporeal ~ 33979
Implant removal ~ see specific anatomical site
Impression, maxillofacial
auricular prosthesis ~ 21086
definitive obturator prosthesis ~ 21080
facial prosthesis ~ 21088
interim obturator ~ 21079
mandibular resection prosthesis ~ 21081
nasal prosthesis ~ 21087
oral surgical splint ~ 21085
orbital prosthesis ~ 21077
palatal augmentation prosthesis ~ 21082
palatal lift prosthesis ~ 21083
speech aid prosthesis ~ 21084
surgical obturator ~ 21076
In situ hybridization ~ see nucleic acid probe, cytogenetic studies, morphometric analysis
IM injection ~ see injection, intramuscular
In vitro fertilization ~ 58321-58322

Incision ~ *continued*
leg, upper fasciotomy ~ 27305
tenotomy ~ 27306-27307, 27390-27392
lip, frenum ~ 40806
liver ~ see hepatotomy
lung
biopsy ~ 32095-32100
decortication
partial ~ 32225
total ~ 32220
lymphatic channels ~ 38308
mastoid ~ see mastoidotomy
medullary tract ~ 61470
mesencephalic tract ~ 61480
metacarpophalangeal joint capsule ~ 26520
mitral valve ~ 33420-33422
muscle ~ see myotomy
nerve ~ 64573-64580, 64585, 64595, 64702-64772
foot ~ 28035
root ~ 63185-63190
sacral ~ 64581
vagus ~ 43640-43641
nose ~ see rhinotomy
orbit ~ see orbitotomy
palm fasciotomy ~ 26040-26045
pancreas sphincter ~ 43262
penis
prepuce ~ 54000-54001
newborn ~ 54000
pericardium
with clot removal ~ 33020
with foreign body removal ~ 33020
with tube ~ 33015
pharynx stoma ~ 42955
pleura biopsy ~ 32095-32100
pleural cavity
empyema ~ 32035-32036
pneumothorax ~ 32020
prostate
exposure
bilateral pelvic lymphadenectomy ~ 55865
insertion radioactive substance ~ 55860
lymph node biopsy ~ 55862
transurethral ~ 52450
pterygomaxillary fossa ~ 31040
pulmonary valve ~ 33470-33474
pyloric sphincter ~ 43520
retina, encircling material ~ 67115
sclera
fistulization
iridencleisis or iridotasis ~ 66165
sclerectomy with punch or scissors with iridectomy ~ 66160
thermocauterization with iridectomy ~ 66155
trabeculectomy ab externo in absence previous surgery ~ 66170
trephination with iridectomy ~ 66150
semicircular canal
fenestration ~ 69820
revision ~ 69840

Incision ~ *continued*
seminal vesicle ~ 55600-55605
complicated ~ 55605
shoulder
bone ~ 23035
capsular contracture release ~ 23020
removal, calcareous deposits ~ 23000
tenomyotomy ~ 23405-23406
shoulder joint ~ 23040-23044
sinus
frontal ~ 31070-31087
maxillary ~ 31020-31032
endoscopic ~ 31256-31267
multiple ~ 31090
sphenoid
sinusotomy ~ 31050-31051
skin ~ 10040-10180
skull ~ 61316, 62148
suture ~ 61550-61552
spinal cord ~ 63200
tract ~ 63170, 63194-63199
stomach
creation, stoma ~ 43830-43832
exploration ~ 43500
pyloric sphincter ~ 43520
synovectomy ~ 26140
temporomandibular joint ~ 21010
tendon, arm, upper ~ 24310
thigh, fasciotomy ~ 27025
thorax
empyema ~ 32035-32036
pneumothorax ~ 32020
thyroid gland ~ see thyrotomy
tibia ~ 27607
toe
capsule ~ 28270-28272
fasciotomy ~ 28008
tendon ~ 28232-28234
tenotomy ~ 28010-28011
tongue, frenum ~ 41010
trachea
emergency ~ 31603-31605
planned ~ 31600-31601
with flaps ~ 31610
tympanic membrane ~ 69420
with anesthesia ~ 69421
ureter ~ 50600
ureterocele ~ 51535
urethra ~ 53000-53010
meatus ~ 53020-53025
uterus, remove lesion ~ 59100
vagina, exploration ~ 57000
vas deferens ~ 55200
for X-ray ~ 55300
vestibule of the mouth ~ see mouth, vestibule
vitreous strands
laser surgery ~ 67031
pars plana approach ~ 67030
wrist ~ 25100-25105
capsule ~ 25085
decompression ~ 25020-25025
tendon sheath ~ 25000-25001

Incisional hernia repair ~ see hernia, repair, incisional
Incision and drainage ~ see also drainage; incision
abdomen
fluid ~ 49080-49081
pancreatitis ~ 48000
abscess
abdomen ~ 49020, 49040
open ~ 49040
percutaneous ~ 49021
anal ~ 46045-46050
ankle ~ 27603
appendix ~ 44900
open ~ 44900
percutaneous ~ 44901
arm, lower ~ 25028
arm, upper ~ 23930-23931
auditory canal, external ~ 69020
Bartholin's gland ~ 56420
bladder ~ 51080
brain ~ 61320-61321
breast ~ 19020
ear, external
complicated ~ 69005
simple ~ 69000
elbow ~ 23930
epididymis ~ 54700
eyelid ~ 67700
finger ~ 26010-26011
gums ~ 41800
hip ~ 26990
kidney ~ 50020
open ~ 50020
percutaneous ~ 50021
knee ~ 27301
leg, lower ~ 27603
leg, upper ~ 27301
liver ~ 47010
open ~ 47010
percutaneous ~ 47011
lung ~ 32200
percutaneous ~ 32201
lymph node ~ 38300-38305
mouth ~ 40800-40801, 41005-41009, 41015-41018
nasal septum ~ 30020
neck ~ 21501-21502
nose ~ 30000-30020
ovary ~ 58820-58822
abdominal approach ~ 58822
palate ~ 42000
paraurethral gland ~ 53060
parotid gland ~ 42300-42305
pelvis ~ 26990, 45000
perineum ~ 56405
peritoneum ~ 49020
percutaneous ~ 49021
prostrate ~ 55720-55725
rectum ~ 45005-45020, 46040, 46050-46060
retroperitoneal ~ 49060
open ~ 49060

Incision and drainage ~ *continued*
abscess ~ *continued*
salivary gland ~ 42300-42320
scrotum ~ 54700, 55100
Skene's gland ~ 53060
skin ~ 10060-10061
subdiaphragmatic, percutaneous ~ 49040-49041
sublingual gland ~ 42310-42320
submaxillary gland ~ 42310-42320
subphrenic, percutaneous ~ 49040-49041
testis ~ 54700
thorax ~ 21501-21502
throat ~ 42700-42725
tongue ~ 41000-41006, 41015
tonsil ~ 42700
urethra ~ 53040
uvula ~ 42000
vagina ~ 57010
vulva ~ 56405
wrist ~ 25028
ankle ~ 27610
bile duct ~ 47420-47425
bladder ~ 51040
bulla, skin, puncture aspiration ~ 10160
bursa
ankle ~ 27604
arm, lower ~ 25031
elbow ~ 23931
foot ~ 28001
hip ~ 26991
knee ~ 27301
leg, lower ~ 27604
leg, upper ~ 27301
palm ~ 26025-26030
pelvis ~ 26991
wrist ~ 25031
carbuncle
skin ~ 10060-10061
carpals ~ 25035, 26034
comedones
skin ~ 10040
cyst
conjunctiva ~ 68020
gums ~ 41800
liver
open ~ 47010
percutaneous ~ 47011
lung ~ 32200
percutaneous ~ 32201
mouth ~ 40800-40801, 41005-41009, 41015-41018
ovarian ~ 58800-58805
skin ~ 10040-10061
pilonidal ~ 10080-10081
puncture aspiration ~ 10160
spinal cord ~ 63172-63173
thyroid gland ~ 60000
tongue ~ 41000-41006, 41015, 60000
elbow
abscess ~ 23935
arthrotomy ~ 24000

Incision and drainage ~ *continued*
femur ~ 27303
fluid collection
skin ~ 10140
foreign body, skin ~ 10120-10121
furuncle ~ 10060-10061
gallbladder ~ 47480
hematoma
ankle ~ 27603
arm, lower ~ 25028
arm, upper ~ 23930
brain ~ 61312-61315
ear, external
complicated ~ 69005
simple ~ 69000
elbow ~ 23930
epididymis ~ 54700
gums ~ 41800
hip ~ 26990
knee ~ 27301
leg, lower ~ 27603
leg, upper ~ 27301
mouth ~ 40800-40801, 41005-41009, 41015-41018
nasal septum ~ 30020
neck ~ 21501-21502
nose ~ 30000-30020
pelvis ~ 26990
scrotum ~ 54700
skin ~ 10140
puncture aspiration ~ 10160
skull ~ 61312-61315
testis ~ 54700
thorax ~ 21501-21502
tongue ~ 41000-41006, 41015
vagina ~ 57022-57023
wrist ~ 25028
hepatic duct ~ 47400
hip bone ~ 26992, 27030
humerus abscess ~ 23935
interphalangeal joint
toe ~ 28024
intertarsal joint ~ 28020
kidney ~ 50040, 50125
knee ~ 27303, 27310
lacrimal gland ~ 68400
lacrimal sac ~ 68420
liver
abscess or cyst ~ 47010-47011
percutaneous ~ 47011
mediastinum ~ 39000-39010
metatarsophalangeal joint ~ 28022
milia, multiple ~ 10040
onychia ~ 10060-10061
orbit ~ 67405, 67440
paronychia ~ 10060-10061
pelvic bone ~ 26992
penis ~ 54015
pericardium ~ 33025
phalanges, finger ~ 26034
pilonidal cyst ~ 10080-10081

Incision and drainage ~ *continued*
pustules, skin ~ 10040
radius ~ 25035
seroma, skin ~ 10140
shoulder
abscess ~ 23030
arthrotomy
acromioclavicular joint ~ 23044
sternoclavicular joint ~ 23044
bursa ~ 23031
hematoma ~ 23030
shoulder joint, arthrotomy, glenohumeral joint ~ 23040
tarsometatarsal joint ~ 28020
tendon sheath
finger ~ 26020
palm ~ 26020
thorax
deep ~ 21510
toe ~ 28024
ulna ~ 25035
ureter ~ 50600
vagina ~ 57020
wound infection, skin ~ 10180
wrist ~ 25028, 25040
Inclusion bodies
fluid ~ 88106
smear ~ 87207-87210
Incomplete abortion ~ see abortion, incomplete
Indicator dilution studies ~ 93561-93562
Induced abortion ~ see abortion
Induced hyperthermia ~ see thermotherapy
Induced hypothermia ~ see hypothermia
Induratio penis plastica ~ see Peyronie disease
Infant, newborn, intensive care ~ see intensive care, neonatal
Infantile paralysis ~ see polio
Infection
actinomyces ~ see actinomycosis
bone ~ see osteomyelitis
filarioidea ~ see filariasis
immunoassay ~ 86317-86318
postoperative wound ~ see postoperative wound infection
rapid test ~ 86403-86406
wound ~ see wound, infection
Infectious agent
antigen detection
direct fluorescence ~ 87265-87272, 87276, 87278, 87280, 87285-87290
bordetella ~ 87265
chlamydia trachomatis ~ 87270
cryptosporidium ~ 87272
cytomegalovirus ~ 87271
enterovirus ~ 87267
giardia ~ 87269
influenza A ~ 87276
legionella pneumophila ~ 87278
respiratory syncytial virus ~ 87280
treponema pallidum ~ 87285
varicella-zoster ~ 87290

Infectious agent ~ *continued*
antigen detection ~ *continued*
enzyme immunoassay
adenovirus ~ 87301
aspergillus ~ 87305
chlamydia trachomatis ~ 87320
clostridium difficile ~ 87324
cryptococcus neoformans ~ 87327
cryptosporidium ~ 87328
cytomegalovirus ~ 87332
entamoeba histolytica dispar group ~ 87336
entamoeba histolytica group ~ 87337
escherichia coli 0157 ~ 87335
giardia ~ 87329
helicobacter pylori ~ 87338-87339
hepatitis B surface antigen (HBsAg) ~ 87340
hepatitis B surface antigen (HBsAg) neutralization ~ 87341
hepatitis Be antigen (HBeAg) ~ 87350
hepatitis, delta agent ~ 87380
histoplasma capsulatum ~ 87385
HIV-1 ~ 87390
HIV-2 ~ 87391
influenza A ~ 87400
influenza B ~ 87400
multiple step method ~ 87301-87449, 87451
not otherwise specified ~ 87449, 87451
respiratory syncytial virus ~ 87420
rotavirus ~ 87425
shiga-like toxin ~ 87427
single step method ~ 87450
streptococcus, group A ~ 87430
immunofluorescence ~ 87260, 87273-87275, 87277, 87279, 87281-87283, 87299-87300
adenovirus ~ 87260
herpes simplex ~ 87273-.87274
influenza B ~ 87275
legionella micdadei ~ 87277
not otherwise specified ~ 87299
parainfluenza virus ~ 87279
pneumocystis carinii ~ 87281
polyvalent ~ 87300
rubeola ~ 87283
concentration ~ 87015
detection
by immunoassay
with direct optical observation ~ 87802-87899
chlamydia trachomatis ~ 87810
clostridium difficile ~ 87803
influenza ~ 87804
neisseria gonorrheae ~ 87850
not otherwise specified ~ 87899
respiratory syncytial virus ~ 87807
streptococcus, group A ~ 87880
streptococcus, group B ~ 87802
trichomonas vaginalis ~ 87808
with direct optical observation ~ 87802-87899

Infectious agent ~ *continued*
detection ~ *continued*
by nucleic acid
bartonella henselae ~ 87470-87472
bartonella quintana ~ 87470-87472
borrelia burgdorferi ~ 87475-87477
candida species ~ 87480-87482
chlamydia pneumoniae ~ 87485-87487
chlamydia trachomatis ~ 87490-87492
cytomegalovirus ~ 87495-87497
enterovirus ~ 87498
gardnerella vaginalis ~ 87510-87512
hepatitis B virus ~ 87515-87517
hepatitis B ~ 87520-87522
hepatitis G ~ 87525-87527
herpes simplex virus ~ 87528-87530
herpes virus-6 (six) ~ 87531-87533
HIV-1 ~ 87534-87536
HIV-2 ~ 87537-87539
legionella pneumophila ~ 87540-87542
multiple organisms ~ 87800-87801
mycobacteria avium-intracellulare ~ 87560-87562
mycobacteria species ~ 87550-87552
mycobacteria tuberculosis ~ 87555-87557
mycoplasma pneumoniae ~ 87580-87582
neisseria gonorrheae ~ 87590-87592
not otherwise specified ~ 87797-87799
papillomavirus, human ~ 87620-87622
staphylococcus aureus ~ 87640-87641
streptococcus, group A ~ 87650-87652
streptococcus, group B ~ 87653
trichomonas vaginalis ~ 87660
urinalysis ~ 0041T
genotype analysis
by nucleic acid
hepatitis C virus ~ 87902
HIV-1 protease/reverse transcriptase ~ 87901
phenotype analysis
by nucleic acid
HIV-1 drug resistance ~ 87903-87904
phenotype prediction
by genetic database
HIV-1 drug resistance ~ 0023T
Infectious mononucleosis virus ~ see Epstein-Barr virus
Inflammatory process
localization
nuclear medicine ~ 78805-78807
Inflation
ear, middle
eustachian tube
with catheterization ~ 69400
without catheterization ~ 69401
eustachian tube
myringotomy ~ 69420
anesthesia ~ 69424
Influenza A
antigen detection
direct fluorescence ~ 87276
enzyme immunoassay ~ 87400

Influenza B
antigen detection
enzyme immunoassay ~ 87400
immunofluorescence ~ 87275
Influenza vaccine ~ see vaccines
Influenza virus
antibody ~ 86710
by immunoassay
with direct optical observation ~ 87804
Infraorbital nerve
avulsion ~ 64734
incision ~ 64734
transection ~ 64734
Infrared light treatment ~ 97026
Infratentorial craniectomy ~ 61520-61521
Infusion
amnion, transabdominal ~ 59072
cerebral, intravenous, for thrombolysis ~ 37195
intraosseous ~ 36680
radioelement ~ 77750
transcatheter therapy ~ 37201-37202
Infusion pump
electronic analysis, spinal cord ~ 62367-62368
insertion, intra-arterial ~ 36260
intra-arterial
removal ~ 36262
revision ~ 36261
intravenous
insertion ~ 36563
repair ~ 36576
replacement ~ 36583
maintenance ~ 95990-95991, 96520-96530
spinal cord ~ 62361-62362
ventricular catheter ~ 61215
Infusion therapy ~ 62350-62351, 62360-62362
arterial catheterization ~ 36640
chemotherapy ~ 96410-96414, 96422-96425
home infusion procedures ~ 99601-99602
intravenous ~ 90780-90781
pain ~ 62360-62362, 62367-62368
transcatheter therapy ~ 75896
Ingestion challenge test ~ 95075
Inguinal hernia repair ~ see hernia, repair, inguinal
INH ~ see drug assay
Inhalation pentamidine ~ 94642
Inhalation provocation tests ~ see bronchial challenge test
Inhalation treatment ~ (see also pulmonology, therapeutic) 94640, 94644-94645, 94664, 99503
Inhibin A ~ 86336
Inhibition test, hemagglutination ~ see hemagglutination inhibition test
Inhibition, fertilization ~ see contraception
Inhibitor, alpha 1-protease ~ see alpha-1 antitrypsin
Inhibitor, alpha 2-plasmin ~ see alpha-2 antiplasmin
Inhibitory concentration, minimum ~ see minimum inhibitory concentration
Initial inpatient consultations ~ see consultation, initial inpatient
Injection ~ see allergen immunotherapy; infusion
abdomen
air ~ 49400
contrast material ~ 49400
angiography, pulmonary ~ 75746
ankle, radial ~ 27648
antibiotic ~ see antibiotic administration
antigen (allergen) ~ 95115-95125
aorta (aortography), radiologic ~ 93544
aponeurosis ~ 20550
bladder, radiologic ~ 51600-51610
brain canal ~ 61070
bronchography, segmental ~ 31656
bursa ~ 20600-20610
cardiac catheterization ~ 93539-93545
carpal tunnel, therapeutic ~ 20526
chemotherapy ~ 96400-96450, 96542
cistern, medication or other ~ 61055
contrast, via catheter ~ 49424
corpora cavernosa ~ 54235
cyst
bone ~ 20615
kidney ~ 50390
pelvis ~ 50390
thyroid ~ 60001
elbow, arthrography, radiologic ~ 24220
epidural ~ see epidural, injection
esophageal varices, endoscopy ~ 43243
esophagus
sclerosing agent ~ 43204
submucosal ~ 43201
extremity, pseudoaneurysm ~ 36002
eye
air ~ 66020
medication ~ 66030
eyelid, subconjunctional ~ 68200
ganglion, anesthetic ~ 64505, 64510
ganglion cyst ~ 20612
gastric secretion stimulant ~ 91052
gastric varices, endoscopy ~ 43243
heart vessels
cardiac catheterization ~ 93539-93545
radiologic ~ 93545
hemorrhoids, sclerosing solution ~ 46500
hip, radiologic ~ 27093-27095
insect venom ~ 95130-95134
intervertebral disk
chemonucleolysis agent ~ 62292
radiological ~ 62290-62291
intraamniotic ~ 59852
intra-arterial
diagnostic ~ 90783
therapeutic ~ 90783
intradermal, for tattooing ~ 11920-11922
intralesional, skin ~ 11900-11901
intramuscular
antibiotic ~ 90788
diagnostic ~ 90782
therapeutic ~ 90782, 99506

Injection ~ *continued*
intravenous
diagnostic ~ 90784
therapeutic ~ 90784
vascular flow check, graft ~ 15860
joint ~ 20600-20610
kidney
drugs ~ 50391
radiologic ~ 50394
knee, radiologic ~ 27370
lacrimal gland, radiologic ~ 68850
left heart, radiologic ~ 93543
lesion, skin ~ 11900-11901
ligament ~ 20550
liver ~ 47015
radiologic ~ 47500-47505
mammary ductogram/galactogram ~ 19030
muscle endplate
cervical spine ~ 64613
extremity ~ 64614
facial ~ 64612
trunk ~ 64614
nerve
anesthetic ~ 01991-01992, 64400-64530
neurolytic agent ~ 64600-64681
orbit
retrobulbar
alcohol ~ 67505
medication ~ 67500
tenon's capsule ~ 67515
pancreatography ~ 48400
paraveretebral facet joint/nerve ~ 64470-64476
penis
for erection ~ 54235
Peyronie disease ~ 54200
with surgical exposure of plague ~ 54205
radiology ~ 54230
vasoactive drugs ~ 54231
peritoneal cavity air ~ see pneumoperitoneum
radiologic, breast ~ 19030
rectum, sclerosing solution ~ 45520
right heart ~ see cardiac catheterization, injection
radiologic ~ 93542
sacroiliac joint, for arthrography ~ 27096
salivary duct ~ 42660
salivary gland, radiologic ~ 42550
sclerosing agent
esophagus ~ 43204
intravenous ~ 36470-36471
sentinel node identification ~ 38792
shoulder, arthrography, radiologic ~ 23350
shunt, peritoneal, venous ~ 49427
sinus tract ~ 20500
diagnostic ~ 20501
spider veins, telangiectasia ~ 36468-36469
spinal artery ~ 62294
spinal cord
anesthetic ~ 62310-62319
blood ~ 62273
neurolytic agent ~ 62280-62282
other ~ 62310-62311

Injection ~ *continued*
radiological ~ 62284
steroids, urethral stricture ~ 52283
subcutaneous
diagnostic ~ 90782
silicone ~ 11950-11954
therapeutic ~ 90782
temporomandibular joint, arthrography ~ 21116
tendon origin, insertion ~ 20551
tendon sheath ~ 20550
therapeutic
extremity pseudoaneurysm ~ 36002
lung ~ 32960
thyroid ~ 60001
turbinate ~ 30200
thoracic cavity ~ see pleurodesis, chemical
trachea ~ 31612
puncture ~ 31612
transtracheal, bronchography ~ 31715
trigger point(s)
one or two muscles ~ 20552
two or more muscles ~ 20553
turbinate ~ 30200
unlisted services and procedures ~ 90799
ureter
drugs ~ 50391
radiologic ~ 50684
venography ~ 36005
ventricle
dye ~ 61120
medication or other ~ 61026
vitreous ~ 67028
fluid substitute ~ 67025
vocal cords, therapeutic ~ 31513, 31570-31571
wrist
carpal tunnel, therapeutic ~ 20526
radiologic ~ 25246
Inkblot test ~ 96101-96103
Inner ear ~ see ear, inner
Innominate arteries ~ see artery, brachiocephalic
Innominate tumor excision ~ 27077
Inorganic sulfates ~ see sulfate
Insemination, artificial ~ 58321-58322, 89268
Insertion ~ see also implantation; intubation; transplantation
baffle, ear, middle ~ 69410
balloon, intra-aortic ~ 33967, 33973
breast implants ~ 19340-19342
cannula
arteriovenous ~ 36810-36815
ECMO ~ 36822
extra corporeal circulation for regional chemotherapy of extremity ~ 36823
thoracic duct ~ 38794
vein to vein ~ 36800
catheter
abdomen ~ 49324, 49419-49421, 49435
abdominal artery ~ 36245-36248
aorta ~ 36200

Insertion ~ *continued*
bile duct ~ 47525-47530, 75982
percutaneous ~ 47510
bladder ~ 51045, 51701-51703
brachiocephalic artery ~ 36215-36218
brain ~ 61210, 61770
breast, for interstitial radioelement application ~ 19296-19298
bronchi ~ 31717
bronchus, for intracavitary radioelement application ~ 31643
cardiac ~ see catheterization, cardiac
flow directed ~ 93503
ear, middle ~ 69405
eustachian tube ~ 69405
gastrointestinal, upper ~ 43241
jejunum ~ 44015
kidney ~ 50392
lower extremity artery ~ 36245-36248
nasotracheal ~ 31720
pelvic artery ~ 36245-36248
pleural cavity ~ 32019
portal vein ~ 36481
prostate ~ 55875
pulmonary artery ~ 36013-36015
right heart ~ 36013
skull ~ 61107
spinal cord ~ 62350-62351
suprapubic ~ 51010
thoracic artery ~ 36215-36218
tracheobronchial ~ 31725
ureter via kidney ~ 50393
urethra ~ 51701-51703
vena cava ~ 36010
venous ~ 36011-36012, 36400-36410, 36420-36425, 36500-36510, 36555-36558, 36568-36569
cervical dilation ~ 59200
cochlear device ~ 69930
contraceptive capsules ~ 11975, 11977
drug delivery implant ~ 11981, 11983
electrode
brain ~ 61531-61533, 61760, 61850-61875
heart ~ 33202-33203, 33210-33211, 33216-33217, 33224-33225, 93620-93622
nerve ~ 64553-64581
sphenoidal ~ 95830
spinal cord ~ 63650-63655
endotracheal tube ~ 31500
gastrostomy tube
laparoscopic ~ 43653
percutaneous ~ 43750
graft
aorta ~ 33330-33335
heart vessel ~ 33330-33335
guide, kidney pelvis ~ 50395
guide wire
endoscopy ~ 43248
esophagoscopy ~ 43248
with dilation ~ 43226

Insertion ~ *continued*
Heyman capsule, uterus
for brachytherapy ~ 58346
iliac artery occlusion device ~ 34808
implant, bone
for external speech processor/cochlear stimulator ~ 69714-69718
infusion pump
intra-arterial ~ 36260
intravenous ~ 36563
spinal cord ~ 62361-62362
intracatheter/needle
aorta ~ 36160
arteriovenous shunt ~ 36145
intra-arterial ~ 36100-36140
intravenous ~ 36000
kidney ~ 50392
intraocular lens ~ 66983
manual or mechanical technique ~ 66982, 66984
not associated with concurrent cataract removal ~ 66985
intrauterine device (IUD) ~ 58300
IVC filter ~ 75940
jejunostomy tube, endoscopy ~ 44372
keel, laryngoplasty ~ 31580
laminaria ~ 59200
mesh, pelvic floor ~ 57267
nasobiliary tube, endoscopy ~ 43267
nasopancreatic tube, endoscopy ~ 43267
needle
bone ~ 36680
intraosseous ~ 36680
prostate ~ 55875-55876
needle wire, trachea ~ 31730
neurostimulator
pulse generator ~ 64590
receiver ~ 64590
nose, septal prosthesis ~ 30220
obturator, larynx ~ 31527
ocular implant
with/without conjunctival graft ~ 65150
with foreign material ~ 65155
muscles attached ~ 65140
muscles, not attached ~ 65135
in scleral shell ~ 65130
orbital transplant ~ 67550
oviduct
chromotubation ~ 58350
hydrotubation ~ 58350
ovoid, vagina, for brachytherapy ~ 57155
pacemaker
fluoroscopy/radiography ~ 71090
heart ~ 33206-33208, 33212-33213
pacing cardio-defibrillator
leads ~ 33216-33220, 33224-33225, 33243-33244
pulse generator only ~ 33240-33241
packing, vagina ~ 57180
penile prosthesis, inflatable ~ see penile prosthesis, insertion, inflatable

Insertion ~ ***continued***
pessary, vagina ~ 57160
pin, skeletal traction ~ 20650
probe, brain ~ 61770
prostaglandin ~ 59200
prostate, radioactive substance ~ 55860
prosthesis
knee ~ 27438, 27445
nasal septal ~ 30220
palate ~ 42281
pelvic floor ~ 57267
penis
inflatable ~ 54401-54405
noninflatable ~ 54400
speech ~ 31611
testis ~ 54660
urethral sphincter ~ 53444-53445
pulse generator
brain ~ 61885-61886
heart ~ 33212-33213
spinal cord ~ 63685
radioactive material
bladder ~ 51020
cystourethroscopy ~ 52250
receiver
brain ~ 61885-61886
spinal cord ~ 63685
reservoir
brain ~ 61210-61215
spinal cord ~ 62360
subcutaneous ~ 49419
sensor, fetal oximetry
cervix ~ 0021T
vagina ~ 0021T
shunt ~ 36835
abdomen
vein ~ 49425
venous ~ 49426
intrahepatic portosystemic ~ 37182
spinal instrument ~ 22849
spinous process ~ 22841
spinal instrumentation
anterior ~ 22845-22847
internal spinal fixation ~ 22841
pelvic fixation ~ 22848
posterior nonsegmental
Harrington rod technique ~ 22840
posterior segmental ~ 22842-22844
prosthetic device ~ 22851
stent
bile duct ~ 43268, 47801
percutaneous ~ 47511
bladder ~ 51045
conjunctiva ~ 68750
coronary ~ 92980-92981
esophagus ~ 43219
gastrointestinal, upper ~ 43256
ileum ~ 44383
indwelling ~ 50605
lacrimal duct ~ 68815

Insertion ~ ***continued***
pancreatic duct ~ 43268
small intestines ~ 44370, 44379
ureter via kidney ~ 50393
ureteral ~ 50947, 52332
urethral ~ 0084T, 52282
tamponade, esophagus ~ 43460
tandem uterus for brachytherapy ~ 57155
tendon graft
finger ~ 26392
hand ~ 26392
testicular prosthesis ~ see prosthesis, testicular, insertion
tissue expanders, skin ~ 11960-11971
tube
bile duct ~ 43268
esophagus ~ 43510
gastrointestinal, upper ~ 43241
ileum ~ 44383
kidney ~ 50398
pancreatic duct ~ 43268
small intestines ~ 44379
trachea ~ 31730
ureter ~ 50688
ureteral guide wire ~ 52334
vascular pedicle, carpal bone ~ 25430
venous access device
central ~ 36560-36566
peripheral ~ 36570-36571
ventilating tube ~ 69433
ventricular assist device ~ 33975
wire, skeletal traction ~ 20650
Inspiratory positive pressure breathing ~ see intermittent positive pressure breathing (IPPB)
Instillation
bladder ~ see bladder, instillation
drugs
bladder ~ 51720
kidney ~ 50391
ureter ~ 50391
Instrumentation ~ see application; bone, fixation; spinal instrumentation
spinal
insertion ~ 22840-22848, 22851
reinsertion ~ 22849
removal ~ 22850, 22852-22855
Insufflation, eustachian tube ~ see eustachian tube, inflation
Insulin ~ 80422, 80432-80435
antibody ~ 86337
blood ~ 83525
free ~ 83527
Insulin C-peptide measurement ~ see C-peptide
Insulin like growth factors ~ see somatomedin
Insurance
basic life and/or disability evaluation services ~ 99450
examination ~ 99450-99456

Integumentary system, surgical procedures ~ 10040-19499
biopsy ~ 11100-11101
breast
excision ~ 19100-19272
incision ~ 19000-19030
metallic localization clip placement ~ 19295
preoperative placement of needle localization ~ 19290-19291
reconstruction ~ 19316-19396
repair ~ 19316-19396
unlisted services and procedures ~ 19499
burns ~ 15002-15005, 15100-15121, 15342-15401
debridement ~ 11000-11006, 11010-11044
destruction ~ see also dermatology
actinotherapy ~ 96900
benign or premalignant lesion ~ 17000-17250
chemical exfoliation ~ 17360
cryotherapy ~ 17340
electrolysis epilation ~ 17380
malignant lesion ~ 17260-17286
by photodynamic therapy ~ 96567
Mohs micrographic surgery ~ 17311-17315
photodynamic therapy ~ 96567-96571
unlisted services and procedures ~ 17999
drainage ~ 10040-10180
excision
benign lesion ~ 11400-11471
debridement ~ 11000-11006, 11010-11044
malignant lesion ~ 11600-11646
incision ~ 10040-10180
introduction ~ 11900-11977
drug delivery implant ~ 11981, 11983
nails ~ 11720-11765
paring ~ 11055-11057
photography ~ 96904
pressure ulcers ~ 15920-15999
removal, drug delivery implant ~ 11982-11983
repair
adjacent tissue transfer/rearrangement ~ 14000-14350
complex ~ 13100-13160
flaps, other ~ 15740-15776
free skin grafts ~ 15050-15136, 15200-15321, 15420-15431
intermediate ~ 12031-12057
other procedures ~ 15780-15879
simple ~ 12001-12021
skin and/or deep tissue ~ 15570-15738
shaving of epidermal or dermal lesion ~ 11300-11313
skin tags, removal ~ 11200-11201
Intelligence test ~ 96100
Intensive care
low birthweight infant, subsequent care ~ 99298-99299
neonatal ~ 99295, 99296
Intercarpal joint
arthrodesis ~ 25820-25825
dislocation, closed treatment ~ 25660
repair ~ 25447
Intercostal nerve
destruction ~ 64620
injection
anesthetic ~ 64420-64421
neurolytic ~ 64620
Interdental fixation
device application ~ 21110
without fracture ~ 21497
mandibular fracture
closed treatment ~ 21453
open treatment ~ 21462
Interdental papilla ~ see gums
Interdental wire fixation
closed treatment craniofacial separation ~ 21431
Interferometry eye, biometry ~ 92136
Intermediate care facility (ICF) visits ~ 99304-99318
Intermittent positive pressure breathing (IPPB) ~ see continuous positive airway pressure (CPAP); continuous negative pressure breathing (CNPB)
Internal breast prostheses ~ see breast, implants
Internal ear ~ see ear, inner
Internal rigid fixation, reconstruction, mandibular rami ~ 21196
Internet E/M service ~ 0074T
Interphalangeal joint
arthrodesis ~ 26860-26863
arthroplasty ~ 26535-26536
arthrotomy ~ 26080, 28054
biopsy, synovium ~ 26110
capsule
excision ~ 26525
incision ~ 26525
dislocation
closed treatment ~ 26770
with manipulation ~ 26340
open treatment ~ 26785
percutaneous fixation ~ 26776
exploration ~ 26080
fracture
closed treatment ~ 26740
with manipulation ~ 26742
open treatment ~ 26746
fusion ~ 26860-26863
great toe
arthrodesis ~ 28755
with tendon transfer ~ 28760
fusion ~ 28755
with tendon transfer ~ 28760
removal of foreign body ~ 26080
repair
collateral ligament ~ 26545
volar plate ~ 26548
synovectomy ~ 26140

Interphalangeal joint ~ *continued*
toe ~ 28272
arthrotomy ~ 28024
dislocation ~ 28660-28665, 28675
percutaneous fixation ~ 28666
excision ~ 28160
exploration ~ 28024
removal
foreign body ~ 28024
loose body ~ 28024
synovial biopsy ~ 28054
Interruption
vein
femoral ~ 37650
iliac ~ 37660
vena cava ~ 37620
Intersex state
clitoroplasty ~ 56805
vaginoplasty ~ 57335
Intersex surgery
female to male ~ 55980
male to female ~ 55970
Interstitial cell stimulating hormone ~ see luteinizing hormone (LH)
Interstitial cystitides, chronic ~ see cystitis, interstitial
Interstitial cystitis ~ see cystitis, interstitial
Interstitial fluid pressure monitoring ~ 20950
Interstitial cell stimulating hormone ~ see luteinizing hormone (LH)
Intertarsal joint
arthrotomy ~ 28020, 28050
exploration ~ 28020
removal
foreign body ~ 28020
loose body ~ 28020
synovial
biopsy ~ 28050
excision ~ 28070
Interthoracoscapular amputation ~ see amputation, interthoracoscapular
Intertrochanteric femur fracture ~ see femur, fracture, intertrochanteric
Intervertebral chemonucleolysis ~ see chemonucleolysis
Intervertebral disk
diskography
cervical ~ 72285
lumbar ~ 72295
thoracic ~ 72285
excision
decompression ~ 63075-63078
herniated ~ 63020-63044, 63055-63066
injection
chemonucleolysis agent ~ 62292
X-ray ~ 62290-62291
Intestinal anastomosis ~ see anastomosis, intestines
Intestinal invagination ~ see intussusception
Intestinal peptide, vasoactive ~ see vasoactive intestinal peptide
Intestine(s)
allotransplantation ~ 44135-44136
removal ~ 44137
anastomosis ~ 44625-44626
biopsy ~ 44100
bleeding tube ~ 91100
closure
enterostomy, large or small ~ 44625-44626
stoma ~ 44620-44625
excision, donor ~ 44132-44133
exclusion ~ 44700
laparoscopic resection, with anastomosis ~ 44202-44208
lesion excision ~ 44110, 44111
lysis of adhesions, laparoscopic ~ 44200
nuclear medicine imaging ~ 78290
reconstruction
bladder ~ 50820
colonic reservoir ~ 45119
repair
diverticula ~ 44605
obstruction ~ 44615
ulcer ~ 44605
wound ~ 44605
suture
diverticula ~ 44605
stoma ~ 44620-44625
ulcer ~ 44605
wound ~ 44605
transplantation
allograft preparation ~ 44715-44721
donor enterectomy ~ 44132-44133
removal of allograft ~ 44137
unlisted services and procedures ~ 44238, 44799
Intestines, large ~ see anus; cecum; colon; rectum
Intestines, small
anastomosis ~ 43845, 44130
biopsy ~ 44020
endoscopy ~ 44361
catheterization jejunum ~ 44015
decompression ~ 44021
destruction lesion ~ 44369
tumor ~ 44369
endoscopy ~ 44364
biopsy ~ 44361, 44377
control of bleeding ~ 44366, 44378
via stoma ~ 44382
destruction
lesion ~ 44369
tumor ~ 44369
diagnostic ~ 44376
exploration ~ 44360
hemorrhage ~ 44366
insertion
stent ~ 44370, 44379
tube ~ 44379
pelvic pouch ~ 44385-44386

Intestine, small ~ *continued*
removal
foreign body ~ 44363
lesion ~ 44365
polyp ~ 44364-44365
tumor ~ 44364-44365
via stoma ~ 44380
tube placement ~ 44372
tube revision ~ 44373
enterostomy ~ 44300
excision ~ 44120-44128
partial with anastomosis ~ 44140
exclusion ~ 44700
exploration ~ 44020
gastrostomy tube ~ 44373
hemorrhage ~ 44378
hemorrhage control ~ 44366
ileostomy ~ 44310-44314, 45136
continent ~ 44316
incision ~ 44020
creation
pouch ~ 44316
stoma ~ 44300-44310, 44314
decompression ~ 44021
exploration ~ 44020
revision
stoma ~ 44312
stoma closure ~ 44620-44626
insertion
catheter ~ 44015
jejunostomy tube ~ 44372
jejunostomy ~ 44310
laparoscopic ~ 44201
lysis adhesions ~ 44005
removal foreign body ~ 44020, 44363
repair
diverticula ~ 44602-44603
enterocele
abdominal approach ~ 57270
vaginal approach ~ 57268
fistula ~ 44640-44661
hernia ~ 44050
malrotation ~ 44055
obstruction ~ 44050
ulcer ~ 44602-44603
volvulus ~ 44050
wound ~ 44602-44603
revision jejunostomy tube ~ 44373
specimen collection ~ 89100-89105
suture
diverticula ~ 44602-44603
fistula ~ 44640-44661
plication ~ 44680
ulcer ~ 44602-44603
wound ~ 44602-44603
X-ray ~ 74245, 74249-74251
guide intubation ~ 74355
Intestinovesical fistula ~ see fistula, enterovesical
Intimectomy ~ see endarterectomy
Intra arterial injections ~ see injection, intra-arterial
Intra-abdominal voiding pressure studies ~ 51797
Intra-osseous infusion ~ see infusion, intraosseous
Intracapsular extraction of lens ~ see extraction, lens, intracapsular
Intracardiac echocardiography ~ 93662
Intracranial arterial perfusion, thrombolysis ~ 61624
biopsy ~ 61140
extracranial ~ 61623
microdissection ~ 69990
neoplasm
acoustic neuroma ~ see brain, tumor, excision
craniopharyngioma ~ see craniopharyngioma
meningioma ~ see meningioma
Intrafallopian transfer, gamete ~ see GIFT
Intraluminal angioplasty ~ see angioplasty
Intramuscular injection ~ see injection, intramuscular
Intraocular lens
exchange ~ 66986
insertion ~ 66983
not associated with concurrent cataract removal ~ 66985
manual or mechanical technique ~ 66982, 66984
Intratracheal intubation ~ see insertion, endotracheal tube
Intrauterine contraceptive device ~ see intrauterine device (IUD)
Intrauterine device (IUD)
insertion ~ 58300
removal ~ 58301
Intrauterine synechiae ~ see adhesions, intrauterine
Intravascular stent ~ see transcatheter, placement, intravascular stents
X-ray ~ 75960
Intravascular ultrasound
intraoperative ~ 37250-37251
Intravenous injection ~ see injection, intravenous
Intravenous pyelogram ~ see urography, intravenous
Intravenous therapy ~ (see also injection, chemotherapy) 90780-90781
pain management ~ 90783-90784
Intravesical instillation ~ see bladder, instillation
Intravitreal injection pharmacologic agent ~ 67028
Intrinsic factor ~ 83528
antibody ~ 86340

Introduction
breast
metallic localization clip placement ~ 19295
preoperative placement, needle ~ 19290-19291
contraceptive capsules
implantable ~ 11975-11977
drug delivery implant ~ 11981, 11983
gastrointestinal tube ~ 44500
with fluoroscopic guidance ~ 74340
tissue expanders, skin ~ 11960-11971
Intubation ~ see insertion
endotracheal tube ~ 31500
eustachian tube ~ see catheterization, eustachian tube
gastric ~ 89130-89141, 91105
specimen collection
esophagus ~ 91000
stomach ~ 91055
Intubation tube ~ see endotracheal tube
Intussusception
barium enema ~ 74283
reduction
laparotomy ~ 44050
Invagination, intestinal ~ see intussusception
Inversion, nipple ~ see nipples, inverted
Iodide test ~ see nuclear medicine, thyroid, uptake
Iodine test ~ see starch granules, feces
Ionization, medical ~ see iontophoresis
Iontophoreses ~ see iontophoresis
Iontophoresis ~ 97033
sweat collection ~ 89230
IP ~ see allergen immunotherapy
Ipecac administration ~ 99175
IPPB ~ see intermittent positive pressure breathing; pulmonology, therapeutic
Iridectomy
with corneoscleral or corneal section ~ 66600
by laser surgery ~ 66761
peripheral for glaucoma ~ 66625
with sclerectomy with punch or scissors ~ 66160
with thermocauterization ~ 66155
with transfixion as for iris bombe ~ 66605
with trephination ~ 66150
Iridencleisis ~ 66165
Iridodialysis ~ 66680
Iridoplasty ~ 66762
Iridotasis ~ 66165
Iridotomy
excision
with corneoscleral or corneal section ~ 66600
with cyclectomy ~ 66605
optical ~ 66635
peripheral ~ 66625
incision
stab ~ 66500
with transfixion as for iris bombe ~ 66505
by laser surgery ~ 66761
Iridotomy ~ *continued*
optical ~ 66635
peripheral ~ 66625
sector ~ 66630
by stab incision ~ 66500
Iris
cyst, destruction ~ 66770
excision
iridectomy
with corneoscleral or corneal section ~ 66600
with cyclectomy ~ 66605
optical ~ 66635
peripheral ~ 66625
sector ~ 66630
incision
iridotomy
stab ~ 66500
with transfixion as for iris bombe ~ 66505
lesion, destruction ~ 66770
repair
with ciliary body ~ 66680
suture ~ 66682
revision
laser surgery ~ 66761
photocoagulation ~ 66762
suture, with ciliary body ~ 66682
Iron ~ 83540
absorption ~ 78162
chelatable total body iron ~ 78172
turnover rate ~ 78160
utilization ~ 78170
Iron binding capacity ~ 83550
Iron hematoxylin stain ~ 88312
Iron stain ~ 85536, 88313
Irradiation blood products ~ 86945
Irrigation
bladder ~ 51700
catheter, brain ~ 62194, 62225
corpora cavernosa, priapism ~ 54220
penis, priapism ~ 54220
peritoneal ~ see peritoneal lavage
rectum, for fecal impaction ~ 91123
shunt, spinal cord ~ 63744
sinus
maxillary ~ 31000
sphenoid ~ 31002
vagina ~ 57150
Irving sterilization (ligation, fallopian tube, oviduct) ~ 58600-58611, 58670
Ischial
bursa excision ~ 27060
tumor excision ~ 27078-27079
Ischiectomy ~ 15941
Islands of Langerhans ~ see Islet cell
Island pedicle flaps ~ 15740
Islet cell
antibody ~ 86341
transplantation ~ 0141T-0143T
Isocitrate dehydrogenase ~ see isocitric dehydrogenase
Isocitric dehydrogenase blood ~ 83570

Isolation sperm ~ 89260-89261
Isomerase, glucose 6 (six) phosphate ~ see phosphohexose isomerase
Isopropanol ~ see isopropyl alcohol
Isopropyl alcohol ~ 84600
Isthmusectomy, thyroid gland ~ 60210-60225
IUD ~ see intrauterine device (IUD)
IV infusion therapy ~ see allergen immunotherapy; chemotherapy; infusion; injection, chemotherapy
IV ~ see injection, chemotherapy; intravenous therapy
IVC filter placement ~ 75940
IVF ~ see artificial insemination; in vitro fertilization
Ivy bleeding time ~ 85002
IV injection ~ see injection, intravenous
IV, coagulation factor ~ see calcium
IX complex, factor ~ see Christmas factor

J

Jaboulay operation ~ 43810, 43850, 43855
Jannetta procedure ~ 61458
Japanese, river fever ~ see scrub typhus
Jatene type procedure~ 33770-33781
Jaw joint ~ see facial bones; mandible; maxilla
jaws
  muscle reduction ~ 21295-21296
  X-ray for orthodontics ~ 70355
Jejunostomy
  catheterization ~ 44015
  insertion, catheter ~ 44015
  laparoscopic ~ 44201
  non-tube ~ 44310
  with pancreatic drain ~ 48001
Jejunum
  creation, stoma
    laparoscopic ~ 44201
  transfer
    with microvascular anastomosis free ~ 43496
Johannsen procedure ~ 53400
Johanson operation ~ see reconstruction, urethra
Joint ~ see specific joint
  arthrocentesis ~ 20600-20610
  aspiration ~ 20600-20610
  dislocation ~ see dislocation
  drainage ~ 20600-20610
  finger ~ see intercarpal joint
    fixation (surgical) ~ see arthrodesis
  injection ~ 20600-20610
  nuclear medicine imaging ~ 78300, 78315
  radiology stress views ~ 77071
  shoulder ~ see glenohumeral joint
  survey ~ 77077
  wrist ~ see radiocarpal joint
Joint syndrome, temporomandibular ~ see temporomandibular joint (TMJ)
Jones and Cantarow test ~ see blood urea nitrogen; urea nitrogen, clearance
Jones procedure ~ 28760
Joplin procedure ~ 28294
Jugal bone ~ see cheek bone
Jugular vein ~ see vein, jugular

K

K-wire fixation, tongue ~ 41500
Kader operation ~ see incision, stomach, creation, stoma; incision and drainage
Kala Azar smear ~ 87207
Kallidin I /Kallidin 9 ~ see Bradykinin
Kallikreinogen ~ see Fletcher factor
Kallikrein HK3 ~ see antigen, prostate specific
Kasai procedure ~ 47701
Kedani fever ~ see scrub typhus
Keel, insertion/removal, laryngoplasty ~ 31580
Keen operation (laminectomy) ~ 63600
Kelikian procedure ~ 28280
Keller procedure ~ 28292
Kelly urethral plication ~ 57220
Keratectomy, partial, for lesion ~ 65400
Keratomileusis ~ 65760
Keratophakia ~ 65765
Keratoplasty
  lamellar ~ 65710
  penetrating ~ 65730
    in aphakia ~ 65750
    in pseudophakia ~ 65755
Keratoprosthesis ~ 65770
Keratotomy, radial ~ 65771

Ketogenic steroids ~ 83582
Ketone body, acetone ~ 82009-82010
Ketosteroids ~ 83586-83593
Kidner procedure ~ 28238
Kidney
  abscess
    incision and drainage
      open ~ 50020
      percutaneous ~ 50021
  anesthesia ~ 00862
  biopsy ~ 50200-50205
    endoscopic ~ 50555-50559, 52354
  catheterization, endoscopic ~ 50572
  cyst
    ablation ~ 50541
    aspiration ~ 50390
    excision ~ 50280-50290
    injection ~ 50390
    X-ray ~ 74470
  destruction
    calculus ~ 50590
    endoscopic ~ 50557, 50576, 52354

Kidney ~ *continued*
dilation ~ 50395
endoscopy
biopsy ~ 50555, 50574-50576, 52354
catheterization ~ 50553, 50572
destruction ~ 50557, 50576, 52354
dilation
intra-renal stricture ~ 52343, 52346
ureter ~ 50553
excision tumor ~ 52355
exploration ~ 52351
lithotripsy ~ 52353
removal
calculus ~ 50561, 50580, 52352
foreign body ~ 50561, 50580
via incision ~ 50562-50580
via stoma ~ 50551-50561
excision
donor ~ 50300-50320, 50547
partial ~ 50240
recipient ~ 50340
transplantation ~ 50370
with ureters ~ 50220-50236
exploration ~ 50010, 50045, 50120
incision ~ 50010, 50045
incision and drainage ~ 50040, 50125
injection
drugs ~ 50391
radiologic ~ 50394
insertion
catheter ~ 50392-50393
guide ~ 50395
intracatheter ~ 50392
stent ~ 50393
tube ~ 50398
instillation drugs ~ 50391
lithotripsy ~ 50590
manometry pressure ~ 50396
mass ablation ~ 50542
needle biopsy ~ 50200
nuclear medicine
function study ~ 78725
imaging ~ 78700-78710
unlisted services and procedures ~ 78799
removal
calculus ~ 50060-50081, 50130, 50561
foreign body ~ 50561, 50580
repair
blood vessels ~ 50100
fistula ~ 50520-50526
horseshoe kidney ~ 50540
renal pelvis ~ 50400-50405
wound ~ 50500
solitary ~ 50405
suture
fistula ~ 50520-50526
horseshoe kidney ~ 50540
transplantation
anesthesia
donor ~ 00862
recipient ~ 00868

Kidney ~ *continued*
allograft preparation ~ 50323-50329
donor ~ 00862
donor nephrectomy ~ 50300-50320, 50547
implantation of graft ~ 50360
recipient nephrectomy ~ 50340, 50365
reimplantation kidney ~ 50380
removal transplant renal autograft ~ 50370
ultrasound ~ 76770-76776
X-ray with contrast guide catheter ~ 74475
Kidney stone ~ see calculus, removal, kidney
Killian operation ~ see sinusotomy, frontal
Kinase, creatine ~ see CPK
Kineplasty ~ see cineplasty
Kinetic therapy ~ 97530
Kininase A ~ see angiotensin converting enzyme (ACE)
Kininogen ~ 85293
Kininogen, high molecular weight ~ see Fitzgerald factor
Kleihauer-Betke test ~ 85460
Kloramfenikol ~ see chloramphenicol
Knee ~ see femur; fibula; patella; tibia
abscess ~ 27301
arthrocentesis ~ 20610
arthrodesis ~ 27580
arthroplasty ~ 27440-27445, 27447
revision ~ 27486-27487
arthroscopy
diagnostic ~ 29870
surgical ~ 29866-29868, 29871-29889
arthrotomy ~ 27310, 27330-27335, 27403
biopsy ~ 27323-27324, 27330-27331
synovium ~ 27330
bone, drainage ~ 27303
bursa ~ 27301
excision ~ 27340
cyst, excision ~ 27345-27347
disarticulation ~ 27598
dislocation ~ 27550-27552, 27560-27562
open treatment ~ 27556-27558, 27566
drainage ~ 27310
excision
cartilage ~ 27332-27333
ganglion ~ 27347
lesion ~ 27347
synovial lung ~ 27334-27335
exploration ~ 27310, 27331
fasciotomy ~ 27305, 27496-27499
fracture ~ 27520-27524
arthroscopic treatment ~ 29850-29851
fusion ~ 27580
hematoma ~ 27301
incision, capsule ~ 27435
injection, X-ray ~ 27370
magnetic resonance imaging (MRI) ~ 73721-73723
manipulation ~ 27570
meniscectomy ~ 27332-27333

Knee ~ *continued*
reconstruction ~ 27437-27438
ligament ~ 27427-27429
with prosthesis ~ 27445
removal
foreign body ~ 27310, 27331, 27372
loose body ~ 27331
prosthesis ~ 27488
repair
ligament ~ 27405-27409
collateral ~ 27405
collateral and cruciate ~ 27409
cruciate ~ 27407-27409
meniscus ~ 27403
tendon ~ 27380-27381
replacement ~ 27447
retinacular release ~ 27425
strapping ~ 29530
suture tendon ~ 27380-27381
transplantation
chondrocytes ~ 27412
meniscus ~ 29868
osteochondral
allograft ~ 27415-29867
autograft ~ 27412-29866
tumor excision ~ 27327-27329, 27365
unlisted services and procedures ~ 27599
X-ray ~ 73560-73564
arthrography ~ 73580
bilateral ~ 73565
X-ray with contrast arthrography ~ 73580
Knee cap
excision ~ 27350
repair, instability ~ 27420-27424
Knee joint arthroplasty ~ 27446
Knee prosthesis ~ see prosthesis, knee
Knock-knee repair ~ 27455-27457
Kocher operation ~ 23650-23680
Kocher pylorectomy ~ see gastrectomy, partial
Kock pouch ~ 44316
formation ~ 50825
Kock procedure ~ 44316
KOH ~ see hair; nails; tissue, examination for fungi
Kraske procedure ~ 45116
Krause operation ~ see gasserian ganglion, sensory root, decompression
Kroenlein procedure ~ 67420
Krukenberg procedure ~ 25915
Kuhlmann test ~ 96100
Kyphectomy
more than two segments ~ 22819
up to two segments ~ 22818

L

L-alanine ~ see aminolevulinic acid (ALA)
L ascorbic acid ~ see ascorbic acid
L aspartate 2 oxoglutarate aminotransferase ~ see transaminase, glutamic oxaloacetic
L glutamine ~ see glutamine
L-leucylnaphthylamidase ~ see leucine aminopeptidase
L/S ratio, amniotic fluid ~ 83661
Labial adhesions, lysis ~ 56441
Laboratory panel
ACTH stimulation panel ~ 80400
acute hepatitis panel ~ 80074
basic metabolic panel ~ 80048
comprehensive metabolic panel ~ 80053
corticotropic releasing hormone (CRH) stimulation panel ~ 80412
electrolyte panel ~ 80051
general health panel ~ 80050
glucagon tolerance panel ~ 80422-80424
gonadotropin releasing hormone stimulation panel ~ 80426
growth hormone
stimulation panel ~ 80428
suppression panel ~ 80430
hepatic function panel ~ 80076
insulin
tolerance panel ~ 80434-80435
induced C-peptide suppression panel ~ 80432
lipid panel ~ 80061
metyrapone panel ~ 80436
obstetric panel ~ 80055
renal function ~ 80069
thyrotropin releasing hormone (TRH) stimulation panel ~ 80438-80440
Laboratory services ~ 8000-8999
anatomic pathology ~ 88000-88999
chemistry ~ 82000-84999
consultations, clinical pathology ~ 80500-80502
cytogenetic studies ~ 88230-88299
cytopathology ~ 88104-88199
drug testing ~ 80100-80103
evocative/suppression testing ~ 80400-80440
hematology and coagulation ~ 85002-85999
immunology ~ 86000-86849
microbiology ~ 87001-87999
organ or disease oriented panels ~ 80048-80076
other pathology and laboratory procedures ~ 89050-89240
reproductive medicine procedures ~ 89250-89356
surgical pathology ~ 88300-88399
therapeutic drug assays ~ 80150-80299
transcutaneous procedures ~ 88400
transfusion medicine ~ 86850-86999
urinalysis ~ 81000-81099

Labyrinth ~ see ear, inner
Labyrinthectomy ~ 69905
with mastoidectomy ~ 69910
with skull base surgery ~ 61596
Labyrinthotomy
with/without cryosurgery ~ 69801
with mastoidectomy ~ 69802
Laceration repair ~ see specific site **
Lacrimal duct
canaliculi, repair ~ 68700
exploration ~ 68810
with anesthesia ~ 68811
canaliculi ~ 68840
stent ~ 68815
insertion, stent ~ 68815
removal
dacryolith ~ 68530
foreign body ~ 68530
X-ray with contrast ~ 70170
Lacrimal gland
biopsy ~ 68510
close fistula ~ 68770
excision
partial ~ 68505
total ~ 68500
fistulization ~ 68720
incision and drainage ~ 68400
injection, X-ray ~ 68850
nuclear medicine, tear flow ~ 78660
removal
dacryolith ~ 68530
foreign body ~ 68530
repair, fistula ~ 68770
tumor
excision
without closure ~ 68540
with osteotomy ~ 68550
Lacrimal punctum
closure
by plug ~ 68761
by thermocauterization, ligation or laser surgery ~ 68760
dilation ~ 68801
incision ~ 68440
repair ~ 68705
Lacrimal sac
biopsy ~ 68525
excision ~ 68520
incision and drainage ~ 68420
Lacrimal system, unlisted services and procedures ~ 68899
Lactase deficiency breath test ~ 91065
Lactate ~ 83605
Lactate dehydrogenase ~ see lactic dehydrogenase
Lactic acid ~ 83605
Lactic acid measurement ~83605
Lactic cytochrome reductase ~ see lactic dehydrogenase
Lactic dehydrogenase ~ 83615-83625
Lactiferous duct
excision ~ 19112
exploration ~ 19110
Lactoferrin, fecal ~ 83630
Lactogen, human placental ~ 83632
Lactogenic hormone ~ see prolactin
Lactose, urine ~ 83633-83634
Ladd procedure ~ 44055
Lagophthalmos, repair ~ 67912
Laki Lorand factor ~ see fibrin stabilizing factor
Lamblia intestinalis ~ see giardia lamblia
Lambrinudi operation ~ see arthrodesis, foot joint
Lamellar keratoplasties ~ see keratoplasty, lamellar
Laminaria, insertion ~ 59200
Laminectomy ~ 62351, 63001, 63005-63011, 63015-63044, 63180-63200, 63265-63290, 63300-63655
with facetectomy ~ 63045-63048
lumbar ~ 22630, 63012
surgical ~ 63170-63172
Laminoplasty, cervical ~ 63050-63051
Langerhans islands ~ see islet cell
Language evaluation ~ 92506
Language therapy ~ 92507-92508
LAP ~ 83670
Laparoscopic appendectomy ~ see appendectomy, laparoscopic
Laparoscopic biopsy of ovary ~ see biopsy, ovary, laparoscopic
Laparoscopy
abdominal ~ 49320-49326, 49329
adrenalectomy ~ 50545
adrenal gland
biopsy ~ 60650
excision ~ 60650
appendectomy ~ 44970
aspiration ~ 49322
biopsy ~ 47561, 49321
lymph nodes ~ 38570
cholangiography ~ 47560-47561
cholecystectomy ~ 47562-47564
cholecystenterostomy ~ 47570
colectomy
partial ~ 44204-44208
total ~ 44210-44212
destruction, lesion ~ 58662
diagnostic ~ 49320
drainage, extraperitoneal lymphocele ~ 49323
ectopic pregnancy ~ 59150
with salpingectomy and/or oophorectomy ~ 59151
electrode implantation
gastric ~ 43647, 0155T
electrode removal
gastric ~ 43648, 0156T
electrode replacement
gastric ~ 43647, 0155T
electrode revision
gastric ~ 43648, 0156T

Laparoscopy ~ *continued*
enterolysis ~ 44200
esophagogastric fundoplasty ~ 43280
fimbrioplasty ~ 58672
gastric restrictive procedures ~ 43644-43645
gastrostomy, temporary ~ 43653
hernia repair
initial ~ 49650
recurrent ~ 49651
hysterectomy ~ 58541-58544
radical ~ 58548
incontinence repair ~ 51990-51992
in vitro fertilization ~ 58976
retrieve oocyte ~ 58970
transfer embryo ~ 58974
transfer gamete ~ 58976
jejunostomy ~ 44201
kidney, ablation ~ 50541-50542
ligation, veins, spermatic ~ 55550
liver ablation, tumor ~ 47370-47371
lymphadenectomy ~ 38571-38572
lymphatic ~ 38570-38589
lysis of adhesions ~ 58660
lysis of intestinal adhesions ~ 44200
nephrectomy ~ 50545-50548
partial ~ 50543
omentopexy ~ 49326
orchiectomy ~ 54690
orchiopexy ~ 54692
oviduct surgery ~ 58670-58671, 58679
pelvis ~ 49320
prostatectomy ~ 55866
pyeloplasty ~ 50544
removal
fallopian tubes ~ 58661
leiomyomata ~ 58545-58546
ovaries ~ 58661
spleen ~ 38120
testis ~ 54690
resection, intestines, with anastomosis ~ 44202-44203
salpingostomy ~ 58673
splenectomy ~ 38120-38129
stomach ~ 43647-43659
gastric bypass ~ 43644-63645
gastroenterostomy ~ 43644-43645
Roux-en-Y ~ 43644
unlisted services and procedures ~ 38129, 38589, 43289, 43659, 44238-44239, 44979, 47379, 47579, 49329, 49659, 50549, 50949, 54699, 55559, 58578-58579, 58679, 59898
ureterolithotomy ~ 50945
ureteroneocystostomy ~ 50947-50948
urethral suspension ~ 51990
vaginal hysterectomy ~ 58550-58554
vaginal suspension ~ 57425
vagus nerves, transection ~ 43651-43652
with X-ray ~ 47560
Laparotomy
with biopsy ~ 49000
exploration ~ 47015, 49000-49002, 58960
Laparotomy ~ *continued*
hemorrhage control ~ 49002
second look ~ 58960
staging ~ 58960
for staging ~ 49220
Laparotomy, exploratory ~ see abdomen, exploration
Lapidus procedure ~ 28297
Large bowel ~ see anus; cecum; rectum
Laroyenne operation ~ see vagina, abscess, incision and drainage, 57010
Laryngeal function study ~ 92520
Laryngeal sensory testing ~ 92614-92617
Laryngectomy ~ 31360-31382
partial ~ 31367-31382
subtotal ~ 31367-31368
Laryngocele, removal ~ 31300
Laryngofissure ~ 31300
Laryngography ~ 70373
Laryngopharyngectomy ~ see excision, larynx, with pharynx, 31390, 31395
Laryngopharynx ~ see hypopharynx
Laryngoplasty
burns ~ 31588
cricoid split ~ 31587
laryngeal stenosis ~ 31582
laryngeal web ~ 31580
open reduction of fracture ~ 31584
Laryngoscopy
diagnostic ~ 31505
direct ~ 31515-31571
exploration ~ 31505, 31520-31526, 31575
fiberoptic ~ 31575-31579
with stroboscopy ~ 31579
indirect ~ 31505-31513
newborn ~ 31520
operative ~ 31530-31561
Laryngotomy ~ 31300
diagnostic ~ 31320
total ~ 31360-31368
Larynx
aspiration, endoscopy ~ 31515
biopsy, endoscopy ~ 31510, 31535-31536, 31576
dilation, endoscopic ~ 31528-31529
endoscopy
direct ~ 31515-31571
excision ~ 31545-31546
exploration ~ 31505, 31520-31526, 31575
fiberoptic ~ 31575-31579
with stroboscopy ~ 31579
indirect ~ 31505-31513
operative ~ 31530-31561
excision
lesion ~ 31512, 31578
endoscopic ~ 31545-31546
partial ~ 31367-31382
with pharynx ~ 31390-31395
total ~ 31360-31365
exploration, endoscopic ~ 31505, 31520-31526, 31575
fracture, closed treatment

Larynx ~ *continued*
with manipulation ~ 31586
without manipulation ~ 31585
open treatment ~ 31584
insertion, obturator ~ 31527
nerve, destruction ~ 31595
reconstruction
burns ~ 31588
cricoid split ~ 31587
other ~ 31588
stenosis ~ 31582
web ~ 31580
removal
foreign body, endoscopic ~ 31511, 31530-31531, 31577
lesion, endoscopic ~ 31512, 31545-31546, 31578
repair, reinnervation neuromuscular pedicle ~ 31590
stroboscopy ~ 31579
tumor
excision ~ 31300
endoscopic ~ 31540-31541
unlisted services and procedures ~ 31599
vocal cord(s), injection ~ 31513, 31570-31571
X-ray ~ 70370
with contrast ~ 70373
Laser surgery
anal ~ 46917
lesion
mouth ~ 40820
nose ~ 30117-30118
penis ~ 54057
Laser treatment ~ see destruction ~ 17000-17286, 96920-96922
Lateral epicondylitis ~ see tennis elbow
Latex fixation ~ 86403-86406
LATS ~ see thyrotropin releasing hormone (TRH)
Latzko operation ~ see repair, vagina, fistula; revision
LAV ~ see HIV
LAV-2 (two) ~ see HIV-2 (two)
LAV antibodies ~ see antibody, HIV
Lavage
colon ~ 44701
lung
bronchial ~ 31624
total ~ 32997
mammary duct ~ 0046T-0047T
peritoneal ~ 49080
LCM ~ see lymphocytic choriomeningitis
LD ~ lactic dehydrogenase, 83615
LDH ~ 83615-83625
LDL ~ 83721
Lead ~ 83655
Leadbetter procedure ~ 53431
Lecithin-sphingomyelin ratio ~ 83661
Lecithinase C ~ see tissue typing
Lee and White test ~ 85345
Leep procedure ~ 57460
Lefort procedure, vagina ~ 57120
Lefort I procedure
midface reconstruction ~ 21141-21147, 21155, 21160
palatal of maxillary fracture ~ 21421-21423
Lefort II procedure
midface reconstruction ~ 21150-21151
nasomaxillary complex fracture ~ 21345-21348
Lefort III procedure
craniofacial separation ~ 21431-21436
midface reconstruction ~ 21154-21159
Left atrioventricular valve ~ see mitral valve
Left heart cardiac catheterization ~ see cardiac catheterization, left heart
Leg
cast
rigid total contact ~ 29445
lower ~ see also ankle; fibula; knee; tibia
abscess, incision and drainage ~ 27603
amputation ~ 27598, 27880-27882
revision ~ 27884-27886
angiography ~ 73706
artery, ligation ~ 37618
biopsy ~ 27613-27614
bursa, incision and drainage ~ 27604
bypass graft ~ 35903
cast ~ 29405-29435, 29450
CAT scan ~ 73700-73706
decompression ~ 27600-27602
exploration, blood vessel ~ 35860
fasciotomy ~ 27600-27602, 27892-27894
hematoma, incision and drainage ~ 27603
lesion, excision ~ 27630
magnetic resonance imaging (MRI) ~ 73718-73720
repair
blood vessel ~ 35226
with other graft ~ 35286
with vein graft ~ 35256
fascia ~ 27656
tendon ~ 27658-27692
splint ~ 29515
strapping ~ 29580
suture, tendon ~ 27658-27665
tumor, excision ~ 27615-27619
ultrasound ~ 76880
unlisted services and procedures ~ 27899
Unna boot ~ 29580
X-ray ~ 73592
upper ~ see femur
abscess ~ 27301
amputation ~ 27590-27592
at hip ~ 27290-27295
revision ~ 27594-27596
angiography ~ 73706, 75635
artery, ligation ~ 37618
biopsy ~ 27323-27324
bursa ~ 27301
bypass graft ~ 35903
cast ~ 29345-29355, 29365, 29450
cast brace ~ 29358
CT scan ~ 73700-73706, 75635

Leg ~ *continued*
exploration, blood vessel ~ 35860
fasciotomy ~ 27305, 27496-27499, 27892-27894
halo application ~ 20663
hematoma ~ 27301
magnetic resonance imaging (MRI) ~ 73718-73720
neurectomy ~ 27325-27326
removal
cast ~ 29705
foreign body ~ 27372
repair
blood vessel with other graft ~ 35286
blood vessel with vein graft ~ 35256
muscle ~ 27385-27386, 27400, 27430
tendon ~ 27393-27400
splint ~ 29505
strapping ~ 29580
suture, muscle ~ 27385-27386
tenotomy ~ 27306-27307, 27390-27392
tumor, excision ~ 27327-27329
ultrasound ~ 76880
unlisted services and procedures ~ 27599
Unna boot ~ 29580
X-ray ~ 73592
wound exploration, penetrating ~ 20103
Legionella
antibody ~ 86713
antigen ~ 87277-87278, 87540-87542
Legionella micdadei antigen detection, immunofluorescence ~ 87277
Legionella pneumophila antigen detection, direct fluorescence ~ 87278
Leg length measurement X-ray ~ see scanogram
Leiomyomata, removal ~ 58140, 58545-58546, 58561
Leishmania, antibody ~ 86717
Lengthening, tendon ~ see tendon, lengthening
Lens
extracapsular ~ 66940
intracapsular ~ 66920
dislocated ~ 66930
intraocular
exchange ~ 66986
reposition ~ 66825
prosthesis, insertion ~ 66983
manual or mechanical technique ~ 66982, 66984
not associated with concurrent cataract removal ~ 66985
removal, lens material
aspiration technique ~ 66840
extracapsular ~ 66940
intracapsular ~ 66920-66930
pars plana approach ~ 66852
phacofragmentation technique ~ 66850
Lens material
aspiration technique ~ 66840
pars plana approach ~ 66852
phacofragmentation technique ~ 66850
Leptomeningioma ~ see meningioma
Leptospira, antibody ~ 86720
Leriche operation ~ (thoracolumbar sympathectomy) 64809
Lesion ~ see tumor
anal
destruction ~ 46900-46917, 46924
excision ~ 45108, 46922
ankle, tendon sheath ~ 27630
arm, lower
tendon sheath
excision ~ 25110
auditory canal, external
excision
exostosis ~ 69140
radical with neck dissection ~ 69155
radical without neck dissection ~ 69150
soft tissue ~ 69145
bladder, destruction ~ 51030
brain
excision ~ 61534, 61536, 61600-61608, 61615-61616
radiation treatment ~ 77432
brainstem, excision ~ 61575-61576
breast, excision ~ 19120-19126
carotid body, excision ~ 60600-60605
chemotherapy ~ 96405-96406
destruction ~ 67220-67225
choroid, destruction ~ 0016T
ciliary body, destruction ~ 66770
colon
destruction ~ 44393, 45383
excision ~ 44110-44111
conjunctiva
destruction ~ 68135
excision ~ 68110-68130
over 1cm ~ 68115
with adjacent sclera ~ 68130
expression ~ 68040
cornea
destruction ~ 65450
excision ~ 65400
of pterygium ~ 65420-65426
destruction, ureter ~ 52341-52342, 52344-52345, 52354
ear, middle, excision ~ 69540
epididymis, excision ~ 54830
esophagus
ablation ~ 43228
excision ~ 43100-43101
removal ~ 43216
excision ~ 59100
bladder ~ 52224
urethra ~ 52224, 53265
eye, excision ~ 65900
eyelid
destruction ~ 67850
excision
under anesthesia ~ 67808
without closure ~ 67840
multiple, different lids ~ 67805
multiple, same lid ~ 67801

Lesion ~ *continued*
eyelid ~ *continued*
single ~ 67800
facial, destruction ~ 17000-17004, 17280-17286
femur, excision ~ 27062
finger, tendon sheath ~ 26160
foot, excision ~ 28080, 28090
gums
destruction ~ 41850
excision ~ 41822-41828
hand tendon sheath ~ 26160
intestines, excision ~ 44110
intestines, small
destruction ~ 44369
excision ~ 44111
iris, destruction ~ 66770
larynx, excision ~ 31545-31546
leg, lower, tendon sheath ~ 27630
lymph node, incision and drainage ~ 38300-38305
mesentery, excision ~ 44820
mouth
destruction ~ 40820
excision ~ 40810-40816, 41116
vestibule
destruction ~ 40820
repair ~ 40830
nerve, excision ~ 64774-64792
nose, intranasal
external approach ~ 30118
internal approach ~ 30117
orbit, excision ~ 61333, 67412
palate
destruction ~ 42160
excision ~ 42104-42120
pancreas, excision ~ 48120
pelvis, destruction ~ 58662
penis
destruction
cryosurgery ~ 54056
electrodesiccation ~ 54055
extensive ~ 54065
laser surgery ~ 54057
simple ~ 54050-54060
surgical excision ~ 54060
excision ~ 54060
penile plague ~ 54110-54112
pharynx
destruction ~ 42808
excision ~ 42808
rectum, excision ~ 45108
removal, larynx ~ 31512, 31578
resection ~ 52354
retina
destruction
extensive ~ 67227-67228
localized ~ 0017T, 67208-67210
radiation by implantation of source ~ 67218
sclera, excision ~ 66130
skin
abrasion ~ 15786-15787

Lesion ~ *continued*
biopsy ~ 11100-11101
destruction
benign ~ 17000-17250
malignant ~ 17260-17286
by photodynamic therapy ~ 96567
excision
benign ~ 11400-11471
malignant ~ 11600-11646
injection ~ 11900-11901
paring or curettement ~ 11055-11057
shaving ~ 11300-11313
skin tags, removal ~ 11200-11201
skull, excision ~ 61500, 61600-61608, 61615-61616
spermatic cord, excision ~ 55520
spinal cord
destruction ~ 62280-62282
excision ~ 63265-63273
stomach, excision ~ 43611
testis, excision ~ 54512
toe, excision ~ 28092
tongue, excision ~ 41110-41114
uvula
destruction ~ 42145
excision ~ 42104-42107
vagina, destruction ~ 57061-57065
vulva
destruction
extensive ~ 56515
simple ~ 56501
wrist tendon, excision ~ 25110
Lesion of sciatic nerve ~ see sciatic nerve, lesion
Leucine aminopeptidase ~ 83670
Leukemia lymphoma virus I (one), adult T cell ~ see HTLV I (one)
Leukemia lymphoma virus II (two) antibodies, human T cell ~ see antibody, HTLV-II (two)
Leukemia lymphoma virus I (one) antibodies, human T cell ~ see antibody, HTLV I (one)
Leukemia virus II (two), hairy cell associated, human T cell ~ see HTLV II (two)
Leukoagglutinins ~ 86021
Leukocyte ~ see also white blood cell
alkaline phosphatase ~ 85540
antibody ~ 86021
count ~ 85032, 85048, 89055
histamine release test ~ 86343
phagocytosis ~ 86344
transfusion ~ 86950
Leu 2 antigens ~ see CD8
Levarterenol ~ see noradrenalin
Levator muscle rep ~ (blepharoptosis, repair) 67901-67909
Leveen shunt
insertion ~ 49425
patency test ~ 78291
revision ~ 49426
Levulose ~ see fructose

LGV ~ (lymphogranuloma venereum) antibody 86729
LH ~ (luteinizing hormone) 80418, 80426, 83002
LHR ~ (leukocyte histamine release test) 86343
Lid suture ~ (blepharoptosis, repair) 67901-67909
Lidocaine, assay ~ 80176
Lift, face ~ see face lift
Ligament ~ see specific site
collateral repair, knee with cruciate ligament ~ 27409
dentate
incision ~ 63180-63182
section ~ 63180-63182
injection ~ 20550
release
coracoacromial ~ 23415
transverse carpal ~ 29848
repair
elbow ~ 24343-24346
knee joint ~ 27405-27409
Ligation
artery
abdomen ~ 37617
carotid ~ 37600-37606
chest ~ 37616
coronary ~ 33502
coronary artery ~ 33502
ethmoidal ~ 30915
extremity ~ 37618
fistula ~ 37607
maxillary ~ 30920
neck ~ 37615
temporal ~ 37609
esophageal varices ~ 43204, 43400
fallopian tube, oviduct ~ 58600-58611, 58670
gastroesophageal ~ 43405
hemorrhoids ~ 46945-46946
oviducts ~ 59100
salivary duct ~ 42665
shunt
aorta, pulmonary ~ 33924
peritoneal, venous ~ 49428
thoracic duct ~ 38380
abdominal approach ~ 38382
thoracic approach ~ 38381
vas deferens ~ 55450
vein
clusters ~ 37785
esophagus ~ 43205, 43244, 43400
femoral ~ 37650
gastric ~ 43244
iliac ~ 37660
jugular, internal ~ 37565
perforate ~ 37760
saphenous ~ 37700-37735, 37780
vena cava ~ 37620
Ligature strangulation, skin tags ~ 11200-11201
Light coagulation ~ see photocoagulation
Light scattering measurement ~ see nephelometry
Light therapy, UV ~ see actinotherapy
Limb ~ see extremity
Limited lymphadenectomy for staging ~ see lymphadenectomy, limited, for staging
Limited neck dissection, with thyroidectomy ~ 60252
Limited resection mastectomies ~ see breast, excision, lesion
Lindholm operation ~ see tenoplasty
Lingual bone ~ see hyoid bone
Lingual frenectomy ~ see excision, tongue, frenum
Lingual nerve
avulsion ~ 64740
incision ~ 64740
transection ~ 64740
Lingual tonsil ~ see tonsils, lingual
Linton procedure ~ 37760
Lip
biopsy ~ 40490
excision ~ 40500-40530
frenum ~ 40819
incision, frenum ~ 40806
reconstruction ~ 40525-40527
repair ~ 40650-40654
cleft lip ~ 40700-40761
fistula ~ 42260
unlisted services and procedures ~ 40799
Lip, cleft ~ see cleft lip
Lipase ~ 83690
Lipectomies, aspiration ~ see liposuction
Lipectomy ~ 15830-15839
suction assisted ~ 15876-15879
Lipids, feces ~ 82705-82710
Lipo-lutin ~ see progesterone
Lipolysis, aspiration ~ see liposuction
Lipophosphodiesterase I (one) ~ see tissue typing
Lipoprotein
blood ~ 0026T, 83715-83719
LDL ~ 83716, 83721
phospholipase A2 ~ 83698
Lipoprotein, alpha ~ see lipoprotein
Lipoprotein, pre-beta ~ see lipoprotein, blood
Liposuction ~ 15876-15879
Lisfranc operation ~ see amputation, foot; radical resection; replantation
Listeria monocytogenes, antibody ~ 86723
Lithium, assay ~ 80178
Litholapaxy ~ 52317-52318
Lithotripsy ~ see extracorporeal shock wave therapy
bile duct calculi (stone), endoscopy ~ 43265
bladder ~ 52353
kidney ~ 50590, 52353
pancreatic duct calculi (stone), endoscopy ~ 43265
ureter ~ 52353
urethra ~ 52353
with cystourethroscopy ~ 52353

Lithotrity ~ see litholapaxy
Liver ~ see hepatic duct
ablation, tumor ~ 47380-47382
laparoscopic ~ 47370-47371
abscess
aspiration ~ 47015
incision and drainage
open ~ 47010
percutaneous ~ 47011
injection ~ 47015
aspiration ~ 47015
biopsy ~ 47100
cyst
aspiration ~ 47015
incision and drainage
open ~ 47010
percutaneous ~ 47011
excision
extensive ~ 47122
partial ~ 47120, 47125-47130, 47140-47142
total ~ 47133
injection ~ 47015
radiologic ~ 47505
X-ray ~ 47500
lobectomy ~ 47125-47130
partial ~ 47120
needle biopsy ~ 47000-47001
nuclear medicine, function study ~ 78220
imaging ~ 78201-78216
vascular flow ~ 78206
repair
abscess ~ 47300
cyst ~ 47300
wound ~ 47350-47362
suture, wound ~ 47350-47362
transplantation ~ 47135-47136
allograft preparation ~ 47143-47147
trisegmentectomy ~ 47122
unlisted services and procedures ~ 47379, 47399
Living activities, daily ~ see activities of daily living
Lobectomy
brain ~ 61323, 61537-61540
contralateral subtotal, thyroid gland ~ 60212, 60225
liver ~ 47120-47130
lung ~ 32480-32482
sleeve ~ 32486
parotid gland ~ 42410-42415
segmental ~ 32663
sleeve ~ 32486
temporal lobe ~ 61537-61538
thyroid gland partial ~ 60210-60212
total ~ 60220-60225
total ~ 32663
Lobotomy, frontal ~ 61490
Localization of nodule, radiographic, breast ~ 77032
Local excision mastectomies ~ see breast, excision, lesion
Local excision of lesion or tissue of femur ~ see excision, lesion, femur
Log hydrogen ion concentration ~ see pH
Lombard test ~ see audiologic function test
Long term care facility visits ~ see nursing facility services
Longmire operation ~ (anastomosis, hepatic duct to intestines) 47765
Long acting thyroid stimulator ~ see thyrotropin releasing hormone (TRH)
Loopogram ~ see urography, antegrade
Loose body
removal
ankle ~ 27620
carpometacarpal joint ~ 26070
elbow ~ 24101
interphalangeal joint ~ 28020
toe ~ 28024
knee joint ~ 27331
metatarsophalangeal joint ~ 28022
tarsometatarsal joint ~ 28020
toe ~ 28022
wrist ~ 25101
Lord procedure ~ (anal sphincter dilation) 45905
Louis Bar syndrome ~ see ataxia telangiectasia
Lower extremities ~ see extremity, lower
Lower GI series ~ see barium enema
Low birth weight intensive care services ~ 99298-99299
Low density lipoprotein ~ see lipoprotein, LDL
Low vision aids ~ see spectacle services
fitting ~ 92354-92355
supply ~ 92392
LRH ~ (luteinizing releasing hormone) 83727
LSD ~ (lysergic acid diethylamide) 80100-80103, 80299
LTH ~ see prolactin
Lumbar ~ see spine
aspiration, disk, percutaneous ~ 62287
Lumbar plexus
decompression ~ 64714
injection, anesthetic ~ 64449
neuroplasty ~ 64714
release ~ 64714
repair/suture ~ 64862
Lumbar puncture ~ see spinal tap
Lumbar spine fracture ~ see fracture, vertebra, lumbar
Lumbar sympathectomy ~ see sympathectomy, lumbar
Lumbar vertebra ~ see vertebra, lumbar
Lumen dilation ~ 74360
Lumpectomy ~ 19301-19302
Lunate
arthroplasty, with implant ~ 25444
dislocation
closed treatment ~ 25690
open treatment ~ 25695

Lung
abscess
incision and drainage
open ~ 32200
percutaneous ~ 32200-32201
aspiration ~ 32420
biopsy ~ 32095-32100
bullae
excision ~ 32141
endoscopic ~ 32655
cyst
incision and drainage
open ~ 32200
removal ~ 32140
decortication
endoscopic ~ 32651-32652
partial ~ 32225
total ~ 32220
with parietal pleurectomy ~ 32320
empyema, excision ~ 32540
excision
bronchus resection ~ 32486
chest resection ~ 32520-32525
completion ~ 32488
donor
heart-lung ~ 33930
lung ~ 32850
emphysematous ~ 32491
lobe ~ 32480-32482
segment ~ 32484
total ~ 32440-32445
wedge resection ~ 32500
endoscopic ~ 32657
foreign body, removal ~ 32151
hemorrhage ~ 32110
lavage
bronchial ~ 31624
total ~ 32997
lysis, adhesions ~ 32124
needle biopsy ~ 32405
nuclear medicine
imaging, perfusion ~ 78580-78585
imaging, ventilation ~ 78586-78594
unlisted services and procedures ~ 78599
pneumocentesis ~ 32420
pneumolysis ~ 32940
pneumothorax ~ 32960
puncture ~ 32420
removal
bronchoplasty ~ 32501
completion pneumonectomy ~ 32488
extrapleural ~ 32445
single lobe ~ 32480
single segment ~ 32484
sleeve lobectomy ~ 32486
sleeve pneumonectomy ~ 32442
total pneumonectomy ~ 32440-32445
two lobes ~ 32482
volume reduction ~ 32491
wedge resection ~ 32500
repair, hernia ~ 32800
segmentectomy ~ 32484

Lung ~ *continued*
tear, repair ~ 32110
thoracotomy
with excision-plication of bullae ~ 32141
with open intrapleural pneumonolysis ~ 32124
biopsy ~ 32095-32100
cardiac massage ~ 32160
for post-op complications ~ 32120
removal
bullae ~ 32141
cyst ~ 32140
intrapleural foreign body ~ 32150
intrapulmonary foreign body ~ 32151
repair ~ 32110
transplantation ~ 32851-32854, 33935
allograft preparation ~ 32855-32856, 33933
donor pneumonectomy
heart-lung ~ 33930
lung ~ 32850
unlisted services and procedures ~ 32999
Lung function tests ~ see pulmonology, diagnostic
Lung volume reduction, emphysematous ~ 32491
Lupus anticoagulant assay ~ 85705
Lupus band test ~ see immunofluorescent study
Luteinizing hormone (LH) ~ 80418, 80426, 83002
Luteinizing releasing factor ~ 83727
Luteotropic hormone ~ see prolactin
Luteotropin ~ see prolactin
Luteotropin, placental ~ see lactogen, human placental
Lyme disease ~ 86617-86618
Lyme disease ab ~ see antibody, Lyme disease
Lyme disease vaccine ~ see vaccination
Lymph duct, injection ~ 38790
Lymph nodes
abscess, incision and drainage ~ 38300-38305
biopsy ~ 38500, 38510-38530, 38570
needle ~ 38505
dissection ~ 38542
excision ~ 38500, 38510-38530
abdominal ~ 38747
inguinofemoral ~ 38760-38765
laparoscopic ~ 38571-38572
limited, for staging
para-aortic ~ 38562
pelvic ~ 38562
retroperitoneal ~ 38564
pelvic ~ 38770
radical
axillary ~ 38740-38745
cervical ~ 38720-38724
suprahyoid ~ 38720-38724
retroperitoneal transabdominal ~ 38780
thoracic ~ 38746
exploration ~ 38542
hygroma, cystic
axillary/cervical excision ~ 38550-38555

Lymph nodes ~ *continued*
nuclear medicine, imaging ~ 78195
removal
abdominal ~ 38747
inguinofemoral ~ 38760-38765
pelvic ~ 38770
retroperitoneal transabdominal ~ 38780
thoracic ~ 38746
Lymph vessels
abdomen, lymphangiography ~ 75805-75807
arm, lymphangiography ~ 75801-75803
leg, lymphangiography ~ 75801-75803
nuclear medicine, imaging ~ 78195
pelvis, lymphangiography ~ 75805-75807
Lymphadenectomy
abdominal ~ 38747
bilateral inguinofemoral ~ 54130, 56632, 56637
bilateral pelvic ~ 51575, 51585, 51595, 54135, 55845, 55865
total ~ 38571-38572, 57531, 58210
diaphragmatic assessment ~ 58960
gastric ~ 38747
inguinofemoral ~ 38760-38765
inguinofemoral, iliac and pelvic ~ 56640
injection, sentinel node ~ 38792
limited para-aortic, resection of ovarian malignancy ~ 58951, 58954
limited pelvic ~ 55842, 55862, 58954
limited, for staging
para-aortic ~ 38562
pelvic ~ 38562
retroperitoneal ~ 38564
mediastinal ~ 21632
para-aortic ~ 58958
pelvic ~ 58958
peripancreatic ~ 38747
portal ~ 38747
radical
axillary ~ 38740-38745
cervical ~ 38720-38724
pelvic ~ 54135, 55845, 58548
suprahyoid ~ 38700
regional ~ 50230
retroperitoneal transabdominal ~ 38780
thoracic ~ 38746
unilateral inguinofemoral ~ 56631, 56634
Lymphadenitis, incision and drainage ~ 38300-38305
Lymphadenopathy associated antibodies ~ see antibody, HIV
Lymphadenopathy associated virus ~ see HIV
Lymphangiogram, abdominal ~ see lymphangiography, abdomen
Lymphangiography
abdomen ~ 75805-75807
arm ~ 75801-75803
injection ~ 38790
leg ~ 75801-75803
pelvis ~ 75805-75807
Lymphangioma, cystic ~ see hygroma
Lymphangiotomy ~ 38308
Lymphatic channels, incision ~ 38308
Lymphatic cyst ~ see lymphocele
Lymphatic system, unlisted procedure ~ 38999
Lymphatics ~ see specific procedure
Lymphoblast transformation ~ see blastogenesis
Lymphocele
drainage, laparoscopic ~ 49323
extraperitoneal, open drainage ~ 49062
Lymphocoele ~ see lymphocele
Lymphocyte
culture ~ 86821-86822
toxicity assay ~ 86805-86806
transformation ~ 86353
Lymphocyte, thymus-dependent ~ see T cells
Lymphocytes, CD4 ~ see CD4
Lymphocytes, CD8 ~ see CD8
Lymphocytic choriomeningitis, antibody ~ 86727
Lymphocytotoxicity ~ 86805-86806
Lymphogranuloma venereum, antibody ~ 86729
Lymphoma virus, Burkitt ~ see Epstein-Barr virus
Lynch procedure ~ 31075
Lysergic acid diethylamide ~ 80102-80103, 80299
Lysergide ~ see lysergic acid diethylamide
Lysis
adhesions
epidural ~ 0027T, 62263-62264
fallopian tube ~ 58740
foreskin ~ 54450
intestinal ~ 44005
labial ~ 56441
lung ~ 32124
nose ~ 30560
ovary ~ 58740
oviduct ~ 58740
penile, post-circumcision ~ 54162
ureter ~ 50715-50725
urethra ~ 53500
uterus ~ 58559
euglobulin ~ 85360
labial, adhesions ~ 56441
nose, intranasal synechia ~ 30560
Lysozyme ~ 85549

M

Macewen operation ~ see hernia, repair, inguinal
Machado test ~ (complement, fixation test) 86171
Maclean-De Wesselow test ~ see blood urea nitrogen; urea nitrogen, clearance
Macrodactylia, repair ~ 26590
Madlener operation ~ (tubal ligation) 58600

Magnesium ~ 83735
Magnet operation ~ see eye, removal of foreign body
Magnetic resonance, unlisted services and procedures ~ 76498
Magnetic resonance angiography (MRA)
abdomen ~ 74185
arm ~ 73225
chest ~ 71555
head ~ 70544-70546
leg ~ 73725
neck ~ 70547-70549
pelvis ~ 72198
spine ~ 72159
Magnetic resonance imaging (MRI)
abdomen ~ 74181-74183
ankle ~ 73721-73723
arm ~ 73218-73220, 73223
bone marrow study ~ 77084
brain ~ 70551-70555
intraoperative ~ 70557-70559
breast ~ 77058-77059
chest ~ 71550-71552
elbow ~ 73221
face ~ 70540-70543
finger joint ~ 73221
foot ~ 73718-73719
foot joints ~ 73721-73723
guidance
needle placement ~ 77021
parenchymal tissue ablation ~ 77022
visceral tissue ablation ~ 76394
hand ~ 73218-73220, 73223
heart ~ 75552
complete study ~ 75554
flow mapping ~ 75556
limited study ~ 75555
morphology ~ 75553
joint
lower extremity ~ 73721-73723
upper extremity ~ 73221-73223
knee ~ 73721-73723
leg ~ 73718-73720
neck ~ 70540-70543
orbit ~ 70540-70543
pelvis ~ 72195-72197
radiology, diagnostic, procedures ~ 76499
spectroscopy ~ 76390
spine
cervical ~ 72141-72142, 72156-72158
lumbar ~ 72148-72158
thoracic ~ 72146-72147, 72156-72158
temporomandibular joint (TMJ) ~ 70336
toe ~ 73721-73723
wrist ~ 73221
Magnetic resonance spectroscopy ~ 76390
Magnetic stimulation, transcranial ~ 0160T, 0161T
Magnetoencephalography (MEG) ~ 95965-95967
Magnuson procedure ~ 23450
Magpi operation ~ (hypospadias, repair) 54322
Major vestibular gland ~ see Bartholin's gland
Malar area
augmentation ~ 21270
bone graft ~ 21210
fracture
with bone graft ~ 21366
with manipulation ~ 21355
open treatment ~ 21360-21366
reconstruction ~ 21270
Malar bone ~ see cheekbone
Malaria antibody ~ 86750
Malaria smear ~ 87207
Malate dehydrogenase ~ 83775
Maldescent, testis ~ see testis, undescended
Male circumcision ~ see circumcision
Male genital system, surgical procedures ~ 54000-55899
Malformation, arteriovenous ~ see arteriovenous malformation
Malic dehydrogenase ~ (malate dehydrogenase) 83775
Malleolus ~ see ankle; fibula; leg, lower; tibia; tibiofibular joint
metatarsophalangeal joint ~ 27889
Mallet finger repair ~ 26432
Maltose, tolerance test ~ 82951-82952
Malunion repair
femur
with graft ~ 27472
without graft ~ 27470
metatarsal ~ 28322
tarsal joint ~ 28320
Mammalian oviduct ~ see fallopian tube
Mammaplasties ~ see breast, reconstruction
Mammary abscess ~ see abscess, breast
Mammary arteries ~ see artery, mammary
Mammary duct
catheter lavage for cytology ~ 0046T-0047T
X-ray with contrast ~ 77053-77054
Mammary ductogram, injection ~ 19030
Mammary stimulating hormone ~ see prolactin
Mammilliplasty ~ see nipples, reconstruction
Mammogram, breast, localization nodule ~ 77032
Mammography ~ 77055-77057
screening ~ 77057
with computer-aided detection ~ 77051-77052
Mammoplasty
augmentation ~ 19324-19325
reduction ~ 19318
Mammotomy ~ see mastotomy
Mammotropic hormone, pituitary ~ see prolactin
Mammotropic hormone, placental ~ see lactogen, human placental
Mammotropin ~ see prolactin
Mandated services, on call services ~ 99027
Mandible ~ see facial bones; maxilla; temporomandibular joint (TMJ)
abscess, excision ~ 21025
bone graft ~ 21215

Mandible ~ *continued*
cyst, excision ~ 21040, 21046-21047
fracture
closed treatment
with interdental fixation ~ 21453
with manipulation ~ 21451
without manipulation ~ 21450
open treatment ~ 21454-21470
external fixation ~ 21454
with interdental fixation ~ 21462
without interdental fixation ~ 21461
percutaneous treatment ~ 21452
osteotomy ~ 21198-21199
reconstruction, with implant ~ 21244-21246, 21248-21249
removal, foreign body ~ 41806
torus mandibularis, excision ~ 21031
tumor, excision ~ 21040-21047
X-ray ~ 70100-70110
Mandibular body
augmentation
with bone graft ~ 21127
with prosthesis ~ 21125
Mandibular condyle, fracture, open treatment ~ 21465
reconstruction ~ 21247
Mandibular condylectomy ~ see condylectomy
Mandibular fracture ~ see fracture, mandible
Mandibular rami
reconstruction
with bone graft ~ 21194
without bone graft ~ 21193
with internal rigid fixation ~ 21196
without internal rigid fixation ~ 21195
Mandibular resection prosthesis ~ 21081
Mandibular staple bone plate, reconstruction, mandible ~ 21244
Manganese ~ 83785
Manipulation
chest wall ~ 94667-94668
chiropractic ~ 98940-98943
dislocation and/or fracture ~ 25535
acetabulum ~ 27222
acromioclavicular ~ 23545
ankle ~ 27810, 27818, 27860
carpometacarpal ~ 26670-26676
clavicular ~ 23505
elbow ~ 24300, 24640
femoral ~ 27232, 27502, 27510, 27517
pertrochanteric ~ 27240
fibula ~ 27781, 27788
finger ~ 26725-26727, 26742, 26755
greater tuberosity, humeral ~ 23625
hand ~ 26670-26676
heel ~ 28405-28406
hip ~ 27257
hip socket ~ 27222
humeral ~ 23605, 24505, 24535, 24577
epicondyle ~ 24565
hyoid ~ 21494
intercarpal ~ 25660
interphalangeal joint ~ 26340, 26770-26776

Manipulation ~ *continued*
dislocation and/or fracture ~ *continued*
larynx ~ 31586
lunate ~ 25690
malar area ~ 21355
mandibular ~ 21451
metacarpal ~ 26605-26607
metacarpophalangeal ~ 26700-26706, 26742
metacarpophlangeal joint ~ 26340
metatarsal ~ 28475-28476
nasal bone ~ 21315-21320
orbit ~ 21401
phalangeal shaft ~ 26727
distal, finger or thumb ~ 26755
phalanges, finger/thumb ~ 26725
phalanges
finger ~ 26742, 26755, 26770-26776
finger/thumb ~ 26727
great toe ~ 28495-28496
toes ~ 28515
radial ~ 24655, 25565
radial shaft ~ 25505
radiocarpal ~ 25660
radioulnar ~ 25675
scapular ~ 23575
shoulder ~ 23650-23655
with greater tuberosity ~ 23665
shoulder dislocation sternoclavicular ~ 23525
with surgical or anatomical neck fracture ~ 23675
talus ~ 28435-28436
tarsal ~ 28455-28456
thumb ~ 26641-26650
tibial ~ 27532, 27752
trans-scaphoperilunar ~ 25680
ulnar ~ 24675, 25535, 25565
vertebral ~ 22315
wrist ~ 25259, 25624, 25635, 25660, 25675, 25680, 25690
foreskin ~ 54450
globe ~ 92018-92019
hip ~ 27275
interphalangeal joint, proximal ~ 26742
knee ~ 27570
osteopathic ~ 98925-98929
shoulder, application of fixation apparatus ~ 23700
spine, with anesthesia ~ 22505
tibial, distal ~ 27762
Manometric studies
kidney, pressure ~ 50396
rectum/anus ~ 91122
ureter, pressure ~ 50686
ureterostomy ~ 50686
Manometry, rectum ~ 90911
Mantoux test ~ (TB skin test) 86580
Manual therapy ~ 97140
Maquet procedure ~ 27418
Marcellation operation ~ (vaginal hysterectomy) 58260-58270, 58550
Marrow, bone ~ see bone marrow

Marshall-Marchetti-Krantz procedure ~ 51840-51841, 58152, 58267, 58293
Marsupialization ~ 10040
Bartholin's gland cyst ~ 56440
cyst, sublingual salivary ~ 42409
liver, cyst or abscess ~ 47300
pancreatic cyst ~ 48500
urethral diverticulum ~ 53240
Mass, kidney, ablation ~ 50542
Massage, cardiac ~ 32160
therapy ~ 97124
Masseter muscle/bone, reduction ~ 21295-21296
Mass spectrometry and tandem mass spectrometry
analyte
qualitative ~ 83788
quantitative ~ 83789
Mastectomy
gynecomastia ~ 19300
modified radical ~ 19307
partial ~ 19301-19302
radical ~ 19305-19306
simple, complete ~ 19303
subcutaneous ~ 19304
Mastectomy, Halsted ~ see radical mastectomy
Mastoid
excision
complete ~ 69502
radical ~ 69511
modified ~ 69505
petrous apicectomy ~ 69530
simple ~ 69501
obliteration ~ 69670
repair
with apicectomy ~ 69605
by excision ~ 69601-69603
fistula ~ 69700
with tympanoplasty ~ 69604
Mastoid cavity, debridement ~ 69220-69222
Mastoidectomy
cochlear device implantation ~ 69930
complete ~ 69502
revision ~ 69601
ossicular chain reconstruction ~ 69605
radical ~ 69511
modified ~ 69505
revision ~ 69602-69603
simple ~ 69501
with apicectomy ~ 69605
with labyrinthectomy ~ 69910
with labyrinthotomy ~ 69802
with petrous apicectomy ~ 69530
with skull base surgery ~ 61590, 61597
decompression ~ 61595
facial nerve ~ 61595
with tympanoplasty ~ 69604, 69641-69646
Mastoidotomy ~ 69635-69637
with tympanoplasty ~ 69635
ossicular chain reconstruction ~ 69636
and synthetic prosthesis ~ 69636
Mastoids
polytomography ~ 76101-76102
X-ray ~ 70120-70130
Mastopexy ~ 19316
Mastotomy ~ 19020
Maternity care and delivery ~ see abortion; cesarean delivery; ectopic pregnancy; obstetrical care
Maxilla ~ see facial bones; mandible
bone graft ~ 21210
CT scan ~ 70486-70488
cyst, excision ~ 21048-21049
excision ~ 21030, 21032-21034
fracture
closed treatment ~ 21345, 21421
open treatment ~ 21346-21348, 21422-21423
with fixation ~ 21345-21347
osteotomy ~ 21206
reconstruction, with implant ~ 21245-21246, 21248-21249
tumor, excision ~ 21048-21049
Maxillary arteries ~ see artery, maxillary
Maxillary sinus ~ see sinus, maxillary
Maxillary torus palatinus, tumor excision ~ 21032
Maxillectomy ~ 31225-31230
Maxillofacial fixation, application, halo type appliance ~ 21100
Maxillofacial impressions
auricular prosthesis ~ 21086
definitive obturator prosthesis ~ 21080
facial prosthesis ~ 21088
interim obturator prosthesis ~ 21079
mandibular resection prosthesis ~ 21081
nasal prosthesis ~ 21087
oral surgical splint ~ 21085
orbital prosthesis ~ 21077
palatal augmentation prosthesis ~ 21082
palatal lift prosthesis ~ 21083
speech aid prosthesis ~ 21084
surgical obturator prosthesis ~ 21076
Maxillofacial procedures, unlisted services and procedures ~ 21299
Maxillofacial prosthesis ~ 21076-21089
unlisted services and procedures ~ 21089
Maydl operation ~ (colostomy) 45563, 50810
Mayo hernia repair ~ 49580-49587
Mayo operation ~ (varicose vein removal) 37700-37735, 37780, 37785
Mayo procedure ~ 28292
MBC ~ (minimum bactericidal concentration) 87181-87190
McBride procedure ~ 28292
McBurney operation ~ (see also hernia, repair, inguinal) 49495-49500, 49505
McCannel procedure ~ 66682
McDonald operation ~ (repair, cervix, cerclage, abdominal; revision) 57700
McIndoe procedure ~ (vagina, construction) 57291
McKissock surgery ~ (breast, reduction) 19318

McVay operation ~ (hernia, repair, inguinal) 49495-49500, 49505
Measles, German ~ see rubella
Measles uncomplicated ~ see rubeola
Measles vaccine ~ see vaccines
Meat fibers, feces ~ 89160
Meatoplasty ~ 69310
Meatotomy ~ 53020-53025
contact laser vaporization with/without transurethral resection of prostate ~ 52648
with cystourethroscopy ~ 52281
infant ~ 53025
non-contact laser coagulation prostate ~ 52647
transurethral electrosurgical resection, prostate ~ 52601
ureter ~ 52290
ureteral, cystourethroscopy ~ 52290-52305
Meckel's diverticulum, excision ~ 44800
unlisted services and procedures ~ 44899
Median nerve
decompression ~ 64721
neuroplasty ~ 64721
release ~ 64721
repair/suture, motor ~ 64835
transposition ~ 64721
Median nerve compression ~ see carpal tunnel syndrome
Mediastinal cyst ~ see cyst, mediastinal
Mediastinoscopy ~ 39400
Mediastinotomy
cervical approach ~ 39000
transthoracic approach ~ 39010
Mediastinum ~ see chest; thorax
cyst, excision ~ 32662, 39200
endoscopy
biopsy ~ 39400
exploration ~ 39400
exploration ~ 39000-39010
incision and drainage ~ 39000-39010
needle biopsy ~ 32405
removal, foreign body ~ 39000-39010
tumor, excision ~ 32662, 39220
unlisted procedures ~ 39499
Mediastinum and diaphragm, surgical procedures ~ 39000-39599
Medical disability evaluation services ~ 99455-99456
Medical genetics ~ 96040
Medical nutrition therapy ~ 97802-97804
Medical testimony ~ 99075
Medicine, preventive ~ see preventive medicine
Medicine, pulmonary ~ see pulmonology
Medicine services ~ 90281-99602
Medulla, tractotomy ~ 61470
Medullary tract
incision ~ 61470
section ~ 61470
Meibomian cyst ~ see chalazion
Membrane, mucous ~ see mucosa
Membrane, tympanic ~ see ear, drum
Membrane oxygenation, extracorporeal ~ see extracorporeal membrane oxygenation
Meninges, tumor, excision ~ 61512, 61519
Meningioma, excision ~ 61512, 61519
tumor, excision ~ 61512, 61519
Meningitis, lymphocytic benign ~ see lymphocytic choriomeningitis
Meningocele repair ~ 63700-63702
Meningococcal vaccine ~ see vaccines
Meningococcus ~ see neisseria meningitidis
Meningomyelocele ~ see myelomeningocele
Meniscectomy
knee joint ~ 27332-27333
temporomandibular joint ~ 21060
Meniscus
knee
excision ~ 27332-27333
repair ~ 27403
transplantation ~ 29868
Mental nerve
avulsion ~ 64736
incision ~ 64736
transection ~ 64736
Meprobamate ~ 83805
Mercury ~ 83015, 83825
Merskey test ~ see fibrin degradation products
Mesencephalic tract
incision ~ 61480
section ~ 61480
Mesencephalon, tractotomy ~ 61480
Mesenteric arteries ~ see artery, mesenteric
Mesentery
lesion, excision ~ 44820
repair ~ 44850
suture ~ 44850
unlisted services and procedures ~ 44899
Mesh
implantation, hernia ~ 49568
insertion, pelvic floor ~ 57267
removal, abdominal infected ~ 11008
Metabisulfite test ~ (red blood cell (RBC), sickling) 85660
Metabolite ~ 82520
Metacarpal
amputation ~ 26910
craterization ~ 26230
cyst, excision ~ 26200-26205
diaphysectomy ~ 26230
excision ~ 26230
radical, for tumor ~ 26250-26255
fracture
closed treatment ~ 26605
with fixation ~ 26607
with manipulation ~ 26605-26607
without manipulation ~ 26600
open treatment ~ 26615
percutaneous fixation ~ 26608
ostectomy, radical, for tumor ~ 26250-26255
repair
lengthening ~ 26568
nonunion ~ 26546
osteotomy ~ 26565
saucerization ~ 26230
tumor, excision ~ 26200-26205

Metacarpophalangeal joint
arthrodesis ~ 26850-26852
arthroplasty ~ 26530-26531
arthroscopy
diagnostic ~ 29900
surgical ~ 29901-29902
arthrotomy ~ 26075
biopsy, synovium ~ 26105
capsule
excision ~ 26520
incision ~ 26520
capsulodesis ~ 26516-26518
dislocation
closed treatment ~ 26700
open treatment ~ 26715
percutaneous fixation ~ 26705-26706
with manipulation ~ 26340
exploration ~ 26075
fracture
closed treatment ~ 26740
open treatment ~ 26746
with manipulation ~ 26742
fusion ~ 26516-26518, 26850-26852
removal of foreign body ~ 26075
repair, collateral ligament ~ 26540-26542
synovectomy ~ 26135
Metadrenaline ~ see metanephrines
Metals, heavy ~ see heavy metal
Metamfetamine ~ see methamphetamine
Metanephrines ~ 83835
Metatarsal ~ see foot
amputation ~ 28810
condyle, excision ~ 28288
craterization ~ 28122
cyst, excision ~ 28104-28107
diaphysectomy ~ 28122
excision ~ 28110-28114, 28122, 28140
fracture
closed treatment
with manipulation ~ 28475-28476
without manipulation ~ 28470
open treatment ~ 28485
percutaneous fixation ~ 28476
free osteocutaneous flap with microvascular anastomosis ~ 20972
repair ~ 28322
lengthening ~ 28306-28307
osteotomy ~ 28306-28309
saucerization ~ 28122
tumor, excision ~ 28104-28107, 28173
Metatarsectomy ~ 28140
Metatarsophalangeal joint
arthrotomy ~ 28022, 28052
cheilectomy ~ 28289
dislocation ~ 28630-28635, 28645
percutaneous fixation ~ 28636
exploration ~ 28022
great toe
arthrodesis ~ 28750
fusion ~ 28750
removal
of foreign body ~ 28022
Metatarsophalangeal joint ~ *continued*
of loose body ~ 28022
repair, hallux rigidus ~ 28289
synovial
biopsy ~ 28052
excision ~ 28072
toe ~ 28270
Methadone ~ 83840
Methaemoglobin ~ see methemoglobin
Methamphetamine, blood or urine ~ 82145
Methanol ~ 84600
Methbipyranone ~ see metyrapone
Methemalbumin ~ 83857
Methemoglobin ~ 83045-83050
Methenamine silver stain ~ 88312
Methopyrapone ~ see metyrapone
Methoxyhydroxymandelic acid ~ see vanillylmandelic acid
Methsuximide ~ 83858
Methylamphetamine ~ see methamphetamine
Methylene bichloride ~ see dichloromethane
Methylfluorprednisolone ~ see dexamethasone
Methylmorphine ~ see codeine
Methyl alcohol ~ (methanol) 84600
Metroplasty ~ see hysteroplasty
Metyrapone ~ 80436
MIC ~ (minimum inhibitory concentration) 87186
Micro-ophthalmia, orbit reconstruction ~ 21256
Microalbumin, urine ~ 82043-82044
Microbiology ~ 0023T, 87001-87999
Microfluorometries, flow ~ see flow cytometry
Microdissection ~ 88380
Microglobulin, beta 2
blood ~ 82232
urine ~ 82232
Micrographic surgery, Mohs technique ~ 17311-17315
Micropigmentation, correction ~ 11920-11922
Microscope, surgical ~ see operating microscope
Microscopic evaluation, hair ~ 96902
Microscopies, electron ~ see electron microscopy
Microscopy, ear exam ~ 92504
Microsomal antibody ~ 86376
Microsomia, hemifacial ~ see hemifacial microsomia
Microsurgery, operating microscope ~ 69990
Microvascular anastomosis
bone graft
fibula ~ 20955
other ~ 20962
fascial flap, free ~ 15758
muscle flap, free ~ 15756
osteocutaneous flap with, ~ 20969-20973
skin flap, free ~ 15757
Microvite A ~ see vitamin A
Microwave therapy ~ (see also physical medicine/therapy/occupational therapy) 97020

Midbrain ~ see brain; brainstem; mesencephalon; skull base surgery
Midcarpal mediocciptal joint, arthrotomy ~ 25040
Middle cerebral artery velocimetry ~ 76821
Middle ear ~ see ear, middle
Midface
reconstruction
with bone graft ~ 21145-21160, 21188
without bone graft ~ 21141-21143
forehead advancement ~ 21159-21160
Migration inhibitory factor (MIF) ~ 86378
Mile operation ~ see colectomy, total, with proctectomy
Milia, multiple, removal ~ 10040
Miller procedure ~ 28737
Miller-Abbott intubation ~ 44500, 74340
Minerva cast ~ 29035
removal ~ 29710
Minimum inhibitory concentration (MIC) ~ 87186
Minimum lethal concentration ~ 87187
Minnesota multiphasic personality inventory ~ see MMPI
Miscarriage
incomplete abortion ~ 59812
missed abortion
first trimester ~ 59820
second trimester ~ 59821
septic abortion ~ 59830
Missed abortion ~ see abortion; miscarriage, missed abortion
Mitchell procedure ~ 28296
Mitogen blastogenesis ~ 86353
Mitral valve
incision ~ 33420-33422
repair ~ 33420-33427
incision ~ 33420-33422
replacement ~ 33430
Mitrofanoff operation ~ (appendico-vesicostomy) 50845
Miyagawanella ~ see Chlamydia
MMPI ~ (Minnesota multiphasic personality inventory) 96100
MMR shots ~ (measles, mumps and rubella vaccines) 90707
Mobilization
splenic flexure ~ 44139
stapes ~ 69650
Modified radical mastectomy ~ see mastectomy, modified radical
Mohs micrographic surgery ~ 17311-17315
Molar pregnancy ~ see hydatidiform mole
Mold, culture ~ 87107
Mole, carneous ~ see abortion
Mole, hydatid ~ see hydatidiform mole
Molecular cytogenetics ~ 88271-88275
interpretation and report ~ 88291
Molecular diagnostics ~ 83890-83914
amplification ~ 83898-83901
dot/slot production ~ 83893
enzymatic digestion ~ 83892
Molecular diagnostics ~ ***continued***
extraction ~ 83890-83891
interpretation ~ 83912
molecular isolation (extraction) ~ 83890
mutation identification ~ 83904-83906
mutation scanning ~ 83903
nucleic acid probe ~ 83896
nucleic acid transfer ~ 83897
polymerase reaction chain ~ 83898
reverse transcription ~ 83902
RNA stabilization ~ 83913
separation ~ 83894
Molecular oxygen saturation ~ see oxygen saturation
Molluscum contagiosum, destruction ~ 17110-17111, 54050-54065
Molteno procedure ~ 66180
Monilia ~ see candida
Monitoring
blood pressure, 24 hour ~ 93784-93790
electrocardiogram ~ (see also electrocardiography) 93224-93237
electroencephalogram ~ 95812-95813, 95950-95953, 95956
with drug activation ~ 95954
with physical activation ~ 95954
with WADA activation ~ 95958
fetal, during labor ~ 59050-59051, 99500
interpretation only ~ 59051
glucose, interstitial fluid ~ 95250
interstitial fluid pressure ~ 20950
pediatric apnea ~ 94774-94777
seizure ~ 61531, 61760
Monitoring, sleep ~ see polysomnography
Monoethylene glycol ~ see ethylene glycol
Mononucleosis virus, infectious ~ see Epstein-Barr virus
Monophosphate
adenosine ~ (adenosine monophosphate (AMP)) 82030
adenosine cyclic ~ (cyclic AMP) 82030
guanosine ~ (guanosine monophosphate (GMP)) 83008
guanosine cyclic ~ (cyclic GMP) 83008
Monospot test ~ (rapid test for infection) 86308
Monoxide, carbon ~ see carbon monoxide
Monteggia fracture ~ 24620-24635
Monticelli procedure ~ (application, bone fixation device) 20690, 20692
Morbilli ~ see rubeola
Morphine methyl ether ~ see codeine
Morphometric analysis
nerve ~ 88356
skeletal muscle ~ 88355
tumor ~ 88358-88361, 88367-88368
Morton's neuroma, excision ~ 28080
Moschcowitz operation ~ see repair, hernia, femoral; revision
Mosenthal test ~ (urinalysis, routine) 81002
Mother cell ~ see stem cell
Motility study, esophagus ~ 91010-91012

Motion analysis
by video and 3-D kinematics ~ 96000, 96004
computer-based ~ 96000, 96004
Mouth
abscess, incision and drainage ~ 40800-40801, 41005-41009, 41015-41018
biopsy ~ 40808, 41108
cyst, incision and drainage ~ 40800-40801, 41005-41009, 41015-41018
excision, frenum ~ 40819
hematoma, incision and drainage ~ 40800-40801, 41005-41009, 41015-41018
lesion
destruction ~ 40820
excision ~ 40810-40816, 41116
vestibule of
destruction ~ 40820
repair ~ 40830
mucosa, excision ~ 40818
reconstruction ~ 40840-40845
removal, foreign body ~ 40804-40805
repair, laceration ~ 40830-40831
unlisted services and procedures ~ 40899, 41599
vestibule of
excision, destruction ~ 40808-40820
incision ~ 40800-40806
other procedures ~ 40899
removal, foreign body ~ 40804
repair ~ 40830-40845
Move ~ see transfer
finger ~ 26555
toe joint ~ 26556
toe to hand ~ 26551-26554
Moynihan test ~ (gastrointestinal tract, X-ray, with contrast) 74246-74249
MPR ~ (multifetal pregnancy reduction) 59866
MRA ~ see magnetic resonance angiography
MRI ~ see magnetic resonance imaging
MR spectroscopy ~ see magnetic resonance spectroscopy
MSLT ~ (multiple sleep latency testing) 95805
Mucin, synovial fluid ~ 83872
Mucocele sinusotomy, frontal ~ 31075
Mucopolysaccharides ~ 83864-83866
Mucormycoses ~ see mucormycosis
Mucormycosis, antibody ~ 86732
Mucosa
ectopic gastric imaging ~ 78290
excision of lesion
alveolar, hyperplastic ~ 41828
vestibule of mouth ~ 40810-40818
via esophagoscopy ~ 43228
via small intestinal endoscopy ~ 44369
via upper gi endoscopy ~ 43258
peridodontal grafting ~ 41870
urethra, mucosal advancement ~ 53450
vaginal biopsy ~ 57100-57105
Mucosa, buccal ~ see mouth, mucosa
Mucous cyst antibody, hand or finger ~ 26160
Mucous membrane ~ see mouth, mucosa
cutaneous
biopsy ~ 11100-11101
excision
benign lesion ~ 11440-11446
malignant lesion ~ 11640-11646
layer closure, wounds ~ 12051-12057
simple repair, wounds ~ 12011-12018
excision, sphenoid sinus ~ 31288
lid margin
correction of trichiasis ~ 67835
nasal test ~ 95065
ophthalmic test ~ 95060
rectum
proctoplasty for prolapse ~ 45505
MUGA (multiple gated acquisition) ~ 78472-78478, 78483
Muller procedure ~ see sleep study
Multifetal pregnancy reduction ~ 59866
Multiple sleep latency testing (MSLT) ~ 95805
Multiple valve procedures ~ see valvuloplasty
Mumford operation ~ (partial claviculectomy, arthroscopic) 29824
Mumps
antibody ~ 86735
immunization ~ 90704, 90707, 90710
vaccine ~ 90704
MMR ~ 90707
MMRV ~ 90710
Muramidase ~ 85549
Murine typhus ~ 86000
Muscle ~ see specific muscle
abdomen ~ see abdominal wall
biopsy ~ 20200-20206
debridement, infected ~ 11004-11006
heart ~ see myocardium
neck ~ see neck muscle
oculomotor ~ see eye muscles
removal, foreign body ~ 20520-20525
repair
extraocular ~ 65290
forearm ~ 25260-25274
wrist ~ 25260-25274
revision, arm, upper ~ 24330-24331
transfer
arm, upper ~ 24301, 24320
elbow ~ 24301
femur ~ 27110
hip ~ 27100-27105, 27111
shoulder ~ 23395-23397, 24301, 24320
Muscle compartment syndrome, detection ~ 20950
Muscle denervation ~ see denervation
Muscle division
scalenus anticus ~ 21700-21705
sternocleidomastoid ~ 21720-21725
Muscle flaps ~ 15732-15738
free ~ 15756
Muscle grafts ~ 15841-15845

Muscle testing
dynamometry, eye ~ 92260
extraocular multiple muscles ~ 92265
manual ~ 95831-95834
Musculo-skeletal system ~ see musculoskeletal system
Musculoplasty ~ see muscle, repair
Musculoskeletal system, surgical procedures ~ 20000-29999
Musculotendinous (rotator) cuff, repair ~ 23410-23412
Mustard procedure ~ (repair, great arteries; revision) 33774-33777
Myasthenia gravis, tensilon test ~ 95857-95858
Mycobacteria
culture ~ 87116
identification ~ 87118
detection ~ 87550-87562
sensitivity studies ~ 87190
Mycoplasma
antibody ~ 86738
culture ~ 87109
detection ~ 87580-87582
Mycota ~ see fungus
Myectomy, anorectal ~ see myomectomy, anorectal
Myelencephalon ~ see medulla
Myelin basic protein, cerebrospinal fluid ~ 83873
Myelography
brain ~ 70010
spine
cervical ~ 72240
lumbosacral ~ 72265
thoracic ~ 72255
total ~ 72270
Myelomeningocele, repair ~ 63704-63706
Myelotomy ~ 63170
Myocardial, perfusion imaging ~ 78460-78465, 78478-78480
positron emission tomography (PET) ~ 78459
Myocardial imaging ~ 78466-78469
positron emission tomography, perfusion study ~ 78491-78492
repair, postinfarction ~ 33542
Myocutaneous flaps ~ 15732-15738, 15756
Myofascial pain dysfunction syndrome ~ see temporomandibular joint (TMJ)
Myofibroma ~ see leiomyomata
Myoglobin ~ 83874
Myomectomy
anorectal ~ 45108
uterus ~ 58140-58146, 58545-58546
Myoplasty ~ see muscle, repair
Myotomy
esophagus ~ 43030
hyoid ~ 21685
Myringoplasty ~ 69620
Myringostomy ~ see myringostomy
Myringotomy ~ 69420-69421
Myxoid cyst ~ see ganglion

N

N. meningitidis ~ see Neisseria meningitidis
Naffziger operation ~ (decompression, orbit; section) 61330
Nagel test ~ (color vision examination) 92283
Nail(s)
avulsion ~ 11730-11732
biopsy ~ 11755
debridement ~ 11720-11721
evacuation, hematoma, subungual ~ 11740
excision ~ 11750-11752
cyst, pilonidal ~ 11770-11772
KOH examination ~ 87220
removal ~ 11730-11732, 11750-11752
trimming ~ 11719
Nail bed, reconstruction ~ 11762
repair ~ 11760
Nail fold, excision wedge ~ 11765
Nail plate separation ~ see onychia
Narcosynthesis, diagnostic and therapeutic ~ 90865
Nasal abscess ~ see nose, abscess
Nasal area, bone graft ~ 21210
Nasal bleeding ~ see epistaxis
Nasal bone
fracture
closed treatment ~ 21310-21320
open treatment ~ 21325-21335
with manipulation ~ 21315-21320
without manipulation ~ 21310
X-ray ~ 70160
Nasal deformity, repair ~ 40700-40761
Nasal function study ~ 92512
Nasal polyp ~ see nose, polyp
Nasal prosthesis, impression ~ 21087
Nasal septum
abscess, incision and drainage ~ 30020
fracture
closed treatment ~ 21337
open treatment ~ 21336
hematoma, incision and drainage ~ 30020
repair ~ 30630
submucous resection ~ 30520
Nasal sinuses ~ see sinus; sinuses
Nasal smear, eosinophils ~ 89190
Nasal turbinate fracture, therapeutic ~ 30930
Nasoethmoid complex
fracture
open treatment ~ 21338-21339
percutaneous treatment ~ 21340
reconstruction ~ 21182-21184
Nasogastric tube, placement ~ 43752
Nasolacrimal duct
exploration ~ 68810
with anesthesia ~ 68811
insertion, stent ~ 68815
X-ray, with contrast ~ 70170

Nasomaxillary
fracture
closed treatment ~ 21345
open treatment ~ 21346-21348
with bone grafting ~ 21348
Nasopharynges ~ see nasopharynx
Nasopharyngoscopy ~ 92511
Nasopharynx ~ see also pharynx
biopsy ~ 42804-42806
hemorrhage ~ 42970-42972
unlisted services and procedures ~ 42999
Natriuretic peptide ~ 83880
Natural ostium sinus
maxillary ~ 31000
sphenoid ~ 31002
Navicular
arthroplasty, with implant ~ 25443
fracture
closed treatment ~ 25622
open treatment ~ 25628
with manipulation ~ 25624
navigation, computer assisted ~ 0054T-0056T
repair ~ 25440
Neck
angiography ~ 70498, 70547-70549
artery, ligation ~ 37615
biopsy ~ 21550
bypass graft ~ 35901
CT scan ~ 70490-70492, 70498
dissection, radical ~ see radical neck dissection
exploration
blood vessel ~ 35800
lymph nodes ~ 38542
incision and drainage
abscess ~ 21501-21502
hematoma ~ 21501-21502
lipectomy, suction assisted ~ 15876
magnetic resonance angiography (MRA) ~ 70547-70549
magnetic resonance imaging(MRI) ~ 70540-70543
nerve, graft ~ 64885-64886
repair, blood vessel ~ 35201
with other graft ~ 35261
with vein graft ~ 35231
skin, revision ~ 15819
tumor
excision ~ 21555-21556
excision/resection ~ 21557
ultrasound exam ~ 76536
unlisted services and procedures, surgery ~ 21899
urinary bladder ~ see bladder, neck
wound exploration, penetrating ~ 20100
X-ray ~ 70360
Neck muscle
division
scalenus anticus ~ 21700-21705
sternocleidomastoid ~ 21720-21725
Necropsy
coroner's exam ~ 88045
forensic exam ~ 88040
gross and micro exam ~ 88020-88029
gross exam ~ 88000-88016
organ ~ 88037
regional ~ 88036
unlisted services and procedures ~ 88099
Needle biopsy ~ see also biopsy
abdomen mass ~ 49180
bone ~ 20220-20225
bone marrow ~ 38221
breast ~ 19100
colon, endoscopy ~ 45392
colon-sigmoid, endoscopy ~ 45342
CT scan guidance ~ 77012
epididymis ~ 54800
esophagus, endoscopy ~ 43232
fluoroscopic guidance ~ 77002
gastrointestinal, upper, endoscopy ~ 43238, 43242
kidney ~ 50200
liver ~ 47000-47001
lung ~ 32405
lymph nodes ~ 38505
mediastinum ~ 32405
muscle ~ 20206
pancreas ~ 48102
pleura ~ 32400
prostate ~ 55700
retroperitoneal mass ~ 49180
salivary gland ~ 42400
spinal cord ~ 62269
testis ~ 54500
thyroid gland ~ 60100
transbronchial ~ 31629, 31633
Needle localization
breast
placement ~ 19290-19291
with lesion excision ~ 19125-19126
magnetic resonance guidance ~ 77021
Needle manometer technique ~ 20950
Needle wire
introduction, trachea ~ 31730
placement, breast ~ 19290-19291
Neer procedure ~ 23470
Neisseria gonorrheae ~ 87590-87592, 87850
Neisseria meningitidis, antibody ~ 86741
Neobladder, construction ~ 51596
Neonatal critical care ~ see also newborn care
initial ~ 99295
subsequent ~ 99296
Neoplasm
cancer photoradiation therapy ~ see photochemotherapy
cardiac ~ see heart, tumor
colon ~ see colon, tumor
esophageal ~ see tumor, esophagus
spinal cord ~ see spinal cord, neoplasm
unspecified nature of brain ~ see brain, tumor
Neoplastic growth ~ see tumor
Nephelometry ~ 83883

Nephrectomy
donor ~ 50300-50320, 50547
laparoscopic ~ 50545-50548
partial ~ 50240
laparoscopic ~ 50543
recipient ~ 50340
with ureters ~ 50220-50236, 50546, 50548
Nephrolith ~ see calculus, removal, kidney
Nephrolithotomy ~ 50060-50075
Nephropexy ~ 50400-50405
Nephroplasty ~ see kidney, repair
Nephropyeloplasty ~ see pyeloplasty
Nephrorrhaphy ~ 50500
Nephroscopy ~ see endoscopy, kidney
Nephrostogram ~ 50394
Nephrostolithotomy, percutaneous ~ 50080-50081
Nephrostomy ~ 50040
change tube ~ 50398
endoscopic ~ 50562-50570
percutaneous ~ 52334
with drainage ~ 50040
X-ray with contrast, guide dilation ~ 74485
Nephrostomy tract, establishment ~ 50395
Nephrotomogram ~ see nephrotomography
Nephrotomography ~ 74415
Nephrotomy ~ 50040-50045
with exploration ~ 50045
Nerve
see also nerves
cranial ~ see cranial nerve
facial ~ see facial nerve
intercostal ~ see intercostal nerve
lingual ~ see lingual nerve
median ~ see median nerve
obturator ~ see obturator nerve
peripheral ~ see peripheral nerve
phrenic ~ see phrenic nerve
sciatic ~ see sciatic nerve
spinal ~ see spinal nerve
tibial ~ see tibial nerve
ulnar ~ see ulnar nerve
vestibular ~ see vestibular nerve
Nerve conduction
motor nerve ~ 95900-95903
sensory nerve or mixed ~ 95904
Nerve II, cranial ~ see optic nerve
Nerve root ~ see also cauda equina; spinal cord
decompression ~ 63020-63048, 63055-63103
incision ~ 63185-63190
section ~ 63185-63190
Nerve stimulation, transcutaneous ~ see application, neurostimulation
Nerve teasing ~ 88362
Nerves
anastomosis
facial to hypoglossal ~ 64868
facial to phrenic ~ 64870
facial to spinal accessory ~ 64866
avulsion ~ 64732-64772
biopsy ~ 64795
decompression ~ 64702-64727
Nerves ~ ***continued***
destruction ~ 64600-64681
laryngeal, recurrent ~ 31595
foot
incision ~ 28035
graft ~ 64885-64907
implantation, electrode ~ 64553-64581
to bone ~ 64787
to muscle ~ 64787
incision ~ 43640-43641, 64732-64772
injection
anesthetic ~ 01991-01992, 64400-64530
neurolytic agent ~ 64600-64681
insertion, electrode ~ 64553-64581
lesion, excision ~ 64774-64792
neurofibroma, excision ~ 64788-64792
neurolemmoma, excision ~ 64788-64792
neurolytic, internal ~ 64727
neuroma, excision ~ 64774-64786
neuroplasty ~ 64702-64721
removal, electrode ~ 64585
repair
graft ~ 64885-64911
microdissection ~ 69990
suture ~ 64831-64876
spinal accessory
incision ~ 63191
section ~ 63191
suture ~ 64831-64876
sympathectomy, excision ~ 64802-64818
transection ~ 43640-43641, 64732-64772
transposition ~ 64718-64721
unlisted services and procedures ~ 64999
Nerve V, cranial ~ see trigeminal nerve
Nerve VII, cranial ~ see facial nerve
Nerve X, cranial ~ see vagus nerve
Nerve XI, cranial ~ see accessory nerve
Nerve XII, cranial ~ see hypoglossal nerve
Nervous system, surgical procedures ~ 61000-64999
Nesidioblast ~ see islet cell
Neural conduction ~ see nerve conduction
Neural ganglion ~ see ganglion
Neurectomy
foot ~ 28055
gastrocnemius ~ 27326
hamstring muscle ~ 27325
leg, upper ~ 27325
popliteal ~ 27326
tympanic ~ 69676
Neuroendoscopy, intracranial ~ 62160-62165
Neurofibroma
cutaneous nerve, excision ~ 64788
extensive, excision ~ 64792
peripheral nerve, excision ~ 64790
Neurolemmoma
cutaneous nerve, excision ~ 64788
extensive, excision ~ 64792
peripheral nerve, excision ~ 64790
Neurologic system ~ see nervous system

Neurology procedures
diagnostic
anal sphincter ~ 51785
autonomic nervous function
heart rate response ~ 95921-95923
pseudomotor response ~ 95921-95923
sympathetic function ~ 95921-95923
brain surface electrode stimulation ~ 95961-95962
central motor transcranial motor stimulation ~ 95928-95929
electrocorticogram, intraoperative ~ 95829
electroencephalogram (EEG) ~ 95812-95827, 95955
brain death ~ 95824
electrode placement ~ 95830
intraoperative ~ 95955
monitoring ~ 95812-95813, 95950-95953, 95956
physical or drug activation ~ 95954
sleep ~ 95822, 95827
standard ~ 95819
WADA activation ~ 95958
electroencephalography (EEG), digital analysis ~ 95957
electromyography
fine wire dynamic ~ 96004
ischemic limb exercise test ~ 95875
needle ~ 51785, 95860-95872
surface dynamic ~ 96002-96004
higher cerebral function
aphasia test ~ 96105
cognitive function tests ~ 96115
developmental tests ~ 96110-96111
magnetoencephalography (MEG) ~ 95965-95967
motion analysis
by video and 3-D kinematics ~ 96000, 96004
computer-based ~ 96000, 96004
muscle testing, manual ~ 95831-95834
nerve conduction
motor nerve ~ 95900-95903
sensory nerve or mixed ~ 95904
neuromuscular junction tests ~ 95937
neurophysiological testing, intraoperative ~ 95920
neuropsychological testing ~ 96117
plantar pressure measurements, dynamic ~ 96001, 96004
polysomnography ~ 95808-95811
range of motion ~ 95851-95852
reflex
blink reflex ~ 95933
H-reflex ~ 95933-95934
sleep study ~ 95807-95810
somatosensory testing ~ 95925-95927
tensilon test ~ 95857-95858
unlisted services and procedures ~ 95999
urethral sphincter ~ 51785
visual evoked potential, CNS ~ 95930

Neurolysis
nerve ~ 64704-64708
internal ~ 64727
Neuroma
acoustic ~ see brain, tumor, excision
cutaneous nerve, excision ~ 64774
digital nerve, excision ~ 64776-64778
excision ~ 64774
foot, excision ~ 28080
foot nerve, excision ~ 64782-64783
hand nerve, excision ~ 64782-64783
interdigital ~ see Morton's neuroma
peripheral nerve, excision ~ 64784
sciatic nerve, excision ~ 64786
Neuromuscular junction tests ~ 95937
Neuromuscular pedicle reinnervation larynx ~ 31590
Neuromuscular reeducation ~ 97112
Neurophysiologic testing
autonomic nervous function
heart rate response ~ 95921-95923
pseudomotor response ~ 95921-95923
sympathetic function ~ 95921-95923
intraoperative, per hour ~ 95920
Neuroplasty ~ 64712
cranial nerve ~ 64716
digital nerve ~ 64702-64704
peripheral nerve ~ 64708-64714, 64718-64721
Neuropsychological testing ~ 96117
Neurorrhaphy ~ 64831-64876
peripheral nerve
conduit ~ 64910-64911
with graft ~ 64885-64907
Neurostimulation, application ~ 64550
Neurostimulators
analysis ~ 95970-95975
implantation ~ 64553-64565
electrodes ~ 43647, 43881
insertion
pulse generator ~ 64590
receiver ~ 64590
removal
electrodes ~ 43648, 43882, 61880
pulse generator ~ 61888, 64595
receiver ~ 61888, 64595
replacement ~ 61885
electrodes ~ 43647, 43881
Neurotomy, sympathetic ~ see gasserian ganglion, sensory root, decompression
Neurovascular pedicle flaps ~ 15750
Neutralization test, virus ~ 86382
New patient
confirmatory consultations ~ 99271-99275
domiciliary or rest home visit ~ 99321-99323
emergency department services ~ 99281-99288
home services ~ 99341-99345
hospital inpatient services ~ 99221-99239
hospital observation services ~ 99217-99220
initial inpatient consultations ~ 99251-99255
initial office visit ~ see evaluation and management
office and other outpatient ~ 99201-99205

New patient ~ *continued*
office and/or other outpatient consultations ~ 99241-99245
Newborn care ~ 99431-99440, 99502
attendance at delivery ~ 99436
birthing room ~ 99431
blood transfusion ~ 36450
circumcision
clamp or other device ~ 54150
surgical excision ~ 54160
history and examination ~ 99431, 99435
laryngoscopy ~ 31520
normal ~ 99431-99433
prepuce slitting ~ 54000
preventive, office ~ 99432
resuscitation ~ 99440
standby for cesarean delivery ~ 99360
subsequent hospital care ~ 99433
umbilical artery catheterization ~ 36660
Nickel ~ 83885
Nicolas-Durand-Favre disease ~ see lymphogranuloma venereum
Nicotine ~ 83887
Nidation ~ see implantation
Nipples ~ see breast
inverted ~ 19355
reconstruction ~ 19350
Nissen operation ~ see fundoplasty, esophagogastric
Nissen procedure ~ 43324
laparoscopic ~ 43280
Nitrate reduction test ~ see urinalysis
Nitric Oxide ~ 95012
Nitroblue tetrazolium dye test ~ 86384
Nitrogen, blood urea ~ see blood urea nitrogen
NMR imaging ~ see magnetic resonance imaging (MRI)
NMR spectroscopies ~ see magnetic resonance spectroscopy
No man's land, tendon repair ~ 26356-26358
Noble procedure ~ see repair; suture
Nocardia, antibody ~ 86744
Nocturnal penile rigidity test ~ 54250
Nocturnal penile tumescence test ~ 54250
Node, lymph ~ see lymph nodes
Nodes ~ see lymph nodes
Node dissection, lymph ~ see dissection, lymph nodes
Non-invasive vascular imaging ~ 93875-93990
Non-office medical services ~ 99056
Non-stress test, fetal ~ 59025
Nonunion repair
femur
with graft ~ 27472
without graft ~ 27470
metatarsal ~ 28322
tarsal joint ~ 28320
Noradrenalin
blood ~ 82383-82384
urine ~ 82384
Norchlorimipramine ~ see imipramine
Norepinephrine ~ see catecholamines
blood ~ 82383-82384
urine ~ 82384
Nortriptyline, assay ~ 80182
Norwood procedure ~ 33611-33612, 33619
Nose
abscess, incision and drainage ~ 30000-30020
artery, incision ~ 30915-30920
biopsy, intranasal ~ 30100
dermoid cyst, excision
complex ~ 30125
simple ~ 30124
displacement therapy ~ 30210
endoscopy
diagnostic ~ 31231-31235
surgical ~ 31237-31294
excision, rhinectomy ~ 30150-30160
fracture
closed treatment ~ 21345
open treatment ~ 21325-21336, 21338-21339, 21346-21347
percutaneous treatment ~ 21340
with fixation ~ 21330, 21340, 21345-21347
hematoma, incision and drainage ~ 30000-30020
hemorrhage, cauterization ~ 30901-30906
insertion, septal prosthesis ~ 30220
intranasal lesion
external approach ~ 30118
internal approach ~ 30117
lysis of adhesions ~ 30560
polyp, excision
extensive ~ 30115
simple ~ 30110
reconstruction
cleft lip/cleft palate ~ 30460-30462
dermatoplasty ~ 30620
primary ~ 30400-30420
secondary ~ 30430-30450
septum ~ 30520
removal
foreign body ~ 30300
anesthesia ~ 30310
lateral rhinotomy ~ 30320
repair
adhesions ~ 30560
cleft lip ~ 40700-40761
fistula ~ 30580-30600, 42260
rhinophyma ~ 30120
septum ~ 30540-30545, 30630
synechia ~ 30560
vestibular stenosis ~ 30465
skin
excision ~ 30120
surgical planing ~ 30120
submucous resection turbinate
excision ~ 30140
turbinate
excision ~ 30130-30140
fracture ~ 30930
injection ~ 30200

Nose ~ *continued*
turbinate mucosa, cauterization ~ 30801-30802
unlisted services and procedures ~ 30999
Nose bleed ~ (hemorrhage, nasal) 30901-30906
NTD ~ (nitroblue tetrazolium dye test) 86384
Nuclear antigen, antibody ~ 86235
Nuclear imaging ~ see nuclear medicine
Nuclear magnetic resonance imaging ~ see magnetic resonance imaging (MRI)
Nuclear magnetic resonance spectroscopy ~ see magnetic resonance spectroscopy
Nuclear medicine ~ 78000-79999
adrenal gland imaging ~ 78075
automated data ~ 78890-78891
bile duct imaging ~ 78223
bladder, residual study ~ 78730
blood
flow imaging ~ 78445
iron
absorption ~ 78162
chelatable ~ 78172
plasma ~ 78160
red cells ~ 78140
utilization ~ 78170
platelet survival ~ 78190-78191
red cells ~ 78120-78121
red cells survival ~ 78130-78135
unlisted services and procedures ~ 78199
whole blood volume ~ 78122
bone
density study ~ 78350-78351
imaging ~ 78300-78320
SPECT ~ 78320
ultrasound ~ 76977
ultrasound services and procedures ~ 78399
bone marrow imaging ~ 78102-78104
brain
blood flow ~ 78610-78615
cerebrospinal flow ~ 78630-78650
imaging ~ 78600-78609
vascular flow ~ 78610
endocrine system, unlisted services and procedures ~ 78099
esophagus
imaging (motility) ~ 78258
reflux study ~ 78262
gallbladder imaging ~ 78223
gastric mucosa imaging ~ 78261
gastrointestinal
blood loss study ~ 78278
protein loss study ~ 78282
shunt testing ~ 78291
unlisted services and procedures ~ 78299
genitourinary system, unlisted services and procedures ~ 78799
heart
blood flow ~ 78414
blood pool imaging ~ 78472-78473, 78481-78483, 78494-78496
myocardial imaging ~ 78459, 78466-78469
myocardial perfusion ~ 78460-78465, 78478-78480

Nuclear medicine ~ *continued*
heart ~ *continued*
shunt detection ~ 78428
unlisted services and procedures ~ 78499
hepatic duct imaging ~ 78223
inflammatory process ~ 78805-78807
intestines imaging ~ 78290
kidney
function study ~ 78725
imaging ~ 78700-78707, 78710
lacrimal gland, tear flow ~ 78660
liver
function study ~ 78220
imaging ~ 78201-78216
vascular flow ~ 78206
lung
imaging perfusion ~ 78580-78585
imaging ventilation ~ 78586-78594
unlisted services and procedures ~ 78599
lymph nodes ~ 78195
lymphatics ~ 78195
unlisted services and procedures ~ 78199
musculoskeletal system, unlisted services and procedures ~ 78399
nervous system, unlisted services and procedures ~ 78699
parathyroid gland imaging ~ 78070
pulmonary perfusion imaging ~ 78588
salivary gland function study ~ 78232
imaging ~ 78230-78231
spleen
imaging ~ 78185, 78215-78216
unlisted services and procedures ~ 78199
stomach
blood loss study ~ 78278
emptying study ~ 78264
protein loss study ~ 78282
reflux study ~ 78262
vitamin B-12 absorption ~ 78270-78272
testes imaging ~ 78761
therapeutic
heart ~ 79440
interstitial ~ 79300
intra-arterial ~ 79445
intra-articular ~ 79440
intracavitary ~ 79200
intravenous ~ 79101
intravenous infusion ~ 79403
oral ~ 79005
thyroid ~ 79200-79300
unlisted services and procedures ~ 79999
thyroid
imaging ~ 78010
imaging with flow ~ 78011
imaging for metastases ~ 78015-78018
imaging with uptake ~ 78006
metastases uptake ~ 78020
uptake ~ 78000-78003
tumor imaging
positron emission tomography (PET) ~ 78811-78816
with computed tomography ~ 78814-78816

Nuclear medicine ~ *continued*
tumor localization ~ 78800-78804
unlisted services and procedures ~ 78999
urea breath test ~ 78267-78268
ureter, reflux study ~ 78740
vein thrombosis imaging ~ 78455-78458
Nucleases, DNA ~ see DNAse
Nucleic acid probe ~ 83896
amplified probe detection, infectious agent
bartonella henselae ~ 87471
bartonella quintana ~ 87471
borrelia burgdorferi ~ 87476
candida species ~ 87481
chlamydia pneumoniae ~ 87486
chlamydia trachomatis ~ 87491
cytomegalovirus ~ 87496
enterovirus ~ 87498
gardnerella vaginalis ~ 87511
hepatitis B virus ~ 87516
hepatitis C ~ 87521
hepatitis G ~ 87526
herpes simplex virus ~ 87529
herpes virus-6 ~ 87532
HIV-1 ~ 87535
HIV-2 ~ 87538
legionella pneumophila ~ 87541
multiple organisms ~ 87801
mycobacteria avium-intracellulare ~ 87561
mycobacteria species ~ 87551
mycobacteria tuberculosis ~ 87556
mycoplasma pneumoniae ~ 87581
neisseria gonorrheae ~ 87591
not otherwise specified ~ 87798, 87801
papillomavirus, human ~ 87621
staphylococcus aureus ~ 87640-87641
streptococcus, group A ~ 87651
streptococcus, group B ~ 87653
direct probe detection, infectious agent
bartonella henselae ~ 87470
bartonella quintana ~ 87470
borrelia burgdorferi ~ 87475
candida species ~ 87480
chlamydia pneumoniae ~ 87485
chlamydia trachomatis ~ 87490
cytomegalovirus ~ 87495
gardnerella vaginalis ~ 87510
hepatitis B virus ~ 87515
hepatitis C ~ 87520
hepatitis G ~ 87525
herpes simplex virus ~ 87528
herpes virus-6 ~ 87531
HIV-1 ~ 87534
HIV-2 ~ 87537
legionella pneumophila ~ 87540
multiple organisms ~ 87800
mycobacteria avium-intracellulare ~ 87560
mycobacteria species ~ 87550
mycobacteria tuberculosis ~ 87555
mycoplasma pneumoniae ~ 87580
neisseria gonorrheae ~ 87590
not otherwise specified ~ 87797
papillomavirus, human ~ 87620

Nucleic acid probe ~ *continued*
streptococcus, group A ~ 87650
trichomonas vaginalis ~ 87660
genotype analysis, infectious agent
HIV-1 ~ 87901
hepatitis C virus ~ 87902
in situ hybridization ~ 88365-88368
phenotype analysis, infectious agent
HIV-1 drug resistance ~ 87903-87904
quantification, infectious agent
bartonella henselae ~ 87472
bartonella quintana ~ 87472
borrelia burgdorferi ~ 87477
candida species ~ 87482
chlamydia pneumoniae ~ 87487
chlamydia trachomatis ~ 87492
cytomegalovirus ~ 87497
gardnerella vaginalis ~ 87512
hepatitis B virus ~ 87517
hepatitis C ~ 87522
hepatitis G ~ 87527
herpes simplex virus ~ 87530
herpes virus-6 ~ 87533
HIV-1 ~ 87536
HIV-2 ~ 87539
legionella pneumophila ~ 87542
mycobacteria avium-intracellulare ~ 87562
mycobacteria species ~ 87552
mycobacteria tuberculosis ~ 87557
mycoplasma pneumoniae ~ 87582
neisseria gonorrheae ~ 87592
not otherwise specified ~ 87799
papillomavirus, human ~ 87622
streptococcus, group A ~ 87652
Nucleolysis, intervertebral disk ~ see chemonucleolysis
Nucleotidase ~ 83915
Nursemaid elbow ~ 24640
Nursing facility discharge services ~ see discharge services, nursing facility
Nursing facility services ~ 99304-99318
care plan oversight services ~ 99379-99380
comprehensive assessments
new or established patient ~ 99301-99303
discharge services ~ 99315-99316
subsequent care
new or established patient ~ see domiciliary services ~ 99311-99313
Nuss procedure
with thoracoscopy ~ 21743
without thoracoscopy ~ 21742
Nutrition therapy
group ~ 97804
home infusion ~ 99601-99602
initial assessment ~ 97802
reassessment ~ 97803
Nystagmus tests ~ see vestibular function tests
optokinetic ~ 92534, 92544
positional ~ 92532, 92542
spontaneous ~ 92531, 92541

O

O2 (two) saturation ~ see oxygen saturation
Ober-Yount procedure ~ (fasciotomy, hip) 27025
Obliteration
mastoid ~ 69670
vagina
total ~ 57110-57112
vault ~ 57120
Oblongata, medulla ~ see medulla
Observation ~ (see evaluation and management; hospital services) 99234-99236
Obstetrical care
abortion
induced
by amniocentesis injection ~ 59850-59852
by dilation and curettage ~ 59840
by dilation and evaluation ~ 59841
missed
first trimester ~ 59820
second trimester ~ 59821
spontaneous ~ 59812
therapeutic ~ 59840-59852
antepartum care ~ 59425-59426
cesarean delivery ~ 59618-59622
only ~ 59514
postpartum care ~ 59515
routine ~ 59510
with hysterectomy ~ 59525
curettage, hydatidiform mole ~ 59870
evacuation, hydatidiform mole ~ 59870
external cephalic version ~ 59412
miscarriage, surgical completion ~ 59812-59821
placenta delivery ~ 59414
postpartum care ~ 59430, 59514
septic abortion ~ 59830
total (global) ~ 59400, 59610, 59618
unlisted services and procedures ~ 59898-59899
vaginal, after cesarean ~ 59610-59614
vaginal delivery ~ 59409-59410
delivery after cesarean ~ 59610-59614
Obstruction ~ see occlusion
Obstruction clearance, venous access device ~ 36595-36596
Obstruction colon ~ see colon, obstruction
Obturator nerve
avulsion ~ 64763-64766
incision ~ 64763-64766
transection ~ 64763-64766
Obturator prosthesis ~ 21076
definitive ~ 21080
insertion, larynx ~ 31527
interim ~ 21079
Occipital nerve, greater
avulsion ~ 64744
incision ~ 64744
injection, anesthetic ~ 64405
transection ~ 64744
Occlusion
extracranial, intracranial ~ 61623
fallopian tube, oviduct ~ 58565, 58615
penis, vein ~ 37790
umbilical cord ~ 59072
Occlusive disease of artery ~ see repair, artery; revision
Occult blood ~ 82270
penis, by hemoglobin immunoassay ~ 82274
Occupational therapy, evaluation ~ 97003-97004
Ocular implant ~ see orbital implant
insertion
in scleral shell ~ 65130
muscles attached ~ 65140
muscles, not attached ~ 65135
modification ~ 65125
reinsertion ~ 65150
with foreign material ~ 65155
removal ~ 65175
Ocular muscle ~ see eye muscles
Ocular orbit ~ see orbit
Ocular photoscreening ~ 0065T
Ocular prostheses ~ see prosthesis, ocular
Oculomotor muscle ~ see eye muscles
Oddi sphincter ~ see sphincter of Oddi
Odontoid dislocation
open treatment/reduction ~ 22318
with grafting ~ 22319
Odontoid fracture
open treatment/reduction ~ 22318
with grafting ~ 22319
Odontoid process, excision ~ 22548
Oesophageal neoplasm ~ see tumor, esophagus
Oesophageal varices ~ see esophageal varices
Oesophagus ~ see esophagus
Oestradiol ~ see estradiol
Office and/or other outpatient services
consultation, confirmatory ~ 99271-99275
established patient ~ 99211-99215
new patient ~ 99201-99205
normal newborn ~ 99432
office visit
established patient ~ 99211-99215
new patient ~ 99201-99205
outpatient visit
established patient ~ 99211-99215
new patient ~ 99201-99205
prolonged services ~ 99354-99355
Office medical services
after hours ~ 99050-99054
emergency care ~ 99058
Office or other outpatient consultations ~ 99241-99245

Olecranon ~ see elbow; humerus; radius; ulna
bursa, arthrocentesis ~ 20605
cyst, excision ~ 24125-24126
tumor
cyst ~ 24120
excision ~ 24125-24126
Olecranon process
craterization ~ 24147
diaphysectomy ~ 24147
excision ~ 24147
abscess ~ 24138
fracture ~ see elbow; humerus; radius
closed treatment ~ 24670-24675
open treatment ~ 24685
osteomyelitis ~ 24138, 24147
saucerization ~ 24147
sequestrectomy ~ 24138
Oligoclonal immunoglobulins ~ 83916
Omentectomy ~ 49255, 58950-58958
laparotomy ~ 58960
oophorectomy ~ 58943
resection ovarian malignancy ~ 58950-58952
resection peritoneal malignancy ~ 58950-58958
resection tubal malignancy ~ 58950-58958
Omentum
excision ~ 49255, 58950-58958
flap ~ 49904-49905
free, with microvascular anastomosis ~ 49906
unlisted services and procedures ~ 49999
Omphalectomy ~ 49250
Omphalocele, repair ~ 49600-49611
Omphalomesenteric duct, excision ~ 44800
Omphalomesenteric duct, persistent ~ see diverticulum, Meckel's
Oncoprotein, HER-2/neu ~ 83950
One stage prothrombin time ~ (see also prothrombin time) 85610-85611
Onychectomy ~ see excision, nails
Onychia, drainage ~ 10060-10061
Oocyte
assisted fertilization, microtechnique ~ 89280-89281
biopsy ~ 89290-89291
cryopreservation ~ 0059T
culture
extended ~ 89272
less than 4 (four) days ~ 89250
with co-culture ~ 89251
identification, follicular fluid ~ 89254
insemination ~ 89268
retrieval, for in vitro fertilization ~ 58970
storage ~ 89346
thawing ~ 89356
Oophorectomy ~ 58262-58263, 58291-58292, 58552, 58554, 58661, 58940-58943
ectopic pregnancy
laparoscopic treatment ~ 59120
surgical treatment ~ 59120
Oophorectomy, partial ~ see excision, ovary, partial
Oophorocystectomy ~ see cystectomy, ovarian
Open biopsy, adrenal gland ~ see adrenal gland, biopsy
Operating microscope ~ 69990
Operation
Blalock-Hanlon ~ see septostomy, atrial
Blalock-Taussig subclavian-pulmonary anastomosis ~ see pulmonary artery, shunt, subclavian
Borthen ~ see iridotasis
Dana ~ see rhizotomy
Dunn ~ see arthrodesis, foot joint
Duvries ~ see tenoplasty
Estes ~ see ovary, transposition
Foley pyeloplasty ~ see pyeloplasty
Fontan ~ see repair, heart, anomaly
Fox ~ see fox operation
Gardner ~ see meningocele repair
Green ~ see scapulopexy
harelip ~ see cleft lip, repair
Heine ~ see cyclodialysis
Heller ~ see esophagomyotomy
iris, inclusion ~ see iridencleisis
Jaboulay gastroduodenostomy ~ see gastroduodenostomy
Johanson ~ see reconstruction, urethra
Keller ~ see keller procedure
Krause ~ see gasserian ganglion, sensory root, decompression
Mumford ~ see claviculectomy, partial
Nissen ~ see fundoplasty, esophagogastric
Peet ~ see nerves, sympathectomy, excision
Ramstedt ~ see pyloromyotomy
Richardson hysterectomy ~ see hysterectomy, abdominal, total
Schanz ~ see femur, osteotomy
Schlatter total gastrectomy ~ see excision, stomach, total
Smithwick ~ see excision, nerve, sympathetic
Winiwarter cholecystoenterostomy ~ see anastomosis, gallbladder to intestines
Operation microscopes ~ see operating microscope
Operculectomy ~ 41821
Operculum ~ see gums
Ophthalmic mucous membrane test ~ (see also allergy tests) 95060
Ophthalmology services ~ 92002-92499
Ophthalmology, diagnostic
color vision exam ~ 92283
computerized scanning ~ 92135
computerized screening ~ 0065T, 99172
dark adaptation ~ 92284
electro-oculography ~ 92270
electromyography, needle ~ 92265
electroretinography ~ 92275
endoscopy ~ 66990
eye exam
established patient ~ 92012-92014
new patient ~ 92002-92004
with anesthesia ~ 92018-92019
glaucoma provocative test ~ 92140

Ophthalmology, diagnostic ~ *continued*
gonioscopy ~ 92020
ocular photography
external ~ 92285
internal ~ 92286-92287
ophthalmoscopy ~ 92225-92226
with dynamometry ~ 92260
with fluorescein angiography ~ 92235
with fluorescein angioscopy ~ 92230
with fundus photography ~ 92250
with indocyanine-green angiography ~ 92240
photoscreening ~ 0065T
refractive determination ~ 92015
sensorimotor exam ~ 92060
tonography ~ 92120
with provocation ~ 92130
tonometry, serial ~ 92100
ultrasound ~ 76511-76529
visual acuity screen ~ 99172-99173
visual field exam ~ 92081-92083
visual function screen ~ 0065T, 99172
Ophthalmoscopy ~ 92225-92226
Opiates ~ 83925
Opinion, second ~ see confirmatory consultations
Optic nerve
decompression ~ 67570
with nasal/sinus endoscopy ~ 31294
Optokinetic nystagmus test ~ see nystagmus tests, optokinetic
Oral lactose tolerance test ~ see glucose, tolerance test ~ 82951-82953
Oral mucosa ~ see mouth, mucosa
Oral surgical splint ~ 21085
Orbit ~ see orbital contents; orbital floor; periorbital region
biopsy ~ 61332
exploration ~ 67450
fine needle aspiration or orbital contents ~ 67415
orbitotomy without bone flap ~ 67400
CT scan ~ 70480-70482
decompression ~ 61330
bone removal ~ 67414, 67445
exploration ~ 61332, 67400, 67450
lesion, excision ~ 61333
fracture
closed treatment
with manipulation ~ 21401
without manipulation ~ 21400
open treatment ~ 21406-21408
blowout fracture ~ 21385-21395
incision and drainage ~ 67405, 67440
injection
retrobulbar ~ 67500-67505
tenon's capsule ~ 67515
insertion, implant ~ 67550
lesion, excision ~ 67412, 67420
magnetic resonance imaging (MRI) ~ 70540-70543
removal
decompression ~ 67445

Orbit ~ *continued*
exploration ~ 61334
foreign body ~ 61334, 67413, 67430
implant ~ 67560
sella turcica ~ 70482
unlisted services and procedures ~ 67599
X-ray ~ 70190-70200
Orbital contents, aspiration ~ 67415
Orbital floor ~ see orbit; periorbital region
fracture, blow out ~ 21385-21395
Orbital hypertelorism, osteotomy
periorbital ~ 21260-21263
Orbital implant ~ see ocular implant
insertion ~ 67550
removal ~ 67560
Orbital prosthesis ~ 21077
Orbital rims, reconstruction ~ 21182-21184
Orbital rim and forehead, reconstruction ~ 21172-21180
Orbital transplant ~ 67560
Orbital walls, reconstruction ~ 21182-21184
Orbitocraniofacial reconstruction, secondary ~ 21275
Orbitotomy
with bone flap
for exploration ~ 67450
lateral approach ~ 67420
with drainage ~ 67440
with removal foreign body ~ 67430
with removal of bone for decompression ~ 67445
without bone flap
for exploration ~ 67400
with drainage only ~ 67405
with removal lesion ~ 67412
with removal foreign body ~ 67413
with removal of bone for decompression ~ 67414
Orbit area reconstruction, secondary ~ 21275
Orbit wall decompression with nasal/sinus endoscopy ~ 31292-31293
Orchidectomies ~ see excision, testis
Orchidopexy ~ see orchiopexy
Orchidoplasty ~ see repair, testis
Orchiectomy
laparoscopic ~ 54690
partial ~ 54522
radical
abdominal exploration ~ 54535
inguinal approach ~ 54530
simple ~ 54520
Orchiopexy
abdominal approach ~ 54650
inguinal approach ~ 54640
intra-abdominal testis ~ 54692
Orchioplasty ~ see repair, testis
Organ or disease oriented panels ~ 80048-80076
electrolyte ~ 80051
general health panel ~ 80050
hepatic function panel ~ 80076
hepatitis panel ~ 80074

Organ or disease oriented panels ~ *continued*
lipid panel ~ 80061
metabolic
basic ~ 80048
comprehensive ~ 80053
obstetric panel ~ 80055
renal function ~ 80069
Organic acids ~ 83918-83921
Organ grafting ~ see transplantation
Organ system, neurologic ~ see nervous system
Ormond disease ~ see retroperitoneal fibrosis
Orogastric tube placement ~ 43752
Oropharynx, biopsy ~ 42800
Orthodontic cephalogram ~ 70350
Orthomyxoviridae ~ see influenza virus
Orthomyxovirus ~ see influenza virus
Orthopantogram ~ 70355
Orthopedic cast ~ see cast
Orthopedic surgery
computer assisted navigation ~ 0054T-0056T
stereotaxis, computer assisted ~ 0054T-0056T
Orthoptic training ~ 92065
Orthoroentgenogram ~ 77073
Orthosis ~ see orthotics
Orthotics
check-out ~ 97703
fitting and training ~ 97504
Osmolality
blood ~ 83930
urine ~ 83935
Osseous survey ~ 77074-77076
Osseous tissue ~ see bone
Ossicles
excision stapes
with footplate drill out ~ 69661
without foreign material ~ 69660-69661
reconstruction ossicular chain
tympanoplasty with antrotomy or mastoidotomy ~ 69636-69637
tympanoplasty with mastoidectomy ~ 69642, 69644, 69646
tympanoplasty without mastoidectomy ~ 69632-69633
release, stapes ~ 69650
replacement, with prosthesis ~ 69633, 69637
Ostectomy
metacarpal ~ 26250-26255
metatarsal ~ 28288
phalanges, finger ~ 26260-26262
pressure ulcer
ischial ~ 15941, 15945
sacral ~ 15933, 15935, 15937
trochanteric ~ 15951, 15953, 15958
scapula ~ 23190
sternum ~ 21620
Osteocalcin ~ 83937
Osteocartilaginous exostoses ~ see exostosis
Osteochondroma ~ see exostosis
Osteocutaneous flap, with microvascular anastomosis ~ 20969-20973
Osteoma sinusotomy, frontal ~ 31075
Osteomyelitis ~ 20000-20005
elbow, incision and drainage ~ 23935
excision
clavicle ~ 23180
facial ~ 21026
humerus, proximal ~ 23184
mandible ~ 21025
scapula ~ 23182
femur/knee, incision and drainage ~ 27303
finger incision ~ 26034
hand incision ~ 26034
hip incision, deep ~ 26992
humerus ~ 24134
incision and drainage ~ 23935
incision
foot ~ 28005
shoulder ~ 23035
thorax ~ 21510
olecranon process ~ 24138, 24147
pelvis incision, deep ~ 26992
radius ~ 24136, 24145
sequestrectomy
clavicle ~ 23170
humeral head ~ 23174
scapula ~ 23172
skull ~ 61501
Osteopathic manipulation ~ 98925-98929
Osteoplasty
carpal bone ~ 25394
facial bones
augmentation ~ 21208
reduction ~ 21209
femoral neck ~ 27179
femur ~ 27179
lengthening ~ 27466-27468
shortening ~ 27465, 27468
fibula, lengthening ~ 27715
humerus ~ 24420
metacarpal ~ 26568
phalanges, finger ~ 26568
radius ~ 25390-25393
tibia, lengthening ~ 27715
ulna ~ 25390-25393
vertebra ~ 72291-72292
lumbar ~ 22521-22522
thoracic ~ 22520-22522
Osteotomy
calcaneus ~ 28300
chin ~ 21121-21123
clavicle ~ 23480-23485
femur ~ 27140, 27151
femoral neck ~ 27161
for slipped epiphysis ~ 27181
with fixation ~ 27165
without fixation ~ 27448-27450
with open reduction of hip ~ 27156
with realignment ~ 27454
fibula ~ 27707-27712
hip ~ 27146-27151
femoral, with open reduction ~ 27156
femur ~ 27151
humerus ~ 24400-24410

Osteotomy ~ *continued*
mandible ~ 21198-21199
extra-oral ~ 21047
intra-oral ~ 21046
maxilla ~ 21206
extra-oral ~ 21049
intra-oral ~ 21048
metacarpal ~ 26565
metatarsal ~ 28306-28309
orbit reconstruction ~ 21256
pelvis ~ 27158
periorbital
orbital hypertelorism ~ 21260-21263
osteotomy with graft ~ 21267-21268
phalanges
finger ~ 26567
toe ~ 28299, 28310-28312
radius
and ulna ~ 25365, 25375
distal third ~ 25350
middle or proximal third ~ 25355
multiple ~ 25370
skull base ~ 61582-61585, 61592
spine
anterior ~ 22220-22226
posterior, posterolateral ~ 22210-22214
talus ~ 28302
tarsal ~ 28304-28305
tibia ~ 27455-27457, 27705, 27709-27712
ulna ~ 25360
multiple ~ 25370
and radius ~ 25365, 25375
vertebra
additional segment, anterior approach ~ 22226
posterior/posterolateral approach ~ 22216
cervical
anterior approach ~ 22220
posterior/posterolateral approach ~ 22210
lumbar
anterior approach ~ 22224
posterior/posterolateral approach ~ 22214
thoracic
anterior approach ~ 22222
posterior/posterolateral approach ~ 22212
with graft reconstruction periorbital region ~ 21267-21268
Os calcis fracture ~ see calcaneus, fracture
Otolaryngology, diagnostic exam under anesthesia ~ 92502
Otomy ~ see incision
Otoplasty ~ 69300
Otorhinolaryngology services ~ 92502-92597
Ouchterlony immunodiffusion ~ 86331
Outer ear ~ see ear, outer
Outpatient visit ~ see history and physical; office and/or other outpatient services
Output, cardiac ~ see cardiac output
Ova, smear ~ 87177
Oval window, repair fistula ~ 69666
Oval window fistula ~ see fistula, oval window
Ovarian cyst ~ see cyst, ovarian; ovary, cyst
Ovarian vein syndrome, ureterolysis ~ 50722
Ovariectomies ~ see oophorectomy
Ovariolysis ~ 58740
Ovary
abscess, incision and drainage ~ 58820-58822
abdominal approach ~ 58822
biopsy ~ 58900
cryopreservation ~ 0058T
cyst, incision and drainage ~ 58800-58805
excision ~ 58662, 58720
cyst ~ 58925
partial
oophorectomy ~ 58661, 58940
ovarian malignancy ~ 58943
peritoneal malignancy ~ 58943
tubal malignancy ~ 58943
wedge resection ~ 58920
total ~ 58940-58943
laparoscopy ~ 58660-58662, 58679
lysis, adhesions ~ 58660, 58740
radical resection ~ 58950-58952
transposition ~ 58825
tumor, resection ~ 58950-58958
unlisted services and procedures ~ 58679, 58999
wedge resection ~ 58920
Oviduct
anastomosis ~ 58750
chromotubation ~ 58350
ectopic pregnancy ~ 59120-59121
excision ~ 58700-58720
fulguration, laparoscopic ~ 58670
hysterosalpingography ~ 74740
laparoscopy ~ 58679
ligation ~ 58600-58611
lysis, adhesions ~ 58740
occlusion ~ 58615
laparoscopic ~ 58671
repair ~ 58752
anastomosis ~ 58750
create stoma ~ 58770
unlisted services and procedures ~ 58679, 58999
X-ray with contrast ~ 74740
Ovocyte ~ see oocyte
Ovulation tests ~ 84830
Ovum implantation ~ see implantation
Ovum transfer surgery ~ see gamete intrafallopian transfer (GIT)
Oxalate ~ 83945
Oxidase, ceruloplasmin ~ see ceruloplasmin
Oxidoreductase, alcohol-nad+ ~ see antidiuretic hormone
Oximetry (noninvasive) ~ see pulmonology, diagnostic
blood O2 saturation, ear or pulse ~ 94760-94762
Oxoisomerase ~ see phosphohexose isomerase
Oxosteroids ~ see ketosteroids
Oxycodinone ~ 80102-80103, 83925
Oxygenation, extracorporeal membrane ~ see extracorporeal membrane oxygenation

Oxygen saturation ~ 82805-82810
Oxyproline ~ see hydroxyproline
Oxytocin stress test, fetal ~ 59020

P

P & P ~ (proconvertin) 85230
P-acetamidophenol ~ see acetaminophen
Pacemaker, heart
  conversion ~ 33214
  electronic analysis ~ 93641-93642
    antitachycardia system ~ 93724
    dual chamber ~ 93731-93732, 93743-93744
    single chamber ~ 93734-93735, 93741-93742
    wearable device ~ 93741-93742, 93745
  insertion ~ 33206-33208
    electrode ~ 33210-33211, 33216-33217, 33224-33225
    pulse generator only ~ 33212-33213
  removal ~ 33233-33237
    via thoracotomy ~ 33236-33237
  repair, electrode ~ 33218-33220
  replacement
    catheter ~ 33210
    electrode ~ 33210-33211
    insertion ~ 33206-33208
    pulse generator ~ 33212-33213
  repositioning, electrode ~ 33215, 33226
  revise pocket, chest ~ 33222
  telephonic analysis ~ 93733, 93736
  upgrade ~ 33214
Pachymetry, eye ~ 76514
Packing, nasal hemorrhage ~ 30901-30906
Pain management
  epidural/intrathecal ~ 62350-62351, 62360-62362, 99601-99602
  intravenous therapy ~ 90783-90784
Palatal augmentation prosthesis ~ 21082
Palatal lift prosthesis ~ 21083
Palate
  abscess, incision and drainage ~ 42000
  biopsy ~ 42100
  excision ~ 42120, 42145
  fracture
    closed treatment ~ 21421
    open treatment ~ 21422-21423
  lesion
    destruction ~ 42160
    excision ~ 42104-42120
  prosthesis ~ 42280-42281
  reconstruction, lengthening ~ 42226-42227
  repair
    cleft palate ~ 42200-42225
    laceration ~ 42180-42182
    Vomer flap ~ 42235
  unlisted services and procedures ~ 42299
Palate, cleft ~ see cleft palate
Palatoplasty ~ 42200-42225
Palatoschisis ~ see cleft palate
Palm
  bursa, incision and drainage ~ 26025-26030
  fasciectomy ~ 26121-26125
  fasciotomy ~ 26040-26045
  tendon, excision ~ 26170
  tendon sheath
    excision ~ 26145
    incision and drainage ~ 26020
Palsy, seventh nerve ~ see facial nerve paralysis
Pancreas
  anastomosis
    with intestines ~ 48520-48540
  anesthesia ~ 00794
  biopsy ~ 48100
    needle biopsy ~ 48102
  cyst
    anastomosis ~ 48520-48540
    repair ~ 48500
  debridement, peripancreatic tissue ~ 48105
  excision
    ampulla of vater ~ 48148
    duct ~ 48148
    partial ~ 48140-48146, 48150, 48154, 48160
    peripancreatic tissue ~ 48105
    total ~ 48155-48160
  lesion, excision ~ 48120
  needle biopsy ~ 48102
  placement, drainage ~ 48000-48001
  pseudocyst
    drainage
      open ~ 48510
      percutaneous ~ 48511
  removal, calculi (stone) ~ 48020
  removal transplanted allograft ~ 48556
  repair, cyst ~ 48500
  suture ~ 48545
  transplantation ~ 48160, 48550, 48554-48556
    allograft preparation ~ 48550-48552
  unlisted services and procedures ~ 48999
  X-ray with contrast ~ 74300-74305
    injection procedure ~ 48400
Pancreas, endocrine only ~ see islet cell
Pancreatectomy
  donor ~ 48550
  partial ~ 48140-48146, 48150-48154, 48160
  total ~ 48155-48160
  with transplantation ~ 48160
Pancreaticojejunostomy ~ 48548
Pancreatic DNAse ~ see DNAse
Pancreatic duct
  destruction, calculi (stone) ~ 43265
  dilation, endoscopy ~ 43271
  endoscopy
    collection, specimen ~ 43260
    destruction
      calculi (stone) ~ 43265
      tumor ~ 43272
    dilation ~ 43271
    removal (endoscopic)
      calculi (stone) ~ 43264

Pancreatic duct ~ *continued*
endoscopy ~ *continued*
foreign body ~ 43269
stent ~ 43269
sphincter pressure ~ 43263
sphincterotomy ~ 43262
tube placement ~ 43267-43268
incision, sphincter ~ 43262
removal
calculi (stone) ~ 43264
foreign body ~ 43269
stent ~ 43269
tube placement
nasopancreatic ~ 43267
stent ~ 43268
tumor, destruction ~ 43272
X-ray with contrast, guide catheter ~ 74329-74330
Pancreatic elastase 1 (PEL1) ~ 82656
Pancreatic islet cell ab ~ see antibody, islet cell
Pancreatitis, incision and drainage ~ 48000
Pancreatography
injection procedure ~ 48400
intraoperative ~ 74300-74301
postoperative ~ 74305
Pancreatojejunostomies ~ see pancreaticojejunostomy
Pancreatorrhaphy ~ 48545
Pancreatotomy ~ see incision, pancreas
Pancreozymin-secretin test ~ 82938
Panel ~ see organ or disease oriented panel
Panniculectomy ~ see lipectomy
Paper, chromatography ~ see chromatography, paper
Paper chromatographies ~ see chromatography, paper
Papilla, interdental ~ see gums
Pap smears ~ 88141-88155, 88164-88167, 88174-88175
Papillectomy ~ 46220
Papilloma
destruction ~ 54050-54065
anus ~ 46900-46924
penis ~ 54050-54065
PAPP D ~ see lactogen, human placental
Para-tyrosine ~ see tyrosine
Paracentesis ~ 49080
abdomen ~ 49080-49081
eye, anterior chamber
with diagnostic aspiration of aqueous ~ 65800
with removal of blood ~ 65815
with removal vitreous and/or discission of anterior hyaloid membrane ~ 65810
with therapeutic release of aqueous ~ 65805
thorax ~ 32000-32002
Paracervical nerve, injection, anesthetic ~ 64435
Paraffin bath therapy ~ 97018
Paraganglioma, medullary ~ see pheochromocytoma
Parainfluenza virus antigen detection, immunofluorescence ~ 87279
Paralysis, facial nerve ~ see facial nerve paralysis
Paralysis, infantile ~ see polio
Paranasal sinuses ~ see sinus; sinuses
Parasites
blood ~ 87207
examination ~ 87169
smear ~ 87177
Parasitic worms ~ see helminth
Parathormone ~ 83970
Parathyrin ~ see parathormone
Parathyroidectomy ~ 60500-60505
Parathyroid autotransplantation ~ 60512
Parathyroid gland
autotransplant ~ 60512
excision ~ 60500-60502
exploration ~ 60500-60505
nuclear medicine, imaging ~ 78070
Parathyroid hormone ~ 83970
Parathyroid hormone measurement ~ see parathormone
Parathyroid transplantation ~ see transplantation, parathyroid
Paraurethral gland
abscess, incision and drainage ~ 53060
Paravertebral nerve
destruction ~ 64622-64627
injection
anesthetic ~ 64470-64484
neurolytic ~ 64622-64627
Parietal cell vagotomies ~ see vagotomy, highly selective
Parietal craniotomy ~ 61556
Paring
skin lesion, benign hyperkeratotic
more than four lesions ~ 11057
single lesion ~ 11055
two to four lesions ~ 11056
Paronychia, incision and drainage ~ 10060-10061
Parotid duct
diversion ~ 42507-42510
reconstruction ~ 42507-42510
Parotid gland
abscess, incision and drainage ~ 42300-42305
calculi (stone), excision ~ 42330, 42340
excision
partial ~ 42410-42415
total ~ 42420-42426
tumor, excision ~ 42410-42426
Parotitides, epidemic ~ see mumps
Pars abdominalis aortae ~ see aorta, abdominal
Partial
colectomy ~ see colectomy, partial
cystectomy ~ see cystectomy, partial
esophagectomy ~ see esophagectomy, partial
gastrectomy ~ see excision, stomach, partial
glossectomy ~ see excision, tongue, partial
hepatectomy ~ see excision, liver, partial

Partial ~ *continued*
mastectomies ~ see breast, excision, lesion
nephrectomy ~ see excision, kidney, partial
pancreatectomy ~ see pancreatectomy, partial
splenectomy ~ see splenectomy, partial
thromboplastin time ~ see thromboplastin, partial, time
ureterectomy ~ see ureterectomy, partial
Particle agglutination ~ 86403-86406
Parvovirus antibody ~ 86747
Patch allergy tests ~ 95044
Patella
dislocation ~ 27560-27566
excision ~ 27350
with reconstruction ~ 27424
fracture ~ 27520-27524
reconstruction ~ 27437-27438
repair
chondromalacia ~ 27418
instability ~ 27420-27424
Patella, chondromalacia ~ see chondromalacia patella
Patellar tendon bearing (PTB) cast ~ 29435
Patellectomy with reconstruction ~ 27424
Paternity testing ~ 86910-86911
Patey's operation ~ see mastectomy, radical
Pathologic dilatation ~ see dilation
Pathology and laboratory services ~ 8000-89999
clinical
consultation ~ 80500-80502
surgical ~ 88355
consultation ~ 88321-88325
intraoperative ~ 88329-88332
decalcification procedure ~ 88311
electron microscopy ~ 88348-88349
gross and micro exam
level II ~ 88302
level III ~ 88304
level IV (four) ~ 88305
level V (five) ~ 88307
level VI (six) ~ 88309
gross exam, level I ~ 88300
histochemistry ~ 88318-88319
immunocytochemistry ~ 88342
immunofluorescent study ~ 88346-88347
morphometry
nerve ~ 88356
skeletal muscle ~ 88355
tumor ~ 88358-88361
nerve teasing ~ 88362
special stain ~ 88312-88314
staining ~ 88312-88314
tissue hybridization ~ 88365
unlisted services and procedures ~ 88399, 89240
Patterson's test ~ see blood urea nitrogen
Paul-Bunnell test ~ see antibody; antibody identification; microsomal antibody
P B antibodies ~ see antibody, heterophile
PBG ~ see porphobilinogen
PCP ~ (phencyclidine) 83992
PCR ~ (polymerase chain reaction) 83898-83902, 83904-83912
Pean's operation ~ (amputation, upper leg, at hip) 27290
Pectoral cavity ~ see chest cavity
Pectus carinatum
reconstructive repair ~ 21740-21742
with thoracoscopy ~ 21743
Pectus excavatum
reconstructive repair ~ 21740-21742
with thoracoscopy ~ 21743
Pediatric critical care ~ 99293-99294
Pediatric intensive care ~ 99293
Pedicle fixation insertion ~ 22842-22844
Pedicle flap
formation ~ 15570-15576
island ~ 15740
neurovascular ~ 15750
transfer ~ 15650
PEEP ~ see pressure breathing, positive
Peet operation ~ see nerves, sympathectomy, excision
Pelvi-ureteroplasty ~ see pyeloplasty
Pelvic adhesions ~ see adhesions, pelvic
Pelvic exam ~ 57410
Pelvic exenteration ~ 51597
Pelvic fixation insertion ~ 22848
Pelvic lymphadenectomy ~ 58240
Pelvimetry ~ 74710
Pelviolithotomy ~ 50130
Pelvis ~ see also hip
abscess, incision and drainage ~ 26990, 45000
angiography ~ 72191
biopsy ~ 27040-27041
bone, drainage ~ 26992
brace application ~ 20662
bursa, incision and drainage ~ 26991
CT scan ~ 72191-72194
cyst
aspiration ~ 50390
injection ~ 50390
destruction, lesion ~ 58662
endoscopy
destruction of lesion ~ 58662
lysis of adhesions ~ 58660
oviduct surgery ~ 58670-58671
exclusion, small intestine ~ 44700
exenteration ~ 45126, 58240
halo ~ 20662
hematoma, incision and drainage ~ 26990
lysis, adhesions ~ 58660
magnetic resonance angiography ~ 72198
magnetic resonance imaging (MRI) ~ 72195-72197
removal, foreign body ~ 27086-27087
repair
osteotomy ~ 27158
tendon ~ 27098
ring
dislocation ~ 27193-27194, 27216-27218
fracture ~ 27216-27218
closed treatment ~ 27193-27194

Pelvis ~ *continued*
tumor, excision ~ 27047-27049
ultrasound ~ 76856-76857
unlisted services and procedures for hips and hip joint ~ 27299
X-ray ~ 72170-72190, 73540
manometry ~ 74710
Pemberton osteotomy of pelvis ~ see osteotomy, pelvis
Penectomy ~ see amputation, penis
Penetration keratoplasties ~ see keratoplasty, penetrating
Penile induration ~ see Peyronie disease
Penile prosthesis
insertion
inflatable ~ 54401-54405
noninflatable ~ 54400
removal
inflatable ~ 54406, 54410-54417
semi-rigid ~ 54415-54417
repair, inflatable ~ 54408
replacement
inflatable ~ 54410-54411, 54416-54417
semi-rigid ~ 54416-54417
Penile rigidity test ~ 54250
Penile tumescence test ~ 54250
Penis
amputation
partial ~ 54120
radical ~ 54130-54135
total ~ 54125
biopsy ~ 54100-54105
circumcision
with clamp or other device ~ 54150
newborn ~ 54150
repair ~ 54163
surgical excision, newborn ~ 54160
excision
partial ~ 54120
prepuce ~ 54150-54161, 54163
total ~ 54125-54135
frenulum, excision ~ 54164
incision, prepuce ~ 54000-54001
incision and drainage ~ 54015
injection
for erection ~ 54235
peyronie disease ~ 54200
surgical exposure plague ~ 54205
vasoactive drugs ~ 54231
X-ray ~ 54230
insertion, prosthesis
inflatable ~ 54401-54405
noninflatable ~ 54400
irrigation, priapism ~ 54220
lesion
destruction
cryosurgery ~ 54056
electrodesiccation ~ 54055
extensive ~ 54065
laser surgery ~ 54057
simple ~ 54050-54060
surgical excision ~ 54060

Penis ~ *continued*
excision ~ 54060
penile plague ~ 54110-54112
nocturnal penile tumescence test ~ 54250
occlusion, vein ~ 37790
plaque, excision ~ 54110-54112
plethysmography ~ 54240
prepuce, stretch ~ 54450
reconstruction
angulation ~ 54360
chordee ~ 54300-54304, 54328
complications ~ 54340-54348
epispadias ~ 54380-54390
hypospadias ~ 54328-54352
injury ~ 54440
removal
foreign body ~ 54115
prosthesis
inflatable ~ 54406, 54410-54417
semi-rigid ~ 54415-54417
repair
fistulization ~ 54435
priapism with shunt ~ 54420-54430
prosthesis, inflatable ~ 54408
replacement, prosthesis
inflatable ~ 54410-54411, 54416-54417
semi-rigid ~ 54416-54417
revascularization ~ 37788
rigidity test ~ 54250
test erection ~ 54250
unlisted services and procedures ~ 55899
venous studies ~ 93980-93981
Penis adhesions
lysis, post-circumcision ~ 54162
Penis prostheses ~ see penile prosthesis
Pentagastrin test ~ see gastric analysis test
Pentamidine ~ see inhalation treatment
Peptidase P ~ see angiotensin converting enzyme (ACE)
Peptidase S ~ see leucine aminopeptidase
Peptide, connecting ~ see C-peptide
Peptide, vasoactive intestinal ~ see vasoactive intestinal peptide
Peptidyl dipeptidase A ~ see angiotensin converting enzyme (ACE)
Percutaneous abdominal paracentesis ~ see abdomen, drainage
Percutaneous atherectomies ~ see artery, atherectomy
Percutaneous biopsy, gallbladder/bile ducts ~ see bile duct, biopsy
Percutaneous discectomies ~ see diskectomy, percutaneous
Percutaneous electric nerve stimulation ~ see application, neurostimulation
Percutaneous fixation ~ 25671
Percutaneous lumbar diskectomy ~ see aspiration, nucleus of disk, lumbar
Percutaneous lysis ~ 62263-62264
Percutaneous nephrostomies ~ see nephrostomy, percutaneous

Percutaneous transluminal angioplasty
artery
aortic ~ 35472
brachiocephalic ~ 35475
coronary ~ 92982-92984
femoral-popliteal ~ 35474
iliac ~ 35473
pulmonary ~ 92997-92998
renal ~ 35471
tibioperoneal ~ 35470
visceral ~ 35471
venous ~ 35476
Percutaneous transluminal coronary angioplasty ~ see percutaneous transluminal angioplasty
Pereyra procedure ~ 51845, 57289, 58267
Performance measures
ACE inhibitor therapy ~ 4009F
anginal symptom assessment ~ 1002F
antiplatelet therapy ~ 4011F
asthma
history
intermittent ~ 1039F
persistent ~ 1038F
pharmacologic therapy ~ 4015F
beta-blocker therapy ~ 4006F
blood pressure ~ 2000F-2010F
diastolic ~ 3078F-3080F
postpartum care visit ~ 0503F
prenatal care visit, initial ~ 0500F
prenatal care visit, subsequent ~ 0502F
prenatal flow sheet ~ 0501F
systolic ~ 3076F-3077F
chronic obstructive pulmonary disease
history
dyspnea ~ 1018F-1019F
pneumococcus immunization ~ 1022F
smokeless tobacco use ~ 1035F
symptom assessment ~ 1015F
tobacco use ~ 1000F
tobacco smoker ~ 1034F
tobacco non-use ~ 1036F
intervention
bronchodilator prescription ~ 4025F
counseling ~ 4000F
influenza immunization ~ 4035, 4037F
oxygen therapy ~ 4030F
pharmacologic therapy ~ 4001F
pneumococcus immunization ~ 4040F
pulmonary rehabilitation ~ 4033F
test results
chest X-ray ~ 3006F
functional expiratory volume ~ 3040F
oxygen saturation ~ 3035F
spirometry ~ 3023F, 3025F
community acquired bacterial pneumonia
care level ~ 6005F
examination
hydration status ~ 2018F
mental status ~ 2014F
vital signs ~ 2010F

Performance measures ~ ***continued***
history
co-morbid conditions ~ 1026F
influenza immunization ~ 1030F
pneumococcus immunization ~ 1022F
pneumonia assessment ~ 0012F
smokeless tobacco use ~ 1035F
tobacco use ~ 1000F
tobacco smoker ~ 1034F
tobacco non-use ~ 1036F
intervention
antibiotic prescription ~ 4045F
test results
oxygen saturation ~ 3028F
composite measures
heart failure assessment ~ 0001F
coronary artery disease
history
smokeless tobacco use ~ 1035F
tobacco use ~ 1000F
tobacco smoker ~ 1034F
tobacco non-use ~ 1036F
intervention
ACE/ARB ~ 4009F
test results
left ventricular ejection fraction ~ 3021F-3022F
lipid panel ~ 3011F
diabetes
examination
eye ~ 2022F, 2024F, 2026F
foot ~ 2028F
history
smokeless tobacco use ~ 1035F
tobacco smoker ~ 1034F
tobacco non-use ~ 1036F
intervention
ACE/ARB ~ 4009F
test results
blood results
diastolic ~ 3078F-3080F
systolic ~ 3076F-3077F
hemoglobin
A1c ~ 3046F, 3047F
lipid ~ 3048F-3050F
macroalbuminuria ~ 3060F-3062F
nephropathy treatment ~ 3066F
retinopathy risk ~ 3072F
urine protein ~ 3060F-3062F
diagnostic/screening processes or results
chest x-ray ~ 3006F
colorectal cancer screening ~ 3017F
diastolic blood pressure ~ 3078F-3080F
functional expiratory volume ~ 3040F, 3042F
hemoglobin A1c ~ 3046F-3047F
LDL cholestorel ~ 3048F-3050F
left ventricular ejection fraction ~ 3021F, 3022F
left ventricular function ~ 3020F
lipid panel ~ 3011F
macroalbuminuria test ~ 3062F
microalbuminuria test 3060F-3061F

Performance measures ~ *continued*
nephropathy treatment ~ 3066F
oxygen saturation ~ 3028F, 3035F-3037F
retinopathy screening ~ 3072F
screening mammography ~ 3014F
spirometry ~ 3023F-3027F
systolic blood pressure ~ 3076F-3077F
patient history, assessment
disease ~ 1015F
co-morbid conditions ~ 1026F
community-acquired bacterial pneumonia ~ 0012F
current smokeless tobacco user ~ 1035F
current tobacco non-user ~ 1036F
current tobacco smoker ~ 1034F
dyspnea assessment ~ 1018F-1019F
influenza immunization status ~ 1030F
intermittent asthma ~ 1039F
non-steroidal anti-inflammatory drug (NSAID) ~ 1008F
osteoarthritis ~ 1006F
persistent asthma ~ 1038F
pneumococcus immunization assessment ~ 1022F
patient safety
level of care rationale ~ 6005F
physical examination
dilated retinal eye exam ~ 2022F
eye imaging ~ 2026F
field stereoscopic photos ~ 2024F
foot ~ 2028F
hydration status ~ 2018F
mental status ~ 2014F
vital signs ~ 2010F
prescribed therapy
ACE inhibitor ~ 4009F
antibiotic ~ 4045F
ARB ~ 4009F
asthma control ~ 4015F
inhaled bronchodilator ~ 4025F
oxygen ~ 4030F
statin therapy ~ 4002F
therapeutic, preventive or other interventions
antibiotic agent ~ 4045F
asthma medication ~ 4015F
hypertension care plan ~ 4050F
influenza immunization ~ 4035F-4037F
inhaled bronchodilator ~ 4025F
oxygen therapy, long term ~ 4030F
pneumococcal immunization ~ 4040F
pulmonary rehabilitation ~ 4033F
tobacco use
assessment ~ 1000F
counseling ~ 4000F
pharmacologic therapy ~ 4001F
Performance test ~ see physical medicine/therapy/occupational therapy
performance test, physical therapy ~ 97750
psychological test ~ 96100
Perfusion
brain, imaging ~ 0042T
myocardial ~ 78460-78465, 78478-78480
imaging ~ 78466-78469
positron emission tomography (PET), myocardial imaging ~ 78491-78492
Perfusion, intracranial arterial thrombolysis ~ 61624
Perfusion pump ~ see infusion pump
Pericardectomies ~ see excision, pericardium
Pericardial cyst ~ see cyst, pericardial
Pericardial sac drainage ~ 32659
Pericardial window for drainage ~ 33025
Pericardial window technic ~ see pericardiostomy
Pericardiectomy
complete ~ 33030-33031
subtotal ~ 33030-33031
total, endoscopic ~ 32660
Pericardiocentesis ~ 33010-33011
ultrasound guidance ~ 76930
Pericardiostomy tube ~ 33015
Pericardiotomy
removal
clot ~ 33020
foreign body ~ 33020

Pericardium
cyst, excision ~ 32661, 33050
excision ~ 32659, 33030-33031
incision
removal
clot ~ 33020
foreign body ~ 33020
with tube ~ 33015
incision and drainage ~ 33025
puncture aspiration ~ 33010-33011
removal
clot, endoscopic ~ 32658
foreign body, endoscopic ~ 32658
tumor, excision ~ 32661, 33050
Peridural anesthesia ~ see anesthesia, epidural
Peridural injection ~ see epidural, injection
Perineal prostatectomy ~ see prostatectomy, perineal
Perineoplasty ~ 56810
Perineorrhaphy
repair, rectocele ~ 57250
Perineum
abscess, incision and drainage ~ 56405
colposcopy ~ 99170
debridement, infected ~ 11004, 11006
removal, prosthesis ~ 53442
repair ~ 56810
X-ray with contrast ~ 74775
Perionychia ~ see paronychia
Periorbital region
reconstruction, osteotomy with graft ~ 21267-21268
repair, osteotomy ~ 21260-21263
Peripheral artery disease (PAD) rehabilitation ~ 93668

Peripheral nerve repair/suture, major ~ 64856, 64859
Periprosthetic capsulectomy breast ~ 19371
Peristaltic pumps ~ see infusion pump
Peritoneal dialysis ~ 90945-90947
Peritoneal free air ~ see pneumoperitoneum
Peritoneal lavage ~ 49080
Peritoneocentesis ~ 49080-49081
Peritoneoscopy ~ see endoscopy, peritoneum
Peritoneum
abscess
incision and drainage ~ 49020
percutaneous ~ 49021
chemotherapy administration ~ 96445
endoscopy
biopsy ~ 47561
drainage, lymphocele ~ 49323
X-ray ~ 47560
exchange, drainage catheter ~ 49423
injection, contrast, via catheter ~ 49424
ligation, shunt ~ 49428
removal
cannula/catheter ~ 49422
foreign body ~ 49402
shunt ~ 49429
tumor, resection ~ 58950-58956
unlisted services and procedures ~ 49999
venous shunt, injection ~ 49427
X-ray ~ 74190
Persistent, omphalomesenteric duct ~ see diverticulum, Meckel's
Persistent truncus arteriosus ~ see truncus arteriosus
Personal care ~ see self care
Pessary insertion ~ 57160
Pesticides chlorinated hydrocarbons ~ 82441
PET ~ see positron emission tomography
Petrous temporal excision, Apex ~ 69530
Peyronie disease
with graft ~ 54110-54112
injection ~ 54200
surgical exposure ~ 54205
pH ~ see blood
other fluid ~ 83986
urine ~ 83986
Phacoemulsification
removal
extracapsular cataract ~ 66982, 66984
secondary membranous cataract ~ 66850
Phagocytosis, white blood cells ~ 86344
Phalangectomy
toe ~ 28150
partial ~ 28160
Phalanges (hand)) ~ see finger, bone
Phalanx, finger
craterization ~ 26235-26236
cyst, excision ~ 26210-26215
diaphysectomy ~ 26235-26236
excision ~ 26235-26236
radical, for tumor ~ 26260-26262
fracture
articular
Phalanx, finger ~ *continued*
closed treatment ~ 26740
with manipulation ~ 26742
open treatment ~ 26746
distal ~ 26755-26756
closed treatment ~ 26750
open treatment ~ 26765
percutaneous fixation ~ 26756
open treatment ~ 26735
distal ~ 26765
shaft ~ 26720-26727
open treatment ~ 26735
incision and drainage ~ 26034
ostectomy, radical, for tumor ~ 26260-26262
repair
lengthening ~ 26568
nonunion ~ 26546
osteotomy ~ 26567
saucerization ~ 26235-26236
thumb fracture, shaft ~ 26720-26727
tumor, excision ~ 26210-26215
Phalanx, great toe ~ see also phalanx, toe
fracture ~ 28490
with manipulation ~ 28495-28496
open treatment ~ 28505
without manipulation ~ 28490
percutaneous fixation ~ 28496
Phalanx, toe
condyle, excision ~ 28126
craterization ~ 28124
cyst, excision ~ 28108
diaphysectomy ~ 28124
excision ~ 28124, 28150-28160
fracture
with manipulation ~ 28515
without manipulation ~ 28510
open treatment ~ 28525
repair, osteotomy ~ 28310-28312
saucerization ~ 28124
tumor, excision ~ 28108, 28175
Pharmaceutic preparations ~ see drug
Pharmacotherapies ~ see chemotherapy
Pharyngeal tonsil ~ see adenoids
Pharyngectomy partial ~ 42890
Pharyngolaryngectomy ~ 31390-31395
Pharyngoplasty ~ 42950
Pharyngorrhaphy ~ see suture, pharynx
Pharyngostomy ~ 42955
Pharyngotomy ~ see incision, pharynx
Pharyngotympanic tube ~ see eustachian tube
Pharynx ~ see also nasopharynx; throat
biopsy ~ 42800-42806
cineradiography ~ 70371, 74230
creation, stoma ~ 42955
excision ~ 42145
with larynx ~ 31390-31395
partial ~ 42890
resection ~ 42892-42894
hemorrhage ~ 42960-42962
lesion
destruction ~ 42808
excision ~ 42808

Pharanx ~ *continued*
reconstruction ~ 42950
removal, foreign body ~ 42809
repair, with esophagus ~ 42953
unlisted services and procedures ~ 42999
video study ~ 70371, 74230
X-ray ~ 70370, 74210
Phencyclidine ~ 83992
Phenobarbital ~ 82205
assay ~ 80184
Phenothiazine ~ 84022
Phenotype
analysis
by nucleic acid, infectious agent
HIV-1 drug resistance ~ 87903-87904
prediction
by genetic database
HIV-1 drug resistance ~ 0023T
Phenylalanine ~ 84030
Phenylalanine-tyrosine ratio ~ 84030
Phenylketones ~ 84035
Phenylketonuria ~ see phenylalanine
Phenytoin assay ~ 80185-80186
Pheochromocytoma ~ 80424
Pheresis ~ see apheresis
Phlebectasia ~ see varicose vein
Phlebectomy varicose veins ~ 37765-37766
Phlebographies ~ see venography
Phleborrhaphy ~ see suture, vein
Phlebotomy therapeutic ~ 99195
Phoria ~ see strabismus
Phosphatase
alkaline ~ 84075, 84080
blood ~ 84078
forensic examination ~ 84061
Phosphatase acid ~ 84060
blood ~ 84066
Phosphate, pyridoxal ~ see pyridoxal phosphate
Phosphatidylcholine cholinephosphohydrolase ~ see tissue typing
Phosphatidylglycerol ~ 84081
Phosphatidyl glycerol ~ see phosphatidylglycerol
Phosphocreatine phosphotransferase, ADP ~ see CPK
Phosphogluconate-6 dehydrogenase ~ 84085
Phosphoglycerides, glycerol ~ see phosphatidylglycerol
Phosphohexose isomerase ~ 84087
Phosphohydrolases ~ see phosphatase
Phosphokinase, creatine ~ see CPK
Phospholipase C ~ see tissue typing
Phospholipid antibody ~ 86147
Phospholipid cofactor antibody ~ 0030T
Phosphomonoesterase ~ see phosphatase
Phosphoric monoester hydrolases ~ see phosphatase
Phosphorus ~ 84100
urine ~ 84105
Phosphotransferase, ADP phosphocreatine ~ see CPK
Photo patch allergy test ~ see allergy tests ~ 95052
Photochemotherapies, extracorporeal ~ see photopheresis
Photochemotherapy ~ see dermatology ~ 96910-96913
endoscopic light ~ 96570-96571
Photocoagulation
endolaser panretinal, vitrectomy ~ 67040
focal endolaser, vitrectomy ~ 67040
iridoplasty ~ 66762
lesion
cornea ~ 65450
retina ~ 0017T, 67210, 67227-67228
retinal detachment
prophylaxis ~ 67145
repair ~ 67105
Photodensity radiographic
absorptiometry ~ 77083
Photodynamic therapy ~ 96567-96571
Photography skin, diagnostic ~ 96904
Photography, ocular ~ see ophthalmoscopy, diagnostic
Photopheresis extracorporeal ~ 36522
Photophoresis ~ see actinotherapy; photochemotherapy
Photoradiation therapies ~ see actinotherapy
Photoscreen ocular ~ 0065T
Photosensitivity testing ~ see allergy tests ~ 95056
Phototherapies ~ see actinotherapy
Phototherapy, ultraviolet ~ see actinotherapy
Phrenic nerve
anastomosis, to facial nerve ~ 64870
avulsion ~ 64746
incision ~ 64746
injection, anesthetic ~ 64410
transection ~ 64746
Physical medicine/therapy/occupational therapy
activities of daily living ~ 97535, 99509
aquatic therapy, with exercises ~ 97113
athletic training
evaluation ~ 97005
re-evaluation ~ 97006
check-out, orthotic/prosthetic ~ 97703
cognitive skills development ~ 97532
community/work reintegration ~ 97537
evaluation ~ 97001-97002
kinetic therapy ~ 97530
manual therapy ~ 97140
modalities
contrast baths ~ 97034
diathermy treatment ~ 97024
electric simulation
unattended ~ 97014
attended, manual ~ 97032
hot or cold pack ~ 97010
hydrotherapy (Hubbard tank) ~ 97036
infrared light treatment ~ 97026
iontophoresis ~ 97033
microwave therapy ~ 97020

Physical medicine/therapy/occupational therapy ~ *continued*
paraffin bath ~ 97018
traction ~ 97012
ultrasound ~ 97035
ultraviolet light ~ 97028
unlisted services and procedures ~ 97039
vasopneumatic device ~ 97016
whirlpool therapy ~ 97022
orthotics training ~ 97504
osteopathic manipulation ~ 98925-98929
procedures
aquatic therapy ~ 97113
gait training ~ 97116
group therapeutic ~ 97150
massage therapy ~ 97124
neuromuscular reeducation ~ 97112
physical performance test ~ 97750
therapeutic exercises ~ 97110
traction therapy ~ 97140
work hardening ~ 97545-97546
prosthetic training ~ 97520
sensory integration ~ 97533
therapeutic activities ~ 97530
unlisted services and procedures ~ 97139, 97799
wheelchair management/propulsion ~ 97542
work reintegration ~ 97537
Physical therapy ~ see physical medicine/therapy/occupational therapy
Physician services
care plan oversight services ~ 99374-99380
home health agency care ~ 99374
hospice ~ 99377-99378
nursing facility ~ 99379-99380
direction, advanced life support ~ 99288
prolonged
with direct patient contact ~ 99354-99357
outpatient/office ~ 99354-99355
with direct patient services inpatient ~ 99356-99357
without direct patient contact ~ 99358-99359
standby ~ 99360
supervision, care plan oversight services ~ 99374-99380
Piercing of ear lobe ~ 69090
Piles ~ see hemorrhoids
Pilonidal cyst
excision ~ 11770-11772
incision and drainage ~ 10080-10081
Pin ~ see also wire
insertion/removal, skeletal traction ~ 20650
prophylactic treatment
femur ~ 27187
humerus ~ 24498
shoulder ~ 23490-23491
Pinch graft ~ 15050
Pinna ~ see ear, external
Pinworms examination ~ 87172
Pirogoff procedure ~ 27888
Pituitary epidermoid tumor ~ see craniopharyngioma
Pituitary gland
excision ~ 61546-61548
tumor, excision ~ 61546-61548, 62165
Pituitary growth hormone ~ see growth hormone
Pituitary lactogenic hormone ~ see prolactin
Pituitectomy ~ see excision, pituitary gland
PKU ~ see phenylalanine
Placement
bronchial stent ~ 31636-31637
catheter
bile duct ~ 75982
breast, for interstitial radioelement application ~ 19296-19298
bronchus, for intracavitary radioelement application (see also catheterization) ~ 31643
catheter, cardiac (see also catheterization, cardiac) ~ 93503
colonic stent ~ 44397, 45327, 45345, 45387
drainage, pancreas ~ 48001
IVC filter ~ 75940
jejunostomy tube, endoscopic ~ 44372
metallic localization clip, breast ~ 19295
nasogastric tube ~ 43752
needle, bone ~ 36680
needle wire, breast ~ 19290-19291
orogastric tube ~ 43752
radiation delivery device, intracoronary artery ~ 92974
seton, anal ~ 46020
tracheal stent ~ 31631
ureteral stent ~ 50947
Placenta delivery ~ 59414
Placental lactogen ~ see lactogen, human placental
Placental villi ~ see chorionic villus
Plagiocephaly ~ 21175
Plague vaccine ~ 90727
Planing nose, skin ~ 30120
Plantar digital nerve decompression ~ 64726
Plantar pressure measurements dynamic ~ 96001, 96004
Plasma frozen preparation ~ 86927
Plasma prokallikrein ~ see Fletcher factor
Plasma protein-A, pregnancy-associated (PAPP-A) ~ 84163
Plasma test volume determination ~ 78110-78111
Plasma thromboplastin
antecedent ~ 85270
component ~ 85250
Plasmin ~ 85400
Plasmin antiactivator ~ see alpha-2 antiplasmin
Plasminogen ~ 85420-85421
Plasmodium antibody ~ 86750
Plastic repair of mouth ~ see mouth, repair
Plate, bone ~ see bone plate

Platelet ~ see also blood cell count, complete blood count
aggregation ~ 85576
antibody ~ 86022-86023
assay ~ 85055
blood ~ 85025
count ~ 85032, 85049
neutralization ~ 85597
Platelet cofactor I ~ see clotting factor
Platelet test survival test ~ 78190-78191
Platysmal flap ~ 15825
PLC ~ see tissue typing
Pleoptic training ~ 92065
Plethysmography ~ see also vascular studies
extremities ~ 93922-93923
veins ~ 93965
penis ~ 54240
total body ~ 93720-93722
Pleura
biopsy ~ 32095-32100, 32400-32402
decortication ~ 32320
empyema, excision ~ 32540
excision ~ 32310-32320
endoscopic ~ 32656
foreign body, removal ~ 32150-32151
needle biopsy ~ 32400
removal, foreign body ~ 32653
repair ~ 32215
thoracotomy ~ 32095-32100
unlisted services and procedures ~ 32999
Pleural cavity
aspiration ~ 32000-32002
catheterization ~ 32019
chemotherapy administration ~ see also chemotherapy ~ 96440
fusion ~ 32005
incision
empyema ~ 32035-32036
pneumothorax ~ 32020
puncture and drainage ~ 32000-32002
thoracostomy ~ 32035-32036
Pleural endoscopies ~ see thoracoscopy
Pleural scarification for repeat pneumothorax ~ 32215
Pleural tap ~ see thoracentesis
Pleurectomy
anesthesia ~ 00542
parietal ~ 32310-32320
endoscopic ~ 32656
Pleuritis, purulent ~ see abscess, thorax
Pleurocentesis ~ see thoracentesis
Pleurodesis
chemical ~ 32005
endoscopic ~ 32650
Pleurosclerosis ~ see pleurodesis
Plexectomy, choroid ~ see choroid plexus, excision
Plexus, choroid ~ see choroid plexus
Plexus brachialis ~ see brachial plexus
Plexus cervicalis ~ see cervical plexus
Plexus coeliacus ~ see celiac plexus
Plexus lumbalis ~ see lumbar plexus
PLGN ~ see plasminogen
Plication, sphincter, urinary bladder ~ see bladder, repair, neck
Pneumocentesis lung ~ 32420
Pneumocisternogram ~ see cisternography
Pneumococcal vaccine ~ 90669, 90732
Pneumocystis carinii antigen detection, immunofluorescence ~ 87281
Pneumogastric nerve ~ see vagus nerve
Pneumogram pediatric ~ 94772
Pneumolysis ~ 32940
Pneumonectomy ~ 32440-32500
completion ~ 32488
donor ~ 32850, 33930
sleeve ~ 32442
total ~ 32440-32445
Pneumonology ~ see pulmonology
Pneumonolysis ~ 32940
intrapleural ~ 32652
open intrapleural ~ 32124
Pneumonostomy ~ 32200-32201
Pneumonotomy ~ see incision, lung
Pneumoperitoneum ~ 49400
Pneumoplethysmography ocular ~ 93875
Pneumothorax
chemical pleurodesis ~ 32005
pleural scarification for repeat ~ 32215
therapeutic, injection intrapleural air ~ 32960
thoracentesis with tube insertion ~ 32002
Polio
antibody ~ 86658
vaccine ~ 90712-90713
Poliovirus vaccine, inactivated ~ see vaccines
Pollicization digit ~ 26550
Polya gastrectomy ~ see gastrectomy, partial
Polydactylism ~ see supernumerary digit
Polydactylous digit
reconstruction ~ 26587
repair ~ 26587
Polydactyly, toes ~ 28344
Polymerase chain reaction ~ 83898
Polyp
antrochoanal, removal ~ 31032
esophagus, ablation ~ 43228
nose, excision
endoscopic ~ 31237-31240
extensive ~ 30115
simple ~ 30110
sphenoid sinus, removal ~ 31051
urethra, excision ~ 53260
Polypectomy
nose, endoscopic ~ 31237
uterus ~ 58558
Polypeptide, vasoactive intestinal ~ see vasoactive intestinal peptide
Polysomnography ~ 95808-95811
Polyuria test ~ see water load test
Pomeroy's operation ~ (tubal ligation) 58600
Pooling blood products ~ 86965
Popliteal arteries ~ see artery, popliteal
Popliteal synovial cyst ~ see Baker's cyst

Poradenitistras ~ see lymphogranuloma venereum
PORP (partial ossicular replacement prosthesis) ~ 69633, 69637
Porphobilinogen urine ~ 84106-84110
Porphyrin precursors ~ 82135
Porphyrins
feces ~ 84126-84127
urine ~ 84119-84120
Portal vein ~ see vein, hepatic portal
Porter-Silber test ~ see corticosteroid, blood
Portoenterostomies, hepatic ~ see hepaticoenterostomy
Port film ~ 77417
Portoenterostomy ~ 47701
Posadas-Wernicke disease ~ see coccidioidomycosis
Positional nystagmus test ~ see nystagmus tests, positional
Positive-pressure breathing, inspiratory ~ see intermittent positive pressure breathing (IPPB)
Positive end expiratory pressure ~ see pressure breathing, positive
Positron emission tomography (PET)
brain ~ 78608-78609
heart ~ 78459
myocardial imaging, perfusion study ~ 78491-78492
tumor ~ 78811-78813
with computed tomography ~ 78814-78816
Post-op visit ~ 99024
Postauricular fistula ~ see fistula, postauricular
Postcaval ureter ~ see retrocaval ureter
Postmortem ~ see autopsy
Postoperative wound infection incision and drainage ~ 10180
Postop vas reconstruction ~ see vasovasorrhaphy
Postpartum care
cesarean delivery ~ 59515
after attempted vaginal delivery ~ 59622
previous ~ 59610, 59614-59618, 59622
vaginal delivery ~ 59430
after previous cesarean delivery ~ 59614
Potassium ~ 84132
urine ~ 84133
Potential, auditory evoked ~ see auditory evoked potentials
Potential, evoked ~ see evoked potential
Potts-Smith procedure ~ 33762
Pouch, Kock ~ see Kock pouch
PPP ~ see fibrin degradation products
PRA ~ see cytotoxic screen
Prealbumin ~ 84134
Prebeta lipoproteins ~ see lipoprotein, blood
Pregl's test ~ (cystourethroscopy, catheterization, urethral) 52005
Pregnancy
abortion
induced ~ 59855-59857
by amniocentesis injection ~ 59850-59852
Pregnancy ~ *continued*
by dilation and curettage ~ 59840
by dilation and evaluation ~ 59841
septic ~ 59830
therapeutic
by dilation and curettage ~ 59851
by hysterectomy ~ 59852
by saline ~ 59850
cesarean delivery ~ 59618-59622
with hysterectomy ~ 59525
only ~ 59514
postpartum care ~ 59514-59515
routine care ~ 59510
vaginal birth after ~ 59610-59614
ectopic
abdominal ~ 59130
cervix ~ 59140
interstitial
partial resection uterus ~ 59136
total hysterectomy ~ 59135
laparoscopy
with salpingectomy and/or oophorectomy ~ 59151
without salpingectomy and/or oophorectomy ~ 59150
tubal ~ 59121
with salpingectomy and/or oophorectomy ~ 59120
miscarriage
surgical completion
any trimester ~ 59812
first trimester ~ 59820
second trimester ~ 59821
molar ~ see also hydatidiform mole
multifetal reduction ~ 59866
placenta delivery ~ 59414
test ~ 84702-84703
urinalysis ~ 81025
vaginal delivery ~ 59409-59410
antepartum care ~ 59425-59426
after cesarean delivery ~ 59610-59614
postpartum care ~ 59430
total obstetrical care ~ 59400, 59610, 59618
Pregnanediol ~ 84135
Pregnanetriol ~ 84138
Pregnenolone ~ 84140
Prekallikrein ~ see Fletcher factor
Prekallikrein factor ~ 85292
Premature, closure, cranial suture ~ see craniosynostosis
Prenatal procedure ~ 59897
amnioinfusion, transabdominal ~ 59070
drainage, fluid ~ 59074
occlusion, umbilical cord ~ 59072
stunt ~ 59076
Prenatal testing
amniocentesis ~ 59000
with amniotic fluid reduction ~ 59001
chorionic villus sampling ~ 59015
cordocentesis ~ 59012
fetal blood sample ~ 59030

Prenatal testing ~ *continued*
fetal monitoring ~ 59050
interpretation only ~ 59051
non-stress test, fetal ~ 59025, 99500
oxytocin stress test ~ 59020
stress test, oxytocin ~ 59020
ultrasound ~ 76801-76817
fetal biophysical profile ~ 76818-76819
fetal heart ~ 76825
Prentiss operation ~ see orchiopexy, inguinal approach
Preparation
for transfer, embryo ~ 89255
thawing
embryo, cryopreserved ~ 89352
oocytes, cryopreserved ~ 89356
reproductive tissue, cryopreserved ~ 89354
sperm, cryopreserved ~ 89353
Presacral sympathectomy ~ see sympathectomy, presacral
Prescription
contact lens (see also contact lens services) ~ 92310-92317
ocular prosthesis (see also prosthesis, ocular) ~ 92330-92335
Pressure, blood ~ see blood pressure
Pressure, venous ~ see blood pressure, venous
Pressure breathing ~ (see also pulmonology, therapeutic)
negative, continuous (CNP) ~ 94662
positive, continuous (CPAP) ~ 94660
Pressure measurement of sphincter of Oddi ~ see sphincter of Oddi, pressure measurement
Pressure ulcer (decubitus) ~ see debridement; skin graft and flap
Pressure ulcers excision ~ 15920-15999
Pretreatment
red blood cell
antibody identification ~ 86970-86972
serum
antibody identification ~ 86975-86978
Prevention & control ~ see prophylaxis
Preventive medicine ~ 99381-99397
administration/interpretation of health risk assessment ~ 99420
counseling and/or risk factor reduction intervention ~ 99401-99429
group counseling ~ 99411-99412
individual counseling ~ 99401-99404
performance measures ~ 0001F-0011F
established patient ~ 99382-99397
new patient ~ 99381-99387
newborn care ~ 99432
respiratory pattern recording ~ 94772
unlisted services and procedures ~ 99429
Priapism
repair
fistulization ~ 54435
with shunt ~ 54420-54430
Primidone assay ~ 80188
PRL ~ see prolactin
Pro-insulin C peptide ~ see C-peptide
Proalbumin ~ see prealbumin
Probes, DNA ~ see nucleic acid probe
Probes, nucleic acid ~ see nucleic acid probe
Procainamide assay ~ 80190-80192
Procedure, Fontan ~ see repair, heart, anomaly
Procedure, maxillofacial ~ see maxillofacial procedures
Process, odontoid ~ see odontoid process
Procidentia
rectum
excision ~ 45130-45135
repair ~ 45900
Procoagulant activity, glomerular ~ see thromboplastin
Proconvertin ~ 85230
Proctectasis ~ see dilation, rectum
Proctectomy
partial ~ 45111, 45113-45116, 45123
total ~ 45110, 45112, 45119-45120
with colon ~ 45121
with colectomy ~ 44157-44158
with ileostomy ~ 44212
Proctocele ~ see rectocele
Proctopexy ~ 45540-45541
with sigmoid excision ~ 45550
Proctoplasty ~ 45500-45505
Proctorrhaphy ~ see rectum, suture
Proctoscopies ~ see anoscopy
Proctosigmoidoscopy
ablation, polyp or lesion ~ 45320
biopsy ~ 45305
destruction, tumor ~ 45320
dilation ~ 45303
exploration ~ 45300
hemorrhage control ~ 45317
placement, stent ~ 45327
removal
foreign body ~ 45307
polyp ~ 45308-45315
tumor ~ 45315
volvulus repair ~ 45321
Products, gene ~ see protein
Proetz therapy nose ~ 30210
Profibrinolysin ~ see plasminogen
Progenitor cell ~ see stem cell
Progesterone ~ 84144
Progesterone receptors ~ 84234
Progestin receptors ~ see progesterone receptors
Proinsulin ~ 84206
Projective test ~ 96100
Prokallikrein ~ see Fletcher factor
Prokallikrein, plasma ~ see Fletcher factor
Prokinogenase ~ see Fletcher factor
Prolactin ~ 80418, 80440, 84146
Prolapse ~ see procidentia
Prolapse, rectal ~ see procidentia, rectum
Prolastin ~ see alpha-1 antitrypsin
Prolonged services ~ 99354-99357, 99360
without direct patient contact ~ 99358-99359

Prophylactic treatment
femur ~ 27495
pinning ~ 27187
humerus
pinning, wiring ~ 24498
radius ~ 25490, 25492
nailing ~ 25490, 25492
pinning ~ 25490, 25492
plating ~ 25490, 25492
wiring ~ 25490, 25492
shoulder
clavicle ~ 23490
humerus ~ 23491
tibia ~ 27745
ulna ~ 25491-25492
nailing ~ 25491-25492
pinning ~ 25491-25492
plating ~ 25491-25492
wiring ~ 25491-25492
Prophylaxis
retina detachment
cryotherapy, diathermy ~ 67141
photocoagulation ~ 67145
Prostaglandin ~ 84150
insertion ~ 59200
Prostanoids ~ see prostaglandin
Prostate
ablation, cryosurgery ~ 55873
abscess, drainage ~ 52700
incision and drainage ~ 55720-55725
biopsy ~ 55700-55705
brachytherapy, needle insertion ~ 55875-55976
coagulation, laser ~ 52647
destruction
cryosurgery ~ 55873
thermotherapy ~ 53850-53852
microwave ~ 53850
radio frequency ~ 53852
excision
partial ~ 55801, 55821-55831
perineal ~ 55801-55815
radical ~ 55810-55815, 55840-55845
retropubic ~ 55831-55845
suprapubic ~ 55821
transurethral ~ 52601, 52612-52614
exploration, exposure ~ 55860
with nodes ~ 55862-55865
incision
exposure ~ 55860-55865
transurethral ~ 52450
insertion, radioactive substance ~ 55860
needle biopsy ~ 55700
thermotherapy, transurethral ~ 53850-53853
ultrasound ~ 76872-76873
unlisted services and procedures ~ 55899
urinary system ~ 53899
urethra, transurethral balloon dilation ~ 52510
vaporization, laser ~ 52648
Prostate specific antigen ~ 84152-84154
Prostatectomy ~ 52601
laparoscopic ~ 55866
perineal
partial ~ 55801
radical ~ 55810-55815
retropubic
partial ~ 55831
radical ~ 55840-55845, 55866
suprapubic, partial ~ 55821
transurethral ~ 52612-52614
Prostatic abscess ~ see abscess, prostate
Prostatotomy ~ 55720-55725
Prosthesis
augmentation, mandibular body ~ 21125
auricular ~ 21086
breast
insertion ~ 19340-19342
removal ~ 19328-19330
supply ~ 19396
check-out ~ see also physical medicine/therapy/occupational therapy ~ 97703
cornea ~ 65770
facial ~ 21088
hernia, mesh ~ 49568
hip, removal ~ 27090-27091
intestines ~ 44700
knee, insertion ~ 27438, 27445
lens
not associated with concurrent cataract removal ~ 66985
insertion ~ 66982-66985
manual or mechanical technique ~ 66982-66984
mandibular resection ~ 21081
nasal ~ 21087
nasal septum, insertion ~ 30220
obturator ~ 21076
definitive ~ 21080
interim ~ 21079
ocular ~ 21077, 65770, 66982-66985, 92330-92335, 92358, 92393
fitting and prescription ~ 92330
loan ~ 92358
prescription ~ 92335
supply ~ 92393
orbital ~ 21077
partial or total ~ 69633, 69637
ossicle reconstruction, chain ~ 69633
palatal augmentation ~ 21082
palatal lift ~ 21083
palate ~ 42280-42281
penile
insertion ~ 54400-54405
removal ~ 54406, 54410-54417
repair ~ 54408
replacement ~ 54410-54411, 54416-54417
perineum, removal ~ 53442
skull plate
removal ~ 62142
replacement ~ 62143

Prosthesis ~ *continued*
spectacle ~ *continued*
fitting ~ 92352-92353
repair ~ 92371
speech aid ~ 21084
spinal, insertion ~ 22851
synthetic ~ 69633, 69637
temporomandibular joint, arthroplasty ~ 21243
testicular, insertion ~ 54660
training ~ 97520
urethral sphincter
insertion ~ 53444-53445
removal ~ 53446-53447
repair ~ 53449
replacement ~ 53448
wrist, removal ~ 25250-25251
Protease F ~ see plasmin
Protein
C-reactive ~ 86140-86141
glycated ~ 82985
myelin basic ~ 83873
osteocalcin ~ 83937
prealbumin ~ 84134
serum ~ 84155, 84165
total ~ 84155-84160
urine ~ 84156
western blot ~ 84181-84182, 88372
Protein analysis, tissue western blot ~ 88371
Protein blotting ~ see western blot
Protein C activator ~ 85337
Protein C antigen ~ 85302
Protein C assay ~ 85303
Protein C resistance assay ~ 85307
Protein S
assay ~ 85306
total ~ 85305
Prothrombase ~ see thrombokinase
Prothrombin ~ 85210
Prothrombinase ~ see thromboplastin
Prothrombin time ~ 85610-85611
Prothrombokinase ~ 85230
Protime ~ see prothrombin time
Proton treatment delivery
complex ~ 77525
intermediate ~ 77523
simple ~ 77520-77522
Protoporphyrin ~ 84202-84203
Protozoa antibody ~ 86753
Provitamin A ~ see vitamin, A
Provocation test ~ see also allergy tests
for glaucoma ~ 92140
Provocation tonography ~ 92130
Prower factor ~ see Stuart-Prower factor
PSA ~ see prostate specific antigen
Pseudocyst, pancreas ~ see pancreas, pseudocyst
PSG ~ see polysomnography
Psoriasis treatment ~ (see also dermatology; photochemotherapy) 96910-96922
Psychiatric diagnosis
evaluation of records or reports ~ 90885
intervention evaluation, interactive ~ 90802
interview and evaluation ~ 90801-90802
psychological testing ~ 96100
unlisted services and procedures ~ 90899
Psychiatric services ~ 90801-90899
biofeedback training ~ 90875-90876
consultation with family ~ 90887
drug management ~ 90862
electroconvulsive therapy ~ 90870-90871
environmental intervention ~ 90882
family ~ 90846-90849, 99510
group ~ 90853-90857
hypnotherapy ~ 90880
individual
insight-oriented
home visit ~ 99510
hospital or residential care ~ 90816-90822
office or outpatient ~ 90804-90809
interactive
home visit ~ 99510
hospital or residential care ~ 90823-90829
office or outpatient ~ 90810-90815
narcosynthesis analysis ~ 90865
psychoanalysis ~ 90845
report preparation ~ 90889
residential, facility care ~ 90816-90829
unlisted services and procedures ~ 90899
Psychoanalysis ~ 90845
Psychophysiologic feedback ~ see biofeedback
Psychotherapy
family ~ 90846-90849, 99510
group ~ 90853-90857
insight-oriented
hospital or residential care ~ 90816-90822
office or outpatient ~ 90804-90809
interactive
hospital or residential care ~ 90823-90829
office or outpatient ~ 90810-90815
PTA (clotting factor XI (eleven)) ~ 85270
PTA (percutaneous transluminal angioplasty) ~ 35470-35476, 85270. 92997, 92998
PTB (patellar tendon bearing) cast ~ 29435
PTC (clotting factor IX (nine); Christmas factor) ~ 85250
PTCA (percutaneous transluminal coronary angioplasty)
aortic ~ 35472
brachiocephalic ~ 35475
coronary ~ 92982-92984
femoral-popliteal ~ 35474
iliac ~ 35473
pulmonary ~ 92997-92998
renal ~ 35471
tibioperoneal ~ 35470
visceral ~ 35471
Pteroylglutamic acid ~ see folic acid
Pterygium
excision ~ 65420
with graft ~ 65426
Pterygomaxillary fossa incision ~ 31040

Pterygopalatine ganglion ~ see sphenopalatine ganglion
PTH ~ see parathormone
Ptosis ~ see blepharoptosis; procidentia
PTT ~ see thromboplastin, partial, time
Ptyalectasis ~ see dilation, salivary duct
Pubic symphysis ~ 27282
Pubis
craterization ~ 27070
cyst, excision ~ 27065-27067
excision ~ 27070
saucerization ~ 27070
tumor, excision ~ 27065-27067
Pudendal nerve
avulsion ~ 64761
destruction ~ 64630
incision ~ 64761
injection
anesthetic ~ 64430
neurolytic ~ 64630
transection ~ 64761
Puestow procedure ~ 48548
Pulled elbow ~ see nursemaid elbow
Pulmonary artery ~ 33690
catheterization ~ see also catheterization, pulmonary artery
embolism ~ 33910-33916
excision ~ 33910-33916
percutaneous transluminal angioplasty ~ 92997-92998
reimplantation ~ 33788
repair ~ 33690, 33917-33920
reimplantation ~ 33788
shunt
from aorta ~ 33755-33762, 33924
subclavian ~ 33750
from vena cava ~ 33766-33767
transection ~ 33922
Pulmonary function test ~ see pulmonology, diagnostic
Pulmonary hemorrhage ~ see hemorrhage, lung
Pulmonary medical services ~ 94010-94799
Pulmonary perfusion imaging nuclear medicine ~ 78588
Pulmonary valve
incision ~ 33470-33474
repair ~ 33470-33474
replacement ~ 33475
Pulmonary vein
repair
complete ~ 33730
partial ~ 33724
stenosis ~ 33726
stenosis
repair ~ 33726
Pulmonology
diagnostic
airway closing volume ~ 94370
bronchodilation ~ 94664
carbon dioxide response curve ~ 94400
carbon monoxide diffusion capacity ~ 94720
Pulmonology ~ *continued*
diagnostic ~ *continued*
expired gas analysis ~ 0043T, 94250
CO2 ~ 94770
O2 and CO2 ~ 94681
O2 update, direct ~ 94680
O2 uptake, indirect ~ 94690
flow-volume loop ~ 94375
function study ~ 78596
functional residual capacity ~ 94240
hemoglobin O2 affinity ~ 82820
hypoxia response curve ~ 94450
inhalation treatment ~ 94640
maldistribution of inspired air ~ 94350
maximum breathing capacity ~ 94200
maximal voluntary ventilation ~ 94200
membrane compliance ~ 94750
membrane diffusion capacity ~ 94725
nitrogen washout curve ~ 94350
oximetry, ear or pulse ~ 94760-94762
resistance to airflow ~ 94360
spirometry ~ 94010-94070
evaluation ~ 94010-94070
patient initiated with bronchospasm ~ 94014-94016
sputum mobilization with inhalants ~ 94664
stress test, pulmonary ~ 94620
stress test ~ 94621
thoracic gas volume ~ 94260
therapeutic
expired gas analysis ~ 94250
inhalation, pentamidine ~ 94642
inhalation treatment ~ 94640, 94644-94645, 94664, 99503
intrapulmonary surfactant administration ~ 94610
manipulation of chest wall ~ 94667-94668
pressure ventilation
negative CNPB ~ 94662
positive CPAP ~ 94660
unlisted services and procedures ~ 94799
ventilation assist ~ 94002-94005, 99504
unlisted services and procedures ~ 94799
Pulse generator
electronic analysis ~ 95970-95971
heart, insertion/replacement ~ 33212-33213
Pulse rate increased ~ see tachycardia
Pulsed magnetic neuromodulation urinary incontinence ~ 0029T
Pump ~ see chemotherapy, pump services; infusion pump
Pump, infusion ~ see infusion pump
Pump services oxygenator/heat exchanger ~ 99190-99192
Pump stomach for poison ~ 91105
Punch graft ~ 15775-15776
Puncture
artery ~ 36600
chest, drainage ~ 32000-32002
cisternal ~ see cisternal puncture
lumbar ~ see spinal tap
lung ~ 32420

Puncture ~ *continued*
pericardium ~ 33010-33011
pleural cavity, drainage ~ 32000-32002
skull, drain fluid ~ 61000-61020
cistern ~ 61050
inject cistern ~ 61055
inject ventricle ~ 61026
shunt
drain fluid ~ 61070
injection ~ 61070
spinal cord
diagnostic ~ 62270
drain fluid ~ 62272
lumbar ~ 62270
tracheal, aspiration and/or injection ~ 31612
Puncture aspiration
abscess, skin ~ 10160
bulla ~ 10160
cyst
breast ~ 19000-19001
skin ~ 10160
hematoma ~ 10160
Pure-tone audiometry ~ 92552, 92553
Pustules removal ~ 10040
Putti-Platt procedure ~ 23450
PUVA ~ (dermatology; photochemotherapy; ultraviolet light therapy) 96912
Pyelogram ~ see urography, intravenous; urography, retrograde
Pyelography ~ 74400, 74425
injection ~ 50394
Pyelolithotomy ~ 50130
anatrophic ~ 50075
coagulum ~ 50130
Pyeloplasty ~ 50400-50405, 50544
repair, horseshoe kidney ~ 50540
secondary ~ 50405
Pyeloscopy
with cystourethroscopy ~ 52351
biopsy ~ 52354
destruction ~ 52354
lithotripsy ~ 52353
removal, calculus ~ 52352
tumor excision ~ 52355
Pyelostogram ~ 50394
Pyelostolithotomy percutaneous ~ 50080-50081
Pyelostomy ~ 50125, 50400-50405
change tube ~ 50398
Pyelotomy
complicated ~ 50135
with drainage ~ 50125
endoscopic ~ 50570
exploration ~ 50120
with removal calculus ~ 50130
Pyeloureterogram antegrade ~ 50394
Pyeloureteroplasty ~ see pyeloplasty
Pyloric sphincter
incision ~ 43520
reconstruction ~ 43800
Pyloromyotomy ~ 43520
with gastrectomy ~ 43639
Pyloroplasty ~ 43800
with gastrectomy ~ 43639
with vagotomy ~ 43640
Pyothorax ~ see abscess, thorax
Pyridoxal phosphate ~ 84207
Pyrophosphate, adenosine ~ see adenosine diphosphate
Pyrophosphorylase, Udp galactose ~ (galactose-one-phosphate, uridyl transferase) 82775, 82776
Pyruvate ~ 84210-84220

Q

Q fever ~ 86000, 86638
Q fever ab ~ see antibody, coxiella burnetii
Quadriceps repair ~ 27430
Quantitative sudomotor axon reflex test (QSART) ~ 95923
Quick test ~ prothrombin time 85610, 85611
Quinidine assay ~ 80194
Quinine ~ 84228

R

Rabies vaccine ~ 90675-90676
Rachicentesis ~ see spinal tap
Radial arteries ~ see artery, radial
Radial head, subluxation ~ see nursemaid elbow
Radial keratotomy ~ 65771
Radiation ~ see irradiation
Radiation physics
consultation ~ 77336-77370
unlisted services and procedures ~ 77399
Radiation therapy ~ 77280-77295
CT scan guidance ~ 77014
consultation, radiation physics ~ 77336-77370
dose plan ~ 77300, 77305-77331
brachytherapy ~ 77326-77328
intensity modulation ~ 77301
teletherapy ~ 77305-77321
field set-up ~ 77280-77295
planning ~ 77261-77263, 77299
special ~ 77470
stereotactic
body ~ 77373
cerebral lesions ~ 77371-77372
guidance ~ 77432
treatment delivery ~ 77371-77373
intensity modulation ~ 77418
proton beam ~ 77520-77525
single ~ 77402-77406
stereotactic ~ 77371-77373
superficial ~ 77401

Radiation therapy ~ *continued*
three or more areas ~ 77412-77416
two areas ~ 77407-77411
weekly ~ 77427
treatment device ~ 77332-77334
treatment management
one or two fractions only ~ 77431
unlisted services and procedures ~ 77499
weekly ~ 77427
Radical excision of lymph nodes ~ see excision, lymph nodes, radical
Radical mastectomies, modified ~ see mastectomy, modified radical
Radical neck dissection
with auditory canal surgery ~ 69155
laryngectomy ~ 31365-31368
pharyngolaryngectomy ~ 31390-31395
with thyroidectomy ~ 60254
with tongue excision ~ 41135, 41145, 41153-41155
Radical resection ~ see also resection, radical
abdomen ~ 51597
acetabulum ~ 27076
ankle ~ 27615
arm, lower ~ 25077
calcaneus ~ 27647
elbow, capsule, soft tissue, bone with contracture release ~ 24149
face ~ 21015
fibula ~ 27646
finger ~ 26117
foot ~ 28046
forearm ~ 25077
hand ~ 26115
hip
soft tissue ~ 27049
tumor or infection ~ 27075-27076
humerus ~ 23220-23222
innominate ~ 27077
ischial ~ 27078-27079
knee ~ 27329
leg
lower ~ 27615
upper ~ 27329
metacarpal ~ 26250-26255
metatarsal ~ 28173
mouth, with tongue excision ~ 41150, 41155
ovarian tumor
bilateral
salpingo-oophorectomy-omentectomy ~ 58950-58954
with radical dissection for debulking ~ 58952-58954
with total abdominal hysterectomy ~ 58951, 58953-58954
pelvis, soft tissue ~ 27049
peritoneal tumor
bilateral
salpingo-oophorectomy-omentectomy ~ 58952-58954
with radical dissection for debulking ~ 58952-58954

Radical resection ~ *continued*
phalanges
fingers ~ 26260-26262
toe ~ 28175
radius ~ 25170
scalp ~ 21015
scapula ~ 23210
shoulder ~ 23077
sternum ~ 21630-21632
talus, tumor ~ 27647
tarsal ~ 28171
tibia ~ 27645
tonsil ~ 42842-42845
tumor
back/flank ~ 21935
femur ~ 27365
knee ~ 27329, 27365
leg, upper ~ 27329
neck ~ 21557
thorax ~ 21557
ulna ~ 25170
wrist ~ 25077
Radical vaginal hysterectomy ~ see hysterectomy, vaginal, radical
Radical vulvectomy ~ see vulvectomy, radical
Radio-cobalt B12 Schilling test ~ see vitamin, B-12, absorption study
Radioactive colloid therapy ~ 79200-79300
Radioactive substance
insertion
kidney ~ 50578
prostate ~ 55860
ureteral endoscopic ~ 50978
urethral endoscopic ~ 50959
Radiocarpal joint
arthrotomy ~ 25040
dislocation, closed treatment ~ 25660
Radiocinematographies ~ see cineradiography
Radioelement
application ~ 77761-77778
surface ~ 77789
with ultrasound ~ 76965
handling ~ 77790
infusion ~ 77750
Radioelement substance
catheter placement, bronchus ~ 31643
catheterization ~ 55875
Radiography ~ see radiology, diagnostic; X-ray
Radioimmunosorbent test ~ see gammaglobulin, blood
Radioisotope brachytherapy ~ see brachytherapy
Radioisotope scan ~ see nuclear medicine
Radiological marker, preoperative placement, excision of breast lesion ~ 19125-19126
Radiology services ~ 70010-79999
diagnostic radiology ~ 70010-76499
diagnostic ultrasound ~ 76506-76999
nuclear medicine ~ 78000-79999
radiation oncology ~ 77261-77799
stress views ~ 77071

Radionuclide CT scan ~ see emission computerized tomography
Radionuclide imaging ~ see nuclear medicine
Radionuclide therapy
intra-articular ~ 79440
intravascular ~ 79420
intravenous infusion ~ 79403
leukemia ~ 79100
other ~ 79400
polycythemia vera ~ 79100
thyroid gland ~ 79000-79035
unlisted services and procedures ~ 79999
Radionuclide tomography, single photon emission- computed ~ see SPECT
Radiopharmaceutical therapy
heart ~ 79440
intravascular ~ 79420
intravenous infusion ~ 79403
leukemia ~ 79100
other ~ 79400
polycythemia vera ~ 79100
thyroid gland ~ 79020-79035
unlisted services and procedures ~ 79999
Radiotherapeutic ~ see radiation therapy
Radiotherapies ~ see irradiation
Radiotherapy, surface ~ see application, radioelement, surface
Radioulnar joint
arthrodesis, with resection of ulna ~ 25830
dislocation
closed treatment ~ 25675
open treatment ~ 25676
Radius ~ see also also arm, lower; elbow; ulna
arthroplasty ~ 24365
with implant ~ 24366, 25441
craterization ~ 24145, 25151
cyst, excision ~ 24125-24126, 25120-25126
diaphysectomy ~ 24145, 25151
dislocation
with fracture
closed treatment ~ 24620
open treatment ~ 24635
partial ~ 24640
subluxate ~ 24640
excision ~ 24130, 24136, 24145, 24152-24153
epiphyseal bar ~ 20150
partial ~ 25145
styloid process ~ 25230
fracture ~ 25605
closed treatment ~ 25500-25505, 25520, 25600-25605
with manipulation ~ 25605
without manipulation ~ 25600
distal ~ 25600-25609
open treatment ~ 25607-25609
head/neck
closed treatment ~ 24650-24655
open treatment ~ 24665-24666
open treatment ~ 25515, 25525-25526, 25574
percutaneous fixation ~ 25606
shaft ~ 25500-25526
Radius ~ *continued*
open treatment ~ 25574
with ulna ~ 25560-25565
open treatment ~ 25575
implant, removal ~ 24164
incision and drainage ~ 25035
osteomyelitis ~ 24136, 24145
osteoplasty ~ 25390-25393
prophylactic treatment ~ 25490, 25492
repair
epiphyseal arrest ~ 25450-25455
epiphyseal separation
closed ~ 25600
closed with manipulation ~ 25605
open treatment ~ 25607-25609
percutaneous fixation ~ 25606
with graft ~ 25405, 25420-25426
malunion or nonunion ~ 25400, 25415
osteotomy ~ 25350-25355, 25370-25375
and ulna ~ 25365
saucerization ~ 24145, 25151
sequestrectomy ~ 24136, 25145
tumor, cyst ~ 24120
excision ~ 24125-24126, 25120-25126, 25170
Ramstedt operation ~ see pyloromyotomy
Ramus anterior, nervus thoracicus ~ see intercostal nerve
Range of motion test
extremities or trunk ~ 95851
eye ~ 92018-92019
hand ~ 95852
Rapid heart rate ~ see tachycardia
Rapid plasma reagin test ~ 86592-86593
Rapid test for infection ~ 86308, 86403-86406
monospot test ~ 86308
Rapoport test ~ 52005
Raskind procedure ~ 33735-33737
Rathke pouch tumor ~ see craniopharyngioma
Rat typhus ~ (Murine typhus) 86000
Rays, roentgen ~ see X-ray
Raz procedure ~ (repair, bladder, neck) 51845
RBC ~ see red blood cell (RBC)
RBC ab ~ see antibody, red blood cell
Reaction lip without reconstruction ~ 40530
Reaction, polymerase chain ~ see polymerase chain reaction (PCR)
Realignment
femur with osteotomy ~ 27454
knee extensor ~ 27422
Receptor ~ see CD4; estrogen, receptor; FC receptor; progesterone receptors
Receptor assay
hormone ~ 84233-84235
non hormone ~ 84238
Recession gastrocnemius leg, lower ~ 27687
Reconstruction ~ see revision
abdominal wall
omental flap ~ 49905
acetabulum ~ 27120-27122

Reconstruction ~ *continued*
anal
congenital absence ~ 46730-46740
fistula ~ 46742
graft ~ 46753
with implant ~ 46762
sphincter ~ 46750-46751, 46760-46762
ankle ~ 27700-27703
apical-aortic conduit ~ 33404
atrial
endoscopic ~ 33265-33266
open ~ 33254-33256
auditory canal, external ~ 69310-69320
bile duct, anastomosis ~ 47800
bladder
from colon ~ 50810
from intestines ~ 50820, 51960
and urethra ~ 51800-51820
breast ~ 19357-19369
augmentation ~ 19324-19325
with free flap ~ 19364
with latissimus dorsi flap ~ 19361
mammoplasty ~ 19318-19325
nipple ~ 19350-19355
with other techniques ~ 19366
revision ~ 19380
with tissue expander ~ 19357
transverse rectus abdominis myocutaneous flap ~ 19367-19369
bronchi ~ 32501
graft repair ~ 31770
stenosis ~ 31775
canthus ~ 67950
carpal ~ 25443
carpal bone ~ 25394, 25430
cheekbone ~ 21270
chest wall, omental flap ~ 49904
trauma ~ 32820
cleft palate ~ 42200-42225
conduit, apical-aortic ~ 33404
conjunctiva ~ 68320-68335
with flap
bridge or partial ~ 68360
total ~ 68362
cranial bone, extracranial ~ 21181-21184
ear, middle
tympanoplasty with antrotomy or mastoidotomy
with ossicular chain reconstruction ~ 69636-69637
tympanoplasty with mastoidectomy ~ 69641
with intact or reconstructed wall ~ 69643-69644
with ossicular chain reconstruction ~ 69642
radical or complete ~ 69644-69645
tympanoplasty without mastoidectomy ~ 69631
with ossicular chain reconstruction ~ 69632-69633

Reconstruction ~ *continued*
elbow ~ 24360
with implant ~ 24361-24362
total replacement ~ 24363
esophagus ~ 43300, 43310, 43313
creation, stoma ~ 43350-43352
esophagostomy ~ 43350
fistula ~ 43305, 43312, 43314
gastrointestinal ~ 43360-43361
eye
graft
conjunctiva ~ 65782
stem cell ~ 65781
transplantation
amniotic membrane ~ 65780
eyelid
canthus ~ 67950
second stage ~ 67975
total ~ 67973-67975
total eyelid
lower, one stage ~ 67973
upper, one stage ~ 67974
transfer tarsoconjunctival flap from opposing eyelid ~ 67971
facial bones, secondary ~ 21275
fallopian tube ~ see repair
femur
lengthening ~ 27466-27468
shortening ~ 27465, 27468
fibula, lengthening ~ 27715
finger, polydactylous ~ 26587
foot, cleft ~ 28360
forehead ~ 21172-21180, 21182-21184
glenoid fossa ~ 21255
gums
alveolus ~ 41874
gingiva ~ 41872
hand
tendon pulley ~ 26390, 26500-26502
toe to finger transfer ~ 26551-26556
heart
atrial ~ 33253
endoscopic ~ 33265-33266
open ~ 33254-33256
atrial septum ~ 33735-33737
pulmonary artery shunt ~ 33924
vena cava ~ 34502
hip
replacement ~ 27130-27132
secondary ~ 27134-27138
hip joint, with prosthesis ~ 27125
interphalangeal joint ~ 26535-26536
collateral ligament ~ 26545
intestines, small, anastomosis ~ 44130
knee ~ 27437-27438
femur ~ 27442-27443, 27446
ligament ~ 27427-27429
prosthesis ~ 27438, 27445
replacement ~ 27447
revision ~ 27486-27487
tibia ~ 27440-27443, 27446
kneecap, instability ~ 27420-27424

Reconstruction ~ *continued*
larynx
burns ~ 31588
cricoid split ~ 31587
other ~ 31588
stenosis ~ 31582
web ~ 31580
lip ~ 40525-40527, 40761
lunate ~ 25444
malar augmentation,
prosthetic material ~ 21270
with bone graft ~ 21210
mandible, with implant ~ 21244-21246, 21248-21249
mandibular condyle ~ 21247
mandibular rami
with bone graft ~ 21194
without bone graft ~ 21193
with internal rigid fixation ~ 21196
without internal rigid fixation ~ 21195
maxilla, with implant ~ 21245-21246, 21248-21249
metacarpophalangeal joint ~ 26530-26531
midface
with bone graft ~ 21145-21160, 21188
without bone graft ~ 21141-21143
forehead advancement ~ 21159-21160
mouth ~ 40840-40845
nail bed ~ 11762
nasoethmoid complex ~ 21182-21184
navicular ~ 25443
nose
cleft lip/cleft palate ~ 30460-30462
dermatoplasty ~ 30620
primary ~ 30400-30420
secondary ~ 30430-30450
septum ~ 30520
orbit ~ 21256
orbit area, secondary ~ 21275
orbit with bone grafting ~ 21182-21184
orbital rim ~ 21172-21180
orbital rims ~ 21182-21184
orbital walls ~ 21182-21184
orbitocraniofacial, secondary revision ~ 21275
oviduct, fimbrioplasty ~ 58760
palate
cleft palate ~ 42200-42225
lengthening ~ 42226-42227
parotid duct, diversion ~ 42507-42510
patella ~ 27437-27438
instability ~ 27420-27424
penis
angulation ~ 54360
chordee ~ 54300-54304
complications ~ 54340-54348
epispadias ~ 54380-54390
hypospadias ~ 54332, 54352
one stage distal with urethroplasty ~ 54324-54328
one stage perineal ~ 54336
periorbital region, osteotomy with graft ~ 21267-21268

Reconstruction ~ *continued*
pharynx ~ 42950
pyloric sphincter ~ 43800
radius ~ 24365, 25390-25393, 25441
arthroplasty, with implant ~ 24366
shoulder joint, with implant ~ 23470-23472
skull ~ 21172-21180
defect ~ 62140-62141, 62145
sternum ~ 21740-21742
with thoracoscopy ~ 21743
stomach
with duodenum ~ 43810, 43850-43855, 43865
gastric bypass ~ 43846
with jejunum ~ 43820-43825, 43860
for obesity ~ 43846-43848
Roux-en-Y ~ 43846
superior-lateral orbital rim and forehead ~ 21172-21175
supraorbital rim and forehead ~ 21179-21180
symblepharon ~ 68335
temporomandibular joint, arthroplasty ~ 21240-21243
throat ~ 42950
thumb
from finger ~ 26550
opponensplasty ~ 26490-26496
tibia
lengthening ~ 27715
tubercle ~ 27418
toe
angle deformity ~ 28313
extra toes ~ 28344
hammertoe ~ 28285-28286
macrodactyly ~ 28340-28341
polydactylous ~ 26587
syndactyly ~ 28345
webbed toe ~ 28345
tongue, frenum ~ 41520
trachea
carina ~ 31766
cervical ~ 31750
fistula ~ 31755
intrathoracic ~ 31760
trapezium ~ 25445
tympanic membrane ~ 69620
ulna ~ 25390-25393, 25442
radioulnar ~ 25337
ureter ~ 50700
with intestines ~ 50840
urethra ~ 53410-53440, 53445
complications ~ 54340-54348
hypospadias
one stage distal with meatal advancement ~ 54322
one stage distal with urethroplasty ~ 54324-54328
suture to bladder ~ 51840-51841
urethroplasty for second stage ~ 54308-54316
urethroplasty for third stage ~ 54318
uterus ~ 58540

Reconstruction ~ *continued*
vas deferens ~ see vasovasorrhaphy
vena cava ~ 34502
with resection ~ 37799
wound repair ~ 13100-13160
wrist ~ 25332
capsulectomy ~ 25320
capsulorrhaphy ~ 25320
realign ~ 25335
zygomatic arch ~ 21255
Rectal bleeding ~ see hemorrhage, rectum
Rectal prolapse ~ see procidentia, rectum
Rectal sphincter dilation ~ 45910
Rectocele repair ~ 45560
Rectopexy ~ see proctopexy
Rectoplasty ~ see proctoplasty
Rectorrhaphy ~ see rectum, suture
Rectovaginal fistula ~ see fistula, rectovaginal
Rectovaginal hernia ~ see rectocele
Rectum ~ see also anus
abscess, incision and drainage ~ 45005-45020, 46040, 46060
biopsy ~ 45100
dilation, endoscopy ~ 45303
endoscopy
destruction, tumor ~ 45320
dilation ~ 45303
exploration ~ 45300
hemorrhage ~ 45317
removal
foreign body ~ 45307
polyp ~ 45308-45315
tumor ~ 45308-45315
volvulus ~ 45321
excision
with colon ~ 45121
partial ~ 45111, 45113-45116, 45123
total ~ 45110, 45112, 45119-45120
exploration, endoscopic ~ 45300
hemorrhage, endoscopic ~ 45317
injection, sclerosing solution ~ 45520
lesion, excision ~ 45108
manometry ~ 91122
prolapse, excision ~ 45130-45135
pulsed irrigation, fecal impaction ~ 91123
removal
fecal impaction ~ 45915
by pulsed irrigation ~ 91123
foreign body ~ 45307, 45915
repair
fistula ~ 45800-45825
injury ~ 45562-45563
prolapse ~ 45505-45541, 45900
rectocele ~ 45560
stenosis ~ 45500
with sigmoid excision ~ 45550
stricture, excision ~ 45150
suture
fistula ~ 45800-45825
prolapse ~ 45540-45541

Rectum ~ *continued*
tumor
destruction ~ 45190, 45320, 46937-46938
excision ~ 45160-45170
unlisted services and procedures ~ 44239, 45999
Reductase, glutathione ~ see glutathione reductase
Reductase, lactic cytochrome ~ see lactic dehydrogenase
Red blood cell (RBC)
antibody ~ 86850-86870
pretreatment ~ 86970-86972
count ~ 85032-85041
fragility
mechanical ~ 85547
osmotic ~ 85555-85557
hematocrit ~ 85014
iron utilization ~ 78170
morphology ~ 85007
platelet estimation ~ 85007
sedimentation rate
automated ~ 85652
manual ~ 85651
sequestration ~ 78140
sickling ~ 85660
survival test ~ 78130-78135
volume determination ~ 78120-78121
Red blood cell ab ~ see antibody, red blood cell
Reduction
forehead ~ 21137-21139
lung volume ~ 32491
mammoplasty ~ 19318
masseter muscle/bone ~ 21295-21296
osteoplasty, facial bones ~ 21209
pregnancy, multifetal ~ 59866
skull, craniomegalic ~ 62115-62117
ventricular septum, non-surgical ~ 0024T
Reflex test
blink reflex ~ 95933
H reflex ~ 95934-95936
Reflux study ~ 78262
Refraction ~ 92015
Rehabilitation
artery, occlusive disease ~ 93668
aural ~ 92510
cardiac ~ 93797-93798
Rehabilitative ~ see rehabilitation
Rehfuss test ~ see gastroenterology diagnostic, stomach
Reichstein's substances ~ see deoxycortisol
Reimplantation
arteries
aorta prosthesis ~ 35697
carotid ~ 35691, 35694-35695
subclavian ~ 35693-35695
vertebral ~ 35691-35693
visceral ~ 35697
kidney ~ 50380
ovary ~ 58825
pulmonary artery ~ 33788

Reimplantation ~ *continued*
ureters ~ 51565
ureter, to bladder ~ 50780-50785
Reinnervation larynx, neuromuscular pedicle ~ 31590
Reinsch test ~ 83015
Reinsertion
drug delivery implant ~ 11983
implantable contraceptive capsules ~ 11977
spinal fixation device ~ 22849
Relative density ~ see specific gravity
Release
carpal tunnel ~ 64721
elbow contracture, with radical release of capsule ~ 24149
flexor muscles, hip ~ 27036
muscle, knee ~ 27422
nerve ~ 64702-64726
neurolytic ~ 64727
retina, encircling material ~ 67115
spinal cord ~ 63200
stapes ~ 69650
tarsal tunnel ~ 28035
tendon ~ 24332, 25295
Release-inhibiting hormone, somatotropin ~ see somatostatin
Removal
allograft, intestinal ~ 44137
balloon, intra-aortic ~ 33974
balloon assist device, intra-aortic ~ 33968, 33971
blood clot, eye ~ 65930
blood component, apheresis ~ 36511-36516
breast
capsules ~ 19371
implants ~ 19328-19330
modified radical ~ 19307
partial ~ 19300-19302
radical ~ 19305-19306
simple, complete ~ 19303
subcutaneous ~ 19304
calcareous deposit, subdeltoid ~ 23000
calculi (stone)
bile duct ~ 43264, 47420-47425
percutaneous ~ 47554, 47630
bladder ~ 51050, 52310-52318, 52352
gallbladder ~ 47480
hepatic duct ~ 47400
kidney ~ 50060-50081, 50130, 50561, 50580, 52352
pancreas ~ 48020
pancreatic duct ~ 43264
salivary gland ~ 42330-42340
ureter ~ 50610-50630, 50961, 50980, 51060-51065, 52320-52330, 52352
urethra ~ 52310-52315, 52352
cardiac event recorder ~ 33284
cast ~ 29700-29715
cataract
with replacement
not associated with concurrent ~ 66983
extracapsular ~ 66982, 66984

Removal ~ *continued*
cataract ~ *continued*
intracapsular ~ 66983
catheter
central venous ~ 36589
fractured ~ 75961
peritoneum ~ 49422
spinal cord ~ 62355
cerclage, cervix ~ 59871
cerumen, auditory canal, external ~ 69210
clot pericardium ~ 33020
endoscopic ~ 32658
comedones ~ 10040
contraceptive capsules ~ 11976-11977
cranial tongs ~ 20665
cyst ~ 10040
dacryolith
lacrimal duct ~ 68530
lacrimal gland ~ 68530
defibrillator
heart ~ 33244
pulse generator only ~ 33241
via thoracotomy ~ 33243
drug delivery implant ~ 11982-11983
ear wax, auditory canal, external ~ 69210
electrode
brain ~ 61535, 61880
heart ~ 33238
nerve ~ 64585
spinal cord ~ 63660
stomach ~ 0156T, 0158T, 43648, 43882
embolus ~ see embolectomy
external fixation system ~ 20694
eye
bone ~ 67414, 67445
with bone ~ 65112
with implant
muscles attached ~ 65105
muscles, not attached ~ 65103
without implant ~ 65101
with muscle or myocutaneous flap ~ 65114
ocular contents
with implant ~ 65093
without implant ~ 65091
orbital contents only ~ 65110
fallopian tube, laparoscopy ~ 58661
fat, lipectomy ~ 15876-15879
fecal impaction, rectum ~ 45915
fibrin deposit ~ 32150
fixation device ~ 20670-20680
foreign bodies ~ 65205-65265
anal ~ 46608
ankle joint ~ 27610, 27620
arm
lower ~ 25248
upper ~ 24200-24201
auditory canal, external ~ 69200
with anesthesia ~ 69205
bile duct ~ 43269
bladder ~ 52310-52315
brain ~ 61570, 62163
bronchi ~ 31635

Removal ~ *continued*
colon ~ 44025, 44390, 45379
colon-sigmoid ~ 45332
conjunctival embedded ~ 65210
cornea
with slit lamp ~ 65222
without slit lamp ~ 65220
duodenum ~ 44010
elbow ~ 24000, 24101, 24200-24201
esophagus ~ 43020, 43045, 43215, 74235
external eye ~ 65205
eyelid ~ 67938
finger ~ 26075-26080
foot ~ 28190-28193
gastrointestinal, upper ~ 43247
gum ~ 41805
hand ~ 26070
hip ~ 27033, 27086-27087
hysteroscopy ~ 58562
interphalangeal joint, toe ~ 28024
intertarsal joint ~ 28020
intestines, small ~ 44020, 44363
intraocular ~ 65235
kidney ~ 50561, 50580
knee joint ~ 27310, 27331, 27372
lacrimal duct ~ 68530
lacrimal gland ~ 68530
larynx ~ 31511, 31530-31531, 31577
leg, upper ~ 27372
lung ~ 32151
mandible ~ 41806
mediastinum ~ 39000-39010
metatarsophalangeal joint ~ 28022
mouth ~ 40804-40805
muscle ~ 20520-20525
nose ~ 30300
anesthesia ~ 30310
lateral rhinotomy ~ 30320
orbit ~ 61334, 67413, 67430
with bone flap ~ 67430
without bone flap ~ 67413
pancreatic duct ~ 43269
patella ~ see patellectomy
pelvis ~ 27086-27087
penile tissue ~ 54115
penis ~ 54115
pericardium ~ 33020
endoscopic ~ 32658
peritoneum ~ 49402
pharynx ~ 42809
pleura ~ 32150-32151
endoscopic ~ 32653
posterior segment
magnetic extraction ~ 65260
nonmagnetic extraction ~ 65265
rectum ~ 45307, 45915
scrotum ~ 55120
shoulder ~ 23040-23044
complicated ~ 23332
deep ~ 23331
subcutaneous ~ 23330
skin, with debridement ~ 11010-11012

Removal ~ *continued*
foreign bodies ~ *continued*
stomach ~ 43500
subcutaneous tissue ~ 10120-10121
with debridement ~ 11010-11012
tarsometatarsal joint ~ 28020
tendon sheath ~ 20520-20525
toe ~ 28022
ureter ~ 50961, 50980
urethra ~ 52310-52315
uterus ~ 58562
vagina ~ 57415
wrist ~ 25040, 25101, 25248
foreign body, elbow ~ 24101
hair, electrolysis ~ 17380
halo ~ 20665
hearing aid, bone conduction ~ 69711
hematoma, brain ~ 61312-61315
implantation ~ 20670-20680
ankle ~ 27704
contraceptive capsules ~ 11976-11977
elbow ~ 24160
eye ~ 67120-67121
finger ~ 26320
hand ~ 26320
radius ~ 24164
wrist ~ 25449
infusion pump
intra-arterial ~ 36262
intravenous ~ 36590
spinal cord ~ 62365
intra-aortic balloon ~ 33974
assist device ~ 33968, 33971
intrauterine device (IUD) ~ 58301
keel, laryngoplasty ~ 31580
lacrimal gland
partial ~ 68505
total ~ 68500
lacrimal sac, excision/(optional) ~ 68520
laryngocele ~ 31300
leiomyomata ~ 58545-58546, 58561
lens ~ 66920-66940
lens material ~ 66840-66852
lesion
conjunctiva ~ 68040
larynx ~ 31512, 31578
endoscopic ~ 31545-31546
loose body
ankle ~ 27620
carpometacarpal joint ~ 26070
elbow ~ 24101
interphalangeal joint, toe ~ 28024
intertarsal joint ~ 28020
knee joint ~ 27331
metatarsophalangeal joint ~ 28022
tarsometatarsal joint ~ 28020
toe ~ 28022
wrist ~ 25101
lung
bronchoplasty ~ 32501
completion pneumonectomy ~ 32488
cyst ~ 32140

Removal ~ *continued*
lung ~ *continued*
extrapleural ~ 32445
single lobe ~ 32480
single segment ~ 32484
sleeve lobectomy ~ 32486
sleeve pneumonectomy ~ 32442
total pneumonectomy ~ 32440-32445
two lobes ~ 32482
volume reduction ~ 32491
wedge resection ~ 32500
lymph nodes
abdominal ~ 38747
inguinofemoral ~ 38760-38765
pelvic ~ 38770
retroperitoneal, transabdominal ~ 38780
thoracic ~ 38746
mammary implant ~ 19328-19330
mastoid, air cells ~ 69670
mesh, abdominal wall ~ 11008
milia, multiple ~ 10040
nails ~ 11730-11732, 11750-11752
neurostimulators
pulse generator ~ 64595
receiver ~ 64595
ocular implant ~ 65175, 65920
orbital implant ~ 67560
ovaries, laparoscopy ~ 58661
pacemaker, heart ~ 33233-33237
patella, complete ~ 27424
plate, skull ~ 62142
polyp
anal ~ 46610, 46612
antrochoanal ~ 31032
colon ~ 44392, 45385
colon-sigmoid ~ 45333
endoscopy ~ 44364-44365, 44394
esophagus ~ 43217, 43250
gastrointestinal, upper ~ 43250-43251
rectum ~ 45315
sphenoid sinus ~ 31051
prosthesis
abdomen ~ 49606
abdominal wall ~ 11008
hip ~ 27090-27091
knee ~ 27488
penis ~ 54406, 54410-54417
perineum ~ 53442
skull ~ 62142
urethral sphincter ~ 53446-53447
wrist ~ 25250-25251
pulse generator
brain ~ 61888
spinal cord ~ 63688
pustules ~ 10040
receiver, brain ~ 61888
spinal cord ~ 63688
reservoir, spinal cord ~ 62365
seton, anal ~ 46030
shoulder joint, foreign or loose body ~ 23107

Removal ~ *continued*
shunt
brain ~ 62256-62258
heart ~ 33924
peritoneum ~ 49429
spinal cord ~ 63746
skin tags ~ 11200-11201
sling
urethra ~ 53442
vagina ~ 57287
spinal instrumentation
anterior ~ 22855
posterior nonsegmental
Harrington rod ~ 22850
posterior segmental ~ 22852
stent
bile duct ~ 43269
pancreatic duct ~ 43269
suture
anal ~ 46754
anesthesia ~ 15850-15851
thrombus ~ see thrombectomy
tissue expanders, skin ~ 11971
transplant intestines ~ 44137
transplant kidney ~ 50370
tube
ear, middle ~ 69424
finger ~ 26392, 26416
hand ~ 26392, 26416
tumor, temporal bone ~ 69970
ureter, ligature ~ 50940
urethral stent
bladder ~ 52310-52315
urethra ~ 52310-52315
vein
clusters ~ 37785
perforation ~ 37760
saphenous ~ 37720-37735, 37780
varicose ~ 37765-37766
venous access device ~ 36590
obstruction ~ 75901-75902
ventilating tube, ear, middle ~ 69424
ventricular assist device ~ 33977-33978
extracorporeal ~ 0050T
intracorporeal ~ 33980
vitreous, anterior approach ~ 67005-67010
wire, anal ~ 46754
Renal ~ (see also kidney)
abscess ~ see abscess, kidney
arteries ~ see artery, renal
autotransplantation ~ see autotransplantation, renal
calculus ~ see calculus, removal, kidney
cyst ~ see cyst, kidney
dialyses ~ see hemodialysis
disease services ~ see dialysis
transplantation ~ see kidney, transplantation
Renin ~ 80408, 80416, 84244
peripheral vein ~ 80417
Renin-converting enzyme ~ 82164

Reoperation
carotid thromboendarterectomy ~ 35390
coronary artery bypass
valve procedure ~ 33530
distal vessel bypass ~ 35700
Repair ~ see also revision
abdomen ~ 49900
hernia ~ 49491-49525, 49565, 49570, 49582-49590
omphalocele ~ 49600-49611
suture ~ 49900
abdominal wall ~ 15830, 15847
anal
anomaly ~ 46744-46748
fistula ~ 46288, 46706-46716
stricture ~ 46700-46705
anastomosis, cyst ~ 47719
aneurysm, aorta ~ 0033T-0040T, 0078T-0081T, 33877, 34800-34805, 34825-34832, 75952-75953
arteriovenous ~ 36834
iliac artery ~ 75954
intracranial artery ~ 61697-61708
ankle
ligament ~ 27695-27698
tendon ~ 27612, 27650-27654, 27680-27687
aorta ~ 33320-33322, 33802-33803
coarctation ~ 33840-33851
graft ~ 33860-33877
sinus of valsalva ~ 33702-33720
aortic arch
with cardiopulmonary bypass ~ 33853
without cardiopulmonary bypass ~ 33852
aortic valve ~ 33400-33403
obstruction, outflow tract ~ 33414
septic hypertrophy ~ 33416
stenosis ~ 33415
arm
lower ~ 25260-25263, 25270
fasciotomy ~ 24495
secondary ~ 25265, 25272-25274
tendon ~ 25290
tendon sheath ~ 25275
muscle ~ 24341
tendon ~ 24332, 24341, 25280, 25295, 25310-25316
upper
muscle revision ~ 24330-24331
muscle transfer ~ 24301, 24320
tendon lengthening ~ 24305
tendon revision ~ 24320
tendon transfer ~ 24301
tenotomy ~ 24310
arteriovenous aneurysm ~ 36834
arteriovenous fistula
abdomen ~ 35182
acquired or traumatic ~ 35189
head ~ 35180
acquired or traumatic ~ 35188
lower extremity ~ 35184
acquired or traumatic ~ 35190
neck ~ 35180

Repair ~ *continued*
arteriovenous fistula
acquired or traumatic ~ 35188
thorax ~ 35182
acquired or traumatic ~ 35189
upper extremity ~ 35184
acquired or traumatic ~ 35190
arteriovenous malformation
intracranial ~ 61680-61692
intracranial artery ~ 61705-61708
spinal artery ~ 62294
spinal cord ~ 63250-63252
artery
angioplasty ~ 75962-75968
aorta ~ 35452, 35472
axillary ~ 35458
brachiocephalic ~ 35458, 35475
bypass graft ~ 35501-35571, 35601-35683, 35691-35695, 35700
bypass in-situ ~ 35582-35587
bypass venous graft ~ 33510-33516, 35510-35525
femoral ~ 35456, 35474
iliac ~ 34900, 35454, 35473
occlusive disease ~ 35001, 35005-35021, 35045-35081, 35091, 35102, 35111, 35121, 35131, 35141, 35151, 35161
popliteal ~ 35456, 35474
pulmonary ~ 33690
renal ~ 35450
renal or visceral ~ 35471
subclavian ~ 35458
thromboendarterectomy ~ 35301-35321, 35341-35390
tibioperoneal ~ 35459, 35470
viscera ~ 35450, 35471
arytenoid cartilage ~ 31400
bile duct ~ 47701
cyst ~ 47719
with intestines ~ 47760, 47780-47785
wound ~ 47900
bladder
exstrophy ~ 51940
fistula ~ 44660-44661, 45800-45805, 51880-51925
neck ~ 51845
resection ~ 52500
wound ~ 51860-51865
blepharoptosis, frontalis muscle technique with fascial sling ~ 67902
blood vessel
abdomen ~ 35221
with other graft ~ 35281
with vein graft ~ 35251
chest ~ 35211-35216
with other graft ~ 35271-35276
with vein graft ~ 35241-35246
finger ~ 35207
graft defect ~ 35870
hand ~ 35207
kidney ~ 50100
lower extremity ~ 35226

Repair ~ *continued*
blood vessel ~ *continued*
with other graft ~ 35286
with vein graft ~ 35256
neck ~ 35201
with other graft ~ 35261
with vein graft ~ 35231
upper extremity ~ 35206
with other graft ~ 35266
with vein graft ~ 35236
body cast ~ 29720
brain, wound ~ 61571
breast, suspension ~ 19316
bronchi, fistula ~ 32815
brow pyrosis ~ 67900
bunion ~ 28290-28299
bypass graft ~ 35901-35907
fistula ~ 35870
calcaneus, osteotomy ~ 28300
cannula ~ 36860-36861
carpal ~ 25440
carpal bone ~ 25431
cervix
cerclage ~ 57700
abdominal ~ 59320-59325
suture ~ 57720
chest wall ~ 32905
closure ~ 32810
fistula ~ 32906
chin
augmentation ~ 21120, 21123
osteotomy ~ 21121-21123
clavicle, osteotomy ~ 23480-23485
cleft hand ~ 26580
cleft lip ~ 40525-40527, 40700-40761
nasal deformity ~ 40700-40701, 40720-40761
cleft palate ~ see cleft palate, repair
colon
fistula ~ 44650-44661
hernia ~ 44050
malrotation ~ 44055
obstruction ~ 44050
cornea ~ see cornea, repair
coronary chamber fistula ~ 33500-33501
cyst
Bartholin's gland ~ 56440
choledochal ~ 47719
liver ~ 47300
diaphragm
for eventration ~ 39545
hernia ~ 39502-39541
laceration ~ 39501
ductus arteriosus ~ 33820-33824
ear, middle
oval window fistula ~ 69666
round window fistula ~ 69667
elbow
fasciotomy ~ 24350-24356
hemiepiphyseal arrest ~ 24470
ligament ~ 24343-24346
muscle ~ 24341

Repair ~ *continued*
muscle transfer ~ 24301
tendon ~ 24340-24342
each ~ 24341
tendon lengthening ~ 24305
tendon transfer ~ 24301
tennis elbow ~ 24350-24356
encephalocele ~ 62121
enterocele
hysterectomy ~ 58270, 58294
epididymis ~ 54900-54901
epispadias ~ 54380-54390
esophagus ~ 43300, 43310, 43313
esophagogastrostomy ~ 43320
esophagojejunostomy ~ 43340-43341
fistula ~ 43305, 43312, 43314, 43420-43425
fundoplasty ~ 43324-43325
muscles ~ 43330-43331
pre-existing perforation ~ 43405
varices ~ 43401
wound ~ 43410-43415
eye
ciliary body ~ 66680
suture ~ 66682
conjunctiva ~ 65270-65273
wound ~ 65270-65273
cornea ~ 65275
astigmatism ~ 65772-65775
with glue ~ 65286
wound ~ 65275-65285
fistula, lacrimal gland ~ 68770
iris
with ciliary body ~ 66680
suture ~ 66682
lacrimal duct, canaliculi ~ 68700
lacrimal punctum ~ 68705
retina, detachment ~ 67101-67112
sclera
with glue ~ 65286
with graft ~ 66225
reinforcement ~ 67250-67255
staphyloma ~ 66220-66225
wound ~ 65286, 66250
strabismus, chemodenervation ~ 67345
symblepharon
division ~ 68340
with graft ~ 68335
without graft ~ 68330
trabeculae ~ 65855
eye muscles
strabismus
adjustable sutures ~ 67335
one horizontal muscle ~ 67311
one vertical muscle ~ 67314
posterior fixation suture technique ~ 67334-67335
previous surgery, not involving extraocular muscles ~ 67331
release extensive scar tissue ~ 67343
superior oblique muscle ~ 67318
two horizontal muscles ~ 67312
two or more vertical muscles ~ 67316

Repair ~ *continued*
eye muscles ~ *continued*
wound, extraocular muscle ~ 65290
eyebrow, ptosis ~ 67900
eyelashes
epilation
by forceps ~ 67820
by other than forceps ~ 67825
incision of lid margin ~ 67830
with free mucous membrane graft ~ 67835
eyelid ~ 21280-21282
ectropion ~ 67916-67917
suture ~ 67914
thermocauterization ~ 67915
entropion ~ 67924
excision tarsal wedge ~ 67923
suture ~ 67921-67924
thermocauterization ~ 67922
excisional ~ 67961-67966
lagophthalmos ~ 67912
ptosis, conjunctivo-tarso-Muller's muscle-levator resection ~ 67908
frontalis muscle technique ~ 67901-67902
levator resection ~ 67903-67904
reduction of overcorrection ~ 67909
superior rectus technique ~ 67906
retraction ~ 67911
wound, suture ~ 67930-67935
facial bones ~ 21208-21209
facial nerve
paralysis ~ 15840-15845
suture, intratemporal, lateral to geniculate ganglion ~ 69740
intratemporal, medial to geniculate ganglion ~ 69745
fallopian tube ~ 58752
anastomosis ~ 58750
create stoma ~ 58770
fascial defect ~ 50728
femur ~ 27470-27472
epiphysis ~ 27475-27485, 27742
arrest ~ 27185
open treatment ~ 27177-27178
osteoplasty ~ 27179
osteotomy ~ 27181
by pinning ~ 27176
by traction ~ 27175
with graft ~ 27170
muscle transfer ~ 27110
osteotomy ~ 27140, 27151, 27450-27454
femoral neck ~ 27161
with fixation ~ 27165
with open reduction ~ 27156
fibula
epiphysis ~ 27477-27485, 27730-27742
osteotomy ~ 27707-27712
finger
claw finger ~ 26499
macrodactylia ~ 26590
polydactylous ~ 26587
syndactyly ~ 26560-26562
tendon

Repair ~ *continued*
finger ~ *continued*
extensor ~ 26415-26434, 26445-26449
flexor ~ 26356-26358, 26440-26442
joint stabilization ~ 26474
pip joint ~ 26471
toe transfer ~ 26551-26556
trigger ~ 26055
volar plate ~ 26548
web finger ~ 26560-26562
fistula
carotid-cavernous ~ 61710
mastoid ~ 69700
rectovaginal ~ 57308
foot
fascia ~ 28250
muscle ~ 28250
tendon ~ 28200-28226, 28238
gallbladder
with gastroenterostomy ~ 47741
with intestines ~ 47720-47740
great arteries ~ 33770-33781
great vessel ~ 33320-33322
hallux valgus ~ 28290-28299
hamstring ~ 27097
hand
cleft hand ~ 26580
muscle ~ 26591-26593
tendon
extensor ~ 26410-26416, 26426-26428, 26433-26437
flexor ~ 26350-26358, 26440
profundus ~ 26370-26373
hearing aid, bone conduction ~ 69711
heart
anomaly ~ 33600-33617
aortic sinus ~ 33702-33722
artificial heart, intracorporeal ~ 0052T-0053T
atrioventricular canal ~ 33660-33665
complete ~ 33670
atrioventricular valve ~ 33660-33665
blood vessel ~ 33320-33322
cor triatriatum ~ 33732
infundibular ~ 33476-33478
mitral valve ~ 33420-33427
myocardium ~ 33542
outflow tract ~ 33476-33478
postinfarction ~ 33542-33545
prosthetic valve ~ 33670, 33852-33853
prosthetic valve dysfunction ~ 33496
pulmonary artery shunt ~ 33924
pulmonary valve ~ 33470-33474
septal defect ~ 33545, 33608-33610, 33681-33688, 33692-33697
atrial and ventricular ~ 33647
atrium ~ 33641
sinus of valsalva ~ 33702-33722
sinus venosus ~ 33645
tetralogy of Fallot ~ 33692-33697
total replacement heart system, intracorporeal ~ 0052T-0053T
tricuspid valve ~ 33465

Repair ~ *continued*
heart ~ *continued*
ventricle ~ 33611-33612
obstruction ~ 33619
ventricular tunnel ~ 33722
wound ~ 33300-33305
hepatic duct, with intestines ~ 47765, 47802
hernia ~ 50728
abdomen ~ 49565, 49590
incisional ~ 49560
epigastric ~ 49570
incarcerated ~ 49572
femoral ~ 49550
incarcerated ~ 49553
recurrent ~ 49555
recurrent incarcerated ~ 49557
reducible recurrent ~ 49555
incisional
incarcerated ~ 49561
recurrent incarcerated ~ 49566
inguinal ~ 49495-49521
initial ~ 49650
recurrent ~ 49651
sliding ~ 49525
intestinal ~ 44025-44050
lumbar ~ 49540
lung ~ 32800
orchiopexy ~ 54640
reducible ~ 49565, 49570
femoral ~ 49550
incisional ~ 49560
inguinal ~ 49500, 49505
recurrent ~ 49520
sliding ~ 49525
with spermatic cord ~ 54640
spigelian ~ 49590
umbilical ~ 49580, 49585
incarcerated ~ 49582, 49587
reducible ~ 49580
hip
muscle transfer ~ 27100-27105, 27111
osteotomy ~ 27146-27156
tendon ~ 27097
humerus ~ 24420-24430
with graft ~ 24435
osteotomy ~ 24400-24410
ileostomy ~ see ileostomy, repair
interphalangeal joint, volar plate ~ 26548
intestines
enterocele
abdominal approach ~ 57270
vaginal approach ~ 57268
obstruction ~ 44615
intestines, large
closure enterostomy ~ 44620-44626
diverticula ~ 44605
ulcer ~ 44605
wound ~ 44605
intestines, small
closure enterostomy ~ 44620-44626
diverticula ~ 44602-44603
fistula ~ 44640-44661

Repair ~ *continued*
intestines, small ~ *continued*
hernia ~ 44050
malrotation ~ 44055
obstruction ~ 44025-44050
ulcer ~ 44602-44603
wound ~ 44602-44603
introitus, vagina ~ 56800
iris, ciliary body ~ 66680
jejunum
free transfer, with microvascular anastomosis ~ 43496
kidney
fistula ~ 50520-50526
horseshoe ~ 50540
renal pelvis ~ 50400-50405
wound ~ 50500
knee
cartilage ~ 27403
instability ~ 27420
ligament ~ 27405-27409
collateral ~ 27405
collateral and cruciate ~ 27409
cruciate ~ 27407-27409
meniscus ~ 27403
tendon ~ 27380-27381
larynx
fracture ~ 31584-31586
reinnervation, neuromuscular pedicle ~ 31590
leg
lower
fascia ~ 27656
tendon ~ 27658-27692
upper
muscle ~ 27385-27386, 27400, 27430
tendon ~ 27393-27400
ligament ~ see ligament, repair
lip ~ 40650-40654
cleft lip ~ 40700-40761
fistula ~ 42260
liver, abscess ~ 47300
cyst ~ 47300
wound ~ 47350-47361
lung
hernia ~ 32800
pneumolysis ~ 32940
tear ~ 32110
mastoidectomy
complete ~ 69601
modified radical ~ 69602
radical ~ 69603
with apicectomy ~ 69605
with tympanoplasty ~ 69604
maxilla, osteotomy ~ 21206
mesentery ~ 44850
metacarpal
lengthening ~ 26568
nonunion ~ 26546
osteotomy ~ 26565

Repair ~ *continued*
metacarpophalangeal joint
capsulodesis ~ 26516-26518
collateral ligament ~ 26540-26542
fusion ~ 26516-26518
metatarsal ~ 28322
osteotomy ~ 28306-28309
microsurgery ~ 69990
mitral valve ~ 33420-33427
mouth
laceration ~ 40830-40831
vestibule of ~ 40830-40845
musculotendinous cuff ~ 23410-23412
nail bed ~ 11760
nasal deformity, cleft lip ~ 40700-40761
nasal septum ~ 30630
navicular ~ 25440
neck muscles
scalenus anticus ~ 21700-21705
sternocleidomastoid ~ 21720-21725
nerve ~ 64876
graft ~ 64885-64907
microrepair ~ 69990
suture ~ 64831-64876
nose
adhesions ~ 30560
fistula ~ 30580-30600, 42260
rhinophyma ~ 30120
septum ~ 30540-30545, 30630
synechia ~ 30560
vestibular stenosis ~ 30465
omphalocele ~ 49600-49611
osteotomy
femoral neck ~ 27161
radius, and ulna ~ 25365
ulna, and radius ~ 25365
vertebra
additional segment ~ 22216, 22226
cervical ~ 22210, 22220
lumbar ~ 22214, 22224
thoracic ~ 22212, 22222
oviduct ~ 58752
create stoma ~ 58770
pacemaker, heart
electrode ~ 33218-33220
palate
laceration ~ 42180-42182
vomer flap ~ 42235
pancreas
cyst ~ 48500
pseudocyst ~ 48510-48511
percutaneous ~ 48511
paravaginal defect ~ 57284
pectus carinatum ~ 21740-21742
with thoracoscopy ~ 21743
pectus excavatum ~ 21740-21742
with thoracoscopy ~ 21743
pelvic floor, prosthetic insertion ~ 57267
pelvis
osteotomy ~ 27158
tendon ~ 27098

Repair ~ *continued*
penis
fistulization ~ 54435
injury ~ 54440
priapism ~ 54420-54435
shunt ~ 54420-54430
perineum ~ 56810
periorbital region, osteotomy ~ 21260-21263
phalanx
finger
lengthening ~ 26568
osteotomy ~ 26567
nonunion ~ 26546
toe, osteotomy ~ 28310-28312
pharynx, with esophagus ~ 42953
pleura ~ 32215
prosthesis, penis ~ 54408
pulmonary artery ~ 33917-33920
reimplantation ~ 33788
pulmonary valve ~ 33470-33474
quadriceps ~ see quadriceps, repair
radius
epiphyseal ~ 25450-25455
malunion or nonunion ~ 25400, 25415
osteotomy ~ 25350-25355, 25370-25375
with graft ~ 25405, 25420-25426
rectocele ~ see rectocele, repair
rectovaginal fistula ~ 57308
rectum
fistula ~ 45800-45825
injury ~ 45562-45563
prolapse ~ 45505-45541, 45900
rectocele ~ 45560
stenosis ~ 45500
with sigmoid excision ~ 45550
retinal detachment with diathermy ~ see diathermy, retinal detachment, repair
rotator cuff ~ see rotator cuff, repair
salivary duct ~ 42500-42505
fistula ~ 42600
scapula
fixation ~ 23400
scapulopexy ~ 23400
sclera ~ see sclera, repair
scrotum ~ 55175-55180
septal defect ~ 33813-33814
shoulder, capsule ~ 23450-23466
cuff ~ 23410-23412
ligament release ~ 23415
muscle transfer ~ 23395-23397
musculotendinous rotator cuff ~ 23415-23420
tendon ~ 23410-23412, 23430-23440
tenomyotomy ~ 23405-23406
simple, integumentary system ~ see integumentary system, repair, simple
sinus
ethmoid, cerebrospinal fluid leak ~ 31290
sphenoid, cerebrospinal fluid leak ~ 31291
sinus of valsalva ~ 33702-33722

Repair ~ *continued*
skin, wound
complex ~ 13100-13160
intermediate ~ 12031-12057
simple ~ 12020-12021
skull
cerebrospinal fluid leak ~ 62100
encephalocele ~ 62120
spica cast ~ 29720
spinal cord ~ 63700
cerebrospinal fluid leak ~ 63707-63709
meningocele ~ 63700-63702
myelomeningocele ~ 63704-63706
spinal meningocele ~ see meningocele, repair
spine, osteotomy ~ 22210-22226
spleen ~ 38115
stomach
esophagogastrostomy ~ 43320
fistula ~ 43880
fundoplasty ~ 43324-43325
laceration ~ 43501-43502
stoma ~ 43870
ulcer ~ 43501
talus, osteotomy ~ 28302
tarsal ~ 28320
osteotomy ~ 28304-28305
testis
injury ~ 54670
suspension ~ 54620-54640
torsion ~ 54600
throat
pharyngoesophageal ~ 42953
wound ~ 42900
thumb
muscle ~ 26508
tendon ~ 26510
tibia ~ 27720-27725
epiphysis ~ 27477-27485, 27730-27742
osteotomy ~ 27455-27457, 27705, 27709-27712
pseudoarthrosis ~ 27727
toe
bunion ~ 28290-28299
muscle ~ 28240
tendon ~ 28240
webbing ~ 28280, 28345
toes
macrodactylia ~ 26590
polydactylous ~ 26587
tongue ~ 41250-41252
fixation ~ 41500
laceration ~ 41250-41252
mechanical ~ 41500
suture ~ 41510
trachea, fistula ~ 31755
stenosis ~ 31780-31781
stoma ~ 31613-31614
scar ~ 31830
with plastic repair ~ 31825
without plastic repair ~ 31820
with plastic repair ~ 31825
without plastic repair ~ 31820

Repair ~ *continued*
trachea, fistula ~ *continued*
wound
cervical ~ 31800
intrathoracic ~ 31805
tricuspid valve ~ 33463-33465
truncus arteriosus, Rastelli type ~ 33786
tunica vaginalis, hydrocele ~ 55060
tympanic membrane ~ 69450, 69610
ulna
epiphyseal ~ 25450-25455
malunion or nonunion ~ 25400, 25415
osteotomy ~ 25360, 25370-25375, 25425-25426
with graft ~ 25405, 25420
umbilicus, omphalocele ~ 49600-49611
ureter
anastomosis ~ 50740-50825
continent diversion ~ 50825
deligation ~ 50940
fistula ~ 50920-50930
lysis adhesions ~ 50715-50725
suture ~ 50900
urinary undiversion ~ 50830
ureterocele ~ 51535
urethra
artificial sphincter ~ 53449
diverticulum ~ 53240, 53400-53405
fistula ~ 45820-45825, 53400-53405, 53520
stoma ~ 53520
stricture ~ 53400-53405
urethrocele ~ 57230
wound ~ 53502-53515
urethral sphincter ~ 57220
urinary incontinence ~ 53431-53440, 57284
uterus
fistula ~ 51920-51925
rupture ~ 58520, 59350
suspension ~ 58400-58410
vagina
anterior ~ see colporrhaphy, anterior
cystocele ~ 57240, 57260
enterocele ~ 57265
fistula ~ 46715-46716, 51900
rectovaginal ~ 57300-57307
transvesical and vaginal approach ~ 57330
urethrovaginal ~ 57310-57311
vesicovaginal ~ 57320-57330
hysterectomy ~ 58267, 58293
incontinence ~ 57284, 57288
pereyra procedure ~ 57289
postpartum ~ 59300
prolapse ~ 57282-57284
rectocele ~ 57250-57260
suspension ~ 57280, 57284
laparoscopic ~ 57425
wound ~ 57200-57210
vaginal wall prolapse ~ see colporrhaphy
vas deferens, suture ~ 55400

Repair ~ *continued*
vein
angioplasty ~ 35460, 35476, 75978
femoral ~ 34501
graft ~ 34520
pulmonary ~ 33730
transposition ~ 34510
vulva, postpartum ~ 59300
wound
complex ~ 13100-13160
intermediate ~ 12031-12057
simple ~ 12001-12021
wound dehiscence
complex ~ 13160
simple ~ 12020-12021
wrist ~ 25260-25263, 25270, 25447
bone ~ 25440
carpal bone ~ 25431
cartilage ~ 25107
removal, implant ~ 25449
secondary ~ 25265, 25272-25274
tendon ~ 25280-25316
tendon sheath ~ 25275
total replacement ~ 25446
Repeat surgeries ~ see reoperation
Replacement
aortic valve ~ 33405-33413
arthroplasties, hip ~ see arthroplasty, hip
artificial heart, intracorporeal ~ 0052T-0053T
cerebrospinal fluid shunt ~ 62160, 62194, 62225-62230
contact lens ~ see contact lens services
elbow, total ~ 24363
electrode
heart ~ 33210-33211, 33216-33217
stomach ~ 0155T, 0157T, 43647
eye, drug delivery system ~ 67121
gastrostomy tube ~ 43760
hearing aid, bone conduction ~ 69710
hip ~ 27130-27132
revision ~ 27134-27138
implant, bone
for external speech processor/cochlear stimulator ~ 69717-69718
knee, total ~ 27447
mitral valve ~ 33430
nephrostomy tube ~ see nephrostomy, change tube
nerve ~ 64726
neurostimulator
pulse generator/receiver
intracranial ~ 61885
peripheral nerve ~ 64590
spinal ~ 63685
ossicles, with prosthesis ~ 69633, 69637
ossicular replacement ~ see TORP (total ossicular replacement prosthesis)
pacemaker ~ 33206-33208
catheter ~ 33210
electrode ~ 33210-33211, 33216-33217
pacing cardioverter-defibrillator
leads ~ 33243-33244

Replacement ~ *continued*
pulse generator only ~ 33241
penile, prosthesis ~ 54410-54411, 54416-54417
prosthesis, skull ~ 62143
urethral sphincter ~ 53448
pulmonary valve ~ 33475
pulse generator
brain ~ 61885
peripheral nerve ~ 64590
spinal cord ~ 63685
receiver
brain ~ 61885
peripheral nerve ~ 64590
spinal cord ~ 63685
skull plate ~ 62143
spinal cord, reservoir ~ 62360
tissue expanders, skin ~ 11970
total replacement ~ see hip, total replacement
total replacement heart system
intracorporeal ~ 0052T-0053T
tricuspid valve ~ 33465
ureter, with intestines ~ 50840
venous access device ~ 36582-36583, 36585
catheter ~ 36578
venous catheter, central ~ 36580-36581, 36584
Replantation
arm, upper ~ 20802
digit ~ 20816-20822
foot ~ 20838
forearm ~ 20805
hand ~ 20808
thumb ~ 20824-20827
Report preparation
extended, medical ~ 99080
psychiatric ~ 90889
Reposition toe to hand ~ 26551-26556
Repositioning
central venous catheter ~ 36597
electrode, heart ~ 33215-33217, 33226
gastrostomy tube ~ 43761
heart, defibrillator leads ~ 33215-33216, 33226, 33249
intraocular lens ~ 66825
tricuspid valve ~ 33468
Reproductive tissue
cryopreservation
embryo(s) ~ 89258
oocyte(s) ~ 0059T
ovarian tissue ~ 0058T
sperm ~ 89259
testicular tissue ~ 89335
thawing of cryopreserved
embryo(s) ~ 89352
oocytes, each aliquot ~ 89356
sperm/semen ~ 89353
testicular/ovarian tissue ~ 89354
storage
oocyte(s) ~ 89346
sperm/semen ~ 89343
testicular/ovarian ~ 89344
Reprogramming, shunt, brain ~ 62252

Reptilase test ~ 85635
Repilase time ~ see thrombin time
Resection
aortic valve, stenosis ~ 33415
bladder diverticulum ~ 52305
bladder neck, transurethral ~ 52500
brain lobe ~ see lobectomy, brain
chest wall ~ 19260-19272
diaphragm ~ 39560-39561
endaural ~ see ear, inner, excision
humeral head ~ 23195
intestines, small, laparoscopic ~ 44202-44203
lung ~ 32520-32525
mouth, with tongue excision ~ 41153
myocardium
aneurysm ~ 33542
septal defect ~ 33545
nasal septum submucous ~ see nasal septum, submucous resection
nose
septum ~ 30520
ovary, wedge ~ see ovary, wedge resection
palate ~ 42120
phalangeal head, toe ~ 28153
prostate transurethral ~ see prostatectomy, transurethral
radical
arm, upper ~ 24077
elbow ~ 24077
with contracture release ~ 24149
foot ~ 28046
humerus ~ 24150-24151
radius ~ 24152-24153
tumor
ankle ~ 27615
calcaneus or talus ~ 27647
clavicle ~ 23200
femur ~ 27365
fibula ~ 27646
humerus ~ 23220
humerus with autograft ~ 23221
humerus with prosthetic replacement ~ 23222
knee ~ 27329, 27365
leg, lower ~ 27615
leg, upper ~ 27329
metatarsal ~ 28173
phalanx, toe ~ 28175
Scapula ~ 23210
tarsal ~ 28171
tibia ~ 27645
ribs ~ 19260-19272, 32900
synovial membrane ~ see synovectomy
temporal bone ~ 69535
tumor
fallopian tube ~ 58957-58958
ovary ~ 58957-58958
peritoneum ~ 58957-58958
ulna, arthrodesis radioulnar joint ~ 25830
ureterocele
ectopic ~ 52301
orthotopic ~ 52300

Resection ~ *continued*
vena cava, with reconstruction ~ 37799
Resonance spectroscopy, magnetic ~ see magnetic resonance spectroscopy
Respiration, positive-pressure ~ see pressure breathing, positive
Respiratory pattern recording, preventive, infant ~ 94772
Respiratory system, surgical procedures ~ 30000-32999
Respiratory syncytial virus (RSV)
antibody ~ 86756
antigen detection
by direct optical observation ~ 87807
by enzyme immunoassay ~ 87420
by immunofluorescence ~ 87280
immune globulins ~ 90378, 90379
Response, auditory evoked ~ see auditory evoked potentials
Rest home visit ~ see domiciliary services
Resuscitation
cardiac ~ see cardiac massage
cardio-pulmonary ~ see cardio-pulmonary resuscitation (CPR)
newborn ~ 99440
Reticulocyte count ~ 85044-85045
Retina
incision, encircling material ~ 67115
lesion
extensive, destruction ~ 67227-67228
localized, destruction ~ 0017T, 67208-67218
repair
detachment
cryotherapy or diathermy ~ 67101
injection of air ~ 67110
photocoagulation ~ 67105
by scleral buckling ~ 67112
scleral dissection ~ 67107
with vitrectomy ~ 67108, 67112
prophylaxis, detachment ~ 67141-67145
retinopathy
destruction
cryotherapy, diathermy ~ 67227
photocoagulation ~ 67228
Retinacular knee release ~ 27425
Retinopathy
destruction
cryotherapy, diathermy ~ 67227
photocoagulation ~ 67228
Retraction, clot ~ see clot retraction
Retrieval transcatheter foreign body ~ 37203
Retrocaval ureter ureterolysis ~ 50725
Retrograde cholangiopancreatographies, endoscopic ~ see cholangiopancreatography
Retrograde cystourethrogram ~ see urethrocystography, retrograde
Retrograde pyelogram ~ see urography, retrograde
Retroperitoneal area
abscess, incision and drainage
open ~ 49060
percutaneous ~ 49061

Retroperitoneal area ~ *continued*
biopsy ~ 49010
cyst, destruction/excision ~ 49200-49201
endometriomas, destruction/excision ~ 49200-49201
exploration ~ 49010
needle biopsy, mass ~ 49180
tumor, destruction/excision ~ 49200-49201
Retroperitoneal fibrosis ureterolysis ~ 50715
Retropubic prostatectomies ~ see prostatectomy, retropubic
Revascularization
distal upper extremity with interval ligation ~ 36838
interval ligation distal upper extremity ~ 36838
penis ~ 37788
transmyocardial ~ 33140-33141
Reversal, vasectomy ~ see vasovasorrhaphy
Reverse T3 ~ see triiodothyronine, reverse
Reverse triiodothyronine ~ see triiodothyronine, reverse
Revision ~ see reconstruction
aorta ~ 33404
blepharoplasty ~ 15820-15823
bronchial stent ~ 31638
bronchus ~ 32501
bypass graft, vein patch ~ 35685
cervicoplasty ~ 15819
colostomy ~ see colostomy, revision
cornea
prosthesis ~ 65770
reshaping
epikeratoplasty ~ 65767
keratomileusis ~ 65760
keratophakia ~ 65765
defibrillator site, chest ~ 33223
ear, middle ~ 69662
external fixation system ~ 20693
eye, aqueous shunt ~ 66185
gastrostomy tube ~ 44373
hip replacement ~ see replacement, hip, revision
hymenal ring ~ 56700
ileostomy ~ see ileostomy, revision
infusion pump
intra-arterial ~ 36261
intravenous ~ 36576-36578, 36582-36583
iris
iridoplasty ~ 66762
iridotomy ~ 66761
jejunostomy tube ~ 44373
lower extremity arterial bypass ~ 35879-35881
pacemaker site, chest ~ 33222
rhytidectomy ~ 15824-15829
semicircular canal, fenestration ~ 69840
shunt, intrahepatic portosystemic ~ 37183
sling ~ 53442
stapedectomy ~ see stapedectomy, revision
stomach, for obesity ~ 43848
tracheostomy, scar ~ 31830
urinary-cutaneous anastomosis ~ 50727-50728

Revision ~ *continued*
vagina
prosthetic graft ~ 57295-57296
sling
stress incontinence ~ 57287
venous access device ~ 36576-36578, 36582-36583, 36585
ventricle
ventriculomyectomy ~ 33416
ventriculomyotomy ~ 33416
Rheumatoid factor ~ 86430-86431
Rhinectomy
partial ~ 30150
total ~ 30160
Rhinomanometry ~ 92512
Rhinopharynx ~ see nasopharynx
Rhinophyma repair ~ 30120
Rhinoplasty
cleft lip/cleft palate ~ 30460-30462
primary ~ 30400-30420
secondary ~ 30430-30450
Rhinoscopy ~ see endoscopy, nose
Rhinotomy lateral ~ 30118, 30320
Rhizotomy ~ 63185-63190
Rho variant du ~ 86905
Rhytidectomy ~ 15824-15829
Rhytidoplasties ~ see face lift
Rh (D) ~ see blood typing
Rh immune globulin ~ see immune globulins, Rho (D)
Rib
cartilage, graft to face ~ 21230
excision ~ 21600-21616, 32900
fracture
closed treatment ~ 21800
external fixation ~ 21810
open treatment ~ 21805
resection ~ 19260-19272, 32900
X-ray ~ 71100-71111
Riboflavin ~ 84252
Richardson operation hysterectomy ~ see hysterectomy, abdominal, total
Richardson procedure ~ 53460
Rickettsia antibody ~ 86757
Ridell operation ~ see sinusotomy, frontal
Ridge, alveolar ~ see alveolar ridge
Right atrioventricular valve ~ see tricuspid valve
Right heart cardiac catheterization ~ see cardiac catheterization, right heart
Ripstein operation ~ see proctopexy
Risk factor reduction intervention ~ see performance measures, preventive medicine
Risser jacket ~ 29010-29015
removal ~ 29710
Rocky mountain spotted fever ~ 86000
Roentgenographic ~ see X-ray
Roentgenography ~ see radiology, diagnostic
Roentgen rays ~ see X-ray
Ropes test ~ 83872
Rorschach test ~ 96100
Ross procedure ~ 33413

Rotation flap ~ see skin, adjacent tissue transfer
Rotator cuff repair ~ 23410-23420
Rotavirus
antibody ~ 86759
antigen detection, enzyme immunoassay ~ 87425
Rotavirus vaccine ~ 90680
Round window repair fistula ~ 69667
Round window fistula ~ see fistula, round window
Roux-en-y procedure ~ 43621, 43633-43634, 43644, 43846, 47740-47741, 47780-47785, 48540
Rpr ~ 86592-86593
RSV (respiratory syncytial virus)
antibody ~ 86756
antigen detection
by immunofluorescence ~ 87280
by enzyme immunoassay ~ 87420
immune globulins ~ 90378, 90379
RT3 ~ see triiodothyronine, reverse
Rubbing alcohol ~ see isopropyl alcohol
Rubella
antibody ~ 86762
vaccine ~ 90706
Rubella/mumps ~ see vaccines
Rubella HI test ~ see hemagglutination inhibition test
Rubeola
antibody ~ 86765
antigen detection, immunofluorescence ~ 87283
Rubeolla ~ see rubeola
Russell viper venom time ~ 85612-85613

S

Sac, endolymphatic ~ see endolymphatic sac
Saccomanno technique ~ 88108
Sacral nerve
implantation, electrode ~ 64561, 64581
insertion, electrode ~ 64561, 64581
Sacroiliac joint
arthrodesis ~ 27280
arthrotomy ~ 27050
biopsy ~ 27050
dislocation, open treatment ~ 27218
fusion ~ 27280
injection for arthrography ~ 27096
X-ray ~ 72200-72202, 73542
Sacrum tumor, excision ~ 49215
X-ray ~ 72220
Sahli test ~ 91055
Salabrasion ~ 15810-15811
Salicylate assay ~ 80196
Saline-solution abortion ~ see abortion, induced, by saline
Salivary duct
catheterization ~ 42660
dilation ~ 42650-42660
ligation ~ 42665
repair ~ 42500-42505
fistula ~ 42600
Salivary gland virus ~ see Cytomegalovirus
Salivary glands
abscess, incision and drainage ~ 42310-42320
biopsy ~ 42405
calculi (stone), excision ~ 42330-42340
cyst
creation, fistula ~ 42325-42326
drainage ~ 42409
excision ~ 42408
injection, X-ray ~ 42550
needle biopsy ~ 42400
nuclear medicine
function study ~ 78232
imaging ~ 78230-78231
parotid, abscess ~ 42300-42305
unlisted services and procedures ~ 42699
X-ray ~ 70380-70390
with contrast ~ 70390
Salmonella antibody ~ 86768
Salpingectomy ~ 58262-58263, 58291-58292, 58552, 58554, 58661, 58700
ectopic pregnancy
laparoscopic treatment ~ 59151
surgical treatment ~ 59120
oophorectomy ~ 58943
Salpingo-oophorectomy ~ 58720
resection ovarian malignancy ~ 58950-58956
resection peritoneal malignancy ~ 58950-58956
resection tubal malignancy ~ 58950-58956
Salpingohysterostomy ~ see implantation, tubouterine
Salpingolysis ~ 58740
Salpingoneostomy ~ 58673, 58770
Salplingoplasty ~ see fallopian tube, repair
Salpingostomy ~ 58673, 58770
laparoscopic ~ 58673
Salter osteotomy of the pelvis ~ see osteotomy, pelvis
Sampling ~ see biopsy; brush biopsy; needle biopsy
Sang-Park procedure ~ 33735-33737
Sao Paulo typhus ~ see Rocky Mountain spotted fever
Saucerization
calcaneus ~ 28120
clavicle ~ 23180
femur ~ 27070, 27360
fibula ~ 27360, 27641
hip ~ 27070
humerus ~ 23184, 24140
ileum ~ 27070
metacarpal ~ 26230
metatarsal ~ 28122
olecranon process ~ 24147
phalanges, finger ~ 26235-26236

Saucerization ~ *continued*
toe ~ 28124
pubis ~ 27070
radius ~ 24145, 25151
scapula ~ 23182
talus ~ 28120
tarsal ~ 28122
tibia ~ 27360, 27640
ulna ~ 24147, 25150
Saundby test ~ see blood, feces
Scabies ~ see tissue, examination for ectoparasites
Scalenotomy ~ see muscle division, scalenus anticus
Scalenus anticus division ~ 21700-21705
Scaling ~ see exfoliation
Scalp tumor resection, radical ~ 21015
Scalp blood sampling ~ 59030
Scan ~ see specific site, nuclear medicine
abdomen ~ see abdomen, CT scan
CT ~ see CT scan
MRI ~ see magnetic resonance imaging
PET ~ see positron emission tomography
radionuclide ~ see emission computerized tomography
Scanning, radioisotope ~ see nuclear medicine
Scanogram ~ 77073
Scaphoid fracture
closed treatment ~ 25622
open treatment ~ 25628
with manipulation ~ 25624
Scapula
craterization ~ 23182
cyst excision ~ 23140
with allograft ~ 23146
with autograft ~ 23145
diaphysectomy ~ 23182
excision ~ 23172, 23190
partial ~ 23182
fracture
closed treatment
with manipulation ~ 23575
without manipulation ~ 23570
open treatment ~ 23585
ostectomy ~ 23190
repair
fixation ~ 23400
scapulopexy ~ 23400
saucerization ~ 23182
sequestrectomy ~ 23172
tumor
excision ~ 23140, 23210
with allograft ~ 23146
with autograft ~ 23145
radical resection ~ 23210
X-ray ~ 73010
Scapulopexy ~ 23400
Scarification pleural ~ 32215
Scarification of pleura ~ see pleurodesis
Schanz operation ~ see femur, osteotomy
Schauta operation ~ see hysterectomy, vaginal, radical
Schede procedure ~ 32905-32906
Scheie procedure ~ see iridectomy
Schilling test ~ see vitamin B-12 absorption study ~ 78270
Schlatter operation total gastrectomy ~ see excision, stomach, total
Schlicter test ~ (bactericidal titer, serum) 87197
Schocket procedure ~ (aqueous shunt) 66180
Schonbein test ~ see blood, feces
Schuchard procedure osteotomy, maxilla ~ 21206
Schwannoma, acoustic ~ see brain, tumor, excision
Sciatic nerve
decompression ~ 64712
injection, anesthetic ~ 64445-64446
lesion, excision ~ 64786
neuroma, excision ~ 64786
neuroplasty ~ 64712
release ~ 64712
repair/suture ~ 64858
Scintigraphy ~ see nuclear medicine
computed tomographic ~ see emission computerized tomography
Scissoring skin tags ~ 11200-11201
Sclera
excision, sclerectomy with punch or scissors ~ 66160
fistulization
iridencleisis or iridotasis ~ 66165
sclerectomy with punch or scissors with iridectomy ~ 66160
thermocauterization with iridectomy ~ 66155
trabeculectomy ab externo in absence of previous surgery ~ 66170
trephination with iridectomy ~ 66150
incision, fistulization
iridencleisis or iridotasis ~ 66165
sclerectomy with punch or scissors with iridectomy ~ 66160
thermocauterization with iridectomy ~ 66155
trabeculectomy ab externo in absence of previous surgery ~ 66170
trephination with iridectomy ~ 66150
lesion, excision ~ 66130
repair
reinforcement
with graft ~ 67255
without graft ~ 67250
staphyloma
with graft ~ 66225
without graft ~ 66220
with glue ~ 65286
wound
operative ~ 66250
tissue glue ~ 65286
Scleral buckling operation ~ see retina, repair, detachment
Scleral ectasia ~ see staphyloma, sclera
Sclerectomy ~ 66160
Sclerotherapy venous ~ 36468-36471
Sclerotomy ~ see incision, sclera

Screening, drug ~ see drug screen
Scribner cannulization ~ 36810
Scrotal varices ~ see varicocele
Scrotoplasty ~ 55175-55180
Scrotum
abscess, incision and drainage ~ 54700, 55100
excision ~ 55150
exploration ~ 55110
hematoma, incision and drainage ~ 54700
removal, foreign body ~ 55120
repair ~ 55175-55180
ultrasound ~ 76870
unlisted services and procedures ~ 55899
Scrub typhus ~ 86000
Second look surgery ~ see reoperation
Second opinion ~ see confirmatory consultations
Section ~ see also decompression
cesarean ~ see cesarean delivery
cranial nerve ~ 61460
spinal access ~ 63191
dentate ligament ~ 63180-63182
gasserian ganglion, sensory root ~ 61450
medullary tract ~ 61470
mesencephalic tract ~ 61480
nerve root ~ 63185-63190
spinal accessory nerve ~ 63191
spinal cord tract ~ 63194-63199
tentorium cerebelli ~ 61440
vestibular nerve
transcranial approach ~ 69950
translabyrinthine approach ~ 69915
Sedation with or without analgesia ~ 99141-99142
Seddon-Brookes procedure ~ 24320
Sedimentation rate
blood cell
automated ~ 85652
manual ~ 85651
Segmentectomy
breast ~ 19301-19302
lung ~ 32484
Seidlitz powder test ~ see X-ray, with contrast
Selective cellular enhancement technique ~ 88112
Selenium ~ 84255
Self care ~ see physical medicine/therapy/occupational therapy
training ~ 97535, 99509
Sella turcica
CT scan ~ 70480-70482
X-ray ~ 70240
Semen ~ see sperm
Semen analysis ~ 89300-89321
sperm analysis, antibodies ~ 89325
with sperm isolation ~ 89260-89261
Semenogelase ~ see antigen, prostate specific
Semicircular canal
incision
fenestration ~ 69820
revised ~ 69840
Semilunar bone ~ see lunate
ganglion ~ see gasserian ganglion
Seminal vesicle(s)
cyst, excision ~ 55680
excision ~ 55650
incision ~ 55600-55605
mullerian duct, excision ~ 55680
unlisted services and procedures ~ 55899
vesiculography ~ 74440
X-ray with contrast ~ 74440
Seminin ~ see antigen, prostate specific
Semiquantitative ~ 81005
Sengstaaken tamponade esophagus ~ 43460
Senning procedure ~ (repair/revision, great arteries) 33774-33777
Senning type ~ 33774-33777
Sensitivity study
antibiotic
agar ~ 87181
disc ~ 87184
enzyme detection ~ 87185
macrobroth ~ 87188
MIC (minimum inhibitory concentration) ~ 87186
microtiter ~ 87186
MLC (minimum lethal concentration) ~ 87187
mycobacteria ~ 87190
antiviral drugs, HIV-1, tissue culture ~ 87904
Sensor, fetal oximetry
cervix ~ 0021T
vagina ~ 0021T
Sensorimotor exam ~ 92060
Sensory nerve common, repair/suture ~ 64834
Sentinel node injection procedure ~ 38792
Separation, craniofacial
closed treatment ~ 21431
open treatment ~ 21432-21436
Septal defect
repair ~ 33813-33814
ventricular
closure ~ 33675-33688
open ~ 33675-33688
Septectomy
atrial ~ 33735-33737
balloon (Rashkind type) ~ 92992
blade method (Park) ~ 92993
closed ~ see septostomy, atrial
submucous nasal ~ see nasal septum, submucous resection
Septic abortion ~ see abortion, septic
Septoplasty ~ 30520
Septostomy, atrial ~ 33735-33737
balloon (Rashkind type) ~ 92992
blade method (Park) ~ 92993
Septum, nasal ~ see nasal septum
Sequestrectomy
carpal ~ 25145
clavicle ~ 23170
humeral head ~ 23174
humerus ~ 24134
olecranon process ~ 24138

Sequestrectomy ~ *continued*
radius ~ 24136, 25145
scapula ~ 23172
skull ~ 61501
ulna ~ 24138, 25145
Serialography aorta ~ 75625
Serodiagnosis, syphilis ~ see serologic test for syphilis
Serologic test for syphilis ~ 86592-86593
Seroma incision and drainage, skin ~ 10140
Serotonin ~ 84260
Serum
albumin ~ see albumin, serum
antibody identification, pretreatment ~ 86975-86978
CPK ~ see creatine kinase, total
serum immune globulin ~ 90281-90283
Sesamoid bone
excision ~ 28315
finger, excision ~ 26185
foot, fracture ~ 28530-28531
thumb, excision ~ 26185
Sesamoidectomy toe ~ 28315
Sever procedure ~ see contracture, palm, release
Severing of blepharorrhaphy ~ see tarsorrhaphy, severing
Sex change operation
female to male ~ 55980
male to female ~ 55970
Sex chromatin identification ~ 88130-88140
Sex hormone binding globulin ~ 84270
Sex-linked ichthyoses ~ see syphilis test
SGOT ~ 84450
SGPT ~ 84460
Shaving skin lesion ~ 11300-11313
SHBG (sex hormone binding globulin) ~ 84270
Shelf procedure ~ (see also osteotomy, hip) 27146-27151
Shiga-like toxin antigen detection, enzyme immunoassay ~ 87427
Shigella antibody ~ 86771
Shirodkar operation ~ (repair, cervix, cerclage, abdominal) 57700
Shock wave (extracorporeal) therapy ~ 0019T-0020T
Shock wave, lithotripsy ~ 50590
Shock wave, ultrasonic ~ see ultrasound
Shop typhus of Malaya ~ see Murine typhus
Shoulder ~ see also clavicle; scapula
abscess, drainage ~ 23030
amputation ~ 23900-23921
arthrocentesis ~ 20610
arthrodesis ~ 23800
with autogenous graft ~ 23802
arthrography, injection, radiologic ~ 23350
arthroscopy
diagnostic ~ 29805
surgical ~ 29806-29827
arthrotomy, with removal loose or foreign body ~ 23107

Shoulder ~ *continued*
biopsy
deep ~ 23066
soft tissue ~ 23065
blade ~ see scapula
bone
excision
acromion ~ 23130
clavicle ~ 23120-23125
incision ~ 23035
tumor, excision ~ 23140-23146
bursa, drainage ~ 23031
capsular contracture release ~ 23020
cast
figure eight ~ 29049
removal ~ 29710
spica ~ 29055
velpeau ~ 29058
disarticulation ~ 23920-23921
dislocation, closed treatment, with manipulation ~ 23650-23655
exploration ~ 23107
hematoma, drainage ~ 23030
manipulation, application of fixation apparatus ~ 23700
prophylactic treatment ~ 23490-23491
radical resection ~ 23077
removal
calcareous deposits ~ 23000
cast ~ 29710
foreign body
complicated ~ 23332
deep ~ 23331
subcutaneous ~ 23330
foreign or loose body ~ 23107
repair
capsule ~ 23450-23466
ligament release ~ 23415
muscle transfer ~ 23395-23397
rotator cuff ~ 23410-23420
tendon ~ 23410-23412, 23430-23440
tenomyotomy ~ 23405-23406
strapping ~ 29240
surgery, unlisted services and procedures ~ 23929
tumor, excision ~ 23075-23077
unlisted services and procedures ~ 23929
X-ray ~ 73020-73030
X-ray with contrast ~ 73040
Shoulder joint ~ see also clavicle; scapula
arthroplasty, with implant ~ 23470-23472
arthrotomy
with biopsy ~ 23100-23101
with synovectomy ~ 23105-23106
dislocation
with greater tuberosity fracture
closed treatment ~ 23665
open treatment ~ 23670
open treatment ~ 23660
with surgical or anatomical neck fracture
closed treatment with manipulation ~ 23675

Shoulder joint ~ *continued*
dislocation ~ *continued*
open treatment ~ 23680
excision, torn cartilage ~ 23101
exploration ~ 23040-23044
incision and drainage ~ 23040-23044
removal, foreign body ~ 23040-23044
X-ray ~ 73050
Shunt(s)
aqueous
to extraocular reservoir ~ 66180
revision ~ 66185
arteriovenous ~ see arteriovenous shunt
brain
creation ~ 62180-62223
removal ~ 62256-62258
replacement ~ 62160, 62194, 62225-62230, 62258
reprogramming ~ 62252
cerebrospinal fluid ~ see cerebrospinal fluid shunt
creation
arteriovenous
direct ~ 36821
ECMO ~ 36822
Thomas shunt ~ 36835
transposition ~ 36818-36820
with bypass graft ~ 35686
with graft ~ 36825-36830
cerebrospinal fluid ~ 62200
Thomas shunt ~ 36835
fetal ~ 59076
great vessel
aorta to pulmonary artery, ascending ~ 33755
descending ~ 33762
central ~ 33764
subclavian pulmonary artery ~ 33750
systemic to pulmonary ~ 33924
vena cava to pulmonary artery ~ 33766-33767
intra-atrial ~ 33735-33737
Levenn
insertion ~ 49425
patency test ~ 78291
revision ~ 49426
nonvascular, X-ray ~ 75809
peritoneal, venous
injection ~ 49427
ligation ~ 49428
removal ~ 49429
peritoneal X-ray ~ 75809
pulmonary artery
from aorta ~ 33755-33762, 33924
subclavian ~ 33750
from vena cava ~ 33766-33767
revision, arteriovenous ~ 36832
spinal cord
creation ~ 63740-63741
irrigation ~ 63744
removal ~ 63746
replacement ~ 63744
Shunt ~ *continued*
superior mesenteric-caval ~ see anastomosis, caval to mesenteric
ureter to colon ~ 50815
ventriculocisternal with valve ~ (ventriculocisternostomy) 62180, 62200, 62201
Shuntogram ~ 75809
Sialic acid ~ 84275
Sialodochoplasty ~ 42500-42505
Sialogram ~ see sialography
Sialography ~ 70390
Sickling electrophoresis ~ 83020
Siderocytes ~ 85536
Siderophilin ~ see transferrin
Sigmoid ~ see colon-sigmoid
Sigmoid bladder cystectomy ~ 51590
Sigmoidoscopy
ablation
polyp ~ 45339
tumor ~ 45339
biopsy ~ 45331
collection, specimen ~ 45331
exploration ~ 45330, 45335
hemorrhage control ~ 45334
injection, submucosal ~ 45335
needle biopsy ~ 45342
placement, stent ~ 45345
removal
foreign body ~ 45332
polyp ~ 45333, 45338
tumor ~ 45333, 45338
repair, volvulus ~ 45337
ultrasound ~ 45341-45342
Signal-averaged electrocardiography ~ see electrocardiogram
Silica ~ 84285
Silicon dioxide ~ see silica
Silicone contouring injections ~ 11950-11954
Silver operation ~ see Keller procedure
Silver procedure ~ 28290
Simple mastectomies ~ see mastectomy
Single photon absorptiometry ~ see absorptiometry, single photon
Single photon emission computed tomography (SPECT) ~ see also emission computed tomography
abscess localization ~ 78807
bone ~ 78320
cerebrospinal fluid ~ 78647
heart
multiple ~ 78465
single ~ 78464
kidney ~ 78710
liver ~ 78205
tumor localization ~ 78803
Sinus
ethmoidectomy, excision ~ 31254
pilonidal ~ see cyst, pilonidal
Sinus of valsalva repair ~ 33702-33722
Sinus venosus repair ~ 33645
Sinusectomy, ethmoid ~ see ethmoidectomy

Sinuses
ethmoid
excision ~ 31200-31205
with nasal/sinus endoscopy ~ 31254-31255
repair of cerebrospinal leak ~ 31290
frontal
destruction ~ 31080-31085
exploration ~ 31070-31075
with nasal/sinus endoscopy ~ 31276
fracture, open treatment ~ 21343-21344
incision ~ 31070-31087
injection ~ 20500
diagnostic ~ 20501
maxillary
antrostomy ~ 31256-31267
excision ~ 31225-31230
exploration ~ 31020-31032
with nasal/sinus endoscopy ~ 31233
incision ~ 31020-31032, 31256-31267
irrigation ~ 31000
skull base ~ 61581
surgery ~ 61581
multiple
incision ~ 31090
paranasal, incision ~ 31090
sphenoid
biopsy ~ 31050-31051
exploration ~ 31050-31051
with nasal/sinus endoscopy ~ 31235
incision ~ 31050-31051
with nasal/sinus endoscopy ~ 31287-31288
irrigation ~ 31002
repair of cerebrospinal leak ~ 31291
sinusotomy ~ 31050-31051
skull base surgery ~ 61580-61581
unlisted services and procedures ~ 31299
X-ray ~ 70210-70220
Sinusoidal rotational testing ~ see ear, nose and throat
Sinusoscopy
maxillary sinus ~ 31233
sphenoid sinus ~ 31235
Sinusotomy ~ see also sinus, multiple
combined ~ 31090
frontal sinus
exploratory ~ 31070-31075
nonobliterative ~ 31086-31087
obliterative ~ 31080-31085
maxillary ~ 31020-31032
multiple, paranasal ~ 31090
sphenoid sinus ~ 31050-31051
Sisi test ~ 92564
Sistrunk operation ~ see cyst, thyroid gland, excision
Size reduction, breast ~ see breast, reduction
Skeletal fixation humeral epicondyle, percutaneous ~ 24566
Skeletal traction, insertion/removal pin/wire ~ 20650
Skene's gland abscess
destruction ~ 53270
excision ~ 53270
incision and drainage ~ 53060
Skilled nursing facilities (SNF) services
initial care ~ 99304-99306
discharge services ~ 99315-99316
other services ~ 99318
subsequent care ~ 99307-99310
Skin
abrasion ~ 15786-15787
chemical peel ~ 15788-15793
dermabrasion ~ 15780-15783
salabrasion ~ 15810-15811
abscess ~ see abscess, skin
adjacent tissue transfer ~ 14000-14350
allografts ~ see allograft, skin
biopsy ~ 11100-11101
chemical exfoliation ~ 17360
cyst ~ see cyst, skin
debridement ~ 11000-11006, 11010-11044
eczematous ~ 11000-11001
full thickness ~ 11041
infected ~ 11000-11006
partial thickness ~ 11040
subcutaneous tissue ~ 11042-11044
infected ~ 11004-11006
with open fracture and/or dislocation ~ 11010-11012
decubitus ulcer(s) ~ see pressure ulcer (decubitus)
desquamation ~ see exfoliation
destruction
benign lesions
fifteen or more lesions ~ 17004
first lesion ~ 17000
two-fourteen lesions ~ 17003
flat warts ~ 17110-17111
lesions ~ 17106-17108
malignant lesions ~ 17260-17286
by photodynamic therapy ~ 96567
premalignant lesions
by photodynamic therapy ~ 96567
fifteen or more lesions ~ 17004
first lesion ~ 17000
two-fourteen lesions ~ 17003
excision
debridement ~ 11000-11006, 11010-11044
excess skin ~ 15830-15839, 15847
hemangioma ~ 11400-11446
lesion
benign ~ 11400-11446
malignant ~ 11600-11646
expanders ~ see tissue, expander
fasciocutaneous flaps ~ 15732-15738
grafts, free ~ 15050-15321, 15340-15366, 15420-15431, 15757
homografts ~ see homograft, skin
incision and drainage ~ see incision, skin ~ 10040-10180
lesion ~ see lesion; tumor
verrucous ~ see warts

Skin ~ *continued*
muscle flaps ~ 15732-15738
myocutaneous flaps ~ 15732-15738
nose, surgical planing ~ 30120
paring ~ 11055-11057
photography, diagnostic ~ 96904
removal, skin tags ~ 11200-11201
revision
blepharoplasty ~ 15820-15823
cervicoplasty ~ 15819
rhytidectomy ~ 15824-15829
shaving ~ 11300-11313
tags, removal ~ 11200-11201
tests ~ see allergy tests
candida ~ 86485
coccidioidomycosis ~ 86490
histoplasmosis ~ 86510
other antigen ~ 86586
tuberculosis ~ 86580-86585
unlisted services and procedures ~ 17999
wound repair
complex ~ 13100-13160
intermediate ~ 12031-12057
simple ~ 12001-12021
Skin graft and flap
allograft ~ 15350-15351
composite graft ~ 15760-15770
cross finger flap ~ 15574
delay ~ 15600-15630
delay of flap ~ 15600-15630
derma-fat-fascia ~ 15570
fascial, free ~ 15758
fasciocutaneous ~ 15732-15738
formation ~ 15570-15576
free, microvascular anastomosis ~ 15756-15758
free skin graft, full thickness ~ 15200-15261
island pedicle flap ~ 15740
muscle ~ 15732-15738, 15842
free ~ 15756
myocutaneous ~ 15732-15738, 15756
pedicle flap
formation ~ 15570-15576
island ~ 15740
neurovascular ~ 15750
transfer ~ 15650
pinch graft ~ 15050
platysmal ~ 15825
punch graft ~ 15775-15776
punch graft for hair transplant ~ 15775-15776
recipient site preparation ~ 15002-15005
skin, free ~ 15757
split graft ~ 15100-15121
superficial musculoaponeurotic system ~ 15829
tissue transfer ~ 14000-14350
tissue-cultured ~ 15100-15121, 15342-15343
transfer ~ 15650
vascular flow check ~ 15860
xenograft ~ 15400-15401
Skull
burr hole
biopsy brain ~ 61140
drainage
abscess ~ 61150-61151
cyst ~ 61150-61151
hematoma ~ 61154-61156
exploration
infratentorial ~ 61253
supratentorial ~ 61250
insertion
catheter ~ 61210
EEG electrode ~ 61210
reservoir ~ 61210
intracranial, biopsy ~ 61140
with injection ~ 61120
decompression ~ 61322-61323, 61340-61345
orbit ~ 61330
drill hole
catheter ~ 61107
drainage hematoma ~ 61108
exploration ~ 61105
excision ~ 61501
exploration, drill hole ~ 61105
fracture ~ 62000-62010
ematoma, drainage ~ 61108
incision, suture ~ 61550-61552
insertion, catheter ~ 61107
lesion, excision ~ 61500, 61600-61608, 61615-61616
orbit
biopsy ~ 61332
excision, lesion ~ 61333
exploration ~ 61332-61334
removal foreign body ~ 61334
puncture
cervical ~ 61050
cisternal ~ 61050
drain fluid ~ 61070
injection ~ 61070
subdural ~ 61000-61001
ventricular fluid ~ 61020
reconstruction ~ 21172-21180
defect ~ 62140-62141, 62145
reduction, craniomegalic ~ 62115-62117
removal
plate ~ 62142
prosthesis ~ 62142
repair
cerebrospinal fluid leak ~ 62100
encephalocele ~ 62120
replacement
plate ~ 62143
prosthesis ~ 62143
tumor, excision ~ 61500
X-ray ~ 70250-70260
Skull base surgery
anterior cranial fossa
bicoronal approach ~ 61586
craniofacial approach ~ 61580-61583
extradural ~ 61600-61601

Skull base surgery ~ *continued*
Lefort 1 osteotomy approach ~ 61586
orbitocranial approach ~ 61584-61585
transzygomatic approach ~ 61586
carotid aneurysm ~ 61613
carotid artery ~ 61610
transection/ligation ~ 61609-61612
craniotomy ~ 62121
dura, repair of cerebrospinal fluid leak ~ 61618-61619
middle cranial fossa
extradural ~ 61605, 61607
infratemporal approach ~ 61590-61591
intradural ~ 61606, 61608
orbitocranial zygomatic approach ~ 61592
posterior cranial fossa
extradural ~ 61615
intradural ~ 61616
transcondylar approach ~ 61596-61597
transpetrosal approach ~ 61598
transtemporal approach ~ 61595
Sleep study ~ 95806-95807
Sliding inlay graft, tibia ~ see ankle; tibia, repair
Sling operation
incontinence ~ 53440
removal ~ 53442
stress incontinence ~ 51992, 57287
vagina ~ 57287-57288
Small bowel ~ see intestines, small
neoplasm ~ see tumor, intestines, small
Smas flap ~ 15829
Smear cervical ~ see cervical smears
Papanicolaou ~ see Pap smears
Smear and stain ~ see also cytopathology, smears
cornea ~ 65430
fluorescent ~ 87206
gram or giesma ~ 87205
ova, parasites ~ 87177
parasites ~ 87207
wet mount ~ 87210
Smith fracture ~ 25600-25605
Smith-Robinson operation ~ see arthrodesis, vertebra
Smithwick operation ~ see excision, nerve, sympathetic
SO4 ~ see sulfate
Soave procedure ~ 45120
Sodium ~ 84295, 84302
urine ~ 84300
Sodium glycinate, theophylline ~ see theophylline
Sofield procedure ~ 24410
Soft tissue ~ see tissue, soft
Solar plexus ~ see celiac plexus
Solitary cyst ~ see bone, cyst
Somatomammotropin, chorionic ~ 83632
Somatomedin ~ 84305
Somatosensory testing
lower limbs ~ 95926
trunk or head ~ 95927
upper limbs ~ 95925
Somatostatin ~ 84307
Somatotropin ~ 83003
Somatotropin release inhibiting hormone ~ see somatostatin
Somatropin ~ see growth hormone, human
Somnographies ~ see polysomnography
Somophyllin T ~ see theophylline
Sonography ~ see echography
Sonohysterography ~ 76831
saline infusion, injection procedure ~ 58340
Sore, bed ~ see pressure ulcer (decubitus)
Spasm eyelid ~ see blepharospasm
Special services, procedures and reports ~ 99000-99091
after hours medical services ~ 99050-99054
analysis, remote physiologic data ~ 99091
computer data analysis ~ 99090
device handling ~ 99002
emergency care in office ~ 99058
group education ~ 99078
hyperbaric oxygen ~ 99183
hypothermia ~ 99185-99186
medical testimony ~ 99075
non-office medical services ~ 99056
on call services ~ 99026-99027
phlebotomy ~ 99199
post-op visit ~ 99024
pump services ~ 99190-99192
reports and forms
medical, extended ~ 99080
psychiatric ~ 90889
specimen handling ~ 99000-99001
supply of materials ~ 99070
educational ~ 99071
unlisted services and procedures ~ 99199
unusual travel ~ 99082
Specific gravity body fluid ~ 84315
Specimen collection
intestines ~ 89100-89105
stomach ~ 89130-89141
Specimen concentration ~ 87015
Specimen handling ~ 99000-99001
SPECT ~ see also emission computerized tomography ~ 78607
abscess localization ~ 78807
bone ~ 78320
cerebrospinal fluid ~ 78647
heart
multiple ~ 78465
single ~ 78464
kidney ~ 78710
liver ~ 78205
tumor localization ~ 78803
Spectacle services
fitting
low vision aid ~ 92354-92355
spectacle prosthesis ~ 92352-92353
spectacles ~ 92340-92342

Spectacle services ~ *continued*
repair ~ 92370-92371
supply
low vision aids ~ 92392
spectacle prosthesis ~ 92395
spectacles ~ 92390
Spectrometry, mass
analyte
qualitative ~ 83788
quantitative ~ 83789
Spectrophotometry ~ 84311
atomic absorption ~ see atomic absorption spectroscopy
Spectroscopy
atomic absorption ~ 82190
expired breath analysis ~ 0064T
magnetic resonance ~ 76390
Spectrum analyses ~ see spectrophotometry
Speculoscopy ~ 0031T
with direct sampling ~ 0032T
Speech evaluation ~ 92506
cine ~ 70371
for prosthesis ~ 92597, 92607-92608
video ~ 70371
Speech prosthesis ~ 21084, 92609
creation ~ 31611
evaluation for speech ~ 92597, 92607-92608
insertion ~ 31611
Speech therapy ~ 92507-92508
Sperm
cryopreservation ~ 89259
storage ~ 89343
thawing ~ 89353
washing ~ 58323
Sperm analysis
antibodies ~ 89325
cervical mucus penetration test ~ 89330
cryopreservation ~ 89259
hamster penetration test ~ 89329
hyaluron binding assay ~ 0087T
identification, aspiration ~ 89257
from testis tissue ~ 89264
isolation ~ 89260-89261
Sperm evaluation, cervical mucus penetration test ~ see Huhner test
Spermatic cord
hydrocele, excision ~ 55500
laparoscopy ~ 55559
lesion, excision ~ 55520
repair, veins ~ 55530-55540
abdominal approach ~ 55535
with hernia repair ~ 55540
varicocele, excision ~ 55530-55540
Spermatic veins
excision ~ 55530-55540
ligation ~ 55550
Spermatocele excision ~ 54840
Spermatocystectomy ~ (spermatocele excision) 54840
Sphenoid sinus ~ see sinuses, sphenoid
Sphenoidotomy excision, with nasal/sinus endoscopy ~ 31287-31288
Sphenopalatine ganglion injection, anesthetic ~ 64505
Sphincter ~ see specific sphincter
anal ~ see anal sphincter
artificial genitourinary ~ see prosthesis, urethral sphincter
pyloric ~ see pyloric sphincter
Sphincter of Oddi pressure measurement, endoscopy ~ 43263
Sphincteroplasty
anal ~ 46750-46751, 46760-46761
with implant ~ 46762
bile duct ~ 47460
bladder neck ~ see bladder, repair, neck
Sphincterotomy ~ 52277
anal ~ 46080
bile duct ~ 47460
Spica cast
hip ~ 29305-29325
repair ~ 29720
shoulder ~ 29055
Spinal accessory nerve
anastomosis to facial nerve ~ 64866
incision ~ 63191
injection, anesthetic ~ 64412
section ~ 63191
Spinal column ~ see spine
Spinal cord ~ see also cauda equina; nerve root
biopsy ~ 63275-63290
cyst
aspiration ~ 62268
incision and drainage ~ 63172-63173
decompression ~ 63001-63103
with cervical laminoplasty ~ 63050-63051
drain fluid ~ 62272
exploration ~ 63001-63044
graft, dura ~ 63710
implantation
electrode ~ 63650-63655
pulse generator ~ 63685
receiver ~ 63685
incision ~ 63200
dentate ligament ~ 63180-63182
tract ~ 63170, 63194-63199
injection
anesthetic ~ 62310-62319
blood ~ 62273
CT scan ~ 62284
neurolytic agent ~ 62280-62282
other ~ 62310-62311
X-ray ~ 62284
insertion
electrode ~ 63650-63655
pulse generator ~ 63685
receiver ~ 63685
lesion
destruction ~ 62280-62282
excision ~ 63265-63273, 63300-63308
needle biopsy ~ 62269
neoplasm, excision ~ 63275-63290

Spinal cord ~ *continued*
puncture (tap) ~ *continued*
diagnostic ~ 62270
drain fluid ~ 62272
lumbar ~ 62270
release ~ 63200
reconstruction, dorsal spine elements ~ 63295
removal
catheter ~ 62355
electrode ~ 63660
pulse generator ~ 63688
pump ~ 62365
receiver ~ 63688
reservoir ~ 62365
repair
cerebrospinal fluid leak ~ 63707-63709
meningocele ~ 63700-63702
myelomeningocele ~ 63704-63706
section
dentate ligament ~ 63180-63182
tract ~ 63194-63199
shunt
create ~ 63740-63741
irrigation ~ 63744
removal ~ 63746
replacement ~ 63744
stereotaxis
aspiration ~ 63615
biopsy ~ 63615
creation lesion ~ 63600
excision lesion ~ 63615
stimulation ~ 63610
syrinx, aspiration ~ 62268
tumor, excision ~ 63275-63290
Spinal fluid ~ see cerebrospinal fluid
Spinal fracture ~ see fracture, vertebra
Spinal instrumentation
anterior ~ 22845-22847
removal ~ 22855
internal fixation ~ 22841
pelvic fixation ~ 22848
posterior nonsegmental, Harrington rod technique ~ 22840
removal ~ 22850
posterior segmental ~ 22842-22844
removal ~ 22852
prosthetic device ~ 22851
reinsertion of spinal fixation device ~ 22849
Spinal manipulation ~ see manipulation, chiropractic
Spinal nerve
avulsion ~ 64772
transection ~ 64772
Spinal tap ~ see cervical puncture; cisternal puncture; subdural tap; ventricular puncture
drainage fluid ~ 62272
lumbar ~ 62270
Spine ~ see also spinal cord; vertebra; vertebral body; vertebral process
allograft
morselized ~ 20930
structural ~ 20931
Spine ~ *continued*
autograft
local ~ 20936
morselized ~ 20937
structural ~ 20938
biopsy ~ 20250-20251
chemotherapy administration ~ (see also chemotherapy) 96450
CT scan
cervical ~ 72125-72127
lumbar ~ 72131-72133
thoracic ~ 72128-72130
fixation ~ 22842
fusion
anterior ~ 22808-22812
anterior approach ~ 22548-22585, 22812
exploration ~ 22830
lateral extracavitary ~ 22532-22534
posterior approach ~ 22590-22802
insertion, instrumentation ~ 22840-22848, 22851
kyphectomy ~ 22818-22819
magnetic resonance angiography ~ 72159
magnetic resonance imaging
cervical ~ 72141-72142, 72156-72158
lumbar ~ 72148-72158
thoracic ~ 72146-72147, 72156-72158
manipulation, with anesthesia ~ 22505
myelography
cervical ~ 72240
lumbosacral ~ 72265
thoracic ~ 72255
total ~ 72270
reconstruction, dorsal spine elements ~ 63295
reinsertion, instrumentation ~ 22849
removal, instrumentation ~ 22850, 22852-22855
repair, osteotomy
anterior ~ 22220-22226
posterior ~ 22210-22214
cervical laminoplasty ~ 63050-63051
posterolateral ~ 22216
ultrasound ~ 76800
unlisted services and procedures, surgery ~ 22899
X-ray ~ 72020, 72090
absorptiometry ~ 77080-77082
cervical ~ 72040-72052
lumbosacral ~ 72100-72120
standing ~ 72069
thoracic ~ 72070-72074
thoracolumbar ~ 72080
total ~ 72010
with contrast
cervical ~ 72240
lumbosacral ~ 72265
thoracic ~ 72255
total ~ 72270
Spirometry ~ (see also pulmonology, diagnostic) 94010-94070
patient initiated ~ 94014-94016

Splanchnicectomy ~ see nerves, sympathectomy, excision
Spleen
excision ~ 38100-38102
laparoscopic ~ 38120
injection, radiologic ~ 38200
nuclear medicine, imaging ~ 78185, 78215-78216
repair ~ 38115
Splenectomy
laparoscopic ~ 38120
partial ~ 38101
partial with repair, ruptured spleen ~ 38115
total ~ 38100
en bloc ~ 38102
Splenoplasty ~ see repair, spleen
Splenoportography ~ 75810
injection procedures ~ 38200
Splenorrhaphy ~ 38115
Splint ~ see casting; strapping
arm
long ~ 29105
short ~ 29125-29126
finger ~ 29130-29131
foot ~ 29590
leg
long ~ 29505
short ~ 29515
oral surgical ~ 21085
ureteral ~ see ureteral splinting
Split grafts ~ 15100-15121
Split renal function test ~ see cystourethroscopy, catheterization, ureteral
Splitting blood products ~ 86985
Spontaneous abortion ~ see abortion
Sprengel's deformity ~ 23400
Spring water cyst ~ see cyst, pericardial
Spur, bone ~ see exostosis
calcaneal ~ see heel spur
Sputum analysis ~ 89220
SRH ~ (somatostatin) 84307
Ssabanejew-Frank operation ~ (incision, stomach, creation, stoma) 43830-43832
Stabilizing factor, fibrin ~ see fibrin stabilizing factor
Stable factor ~ 85230
Stallard procedure ~ see conjunctivorhinostomy
Stamey procedure ~ (repair, bladder, neck) 51845
Standby services physician ~ 99360
Stanford-Binet test ~ see psychiatric diagnosis
Stanftan ~ (Binet test) 96101-96103
Stapedectomy
revision ~ 69662
with footplate drill out ~ 69661
without foreign material ~ 69660
Stapedotomy
revision ~ 69662
with footplate drill out ~ 69661
without foreign material ~ 69660
Stapes
excision
with footplate drill out ~ 69661
without foreign material ~ 69660
mobilization ~ see mobilization, stapes
release ~ 69650
revision ~ 69662
Staphyloma
sclera repair
with graft ~ 66225
without graft ~ 66220
Starch granules feces ~ 89225
State operation ~ see proctectomy
Statin therapy ~ see performance measures
Statistics/biometry ~ see biometry
Steindler stripping ~ 28250
Stellate ganglion injection, anesthetic ~ 64510
Stem cell
concentration ~ 38215
count ~ 86587
cryopreservation ~ 38207, 88240
donor search ~ 38204
harvesting ~ 38205-38206
limbal, allograft ~ 65781
plasma depletion ~ 38214
platelet depletion ~ 38213
red blood cell depletion ~ 38212
T-cell depletion ~ 38210
thawing ~ 38208-38209, 88241
transplantation ~ 38240-38242
tumor cell depletion ~ 38211
washing ~ 38209
Stem, brain ~ see brainstem
Stenger test ~ (audiologic function test; ear, nose and throat) 92565, 92577
Stenosis
aortic ~ see aortic stenosis
bronchi ~ 31641
reconstruction ~ 31775
excision, trachea ~ 31780-31781
laryngoplasty ~ 31582
reconstruction, auditory canal, external ~ 69310
repair, trachea ~ 31780-31781
tracheal ~ see trachea stenosis
urethral ~ see urethral stenosis
Stensen duct ~ see parotid duct
Stent
indwelling
insertion, ureter ~ 50605
placement
bronchoscopy ~ 31631, 31636-31637
colonoscopy ~ 45387
via stoma ~ 44397
endoscopy, gastrointestinal, upper ~ 43256
enteroscopy ~ 44370
proctosigmoidoscopy ~ 45327
sigmoidoscopy ~ 45345
transcatheter, intravascular ~ 37205-37208, 37215, 37216
extracranial ~ 0075T-0076T
ureteroneocystomy ~ 50947-50948

Stent ~ *continued*
revision, bronchoscopy ~ 31638
urethra ~ 52282
prostatic ~ 0084T
Stent, intravascular ~ see transcatheter, placement, intravascular stents
Stents, tracheal ~ see tracheal stent
Stereotactic frame application/removal ~ 20660
Stereotaxis
aspiration
brain lesion ~ 61750
with CT scan and/or MRI ~ 61751
spinal cord ~ 63615
biopsy
aspiration, brain lesion ~ 61750
brain ~ 61750
with CT scan and/or MRI ~ 61751
breast ~ 77031
spinal cord ~ 63615
computer assisted
brain surgery ~ 61795
orthopedic surgery ~ 0054T-0056T
creation lesion
brain
deep ~ 61720-61735
percutaneous ~ 61790
gasserian ganglion ~ 61790
spinal cord ~ 63600
trigeminal tract ~ 61791
CT scan
aspiration ~ 61751
biopsy ~ 61751
excision lesion
brain ~ 61750
spinal cord ~ 63615
focus beam, radiosurgery ~ 61793
localization, brain ~ 61770
radiation therapy ~ 77421, 77432-77435
stimulation, spinal cord ~ 63610
Sterile coverings ~ see dressings
Sternal fracture ~ see fracture, sternum
Sternoclavicular joint
arthrotomy ~ 23044
with biopsy ~ 23101
with synovectomy ~ 23106
dislocation
closed treatment
with manipulation ~ 23525
without manipulation ~ 23520
open treatment ~ 23530-23532
with fascial graft ~ 23532
Sternocleidomastoid division ~ 21720-21725
Sternotomy closure ~ 21750
Sternum
debridement ~ 21627
excision ~ 21620, 21630-21632
fracture
closed treatment ~ 21820
open treatment ~ 21825
ostectomy ~ 21620
radical resection ~ 21630-21632

Sternum ~ *continued*
reconstruction ~ 21740-21742, 21750
with thoracoscopy ~ 21743
X-ray ~ 71120-71130
Steroid-binding protein, sex ~ see globulin, sex hormone binding
Steroids
anabolic ~ see androstenedione
injection, urethral stricture ~ 52283
ketogenic, urine ~ 83582
STH (somatotropic hormone) ~ see growth hormone
Stimulating antibody, thyroid ~ see immunoglobulin, thyroid stimulating
Stimulation
electric ~ see electrical stimulation
lymphocyte ~ see blastogenesis
spinal cord, stereotaxis ~ 63610
transcutaneous electric ~ see application, neurostimulation
Stimulator, long-acting thyroid ~ see thyrotropin releasing hormone (TRH)
Stimulators, cardiac ~ see heart, pacemaker
Stimulus evoked response ~ 51792
Stoffel operation ~ (rhizotomy) 63185, 63190
Stoma
creation
bladder ~ 51980
kidney ~ 50551-50561
stomach
neonatal ~ 43831
temporary ~ 43830-43831
ureter ~ 50860
ureter, endoscopy via ~ 50951-50961
Stomach
anastomosis
with duodenum ~ 43810, 43850-43855
with jejunum ~ 43820-43825, 43860-43865
biopsy ~ 43600-43605
creation
stoma
temporary ~ 43830-43831
laparoscopic ~ 43653
electrogastrography ~ 91132-91133
excision
partial ~ 43631-43639, 43845
total ~ 43620-43622
exploration ~ 43500
gastric bypass ~ 43644-43645, 43846
revision ~ 43848
incision ~ 43830-43832
exploration ~ 43500
pyloric sphincter ~ 43520
removal, foreign body ~ 43500
intubation with specimen prep ~ 91055
nuclear medicine
blood loss study ~ 78278
emptying study ~ 78264
imaging ~ 78261
protein loss study ~ 78282
reflux study ~ 78262
vitamin B-12 absorption ~ 78270-78272

Stomach ~ *continued*
reconstruction
for obesity ~ 43644-43645, 43842-43847
Roux-en-Y ~ 43644, 43846
removal, foreign body ~ 43500
repair ~ 48547
fistula ~ 43880
fundoplasty ~ 43324-43325
laparoscopic ~ 43280
laceration ~ 43501-43502
stoma ~ 43870
ulcer ~ 43501
specimen collection ~ 89130-89141
stimulation of secretion ~ 91052
suture
fistula ~ 43880
for obesity ~ 43842-43843
stoma ~ 43870
ulcer ~ 43840
wound ~ 43840
tumor, excision ~ 43610-43611
ulcer, excision ~ 43610
unlisted services and procedures ~ 43659, 43999
Stomatoplasty ~ see mouth, repair
Stone, kidney ~ see calculus, removal, kidney
Stookey-Scarff procedure ~ (ventriculocisternostomy) 62200
Stool blood ~ see blood, feces
Storage
embryo ~ 89342
oocyte ~ 89346
reproductive tissue ~ 89344
sperm ~ 89343
Strabismus
chemodenervation ~ 67345
repair
adjustable sutures ~ 67335
extraocular muscles ~ 67340
one horizontal muscle ~ 67311
one vertical muscle ~ 67314
posterior fixation suture technique ~ 67334-67335
previous surgery, not involving extraocular muscles ~ 67331
release extensive scar tissue ~ 67343
superior oblique muscle ~ 67318
transposition ~ 67320
two horizontal muscles ~ 67312
two or more vertical muscles ~ 67316
Strapping ~ see cast; splint
ankle ~ 29540
back ~ 29220
chest ~ 29200
elbow ~ 29260
finger ~ 29280
foot ~ 29540, 29590
hand ~ 29280
hip ~ 29520
knee ~ 29530
shoulder ~ 29240
Strapping ~ *continued*
thorax ~ 29200
toes ~ 29550
unlisted services and procedures ~ 29799
Unna boot ~ 29580
wrist ~ 29260
Strassman procedure ~ 58540
Strayer procedure leg, lower ~ 27687
Streptococcus pneumoniae vaccine ~ see vaccines
Streptococcus
group A
antigen detection
enzyme immunoassay ~ 87430
nucleic acid ~ 87650-87652
direct optical observation ~ 87880
group B
antigen detection, immunoassay with direct optical observation ~ 87802
Streptokinase, antibody ~ 86590
Stress tests
cardiovascular ~ 93015-93024
multiple gated acquisition (MUGA) ~ 78472-78473
myocardial perfusion imaging ~ 78460-78465
pulmonary ~ see pulmonology, diagnostic ~ 94620-94621
Stricture repair, urethra ~ 53400-53405
Stricturoplasty intestines ~ 44615
Stroboscopy larynx ~ 31579
STS ~ (syphilis test) 86592-86593
Stuart-Prower factor ~ 85260
Study, color vision ~ see color vision examination
Sturmdorf procedure ~ 57520
Styloid process radial, excision ~ 25230
Styloidectomy radial ~ 25230
Stypven time ~ see Russell viper venom time
Subacromial bursa arthrocentesis ~ 20610
Subclavian arteries ~ see artery, subclavian
Subcutaneous injection ~ see injection, subcutaneous
Subcutaneous mastectomies ~ see mastectomy, subcutaneous
Subcutaneous tissue excision ~ 15830-15839, 15847
Subdiaphragmatic abscess ~ see abscess, subdiaphragmatic
Subdural electrode
insertion ~ 61531-61533
removal ~ 61535
Subdural hematoma ~ see hematoma, subdural
Subdural puncture ~ 61105-61108
Subdural tap ~ 61000-61001
Sublingual gland
abscess, incision and drainage ~ 42310-42320
calculi (stone), excision ~ 42330
cyst
drainage ~ 42409
excision ~ 42408
excision ~ 42450
Subluxation elbow ~ 24640

Submandibular gland
calculi (stone), excision ~ 42330-42335
excision ~ 42440
Submaxillary gland abscess, incision and drainage ~ 42310-42320
Submucous resection of nasal septum ~ see nasal septum, submucous resection
Subperiosteal implant reconstruction
mandible ~ 21245-21246
maxilla ~ 21245-21246
Subphrenic abscess ~ see abscess, subdiaphragmatic
Substance S, Reichstein's ~ see deoxycortisol
Subtrochanteric fracture ~ see femur, fracture, subtrochanteric
Sucrose hemolysis test ~ see red blood cell (RBC), fragility, osmotic
Suction lipectomies ~ see liposuction
Sudiferous gland ~ see sweat gland
Sugar water test ~ see red blood cell (RBC), fragility, osmotic
Sugars ~ 84375-84379
Sugiura procedure ~ see esophagus, repair, varices
Sulfate
chondroitin ~ see chondroitin sulfate
DHA ~ see dehydroepiandrosterone sulfate
urine ~ 84392
Sulfation factor ~ see somatomedin
Sulphates ~ see sulfate
Sumatran mite fever ~ see scrub typhus
Superficial musculoaponeurotic system (SMAS) flap rhytidectomy ~ 15829
Supernumerary digit
reconstruction ~ 26587
repair ~ 26587
Supply
chemotherapeutic agent ~ (see also chemotherapy) 96545
contact lenses ~ 92391, 92396
educational materials ~ 99071
low vision aids ~ (see also spectacle services) 92392
materials ~ 99070
ocular prosthesis ~ 92393
prosthesis, breast ~ 19396
spectacle prosthesis ~ 92395
spectacles ~ 92390
Suppositories, vaginal ~ see pessary
Suppression ~ 80400-80408
Suppression/testing ~ see evocative/suppression test
Suppressor T lymphocyte marker ~ see CD8
Suppurative hidradenitides ~ see hidradenitis, suppurative
Suprahyoid lymphadenectomy ~ 38700
Supraorbital nerve
avulsion ~ 64732
incision ~ 64732
transection ~ 64732
Supraorbital rim and forehead reconstruction ~ 21179-21180
Suprapubic prostatectomies ~ see prostatectomy, suprapubic
Suprarenal
gland ~ see adrenal gland
vein ~ see vein, adrenal
Suprascapular nerve injection, anesthetic ~ 64418
Suprasellar cyst ~ see craniopharyngioma
Surface CD4 receptor ~ see CD4
Surface radiotherapy ~ see application, radioelement, surface
Surgeries
breast-conserving ~ see breast, excision, lesion
conventional ~ see celiotomy
laser ~ see laser surgery
Mohs ~ see Mohs micrographic surgery
repeat ~ see reoperation
Surgery services ~ 10000-69999
auditory system ~ 69000-69979
cardiovascular system ~ 33000-37799
digestive system ~ 40490-49999
endocrine system ~ 60000-60699
eye and ocular adnexa ~ 65091-68899
female genital system ~ 56405-58999
hemic and lymphatic systems ~ 38100-38999
integumentary system ~ 10000-19999
intersex surgery ~ 55970-55980
male genital system ~ 54000-55899
maternity care and delivery ~ 59000-59899
mediastinum and diaphragm ~ 39000-39599
musculoskeletal system ~ 20000-29999
nervous system ~ 61000-64999
respiratory system ~ 30000-32999
urinary system ~ 50010-53899
Surgical
avulsion ~ see avulsion
cataract removal ~ see cataract, excision
collapse therapy; thoracoplasty ~ see thoracoplasty
diathermy ~ see electrocautery
galvanism ~ see electrolysis
incision ~ see incision
microscopes ~ see operating microscope
pathology ~ 88300-88309
planing, nose, skin ~ 30120
pneumoperitoneum ~ see pneumoperitoneum
removal, eye ~ see enucleation, eye
revision ~ see reoperation
services, post-op visit ~ 99024
Surveillance ~ see monitoring
Suspension
aorta ~ 33800
kidney ~ see nephropexy
muscle, hyoid ~ 21865
vagina ~ see colpopexy
Suture ~ see repair
abdomen ~ 49900
aorta ~ 33320-33322
bile duct, wound ~ 47900
bladder
fistulization ~ 44660-44661, 45800-45805, 51880-51925

Suture ~ *continued*
vesicouterine ~ 51920-51925
vesicovaginal ~ 51900
wound ~ 51860-51865
cervix ~ 57720
colon
diverticula ~ 44604-44605
fistula ~ 44650-44661
plication ~ 44680
stoma ~ 44620-44625
ulcer ~ 44604-44605
wound ~ 44604-44605
esophagus, wound ~ 43410-43415
eyelid ~ 67880
closure of ~ 67875
with transposition of tarsal plate ~ 67882
wound
full thickness ~ 67935
partial thickness ~ 67930
facial nerve, intratemporal
lateral to geniculate ganglion ~ 69740
medial to geniculate ganglion ~ 69745
foot, tendon ~ 28200-28210
gastroesophageal ~ 0008T, 43405
great vessel ~ 33320-33322
hemorrhoids ~ 46945-46946
hepatic duct ~ see hepatic duct, repair
intestine, large
diverticula ~ 44605
ulcer ~ 44605
wound ~ 44605
intestines
large
diverticula ~ 44604
ulcer ~ 44604
wound ~ 44604
small
diverticula ~ 44602-44603
fistula ~ 44640-44661
plication ~ 44680
ulcer ~ 44602-44603
wound ~ 44602-44603
stoma ~ 44620-44625
iris, with ciliary body ~ 66682
kidney
fistula ~ 50520-50526
horseshoe ~ 50540
wound ~ 50500
leg, lower, tendon ~ 27658-27665
leg, upper, muscle ~ 27385-27386
liver, wound ~ 47350-47361
mesentery ~ 44850
nerve ~ 64831-64876
pancreas ~ 48545
pharynx, wound ~ 42900
rectum
fistula ~ 45800-45825
prolapse ~ 45540-45541
removal, anesthesia ~ 15850-15851
spleen ~ see splenorrhaphy
stomach
fistula ~ 43880

Suture ~ *continued*
laceration ~ 43501-43502
stoma ~ 43870
ulcer ~ 43501, 43840
wound ~ 43840
tendon
foot ~ 28200-28210
knee ~ 27380-27381
testis
injury ~ 54670
suspension ~ 54620-54640
thoracic duct
abdominal approach ~ 38382
cervical approach ~ 38380
thoracic approach ~ 38381
throat, wound ~ 42900
tongue, to lip ~ 41510
trachea
fistula
with plastic repair ~ 31825
without plastic repair ~ 31820
stoma
with plastic repair ~ 31825
without plastic repair ~ 31820
wound
cervical ~ 31800
intrathoracic ~ 31805
ulcer ~ 44604-44605
ureter ~ 50900
deligation ~ 50940
fistula ~ 50920-50930
urethra
fistula ~ 45820-45825, 53520
stoma ~ 53520
to bladder ~ 51840-51841
wound ~ 53502-53515
uterus
fistula ~ 51920-51925
rupture ~ 58520, 59350
suspension ~ 58400-58410
vagina
cystocele ~ 57240, 57260
enterocele ~ 57265
fistula
rectovaginal ~ 57300-57307
transvesical and vaginal approach ~ 57330
urethrovaginal ~ 57310-57311
vesicovaginal ~ 51900, 57320-57330
rectocele ~ 57250-57260
suspension ~ 57280, 57283
wound ~ 57200-57210
vas deferens ~ 55400
vein, femoral ~ 37650
iliac ~ 37660
vena cava ~ 37620
wound ~ 44604-44605
Swallowing evaluation ~ 92526, 92610-92613, 92616-92617
cine ~ 74230
treatment ~ 92526
video ~ 74230
Swanson procedure ~ 28309

Sweat collection iontophoresis ~ 89230
Sweat glands, excision
axillary ~ 11450-11451
inguinal ~ 11462-11463
perianal ~ 11470-11471
perineal ~ 11470-11471
umbilical ~ 11470-11471
Sweat test ~ (chloride, blood) 82435
Swenson procedure ~ 45120
Syme procedure ~ 27888
Sympathectomy
artery
digital ~ 64820
radial ~ 64821
superficial palmar arch ~ 64823
ulnar ~ 64822
cervical ~ 64802
cervicothoracic ~ 64804
digital artery, with magnification ~ 64820
lumbar ~ 64818
presacral ~ 58410
thoracic ~ 32664
thoracolumbar ~ 64809
with rib excision ~ 21616
Sympathetic nerve
excision ~ 64802-64818
injection, anesthetic ~ 64508, 64520-64530
Sympathins ~ see catecholamines
Symphysiotomy horseshoe kidney ~ 50540
Symphysis, pubic ~ see pubic symphysis
Syncytial virus, respiratory ~ see respiratory syncytial virus
Syndactylism, toes ~ see webbed, toe
Syndactyly repair ~ 26560-26562
Syndesmotomy ~ see ligament, release
Syndrome
andrenogenital ~ see adrenogenital syndrome
ataxia-telangiectasia ~ see ataxia telangiectasia
Bloom ~ see Bloom syndrome
carpal tunnel ~ see carpal tunnel syndrome
Costen's ~ see temporomandibular joint (TMJ)
Eerb-Goldflam ~ see myasthenia gravis
ovarian vein ~ see ovarian vein syndrome
synechiae, intrauterine ~ see adhesions, intrauterine
Treacher Collins ~ see Treacher-Collins syndrome
urethral ~ see urethral syndrome
Syngesterone ~ see progesterone
Synostosis (cranial) ~ see craniosynostosis
Synovectomy
arthrotomy with, glenohumeral joint ~ 23105
sternoclavicular joint ~ 23106
elbow ~ 24102
excision
carpometacarpal joint ~ 26130
finger joint ~ 26135-26140
hip joint ~ 27054
interphalangeal joint ~ 26140
knee joint ~ 27334-27335
metacarpophalangeal joint ~ 26135
palm ~ 26145
Synovectomy ~ *continued*
wrist ~ 25105, 25118-25119
radical ~ 25115-25116
Synovial
bursa ~ see bursa
cyst ~ see ganglion
membrane ~ see synovium
popliteal space ~ see baker's cyst
Synovium
biopsy
carpometacarpal joint ~ 26100
interphalangeal joint ~ 26110
knee joint ~ 27330
metacarpophalangeal joint, with synovial biopsy ~ 26105
excision
carpometacarpal joint ~ 26130
finger joint ~ 26135-26140
hip joint ~ 27054
interphalangeal joint ~ 26140
knee joint ~ 27334-27335
Syphilis ab ~ see antibody, Treponema pallidum
Syphilis test ~ 86592-86593
Syrinx spinal cord, aspiration ~ 62268
System
endocrine ~ see endocrine system
hemic ~ see hemic system
lymphatic ~ see lymphatic system
musculoskeletal ~ see musculoskeletal system
nervous ~ see nervous system

T

T cell leukemia virus I antibodies, adult ~ 86687, 86689
T cell leukemia virus, I, human ~ 86687, 86689
T cell leukemia virus II antibodies, human ~ 86688
T cell leukemia virus II , human ~ 86688
T lymphotropic virus type III antibodies, human ~ 86689, 86701-86703
T-3 ~ see triiodothyronine
T-4 ~ 84436-84439, 86360
T-7 index ~ 84436
T-8 ~ 86360
T-cells CD4, absolute ~ 86361
count ~ 86359
ratio ~ 86360
T- cell T8 antigens ~ 86360
T- phyl ~ 80198
T3 free ~ 84481
T4 molecule ~ 86360
T4 total ~ 84436
Taarnhoj Procedure ~ see section ~ 61450
Tachycardia heart, recording ~ 93609
Tacrolimus drug assay ~ 80197
Tag, skin ~ see skin, tags

Tail bone
excision ~ 27080
fracture ~ 27200-27202
Takeuchi Procedure ~ 33505
Talectomy ~ see astragalectomy
Talotarsal joint dislocation ~ 28570-28575, 28585
percutaneous fixation ~ 28576
Talus
arthrodesis
pantalar ~ 28705
subtalar ~ 28725
triple ~ 28715
arthroscopy
surgical ~ 29891-29892
craterization ~ 28120
cyst, excision ~ 28100-28103
diaphysectomy ~ 28120
excision ~ 28120, 28130
fracture
open treatment ~ 28445
percutaneous fixation ~ 28436
with manipulation ~ 28435-28436
without manipulation ~ 28430
repair
osteochondritis dissecans ~ 29892
osteotomy ~ 28302
saucerization ~ 28120
tumor, excision ~ 27647, 28100-28103
Tap
cisternal ~ see cisternal puncture
lumbar diagnostic ~ see spinal tap
Tarsal fracture
percutaneous fixation ~ 28456
Tarsal bone ~ see ankle bone
Tarsal joint ~ see foot
arthrodesis ~ 28730-28735, 28740
with advancement ~ 28737
with lengthening ~ 28737
craterization ~ 28122
cyst, excision ~ 28104-28107
diaphysectomy ~ 28122
dislocation ~ 28540-28545, 28555
percutaneous fixation ~ 28545-28546
excision ~ 28116, 28122
fracture
open treatment ~ 28465
with manipulation ~ 28455-28456
without manipulation ~ 28450
fusion ~ 28730-28735, 28740
with advancement ~ 28737
with lengthening ~ 28737
repair ~ 28320
osteotomy ~ 28304-28305
saucerization ~ 28122
tumor, excision ~ 28104-28107, 28171
Tarsal strip procedure ~ 67917-67924
Tarsal tunnel release ~ 28035
Tarsal wedge procedure ~ 67916-67923
Tarsometatarsal joint
arthrodesis ~ 28730-28735, 28740
arthrotomy ~ 28020, 28050
dislocation ~ 28600-28605, 28615
percutaneous fixation ~ 28606
exploration ~ 28020
fusion ~ 28730-28735, 28740
removal
foreign body ~ 28020
loose body ~ 28020
synovial
biopsy ~ 28050
excision ~ 28070
Tarsorrhaphy ~ 67875
median ~ 67880
severing ~ 67710
with transposition of tarsal plate ~ 67882
Tattoo
cornea ~ 65600
skin ~ 11920-11922
TB test, antigen response ~ 0010T
skin test ~ 86580-86585
TBG ~ see thyroxine binding globulin
TBS ~ see Bethesda system
TCT ~ see thrombin time
TD shots ~ see tetanus immunization; vaccines
Team conference case management services ~ 99361-99373
Tear duct ~ see lacrimal duct
Tear gland ~ see lacrimal gland
Technique
pericardial window ~ see pericardiostomy
projective ~ see projective test
Teeth X-ray ~ 70300-70320
Telangiectasia
chromosome analysis ~ 88248
injection ~ 36468
Telangiectasia, cerebello-oculocutaneous ~ see ataxia telangiectasia
Telephone
case management services ~ 99361-99373
pacemaker analysis ~ 93733, 93736
transmission of ECG ~ 93012
Teletherapy dose plan ~ 77305-77321
Temperature gradient studies ~ 93740
Temporal arteries ~ 37609
Temporal bone
electromagnetic bone conduction hearing device
implantation/replacement ~ 69710
removal/repair ~ 69711
excision ~ 69535
resection ~ 69535
tumor, removal ~ 69970
unlisted services and procedures ~ 69979
Temporal, petrous
excision, apex ~ 69530
Temporomandibular joint (TMJ)
arthrocentesis ~ 20605
arthrography ~ 70328-70332
injection ~ 21116
arthroplasty ~ 21240-21243

Temporomandibular joint (TMJ) ~ *continued*
arthroscopy
diagnostic ~ 29800
surgical ~ 29804
arthrotomy ~ 21010
cartilage, excision ~ 21060
condylectomy ~ 21050
coronoidectomy ~ 21070
dislocation
closed treatment ~ 21480-21485
open treatment ~ 21490
injection, radiologic ~ 21116
magnetic resonance imaging (MRI) ~ 70336
meniscectomy ~ 21060
prostheses ~ see prosthesis, temporomandibular joint
reconstruction ~ see reconstruction, temporomandibular joint
X-ray with contrast ~ 70328-70332
Tenago Procedure ~ 53431
Tendinosuture ~ see suture, tendon
Tendon
Achilles ~ see Achilles tendon
arm, upper, revision ~ 24320
excision
forearm ~ 25109
finger, excision ~ 26180
forearm, repair ~ 25260-25274
graft, harvesting ~ 20924
insertion, biceps tendon ~ 24342
lengthening
ankle ~ 27685-27686
arm, upper ~ 24305
elbow ~ 24305
finger ~ 26476, 26478
forearm ~ 25280
hand ~ 26476, 26478
leg, lower ~ 27685-27686
leg, upper ~ 27393-27395
toe ~ 28240
wrist ~ 25280
palm, excision ~ 26170
release
arm, lower ~ 25295
arm, upper ~ 24332
wrist ~ 25295
shortening
ankle ~ 27685-27686
finger ~ 26477, 26479
hand ~ 26477, 26479
leg, lower ~ 27685-27686
transfer
arm, lower ~ 25310-25312, 25316
arm, upper ~ 24301
elbow ~ 24301
finger ~ 26497-26498
hand ~ 26480-26489
leg, lower ~ 27690-27692
leg, upper ~ 27400
pelvis ~ 27098
thumb ~ 26490-26492, 26510
wrist ~ 25310-25312, 25316
Tendon ~ *continued*
transplant, leg, upper ~ 27396-27397
wrist, repair ~ 25260-25274
Tendon origin insertion, injection ~ 20551
Tendon pulley reconstruction of hand ~ see hand, reconstruction, tendon pulley
Tendon sheath
arm
lower
repair ~ 25275
finger
incision ~ 26055
incision and drainage ~ 26020
lesion ~ 26160
foot
excision ~ 28086-28088
hand lesion ~ 26160
injection ~ 20550
palm, incision and drainage ~ 26020
removal, foreign body ~ 20520-20525
wrist
excision, radical ~ 25115-25116
incision ~ 25000-25001
repair ~ 25275
Tenectomy, tendon sheath ~ 25110
Tennis elbow repair ~ 24350-24356
Tenodesis
biceps tendon
at elbow ~ 24340
shoulder ~ 23430
finger ~ 26471-26474
wrist ~ 25300-25301
Tenolysis
ankle ~ 27680-27681
arm, lower ~ 25295
arm, upper ~ 24332
finger
extensor ~ 26445-26449
flexor ~ 26440-26442
foot ~ 28220-28226
hand extensor ~ 26445-26449
flexor ~ 26440-26442
leg, lower ~ 27680-27681
wrist ~ 25295
Tenomyotomy, shoulder ~ 23405-23406
Tenon's capsule injection ~ 67515
Tenoplasty anesthesia ~ 01714
Tenorrhaphy ~ see suture, tendon
Tenosuspension ~ see tenodesis
Tenosuture ~ see suture, tendon
Tenotomy
Achilles tendon ~ 27605-27606
ankle ~ 27605-27606
arm, lower ~ 25290
arm, upper ~ 24310
finger ~ 26060, 26455-26460
foot ~ 28230, 28234
hand ~ 26450, 26460
hip, iliopsoas tendon ~ 27005
hip, abductor ~ 27006
hip, adductor ~ 27000-27003
leg, upper ~ 27306-27307, 27390-27392

Tenotomy ~ *continued*
toe ~ 28010-28011, 28232-28234, 28240
wrist ~ 25290
TENS ~ see physical medicine/therapy/occupational therapy ~ 64550
Tensilon test ~ 95857-95858
Tension, ocular ~ see glaucoma
Tentorium cerebelli section ~ 61440
Terman-Merrill test ~ 96100
Termination, pregnancy ~ see abortion
Test
antiglobulin ~ 86880
aphasia ~ 96105
Bender visual-motor Gestalt ~ 96101-96103
Binet ~ 96101-96103
blood ~ see blood tests
blood coagulation ~ see coagulation
breath ~ see breath test
cervical mucus penetration ~ 89330
clinical chemistry ~ 84999
complement fixation ~ 86171
exercise ~ 93015-93018
fern ~ 87210
fetal, nonstress ~ 59025
function, vestibular ~ see vestibular function tests
gel diffusion ~ 86329-86331
glucose tolerance ~ 82951-82952
hearing ~ see audiologic function tests
hemagglutination inhibition ~ 86280
ink blot ~ see inkblot test
intelligence ~ 96101-96102
lung function ~ see pulmonology, diagnostic
neutralization ~ 86382
Papanicolaou ~ 88141-88155, 88164-88167, 88174-88175
pregnancy ~ 84702-84703
quick ~ 85610-85611
radioimmunosorbent ~ 82784-82787
Rorschach ~ 96101
Schilling ~ 78270
skin ~ see skin, tests
Stanford-Binet ~ see psychiatric diagnosis
tuberculin ~ 86580
Test tube fertilization ~ 58321-58322
Tester, color vision ~ 92283
Testes
cryopreservation ~ 89335
nuclear medicine
imaging ~ 78761
undescended ~ 54550-54560
Testicular vein ~ 55530-55540
Testimony, medical ~ 99075
Testing, histocompatibility ~ see tissue typing
Testing, neurophysiologic intraoperative ~ 95920
Testing, neuropsychological ~ 96117
Testing, range of motion ~ see range of motion test
Testis
abscess, incision and drainage ~ 54700
biopsy ~ 54500-54505
excision
laparoscopic ~ 54690
partial ~ 54522
radical ~ 54530-54535
simple ~ 54520
hematoma, incision and drainage ~ 54700
insertion, prosthesis ~ 54660
lesion, excision ~ 54512
needle biopsy ~ 54500
repair
injury ~ 54670
suspension ~ 54620-54640
torsion ~ 54600
suture
injury ~ 54670
suspension ~ 54620-54640
transplantation, to thigh ~ 54680
tumor, excision ~ 54530-54535
undescended, exploration ~ 54550-54560
unlisted services and procedures ~ 54699, 55899
Testosterone ~ 84402
response ~ 80414
stimulation ~ 80414-80415
total ~ 84403
Testosterone estradiol binding globulin ~ 84270
Tetanus ~ 86280
antibody ~ 86774
immunoglobulin ~ 90389
vaccine ~ 90703
Tetrachloride, carbon ~ 84600
Tetralogy of Fallot ~ 33692-33697, 33924
Thal-Nissen Procedure ~ 43325
Thawing ~ 86930-86932
cryopreserved
embryo ~ 89352
oocytes ~ 89356
reproductive tissue ~ 89354
sperm ~ 89353
previously frozen cells ~ 38208-38209
Thawing and expansion of frozen cell ~ 88241
THBR ~ 84479
Theleplasty ~ 19350
Theophylline assay ~ 80198
Therapeutic
abortion ~ 59850-59852
apheresis ~ 36511-36516
drug assays ~ 80150-80299
mobilization ~ see mobilization
photopheresis ~ 36522
radiology ~ see radiology, therapeutic
Therapies
cold ~ see cryotherapy
exercise ~ 97110-97113
family ~ 90846-90849, 99510
language ~ 92507-92508
milieu ~ 90882

Therapies ~ *continued*
occupational ~ 97003-97004
photodynamic ~ 96910-96913
photoradiation ~ 96900
physical ~ see physical medicine/therapy/occupational therapy
speech ~ 92507-92508
tocolytic ~ 59412
ultraviolet ~ 96900
Therapy
ACE inhibitor therapy ~ 4009F
beta blocker therapy ~ 4009F
desensitization ~ 95180
hemodialysis ~ 90935-90937
hot pack ~ 97010
pharmacologic; for cessation of tobacco use ~ 4009F
radiation ~ 86945
speech ~ 92507-92508
satin therapy, prescribed ~ 4009F
Thermocauterization
ectropion, repair ~ 67922
lesion, cornea ~ 65450
Thermocoagulation ~ 17000-17286
Thermogram
cephalic ~ 93760
peripheral ~ 93762
Thermographies ~ 93760, 93762
Thermography, cerebral ~ 93760
Thermotherapy
prostate ~ 53850-53853
microwave ~ 53850
radiofrequency ~ 53852
Thiamine ~ 84425
Thiersch Operation ~ 15050
Thiersch Procedure ~ 46753
Thigh fasciotomy ~ see femur; leg, upper ~ 27025
Thin layer chromatographies ~ 82489
Thiocyanate ~ 84430
Third disease ~ 86762, 90706
Third opinion ~ see confirmatory consultations
Thompson Procedure ~ 27430
Thompson test ~ see smear and stain, routine
Thoracectomy ~ 32905
Thoracentesis ~ 32000-32002
Thoracic
anterior ramus ~ see intercostal nerve
arteries ~ 36215-36218
cavity ~ see chest cavity
duct ~ see lymphatics
cannulation ~ 38794
ligation ~ 38380
abdominal approach ~ 38382
thoracic approach ~ 38381
suture
abdominal approach ~ 38382
cervical approach ~ 38380
thoracic approach ~ 38381

Thoracic ~ *continued*
empyema ~ 21501-21502
surgery, video-assisted ~ see thoracoscopy
vertebra ~ 22101, 22112
wall ~ see chest wall
Thoracocentesis ~ 32000-32002
Thoracoplasty ~ 32905
with closure bronchopleural fistula ~ 32906
Thoracoscopy
diagnostic ~ 32601-32606
with biopsy ~ 32602, 32604, 32606
without biopsy ~ 32601, 32603, 32605
surgical ~ 32650-32665
with control traumatic hemorrhage ~ 32654
with creation pericardial window ~ 32659
with esophagomyotomy ~ 32665
with excision mediastinal cyst, tumor and/or mass ~ 32662
with excision pericardial cyst, tumor and/or mass ~ 32661
with excision-plication of bullae ~ 32655
with lobectomy ~ 32663
with parietal pleurectomy ~ 32656
with partial pulmonary decortication ~ 32651
with pleurodesis ~ 32650
with removal intrapleural foreign body ~ 32653
with removal of clot/foreign body ~ 32658
with sternum reconstruction ~ 21743
with thoracic sympathectomy ~ 32664
with total pericardiectomy ~ 32660
with total pulmonary decortication ~ 32652
with wedge resection of lung ~ 32657
Thoracostomy empyema ~ 32035-32036
tube, with/without water seal ~ 32020
Thoracotomy
cardiac massage ~ 32160
for post-op complications ~ 32120
hemorrhage ~ 32110
removal
bullae ~ 32141
cyst ~ 32140
defibrillator ~ 33243
electrodes ~ 33238
foreign body
intrapleural ~ 32150
intrapulmonary ~ 32151
pacemaker ~ 33236-33237
with biopsy ~ 32095-32100
with excision-plication of bullae ~ 32141
with lung repair ~ 32110
with open intrapleural pneumolysis ~ 32124
transmyocardial laser revascularization ~ 33140-33141
Thorax ~ see chest; chest cavity; mediastinum
angiography ~ 71275
bioimpedance ~ 93701
biopsy ~ 21550
CT scan ~ 71250-71275

Thorax ~ *continued*
incision, empyema ~ 32035-32036
pneumothorax ~ 32020
incision and drainage
abscess ~ 21501-21502
deep ~ 21510
hematoma ~ 21501-21502
strapping ~ 29200
tumor
excision ~ 21555-21556
excision/resection ~ 21557
unlisted services and procedures, surgery ~ 21899
Three glass test ~ 81020
Three-day measles ~ 86762, 90706
Throat ~ see pharynx
abscess, incision and drainage ~ 42700-42725
biopsy ~ 42800-42806
hemorrhage ~ 42960-42962
reconstruction ~ 42950
removal, foreign body ~ 42809
repair
pharyngoesophageal ~ 42953
wound ~ 42900
suture, wound ~ 42900
unlisted services and procedures ~ 42999
Thrombectomy ~ see also thromboendarterectomy
aortoiliac artery ~ 34151-34201
arteriovenous fistula, graft ~ 36870
axillary artery ~ 34101
axillary vein ~ 34490
brachial artery ~ 34101
bypass graft, other than hemodialysis graft or fistula ~ 35875-35876
carotid artery ~ 34001
celiac artery ~ 34151
dialysis graft, without revision ~ 36831
femoral ~ 34201
femoropopliteal vein ~ 34421-34451
iliac ~ 34151-34201
iliac vein ~ 34401-34451
innominate artery ~ 34001-34101
mesenteric artery ~ 34151
percutaneous, coronary artery ~ 92973
peroneal artery ~ 34203
popliteal artery ~ 34203
radial artery ~ 34111
renal artery ~ 34151
subclavian artery ~ 34001-34101
subclavian vein ~ 34471-34490
tibial artery ~ 34203
ulnar artery ~ 34111
vena cava ~ 34401-34451
vena caval ~ 50230
Thrombin inhibitor I ~ 85300-85301
Thrombin time ~ 85670-85675
Thrombocyte (platelet) ~ see blood, platelet
Thrombocyte AB ~ 86022-86023
Thromboendarterectomy ~ see thrombectomy
aorta, abdominal ~ 35331
aortoiliofemoral artery ~ 35363
axillary artery ~ 35321
brachial artery ~ 35321
carotid artery ~ 35301, 35390
celiac artery ~ 35341
femoral artery ~ 35371-35372
iliac artery ~ 35351, 35361-35363
iliofemoral artery ~ 35355, 35363
innominate artery ~ 35311
mesenteric artery ~ 35341
peroneal artery ~ 35305-35306
popliteal artery ~ 35303
renal artery ~ 35341
subclavian artery ~ 35301-35311
superficial femoral artery ~ 35302
tibial artery ~ 35305-35306
tibioperoneal trunk artery ~ 35304
vertebral artery ~ 35301
Thrombokinase ~ 85260
Thrombolysin ~ 85400
Thrombolysis
catheter exchange, arterial ~ 37209, 75900
cerebral, intravenous infusion ~ 37195
coronary vessels ~ 92975-92977
cranial vessels ~ 37195
Thrombolysis biopsy intracranial arterial perfusion ~ 61624
Thrombolysis intracranial ~ see ciliary body; cornea; eye, removal, foreign body; iris; lens; retina; sclera; vitreous ~ 65205
Thrombomodulin ~ 85337
Thromboplastin
inhibition ~ 85705
inhibition test ~ 85347
partial time ~ 85730-85732
Thromboplastin antecedent, plasma ~ 85270
Thromboplastinogen ~ 85210-85293
Thromboplastinogen B ~ 85250
Thumb ~ 26720-26727
amputation ~ 26910, 26952
arthrodesis, carpometacarpal joint ~ 26841-26842
dislocation
with fracture ~ 26645-26650
open treatment ~ 26665
with manipulation ~ 26641
fracture
with dislocation ~ 26645-26650
open treatment ~ 26665
fusion, in opposition ~ 26820
reconstruction
from finger ~ 26550
opponensplasty ~ 26490-26496
repair
muscle ~ 26508
muscle transfer ~ 26494
tendon transfer ~ 26510
replantation ~ 20824-20827
sesamoidectomy ~ 26185
unlisted services and procedures ~ 26989

Thymectomy ~ 60520-60521
sternal split/transthoracic approach ~ 60521-60522
transcervical approach ~ 60520
Thymotaxin ~ 82232
Thymus gland ~ 60520
excision ~ 60520-60521
Thyramine ~ 82145
Thyrocalcitonin ~ 80410, 82308
Thyroglobulin ~ 84432
antibody ~ 86800
Thyroglossal duct cyst, excision ~ 60280-60281
Thyroid gland
cyst
aspiration ~ 60001
excision ~ 60200
incision and drainage ~ 60000
injection ~ 60001
excision
for malignancy
limited neck dissection ~ 60252
radical neck dissection ~ 60254
partial ~ 60210-60225
secondary ~ 60260
total ~ 60240, 60271
cervical approach ~ 60271
removal all thyroid tissue ~ 60260
sternal split/transthoracic approach ~ 60270
transcervical approach ~ 60520
metastatic cancer, nuclear imaging ~ 78015-78018
needle biopsy ~ 60100
nuclear medicine
imaging ~ 78010
imaging for metastases ~ 78015-78018
imaging with flow ~ 78011
imaging with uptake ~ 78006-78007
metastases uptake ~ 78020
uptake ~ 78000-78003
tumor, excision ~ 60200
Thyroid hormone binding ratio ~ 84479
Thyroid hormone uptake ~ 84479
Thyroid stimulating hormone (TSH) ~ 80418, 80438-80440, 84443
Thyroid stimulating hormone receptor AB ~ 80438-80439
Thyroid stimulating immune globulins ~ 84445
Thyroid stimulator, long acting ~ 80438-80439
Thyroid suppression test ~ 78000-78003
Thyroidectomy
partial ~ 60210-60225
secondary ~ 60260
total ~ 60240, 60271
cervical approach ~ 60271
for malignancy
limited neck dissection ~ 60252
radical neck dissection ~ 60254
removal all thyroid tissue ~ 60260
sternal split/transthoracic approach ~ 60270
Thyrolingual cyst ~ 60000, 60280-60281
Thyrotomy ~ 31300
Thyrotropin receptor AB ~ 80438-80439
Thyrotropin releasing hormone (TRH) ~ 80438-80439
Thyroxine
free ~ 84439
neonatal ~ 84437
total ~ 84436
true ~ 84436
Thyroxine binding globulin ~ 84442
Tibia ~ see ankle
arthroscopy surgical ~ 29891-29892
craterization ~ 27360, 27640
cyst, excision ~ 27635-27638
diaphysectomy ~ 27360, 27640
excision ~ 27360, 27640
epiphyseal bar ~ 20150
fracture ~ 27759
fracture
arthroscopic treatment ~ 29855-29856
plafond ~ 29892
closed treatment ~ 27824-27825
distal ~ 27824-27828
intercondylar ~ 27538-27540
malleolus ~ 27760-27766, 27808-27814
open treatment ~ 27535-27536, 27758-27759, 27826-27828
plateau ~ 29855-29856
closed treatment ~ 27530-27536
shaft ~ 27752-27759
with manipulation ~ 27825
without manipulation ~ 27824
incision ~ 27607
osteoplasty, lengthening ~ 27715
prophylactic treatment ~ 27745
reconstruction ~ 27418
at knee ~ 27440-27443, 27446
repair ~ 27720-27725
epiphysis ~ 27477-27485, 27730-27742
osteochondritis dissecans arthroscopy ~ 29892
osteotomy ~ 27455-27457, 27705, 27709-27712
pseudoarthrosis ~ 27727
saucerization ~ 27360, 27640
tumor, excision ~ 27635-27638, 27645
X-ray ~ 73590
Tibial
arteries ~ see artery, tibial
nerve, repair/suture, posterior ~ 64840
Tibiofibular joint
arthrodesis ~ 27871
dislocation ~ 27830-27832
disruption, open treatment ~ 27829
fusion ~ 27871
TIG ~ see immune globulins, tetanus
Time
bleeding ~ 85002
prothrombin ~ 85610-85611
reptilase ~ 85670-85675
Tinnitus assessment ~ 92625

Tissue
culture
chromosome analysis ~ 88230-88239
homogenization ~ 87176
non-neoplastic disorder ~ 88230, 88237
skin grafts ~ 15100-15121, 15342-15343
solid tumor ~ 88239
toxin/antitoxin ~ 87230
virus ~ 87252-87253
enzyme activity ~ 82657
examination for ectoparasites ~ 87220
examination for fungi ~ 87220
expander
breast reconstruction with ~ 19357
insertion, skin ~ 11960
removal, skin ~ 11971
replacement, skin ~ 11970
grafts, harvesting ~ 20926
granulation ~ 17250
homogenization ~ 87176
hybridization in situ ~ 88365-88368
mucosal ~ see mucosa
preparation, drug analysis ~ 80103
soft, abscess ~ 20000-20005
transfer
adjacent
eyelids ~ 67961
skin ~ 14000-14350
facial muscles ~ 15845
finger flap ~ 14350
toe flap ~ 14350
typing
HLA antibodies ~ 86812-86817
lymphocyte culture ~ 86821-86822
Tissue factor ~ see thromboplastin
TLC ~ 82489
screen ~ 84375
TMJ ~ see temporomandibular joint (TMJ)
prostheses ~ 21243
Tobacco ~ 4009F
Tobramycin assay ~ 80200
Tocolysis ~ 59412
Tocopherol ~ 84446
Toe ~ see phalanx ~ 28270, 28272
amputation ~ 28810-28825
capsulotomy ~ 28270-28272
fasciotomy ~ 28008
fracture ~ see fracture, phalanges, toe
lesion, excision ~ 28092
reconstruction
angle deformity ~ 28313
extra toes ~ 28344
hammer toe ~ 28285-28286
macrodactyly ~ 28340-28341
syndactyly ~ 28345
webbed toe ~ 28345
repair
bunion ~ 28290-28299
muscle ~ 28240
tendon ~ 28232-28234, 28240
webbed ~ 28280
webbed toe ~ 28345
Toe ~ *continued*
tenotomy ~ 28010-28011, 28232-28234
unlisted services and procedures ~ 28899
Toe flap tissue transfer ~ 14350
Toes
arthrocentesis ~ 20600
dislocation ~ see specific joint**
magnetic resonance imaging (MRI) ~ 73721-73723
reconstruction, extra digit ~ 26587
repair
extra digit ~ 26587
macrodactylia ~ 26590
reposition to hand ~ 26551-26556
strapping ~ 29550
X-ray ~ 73660
Tolbutamide tolerance test ~ 82953
Tolerance test
glucagon ~ 82946
glucose ~ 82951-82952
with tolbutamide ~ 82953
heparin-protamine ~ 85530
insulin ~ 80434-80435
maltose ~ 82951-82952
tolbutamide ~ 82953
Tomodensitometries ~ see CT scan
Tomographic scintigraphy, computed ~ 78607
Tomographic spect myocardial imaging ~ 78469
Tomographies, computed X-ray ~ see CT scan
Tomography, computerized axial abdomen ~ 74150-74175, 75635
head ~ 70450-70470, 70496
Tomography, emission computed ~ see positron emission tomography
single photon ~ 78607
Tompkins metroplasty ~ 58540
Tongue
abscess, incision and drainage ~ 41000-41006, 41015
biopsy ~ 41100-41105
cyst, incision and drainage ~ 41000-41006, 41015, 60000
excision
complete ~ 41140-41155
frenum ~ 41115
partial ~ 41120-41135
with mouth resection ~ 41150-41153
with radical neck ~ 41135, 41145, 41153-41155
fixation ~ 41500
hematoma, incision and drainage ~ 41000-41006, 41015
incision, frenum ~ 41010
lesion, excision ~ 41110-41114
reconstruction, frenum ~ 41520
reduction for sleep apnea ~ 0088T
repair ~ 41250-41252
laceration ~ 41250-41252
suture ~ 41510
suture ~ 41510
unlisted services and procedures ~ 41599

Tonography ~ 92120
with provocation ~ 92130
Tonometry, serial ~ 92100
Tonsil, pharyngeal ~ see adenoids
Tonsillectomy ~ 42820-42826
Tonsils
abscess, incision and drainage ~ 42700
excision ~ 42825-42826
lingual ~ 42870
radical ~ 42842-42845
tag ~ 42860
with adenoids ~ 42820-42821
lingual, destruction ~ 42870
unlisted services and procedures ~ 42999
Topiramate assay ~ 80201
Torek Procedure ~ see orchiopexy
Torkildsen Procedure ~ 62180
TORP (total ossicular replacement prosthesis) ~ 69633, 69637
Torsion swing test ~ 92546
Torula ~ see cryptococcus
Torus mandibularis tumor excision ~ 21031
Total
abdominal hysterectomy ~ 58150, 58200, 58956
bilirubin level ~ 82247-82248, 88400
catecholamines ~ 82382
cystectomy ~ 51570, 51580, 51590-51597
dacryoadenectomy ~ 68500
elbow replacement ~ 24363
esophagectomy ~ 43107-43113, 43124
gastrectomy ~ 43620-43622
hemolytic complement ~ 86162
hip arthroplasty ~ 27130-27132
knee arthroplasty ~ 27438, 27445
mastectomies ~ see mastectomy
ostectomy of patella ~ 27424
splenectomy ~ 38100
Touroff Operation ~ 37615
Toxicology screen ~ 80100-80103
Toxin assay ~ 87230
Toxin, botulinum ~ see chemodenervation
Toxoplasma antibody ~ 86777-86778
Trabeculectomies ~ 65855
Trabeculectomy ab externo
in absence of previous surgery ~ 66170
with scarring previous surgery ~ 66172
Trabeculoplasty by laser surgery ~ 65855
Trabeculotomy AB externo eye ~ 65850
Trachea
aspiration ~ 31720
catheter ~ 31720-31725
dilation ~ 31630-31631, 31636-31638
endoscopy, via tracheostomy ~ 31615
excision, stenosis ~ 31780-31781
fistula
with plastic repair ~ 31825
without plastic repair ~ 31820
fracture, endoscopy ~ 31630
Trachea ~ ***continued***
incision
emergency ~ 31603-31605
planned ~ 31600-31601
with flaps ~ 31610
introduction, needle wire ~ 31730
puncture, aspiration and/or injection ~ 31612
reconstruction
carina ~ 31766
cervical ~ 31750
fistula ~ 31755
intrathoracic ~ 31760
repair
cervical ~ 31750
fistula ~ 31755
intrathoracic ~ 31760
stoma ~ 31613-31614
revision, stoma, scars ~ 31830
scar, revision ~ 31830
stenosis
excision ~ 31780-31781
repair ~ 31780-31781
stoma
repair
with plastic repair ~ 31825
without plastic repair ~ 31820
revision, scars ~ 31830
tumor
excision
cervical ~ 31785
thoracic ~ 31786
unlisted services and procedures, bronchi ~ 31899
wound, suture
cervical ~ 31800
intrathoracic ~ 31805
Tracheal stent, placement ~ 31631
tubes ~ 31500
Trachelectomy ~ 57530
radical ~ 57531
Tracheloplasty ~ 15819
Trachelorrhaphy ~ 57720
Tracheo-esophageal fistula ~ see fistula, tracheoesophageal
Tracheobronchoscopy through tracheostomy ~ 31615
Tracheoplasty
cervical ~ 31750
intrathoracic ~ 31760
tracheopharyngeal fistulization ~ 31755
Tracheostoma revision ~ 31613-31614
Tracheostomy
emergency ~ 31603-31605
planned ~ 31600-31601
revision, scar ~ 31830
surgical closure
with plastic repair ~ 31825
without plastic repair ~ 31820
tracheobronchoscopy through ~ 31615
with flaps ~ 31610
Tracheotomy tube change ~ 31502
Tracking tests (ocular) ~ 92545

Tract, urinary ~ 74400-74425
Traction therapy ~ 97140
manual ~ 97140
mechanical ~ 97012
Tractotomy
medulla ~ 61470
mesencephalon ~ 61480
Training
activities of daily living ~ 97535, 99509
biofeedback ~ 90901-90911
cognitive skills ~ 97532
community/work reintegration ~ 97537
home management ~ 97535, 99509
orthoptic/pleoptic ~ 92065
orthotics ~ 97504
prosthetics ~ 97520
self care ~ 97535, 99509
sensory integration ~ 97533
walking (physical therapy) ~ 97116
wheelchair management/propulsion ~ 97542
Tram flap
breast reconstruction ~ 19367-19369
Trans-scaphoperilunar fracture/dislocation
closed treatment ~ 25680
open treatment ~ 25685
Transaminase
glutamic oxaloacetic ~ 84450
glutamic pyruvic ~ 84460
Transcatheter
biopsy ~ 37200
closure
percutaneous
heart ~ 93580-93581
transmyocardial
heart ~ 0166T, 0167T
embolization, percutaneous ~ 37204
cranial ~ 61624-61626
occlusion, percutaneous ~ 37204
cranial ~ 61624-61626
placement
intravascular stents ~ 0075T-0076T, 37205-37208, 37215-37216
sensor, pressure ~ 0153T
therapy
embolization ~ 75894
infusion ~ 37201-37202, 75896-75898
perfusion, cranial ~ 61624-61626
retrieval ~ 75961
Transcatheter foreign body retrieval ~ 37203
Transcortin ~ 84449
Transcranial Doppler study (TCP) ~ 93886-93893
stimulation, motor ~ 95928-95929
Transcutaneous electric nerve stimulation ~ 64550
Transdermal electrostimulation ~ 64550
Transection
artery, carotid ~ 61610, 61612
blood vessel, kidney ~ 50100
brain, subpial ~ 61567
carotid, with skill base surgery ~ 61609
Transection ~ *continued*
nerve ~ 64732-64772
vagus ~ 43640-43641
pulmonary artery ~ 33922
Transesophageal Doppler echocardiography ~ 93312-93318
Transfer
blastocyst ~ 58974-58976
gamete intrafallopian ~ see GIFT
jejunum, with microvascular anastomosis, free ~ 43496
preparation, embryo ~ 89255
cryopreserved ~ 89352
surgical ~ see transposition
tendon ~ see tendon, transfer
toe to hand ~ 26551-26556
Transferase
aspartate amino ~ 84450
glutamic oxaloacetic ~ 84450
Transferrin ~ 84466
Transformation lymphocyte ~ 86353
Transfusion blood ~ 36430
exchange ~ 36450-36455
fetal ~ 36460
push, infant ~ 36440
blood parts, exchange ~ 36511-36516
unlisted services and procedures ~ 86999
white blood cells ~ 86950
Transfusion medicine ~ 86850-86999
Transluminal
angioplasty, arterial ~ 75962-75968
atherectomies ~ 35480-35495
coronary balloon dilatation ~ 92982-92984
Transmyocardial laser revascularization ~ 33140-33141
Transosteal bone plate reconstruction, mandible ~ 21244
Transpeptidase, gamma-glutamyl ~ 82977
Transplant ~ see graft
bone ~ see bone graft
hair ~ see hair, transplant
Transplantation ~ see graft
allogenic ~ 15300-15336
autologous ~ see autograft
bone marrow ~ 38240-38242
cartilage, knee
allograft ~ 27415, 29867
autograft ~ 27412, 29866
chondrocytes, knee ~ 27412
conjunctiva ~ 65782
cornea
autograft/homograft
lamellar ~ 65710
penetrating ~ 65730-65755
for aphakia ~ 65750
eye
amniotic membrane ~ 65780
conjunctiva ~ 65782
stem cell ~ 65781
hair
punch graft ~ 15775-15776
strip ~ 15220-15221

Transplantation ~ *continued*
heart ~ 33945
allograft preparation ~ 33933, 33944
heart-lung ~ 33935
heterologous ~ 15400-15401, 15420-15421
intestines
allograft preparation ~ 44715-44721
allotransplantation ~ 44135-44136
donor enterectomy ~ 44132-44133
removal of allograft ~ 44137
liver ~ 47135
allograft preparation ~ 47143-47147
heterotopic ~ 47136
lung
allograft preparation ~ 32855-32856, 33933
anesthesia ~ 00580
donor pneumonectomy ~ 32850
double, with cardiopulmonary bypass ~ 32854
double, without cardiopulmonary bypass ~ 32853
single, with cardiopulmonary bypass ~ 32852
single, without cardiopulmonary bypass ~ 32851
meniscus, knee ~ 29868
muscle ~ 15732-15738
pancreas ~ 48160, 48550, 48554-48556
allograft preparation ~ 48551-48552
parathyroid ~ 60512
renal
allograft preparation ~ 50323-50329
allotransplantation ~ 50360
with recipient nephrectomy ~ 50365
autotransplantation ~ 50380
donor nephrectomy ~ 50300-50320, 50547
recipient nephrectomy ~ 50340
removal transplanted renal allograft ~ 50370
skin ~ see dermatology
stem cells ~ 38240-38241
cell concentration ~ 38215
cryopreservation ~ 38207
harvesting ~ 38205-38206
plasma depletion ~ 38214
platelet depletion ~ 38213
red blood cell depletion ~ 38212
T-cell depletion ~ 38210
thawing ~ 38208
tumor cell depletion ~ 38211
washing ~ 38209
testis ~ 38208
to thigh ~ 54680
tissue, harvesting ~ 20926
Transpleural thoracoscopy ~ see thoracoscopy
Transposition
arteries
carotid ~ 0037T, 35691, 35694-35695
subclavian ~ 0037T, 35693-35695
vertebral ~ 35691-35693
cranial nerve ~ 64716
eye muscles ~ 67320
great arteries, repair ~ 33770-33781
Transposition ~ *continued*
nerve ~ 64718-64721
ovary ~ 58825
peripheral nerve
major ~ 64856
vein valve ~ 34510
Transthoracic echocardiography ~ 93303-93318, 93350
Transthyretin ~ 84134
Transureteroureterostomy ~ 50770
Transurethral balloon dilation prostatic urethra ~ 52510
Transurethral fulguration postoperative bleeding ~ 52606
Transurethral procedure ~ see specific procedure**
prostate
incision ~ 52450
resection ~ 52612-52614
thermotherapy ~ 53850-53853
microwave ~ 53850
radiofrequency ~ 53852
Trapezium arthroplasty with implant ~ 25445
Travel, unusual ~ 99082
Treacher-Collins syndrome midface reconstruction ~ 21150-21151
Treatment, tocolytic ~ 59412
Trendelenburg Operation ~ 37785
Trephine procedure sinusotomy, frontal ~ 31070
Treponema pallidum
antibody, confirmation test ~ 86781
antigen detection, direct fluorescence ~ 87285
TRH ~ see thyrotropin releasing hormone (TRH)
Triacylglycerol ~ 84478
Triacylglycerol hydrolase ~ 83690
Tributyrinase ~ 83690
Trichiasis repair ~ 67825
epilation, by forceps ~ 67820
epilation, by other than forceps ~ 67825
incision of lid margin ~ 67830
with free mucous membrane graft ~ 67835
Trichina ~ 86784, 96902
Trichinella
antibody ~ 86784
trichogram ~ 96902
Trichomonas vaginalis
antigen detection
nucleic acid ~ 87660
by immunoassay with direct optical observation ~ 87808
Trichrome stain ~ 88313
Tricuspid valve
excision ~ 33460
repair ~ 33463-33465
replacement ~ 33465
repositioning ~ 33468
Tridymite ~ 84285
Trigeminal ganglia ~ see Gasserian ganglion

Trigeminal nerve
destruction ~ 64600-64610
injection
anesthetic ~ 64400
neurolytic ~ 64600-64610
Trigeminal tract stereotactic, create lesion ~ 61791
Trigger finger repair ~ 26055
Trigger point injection
one or two muscles ~ 20552
two or more muscles ~ 20553
Triglyceridase ~ 83690
Triglyceride lipase ~ 83690
Triglycerides ~ 84478
Trigonocephaly ~ 21175
Triiodothyronine
free ~ 84481
reverse ~ 84482
total ~ 84480
true ~ 84480
Triolean hydrolase ~ 83690
Trioxopurine ~ 84550, 84560
Tripcellim ~ 84485, 84488-84490
Trisegmentectomy ~ 47122
Trocar biopsy bone marrow ~ 38221
Trochanteric femur fracture ~ 27246, 27248
Trophoblastic tumor GTT ~ 59100, 59870
Troponin ~ 84484
qualitative ~ 84512
quantitative ~ 84484
Truncal vagotomies ~ 43640
Truncus arteriosus repair ~ 33786
Truncus brachiocephalicus ~ see artery, brachiocephalic
Trunk, brachiocephalic ~ see artery, brachiocephalic
Trypanosomiases ~ 86171, 86280
Trypanosomiasis ~ 86171, 86280
Trypsin
duodenum ~ 84485
feces ~ 84488-84490
Trypsin inhibitor, alpha 1-antirypsin ~ see alpha-1 antitrypsin
Trypure ~ 84485, 84488-84490
Tsalicylate intoxication ~ 80196
TSH ~ see thyroid stimulating hormone
TSI ~ see thyroid stimulating immunoglobulin
Tsutsugamushi disease ~ 86000
TT ~ see thrombin time
TT-3 ~ see triiodothyronine, true
TT-4 ~ see thyroxine, true
Tuba auditoria (auditiva) ~ see eustachian tube
Tubal embryo stage transfer ~ see embryo transfer
Tubal ligation ~ 58600
laparoscopic ~ 58670
with cesarean section ~ 58611
Tubal occlusion ~ 58615
with cesarean delivery ~ see occlusion ~ 58615
creat lesion ~ 58565, 58615
Tubal pregnancy ~ 59121
with salpingectomy and/or oophorectomy ~ 59120
Tube change tracheotomy ~ 31502
Tube placement
endoscopic
bile duct, pancreatic duct ~ 43268
nasobiliary, nasopancreatic for drainage ~ 43267
gastrostomy tube ~ 43750
nasogastric tube ~ 43752
orogastric tube ~ 43752
Tube, fallopian ~ see fallopian tube
Tubectomy ~ 58700, 58720
Tubed pedicle flap formation ~ 15570-15576
Tubercle bacilli culture ~ 87116
Tubercleplasty tibia, anterior ~ 27418
Tuberculin test ~ 85480
Tuberculosis
antigen response test ~ 0010T
culture ~ 87116
skin test ~ 86580-86585
Tuberculosis vaccine (BCG) ~ 90585-90586
Tubes
endotracheal ~ 31500
gastrostomy ~ 43246, 43750, 43760-43761
Tudor "rabbit ear" ~ see urethra, repair
Tuffier vaginal hysterectomy ~ 58260-58270, 58290-58294, 58550-58554
Tumor
abdomen, destruction/excision ~ 49200-49201
abdominal wall, excision ~ 22900
acetabulum, excision ~ 27076
ankle ~ 27615-27619
arm, lower ~ 25075-25077
arm, upper, excision ~ 24075-24077
back/flank
excision ~ 21930
radical resection ~ 21935
bile duct
destruction ~ 43272
extrahepatic ~ 47711
intrahepatic ~ 47712
bladder ~ 52234-52240
excision ~ 51530, 52355
bone, ablation ~ 20982
brain ~ 61510
excision ~ 61518, 61520-61521, 61526-61530, 61545, 62164
breast, excision ~ 19120-19126
bronchi, excision ~ 31640
calcaneus ~ 28100-28103
excision ~ 27647
carpal ~ 25130-25136
cheekbone ~ 21030, 21034
chest wall, excision ~ 19260-19272
clavicle excision ~ 23140, 23200
with allograft ~ 23146
with autograft ~ 23145
coccyx ~ 49215
colon, destruction ~ 44393, 45383
cranial bone, reconstruction ~ 21181-21184

Tumor ~ *continued*
destruction
chemosurgery ~ 17311-17315
urethra ~ 53220
ear, middle
extended ~ 69554
transcanal ~ 69550
transmastoid ~ 69552
elbow, excision ~ 24075-24077
esophagus, ablation ~ 43228
excision, femur ~ 27355-27358
facial bone ~ 21029-21030, 21034
fallopian tube, resection ~ 58950, 58952-58958
femoral ~ 27355-27358
femur ~ 27065-27067
excision ~ 27365
fibroid ~ 58140, 58545-58546, 58561
fibula ~ 27635-27638
excision ~ 27646
finger, excision ~ 26115-26117
foot ~ 28043-28046
forearm, radical resection ~ 25077
gastrostomy ~ see lesion
gums, excision ~ 41825-41827
hand, excision ~ 26115-26117
heart, excision ~ 33120-33130
hip ~ 27047-27049, 27065-27067
excision ~ 27075-27076
humerus excision ~ 23150, 23220-23222, 24110
with allograft ~ 23156, 24116
with autograft ~ 23155, 24115
ileum ~ 27065-27067
immunoassay for antigen ~ 86294, 86316
CA 125 ~ 86304
CA 15-3 ~ 86300
CA 19-9 ~ 86301
innominate, excision ~ 27077
intestines, small, destruction ~ 44369
ischial, excision ~ 27078-27079
kidney, excision ~ 50562, 52355
knee, excision ~ 27327-27329, 27365
lacrimal gland, excision
frontal approach ~ 68540
with osteotomy ~ 68550
larynx
excision ~ 31300
endoscopic ~ 31540-31541, 31578
incision ~ 31300
leg, lower ~ 27615-27619
leg, upper, excision ~ 27327-27329
localization, nuclear medicine ~ 78800-78804
mandible ~ 21044-21047
maxilla ~ 21030, 21034, 21048-21049
maxillary torus palatinus ~ 21032
mediastinal, excision ~ 39220
mediastinum ~ 32662
meningioma ~ 61512
excision ~ 61519
metacarpal ~ 26200-26205, 26250-26255
metatarsal ~ 28104-28107

Tumor ~ *continued*
excision ~ 28173
neck
excision ~ 21555-21556
radical resection ~ 21557
olecranon, excision ~ 24120
olecranon process
with allograft, excision ~ 24126
with autograft, excision ~ 24125
ovary, resection ~ 58950-58958
pancreatic duct, destruction ~ 43272
parotid gland, excision ~ 42410-42426
pelvis ~ 27047-27049
pericardial
endoscopic ~ 32661
excision ~ 33050
peritoneum, resection ~ 58950-58958
phalanges
finger ~ 26210-26215, 26260-26262
toe ~ 28108
excision ~ 28175
pituitary gland, excision ~ 61546-61548, 62165
positron emission tomography (PET) ~ 78811-78816
pubis ~ 27065-27067
pulmonary
ablation ~ 32998
radiation therapy ~ 77295
radius ~ 25120-25126, 25170
excision ~ 24120
with allograft, excision ~ 24126
with autograft, excision ~ 24125
rectum
destruction ~ 45190, 45320, 46937-46938
excision ~ 45160-45170
resection
face ~ 21015
scalp ~ 21015
with cystourethroscopy ~ 52355
retroperitoneal, destruction/excision ~ 49200-49201
sacrum ~ 49215
scapula
excision ~ 23140, 23210
with allograft ~ 23146
with autograft ~ 23145
shoulder, excision ~ 23075-23077
skull, excision ~ 61500
soft tissue
elbow, excision ~ 24075
finger, excision ~ 26115
forearm, radical resection ~ 25077
hand, excision ~ 26115
wrist
excision ~ 25075
radical resection ~ 25077
spinal cord, excision ~ 63275-63290
stomach, excision ~ 43610-43611
talus ~ 28100-28103
excision ~ 27647

Tumor ~ *continued*
tarsal ~ 28104-28107
excision ~ 28171
temporal bone, removal ~ 69970
testis, excision ~ 54530-54535
thorax
excision ~ 21555-21556
radical resection ~ 21557
thyroid, excision ~ 60200
tibia ~ 27365, 27635-27638
excision ~ 27645
torus mandibularis ~ 21031
trachea, excision
cervical ~ 31785
thoracic ~ 31786
ulna ~ 25120-25126, 25170
excision ~ 24120
with allograft, excision ~ 24126
with autograft, excision ~ 24125
ureter, excision ~ 52355
urethra ~ 52234-52240, 53220
excision ~ 52355
uterus
excision ~ 58140-58146
resection ~ 58950-58958
vagina, excision ~ 57135
vertebra, additional segment
excision ~ 22116
cervical, excision ~ 22100
lumbar ~ 22102
thoracic, excision ~ 22101
wrist ~ 25075-25077, 25135-25136
radical resection ~ 25077
Tunica vaginalis hydrocele
aspiration ~ 55000
excision ~ 55040-55041
repair ~ 55060
Turbinate
excision ~ 30130-30140
fracture, therapeutic ~ 30930
injection ~ 30200
submucous resection, nose excision ~ 30140
Turbinate mucosa cauterization ~ 30801-30802
Turcica, sella ~ 70240, 70480-70482
Turnbuckle jacket ~ 29020-29025
removal ~ 29715
TURP ~ 52612-52614
Tylectomy ~ *see* breast, excision, lesion
Tylenol urine ~ 82003
Tympanic membrane
create stoma ~ 69433-69436
incision ~ 69420-69421
reconstruction ~ 69620
repair ~ 69450, 69610
Tympanic nerve excision ~ 69676
Tympanolysis ~ 69450
Tympanomastoidectomy ~ see tympanoplasty
Tympanometry ~ see audiologic function tests ~ 92567
Tympanoplasty ~ 69620
radical or complete ~ 69645
with ossicular chain reconstruction ~ 69646
with antrotomy or mastoidotomy ~ 69635
with ossicular chain reconstruction ~ 69636
and synthetic prosthesis ~ 69637
with mastoidectomy ~ 69641
with intact or reconstructed wall ~ 69643
and ossicular chain reconstruction ~ 69644
with ossicular chain reconstruction ~ 69642
without mastoidectomy ~ 69631
with ossicular chain reconstruction ~ 69632
and synthetic prosthesis ~ 69633
Tympanostomy ~ 69433-69436
Tympanotomy ~ 69420-69421
Typhoid vaccine ~ 90690-90693
AKD ~ 90693
oral ~ 90690
polysaccharide ~ 90691
Typhus
endemic ~ 86000
mite-bone ~ 86000
Sno Paulo ~ 86000
tropical ~ 86000
Typing, blood ~ see blood typing
Typing, HLA ~ 86812-86817
Typing, tissue ~ see tissue typing
Tyrosine ~ 84510
Tzank smear ~ 87207

U

Uchida Procedure ~ 58600
UDP galactose pyrophosphorylase ~ 82775-82776
UFR ~ 51736-51741
Ulcer
anal ~ 46200, 46940-46942
decubitus ~ see debridement; skin graft and flap ~ 15920-15999
pinch graft ~ 15050
pressure ~ 15920-15999
stomach, excision ~ 43610
Ulcerative, cystitis ~ 52260-52265
Ulna ~ see arm, lower; elbow; humerus; radius
arthrodesis, radioulnar joint, with resection ~ 25830
arthroplasty, with implant ~ 25442
centralization or wrist ~ 25335
craterization ~ 24147, 25150-25151
cyst, excision ~ 24125-24126, 25120-25126
diaphysectomy ~ 24147, 25150-25151
excision ~ 24147
abscess ~ 24138
complete ~ 25240
epiphyseal bar ~ 20150
partial ~ 25145..2515, 1, 25240

Ulna ~ *continued*
fracture
closed treatment ~ 25530-25535
olecranon ~ 24670-24675
open treatment ~ 24685
open treatment ~ 25545
shaft ~ 25530-25545
open treatment ~ 25574
styloid
closed treatment ~ 25650
open treatment ~ 25652
percutaneous fixation ~ 25651
with dislocation
closed treatment ~ 24620
open treatment ~ 24635
with manipulation ~ 25535
with radius ~ 25560-25565
open treatment ~ 25575
without manipulation ~ 25530
incision and drainage ~ 25035
osteoplasty ~ 25390-25393
prophylactic treatment ~ 25491-25492
reconstruction, radioulnar ~ 25337
repair
epiphyseal arrest ~ 25450-25455
malunion or nonunion ~ 25400, 25415
osteotomy ~ 25360, 25370-25375
and radius ~ 25365
with graft ~ 25405, 25420-25426
saucerization ~ 24147, 25150-25151
sequestrectomy ~ 24138, 25145
tumor
cyst ~ 24120
excision ~ 24125-24126, 25120-25126, 25170
Ulnar arteries ~ see artery, ulnar
Ulnar nerve
decompression ~ 64718
neuroplasty ~ 64718-64719
reconstruction ~ 64718-64719
release ~ 64718-64719
repair/suture, motor ~ 64836
transposition ~ 64718-64719
Ultrasonic ~ see ultrasound
Ultrasonic cardiography ~ see echocardiography
Ultrasonic procedure ~ 52325
Ultrasonography ~ see echography
Ultrasound ~ see echocardiography; echography
abdomen ~ 76700-76705
arm ~ 76880
artery
intracranial ~ 93886-93893
middle cerebral ~ 76821
umbilical ~ 76820
bladder ~ 51798
bone density study ~ 76977
breast ~ 76645
bronchi, endoscopy ~ 31620
chest ~ 76604
colon, endoscopic ~ 45391-45392
colon-sigmoid, endoscopic ~ 45341-45342

Ultrasound ~ *continued*
drainage, abscess ~ 75989
echoencephalography ~ 76506
esophagus, endoscopy ~ 43231-43232
eye ~ 76510-76513
arteries ~ 93875
biometry ~ 76516-76519
foreign body ~ 76529
pachymetry ~ 76514
fetus ~ 76818-76828
follow-up ~ 76970
for physical therapy ~ 97035
gastrointestinal ~ 76975
gastrointestinal, upper, endoscopic ~ 43237-43238, 43242, 43259
guidance
amniocentesis ~ 59001, 76946
amnioinfusion ~ 59070
arteriovenous fistulae ~ 76936
chorionic villus sampling ~ 76945
cryosurgery ~ 55873
drainage, fetal fluid ~ 59074
endometrial ablation ~ 58356
fetal cordocentesis ~ 76941
fetal transfusion ~ 76941
heart biopsy ~ 76932
needle biopsy ~ 43232, 43238, 43242, 45342, 45392, 76942
occlusion, umbilical cord ~ 59072
ova retrieval ~ 76948
pericardiocentesis ~ 76930
pseudoaneurysm ~ 76936
radiation therapy ~ 76950
radioelement ~ 76965
shunt placement, fetal ~ 59076
thoracentesis ~ 76942
tissue ablation ~ 76490
vascular access ~ 76937
head ~ 76506, 76536
heart, fetal ~ 76825
hips, infant ~ 76885-76886
hysteronsonography ~ 76831
intraoperative ~ 76998
intravascular, intraoperative ~ 37250-37251
kidney ~ 76770-76776
leg ~ 76880
neck ~ 76536
non-coronary, intravascular ~ 75945-75946
pelvis ~ 76856-76857
pregnant uterus ~ 76801-76817
prostate ~ 76873
rectal ~ 76872-76873
retroperitoneal ~ 76770-76775
scrotum ~ 76870
sonohysterography ~ 76831
spine ~ 76800
stimulation to aid bone healing ~ 20979
umbilical artery ~ 76820
unlisted services and procedures ~ 76999
uterus, tumor ablation ~ 0071T-0072T
vagina ~ 76830

Ultraviolet light therapy dermatology
ultraviolet A ~ 96912
ultraviolet B ~ 96910
for dermatology ~ 96900
for physical medicine ~ 97028
Umbilectomy ~ 49250
Umbilical
artery ultrasound ~ 76820
hernia ~ 49600-49611
vein catheterization ~ 36510
Umbilical cord occlusion ~ 59072
Umbilicus
excision ~ 49250
repair
hernia ~ 49580-49587
omphalocele ~ 49600-49611
Undescended testicle ~ 54550-54560
Unfertilized egg ~ 87177
Unguis ~ see nails
Unilateral simple mastectomy ~ see mastectomy
Unlisted services and procedures ~ **99499, 99600**
abdomen ~ 22999, 49329, 49999
allergy/immunology ~ 95199
anal ~ 46999
anesthesia ~ 01999
arm ~ 25999
arthroscopy ~ 29999
autopsy ~ 88099
bile duct ~ 47999
brachytherapy ~ 77799
breast ~ 19499
bronchi ~ 31899
cardiac ~ 33999
cardiovascular studies ~ 93799
casting ~ 29799
cervix ~ 58999
chemistry procedure ~ 84999
chemotherapy ~ 96549
chest ~ 32999
coagulation ~ 85999
colon ~ 44799
conjunctiva surgery ~ 68399
craniofacial ~ 21299
CT scan ~ 76497
cytogenetic study ~ 88299
cytopathology ~ 88199
pdermatology ~ 96999
dialysis ~ 90999
diaphragm ~ 39599
ear, external ~ 69399
inner ~ 69949
middle ~ 69799
endocrine system ~ 60699
epididymis ~ 55899
esophagus ~ 43289, 43499
evaluation and management services ~ 99499
eye muscle ~ 67399
eye surgery
anterior segment ~ 66999
posterior segment ~ 67299

Unlisted services and procedures ~ *continued*
eyelid ~ 67999
fluoroscopy ~ 76496
forearm ~ 25999
gallbladder ~ 47999
gastroenterology test ~ 91299
gum ~ 41899
hand ~ 26989
hemic system ~ 38999
hepatic duct ~ 47999
hip joint ~ 27299
home services ~ 99600
hysteroscopy ~ 58579
immunization ~ 90749
immunology ~ 86849
injection ~ 90799
injection of medication ~ 90799
intestine ~ 44238, 44799
kidney ~ 49659
lacrimal system ~ 68899
laparoscopy ~ 38129, 38589, 43289, 43659, 44238-44239, 44979, 47379, 47579, 49329, 49659, 50549, 50949, 54699, 55559, 58578, 58679, 59898, 60659
larynx ~ 31599
lip ~ 40799
liver ~ 47379, 47399
lungs ~ 32999
lymphatic system ~ 38999
magnetic resonance ~ 76498
maxillofacial ~ 21299
maxillofacial prosthetics ~ 21089
Meckel's diverticulum ~ 44899
mediastinum ~ 39499
mesentery surgery ~ 44899
microbiology ~ 87999
mouth ~ 40899, 41599
musculoskeletal ~ 25999, 26989
musculoskeletal surgery, abdominal wall ~ 22999
neck ~ 21899
spine ~ 22899
thorax ~ 21899
musculoskeletal system ~ 20999
ankle ~ 27899
arm, upper ~ 24999
elbow ~ 24999
head ~ 21499
knee ~ 27599
leg, lower ~ 27899
leg, upper ~ 27599
necropsy ~ 88099
nervous system surgery ~ 64999
neurology/neuromuscular testing ~ 95999
nose ~ 30999
nuclear medicine ~ 78999
blood ~ 78199
bone ~ 78399
endocrine system ~ 78099
genitourinary system ~ 78799
heart ~ 78499
hematopoietic system ~ 78199

Unlisted services and procedures ~ *continued*
lymphatic system ~ 78199
musculoskeletal system ~ 78399
nervous system ~ 78699
therapeutic ~ 79999
obstetrical care ~ 59898-59899
omentum ~ 49329, 49999
ophthalmology ~ 92499
orbit ~ 67599
otorhinolaryngology ~ 92700
ovary ~ 58679, 58999
oviduct ~ 58679, 58999
palate ~ 42299
pancreas surgery ~ 48999
pathology ~ 89240
pelvis ~ 27299
penis ~ 55899
peritoneum ~ 49329, 49999
pharynx ~ 42999
physical therapy ~ 97039, 97139, 97799
pleura ~ 32999
pressure ulcer ~ 15999
preventive medicine ~ 99429
prostate ~ 55899
psychiatric ~ 90899
pulmonology ~ 94799
radiation physics ~ 77399
radiation therapy ~ 77499
planning ~ 77299
radiology, diagnostic ~ 76499
radionuclide therapy ~ 79999
radiopharmaceutical therapy ~ 79999
rectum ~ 44239, 45999
salivary gland ~ 42699
scrotum ~ 55899
seminal vesicle ~ 55899
shoulder surgery ~ 23929
sinuses ~ 31299
skin ~ 17999
special services and reports ~ 99199
spine ~ 22899
stomach ~ 43659, 43999
strapping ~ 29799
surgical pathology ~ 88399
temporal bone ~ 69979
testis ~ 54699, 55899
throat ~ 42999
tongue ~ 41599
tonsil/adenoid ~ 42999
trachea ~ 31899
transfusion ~ 86999
ultrasound ~ 76999
ureter ~ 50949
urinary system ~ 53899
uterus ~ 58578-58579, 58999
uvula ~ 42299
vagina ~ 58999
vas deferens ~ 55899
vascular ~ 37799
vascular endoscopy ~ 37501
vascular injection ~ 36299

Unlisted services and procedures ~ *continued*
vascular studies ~ 93799
wrist ~ 25999
Unna paste boot ~ 29580
removal ~ 29700
UPP ~ 51772
Upper
digestive system endoscopy ~ see endoscopy, gastrointestinal, upper
extremity ~ see arm, upper; elbow; humerus
gastrointestinal bleeding ~ 43255
gastrointestinal endoscopy, biopsy ~ 43239
planning ~ 43239
GI tract ~ 43249
Urachal cyst ~ 51500
Urea breath test ~ 78267-78268, 83014
Urea nitrogen ~ 84520-84525
clearance ~ 84545
quantitative ~ 84520
semiquantitative ~ 84525
urine ~ 84540
Urea nitrogen, blood ~ 84520-84525
Urecholine supersensitivity test ~ 51725-51726
Ureter
anastomosis
to bladder ~ 50780-50785
to colon ~ 50810-50815
to intestine ~ 50800, 50820-50825
to kidney ~ 50740-50750
to ureter ~ 50760-50770
biopsy ~ 50955-50957, 50974-50976, 52007
catheterization ~ 52005
continent diversion ~ 50825
creation, stoma ~ 50860
destruction
endoscopic ~ 50957, 50976
dilation ~ 52341-52342, 52344-52345
endoscopic ~ 50553, 50572, 50953, 50972
endoscopy
biopsy ~ 50955-50957, 50974-50976, 52007, 52354
catheterization ~ 50953, 50972, 52005
destruction ~ 50957, 50976, 52354
dilation ~ 52341-52342, 52344-52345
excision, tumor ~ 52355
exploration ~ 52351
injection of implant material ~ 52327
insertion, stent ~ 50947, 52332-52334
lithotripsy ~ 52353
tmanipulation of ureteral calculus ~ 52330
removal
calculus ~ 50961, 50980, 52320-52325, 52352
foreign body ~ 50961, 50980
resection ~ 52355
via incision ~ 50970-50980
via stoma ~ 50951-50961
exploration ~ 50600
incision and drainage ~ 50600
injection, radiologic ~ 50684, 50690

Ureter ~ *continued*
insertion
catheter ~ 50393
stent ~ 50393, 50947, 52332-52334
tube ~ 50688
instillation, drugs ~ 50391
lesion, destruction ~ 52354
lithotripsy ~ 52353
lysis, adhesions ~ 50715-50725
manometric studies, pressure ~ 50686
meatotomy ~ 52290
nuclear medicine, reflux study ~ 78740
postcaval ~ 50725
reconstruction ~ 50700
with intestines ~ 50840
reflux study ~ 78740
reimplantation ~ 51565
removal
anastomosis ~ 50830
calculus ~ 50610-50630, 50961, 51060-51065, 52320-52325
foreign body ~ 50961
repair ~ 50900
anastomosis ~ 50740-50825
continent diversion ~ 50825
deligation ~ 50940
fistula ~ 50920-50930
lysis adhesions ~ 50715-50725
ureterocele ~ 51535
ectopic ~ 52301
orthotopic ~ 52300
urinary undiversion ~ 50830
replacement, with intestines ~ 50840
resection ~ 52355
revision, anastomosis ~ 50727-50728
suture ~ 50900
deligation ~ 50940
fistula ~ 50920-50930
tube
change ~ 50688
insertion ~ 50688
tumor resection ~ 52355
unlisted services and procedures ~ 50949, 53899
X-ray with contrast
guide catheter ~ 74480
guide dilation ~ 74485
Ureteral
catheterization ~ see catheterization, ureter
guide wire insertion ~ 52334
meatotomy ~ 52290
splinting ~ 50400-50405
stent insertion ~ 52332
Ureterectomy ~ 50650-50660
partial ~ 50220, 50546
total ~ 50548
Ureterocalycostomy ~ 50750
Ureterocele
excision ~ 51535
fulguration
ectopic ~ 52301
orthotopic ~ 52300
Ureterocele ~ *continued*
incision ~ 51535
repair ~ 51535
resection, ectopic ~ 52301
orthotopic ~ 52300
Ureterocolon conduit ~ 50815
Ureteroenterostomy ~ 50800
revision ~ 50830
Ureterography injection procedure ~ 50684
Ureteroileal conduit ~ 50820
cystectomy ~ 51590
removal ~ 50830
Ureterolithotomy ~ 50610-50630
laparoscopy ~ 50945
transvesical ~ 51060
Ureterolysis
for ovarian vein syndrome ~ 50722
for retrocaval ureter ~ 50725
for retroperitoneal fibrosis ~ 50715
Ureteroneocystostomy ~ 50780-50785, 50830, 51565
laparoscopic ~ 50947-50948
Ureteroplasty ~ 50700
Ureteropyelography ~ 50951, 52005
injection procedure ~ 50684, 50690
Ureteropyelostomy ~ 50740
Ureteroscopy
dilation
intra-renal stricture ~ 52346
ureter ~ 52344-52345
third stage with cystourethroscopy ~ 52351
biopsy ~ 52354
destruction ~ 52354
lithotripsy ~ 52353
removal, calculus ~ 52352
tumor excision ~ 52355
Ureterosigmoidostomy ~ 50810
revision ~ 50830
Ureterostomy ~ 50860, 50951
injection procedure ~ 50684
manometric studies ~ 50686
Ureterostomy tube change ~ 50688
Ureterotomy ~ 50600
insertion indwelling stent ~ 50605
Ureteroureterostomy ~ 50760-50770, 50830
Urethra
abscess, incision and drainage ~ 53040
adhesions, lysis ~ 53500
artificial sphincter, repair ~ 53449
biopsy ~ 52204, 53200
destruction ~ 52214-52224
dilation ~ 52260-52265, 53600-53621
general ~ 53665
suppository and/or instillation ~ 53660-53661
diverticulum ~ 53240
drainage, extravasation ~ 53080-53085
endoscopy ~ 52000
biopsy ~ 52204, 52354
catheterization ~ 52010
destruction ~ 52354, 52400
evacuation, clot ~ 52001

Urethra ~ *continued*
endoscopy ~ *continued*
excision, tumor ~ 52355
exploration ~ 52351
incision, ejaculatory duct ~ 52402
injection of implant material ~ 51715
lithotripsy ~ 52353
removal, calculus ~ 52352
resection, ejaculatory duct ~ 52402
vasectomy ~ 52402
vasotomy ~ 52402
excision
diverticulum ~ 53230-53235
total
female ~ 53210
male ~ 53215
incision ~ 53000-53010
meatus ~ 53020-53025
incision and drainage ~ 53060
insertion, stent ~ 0084T, 52282
lesion
destruction ~ 53265
excision ~ 53260
paraurethral gland, incision and drainage ~ 53060
polyp
destruction ~ 53260
excision ~ 53260
pressure profile ~ 51772
prolapse
destruction ~ 53275
excision ~ 53275
repair ~ 53275
prostate, transurethral balloon dilation ~ 52510
radiotracer ~ 52250
reconstruction ~ 53410-53440, 53445
and bladder ~ 51800-51820
complications ~ 54340-54348
hypospadias
one stage ~ 54322-54328
second stage ~ 54308-54316
third stage ~ 54318
meatus ~ 53450-53460
removal
calculus ~ 52310-52315
foreign body ~ 52310-52315
sling ~ 53442
urethral stent ~ 52310-52315
repair
diverticulum ~ 53240, 53400-53405
fistula ~ 45820-45825, 53400-53405, 53520
sphincter ~ 57220
stricture ~ 53400-53405
urethrocele ~ 57230
wound ~ 53502-53515
Skene's gland, incision and drainage ~ 53060
sphincter ~ 52277
electromyography ~ 51784-51785
needle ~ 51785
insertion, prosthesis ~ 53444
reconstruction ~ 53445
removal, prosthesis ~ 53446-53447

Urethra ~ *continued*
sphincter ~ *continued*
repair, prosthesis ~ 53449
replacement, prosthesis ~ 53448
suture
fistula ~ 45820-45825, 53520
to bladder ~ 51840-51841
wound ~ 53502-53515
tumor
destruction ~ 53220
excision ~ 53220
unlisted services and procedures ~ 53899
urethrocystography ~ 74450-74455
urethrotomy ~ 52270-52276
X-ray with contrast ~ 74450-74455
Urethral
diverticulum
marsupialization ~ 53240
meatus, dorsal ~ see epispadias
sphincter
biofeedback training ~ 90911
insertion, prosthesis ~ 53444
removal, prosthesis ~ 53446-53447
replacement, prosthesis ~ 53448
stenosis, dilation ~ 52281
stent
insertion ~ 0084T, 52282
removal
bladder ~ 52310-52315
urethra ~ 52310-52315
stricture
dilation ~ 52281, 53600-53621
injection, steroids ~ 52283
syndrome, cystourethroscopy ~ 52285
Urethrectomy total
female ~ 53210
male ~ 53215
Urethrocele ~ 53275
Urethrocystography ~ 74450-74455
contrast and/or chain ~ 51605
retrograde ~ 51610
voiding ~ 51600
Urethrocystopexy ~ 51840-51841
Urethromeatoplasty ~ 53450-53460
Urethropexy ~ 51840-51841
Urethroplasty ~ 46744-46746
first stage ~ 53400
one stage, hypospadias ~ 54322-54328
reconstruction
female urethra ~ 53430
male anterior urethra ~ 53410
prostatic/membranous urethra
first stage ~ 53420
one stage ~ 53415
second stage ~ 53425
second stage ~ 53405
hypospadias ~ 54308-54316
third stage, hypospadias ~ 54318
Urethrorrhaphy ~ 53502-53515
Urethroscopy ~ 52000
Urethrostomy ~ 53000-53010

Urethrotomy ~ 53000-53010
direct vision, with cystourethroscopy ~ 52276
internal ~ 52601, 52647-52648
with cystourethroscopy
female ~ 52270
male ~ 52275
Uric acid
blood ~ 84550
other source ~ 84560
urine ~ 84560
Uridyltransferase, galactose-1-phosphate ~ 82775-82776
Uridylyltransferase, galactosephosphate ~ 82775-82776
Urinalysis ~ 0041T, 81000-81099
automated ~ 81001, 81003
glass test ~ 81020
microalbumin ~ 82043-82044
microscopic ~ 81015
pregnancy test ~ 81025
qualitative ~ 81005
routine ~ 81002
screen ~ 81007
semiquantitative ~ 0041T, 81005
unlisted services and procedures ~ 81099
volume measurement ~ 81050
without microscopy ~ 81002
Urinary bladder ~ see bladder
Urinary catheter irrigation ~ 62194, 62225
Urinary concentration test ~ 89235
Urinary sphincter, artificial ~ 53444-53449
Urinary system, surgical procedures ~ 50010-53899
Urinary tract X-ray with contrast ~ 74400-74425
Urine
albumin ~ 82042-82044
blood ~ 83491
colony count ~ 87086
pregnancy test ~ 81025
tests ~ 81001
Urobilinogen
feces ~ 84577
urine ~ 84578-84583
Urodynamic tests
bladder capacity, ultrasound ~ 51798
cystometrogram ~ 51725-51726
electromyography studies, needle ~ 51785
residual urine, ultrasound ~ 51798
stimulus evoked response ~ 51792
urethra pressure profile ~ 51772
uroflowmetry ~ 51736-51741
voiding pressure studies
bladder ~ 51795
intra-abdominal ~ 51797
Uroflowmetry ~ 51736-51741
Urography
antegrade ~ 74425
infusion ~ 74410-74415
intravenous ~ 74400-74415
retrograde ~ 74420
Uroporphyrin ~ 84120
Urothromboplastin ~ see thromboplastin
Uterine
adhesion ~ 58559
cervix ~ see cervix
endoscopies ~ see endoscopy, uterus
haemorrhage ~ 59160
Uterus, ablation
endometrium ~ 58353-58356
tumor, ultrasound, focused ~ 0071T-0072T
biopsy
endometrium ~ 58100
endoscopic ~ 58558
catheterization, X-ray ~ 58340
chromotubation ~ 58350
curettage ~ 58356
postpartum ~ 59160
dilation and curettage ~ 58120
postpartum ~ 59160
ectopic pregnancy
interstitial
partial resection uterus ~ 59136
total hysterectomy ~ 59135
endoscopy
endometrial ablation ~ 58563
exploration ~ 58555
surgery ~ 58558-58565
treatment ~ 58558-58565
excision
laparoscopic ~ 58541-58544, 58550
partial ~ 58180
radical ~ 58210, 58285
removal of tubes and/or ovaries ~ 58262-58263, 58291-58293, 58552, 58554
total ~ 58150-58152, 58200, 58953-58956
vaginal ~ 58260-58270, 58290-58294, 58550-58554
with colpectomy ~ 58275-58280
with colpo-urethrocystopexy ~ 58267
with repair of enterocele ~ 58270, 58294
hemorrhage, postpartum ~ 59160
hydatidiform mole, excision ~ 59100
hydrotubation ~ 58350
hysterosalpingography ~ 74740
incision, removal lesion ~ 59100
insertion
Heyman capsule, for brachytherapy ~ 58346
intrauterine device (IUD) ~ 58300
tandem, for brachytherapy ~ 57155
laparoscopy ~ 58578
lesion, excision ~ 58545-58546, 59100
reconstruction ~ 58540
removal, intrauterine device (IUD) ~ 58301
repair
fistula ~ 51920-51925
rupture ~ 58520, 59350
suspension ~ 58400
with presacral sympathectomy ~ 58410
sonohysterography ~ 76831
suture, rupture ~ 59350

Uterus, ablation ~ *continued*
tumor
ablation
ultrasound, focused ~ 0071T-0072T
excision
abdominal approach ~ 58140, 58146
vaginal approach ~ 58145
unlisted services and procedures ~ 58578, 58999
X-ray with contrast ~ 74740
UTP hexose 1 phosphate uridylyltransferase ~ 82775-82776
UV light therapy ~ 96900
Uvula
abscess, incision and drainage ~ 42000
biopsy ~ 42100
excision ~ 42140-42145
lesion
destruction ~ 42145
excision ~ 42104-42107
unlisted services and procedures ~ 42299
Uvulectomy ~ 42140

V

V flap procedure one stage distal hypospadias repair ~ 54322
V, cranial nerve ~ see trigeminal nerve
V-Y operation, bladder, neck ~ 51845
V-Y plasty ~ 14000-14350
Vaccination ~ see allergen immunotherapy; immunization; vaccines
Vaccines and toxoids ~ 90476-90749
adenovirus ~ 90476-90477
anthrax ~ 90581
chicken pox ~ 90716
cholera, injectable ~ 90725
diphtheria toxoid ~ 90719
diphtheria, tetanus (DT) ~ 90702
diphtheria, tetanus, acellular pertussis (DTAP) ~ 90700
diphtheria, tetanus, acellular pertussis and hemophilus influenza B (HIB) (DTAP-HIB) ~ 90721
diphtheria, tetanus, acellular pertussis, haemophilus influenza type B, and inactivated poliovirus (DTAP-HIB-IPV) ~ 90698
diphtheria, tetanus, acellular pertussis, hepatitis B, and inactivated poliovirus (DTAP-HepB-IPV) ~ 90723
diphtheria, tetanus, and acellular pertussis (TDAP) ~ 90715
diphtheria, tetanus, whole cell pertussis (DTP) ~ 90701
diphtheria, tetanus, whole cell pertussis and hemophilus influenza B (HIB) (DTP-HIB) ~ 90720
encephalitis, Japanese ~ 90735

Vaccines and toxoids ~ *continued*
hemophilus influenza B ~ 90645-90648
hepatitis A ~ 90632-90634
hepatitis A and hepatitis B ~ 90636
hepatitis B ~ 90740-90747
hepatitis B and hemophilus influenza B (HepB-HIB) ~ 90748
influenza ~ 90655-90660
Lyme disease ~ 90665
measles ~ 90705
measles and rubella ~ 90708
measles, mumps and rubella (MMR) ~ 90707
measles, mumps and rubella and varicella (MMRV) ~ 90710
meningococcal ~ 90733-90734
mumps ~ 90704
plague ~ 90727
pneumococcal ~ 90669, 90732
poliovirus, inactivated, subcutaneous ~ 90713
poliovirus, live, oral ~ 90712
rabies ~ 90675-90676
rotavirus ~ 90680
rubella ~ 90706
tetanus and diphtheria ~ 90718
tetanus toxoid ~ 90703
tetanus, diphtheria, and acellular pertussis (TDAP) ~ 90715
tuberculosis (BCG) ~ 90585-90586
typhoid ~ 90690-90693
unlisted vaccine/toxoid ~ 90749
varicella (chicken pox) ~ 90716
yellow fever ~ 90717
Vagina
abscess, incision and drainage ~ 57010
amines test ~ 82120
biopsy
colposcopy ~ 57421
endocervical ~ 57454
extensive ~ 57105
simple ~ 57100
closure ~ 57120
colposcopy ~ 57420-57421, 57455-57456, 57461
construction
without graft ~ 57291
with graft ~ 57292
cyst, excision ~ 57135
dilation ~ 57400
endocervical
biopsy ~ 57454
exploration ~ 57452
excision
closure ~ 57120
complete
with removal of paravaginal tissue ~ 57111
with removal of paravaginal tissue with lymphadenectomy ~ 57112
with removal of vaginal wall ~ 57110
partial
with removal of paravaginal tissue ~ 57107

Vagina ~ *continued*
excision ~ *continued*
with removal of paravaginal tissue with lymphadenectomy ~ 57109
with removal of vaginal wall ~ 57106
total ~ 57110
with hysterectomy ~ 58275-58280
with repair of enterocele ~ 58280
exploration
endocervical ~ 57452
incision ~ 57000
hematoma, incision and drainage ~ 57022-57023
hemorrhage ~ 57180
hysterectomy ~ 58290, 58550-58554
incision and drainage ~ 57020
insertion
ovoid, for brachytherapy ~ 57155
packing for bleeding ~ 57180
pessary ~ 57160
sensor, fetal oximetry ~ 0021T
irrigation ~ 57150
lesion
destruction ~ 57061-57065
extensive ~ 57065
simple ~ 57061
prolapse, sacrospinous ligament fixation ~ 57282
removal
foreign body ~ 57415
sling, stress incontinence ~ 57287
repair ~ 56800
cystocele ~ 57240, 57260
combined anteroposterior ~ 57260-57265
posterior ~ 57240
enterocele ~ 57265
fistula ~ 51900
rectovaginal ~ 57300-57308
transvesical and vaginal approach ~ 57330
urethrovaginal ~ 57310-57311
vesicovaginal ~ 51900, 57320-57330
hysterectomy ~ 58267, 58293
incontinence ~ 57284, 57288
obstetric ~ 59300
paravaginal defect ~ 57284
Pereyra Procedure ~ 57289
prolapse ~ 57282-57284
rectocele
combined anteroposterior ~ 57260-57265
posterior ~ 57250
prosthesis insertion ~ 57267
suspension ~ 57280-57283
laparoscopic ~ 57425
urethral sphincter ~ 57220
wound ~ 57200-57210
colpoperineorrhaphy ~ 57210
colporrhaphy ~ 57200
revision
sling
stress incontinence ~ 57287
septum, excision ~ 57130

Vagina ~ *continued*
suspension ~ 57280-57283
laparoscopic ~ 57425
suture
cystocele ~ 57240, 57260
enterocele ~ 57265
fistula ~ 51900, 57300-57330
rectocele ~ 57250-57260
wound ~ 57200-57210
tumor, excision ~ 57135
ultrasound ~ 76830
unlisted services and procedures ~ 58999
X-ray with contrast ~ 74775
Vaginal delivery ~ 59400, 59610-59614
after previous cesarean delivery ~ 59610-59612
attempted ~ 59618-59622
antepartum care ~ 59400
cesarean delivery after attempted ~ 59618
delivery only ~ 59620
postpartum care ~ 59622
delivery after previous, vaginal delivery only, postpartum care ~ 59614
delivery only ~ 59409
external cephalic version ~ 59412
placenta ~ 59414
postpartum care ~ 59410
routine care ~ 59400
Vaginal hysterectomy ~ 58552-58554
Vaginal smear ~ 88141-88155, 88164-88167, 88174-88175
Vaginal suppositories
induced abortion ~ 59855
with dilation and curettage ~ 59856
with hysterectomy ~ 59857
Vaginectomy ~ see colpectomy
Vaginoplasty intersex state ~ 57335
Vaginorrhaphy ~ see colporrhaphy
Vaginoscopy
biopsy ~ 57454
exploration ~ 57452
Vaginotomy ~ see colpotomy
Vagotomy
abdominal ~ 64760
highly selective ~ 43641
parietal cell ~ 43641, 64755
selective ~ 43640
transthoracic ~ 64752
truncal ~ 43640
with gastroduodenostomy revision, reconstruction ~ 43855
with gastrojejunostomy revision, reconstruction ~ 43865
with partial distal gastrectomy ~ 43635
Vagus nerve
avulsion
abdominal ~ 64760
selective ~ 64755
thoracic ~ 64752
incision ~ 43640-43641
abdominal ~ 64760
selective ~ 64755

Vagus nerve ~ *continued*
incision ~ *continued*
thoracic ~ 64752
injection, anesthetic ~ 64408
transection ~ 43640-43641
abdominal ~ 64760
selective ~ 43652, 64755
thoracic ~ 64752
truncal ~ 43651
Valentine's test ~ 81020
Valproic acid ~ 80164
Valproic acid measurement ~ 80164
Valsalva sinus ~ 33702-33722
Valva atrioventricularis sinistra (valva mitralis) ~ see mitral valve
Valve
aortic ~ 33405-33414
bicuspid ~ see mitral valve
mitral ~ see mitral valve
pulmonary ~ 33470-33475
tricuspid ~ 33460, 33463-33465, 33468
Valve stenoses, aortic ~ 33415, 33417
Valvectomy tricuspid valve ~ 33460
Valvotomy
mitral valve ~ 33420-33422
pulmonary valve ~ 33470-33474
reoperation ~ 33530
Valvuloplasty
aortic valve ~ 33400-33403
femoral vein ~ 34501
mitral valve ~ 33425-33427
percutaneous balloon
aortic valve ~ 92986
mitral valve ~ 92987
pulmonary valve ~ 92990
prosthetic valve ~ 33496
reoperation ~ 33530
tricuspid valve ~ 33463-33465
Van Deen test ~ 82270, 82272
Van Den Bergh test ~ 82247-82248
Vancomycin assay ~ 80202
Vanillylmandelic acid urine ~ 84585
Vanilmandelic acid ~ 84585
Varicella (chicken pox) ~ 90716
Varicella-zoster
antibody ~ 86787
antigen detection, direct fluorescence ~ 87290
Varices esophageal ~ 43205, 43400-43401
Varicocele spermatic cord, excision ~ 55530-55540
Varicose vein
ablation ~ 36475-36479
removal ~ 37720-37730, 37765-37785
secondary varicosity ~ 37785
with tissue excision ~ 37735-37760
Vas deferens
anastomosis
to epididymis ~ 54900-54901
excision ~ 55250
incision ~ 55200
for X-ray ~ 55300
ligation ~ 55450
Vas deferens ~ *continued*
repair, suture ~ 55400
unlisted services and procedures ~ 55899
vasography ~ 74440
X-ray with contrast ~ 74440
Vascular flow check, graft ~ 15860
Vascular injection unlisted services and procedures ~ 36299
Vascular lesion
cranial, excision ~ 61600-61608, 61615-61616
cutaneous, destruction ~ 17106-17108
Vascular malformation
cerebral, repair ~ 61710
finger, excision ~ 26115
hand, excision ~ 26115
Vascular procedure(s)
angioscopy, non-coronary vessels ~ 35400
brachytherapy, intracoronary artery ~ 92974
endoscopy, surgical ~ 37500
harvest, lower extremity vein ~ 35572
intravascular ultrasound
coronary vessels ~ 92978-92979
non-coronary vessels ~ 75945-75946
stent, intracoronary ~ 92980-92981
thrombolysis
coronary vessels ~ 92975-92977
cranial vessels ~ 37195
Vascular rehabilitation ~ 93668
Vascular studies ~ see Doppler scan, duplex, plethysmography
angioscopy, non-coronary vessels ~ 35400
aorta ~ 93978-93979
arterial studies (non-invasive)
extracranial ~ 93875-93882
extremities ~ 93922-93924
intracranial ~ 93886-93891
lower extremity ~ 93925-93926
middle cerebral artery, fetal ~ 76821
umbilical artery, fetal ~ 76820
artery studies, upper extremity ~ 93930-93931
blood pressure monitoring, 24 hour ~ 93784-93790
cardiac catheterization, imaging ~ 93555-93556
hemodialysis access ~ 93990
kidney
multiple study, with pharmacological intervention ~ 78709
single study, with pharmacological intervention ~ 78708
penile vessels ~ 93980-93981
plethysmography, total body ~ 93720-93722
temperature gradient ~ 93740
thermogram
cephalic ~ 93760
peripheral ~ 93762
unlisted services and procedures ~ 93799
venous studies
extremity ~ 93965-93971
venous pressure ~ 93770
visceral studies ~ 93975-93979

Vascular surgery
arm, upper, anesthesia ~ 01770-01782
elbow, anesthesia ~ 01770-01782
endoscopy ~ 37500
unlisted services and procedures ~ 37799
Vasectomy ~ 55250
contact laser vaporization with/without transurethral resection, of prostate ~ 52648
non-contact laser coagulation of prostate ~ 52647
reversal ~ 55400
transurethral, cystourethroscopic ~ 52402
transurethral electrosurgical resection of prostate ~ 52601, 52648
Vasoactive drugs injection, penis ~ 54231
Vasoactive intestinal peptide ~ 84586
Vasogram ~ 74440
Vasography ~ 74440
Vasointestinal peptide ~ 84586
Vasopneumatic device therapy ~ see physical medicine/therapy/occupational therapy ~ 97016
Vasopressin ~ 84588
Vasotomy ~ 55200, 55300
transurethral, cystourethroscopic ~ 52402
Vasovasorrhaphy ~ 55400
Vasovasostomy ~ 55400
VATS ~ see thoracoscopy
VDRL ~ 86592-86593
Vein
ablation, endovenous ~ 36475-36479
adrenal, venography ~ 75840-75842
anastomosis
caval to mesenteric ~ 37160
intrahepatic portosystemic ~ 37182-37183
portocaval ~ 37140
reniportal ~ 37145
saphenopopliteal ~ 34530
splenorenal ~ 37180-37181
to vein ~ 37140-37160, 37182-37183
angioplasty ~ 75978
transluminal ~ 35460
arm
harvest of vein for bypass graft ~ 35500
venography ~ 75820-75822
axillary, thrombectomy ~ 34490
biopsy, transcatheter ~ 75970
cannulization
to artery ~ 36810-36815
to vein ~ 36800
catheterization
central insertion ~ 36555-36558
organ blood ~ 36500
peripheral insertion ~ 36568-36569
removal ~ 36589
repair ~ 36575
replacement ~ 36578-36581, 36584
umbilical ~ 36510
endoscopic harvest, for bypass graft ~ 33508
external cannula, declotting ~ 36860-36861
extremity, non-invasive studies ~ 93965-93971
femoral, repair ~ 34501

Vein ~ *continued*
femoropopliteal, thrombectomy ~ 34421-34451
guidance
fluoroscopic ~ 77001
ultrasound ~ 76937
hepatic portal
splenoportography ~ 75810
venography ~ 75885-75887
iliac, thrombectomy ~ 34401-34451
injection, sclerosing agent ~ 36468-36471
insertion, IVC filter ~ 75940
interrupt
femoral ~ 37650
iliac ~ 37660
vena cava ~ 37620
jugular, venography ~ 75860
leg
harvest for vascular reconstruction ~ 35572
venography ~ 75820-75822
ligation
clusters ~ 37785
esophagus ~ 43205
jugular ~ 37565
perforation ~ 37760
saphenous ~ 37700-37735, 37780
secondary ~ 37785
liver, venography ~ 75889-75891
neck, venography ~ 75860
nuclear medicine, thrombosis imaging ~ 78455-78458
orbit, venography ~ 75880
placement, IVC filter ~ 75940
portal, catheterization ~ 36481
pulmonary, repair ~ 33730
removal
clusters ~ 37785
saphenous ~ 37720-37735, 37780
varicose ~ 37765-37766
renal, venography ~ 75831-75833
repair
aneurysm ~ 36834
angioplasty ~ 75978
graft ~ 34520
sampling, venography ~ 75893
sinus, venography ~ 75870
skull, venography ~ 75870-75872
spermatic
excision ~ 55530-55540
ligation ~ 55550
splenic, splenoportography ~ 75810
stripping, saphenous ~ 37720-37735
subclavian, thrombectomy ~ 34471-34490
thrombectomy, other than hemodialysis graft or fistula ~ 35875-35876
unlisted services and procedures ~ 37799
valve transposition ~ 34510
varicose ~ see varicose vein
vena cava
thrombectomy ~ 34401-34451
venography ~ 75825-75827
Velpeau cast ~ 29058

Vena cava
catheterization ~ 36010
reconstruction ~ 34502
resection with reconstruction ~ 37799
Vena caval thrombectomy ~ 50230
Venereal disease research laboratory ~ see VDRL
Venesection ~ 99195
Venipuncture ~ see catheterization ~ 36821
child/adult
cutdown ~ 36425
percutaneous ~ 36410
infant
cutdown ~ 36420
percutaneous ~ 36400-36406
routine ~ 36415
Venography
adrenal ~ 75840-75842
arm ~ 75820-75822
epidural ~ 75872
hepatic portal ~ 75885-75887
injection ~ 36005
jugular ~ 75860
leg ~ 75820-75822
liver ~ 75889-75891
neck ~ 75860
nuclear medicine ~ 78445, 78457-78458
orbit ~ 75880
renal ~ 75831-75833
sagittal sinus ~ 75870
vena cava ~ 75825-75827
venous sampling ~ 75893
Venorrhaphy ~ see suture, vein
Venotomy ~ 99195
Venous access device
fluoroscopic guidance ~ 77001
insertion, central ~ 36560-36566
peripheral ~ 36570-36571
obstruction clearance ~ 36595-36596
guidance ~ 75901-75902
removal ~ 36590
repair ~ 36576
replacement ~ 36582-36583, 36585
catheter only ~ 36578
Venous blood pressure ~ 93770
Venovenostomy ~ 34530
Ventilating tube
insertion ~ 69433
removal ~ 69424
Ventilation assist ~ 94002-94005, 99504
Ventricular puncture ~ 61020-61026, 61105-61120
Ventriculocisternostomy ~ 62180, 62200-62201
Ventriculography
anesthesia
brain ~ 00214
cardiac ~ 01920
nuclear imaging ~ 78635
Ventriculomyectomy ~ 33416
Ventriculomyotomy ~ 33416
Vermiform appendix ~ see appendix
Vermilionectomy ~ 40500
Verruca plana ~ 17110-17111
Verruca(e) ~ 17110-17111
Version, cephalic ~ 59412
Vertebra ~ see spinal cord; spine; vertebral body ~ 22315
additional segment, excision ~ 22103, 22116
arthrodesis
anterior ~ 22548-22585
exploration ~ 22830
lateral extracavitary ~ 22532-22534
posterior ~ 22590-22802
spinal deformity
anterior approach ~ 22808-22812
posterior approach ~ 22800-22804
cervical, excision, for tumor ~ 22100, 22110
fracture ~ 23675-23680
fracture/dislocation
additional segment, open treatment ~ 22328
cervical, open treatment ~ 22326
lumbar, open treatment ~ 22325
thoracic, open treatment ~ 22327
kyphectomy ~ 22818-22819
lumbar, excision, for tumor ~ 22102, 22114
osteoplasty, CT scan ~ 72292
fluoroscopy ~ 72291
lumbar ~ 22521-22522
thoracic ~ 22520-22522
osteotomy, additional segment, anterior approach ~ 22226
posterior/posterolateral approach ~ 22216
cervical, anterior approach ~ 22220
posterior/posterolateral approach ~ 22210
lumbar,
anterior approach ~ 22224
posterior/posterolateral approach ~ 22214
thoracic, anterior approach ~ 22222
posterior/posterolateral approach ~ 22212
thoracic, excision, for tumor ~ 22101, 22112
Vertebrae ~ see vertebra
arthrodesis, anterior ~ 22548-22585
lateral extracavitary ~ 22532-22534
spinal deformity ~ 22818-22819
Vertebral arteries ~ see artery, vertebral
body
biopsy ~ 20250-20251
excision
decompression ~ 63081-63103
lesion ~ 63300-63308
with skull base surgery ~ 61597
fracture/dislocation
closed treatment ~ 22305
without manipulation ~ 22310
kyphectomy ~ 22818-22819
column ~ see spine
corpectomy ~ 63081-63103, 63300-63308
fracture ~ see fracture, vertebra
process
fracture/dislocation
closed treatment
with manipulation, casting and/or bracing ~ 22315

Very low density lipoprotein ~ 0026T, 83695-83721
Vesication ~ see bulla
Vesicle, seminal ~ see seminal vesicle
Vesico-psoas hitch ~ 50785
Vesicostomy cutaneous ~ 51980
Vesicourethropexy ~ 51840-51841
Vesicovaginal fistula ~ 51900, 57320, 57330
Vesiculectomy ~ 55650
Vesiculogram, seminal ~ 55300, 74440
Vesiculography ~ 55300, 74440
Vesiculotomy ~ 55600-55605
complicated ~ 55605
Vessel, blood ~ see blood vessels
Vessels transposition, great ~ 33770-33781
Vestibular function tests ~ see ear, nose and throat
additional electrodes ~ 92547
caloric test ~ 92533
caloric vestibular tests ~ 92543
nystagmus
optokinetic ~ 92534, 92544
positional ~ 92532, 92542
spontaneous ~ 92531, 92541
posturography ~ 92548
sinusoidal rotational testing ~ 92546
torsion swing test ~ 92546
tracking test ~ 92545
Vestibular nerve
section
transcranial approach ~ 69950
translabyrinthine approach ~ 69915
Vestibule of mouth ~ see mouth, vestibule of
Vestibuloplasty ~ 40840-40845
Vidal Procedure ~ 55530-55540
Video
esophagus ~ 74230
pharynx ~ 70371, 74230
speech evaluation ~ 70371
swallowing evaluation ~ 74230
Video-assisted thoracoscopic surgery ~ see thoracoscopy
Videoradiography unlisted services and procedures ~ 76120-76125
VII, coagulation factor ~ 85230
VII, cranial nerve ~ see facial nerve
VIII, coagulation factor ~ 85210-85293
Villus, chorionic ~ 59015
Villusectomy ~ see synovectomy
VIP ~ see vasoactive intestinal peptide
Viral antibodies ~ 86280
Viral warts ~ 17110-17111
Virtual colonoscopy
diagnostic ~ 0067T
screening ~ 0066T
Virus
AIDS ~ 87390
Burkitt lymphoma ~ 86663-86665
human immunodeficiency ~ 86689, 86701-86703
influenza ~ 86710, 87804
Virus ~ *continued*
respiratory syncytial ~ see respiratory syncytial virus
salivary gland ~ see cytomegalovirus
Virus identification immunofluorescence ~ 87254
Virus isolation ~ 87250-87255
Visceral larval migrans ~ 86280
Viscosities, blood ~ 85810
Visit, home ~ 99341-99350
Visual acuity screen ~ 99172-99173
Visual field exam ~ 92081-92083
Visual function screen ~ 0065T, **99172**
Visual reinforcement audiometry ~ see audiologic function tests ~ 92579
Visualization ileal conduit ~ 50690
Vital capacity measurement ~ 94150
Vitamin ~ 84591
A ~ 84590
B complex ~ 78270-78272
B-1 ~ 84425
B-12 ~ 82607-82608
absorption study ~ 78270-78272
B-2 ~ 84252
B-6 ~ 84207
B-6 measurement ~ 84207
BC ~ 82747
C ~ 82180
D ~ 82307, 82652
D, 25-hydroxy measurement ~ 82307
D-2 ~ 82307
D-3 ~ 82306
E ~ 84446
K ~ 84597
K dependent bone protein ~ 83937
K-dependent protein S ~ 85305-85306
Vitelline duct ~ 44800
Vitrectomy
anterior approach, partial ~ 67005
pars plana approach ~ 67036
subtotal ~ 67010
with endolaser panretinal photocoagulation ~ 67040
with epiretinal membrane stripping ~ 67038
with focal endolaser photocoagulation ~ 67039
with implantation or replacement, drug delivery system ~ 67027
Vitreous
aspiration ~ 67015
excision
pars planta approach ~ 67036
with epiretinal membrane stripping ~ 67038
with focal endolaser photocoagulation ~ 67039
implantation, drug delivery system ~ 67027
incision, strands ~ 67030-67031
injection
fluid substitute ~ 67025
pharmacologic agent ~ 67028
removal
anterior approach ~ 67005
subtotal ~ 67010

Vitreous ~ *continued*
replacement, drug delivery system ~ 67027
strands
discission ~ 67030
severing ~ 67031
subtotal ~ 67010
VLDL ~ 0026T, 83695-83721
VMA ~ 84585
Vocal cords
injection, endoscopy ~ 31513
therapeutic ~ 31570-31571
Voice box ~ see larynx
Voice button ~ 31611
Voiding pressure studies
abdominal ~ 51797
bladder ~ 51795
Volatiles ~ 84600
Volhard's test ~ 89235
Volkman contracture ~ 25315-25316
Volume reduction, lung ~ 32491
Von Kraske proctectomy ~ 45111, 45113-45116, 45123
VP ~ see voiding pressure studies
Vulva
abscess, incision and drainage ~ 56405
colposcopy ~ 56820
biopsy ~ 56821
excision
complete ~ 56625, 56633-56640
partial ~ 56620, 56630-56632
radical ~ 56630-56631, 56633-56640
complete ~ 56633-56640
partial ~ 56630-56632
simple
complete ~ 56625
partial ~ 56620
lesion, destruction ~ 56501-56515
perineum
biopsy ~ 56605-56606
incision and drainage ~ 56405
repair, obstetric ~ 59300
Vulvectomy
complete ~ 56625, 56633-56640
partial ~ 56620, 56630-56632
radical ~ 56630-56631, 56633-56640
complete
with bilateral inguinofemoral lymphadenectomy ~ 56637
with inguinofemoral, iliac, and pelvic lymphadenectomy ~ 56640
with unilateral inguinofemoral lymphadenectomy ~ 56634
partial
with bilateral inguinofemoral lymphadenectomy ~ 56632
with unilateral inguinofemoral lymphadenectomy ~ 56631
simple
complete ~ 56625
partial ~ 56620
VZIG ~ 90396

W

W-plasty ~ see skin, adjacent tissue transfer
WADA activation test ~ 95958
WAIS-R ~ 96100
Waldius Procedure ~ 27445
Wall, abdominal ~ see abdominal wall
Walsh modified radical prostatectomy ~ 52601
Warts, flat, destruction ~ 17110-17111
Washing sperm ~ 58323
Wasserman test ~ 86592-86593
Wassmund Procedure osteotomy, maxilla ~ 21206
Water load test ~ 89235
Water wart ~ 17110-17111, 54050-54065
Waterston Procedure ~ 33755
Watson-Jones Procedure ~ 27695-27698
Wave, ultrasonic shock ~ see ultrasound
WBC ~ see white blood cell
Webbed toe, repair ~ 28280
Wedge excision osteotomy ~ 21122
Wedge resection ovary ~ 58920
Well-baby care ~ 99381, 99391, 99432
Wellness behavior ~ see evaluation and management, health behavior
Wernicke-posadas disease ~ 86490
West Nile virus ~ 86788-86789
Westergren test ~ 85651-85652
Western blot
HIV ~ 86689
protein ~ 84181-84182
tissue analysis ~ 88371-88372
Wheelchair management/propulsion ~ 97542
training ~ 97542
Wheeler knife procedure ~ 66820-66821
Wheeler Procedure ~ 15820-15823
discission secondary membranous cataract ~ 66820
Whipple Procedure ~ 48150
Whirlpool therapy ~ 97022
White blood cell
alkaline phosphatase ~ 85540
antibody ~ 86021
count ~ 85032, 85048, 89055
differential ~ 85004-85007, 85009
histamine release test ~ 86343
phagocytosis ~ 86344
transfusion ~ 86950
Whitemead Operation ~ 46260
Whitman astragalectomy ~ 28120, 28130
Whitman Procedure ~ 27120
Wick catheter technique ~ 20950
Widal serum test ~ 86000
Window
oval ~ 69666
round ~ 69667
Window technic, pericardial ~ 33015
Windpipe ~ see trachea

Winiwarter Operation ~ 47720-47740
Winter Procedure ~ 54435
Wintrobe test ~ 85651-85652
Wire ~ see pin
insertion/removal, skeletal traction ~ 20650
interdental, without fracture ~ 21497
Wiring prophylactic treatment, humerus ~ 24498
Wirsung duct ~ see pancreatic duct
Witzel Operation ~ see incision, stomach, creation, stoma; incision and drainage ~ 43500, 43520, 43830-43832
Womb ~ see uterus
Wood alcohol ~ 84600
Work hardening ~ see physical medicine/therapy/occupational therapy ~ 97545-97546
Work related evaluation services ~ 99455-99456
Worm ~ 86682
Wound
debridement
non-selective ~ 97602
selective ~ 97597-97598
dehiscence, repair ~ 12020-12021, 13160
exploration
penetrating
abdomen/flank/back ~ 20102
chest ~ 20101
extremity ~ 20103
neck ~ 20100
penetrating trauma ~ 20100-20103
infection, incision and drainage, postoperative ~ 10180
negative pressure therapy ~ 97605-97606
repair
complex ~ 13100-13160
intermediate ~ 12031-12057
simple ~ 12001-12021
urethra ~ 53502-53515
suture
bladder ~ 51860-51865
kidney ~ 50500
trachea
cervical ~ 31800
intrathoracic ~ 31805
urethra ~ 53502-53515
vagina repair ~ 57200-57210
Wrist ~ see arm, lower; carpal bone
abscess ~ 25028
arthrocentesis ~ 20605
arthrodesis ~ 25800
with graft ~ 25810
with sliding graft ~ 25805
arthrography ~ 73115
arthroplasty ~ 25332, 25443, 25447
revision ~ 25449
total replacement ~ 25446
with implant ~ 25441-25442, 25444-25445
arthroscopy, diagnostic ~ 29840
surgical ~ 29843-29848
Wrist ~ *continued*
arthrotomy ~ 25040, 25100-25105
for repair ~ 25107
biopsy ~ 25065-25066, 25100-25101
bursa
excision ~ 25115-25116
incision and drainage ~ 25031
capsule, incision ~ 25085
cast ~ 29085
cyst ~ 25130-25136
decompression ~ 25020-25025
disarticulation ~ 25920
reamputation ~ 25924
revision ~ 25922
dislocation
closed treatment ~ 25660
intercarpal ~ 25660
open treatment ~ 25670
open treatment ~ 25670, 25676
percutaneous fixation ~ 25671
radiocarpal ~ 25660
open treatment ~ 25670
radioulnar
closed treatment ~ 25675
percutaneous fixation ~ 25671
with fracture
closed treatment ~ 25680
open treatment ~ 25685
with manipulation ~ 25259, 25660, 25675
excision
carpal ~ 25210-25215
cartilage ~ 25107
exploration ~ 25040, 25101
fasciotomy ~ 25020-25025
fracture ~ 25645
closed treatment ~ 25622, 25630
open treatment ~ 25628
with dislocation ~ 25680-25685
with manipulation ~ 25259, 25624, 25635
ganglion cyst, excision ~ 25111-25112
hematoma ~ 25028
incision ~ 25040, 25100-25105
tendon sheath ~ 25000-25001
injection
carpal tunnel, therapeutic ~ 20526
X-ray ~ 25246
joint ~ 25040, 25660
lesion, tendon sheath, excision ~ 25110
magnetic resonance imaging (MRI) ~ 73221
reconstruction
capsulectomy ~ 25320
capsulorrhaphy ~ 25320
carpal bone ~ 25394, 25430
realign ~ 25335
removal
foreign body ~ 25040, 25101, 25248
implant ~ 25449
loose body ~ 25101
prosthesis ~ 25250-25251

Wrist ~ ***continued***
repair ~ 25447
bone ~ 25440
carpal bone ~ 25431
muscle ~ 25260, 25270
secondary ~ 25263-25265, 25272-25274
tendon ~ 25260, 25270, 25280-25316
secondary ~ 25263-25265, 25272-25274
tendon sheath ~ 25275
strapping ~ 29260
synovium, excision ~ 25105, 25115-25119
tendon sheath, excision ~ 25115-25116
tenodesis ~ 25300-25301
tenotomy ~ 25290
tumor ~ 25130-25136
excision ~ 25075-25077
unlisted services and procedures ~ 25999
X-ray ~ 73100-73110
with contrast ~ 73115

X

X, coagulation factor ~ 85260
X, cranial nerve ~ see vagus nerve
X-linked ichthyoses ~ 86592-86593
X-ray
abdomen ~ 74000-74022
abscess ~ 76080
acromioclavicular joint ~ 73050
ankle ~ 73600-73610
arm, lower ~ 73090
arm, upper ~ 73092
artery, atherectomy ~ 75992-75996
auditory meatus ~ 70134
bile duct, guide dilation ~ 74360
body composition, dual energy absorptiometry ~ 0028T
body section ~ 76100
motion ~ 76101-76102
bone
age study ~ 77072
dual energy absorptiometry ~ 77080-77081
length study ~ 77073
osseous survey ~ 77074-77077
ultrasound ~ 76977
breast ~ 77055-77057
localization nodule ~ 77032
with computer-aided detection ~ 77051-77052
calcaneus ~ 73650
chest ~ 71010-71035
complete (four views), with fluoroscopy ~ 71034
insert pacemaker ~ 71090
partial (two views), with fluoroscopy ~ 71023
stereo ~ 71015
with fluoroscopy ~ 71090
clavicle ~ 73000

X-ray ~ ***continued***
coccyx ~ 72220
consultation ~ 76140
with contrast
ankle ~ 73615
aorta ~ 0080T-0081T, 75600-75630, 75952-75953
artery
abdominal ~ 75726
additional vessels ~ 75774
adrenal ~ 75731-75733
arm ~ 75710-75716
arteriovenous shunt ~ 75790
brachial ~ 75658
carotid ~ 75660-75680
coronary ~ 93556
coronary bypass ~ 93556
head and neck ~ 75650
iliac ~ 75953
leg ~ 75710-75716
mammary ~ 75756
pelvic ~ 75736
pulmonary ~ 75741-75746
renal ~ 75722-75724
spine ~ 75705
transcatheter therapy ~ 75894-75898
vertebral ~ 75685
bile duct ~ 74300-74320
calculus removal ~ 74327
catheterization ~ 75982-75984
drainage ~ 75980-75982
guide catheter ~ 74328, 74330
bladder ~ 74430, 74450-74455
brain ~ 70010-70015
bronchi ~ 71040-71060
colon, barium enema ~ 74270-74280
corpora cavernosa ~ 74445
elbow ~ 73085
epididymis ~ 74440
gallbladder ~ 74290-74291
gastrointestinal tract ~ 74246-74249
hip ~ 73525
iliofemoral artery ~ 75630
intervertebral disk
cervical ~ 72285
lumbar ~ 72295
thoracic ~ 72285
joint, stress views ~ 77071
kidney
cyst ~ 74470
guide catheter ~ 74475
knee ~ 73560-73564, 73580
lacrimal duct ~ 70170
larynx ~ 70373
lymph vessel
abdomen ~ 75805-75807
arm ~ 75801-75803
leg ~ 75801-75803
nasolacrimal duct ~ 70170
guide dilation ~ 74485
oviduct ~ 74740
pancreas ~ 74300-74305

X-ray ~ *continued*
pancreatic duct, guide catheter ~ 74329-74330
perineum ~ 74775
peritoneum ~ 74190
salivary gland ~ 70390
seminal vesicles ~ 74440
shoulder ~ 73040
spine
cervical ~ 72240
lumbosacral ~ 72265
thoracic ~ 72255
total ~ 72270
subtraction method ~ 76350
temporomandibular joint (TMJ) ~ 70328-70332
ureter
guide catheter ~ 74480
guide dilation ~ 74485
urethra ~ 74450-74455
urinary tract ~ 74400-74425
uterus ~ 74740
vas deferens ~ 74440
vein
adrenal ~ 75840-75842
arm ~ 75820-75822
hepatic portal ~ 75810, 75885-75887
jugular ~ 75860
leg ~ 75820-75822
liver ~ 75889-75891
neck ~ 75860
orbit ~ 75880
renal ~ 75831-75833
sampling ~ 75893
sinus ~ 75870
skull ~ 75870-75872
splenic ~ 75810
vena cava ~ 75825-75827
wrist ~ 73115
duodenum ~ 74260
elbow ~ 73070-73080
esophagus ~ 74220
eye ~ 70030
facial bones ~ 70140-70150
fallopian tube ~ 74742
femur ~ 73550
fibula ~ 73590
finger ~ 73140
fistula ~ 76080
foot ~ 73620-73630
gastrointestinal tract ~ 74240-74245
guide dilation ~ 74360
guide intubation ~ 74340-74350
hand ~ 73120-73130
head ~ 70350
heel ~ 73650
hip ~ 73500-73520, 73540
intraoperative ~ 73530
humerus ~ 73060
intestines, small ~ 74245, 74249-74251
guide intubation ~ 74355
intravascular stent ~ 75960

X-ray ~ *continued*
jaws ~ 70355
joint, stress views ~ 77071
knee ~ 73560-73564, 73580
bilateral ~ 73565
larynx ~ 70370
leg ~ 73592
lumen dilator ~ 74360
mandible ~ 70100-70110
mastoids ~ 70120-70130
nasal bone ~ 70160
neck ~ 70360
nose to rectum, foreign body ~ 76010
orbit ~ 70190-70200
pelvis ~ 72170-72190, 73540
manometry ~ 74710
peritoneum ~ 74190
pharynx ~ 70370, 74210
ribs ~ 71100-71111
sacroiliac joint ~ 72200-72202, 73542
sacrum ~ 72220
salivary gland ~ 70380
scapula ~ 73010
sella turcica ~ 70240
shoulder ~ 73020-73030, 73050
sinus tract ~ 76080
sinuses ~ 70210-70220
skull ~ 70250-70260
specimen/surgical ~ 76098
spine ~ 72020, 72090
cervical ~ 72040-72052
lumbosacral ~ 72100-72120
thoracic ~ 72070-72074
thoracolumbar ~ 72080
total ~ 72010
standing, spine ~ 72069
sternum ~ 71120-71130
teeth ~ 70300-70320
tibia ~ 73590
toe ~ 73660
total body, foreign body ~ 76010
unlisted services and procedures ~ 76120-76125
wrist ~ 73100-73110
X-ray tomography, computed ~ see CT scan
XA, coagulation factor ~ 85260
Xenoantibodies ~ 86308-86310
Xenograft ~ 15400-15401
Xenografts, skin ~ 15400-15401, 15420-15421
Xenotransplantation ~ 15400-15401, 15420-15421
Xerography ~ 76150
Xeroradiography ~ 76150
XI, coagulation factor ~ 85270
XI, cranial nerve ~ see accessory nerve
XII, coagulation factor ~ 85280
XII, cranial nerve ~ see hypoglossal nerve
XIII, coagulation factor ~ 85290-85291
Xylose absorption test
blood ~ 84620
urine ~ 84620

Y

Yeast culture ~ 87106
Yellow fever vaccine ~ 90717
Yersinia antibody ~ 86793

Z

Ziegler Procedure discission secondary membranous cataract ~ 66820
Zinc ~ 84630
Zinc manganese leucine aminopeptidase ~ 83670
Zygoma ~ see cheekbone
Zygomatic arch fracture
open treatment ~ 21356-21366
with manipulation ~ 21355